KU-266-182

Synopsis of Pediatric Emergency Medicine

Revised Edition

Synopsis of Pediatric Emergency Medicine

Revised Edition

Editors

Gary R. Fleisher, M.D.

Professor
Department of Pediatrics
Harvard Medical School;
Chief, Division of Emergency Medicine
Children's Hospital
Boston, Massachusetts

Stephen Ludwig, M.D.

Professor
Departments of Pediatrics and Emergency Medicine
The University of Pennsylvania School of Medicine;
Associate Physician-in-Chief, John H. and Hortense Cassel
Jensen Endowed Chair
Division of Pediatric Emergency Medicine
The Children's Hospital of Philadelphia
Philadelphia, Pennsylvania

Senior Associate Editor

Benjamin K. Silverman, M.D.

Professor
Department of Pediatrics
Attending Physician, Emergency Services
UCLA/Harbor Medical Center
Children's Hospital of Orange County
Orange, California

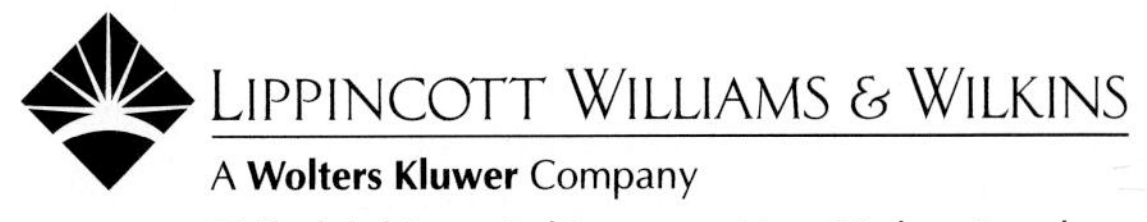

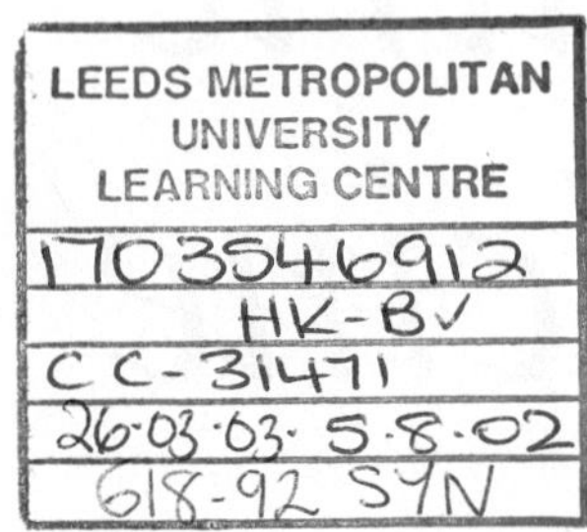

Acquisitions Editor: Anne M. Sydor
Developmental Editor: Tanya Lazar
Production Manager: Toni Ann Scaramuzzo
Production Editor: Michael Mallard
Manufacturing Manager: Tim Reynolds
Cover Designer: Christine Jenny
Compositor: Maryland Composition
Printer: Courier Westford

© 2002 by LIPPINCOTT WILLIAMS & WILKINS
530 Walnut Street
Philadelphia, PA 19106 USA
LWW.com

All rights reserved. This book is protected by copyright. No part of this book may be reproduced in any form or by any means, including photocopying, or utilized by any information storage and retrieval system without written permission from the copyright owner, except for brief quotations embodied in critical articles and reviews. Materials appearing in this book prepared by individuals as part of their official duties as U.S. government employees are not covered by the above-mentioned copyright.

Printed in the USA

Library of Congress Cataloging-in-Publication Data

Synopsis of pediatric emergency medicine / editors, Gary R. Fleisher, Stephen Ludwig–
2nd ed.
p. ; cm.
Includes bibliographical references and index.
ISBN 0-7817-3274-3
1. Pediatric emergencies. I. Fleisher, Gary R. (Gary Robert), 1951- II. Ludwig, Stephen, 1945–
[DNLM: 1. Emergencies–Child. 2. Emergencies–Infant. WS 205 S992 2002]
RJ370 .S97 2002
618.92′0025–dc21 2001050399

Care has been taken to confirm the accuracy of the information presented and to describe generally accepted practices. However, the authors, editors, and publisher are not responsible for errors or omissions or for any consequences from application of the information in this book and make no warranty, expressed or implied, with respect to the currency, completeness, or accuracy of the contents of the publication. Application of this information in a particular situation remains the professional responsibility of the practitioner.

The authors, editors, and publisher have exerted every effort to ensure that drug selection and dosage set forth in this text are in accordance with current recommendations and practice at the time of publication. However, in view of ongoing research, changes in government regulations, and the constant flow of information relating to drug therapy and drug reactions, the reader is urged to check the package insert for each drug for any change in indications and dosage and for added warnings and precautions. This is particularly important when the recommended agent is a new or infrequently employed drug.

Some drugs and medical devices presented in this publication have Food and Drug Administration (FDA) clearance for limited use in restricted research settings. It is the responsibility of the health care provider to ascertain the FDA status of each drug or device planned for use in their clinical practice.

10 9 8 7 6 5 4 3 2 1

Dedicated To Our Families;
Those who gave birth to and reared us
Those with whom we have bonded as life partners
Those with whom we work
Those who call us doctor

Contents

Section III: MEDICAL EMERGENCIES

Section IV: TRAUMA

Section V: SURGICAL EMERGENCIES

Section VI: PSYCHOSOCIAL EMERGENCIES

Contributing Authors

Evaline A. Alessandrini, M.D.
Assistant Professor
Departments of Pediatrics, Emergency Medicine, and Epidemiology
The University of Pennsylvania School of Medicine;
Attending Physician
Division of Emergency Medicine
The Children's Hospital of Philadelphia
Philadelphia, Pennsylvania

Elizabeth R. Alpern, M.D.
Assistant Professor
Department of Pediatrics
The University of Pennsylvania School of Medicine;
Attending Physician
Department of Emergency Medicine
The Children's Hospital of Philadelphia
Philadelphia, Pennsylvania

Angela C. Anderson, M.D.
Assistant Professor
Department of Pediatrics
Brown University School of Medicine;
Attending Physician
Department of Pediatric Emergency Medicine
Rhode Island Hospital
Providence, Rhode Island

Amy M. Arnett, M.D.
Assistant Professor
Department of Pediatrics
Boston University School of Medicine;
Attending Physician
Department of Pediatric Emergency Medicine
Boston Medical Center
Boston, Massachusetts

Magdy Attia, M.D.
Clinical Assistant Professor
Department of Pediatrics
Jefferson Medical College
Philadelphia, Pennsylvania;
Director, PEM Fellowship Program
Division of Emergency Medicine
Alfred I. duPont Hospital for Children
Wilmington, Delaware

David Bachman, M.D.
Associate Professor
Department of Pediatrics
University of Vermont School of Medicine
Burlington, Vermont;
Director, Pediatric and Adult Emergency Services
Portland, Maine

Richard Bachur, M.D.
Instructor
Department of Medicine
Harvard Medical School;
Attending Physician
Division of Emergency Medicine
Children's Hospital
Boston, Massachusetts

M. Douglas Baker, M.D.
Professor
Department of Pediatrics
Yale University School of Medicine;
Chief
Department of Pediatric Emergency Medicine
Yale–New Haven Children's Hospital
New Haven, Connecticut

Marc N. Baskin, M.D.
Assistant Professor
Department of Pediatrics
Harvard Medical School;
Attending Physician
Department of Pediatric Emergency Medicine;
Service Chief, Short Stay Unit
Children's Hospital
Boston, Massachusetts

Carl R. Baum, M.D.
Assistant Professor
Department of Pediatrics Emergency Medicine
Yale University;
Attending Physician
Pediatric Emergency Medicine
Yale–New Haven Hospital
New Haven, Connecticut

Louis M. Bell, M.D.
Professor
Department of Pediatrics
The University of Pennsylvania School of Medicine;
Chief
Division of General Pediatrics
The Children's Hospital of Philadelphia
Philadelphia, Pennsylvania

Robert G. Bolte, M.D.
Professor
Department of Pediatrics
University of Utah School of Medicine;
Director, Emergency Services
Primary Children's Medical Center
Salt Lake City, Utah

Vincent W. Chiang, M.D.
Instructor
Department of Pediatrics
Harvard Medical School;
Attending Physician
Division of Emergency Medicine
Children's Hospital
Boston, Massachusetts

Lydia Ciarallo, M.D.
Assistant Professor
Department of Pediatrics
Brown University School of Medicine
Providence, Rhode Island

Alan R. Cohen, M.D.
Professor and Chairman
Department of Pediatrics
The University of Pennsylvania School of Medicine;
Physician-in-Chief
The Children's Hospital of Philadelphia
Philadelphia, Pennsylvania

Howard M. Corneli, M.D.
Associate Professor
Department of Pediatrics
University of Utah School of Medicine;
Emergency Physician
Primary Children's Medical Center
Salt Lake City, Utah

Kate Cronan, M.D.
Clinical Assistant Professor
Department of Pediatrics
Thomas Jefferson University
Philadelphia, Pennsylvania;
Chief, Emergency Department
A. I. duPont Hospital for Children
Wilmington, Delaware

Joanne M. Decker, M.D.
Clinical Assistant Professor
Department of Pediatrics
The University of Pennsylvania School of Medicine;
Attending Physician
Division of Emergency Medicine
The Children's Hospital of Philadelphia
Philadelphia, Pennsylvania

Carlos A. Delgado, M.D.
Assistant Professor
Department of Pediatrics
Emory University School of Medicine;
Associate Fellowship Director and Attending Physician
Division of Pediatric Emergency Medicine
Egleston Children's Hospital
Atlanta, Georgia

Dennis R. Durbin, M.D., M.S.C.E.
Assistant Professor
Departments of Pediatrics and Epidemiology
Division of Emergency Medicine
The University of Pennsylvania School of Medicine;
Attending Physician
The Children's Hospital of Philadelphia
Philadelphia, Pennsylvania

Robert A. Felter, M.D.
Professor
Department of Pediatrics
Northeast Ohio University;
Chairman
Departments of Pediatrics and Adolescent Medicine;
Medical Director, Tod Children's Hospital;
Vice-Chairman, Pediatrics, NEOUCOM;
Chairman, EMS Board
State of Ohio Department of Public Safety
Youngstown, Ohio

Gary R. Fleisher, M.D.
Professor
Department of Pediatrics
Harvard Medical School;
Chief, Division of Emergency Medicine
Children's Hospital
Boston, Massachusetts

Janet H. Friday, M.D.
Assistant Professor
Department of Pediatrics
University of California, San Diego School of Medicine;
Attending Physician
Division of Emergency Medicine
Children's Hospital
San Diego, California

Ronald A. Furnival, M.D.
Associate Professor
Department of Pediatrics
University of Utah School of Medicine;
Attending Physician
Department of Pediatric Emergency Medicine
Primary Children's Medical Center
Salt Lake City, Utah

Carmen Teresa Garcia, M.D.
Attending Physician
Pediatric Emergency Department
Jackson Memorial Hospital
Miami, Florida

Michael H. Gewitz, M.D.
Professor and Vice Chairman
Department of Pediatrics
New York Medical College;
Director of Pediatrics and Chief, Pediatric Cardiology
Children's Hospital at Westchester Medical Center
Valhalla, New York

Javier A. Gonzalez del Rey, M.D.
Associate Professor
Department of Pediatrics
University of Cincinnati College of Medicine;
Associate Director
Division of Emergency Medicine
Children's Hospital Medical Center
Cincinnati, Ohio

Marc H. Gorelick, M.D., M.S.C.E.
Director
Department of Emergency Medicine
Children's Hospital
Milwaukee, Wisconsin;
Department of Pediatrics
Jefferson Medical College
Philadelphia, Pennsylvania

David S. Greenes, M.D.
Instructor
Department of Pediatrics
Harvard Medical School;
Staff Physician
Division of Emergency Medicine
Children's Hospital
Boston, Massachusetts

Karen Gruskin, M.D.
Instructor
Department of Pediatrics
Harvard Medical School;
Assistant in Medicine
Children's Hospital
Boston;
Director
Department of Pediatrics
Winchester Hospital
Winchester, Massachusetts

Daniel E. Hale, M.D.
Associate Professor
Department of Pediatrics
The University of Texas Health Science Center at San Antonio;
Senior Physician, Pediatric Endocrinology
Santa Rosa Children's Hospital
San Antonio, Texas

Steven D. Handler, M.D.
Professor
Department of Otorhinolaryngology: Head and Neck Surgery
The University of Pennsylvania School of Medicine;
Associate Director
Division of Pediatric Otolaryngology
The Children's Hospital of Philadelphia
Philadelphia, Pennsylvania

Marvin B. Harper, M.D.
Assistant Professor
Department of Pediatrics
Harvard Medical School;
Assistant in Medicine
Divisions of Emergency Medicine and Infectious Diseases
Children's Hospital
Boston, Massachusetts

Fred M. Henretig, M.D.
Professor
Department of Pediatrics and Emergency Medicine
The University of Pennsylvania School of Medicine;
Director
Section of Clinical Toxicology
The Children's Hospital of Philadelphia;
Medical Director, The Poison Control Center
Philadelphia, Pennsylvania

Gordon R. Hodas, M.D.
Clinical Associate Professor
Department of Psychiatry
The University of Pennsylvania School of Medicine;
Statewide Child Psychiatric Consultant
Office of Mental Health and Substance Abuse Services
Pennsylvania Department of Public Welfare
Philadelphia, Pennsylvania

Dee Hodge III, M.D.
Associate Professor
Department of Pediatrics
Washington University School of Medicine;
Associate Director
Clinical Affairs, Emergency Services
St. Louis Children's Hospital
St. Louis, Missouri

Michael D. Hogarty, M.D.
Clinical Associate
Department of Pediatrics
The University of Pennsylvania School of Medicine;
Division of Oncology
The Children's Hospital of Philadelphia
Philadelphia, Pennsylvania

Paul J. Honig, M.D.
Professor
Departments of Pediatrics and Dermatology
The University of Pennsylvania School of Medicine;
Director
Department of Pediatric Dermatology
The Children's Hospital of Philadelphia
Philadelphia, Pennsylvania

Daniel J. Isaacman, M.D.
Professor
Department of Pediatrics
Eastern Virginia Medical School;
Director, Division of Pediatric Emergency Medicine
Children's Hospital of The King's Daughters
Norfolk, Virginia

Mark D. Joffe, M.D.
Associate Professor
Department of Pediatrics
The University of Pennsylvania School of Medicine;
Director, Community Pediatric Medicine;
Attending Physician
Pediatric Emergency Medicine
The Children's Hospital of Philadelphia
Philadelphia, Pennsylvania

Howard Kadish, M.D.
Associate Professor
Department of Pediatrics
The University of Utah School of Medicine;
Attending Physician, Emergency Department
Primary Children's Medical Center
Salt Lake City, Utah

Robert E. Kelly Jr, M.D.
Assistant Clinical Professor
Departments of Surgery and Pediatrics
Eastern Virginia Medical School;
Chief
Department of Surgery
Children's Hospital of The King's Daughters
Norfolk, Virginia

Sigmund J. Kharasch, M.D.
Assistant Professor
Department of Pediatrics
Boston University School of Medicine;
Director
Division of Pediatric Emergency Medicine
Boston Medical Center
Boston, Massachusetts

Christopher King, M.D.
Assistant Professor
Departments of Emergency Medicine and Pediatrics
University of Pittsburgh School of Medicine;
Attending Physician
Department of Emergency Medicine
University of Pittsburgh Medical Center (UPMC) Presbyterian Hospital
Children's Hospital of Pittsburgh
Pittsburgh, Pennsylvania

Bruce L. Klein, M.D.
Associate Professor
Departments of Pediatrics and Emergency Medicine
The George Washington University School of Medicine and Health Sciences;
Associate Medical Director
Department of Emergency Medicine
Children's National Medical Center
Washington, D.C.

Susanne Kost, M.D.
Clinical Assistant Professor
Jefferson Medical College
Philadelphia, Pennsylvania;
Attending Physician
A. I. duPont Hospital for Children
Wilmington, Delaware

Roy M. Kulick, M.D.
Staff Physician
Division of Emergency Medicine
Children's Hospital Medical Center
Cincinnati, Ohio

Nathan Kuppermann, M.D., M.P.H.
Associate Professor
Departments of Emergency Medicine and Pediatrics;
Director of Research
Emergency Medicine
University of California at Davis School of Medicine
Sacramento, California

Beverly J. Lange, M.D.
Professor
Department of Pediatrics
The University of Pennsylvania School of Medicine;
Medical Director, Pediatric Oncology
The Children's Hospital of Philadelphia
Philadelphia, Pennsylvania

Alex V. Levin, M.D.
Assistant Professor
Departments of Pediatrics, Genetics, and Ophthalmology
University of Toronto;
Staff Ophthalmologist
The Hospital for Sick Children
Toronto, Ontario
Canada

William J. Lewander, M.D.
Associate Professor
Department of Pediatrics
Brown University School of Medicine;
Director
Department of Pediatric Emergency Medicine
Hasbro Children's Hospital
Rhode Island Hospital
Providence, Rhode Island

Chris A. Liacouras, M.D.
Assistant Professor
Division of Gastroenterology and Nutrition
The University of Pennsylvania School of Medicine;
Attending Physician
Department of Pediatrics
Children's Hospital of Philadelphia
Philadelphia, Pennsylvania

Erica L. Liebelt, M.D.
Director, Pediatric Residency Program
Geisinger Medical Center
Danville, Pennsylvania

James G. Linakis, M.D., Ph.D.
Associate Professor
Department of Pediatrics
Brown University School of Medicine;
Associate Director, Pediatric Emergency Medicine
Hasbro Children's Hospital
Rhode Island Hospital
Providence, Rhode Island

John Loiselle, M.D.
Assistant Director
Emergency Services
A. I. duPont Institute
Wilmington, Delaware

Stephen Ludwig, M.D.
Professor
Departments of Pediatrics and Emergency Medicine
The University of Pennsylvania School of Medicine;
Associate Physician-in-Chief, John H. and Hortense Cassel Jensen Endowed Chair
Division of Pediatric Emergency Medicine
The Children's Hospital of Philadelphia
Philadelphia, Pennsylvania

Dennis P. Lund, M.D.
Assistant Professor
Department of Surgery
University of Wisconsin;
Chief
Pediatric Surgery
Children's Hospital of the University of Wisconsin
Madison, Wisconsin

Joseph R. Madsen, M.D.
Assistant Professor
Department of Surgery
Harvard Medical School;
Neurosurgeon
Department of Neurosurgery
Children's Hospital
Boston, Massachusetts

Soroosh Mahboubi, M.D.
Professor
Departments of Radiology and Pediatrics
The University of Pennsylvania School of Medicine;
Director, Body CT
The Children's Hospital of Philadelphia
Philadelphia, Pennsylvania

Richard Malley, M.D.
Assistant Professor
Department of Pediatrics
Harvard Medical School;
Assistant in Medicine
Divisions of Emergency Medicine and Infectious Diseases
Children's Hospital
Boston, Massachusetts

Kenneth D. Mandl, M.D., M.P.H.
Assistant Professor
Department of Pediatrics
Harvard Medical School;
Director of Clinical Research
Division of Emergency Medicine
Children's Hospital
Boston, Massachusetts

Jonathan Markowitz, M.D.
Instructor
Department of Pediatrics
The University of Pennsylvania School of Medicine;
Fellow
Departments of Gastroenterology and Nutrition
The Children's Hospital of Philadelphia
Philadelphia, Pennsylvania

Constance M. McAneney, M.D.
Associate Professor
Department of Pediatrics
University of Cincinnati College of Medicine;
Associate Director
Division of Emergency Medicine
Children's Hospital Medical Center
Cincinnati, Ohio

Fran Nadel, M.D.
Assistant Professor
Department of Pediatrics
The University of Pennsylvania School of Medicine;
Attending Physician
Division of Emergency Medicine
The Children's Hospital of Philadelphia
Philadelphia, Pennsylvania

Howard L. Needleman, D.M.D.
Clinical Professor and Associate Chairman
Department of Pediatric Dentistry
Harvard School of Dental Medicine;
Associate Dentist-in-Chief
Children's Hospital
Boston, Massachusetts

Douglas S. Nelson, M.D.
Assistant Professor
Departments of Pediatrics and Emergency Medicine
University of Utah School of Medicine;
Attending Physician
Primary Children's Medical Center
Salt Lake City, Utah

Linda P. Nelson, D.M.D., M.Sc.D.
Assistant Professor
Department of Pediatric Dentistry
Harvard School of Dental Medicine;
Associate in Pediatric Dentistry
Children's Hospital
Boston, Massachusetts

Michael E. Norman, M.D.
Clinical Professor
Department of Pediatrics
University of North Carolina School of Medicine
Chapel Hill;
Chairman and Residency Program Director
Department of Pediatrics
Carolinas Medical Center
Charlotte, North Carolina

Daniel W. Ochsenschlager, M.D.
Associate Professor
Department of Pediatrics
Department of Child Health and Development
George Washington University Medical Center;
Medical Director, Emergency Medical Trauma Center
Children's Hospital Medical Center
Washington, D.C.

Kevin C. Osterhoudt, M.D.
Assistant Professor
Department of Pediatrics
The University of Pennsylvania School of Medicine;
Attending Physician
Division of Emergency Medicine
The Children's Hospital of Philadelphia
Philadelphia, Pennsylvania

Bonnie L. Padwa, D.M.D, M.D.
Assistant Professor
Oral and Maxillofacial Surgery
Harvard School of Dental Medicine;
Associate in Surgery
Division of Plastic and Oral Surgery
Children's Hospital
Boston, Massachusetts

Jan E. Paradise, M.D.
Bridgewater Goddard Park Medical Associates
Brockton, Massachusetts

Mary D. Patterson, M.D.
Assistant Professor
Department of Pediatrics
University of Cincinnati College of Medicine;
Attending Physician
Division of Emergency Medicine
Children's Hospital Medical Center
Cincinnati, Ohio

Ronald I. Paul, M.D.
Associate Professor and Chief
Division of Pediatric Emergency Medicine
Department of Pediatrics
University of Louisville School of Medicine;
Medical Director, Emergency Department
Kosair Children's Hospital
Louisville, Kentucky

Barbara B. Pawel, M.D.
Clinical Assistant Professor
Department of Pediatrics
The University of Pennsylvania School of Medicine;
Attending Physician
Division of Emergency Medicine
The Children's Hospital of Philadelphia
Philadelphia, Pennsylvania

Catherine E. Perron, M.D.
Instructor
Department of Pediatrics
Harvard Medical School;
Attending Physician
Division of Emergency Medicine
Children's Hospital
Boston, Massachusetts

Holly Perry, M.D.
Assistant Professor
Department of Pediatrics
Division of Emergency Medicine
University of Connecticut School of Medicine
Farmington;
Attending Physician
Pediatric Emergency Department
Connecticut Children's Medical Center
Hartford, Connecticut

William P. Potsic, M.D.
Newlin Professor of Pediatric Otorhinolaryngology: Head and Neck Surgery
The University of Pennsylvania School of Medicine;
Director, Pediatric Otolaryngology and Human Communication
The Children's Hospital of Philadelphia
Philadelphia, Pennsylvania

Mark G. Roback, M.D.
Associate Professor
Department of Pediatrics
University of Colorado Health Sciences Center;
Fellowship Director
Department of Pediatric Emergency Medicine
The Children's Hospital
Denver, Colorado

Bruce Rosenthal, M.D.
Associate Professor
Division of Pediatric Emergency Medicine
Children's Hospital;
University of Pittsburg
Pittsburgh, Pennsylvania

Richard M. Ruddy, M.D.
Professor of Clinical Pediatrics
Department of Pediatrics
University of Cincinnati College of Medicine;
Director
Division of Emergency Medicine
Children's Hospital Medical Center
Cincinnati, Ohio

Richard A. Saladino, M.D.
Associate Professor
Department of Pediatrics
University of Pittsburg;
Chief
Division of Emergency Medicine
Children's Hospital
Pittsburg, Pennsylvania

Stephen Santora, M.D.
Associate Clinical Professor
Department of Orthopedics
University of Utah School of Medicine;
Pediatric Orthopedist
Primary Children's Medical Center
Salt Lake City, Utah

John Sargent, M.D.
Professor and Dean
Department of Psychiatry
Karl Menninger School of Psychiatry and Mental Health Sciences;
Director, Education and Research
The Menninger Clinic
Topeka, Kansas

Thomas F. Scanlin, M.D.
Professor
Department of Pediatrics
The University of Pennsylvania School of Medicine;
Director, Cystic Fibrosis Center
The Children's Hospital of Philadelphia
Philadelphia, Pennsylvania

Richard J. Scarfone, M.D., M.C.P.
Assistant Professor
Department of Pediatrics
The University of Pennsylvania School of Medicine;
Attending Physician
Department of Pediatric Emergency Medicine
The Children's Hospital of Philadelphia
Philadelphia, Pennsylvania

Louise Schnaufer, M.D.
Professor
Department of Pediatric Surgery
The University of Pennsylvania School of Medicine;
Senior Surgeon
The Children's Hospital of Philadelphia
Philadelphia, Pennsylvania

Jeff E. Schunk, M.D.
Associate Professor and Chief
Division of Pediatric Emergency Medicine
University of Utah School of Medicine;
Attending Physician
Emergency Department
Primary Children's Medical Center
Salt Lake City, Utah

Sara A. Schutzman, M.D.
Assistant Professor
Department of Pediatrics
Harvard Medical School;
Assistant in Medicine
Division of Emergency Medicine
Children's Hospital
Boston, Massachusetts

Steven M. Selbst, M.D.
Professor
Department of Pediatrics
Thomas Jefferson University;
Attending Physician
Division of Emergency Medicine
A. I. duPont Hospital for Children
Wilmington, Delaware

Michael Shannon, M.D., M.P.H.
Associate Professor
Department of Pediatrics
Harvard Medical School;
Associate Chief and Fellowship Director
Division of Emergency Medicine
Boston, Massachusetts

Kathy N. Shaw, M.D.
Associate Professor
Department of Pediatrics
The University of Pennsylvania School of Medicine;
Chief, Emergency Medical Services
The Children's Hospital of Philadelphia
Philadelphia, Pennsylvania

Stephen Shusterman, D.M.D.
Associate Clinical Professor
Department of Pediatric Dentistry
Harvard School of Dental Medicine
Dentist-in-Chief
Children's Hospital
Boston, Massachusetts

Benjamin K. Silverman, M.D.
Professor
Department of Pediatrics
Attending Physician
Emergency Services
UCLA/Harbor Medical Center
Children's Hospital of Orange County
Orange, California

Joseph E. Simon, M.D.
Medical Director, Care Delivery
Scottish Rite Children's Medical Center
Atlanta, Georgia

Howard M. Snyder III, M.D.
Professor
Department of Surgery in Urology
The University of Pennsylvania School of Medicine;
Associate Director/Academic Chief, Pediatric Urology
The Children's Hospital of Philadelphia
Philadelphia, Pennsylvania

Jonathan I. Singer, M.D.
Professor
Departments of Emergency Medicine and Pediatrics;
Vice Chairman and Program Director
Department of Emergency Medicine
Wright State University School of Medicine
Dayton, Ohio

Anne M. Stack, M.D.
Assistant Professor
Department of Pediatrics
Harvard Medical School;
Attending Physician
Division of Emergency Medicine
Children's Hospital
Boston, Massachusetts

Dale W. Steele, M.D.
Assistant Professor
Department of Pediatrics
Section of Emergency Medicine
Brown University;
Attending Physician
Emergency Department
Hasbro Children's Hospital
Providence, Rhode Island

Molly W. Stevens, M.D.
Assistant Professor
Department of Pediatrics
The University of Pennsylvania School of Medicine;
Attending Physician
Division of Emergency Medicine
The Children's Hospital of Philadelphia
Philadelphia, Pennsylvania

Stephen J. Teach, M.D., M.P.H.
Assistant Professor
Department of Pediatrics
George Washington University School of Medicine;
Department of Emergency
Children's National Medical Center
Washington, D.C.

Frederick W. Tecklenburg, M.D.
Associate Professor
Department of Pediatrics
The Medical University of South Carolina;
Director
Division of Emergency/Critical Care
MUSC Children's Hospital
Charleston, South Carolina

Susan B. Torrey, M.D.
Assistant Professor
Department of Pediatrics
Harvard Medical School;
Attending Physician
Division of Emergency Medicine
Children's Hospital
Boston, Massachusetts

Victoria L. Vetter, M.D.
Professor
Department of Pediatrics
The University of Pennsylvania School of Medicine;
Chief
Division of Cardiology
The Children's Hospital of Philadelphia
Philadelphia, Pennsylvania

Robert J. Vinci, M.D.
Associate Professor
Department of Pediatrics
Boston University School of Medicine;
Vice Chairman
Department of Pediatrics
Boston Medical Center
Boston, Massachusetts

Debra L. Weiner, M.D., Ph.D.
Instructor
Department of Pediatrics
Harvard Medical School;
Attending Physician
Department of Emergency Medicine
Children's Hospital
Boston, Massachusetts

James F. Wiley II, M.D.
Associate Professor
Departments of Pediatrics and Emergency Medicine
The School of Medicine at the University of Connecticut Health Center;
Director, Emergency Medical Services
Connecticut Children's Medical Center
Hartford, Connecticut

Loren G. Yamamoto, M.D., M.P.H., M.B.A.
Professor
Department of Pediatrics
University of Hawaii
John A. Burns School of Medicine;
Vice-Chief of Staff
Kapiolani Medical Center for Women and Children
Honolulu, Hawaii

Marc Yudkoff, M.D.
Grant Professor of Pediatrics
The University of Pennsylvania School of Medicine;
Chief, Child Development
The Children's Hospital of Philadelphia
Philadelphia, Pennsylvania

Moritz M. Ziegler, M.D.
Professor
Department of Surgery
Harvard Medical School;
Chairman
Department of Surgery
Children's Hospital
Boston, Massachusetts

Preface

The *Textbook of Pediatric Emergency Medicine* was published in its 4th edition in 2000. This abbreviated version, *Synopsis of Pediatric Emergency Medicine*, represents a synopsis of that text. Why a synopsis? We and our many supportive colleagues and fellowship program graduates wrote *Textbook of Pediatric Emergency Medicine* to be an aid to those who deliver emergency care to children. The first edition of the text appeared in 1983 before the field of Pediatric Emergency Medicine was even recognized as a formal subspecialty. Now there are over 1,000 board certified Pediatric Emergency Medicine specialists who come from either pediatric or emergency medicine backgrounds. They have consulted *Textbook of Pediatric Emergency Medicine* for almost 20 years over four editions. As users of the textbook, they have communicated to us that they like the direct applicability of the information the textbook provides. The textbook tells them what to do. They rely on the ease of finding important information and they appreciate the Signs and Symptoms chapters as a way to quickly review differential diagnoses and make certain that they are not overlooking an important patient problem. Many colleagues have told us, "I don't go to a night on-call in the ED without my copy." Many have described how the book directly helped them save a child's life. The synopsis is our way of acknowledging these comments and making the core of the textbook available to more readers, particularly to students, residents, and fellows in training, and to those who do not need or lack the time to pursue an in-depth background on what they read. We have included all the essentials and maintained the essence of the textbook in a form that is more usable, more portable, and more affordable. We hope it will further our original goal, helping ill and injured children throughout the world.

We thank all the chapter authors for allowing us to synthesize their work. Their original chapters, as they appear in the textbook, are well worth reading, and we hope that if the synopsis stimulates your thinking, you will go back to the full text at a convenient moment. We thank our Associate Editors of the textbook, Fred Henretig and Rich Ruddy, whose contributions to that book were vital to the production of the synopsis. We also thank Ben Silverman, who has always served as our Associate Editor and technical advisor. Our office assistants, Cindy Chow and Carolyn Trojan, have provided invaluable assistance and made the preparation of the book easy. Another round of thanks goes to those staff members at Lippincott Williams & Wilkins for their efforts, especially Anne Sydor, Tim Hiscock, Michael Mallard, and Tanya Lazar.

Our families deserve our final note of appreciation. When we started this process, we were young married couples with kids in diapers. Now our children are finishing their education and starting careers on their own. It is hard enough to be a wife or child of a physician, harder yet to have to cope with the night and weekend call of a pediatric emergency medicine physician, and hardest to be related to those who write and edit. We love them and thank them for their indulgence and forbearance.

Stephen Ludwig, M.D.
Philadelphia, Pennsylvania

Gary R. Fleisher, M.D.
Boston, Massachusetts

SECTION

I

Life-Threatening Emergencies

CHAPTER 1

Resuscitation—Pediatric Basic and Advanced Life Support

Stephen Ludwig, M.D.

Cardiopulmonary resuscitation (CPR) is a series of interventions aimed at restoring and supporting vital function after apparent death. The urgent and immediate goal of resuscitation is to reestablish substrate delivery to meet the metabolic needs of the myocardium, brain, and other vital organs. The overall goal is to return the child to society without morbidity related either to the underlying disease process or to the resuscitation process.

Instruction in CPR techniques has come from two widely disseminated national courses: Pediatric Advanced Life Support (PALS) and Advanced Pediatric Life Support (APLS). Both of these courses have been successful in training health care providers in the appropriate resuscitative techniques. Both courses stress the early recognition of the child who is in need of resuscitative efforts. The outcome of resuscitation in situations in which there has been prolonged asystolic arrest is poor. As in many conditions we manage in pediatric patients, primary prevention, or at least early recognition, is the most successful strategy.

TREATMENT

Pediatric CPR presents the emergency physician with several complexities and frustrations. The first difficulty often encountered is that the patient has received only minimal prehospital care. In many locales, paramedics are trained and equipped primarily to provide adult life support; however, they may be forced to initiate pediatric life support at the most basic level. In other areas, paramedics are limited by laws, regulations, or negative attitudes. Absent or inadequate prehospital care leads to longer periods of hypoxia and hypoperfusion, which directly affect prognosis and central nervous system (CNS) morbidity. The wide spectrum of age and diagnoses adds additional complexity. The resuscitation team must provide an array of technical skills, drugs, and equipment. Without delay, the team must have the flexibility to adjust to the correct sizes and drug dosages for children.

One of the common frustrations when administering drugs is establishing an i.v. line. This technical skill continues to be the most common obstacle toward achieving successful CPR. However, the use of intraosseous technique and central line placement have been great advances in the solution of the access problem.

Arrhythmia management is generally not a problem in pediatric life support. The absence of atherosclerotic vascular disease makes the child's myocardium less susceptible to arrhythmia. As a result, antiarrhythmic medications and defibrillation are used infrequently. The most common cardiac rhythms to be recognized and managed are sinus bradycardia, supraventricular tachycardia, and asystole. The exceptions to this are those children with congenital heart disease (preoperative and postoperative) and those who have sustained direct myocardial trauma (see Chapter 72).

PROGNOSIS

The outlook for survival after CPR is very good for pediatric patients. If the arrest is recognized rapidly and managed skillfully, immediate survival may be as high as 90% and the survival to discharge rate 60%. These figures are based on a hospitalized population of children who require resuscitation. For patients in the emergency department, the outcome is not as good. Children who arrive in the emergency department in asystolic arrest have a poor prognosis. The poorer prognosis for patients in the emergency department may be attributed to delayed recognition of the arrest and to limited prehospital care. Other series have documented an even more grim prognosis as shown in Table 1.1.

CLINICAL MANIFESTATIONS

Infants and children who have experienced disruption of oxygen or glucose delivery to the brain may benefit from the various elements of basic or advanced cardiac life support. The clinical manifestations of those requiring immediate life support are most often related to failure of oxygen delivery to the skin, brain, kidneys, and cardiovascular system. Cutaneous manifestations of oxygen deprivation include circumoral pallor, grayish hue, cyanosis, diaphoresis, mottling, and poor capillary refill. Manifestations of CNS hypoxia include irritability, confusion, delirium, seizures, and unresponsiveness. Cardiovascular manifestations include tachycardia, diaphoresis, bradycardia, and hypotension. Figure 1.1 shows the sequential development of signs and symptoms when there is failure of substrate delivery to different oxygen systems.

Glucose is the second essential substrate necessary for maintenance of CNS integrity. Severe hypoglycemia may be just as devastating as severe hypoxemia. Clinical manifestations are often similar to hypoxemia because the primary effect on the CNS is coma. In addition, the effect of hypoglycemia on the cardiovascular system may lead to a secondary failure of oxygen delivery because of hypotension and related hypoperfusion.

TABLE 1.1. Case Series and Outcomes of Pediatric Cardiopulmonary Resuscitation (CPR)

Lead author	Year of publication	Patient location at time of CPR	Age of patients	Sample size	Immediate survival ROSC	Discharge from hospital	Other
Slonim	1997	PICU	<1 mo to >12 yr Mean 30.8 mo	N = 205 (32 centers)	24.3%	13.7%	PICU population
Torres	1997	IP	<18 yr	N = 92	36%		10% alive at 1 yr
Schindler	1996	ED	Median 2 yr	N = 101	63%	15%	Included respiratory and asystolic arrest
Hickey	1995	ED		N = 95	48%	27%	Most survivors responded to prehospital therapy
Kuisma	1995	ED	<16 yr Mean 2.9 yr	N = 79	14.7%	9.6%	
Teach	1995	ED	0–17.9 yr	N = 32	73%	50%	Arrest while in ED
Fiser	1987	ED	1 day to 21 yr	N = 35	61%	22%	
Zaritsky	1987	IP	55% <1 yr	N = 113		10% CA 27.5 RA	Differentiated CA and RA
O'Rourke	1986	ED		N = 34		21%	Survivors had significant neurologic impairment
Ludwig	1984	IP ED	<1 mo to >16 yr Mean 23 mo	N = 130 ED: 56%	IP: 90% ED: 29%	IP: 65%	Included respiratory and asystolic arrest
Rosenberg	1984	ED	Median 1 yr	N = 26	50%	15%	Asystole
Torphy	1984	ED	Median 2 yr	N = 91	36%	5%	Respiratory arrest excluded
Friesen	1982	IP ED	1 mo to 16 yr 36 <1 yr	N = 66	36%	9%	

CPR, cardiopulmonary resuscitation; PICU, pediatric intensive care unit; IP, inpatients; ED, emergency department; ROSC, return of spontaneous circulation; CA, cardiac arrest; RA, respiratory arrest.

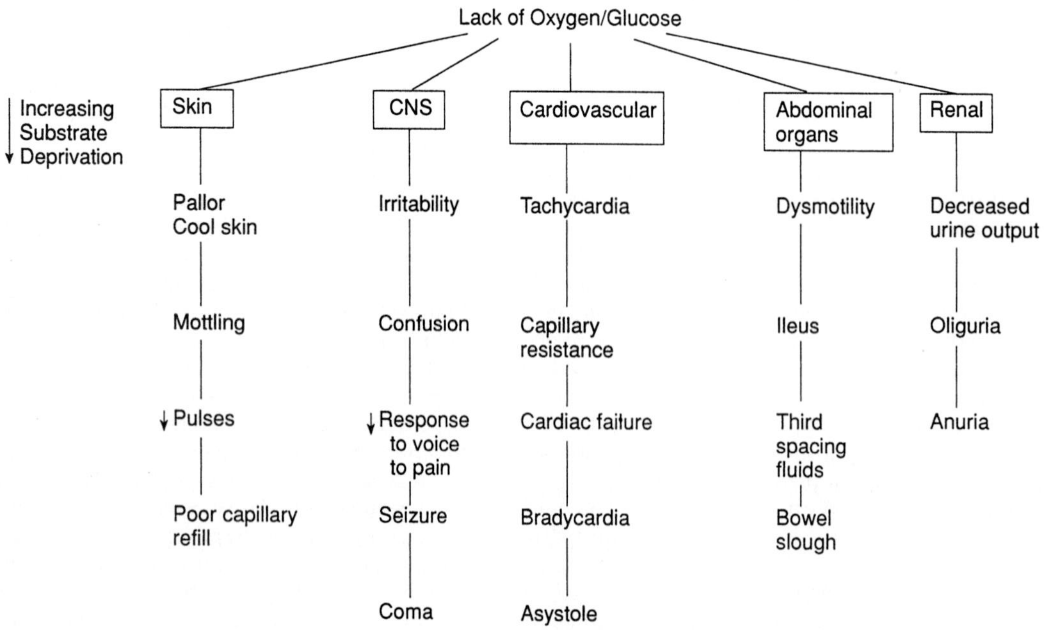

Lack of Oxygen/Glucose

↓ Increasing Substrate Deprivation

Skin: Pallor, Cool skin → Mottling → ↓ Pulses → Poor capillary refill

CNS: Irritability → Confusion → ↓ Response to voice to pain → Seizure → Coma

Cardiovascular: Tachycardia → Capillary resistance → Cardiac failure → Bradycardia → Asystole

Abdominal organs: Dysmotility → Ileus → Third spacing fluids → Bowel slough

Renal: Decreased urine output → Oliguria → Anuria

Figure 1.1. Signs and symptoms of lack of substrate delivery to vital organ systems.

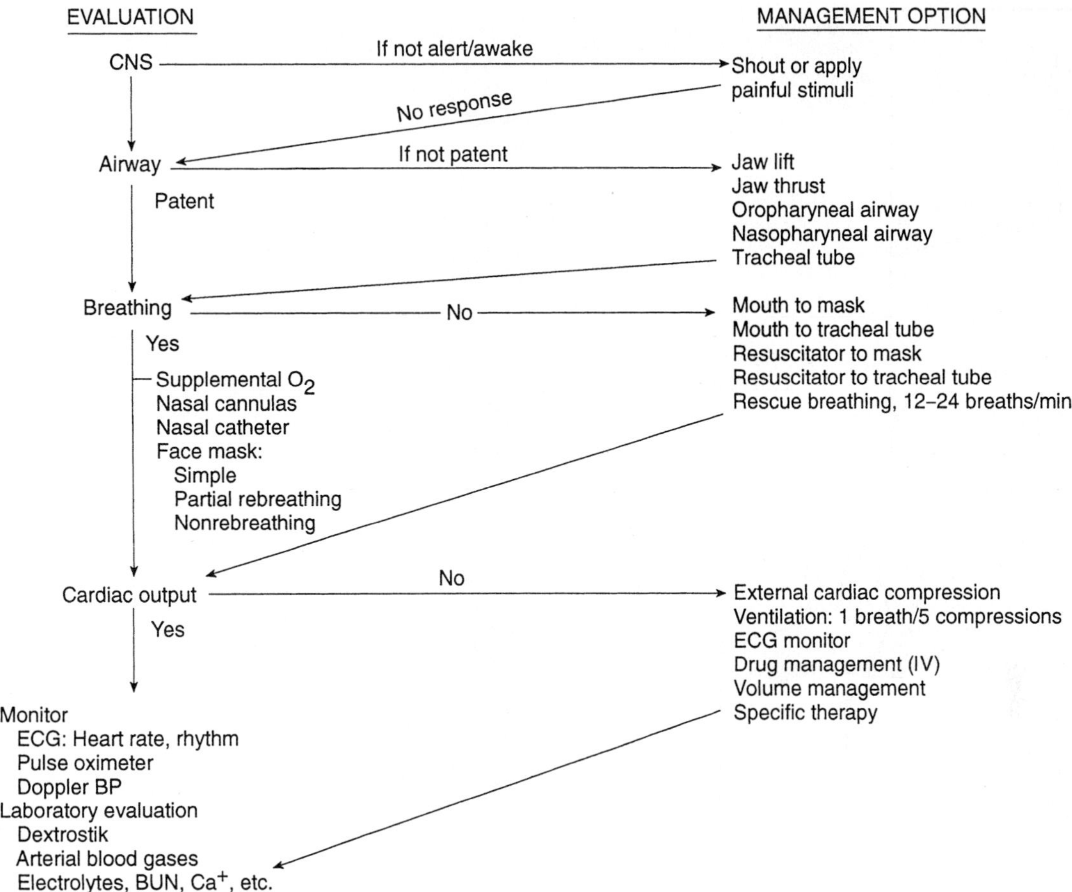

Figure 1.2. Management sequence for pediatric life support.

MANAGEMENT

Management Sequence

Once a child has been identified as requiring life support, a sequence of evaluations and interventions should be accomplished (Fig. 1.2). Initially, CNS integrity must be evaluated: Is the patient alert? Does he or she respond to a shout or painful stimulus? If there is no response, the physician assumes that the brain is no longer receiving an adequate amount of oxygen, and the three basic sequences of evaluation and management are initiated.

First, the airway is maneuvered to move the mandibular block of tissue up and off the posterior pharyngeal wall. The physician places his or her cheek next to the mouth and nose while listening and feeling for movement of air. At the same time, the physician is watching the chest for any evidence of chest wall movement. If the patient is moving air independently, the physician simply continues to support the airway and looks to provide a mechanism for delivering supplemental oxygen. If the patient is not breathing spontaneously, the physician must breathe for the patient, using an expired air technique when a manual resuscitator is not available. As soon as advanced life support breathing technology is available, it should be used. With the recognition that the airway is open and ventilation is occurring, the third phase of oxygen delivery is evaluated by feeling for arterial pulsations. The physician should palpate the brachial, carotid, or femoral arteries. If palpable pulses are not present after a 15-second evaluation, external cardiac compression (ECC) is initiated to provide a circulation. The adequacy of ECC is initially determined by feeling for pulses. In determining whether the oxygen delivery system has been reestablished, the physician should look for improvement in the level of consciousness or a return to spontaneous breathing or an inherent cardiac rhythm.

More specific management sequences are offered at the end of this chapter.

Airway

EVALUATION

The first priority is evaluation and treatment of the airway. The physician should look, listen, and feel for evidence of gas exchange. The physician should *look* at the chest to see whether there is chest wall or abdominal movement suggestive of breathing effort. The physician should *listen* over the mouth and nose for the sound of air movement. With a stethoscope, the physician should listen over the trachea and the axilla for air entry. The physician should *feel* with his or her cheek for evidence of air movement. If there is evidence of spontaneous breathing and no evidence of gas movement through the central airway, the presumptive diagnosis is that of airway obstruction.

MANAGEMENT

If trauma is suspected, the head and cervical spine must be stabilized during evaluation and management of the airway. Someone must be assigned to hold the head in the midline position while applying gentle cephalad traction. The most effective noninvasive maneuver for clearing an obstructed airway in-

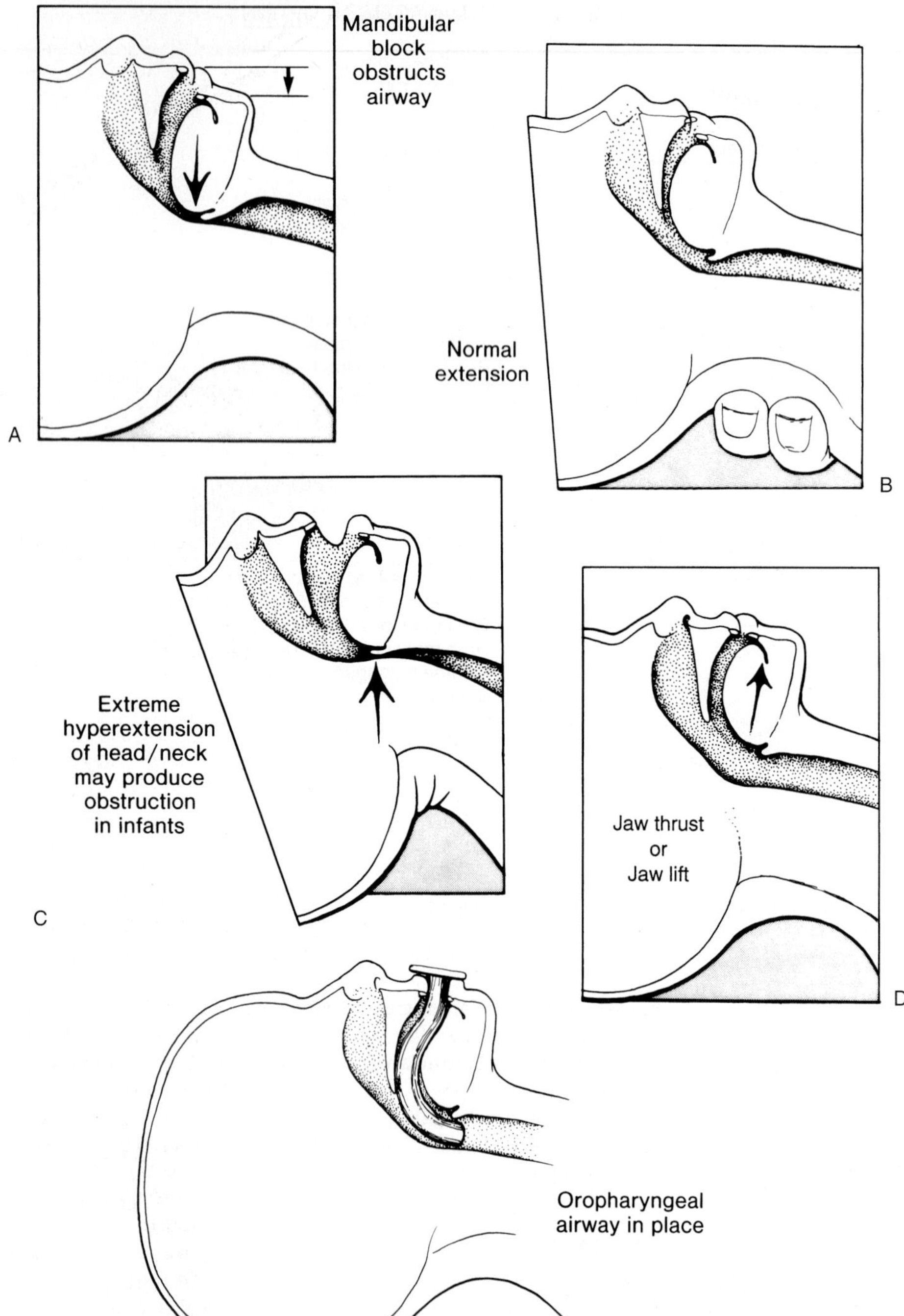

Figure 1.3. **A**: Upper airway obstruction related to hypotonia. **B**: Partial relief of airway obstruction by means of head extension (danger of cervical spine injury in cases of trauma). **C**: Extreme hyperextension causing upper airway obstruction. **D**: Fully open airway through use of jaw thrust or jaw lift. **E**: Oropharyngeal airway stenting mandibular block off of posterior pharyngeal wall.

volves tilting the head back slightly and lifting the chin forward by pulling or pushing the mandibular block of tissue forward (Fig. 1.3). The traditional mechanism of gentle flexion of the cervical spine on the thoracic spine may open the airway, but it provides less efficient ventilation and is hazardous if cervical spine trauma has occurred.

Most airway obstruction is related to the mandibular block of tissue falling posteriorly and lying against the posterior wall of the hypopharynx. This can be relieved by physically grasping the mandibular block and pulling it forward so that the lower anterior central incisors are anterior to the maxillary central incisors. The same result can be obtained by pushing the mandibular block of tissue forward. The fingers should be placed behind the angle of the jaw and the jaw pushed forward so that the lower central incisors are in a plane anterior to the upper central incisors. These noninvasive maneuvers should be attempted before any of the more invasive airway adjuncts are tried. Table 1.2 lists rates of respiration to be achieved by providing CPR for pediatric life support.

TABLE 1.2. Rate of Respiration

Infant:	20–24 breaths/min
Child:	16–20 breaths/min
Adolescent:	12–16 breaths/min

ARTIFICIAL AIRWAYS

Oropharyngeal Airways

Oropharyngeal airways are used when manual manipulation of the airway cannot maintain airway patency. The purpose of the oropharyngeal airway is to stent or support the mandibular block of tissue off of the posterior pharyngeal wall. There are three basic parts to this airway. The flange is used to prevent the airway from falling back into the mouth. It also serves as a point of fixation for adhesive tape. The bite block portion is designed to prevent approximation of the central incisors. A forceful bite may produce obstruction of an oral tracheal tube. The stent of the oropharyngeal airway is designed specifically to hold the tongue away from the posterior pharyngeal wall. Secondarily, the stent may provide an air channel or suction conduit through the mouth. The proper size oropharyngeal airway can be estimated by placing the airway alongside the face so that the bite block portion is parallel to the palate. The tip of the airway should just approximate the angle of the mandible.

The primary use of the airway is in the unconscious patient. The airway should be placed by using a wooden spatula or tongue depressor to press the tongue into the floor of the mouth. The airway is then passed so that the stent conforms to the contour of the tongue. If the oropharyngeal airway is not inserted properly, it may push the tongue backward into the posterior pharynx, aggravating or creating upper airway obstruction. If the airway is too long, it may touch the larynx and stimulate vomiting or laryngospasm.

Nasopharyngeal Airways

The purpose of nasopharyngeal airways is to stent the tongue from the posterior pharyngeal wall. It may also be used to facilitate nasotracheal suctioning. The length of the nasopharyngeal airway is estimated by measuring the distance from the nares to the tragus of the ear. The outside diameter of the airway should not be so large that it produces sustained blanching of the skin of the ala nasae. The nasopharyngeal airway is inserted through the nares and passed along the floor of the nostril into the nasopharynx and oropharynx so that it rests between the tongue and the posterior pharyngeal wall. Nasopharyngeal airways may lacerate the vascular adenoidal tissue found in the nasopharynx of children. Therefore, adenoidal hypertrophy and bleeding diatheses are relative contraindications to the use of these airways.

Endotracheal Tubes

The purpose of the endotracheal (ET) tube is to supply a stable alternate airway. ET tubes are used to (1) overcome upper airway obstruction, (2) isolate the larynx from the pharynx, (3) allow mechanical aspiration of secretions from the tracheal bronchial tree, and (4) facilitate mechanical ventilation or end-expiratory pressure. The correct tube size can be approximated by using a simple formula based on the patient's age:

$$\text{Inside diameter (ID) in mm} = 16 + \text{Age in years}/4$$

Because this is an estimate, it is prudent to have the next smaller and larger size ET tube available. Estimation of tube size based on the size of the patient's fifth finger is not accurate. Tube size may also need to be modified based on the cause of the arrest (e.g., croup). In the pediatric patient, uncuffed tubes are used and are compatible with positive-pressure ventilation. This is because there is a normal narrowing of the trachea at the level of the cricoid ring in children. With proper tube selection, this narrowing serves as a functional seal. With patients 10 years of age and older, cuffed ET tubes should be used. By using a cuffed tube, one essentially adds 0.5 mm to the tube size.

A variety of ET tubes are available. Tracheal tubes should be translucent to facilitate inspection of internal debris or occlusion, have a radiopaque tip marker, have the internal diameter noted proximally so that it is visible after intubation, have a distal vocal cord marker so that when the marker is placed at the level of the vocal cords the tip of the tube is in a midtracheal position, and have centimeter markings along the course of the tube to be used as reference points for detecting tube movement.

Other Techniques

Alternative airway management systems, including esophageal/tracheal tubes, laryngeal mask airways, and transtracheal ventilation systems, have all been used with adult patients with varying degrees of success. All of the methods have been approved by government agencies and professional societies, but their use in children has not been well tested or researched. Thus, they remain techniques worth consideration in a setting where standard methods have failed.

Laryngoscopy and Intubation

The purpose of laryngoscopy is to create a spatial plane through the mouth to the larynx through which an ET tube can be passed into the trachea. The laryngoscope consists of a blade and a handle. It is used to identify the glottis and to compress the intervening soft tissue structures into the floor of the mouth. The three components of the laryngoscope blade are the spatula, the tip, and the flange. The spatula may be curved or straight and is used to compress tissue. The tip of the blade is used for positioning the spatula so that an optimal compression of the mandibular block or soft tissue can be achieved. The purpose of the flange is to keep the tongue out of the way of the intubating channel. The laryngoscope is introduced into the mouth so that the tip of the blade slides down the right side of the tongue. As the tip of the blade follows the tongue posteriorly, it bumps into the anterior pillars of the tonsils. The tip is moved around the pillars of the tonsils until it bumps into the epiglottis. When using a curved spatula, the tip is placed in the vallecula, the space between the tongue and epiglottis. When using a straight spatula, the tip is placed under the epiglottis with the leading edge resting on the aryepiglottic folds. Once the tip is properly placed, the spatula is shifted from the right side of the mouth to the middle of the mouth. This left lateral movement of the spatula allows the flange to push the tongue ahead of it so that the tongue eventually occupies the middle third of the mouth. The right one-third of the mouth is then available as a channel through which the tracheal tube can pass. Once the tip of the blade is properly positioned and the flange has moved the tongue into the left corner of the mouth, the full surface of the spatula is used to compress the tongue into the floor of the mouth. With compression of the soft tissue of the mouth, the glottis should be exposed and the tracheal tube can be passed. The tracheal tube should be fitted with a stylet. The purpose of the stylet is to provide some degree of curvature to the tube for those circumstances where a totally straight channel cannot be achieved. The tracheal tube is passed through the glottis so that the ring marker near the tip of the tube is aligned with the vocal cords. If the tube selected is the proper size and the ring marker is placed directly at the vocal cords, the tip of the tube should be at a midtracheal position.

Proper positioning of the tube is confirmed most accurately by end-tidal CO_2 monitoring (Fig. 1.4) and by auscultating for breath sounds and observing for symmetric chest movement. The child's small chest wall may transmit sounds widely and thus mislead the physician into thinking that positioning is correct. The physician should listen carefully. He or she should listen over the stomach and both axillae, and look for improved color of the patient. If

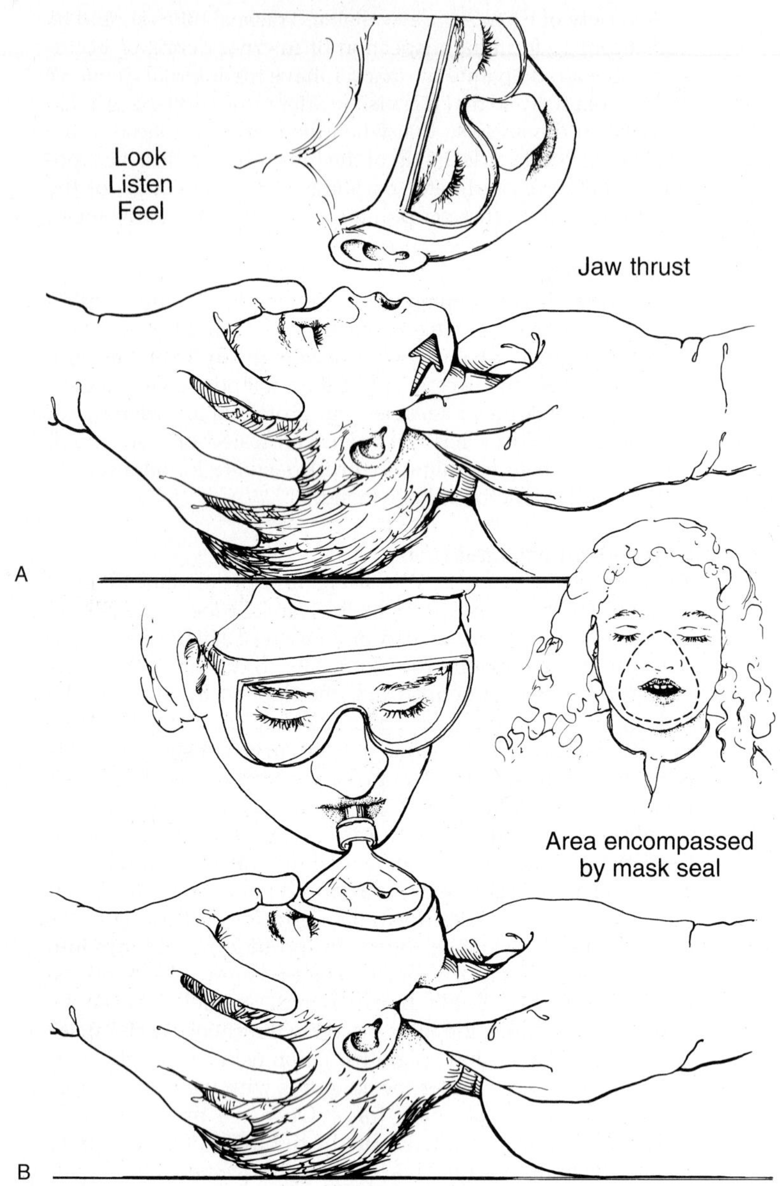

Figure 1.4. Basic life support—airway and breathing. **A**: Positioning of head to open airway and evaluation for spontaneous ventilation. **B**: Expired air (mouth- to-mask) ventilation.

breath sounds are not equal or end-tidal CO_2 monitoring is not available, the tube should be withdrawn slightly and the breath sounds and chest movement reevaluated. When circumstances allow, tube position should be confirmed with an anteroposterior (AP) chest roentgenogram. On the AP film, the tip of the tracheal tube should be at a T2 to T3 vertebral level or directly between the lower edges of the medial aspect of the clavicles.

Depth of insertion in cm for children > 2 years
= Age in years + 12/2

or

depth of insertion = internal diameter (ID) of tube (mm) × 3

Breathing

EVALUATION

When a clear and stable airway has been established, the patient should be reassessed. The physician should look, listen, and feel for evidence of gas exchange. In infants, adequacy of ventilation is assessed by observing free uniform expansion of the lower chest and upper abdomen. This is in contrast to older children and adolescents in whom one looks for uniform upper chest expansion as a sign of adequate ventilation. Gas exchanges should be confirmed by auscultation and by electronic monitoring of end-tidal CO_2 and pulse oximetry. First, the physician should listen over the trachea to establish quickly that gas exchange is occurring through the central airway. Then, he or she should listen to breath sounds bilaterally to assess for peripheral aeration and symmetric lung expansion.

MANAGEMENT

Spontaneous Ventilation

If the airway has been established and the patient is breathing spontaneously, supplemental oxygen should be administered. Although elimination of CO_2 is important, it is not nearly as important as delivery of oxygen. Children are quite resistant to the effects of severe hypercarbia and respiratory acidosis. They do not tolerate even short periods of oxygen deprivation.

Oxygen Delivery Devices

A variety of oxygen delivery devices are available for use in patients who have stable airways without ET tubes.

Nasal Cannulas. Nasal cannulas have two hollow plastic prongs that arise from a flexible hollow face piece. Humidified oxygen delivered through the hollow tubing is directed to the nostrils. One hundred percent oxygen is run through a bubbler into the cannula system at a flow of 4 to 6 L per minute. Because of oropharyngeal and nasopharyngeal entrainment of air, the final oxygen delivery is usually 30% to 40%. The advantages of cannulas are that they are easy to apply, lightweight, economical, and disposable. Inefficiency of the bubbler humidifier is compensated for by the fact that the normal humidification and warming systems of the upper airway are not bypassed. The use of this device presumes that the patient's oxygen needs can be met with substantially less than 100% oxygen. This method of oxygen delivery is best tolerated by the older child.

Oxygen Hoods. Oxygen hoods are clear plastic cylinders with removable lids or clear, soft, plastic tents just large enough to accommodate the infant's head. They are used for delivery of oxygen to infants and come in a variety of sizes. They usually have a gas inlet system for wide-bore tubing and a port for positioning the cylinder across the neck. Their purpose is to maintain a controlled environment for oxygen, humidity, and temperature. This can be done without producing a tight seal at the neck. Hoods are best used for newborns and infants. One can, without difficulty, deliver oxygen concentrations in the 80% to 90% range simply by increasing the oxygen flow to flood the canister. Another advantage is that the oxygen may be well humidified. Because of their potential for delivering concentrations of oxygen that may be toxic to the eyes or lungs of the infant, it is imperative to monitor both the fraction of inspired oxygen (FiO_2) and the PaO_2.

Oxygen Tents. The basic purpose of the oxygen tent is to provide a controlled and stable environment for humidity, temperature, and oxygen. Tents are useful for delivery of oxygen between 21% and 50%. Oxygen concentration may be variable because of a poor seal and frequent entry. Therefore, a tight fit and only necessary entry should be allowed. Tents potentially impede access to the patient, and if mist is used, the patient may be hidden in a cloud that makes skin color difficult to evaluate.

Oxygen Masks. The most often used equipment for the spontaneously breathing patient is the oxygen mask. Several types of oxygen masks can be used to offer the patient a wide range of inspired oxygen concentrations. Masks seem to be better tolerated than nasal cannula by the young child, particularly when the mask is held by a calm parent or by emergency department personnel. There are several mask types from which to select. As with all equipment, even masks have associated hazards. In patients prone to vomit, the mask can block the flow of vomit and increase the risk of aspiration. The obtunded patient wearing a mask must always be observed.

SIMPLE MASKS. The purpose of the simple face mask is to deliver a moderate concentration of oxygen. These masks are lightweight and inexpensive. They should be clear to allow observation of the child's color. They can be used in a loose-fitting fashion and are relatively comfortable. If the flow of oxygen is inadvertently disrupted, the child can breathe through side ports. A minimal flow of oxygen is necessary to flush potential dead space. This type of oxygen delivery device does not bypass the upper airway mechanisms for warming and humidification of inspired gas. The disadvantages of the simple mask lie in the fact that it is difficult to provide a known and stable FiO_2. The FiO_2 will vary with the inspiratory flow rate of the patient and with the oxygen flow into the system. The actual pharyngeal FiO_2 may be difficult to predict or measure.

PARTIAL REBREATHING MASKS. Partial rebreathing masks allow delivery of a higher oxygen concentration than simple masks do. They are also helpful in conserving oxygen. This system is a combined face mask and reservoir bag. When the flow rate into the bag is greater than the patient's minute ventilation and when the oxygen is adjusted so that the bag does not collapse during inhalation, there is negligible CO_2 rebreathing. Partial rebreathing masks are usually used for midrange oxygen delivery. We use one when we are trying to maintain an FiO_2 between 35% and 60%.

NONREBREATHING MASKS. Nonrebreathing masks are combined face mask and reservoir bag devices that have nonrebreathing valves incorporated into the face mask. They are useful for giving oxygen concentrations up to 100%.

Assisted Ventilation

If the airway has been established and the child is not breathing spontaneously or gas exchange is not adequate, artificial ventilation should be started.

If adjuncts for mechanical ventilatory support are not available, an expired air technique may be used. Patient size, type of available airway, and trial will determine which type should be used. Because of risk of human immunodeficiency virus (HIV) transmission, mouth-to-mouth resuscitation is no longer recommended. Instead, rescue breathing should be done with a pocket mask that contains an appropriate Millipore filter (Fig. 1.5). Placement of the mask over the mouth alone, over the mouth and nose, or over a tracheostomy site depends on the patient and the equipment available (Fig. 1.5).

Expired Air Techniques

Hand-Squeezed, Self-Inflating Resuscitators. Hand-squeezed, self-inflating resuscitators are the most commonly used resuscitators for infants and children. The elasticity of a self-inflating bag allows the bag to refill independently of gas flow. This feature makes the self-inflating bag easy to use for the inexperi-

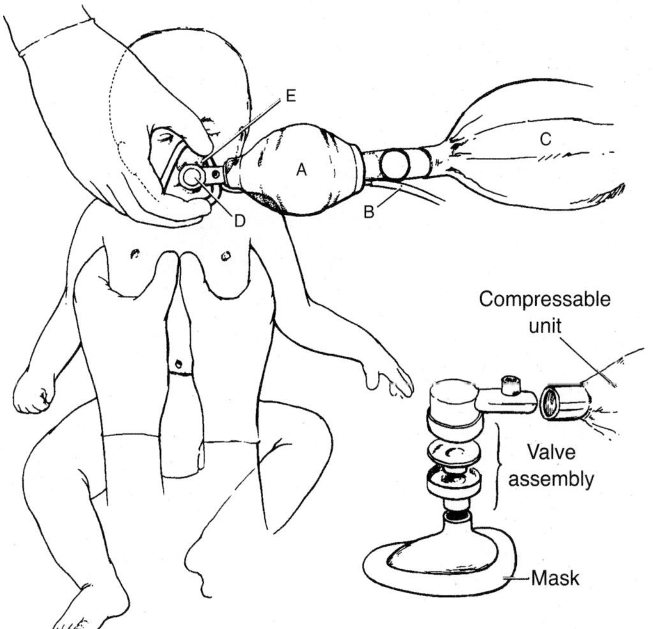

Figure 1.5. Self-inflating, hand-powered resuscitator: compressible unit *(A)*; oxygen source *(B)*; oxygen reservoir *(C)*; one-way valve assembly *(D)*; and mask with transparent body *(E)*.

enced operator. Many of the self-inflating bags are equipped with a pressure-limiting pop-off valve that is usually preset at 30 to 35 cm H_2O to prevent delivery of high pressures. Self-inflating bags that are not pressure-limited should have a manometer in line. For gas to flow, the bag must be squeezed. Thus, for the patient who is breathing spontaneously, the operator must time the bag compressions to the patient's efforts. These resuscitators should be adapted to deliver high concentrations of oxygen. In most cases, this involves using an oxygen reservoir adaptation with the unit. Recent research has shown that even with an attached reservoir, only oxygen concentrations of 60% to 90% were obtainable. Units without oxygen reservoir adaptations often deliver low concentrations of supplemental oxygen and therefore should be avoided. The resuscitator may be used with a mask. When selecting a family of mask sizes, select a mask type that seals a variety of facial contours. Also, the body of the mask should be sufficiently transparent so that vomit can be recognized easily through the mask. Masks with a pneumatic cuff design allow for easiest and most efficient fit to avoid air leaks around the mask. Resuscitators, masks, and ET tubes should be standardized so that any resuscitator can connect with any mask or ET tube.

Anesthesia Bags. Anesthesia bags depend on an adequate gas flow to maintain a compressible unit that propels gas toward the patient. An exit port must also be present so that the bag does not become a CO_2 reservoir. When used with an oxygen blender, any desired concentration of oxygen may be provided for the patient because this system delivers directly the gas flowing into it. When used correctly, this device allows 100% oxygen to be delivered as well as maintaining end-expiratory pressure. However, the major disadvantage of this type of bag is that considerable experience is needed to use it effectively, which has prompted some to recommend the use of the self-inflating bag as the primary mode of ventilation. One must be able to judge accurately the rate of gas flow into the bag and the rate of gas escape from the exit port so that underfilling or overfilling does not occur. If the bag is removed from a leak-tight patient application, it promptly deflates and one must wait for the reservoir to refill. Overfilling the bag is dangerous because high pressures can be transmitted to the lung and stomach.

Circulation

As with the other components of CPR, the circulation must be first assessed and then managed.

EVALUATION

Once the airway has been opened and gas exchange ensured, the physician must evaluate the effectiveness of circulation by (1) observing skin and mucous membrane color and (2) palpating a peripheral pulse and checking capillary refill. If the patient's color is ashen or cyanotic, the circulation will need to be treated.

The palpation of a peripheral pulse and assessment of capillary refill is mandatory. Often, ineffective cardiac activity can be palpated over the child's thin chest wall. Thus, the presence of an apical pulse may not be meaningful. The palpation of a strong femoral or brachial pulse indicates presumptively that the cardiac output is adequate. Capillary refill should be assessed repeatedly.

Most modern defibrillators have a "quick-look" paddle configuration that allows a rapid evaluation of cardiac rhythm to be

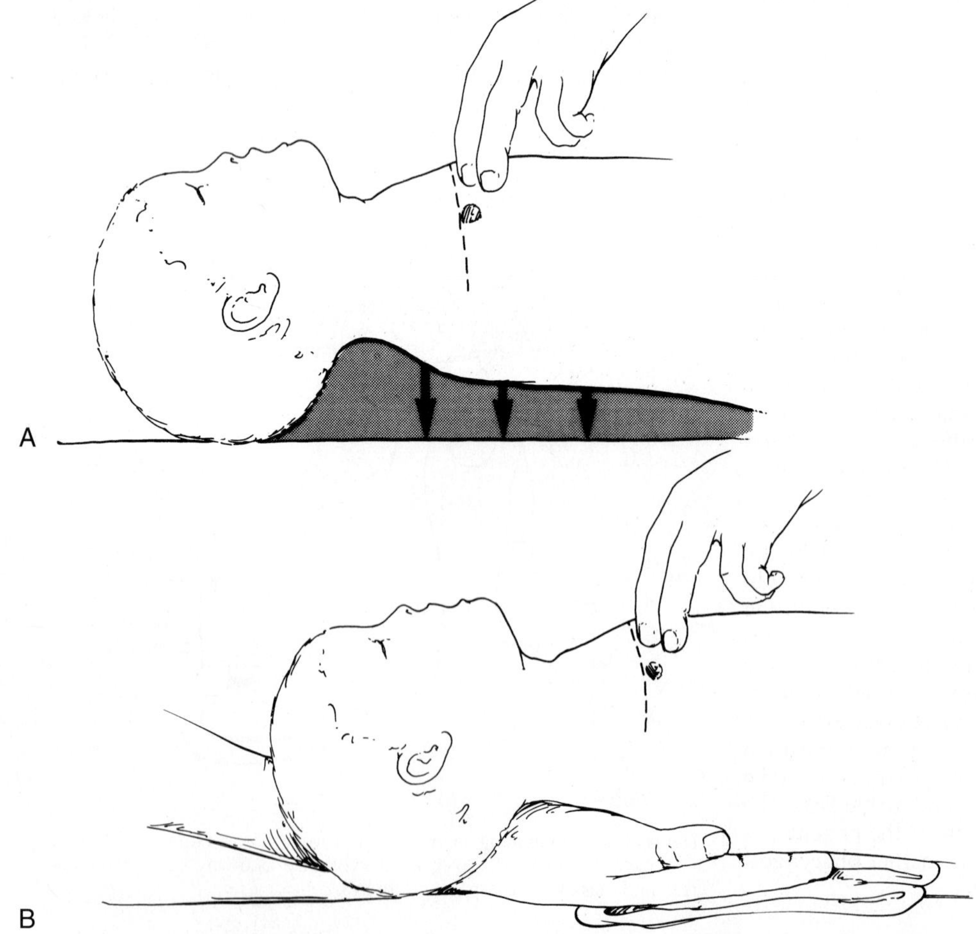

Figure 1.6. Thoracic cage support for external cardiac compression. **A**: Dead space created by prominent occiput. **B**: Hand providing thoracic support.

made by placing the defibrillation paddles on the chest and using them as monitoring electrodes.

The resuscitation team will also find it helpful to have continuous blood pressure monitoring. Blood pressure measurements will help quantify the effectiveness of cardiac function. An ultrasound or portable Doppler device may be necessary to detect systolic pressure at low levels in small infants.

As soon as possible, the team will also require continuous electrocardiogram (ECG) monitoring to assess the development of arrhythmia as the resuscitation proceeds.

TABLE 1.3. Ventilation/Compression Schedule for Pediatric Resuscitation

	Infant	Child	Adult[a]
Compression (rate/min)	100	80	60
Depth of compression (inches)	0.5–1	1–1.5	1.5–2
Ventilation (rate/min)	20	16	12

[a] Two-person rescue.

MANAGEMENT

Management may be divided into five phases: (1) cardiac compression, (2) establishment of an intravascular route, (3) use of primary drugs, (4) use of secondary drugs, and (5) defibrillation.

Cardiac Compression

Absence of a peripheral pulse requires immediate institution of cardiac compression (CC) to establish at least a minimum circulation to the brain. ECC has the advantage of immediate applicability. The technique of ECC is also widely known and can be applied in almost any setting. However, several recent reports have pointed to the potential advantages of open cardiac compression (OCC). This technique is obviously more difficult to apply. OCC may produce better coronary and cerebral perfusion pressures. Survival rates may also be higher in studies comparing OCC with ECC. The role of OCC may become more important as future studies evolve. For now, OCC is indicated primarily in the selected traumatized patient (see Chapters 91 and 94).

The mechanism by which blood moves during ECC has been the subject of ongoing investigation. The traditional view assumes that chest compressions move blood by direct CC. Therefore, it was believed to be important to compress directly over the ventricles that were assumed to be located under the middle one-third of a child's sternum. However, another model suggests that the movement of blood is caused by an increased intrathoracic pressure and expulsion of blood from the lungs through the left heart and simultaneous openings of both the mitral and aortic valves. This proposed thoracic pump mechanism quiets the controversy concerning the relative position of the child's heart within the thorax and its relation to the sternum. The intrathoracic pressure pump model for the production of blood flow has sparked the investigation of several alternative methods for achieving flow. Probably both models of ECC-produced blood flow play a part in the actual mechanism in children.

For now, we continue to recommend that compression be applied evenly over the midsternum of the child. This standard technique has proved effective. Compression over the lower one-third of the sternum should be avoided because of a potential risk of liver trauma.

The midsternal location for ECC can be found by spanning the sternum between the thumb and fifth finger and then measuring or judging the midpoint. Another method used in locating the midsternum is to find the point where the transnipple line intersects the sternum. Finger or hand position should be just caudal (toward the feet) to the transnipple line.

The depth and rate of compression are based on the child's age. Suggested rates and depths are shown in Table 1.3. Compression should be smooth, continuous, and uninterrupted. The compression phase should consume 60% of the time for the compression–release cycle. Jabbing, jerky, brief compressions may produce pressure pulses of adequate amplitude on a monitor, but blood flow will be inadequate for cerebral perfusion.

Because the child has a relatively large occiput, neck extension may elevate the shoulders and upper thorax off of the firm resuscitation surface. The resultant wedge-shaped dead space beneath the upper thorax may absorb the force of compression (Fig. 1.6A). The dead space must be filled with a firm substance

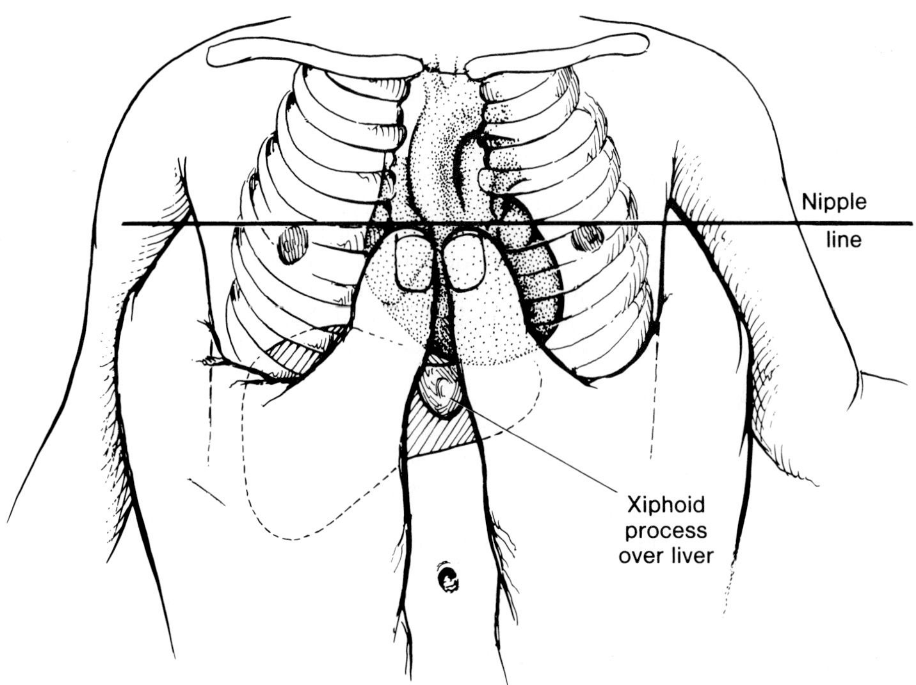

Figure 1.7. External cardiac compression—Thaler technique for infants.

so that the work of compression will not be lost. A firm towel or the rescuer's hand should be placed beneath the upper thoracic spine (Fig. 1.6B). Compressions may then be applied with one or two fingers in the infant or with one hand in the older child. When using the technique developed by Thaler, the rescuer links his or her fingers beneath the thoracic spine and compresses with the thumbs (Fig. 1.7). This method is comfortable when using external cardiac compression on a newborn patient. With older children, an effort should be made not to allow the encircling hands to limit the respiratory movements of the thorax.

Mechanical chest compressors should not be used for children. There is insufficient information about their effectiveness or safety for this patient population.

Intravenous Lines

The placement of an intravenous (i.v.) line is often the most difficult and time-consuming aspect of pediatric life support. The resuscitation team should have a set protocol for the attainment of i.v. access (an example is shown in Table 1.4). This protocol should outline which personnel should attempt which form of access for a finite period as well as when to move on to more advanced forms of access. When possible, a short, large-gauge i.v. line should be obtained. Peripheral sites are an acceptable choice and may be readily available. Central lines are useful for getting drugs and a large volume of fluids into the central circulation. Intraosseous (into the bone) infusion is an old technique that has been revived and widely promulgated. Spivey and colleagues have shown it to be an excellent route for fluid and drug administration. While waiting for an i.v. line to be secured, some drugs may be given through the ET tube as they are absorbed at an alveolar level and circulated rapidly. The drugs should be administered through a small-gauge catheter inserted through the ET tube into the distal trachea or one of the mainstream bronchi and followed by several positive pressure ventilations. Table 1.5 lists the drugs that may be given through this route.

When using an ET route, the physician should dilute the medications with normal saline to a volume of 3 to 5 mL, lest they remain on the tube surface and fail to reach the lung.

Intravenous cut down over the saphenous vein is another acceptable method but seems to be time-consuming even in experienced hands. Intracardiac administration of drugs is dangerous and should be avoided. In the circumstance of CPR, the cannulation of the subclavian vessel may also be difficult and associated with pneumothorax and hemothorax.

Three vessels that are easily cannulated and give access to the central circulation are the femoral, internal jugular, and external jugular veins. Our vein of first choice is the femoral because its cannulation does not interfere with ongoing CPR. The femoral vein is located by palpating the femoral artery pulsation and moving just medial to it. If good external cardiac compression is being accomplished, the pulsation should be present. When the pulse is not palpable, the physician should find the midpoint between the symphysis pubis and the anterior-superior iliac spine on the plane of the inguinal ligament. The vein should be approached at a 45-degree angle to the skin 2 to 3 cm below the inguinal ligament at the defined midpoint. The needle must not pass cephalad to the inguinal ligament because it may enter the peritoneal cavity and pierce the bowel.

TABLE 1.4. Sample Protocol for Intravenous Access

1. First 1.5 min
   Peripheral i.v. catheter, two sites
2. 1.5–5 min
   a. If intubated: give drugs via endotracheal tube (including epinephrine/atropine/lidocaine)
   b. If not intubated: intraosseous—one site
   Continued peripheral i.v.—one site
3. Longer than 5 min
   a. Femoral vein percutaneous
   b. External/internal jugular percutaneous
   c. Subclavian vein percutaneous
   d. Saphenous vein cutdown

Adapted from Kanter RK, Zimmerman JJ, Strauss RH, et al. *Am J Dis Child* 1986; 140:144, with permission.

TABLE 1.5. Resuscitation Drugs That May Be Given Intratracheally

Epinephrine
Atropine
Lidocaine

The internal jugular is best approached by finding the triangle created by the medial one-third of the clavicle and the two heads of the sternocleidomastoid muscle—the sternum and clavicular. The internal jugular vein courses within the triangle. The physician should puncture the skin at the apex of the triangle and direct the needle toward the ipsilateral nipple at a 45-degree angle to the frontal plane. The external jugular vein is located by placing the child in a 20-degree head-down position. With the patient at this angle, the vein will fill and be seen as it courses over the midportion of the sternocleidomastoid muscle.

In cannulating either the femoral or internal jugular vein, the Seldinger technique is recommended. This method uses a 20- to 22-gauge, short-beveled, thin-walled needle for the small child. Larger needles should be used for older children. The needle is attached to a syringe, and the vein is punctured and aspirated so that free blood flow into the syringe is seen. The syringe is then removed, and blood is sent for appropriate laboratory studies. A braided wire is introduced through the needle and positioned in the lumen of the vein. The needle is withdrawn over the free end of the wire. Next, a flexible Teflon catheter is passed over the wire and into the vein. Finally, the wire is removed from the lumen of the catheter, and the catheter is secured with suture. Although this technique requires several steps, it represents a safe and effective way to secure an i.v. line. It allows a small initial puncture to result in the placement of a larger-bore catheter. It is particularly useful for the femoral and internal jugular veins.

If the Seldinger technique is unsuccessful, an acceptable alternative is to cut down over the lesser saphenous vein just above and anterior to the medial malleolus. In extreme circumstances, cut down over the femoral vein may be attempted. This technique is more difficult and fraught with more complications. Remember also that in newborns during the first 2 weeks, it may be easy to cannulate the umbilical vein.

Primary Drugs

The primary drugs for advanced life support are oxygen, epinephrine, sodium bicarbonate, atropine, and glucose (Table 1.6). Each agent has specific actions, indications, dosages, and untoward effects. The primary drugs are those that are used first in the resuscitation. Our recommended drug dosages are based on kilograms of body weight. The resuscitation team must be able to determine the weight of the child accurately. If estimates prove too difficult, a standardized growth curve should be posted in the resuscitation area so that the fiftieth percentile

TABLE 1.6. Primary Life Support Drugs and Dosages

Drug	Dosage
Epinephrine	10–200 μg/kg i.v. or intratracheally
Sodium bicarbonate	1 mEq/kg i.v.
Atropine	0.02 mg/kg i.v. or intratracheally (min 0.2 mg)
Glucose	0.5–1.0 g/kg i.v.

weight for the child's age may be used. Another method for establishing the correct dosage schedule has been proposed by Broselow in the invention of the Broselow Tape. This method bases dosage on the patient's length, which is determined by placing the tape alongside the child in the supine position (Fig. 1.8A). An appropriate drug dosage schedule has been printed on the tape (Fig. 1.8B) at intervals. Using this method eliminates the estimation of patient weights and the need to cross-reference to a drug dosage chart or to memorize the dosage schedule. If the pediatric drug dosage schedule is not used often, it is advisable to prominently display the schedule on the emergency department wall.

Oxygen. In the patient in cardiac arrest, there are many factors that contribute to the pathophysiologic disruption of oxygen delivery (i.e., hypoxemia). A fundamental goal of basic and advanced life support is to correct cerebral and myocardial hypoxia before irreversible injury occurs.

During resuscitation, the initial dosage of oxygen for the patient needing oxygen is 100%. The potential negative effects of high oxygen concentration are not a consideration in the life-or-death setting of CPR.

The physician should be familiar with the different oxygen delivery systems mentioned previously in this chapter in the sections on airway and breathing. Oxygen concentrations delivered by mouth-to-mask breathing vary from 17% to 21%. Bag-valve-mask devices deliver 21%. When an oxygen source is attached, bag-valve-mask devices may deliver 30% to 60%, and when a reservoir is added, 70% to 90% may be achieved. An anesthesia bag may deliver 100%. Oxygen should be ordered like other drugs. The order should clearly specify the dose, mechanism, and duration of treatment.

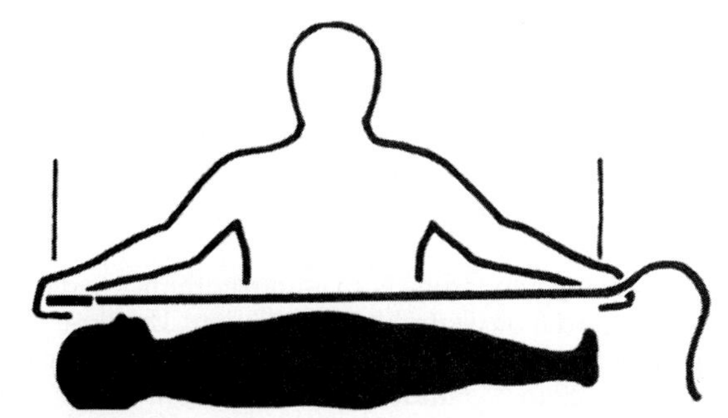

A

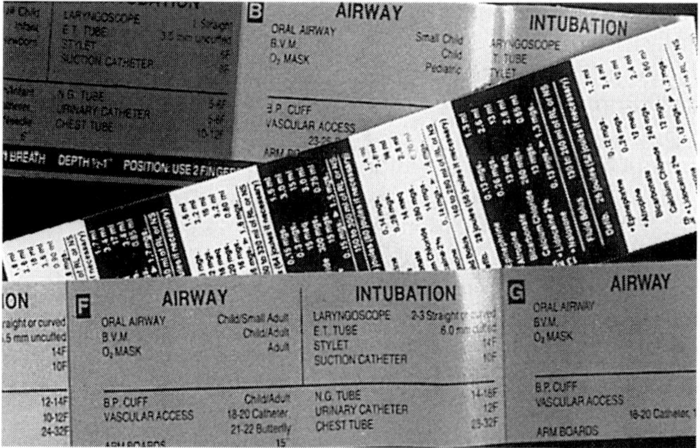

B

Figure 1.8. Broselow Tape for determining drug dosage schedule based on patient length. **A**: Placement of tape. **B**: Equipment size and drug dosage schedule printed on tape.

Epinephrine. Despite the development of many new exogenous catecholamines, epinephrine remains the essential cardiac stimulant. Epinephrine actions include α- and β-adrenergic stimulation. The primary α effect is vasoconstriction and a resultant increase in systolic and diastolic blood pressure. The β-adrenergic action of the drug is also beneficial in producing an increased inotropic (contractile force) and chronotropic (cardiac rate) effect. In addition, the β effect produces vasodilation of the coronary and cerebral vasculature. All of these actions are beneficial to the resuscitative effort.

Indications for the use of epinephrine include asystole, symptomatic bradycardia, and hypotension not related to volume depletion. Epinephrine is also used to try to change a fine fibrillation pattern to a coarse one before a defibrillation attempt. There is belief that a coarse fibrillation pattern is more easily converted.

The recommended initial dose of epinephrine for asystole or electromechanical dissociation is 10 μg per kg i.v. Recently, several investigators have looked at the scientific basis for current epinephrine dose recommendations and have used doses 10 to 20 times greater (i.e., 0.1 to 0.2 mg per kg). Thus far, higher-dose therapy with epinephrine (HDE) has not been proved to be of greater efficacy. In the experimental situations in which it has been used, HDE has resulted in no adverse effects. We continue to support a dose-response method of epinephrine administration. We initiate therapy with the currently recommended dose (0.01 mg per kg). Subsequent doses are given by a dose–response method of titration. With this method, the second dose is increased tenfold to 0.1 mg per kg, and the physician observes the patient for the desired response. If an inadequate response occurs, the dose should be doubled to 0.2 mg per kg. In the absence of underlying cardiovascular disease, this is a safe and effective approach. The dose of epinephrine for hypotension is 1 μg per kg i.v. An epinephrine infusion may be prepared by adding 6 mg of epinephrine to 100 mL of 5% dextrose in water (D5W). This creates a solution that has 60 μg per mL. When this solution is infused at 1 mL per kg per hour, the patient receives a dose of 1 μg per kg per minute. If an i.v. or intraosseous line has not been established, epinephrine can be given endotracheally. The dose and concentration of the drug (1:10,000) should be the same. The drug is instilled past the tracheal tube via a smaller-gauge catheter and is followed by several positive-pressure ventilations.

Epinephrine is a relatively safe drug, and few untoward effects are seen in pediatric patients. Ischemia of the myocardium rarely occurs and has not been reported even with high-dose epinephrine. There is the hazard of producing supraventricular or ventricular tachycardia, premature ventricular contractions, or ventricular fibrillation. When possible, the physician should avoid intracardiac injection of epinephrine because this route is associated with greater risk and complications. As previously noted, mixing bicarbonate with epinephrine inactivates the epinephrine.

Sodium Bicarbonate. With the onset of respiratory failure, the patient develops respiratory acidosis. Rising levels of CO_2 in the blood produce a fall in pH. The immediate treatment for this type of acidosis is adequate ventilation. As the patient's circulation begins to fail, there is production of lactic acid and a metabolic acidosis. Sodium bicarbonate corrects the metabolic acidosis by combining with hydrogen to form CO_2 and water. This additional production of CO_2 must also be eliminated through ventilation.

Metabolic acidosis is a harmful byproduct of the arrest because acidosis further impairs cardiac and circulatory function. Acidosis depresses spontaneous cardiac activity, decreases the contractile force of the ventricle, and predisposes the patient to ventricular fibrillation. In addition, catecholamines such as epinephrine will be less effective in a patient whose metabolic acidosis is uncorrected.

It is not necessary to prove a diagnosis of metabolic acidosis before beginning the first steps in treatment. Sodium bicarbonate is also indicated for the correction of suspected metabolic acidosis. This includes any patient who has arrested for more than a few minutes.

For the patient whose arrest was not witnessed, the initial dose of sodium bicarbonate is 1 mEq per kg i.v. This should be given as full-strength bicarbonate (1.0 mEq per mL) for children older than 6 months of age. For infants less than 6 months of age, we recommend that the same dose be given, but in the form of half-strength bicarbonate (0.5 mEq per mL) to lessen the osmotic load of the drug.

After the initial dose of bicarbonate, subsequent doses are best determined by measuring arterial pH and calculating the dosage using the base deficit.

The factor of 0.4 represents the bicarbonate distribution space, which is 40% of the total body weight. The formula divides the dose by 2 to prevent overcorrection with bicarbonate and produce alkalemia. If blood gas analysis is impossible, doses of 0.5 mEq per kg may be administered every 10 to 15 minutes.

Untoward effects of bicarbonate include alkalosis, hypernatremia, and hyperosmolar states. Each of these effects is significant and can in themselves lessen survival. In the context of inadequate ventilation, bicarbonate administration may result in rapid increase in P_{CO_2} levels. Because CO_2 is readily permeable across cell membranes and sodium bicarbonate is not, rapid elevation in CO_2 can exacerbate intracellular acidosis. This intracellular acidosis depresses myocardial function in animal studies. Hypernatremia and hyperosmolar states are most easily produced in the young infant. Alkalosis is tolerated poorly by the body. Thus, it is important to determine the exact need for bicarbonate as quickly as possible. Bicarbonate administration must always be secondary to the establishment of an airway and ventilations that are important for correcting the acidosis of respiratory origin.

There are other potential untoward effects of bicarbonate: the precipitation of bicarbonate and calcium in the i.v. line and the inactivation of catecholamines. To avoid these two problems, we discourage the addition of bicarbonate to i.v. fluid reservoirs during the resuscitation. Bicarbonate should be given by direct i.v. administration and followed with a saline flush solution before giving subsequent medication, such as calcium or epinephrine. ET administration of bicarbonate can be hazardous. Bicarbonate is irritating to the airways, destroys lung surfactant, and can produce massive atelectasis. Also, the large volume of bicarbonate usually required will virtually drown the patient.

Atropine. The actions of atropine are parasympatholytic. Atropine has both peripheral and central effects. The peripheral effect is vagolytic and thus increases heart rate by increasing the rate of discharge from the sinoatrial node, while increasing conduction through the atrioventricular node. The central effect of atropine is to stimulate the medullary vagal nucleus and is produced with low dosage of the drug. The actions are opposite to those desired for resuscitation therapy.

The indication for atropine is bradycardia associated with hypotension, premature ventricular ectopic beats, or symptoms of poor CNS or myocardial perfusion. Atropine may be used for second- or third-degree heart block, although its actions may be only temporary for these arrhythmias.

The dose of atropine is 0.02 mg per kg i.v. There is a minimum dose of 0.10 mg repeated every 5 to 10 minutes to a maximum total dose of 1.0 mg in a child and in an adolescent. Atropine may be given intratracheally if an i.v. route is not available.

The untoward reactions associated with atropine include paradoxic bradycardia, atrial and ventricular tachyarrhythmias, and myocardial ischemia. Paradoxic bradycardia is caused by the central action of atropine. This side effect can be avoided by using at least 0.2 mg for any patient being treated with atropine. Tachyarrhythmias occur but are not usually hemodynamically significant in the pediatric patient. Myocardial ischemia is rare in the absence of existing cardiac disease.

Glucose. The action of glucose is to correct hypoglycemia. Glucose should be considered a primary drug. Infants have minimal glycogen stores for rapid conversion to glucose. Moreover, many infants may have had decreased caloric intake and excessive losses (diarrhea and vomiting) in the days before the arrest.

The dose of glucose is 0.5 to 1.0 g per kg i.v. Either a 10% or a 25% solution may be used except in the neonatal period when 10% glucose is indicated. Doses of glucose should be based on a rapid serum glucose determination.

Untoward effects include hyperglycemia and hyperosmolality, but these should not occur if the initial dose of glucose is based on a documented need. Some studies have found a correlation between mortality and high serum glucose levels in pediatric patients with head trauma.

Secondary Drugs

A number of useful second line drugs should be available in the emergency department for resuscitations. These secondary drugs are listed in Table 1.7.

Amiodarone. Amiodarone is an antiarrhythmic used for ventricular tachycardia or ventricular fibrillation. The dose is 5 mg per kg given i.v. bolus. For perfusion supraventricular tachycardia infuse over 20 to 60 minutes. The indications are for a wide range of atrial and ventricular arrhythmias, particularly ectopic atrial tachycardia, junctional ectopic tachycardia, and ventricular tachycardia.

The untoward effects include hypotension. It may prolong the Q-T interval and should not be used with procainamide.

Lidocaine. Lidocaine works by reducing the automaticity of ventricular pacemakers. Thus, it increases the fibrillation threshold. Ventricular fibrillation is a relatively uncommon event in pediatric resuscitations. However, when it occurs, lidocaine is the drug of choice. The initial dose is 1 mg per kg i.v. This dose may be repeated three times at 5-minute intervals. Once the initial bolus has been given, an infusion of lidocaine 20 to 50 μg per kg per minute should be initiated (Table 1.8). If an i.v. line cannot be established, the initial dose of lidocaine may be administered by the tracheal route.

The adverse reactions of lidocaine include nausea, vomiting, lethargy, paresthesias, tinnitus, disorientation, and seizures. CNS symptoms may be the first to appear. Later, symptoms of

TABLE 1.7. Secondary Useful Life Support Drugs

Drug	Initial	Subsequent
Lidocaine	1 mg/kg i.v. or intratracheally	10–20 μg/kg/min i.v.
Amiodarone	5 mg/kg i.v.	5–15 mg/kg/d
Adenosine	0.1 mg/kg i.v. bolus	0.2 mg/kg i.v.
Dopamine	10 μg/kg/min i.v.	
Isoproterenol	0.1 μg/kg/min i.v.	
Calcium chloride	10–20 mg/kg/min i.v.	
Calcium gluconate	30 mg/kg i.v.	
Furosemide	1 mg/kg i.v.	2 mg/kg i.v.
Naloxone	1 mg, child; 2 mg, adolescent	Repeat
Methylprednisolone	30 mg/kg i.v.	
Dexamethasone	1 mg/kg i.v.	
Difibrillation current	2 watt-sec/kg	4 watt-sec/kg

cardiac toxicity may appear and include depression of myocardial contractility and ventricular irritability. Heart block and eventual drug-induced asystole may occur. The metabolism of lidocaine depends on normal liver function. Thus, the dose must be modified for children with chronic congestive heart failure, hepatitis, or cirrhosis.

Adenosine. Adenosine is an endogenous purine nucleoside. It was first noted to have an effect on cardiac condition in the early part of the twentieth century. In the mid-1950s, it was first successfully used for treatment of supraventricular tachycardia (SVT). Adenosine seems to exert a strong but brief depressant effect on the sinus and atrioventricular (AV) nodes, resulting in slowed conduction and interruption of the reentry pathway. The indication for the use of adenosine is SVT with hemodynamic compromise.

The dose of adenosine is 0.1 to 0.2 mg per kg (maximum dose is 12 mg). The half-life of the drug is estimated to be less than 10 seconds. If an initial lower dose is chosen and is unsuccessful, the dose may be doubled and repeated. The agent must be given in an i.v. bolus.

The untoward effects of adenosine are flushing and dyspnea, but these are short-lived. In patients with "sick sinus syndrome," long sinus pauses may occur. Adenosine has been used successfully in infants and children of all ages.

Dopamine. Dopamine is a precursor of epinephrine. It acts on both α- and β-adrenergic receptors. Dopamine has a unique "dopaminergic" effect that increases blood flow to renal and mesenteric blood vessels. The dopaminergic effect occurs over the low-dose range, 2 to 10 μ/kg per minute. The cardiac actions of dopamine are similar to those of epinephrine and include a positive inotropic and chronotropic effect. There is also an increase in peripheral vascular resistance, which causes an increase in blood pressure at moderate doses, 5 to 20 μ/kg per minute (Table 1.8). At high doses, greater than 20 μ/kg per minute, there is a marked increase in peripheral vascular resistance and a decrease in the renal and mesenteric blood flow.

Dopamine is indicated for the patient with hypotension and inadequate renal perfusion. The dose of dopamine is 10 μg/kg per minute, which is within the range for desired cardiac action. The standard infusion may be made by mixing 60 mg of dopamine in 100 mL of D5W. This solution is infused at 1 mL/kg/hr. Thus, the rate in milliliters per hour is equal to the patient's body weight (e.g., in a 20-kg patient, the solution is infused at a rate of 20 mL per hour) (Table 1.8). This simple method is appropriate for emergency department use because minimal calculation is required. When the patient reaches an inpatient critical care unit, an infusion better suited for precision drug titration can be prepared. Dopamine may produce tachyarrhythmias as an untoward reaction. Ectopic cardiac beats, nausea, and vomiting may occur. Myocardial ischemia is a rare event in children. The drug must be used with careful monitoring. Rapid increases or decreases in the dosage must be avoided. At low dosages, the dopaminergic effect may result in hypotension that must be supported with intravascular volume expansion. Extravasation of the drug into subcutaneous tissue may cause tissue necrosis. Thus, it should be given through a central line when possible. As with other catecholamines, dopamine should not be mixed with bicarbonate because this will inactivate the drug.

Isoproterenol. Isoproterenol is a synthetic catecholamine. The action of this drug is almost entirely through β-adrenergic receptors. The effects on the cardiovascular system are due to an increase in heart rate, an increased contractile force, and an increase in venous return to the heart. Unlike epinephrine, isoproterenol produces peripheral arterial dilation. Despite the decrease in vascular resistance, the drug usually produces an increase in blood pressure due to increased cardiac output.

Isoproterenol can be used for bradyarrhythmias that are not responsive to atropine. Heart block, sinus bradycardia, or nodal

TABLE 1.8. Drugs for Intravenous Infusion

Drug	Add to 5% dextrose in water to make 100 mL	Infuse	Dosage delivers
Lidocaine	120 mg (3 mL)	1 mL/kg/hr	20 μg/kg/min
Dopamine	60 mg (1.5 mL)	1 mL/kg/hr	10 μg/kg/min
Epinephrine	6 mg (6 mL)	1 mL/kg/hr	1 μg/kg/min
Isoproterenol	0.6 mg (3 mL)	1 mL/kg/hr	0.1 μg/kg/min

bradycardia may be treated while the more definitive therapy of electrical pacing is arranged.

The dose of isoproterenol is variable. A simple infusion can be prepared by adding 0.6 mg of isoproterenol to 100 mL of D5W. Infusing the solution at 1 mL per kg per hour will deliver 0.1 μg per kg per minute (Table 1.8).

The adverse reactions of isoproterenol include tachyarrhythmias and myocardial ischemia. It should be used with extreme caution in children receiving digitalis. In dehydrated or hypovolemic patients, isoproterenol may produce or aggravate existing hypotension. Thus, the physician must be prepared to support a further drop in blood pressure with intravascular volume repletion.

Calcium. The actions of calcium are to increase myocardial contractibility, increase ventricular excitability, and increase conduction velocity through the ventricular muscle. There is currently a trend against the use of calcium in CPR because of possible cytotoxic effects, but for pediatric patients, the positive cardiac stimulant effects require that it remain on the list of secondary drugs.

The indications for calcium include asystole and electromechanical dissociation, but there is no good scientific support for this. Further indications include documented hypocalcemia, hyperkalemia, hypermagnesemia, and calcium channel blocker overdose.

The dose of calcium depends on the form of calcium used. Calcium chloride should be given as 10 to 20 mg per kg i.v. (to deliver 3 to 5 mg per kg of elemental calcium). In the chloride form, calcium should be given only through a central venous line. Calcium gluconate has properties that make the calcium ion less available. Thus, the dose is 30 mg per kg i.v. Calcium gluconate may be given through a peripheral vein. When giving either form of calcium, the physician should infuse it slowly while watching the cardiac monitor for the appearance of bradycardia. The initial dose of calcium may be repeated once. However, subsequent doses should be guided by a serum-ionized calcium level.

The untoward effects of calcium are significant. The patient who is made hypercalcemic may experience an arrest in systole. This is an untreatable situation in which even ECC will not be beneficial. Calcium must always be given slowly, particularly to the patient receiving digitalis who is more prone to develop arrhythmias.

Furosemide. Furosemide is fast-acting and thus is the agent of choice for treating acute pulmonary edema and congestive heart failure. Furosemide works by inhibiting reabsorption of sodium in the proximal and distal tubules and in the loop of Henle. In addition to its action as a diuretic, furosemide also acts to increase blood flow to renal vasculature.

The initial dose of furosemide is 1 mg per kg i.v. If there is not adequate urine output within 20 to 30 minutes, a repeat dose may be given or the dose may be doubled. If the patient is hypovolemic, the administration of furosemide may result in worsening of hypotension. Other adverse reactions include hypokalemia and hyperosmolality. Hypokalemia in the patient receiving digitalis therapy may result in the development of life-threatening arrhythmias.

Naloxone. Naloxone is a narcotic antagonist. It works to block the action of both synthetic and natural narcotics. Naloxone reverses the actions of codeine, morphine, heroin, hydromorphone, and methadone. Children who have overdosed on these drugs may have signs and symptoms of respiratory or cardiorespiratory arrest. The details of management of these poisonings are discussed in Chapter 78.

If narcotic overdose is suspected as the cause of the arrest, naloxone should be administered at 2 mg in a child older than 5 years of age or an adolescent, or at 0.1 mg per kg of body weight in a child less than 5 years of age or an infant. This drug has a rapid onset of action and a short half-life. If a positive reaction to the agent is noted, a repeat dose of 0.1 mg per kg should be given as often as every 3 to 5 minutes up to a total of 10 to 20 mg. After three to five doses, a sustained effect should be apparent. No significant adverse reactions are noted with naloxone.

Corticosteroids. There continues to be great controversy about the specific indications for the use of corticosteroids. There is a general belief that steroids exert a positive effect on the shock state by stabilizing lysosomal membranes and preventing the release of histamine interleukin, tumor necrosis factor, and bradykinin. The possible clinical indications for the use of steroids include adrenal insufficiency either primary or due to adrenal suppression secondary to prolonged steroid use, anaphylaxis, and asthma.

The dose of corticosteroids is also controversial. However, current recommendations include methylprednisolone 30 mg per kg i.v., or dexamethasone 1 mg per kg i.v. The adverse reactions with short-term administration of corticosteroids are minimal. There may be worsening of hyperglycemia and retention of sodium and water. The worsening of a bacterial infection is a theoretical risk that should not inhibit the short-term use of steroids in a life-threatening situation.

Defibrillation

Defibrillation is a relatively uncommon intervention in pediatric resuscitation. It is unusual for a child's heart to fibrillate, and thus there should be careful confirmation of the rhythm before attempted defibrillation. Unmonitored defibrillation of a child is discouraged. However, if the onset of fibrillation was monitored and the defibrillator is at the bedside, direct defibrillation should be attempted. Precordial thump is not recommended for use in children.

Defibrillation works by producing a mass polarization of myocardial cells with the intent that a spontaneous sinus rhythm returns.

Once the diagnosis of ventricular fibrillation has been made, the patient should be prepared for defibrillation. Acidosis and hypoxemia should be corrected. If the patient was unobserved or if a long interval of poor perfusion has elapsed, 100% oxygen and sodium bicarbonate (1 mEq per kg) should be administered. Coarse (high-amplitude) fibrillation is treated more easily than fine (low- amplitude) fibrillation. Fibrillation can be coarsened with the administration of epinephrine. Defibrillation doses are given two at a time. If the first dose is ineffective, a second dose at the same energy level is given immediately. The first dose will lessen resistance; thus, the second may be more effective.

Standard adult paddles are 8 cm in diameter. Pediatric paddles that are 4.5 cm in diameter are also available for most defibrillators. The correct size paddle is that which makes complete uniform contact with the chest wall. If the large size paddle fits entirely on the chest wall, it is preferred because the larger the paddle the lower the intrathoracic impedance and the more effective the defibrillation current. The electrodes should be prepared with electrode paste or saline-soaked pads. Placement of the paste or pads must be meticulous. The small size of the child's chest wall predisposes to bridging of the electric current. Electrical bridging will result in ineffective defibrillation and possible burning of the skin surface.

Once the correct paddles are selected and the electrode skin interface carefully prepared, the electrodes are ready to be placed on the chest wall. Both electrodes may be placed on the anterior chest wall, one at the right of the sternum below the clavicle and the other at the level of the xiphoid along the left midclavicular line. An AP placement of the electrodes is also acceptable; however, this is cumbersome in the usual resuscitation situation. Using either method of electrode placement, the physician should apply firm pressure to the paddles to hold them in contact with the skin. Personnel should be cleared from contact with the patient and the bed.

A dose of current for the initial two shocks is 2 J per kg. If the first defibrillation couplet is unsuccessful, CPR is continued for 3 to 5 minutes and then the dose of current is doubled to 4 J per kg and repeated twice if needed. If a third defibrillation round is needed, the dose is again doubled to 8 J per kg. Defibrillation should not be confused with synchronous cardioversion, which is a treatment for ventricular tachycardia or resistant supraventricular tachycardia. With cardioversion, the synchronous switch of the defibrillator must be activated and a low dose of current used (see Chapter 72 for more details).

Adverse reactions from defibrillation include myocardial injury from excessive current or from multiple discharges delivered in rapid succession (less than 3-minute intervals). Another adverse reaction is the damage to skin and subcutaneous tissue that occurs when the electrode skin interfaces are inadequate. Alcohol pads should never be used as an electrode interface because they are flammable.

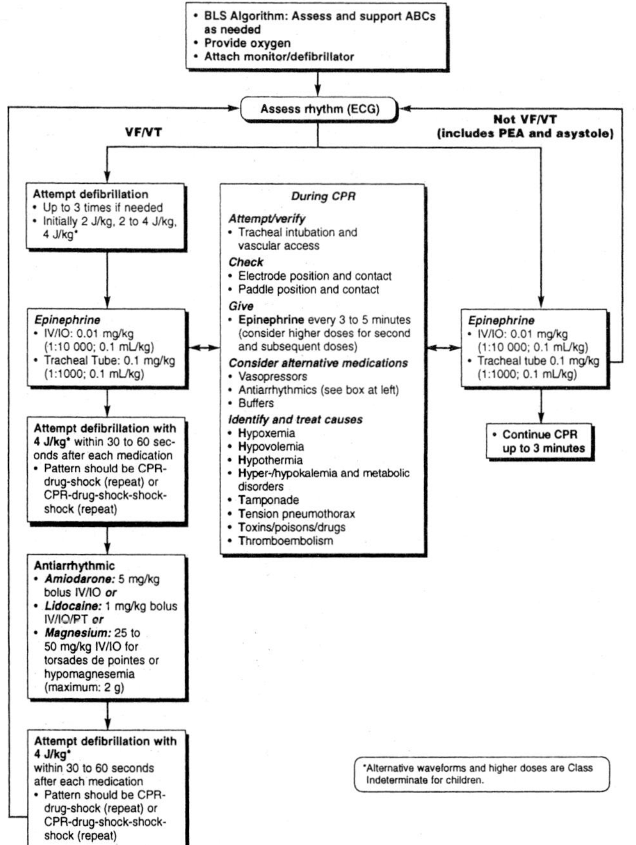

Figure 1.9. Pediatric pulseless arrest algorithm. (From Emergency Cardiac Care Committee and Subcommittees, American Heart Association. Guidelines for cardiopulmonary resuscitation and emergency cardiac care. VI. Pediatric advanced life support. *JAMA* 1992;268: 2262–2275, with permission.)

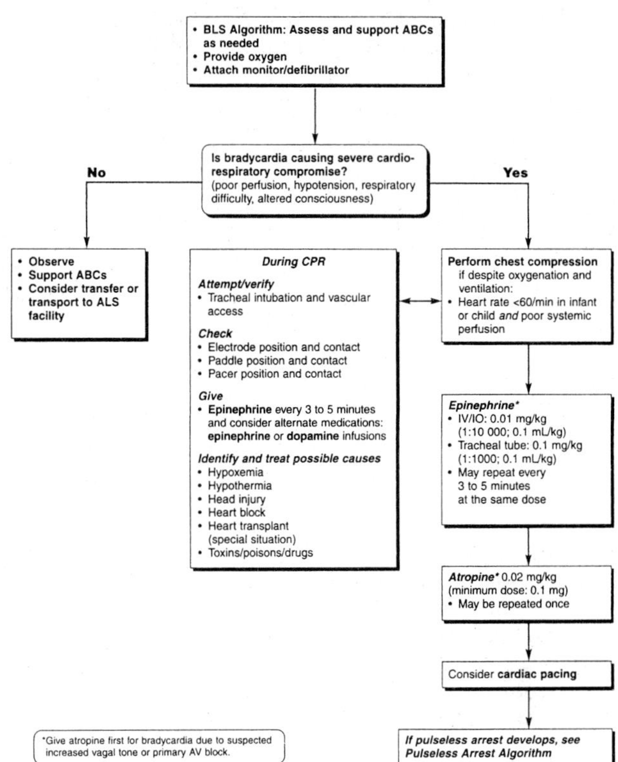

Figure 1.10. Pediatric bradycardia algorithm. (From Emergency Cardiac Care Committee and Subcommittees, American Heart Association. Guidelines for cardiopulmonary resuscitation and emergency cardiac care. VI. Pediatric advanced life support. *JAMA* 1992;268: 2262–2275, with permission.)

Specific Resuscitation Situations

PEDIATRIC PULSELESS ARREST

For the treatment of asystole, we suggest the algorithm presented in Fig. 1.9. No algorithm can cover every clinical situation, thus those presented in this chapter represent guidelines for treatment and not absolute treatment regimens. The physician must keep in mind the possible etiology of the arrest in order to modify treatment in some cases. It should be noted that asystole can be diagnosed clinically or by monitor. The monitor tracing may be confused with ventricular fibrillation. If there is a doubt that it is asystole, the resuscitation leader may want to follow the protocol for ventricular fibrillation.

BRADYCARDIA

The algorithm for bradycardia management is shown in Fig. 1.10. As with other algorithms, this represents only a treatment guideline and not an absolute treatment. Remember that bradycardia may result from hypoxemia and that the patient should first have assessment of the airway and breathing. Other causes of bradycardia include intrinsic node disease, increased intracardiac pressure, hypoglycemia, hypercalcemia, drug effect (e.g., digitalis, propranolol), increased parasympathetic tone (e.g., distended abdomen), or hypothermia. An athletic adolescent may have a resting heart rate of 48 to 60 beats per minute. Treatment must be clinically indicated by signs of cardiovascular failure. There are many forms of bradycardia, including sinus bradycardia, the most common form, and bradycardia from second- and third-degree heart blocks. The differentiation of these forms of heart block is covered in Chapter 72.

Ventricular Fibrillation

Ventricular fibrillation initially may be mistaken for asystole. This depends on the sensitivity setting of the cardiac monitor and the coarseness (amplitudes) of the fibrillation. It is essential that fibrillation be diagnosed correctly. Loose electrodes can readily simulate fibrillation; thus it is important to check the leads and correlate the monitor with the clinical appearance of the patient. It may be difficult to differentiate ventricular fibrillation from ventricular tachycardia with hypotension. This differentiation is moot because the same treatment protocol should be followed in either case.

If the onset of fibrillation is witnessed, the immediate response is to attempt defibrillation. If the arrest was not witnessed, basic CPR must be initiated and the patient prepared before defibrillation is attempted. We do not recommend precordial thump for the pediatric patient.

Rarely is ventricular fibrillation an agonal rhythm in the pediatric patient. Its presence usually indicates some underlying cardiac pathology such as myocarditis, cardiomyopathy, prolonged Q-T syndrome, cardiac trauma, electrical shock, or intoxication with digitalis.

TACHYCARDIA WITH POOR PERFUSION

Tachycardia with poor perfusion is a condition that requires resuscitative effort. The underlying rhythm is usually SVT caused by aberrant reentry pathways due to defects in the normal cardiac conduction system. Most often, SVT is reasonably well tolerated by the infant or young child whose only manifestation may be increased restlessness, pallor, sweating, or poor feeding (see Chapter 72). Sometimes, however, SVT can result in cardiovascular collapse and circulatory failure requiring resuscitation. For the physician, the major point of caution is differentiation between SVT and sinus tachycardia. With SVT, heart rates are usually 230 beats per minute or higher. The P wave axis is usually abnormal (if P waves can be found) and there is little beat-to-beat variation. In sinus tachycardia, there is more rate variation, P waves have a normal axis, and the rate is usually less than 200 beats per minute. The causes for sinus tachycardia—dehydration, hypoxemia, fever, shock, pneumothorax, cardiac tamponade, or drug-induced—should also be considered.

At times, it may also be difficult to differentiate SVT from ventricular tachycardia, particularly if the SVT is associated with aberrant conduction that widens the QRS waves of the ECG. Usually in SVT, the QRS is less than 0.08 seconds. Figure 1.11 outlines the treatment strategy for tachycardia with poor perfusion. If there is no pulse present, the physician should follow the asystole management scheme.

UPPER AIRWAY OBSTRUCTION

A number of tasks must be accomplished as quickly as possible once the patient has been identified as being at high risk for total airway obstruction. The child should receive supplemental oxygen and have his or her heart rate and blood pressure monitored. Equipment for managing an obstructed airway should be immediately available. The hospital's identified airway specialist should be notified of the child's condition and should move as quickly as possible to the emergency department. Beyond the emergency physician, if additional expertise is needed, specialty groups commonly identified as having airway expertise include anesthesiologists, otorhinolaryngologists, nurse anesthetists, general surgeons, respiratory therapists, and cardiothoracic surgeons. It is important to keep in mind that the two important elements for successful management are technical expertise and judgment. These attributes are not necessarily found in the same individual. What may be necessary is a cooperative effort between those with technical expertise and those with clinical experience and judgment.

If obstruction is not imminent, there is usually time to obtain a history and to perform an abbreviated physical examination. In addition, a chest radiograph and lateral neck radiographs may help to define more specifically the pathophysiologic process. These evaluations should occur only if there is no obvious evolution of the airway obstruction and if the natural history of the disease under consideration suggests further diagnostic studies.

If the patient is obtunded, the team must initiate the formal sequence of evaluation and management as described previously. The airway should be opened by flexing the cervical spine on the thoracic spine and tilting the head backward so that the skull is extended on the cervical spine. In addition to this maneuver, the jaw thrust or jaw pull may be used by pushing or pulling the mandibular block of tissue forward off of the posterior pharyngeal wall. At this time, the examiner evaluates the respiratory effort by looking, listening, and feeling for air flow. If the patient is breathing and there is gas exchange, the patient should receive supplemental oxygen and the sequence should progress toward an evaluation of the cardiovascular system. If the patient is not breathing, the oropharynx should be suctioned and an oropharyngeal or nasopharyngeal airway placed in an effort to open the airway. With the airway in place, the physician should reevaluate for gas exchange. If there is now gas exchange, supplemental oxygen should be administered. If there is no gas exchange, the physician should proceed immediately to laryngoscopy.

The purpose of laryngoscopy is twofold: the first priority is placement of an ET tube; second, the laryngoscopy may provide diagnostic information. If a foreign body is evident, the physician should try to intubate before attempting removal.

If the tracheal tube can be placed, the child should be oxygenated and ventilated. Then the cause of the upper airway obstruction should be evaluated and treated. If the child cannot be intubated, a transcricothyroid membrane catheter should be inserted for delivery of supplemental oxygen. Jet ventilation may be accomplished through the catheter oxygenation system. Once the catheter is in place and oxygen is being administered, it is appropriate to reexamine the upper airway, to look for a cause of the obstruction, and to reattempt placement of an ET tube. If the airway cannot be secured at this time, a surgical team should be mobilized to perform a tracheostomy. Effective needle oxygenation and ventilation may permit transfer of the child to the operating room for tracheostomy. If circumstances do not allow oxygenation and ventilation, a formal tracheostomy may have to be performed in the emergency department.

DISCONTINUATION OF LIFE SUPPORT

Termination of life support in the emergency department is usually determined by whether the cardiovascular system can be supported with other than closed-chest massage. If the heart and supporting technology applied to it cannot sustain brain function, resuscitative effort should be discontinued. Obviously, time must be allowed to mobilize and implement for appropriate technology and therefore most unsuccessful resuscitations often go beyond 1 hour. There is growing evidence that if the cardiac muscle is not responsive to the first three doses of epinephrine in the state of adequate oxygenation and ventilation, there is no hope for a successful resuscitation. Additional research will be needed to confirm this as an absolute indicator of when to stop.

Respiratory functions are easily supported mechanically and therefore are not used as markers for continuation or discontinuation of effort.

Brain death is becoming widely accepted as the ultimate determinant of death. It is a clinical diagnosis that should be con-

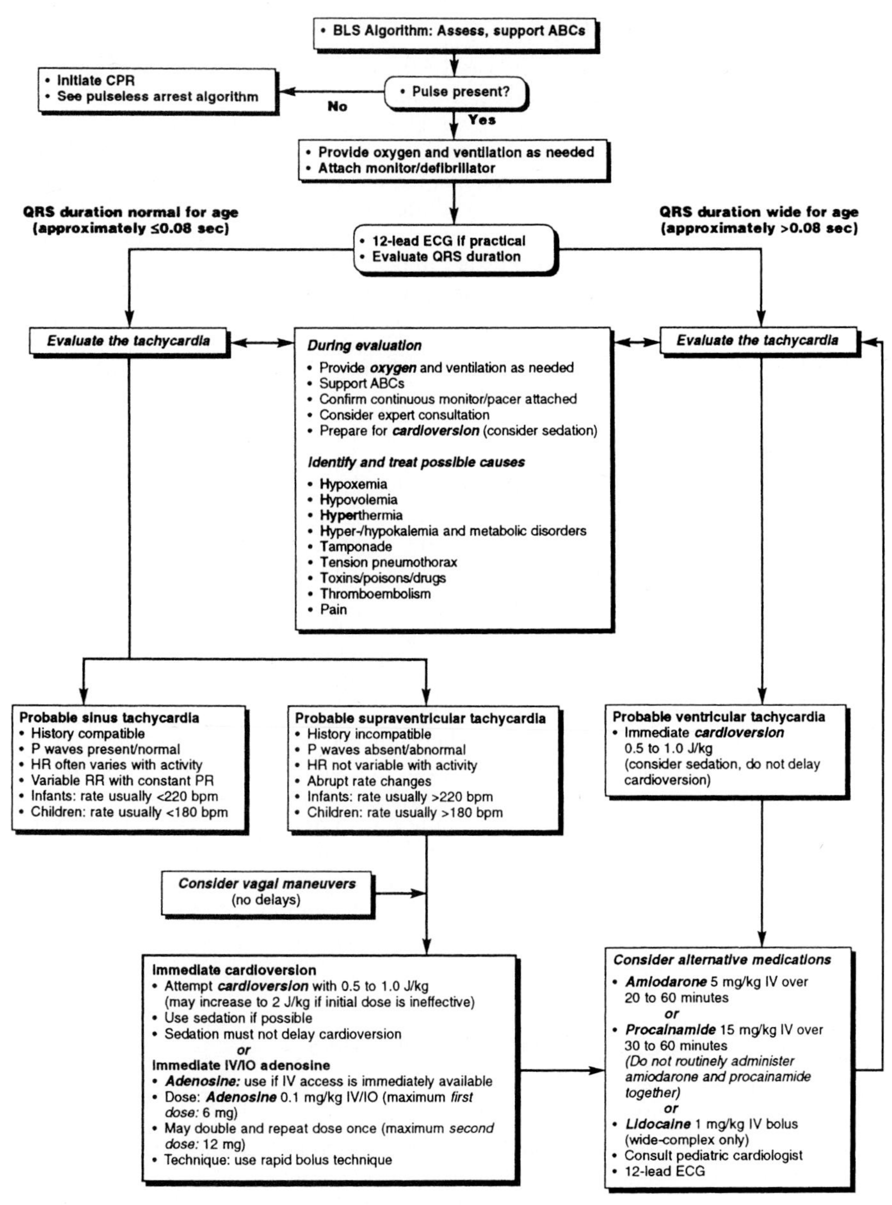

Figure 1.11. Algorithm for pediatric tachycardia with poor perfusion. (From Emergency Cardiac Care Committee and Subcommittees, American Heart Association. Guidelines for cardiopulmonary resuscitation and emergency cardiac care. VI. Pediatric advanced life support. *JAMA* 1992; 268:2262–2275, with permission.)

firmed by observations over time or by studies documenting absence of cerebral blood flow or cerebral metabolic activity. We have seen infant botulism and postictal depression misdiagnosed as brain death and are therefore extremely cautious of making this diagnosis in the emergency department.

Ultimately, the diagnosis of death and subsequent discontinuation of resuscitative effort is a judgment that should be made by the senior physician who is directly attending the child. A decision not to begin resuscitation is generally not made in the emergency department unless there is a clear plan made with parents and written documentation of the plan transmitted by the child's primary attending physician.

SUMMARY

In most circumstances, resuscitation of the pediatric patient can be approached with a sense of optimism for reversing the process that acutely threatens the child's life. Well-organized and well-qualified personnel can effect a high rate of successful resuscitation. However, organization and qualification require advanced planning, training, and preparation. Inherent in this preparation is the development of personnel disciplined to follow the sequence of evaluation and management for airway, breathing, and circulation. In addition, personnel must be familiar with the nuances of resuscitation peculiar to the age and size ranges of the pediatric population.

CHAPTER 2

Neonatal Resuscitation

Evaline A. Alessandrini, M.D.

EMERGENCY DEPARTMENT PREPAREDNESS

The best place for the birth of a newborn infant is in the delivery suite. However, because of varying circumstances, infants are born at home, in the prehospital setting, and in the emergency department (ED). Most neonatal resuscitations in the ED occur without prior notice. Any knowledge that can be obtained before arrival of the laboring mother or recently born infant will aid in the success of the resuscitation. Education of staff, available and functioning equipment, and familiar policies and procedures are critical for preparedness.

Equipment

In addition to a standard obstetric tray, every ED should have a newborn resuscitation kit that is readily accessible, maintained meticulously with other emergency equipment, and rapidly replenished after use. Necessary equipment and medications are listed in Table 2.1. A medication dosing chart by weight and a radiant warmer are invaluable to a neonatal resuscitation.

TABLE 2.1. Neonatal Resuscitation Equipment and Drugs

Equipment
Gowns, gloves, and masks for universal precautions
Radiant warmer
Warm towels and blankets
Bulb syringe
Suction equipment with manometer
Suction catheters (5, 8, and 10 French)
Meconium aspirator
Oxygen with flow meter and tubing
Self-inflating resuscitation bag (500 mL) with oxygen reservoir or anesthesia bag with manometer
Face masks (premature, newborn, and infant sizes)
Oral airways (sizes 000, 00, and 0)
Endotracheal tubes (2.5, 3.0, 3.5, and 4.0) and small stylets
Laryngoscope handles and straight blades (nos. 0 and 1)
Extra batteries and laryngoscope bulbs
Stethoscope
Tape
Sterile umbilical catheterization tray
Umbilical catheters (3.5 and 5 French)
Three-way stopcocks
Needles and syringes
Nasogastric feeding tubes (8 and 10 French)
Cardiorespiratory monitor
Small electrocardiographic leads
Pulse oximeter with newborn probe
Chest tubes (8 and 10 French)
Magill forceps, small
Drugs
Weight-based resuscitation chart
Epinephrine 1:10,000
Dextrose in water, 10%
Naloxone (1 mg/mL or 0.4 mg/mL)
Sodium bicarbonate (0.5 mEq/mL)
Normal saline, Ringer's lactate, 5% albumin

Asphyxia

Asphyxia is defined as the failure to provide the cell with oxygen and remove carbon dioxide, resulting in metabolic acidemia. Both circulation and ventilation are essential to avoid asphyxia. There are multiple stimuli at birth to alter the prenatal circulation and initiate respirations. The actual stimuli for initiating respirations are thought to include a rise in $Paco_2$, interruption of umbilical circulation, and tactile and temperature stimulation.

Neonatal asphyxia can result from multiple factors, as listed in Table 2.2. The initial response to asphyxia will be hyperpnea for 2 to 3 minutes and sinus tachycardia. If there is no significant increase in Pao_2, respirations will stop for 1 to 1 minutes (primary apnea). The infant loses muscle tone and becomes mottled, pale, and then cyanotic. The infant may attempt gasping, nonrhythmic respiratory efforts of 6 to 10 times per minute for several minutes, while the heart rate falls below 100 beats per minute. Soon thereafter, the child ceases to gasp (secondary apnea). At this point, ventilatory and circulatory support must be aggressively provided for the newborn to survive. Brain and other organ damage progresses rapidly beyond this point.

It is important to realize that when one evaluates a neonate in distress or full arrest, the asphyxial event may have begun in utero. It is difficult to document the beginning of the hypoxic period. Indeed, the infant may have passed through both stages of apnea in utero. Thus, there must be aggressive intervention if the infant is to survive. The rule of thumb is that for every minute of secondary apnea, the infant will require 4 minutes of artificial ventilation before rhythmic breathing is reestablished. An apneic infant must be treated as if he or she is in a secondary apneic stage, and resuscitation must begin immediately. If hypoxemia is not treated, there may be further pulmonary vasoconstriction and increased right-to-left shunting through the ductus arteriosus and foramen ovale and a persistence of fetal circulation.

CLINICAL MANIFESTATIONS

Temperature

Particular attention must be paid to the thermoregulation of all infants, especially those born in a prehospital setting or in a cool ED. As the patient is dried and placed under a radiant warmer, the temperature should be monitored via the axillary route using electronic thermometers with a disposable tip. Normal axillary temperatures fall between 36.5° and 37.4°C. Rectal temperatures are reserved for infants whose core temperature may be in question. Recovery from acidosis is delayed by hypothermia. In addition, hypothermia increases metabolic needs and pro-

TABLE 2.2. Causes of Neonatal Asphyxia

Maternal	Fetal
Diabetes	Abnormal presentation
Hypertension	Meconium aspiration
Toxemia	Sepsis
Preeclampsia	Hypovolemia
Eclampsia	Prolapsed cord
Treatment with alcohol, magnesium, β-adrenergic agents, narcotics	Congenital anomalies
Isoimmunization	
Infection	
Abruptio placenta	
Placenta previa	

duces hypoxia, hypercarbia, metabolic acidosis, and hypoglycemia. Thus, efforts to maintain a normal body temperature are crucial to a successful resuscitation.

Respiratory Effort

Most newborns will begin to breathe effectively in response to mild stimulation. The infant should be assessed for respiratory rate (between 35 and 60 breaths per minute is normal). Adequacy of respirations is noted by evaluating chest rise, auscultating good air movement, and confirming a heart rate above 100 beats per minute with improving color of the infant. Observation of tachypnea, retractions, or grunting warrants close evaluation and management. A gasping, cyanotic, or unresponsive infant requires immediate respiratory support with oxygenation and ventilation (see "Management" section following).

Heart Rate

The newborn's heart rate is an excellent objective measurement of the success of the resuscitation and should be monitored closely after assessment of respiratory effort. The heart rate may be determined by one of many ways: (1) palpation of the pulse at the base of the umbilical cord; (2) auscultation of heart tones with a stethoscope; (3) palpation of the femoral or brachial pulse; or (4) placement of a cardiac monitor. Auscultation of the apical heart rate is often difficult in a noisy environment, and the electrodes of a cardiac monitor may be difficult to place while vernix covers the newborn's body. The normal infant's heart rate is greater than 100 beats per minute at birth. The average awake infant's heart rate is between 120 and 150 beats per minute shortly after birth. Variations in heart rate commonly occur with hypoxia, hypovolemia, hypothermia, and maternal drug use. Trends in heart rate are followed closely during resuscitation and postresuscitation stabilization.

The average mean arterial pressure of term infants in the first 12 hours of life is between 50 and 55 mm Hg.

Color

As respirations begin and pulmonary vascular pressures fall, the newborn rapidly becomes pink. Acrocyanosis, or persistent cyanosis of the distal extremities, may persist for several hours after birth. Acrocyanosis is not a reflection of inadequate oxygenation, but it may indicate hypothermia if persistent. Pallor may be a sign of decreased cardiac output, anemia, hypovolemia, hypothermia, or acidosis. Its cause should be investigated and corrected promptly. Central cyanosis that has not resolved with administration of oxygen and ventilation within the first minute of life must be emergently evaluated for heart disease, sepsis, diaphragmatic hernia, other congenital anomalies, or other causes.

Apgar Score

The Apgar score is a useful guide to evaluate the newborn at specific intervals after birth. Five objective signs—heart rate, respirations, muscle tone, grimace, and color—are assessed 1 minute and 5 minutes after birth. Each sign receives a score between 0 and 2, and the points are then totaled for the final score (Table 2.3). If the 5-minute Apgar score is less than 7, additional scores are obtained every 5 minutes until the infant is 20 minutes old. The Apgar score has been used as an indicator of responsiveness to resuscitative efforts. The score at 5 minutes and beyond is more predictive of survival and neurologic status. Although experienced physicians have developed these guidelines, they have not undergone rigorous clinical trials. Thus, if resuscitative efforts are needed for a newborn infant, they should be started immediately and not be delayed while the Apgar score is obtained.

MANAGEMENT

The initial steps of neonatal resuscitation include prevention of heat loss, stimulation, clearing of the airway, initiation of respirations, and evaluation of circulation. When possible, all resuscitation equipment should be ready for use, the radiant warmer on, and a team with preassigned roles assembled.

When and if to begin resuscitative efforts on a newborn is fraught with emotion and difficult to objectively study. Studies have shown that between 40% and 50% of term newborns who were stillborn survived. Approximately two-thirds of these infants had a normal neurologic outcome. It thus seems obvious that resuscitative efforts should be performed on any term infant. A difficult decision is when to stop resuscitation. One predictor is the Apgar score. Survival is extremely unlikely if the 10-minute Apgar score remains zero. There are multiple ethical issues regarding initiation of resuscitation of the very low–birth weight infant. However, with surfactant therapy and improved management of these infants, outcomes have improved over time and the controversy of resuscitation remains. At the stressful time of an emergency delivery, if there is any question of viability, it is probably best to initiate resuscitative efforts.

Thermoregulation

The initial step of drying the infant to minimize heat loss is extremely important, and further resuscitation is continued after warming has begun. As previously stated, recovery from acidosis is delayed by hypothermia, and hypothermia is a special problem for the infant born outside of the hospital. Thus, simply resuscitating the baby in a warm environment, under a prewarmed radiant warmer while drying the amniotic fluid from the infant and removing wet linens from contact with the skin

TABLE 2.3. Apgar Score

	Score		
Sign	0	1	2
Heart rate	Absent	<100 beats/min	≥100 beats/min
Respirations	Absent	Slow, irregular	Good, crying
Muscle tone	Limp	Some flexion	Active motion
Reflex irritability	None	Grimace	Cough, sneeze, cry
Color	Blue or pale	Pink body, blue hands and feet	Completely pink

will markedly decrease heat loss. These maneuvers will maximize the infant's chance at recovery. Alternative methods of warming infants, particularly while awaiting a radiant warmer in the case of an unexpected delivery, include warm blankets and towels. Placing the infant naked against the mother's body and covering both mother and infant with blankets may also warm the stable infant.

TABLE 2.4. Indications for Positive-Pressure Ventilation

Apnea or gasping respirations
Heart rate <100 beats/min
Persistent central cyanosis despite administration of 100% oxygen

Suctioning

Many newborns have excessive secretions, including amniotic fluid, cervical mucus, and meconium, which may obstruct their airways. (Meconium is a special situation discussed in the section on "Meconium" later in this chapter.) These secretions can generally be removed by placing the infant on his or her side and gently suctioning the buccal pouch with a bulb syringe. Mechanical suction with an 8- or 10-Fr suction catheter may also be used. To avoid soft tissue injury, negative pressure from mechanical suctioning should not exceed −100 mm Hg. Deep suctioning of the oropharynx in a newborn is likely to cause vagally mediated bradycardia and/or apnea. Excessive suctioning may also contribute to atelectasis. Most clear fluid is resorbed by the lungs into the arterial system. Consequently, suctioning should be gentle and limited to 5 seconds per pass. Adequate time must be allowed between necessary suctioning attempts for spontaneous or assisted ventilation.

Stimulation

Most newborns will begin effective breathing during routine drying and suctioning. Other methods of safe stimulation include flicking the heels and rubbing the back of the newborn infant. More vigorous methods of stimulation are unnecessary. If after 10 to 15 seconds of stimulation, effective respirations have not been established, positive-pressure ventilation (PPV) is initiated.

Airway and Breathing

OXYGEN ADMINISTRATION AND AIRWAY POSITIONING

Most infants require only warming, drying, stimulation, and suctioning after birth for a smooth transition to their extrauterine environment. If a newborn is exhibiting signs and symptoms of airway obstruction after routine suctioning, the airway should be repositioned. This maneuver is often accomplished by placing a towel or blanket beneath the shoulders and upper back of the supine infant. By elevating the shoulders and upper back approximately 1 inch, the airway is slightly extended into a neutral position, compensating for the infant's relatively large occiput. Avoid flexion or hyperextension of the newborn's neck, which is likely to exacerbate airway obstruction.

An infant who exhibits central cyanosis, yet is making adequate, spontaneous respirations and has a heart rate above 100 beats per minute, needs supplemental oxygen. Oxygen is delivered at 100% and a flow rate of at least 5 L per minute by blow-by through tubing, a face mask attached to an anesthesia bag, an appropriately sized simple mask, or an oxygen hood. Ideally, oxygen should be warmed and humidified. Although this may not always be possible initially in an emergency setting, efforts to warm and humidify oxygen delivered to a newborn should be made as soon as possible.

BAG-VALVE-MASK VENTILATION

Adequate expansion of the lung is often the only measure needed for successful resuscitation of the newborn. The fluid-filled lungs must be inflated with air. Adequate inflation stimulates surfactant secretion and also allows some gas trapping during exhalation to create a functional residual capacity. Although this is best done by negative pressure generated by a vigorous term infant with a strong chest wall, some infants require PPV to initiate lung expansion. Indications for PPV are listed in Table 2.4.

Lung expansion is best achieved with a well-fitted face mask, which covers the infant's nose and mouth but does not place pressure on the eyes. A cushioned rim on the face mask allows the best possible seal.

A relatively high inflation pressure, between 25 and 40 cm H_2O, delivered slowly over several seconds is necessary for the infant's first breath. Subsequent ventilations typically require less pressure and are best judged by good chest wall rise and breath sounds. If effective ventilation does not result, the airway should be repositioned and suctioning of the oropharynx considered. An assisted ventilatory rate of 40 to 60 breaths per minute will provide effective oxygenation and ventilation. Typically 100% oxygen is delivered via PPV. However, some authors advocate resuscitation with room air because of concerns about the generation of free radicals from high concentrations of oxygen, which may exacerbate brain injury. Although current findings do not justify changes in guidelines for resuscitation, further work in this area may have implications for neonatal resuscitation in the future.

PPV may be delivered by a self-inflating bag or an anesthesia bag. Although self-inflating bags do not require a gas source to operate, they must be used with an oxygen source and a reservoir to deliver high concentrations of oxygen. They are straightforward and easy to use, but several caveats must be kept in mind. First, relatively small volumes of air (approximately 6 to 8 mL per kg) are delivered to newborns during PPV. A 450-mL self-inflating bag rather than the larger bags should be used to avoid complications from barotrauma such as a pneumothorax. In addition, many self-inflating bags have a pressure-limiting pop-off valve set at 30 to 45 cm H_2O. In some circumstances, when an infant requires higher initial inflation pressures, the bag may not allow the resuscitator to deliver enough pressure to the newborn for an adequate first breath. Unless the valve is occluded, effective inflation may be prevented.

Anesthesia bags require air flow into them as well as a good mask seal to inflate. Consequently, the resuscitator must be facile at positioning the airway and mask, controlling the flow valves, and monitoring the manometer, which is needed to monitor peak ventilatory pressures delivered to the infant. Benefits of the anesthesia bag include the ability to deliver a wide range of peak inspiratory pressures, positive end-expiratory pressure, and high concentrations of oxygen compared with the self-inflating bag. Proper use requires training and practice.

If bag-valve-mask ventilation is prolonged or results in gastric distension, an orogastric tube should be placed to decompress the stomach so that further effective ventilation is not inhibited. The infant should be reevaluated after 30 seconds of PPV for spontaneous respirations and heart rate. If the infant has begun breathing and the heart rate is above 100 beats per minute, PPV may be slowly discontinued. If respirations are in-

TABLE 2.5. Indications for Endotracheal Intubation

Ineffective bag-valve-mask ventilation
Prolonged need for positive-pressure ventilation
Suctioning of meconium
Administration of resuscitation medications

TABLE 2.7. Indications for Chest Compressions

Heart rate <60 beats/min
Heart rate 60–80 beats/min and not rapidly increasing despite positive-pressure ventilation with 100% oxygen for 30 seconds

adequate or the heart rate remains less than 100 beats per minute, assisted ventilation must be continued and endotracheal (ET) intubation must be considered.

ENDOTRACHEAL INTUBATION

Most resuscitative efforts succeed with bag-valve-mask ventilation alone. Indications for ET intubation are listed in Table 2.5. Once the decision to intubate the trachea has been made, supplies from the newborn resuscitation tray are organized. Sizes of airway equipment can be determined by birth weight (Table 2.6). ET tube size can also be estimated by gestational age:

$$\text{ET tube size in mm} = \text{Gestational age in weeks}/10$$

Thus, a 35-week premature infant would require a 3.5-mm ET tube.

ET intubation is typically performed via the orotracheal route during direct laryngoscopy. Laryngoscopy in the newborn is challenging because of the infant's large tongue and secretions, which may obscure airway landmarks. Hancock and colleagues advocate finger intubation of the trachea in newborns. They successfully and quickly used this method to intubate 37 infants and had no complications. The technique requires some practice, as does laryngoscopic intubation.

Successful ET intubation also requires proper tube positioning. Most neonatal ET tubes have a black vocal cord line near the tip. When this guide is placed at the level of the vocal cords, the tip of the tube is likely to be positioned properly in the trachea. Another estimate for the insertion distance of the ET tube is:

$$\text{Total cm at gum line} = 6 + \text{Weight of the infant in kg}$$

Proper positioning of the ET tube must be confirmed by auscultation of equal breath sounds in both axillae; good, symmetric chest wall movement; improvement of the infant's cardiorespiratory status; and detection of exhaled carbon dioxide. Once positioning is clinically verified, the ET tube must be securely taped in place, and positioning may then be confirmed with a radiograph as indicated.

Circulation

CHEST COMPRESSIONS

Chest compressions are rarely needed during neonatal resuscitation. In 1993, Jain reported that 0.03% of newborns delivered required chest compressions. (In 1995, Perlman demonstrated a need in 0.12%.) Bradycardia and asystole in the newborn are virtually always a result of respiratory failure, hypoxemia, and tissue acidosis. Consequently, oxygenation and ventilation are critical to successful resuscitation even of the infant's circulation. Indications for chest compressions, which are always performed simultaneously with PPV with 100% oxygen, are listed in Table 2.7.

Current recommendations state that three chest compressions are followed by a brief pause for one ventilation. Thus, in 1 minute, the newborn should receive 90 chest compressions and 30 ventilations. This technique, when compared with previous recommendations of 120 compressions and 40 to 60 simultaneous respirations per minute, allows for optimal lung expansion by not compressing the chest during PPV. The most important aspect of reversing neonatal asphyxia, good oxygenation, and ventilation is maximized.

Two techniques of performing chest compressions in the neonate or young infant are recommended. The preferred method involves placing the thumbs on the middle third of the sternum, encircling the chest, and supporting the back with the fingers (Fig. 2.1). Ultimately, the thumbs should be placed side by side just below the nipple line. However, if the neonate is very small or if the resuscitator is large, the thumbs may need to be superimposed. Pressure must be placed on the sternum and not the adjacent ribs. In the event that the resuscitator's hands are too small to encircle the newborn's chest, or encircling the chest obstructs other resuscitative efforts such as umbilical line placement, then the two-finger technique may be used. This method entails placing the ring and middle fingers on the sternum just below the nipple line for chest compressions.

With either method of chest compression, the resuscitator should compress the chest approximately 1/2 to 3/4 of an inch in a smooth fashion. The compression and relaxation phases should be equal in duration, and the fingers or thumbs should not be lifted off of the chest at any time. The spontaneous heart rate should be checked periodically during the resuscitation, and chest compressions discontinued when the heart rate exceeds 80 beats per minute.

VASCULAR ACCESS

A newborn requires vascular access for administration of medications or volume expansion. Bradycardia or asystole unresponsive to effective oxygenation, ventilation, and chest compressions warrant pharmacologic therapy. Infants exhibiting signs of poor perfusion, particularly those with risk for hypo-

TABLE 2.6. Selection of Airway Equipment by Weight

Weight (g)	Endotracheal tube size (mm)	Suction catheter (French)	Oral airway	Laryngoscope straight blade
<1000	2.5	5	000	0
1,000–1,250	2.5, 3.0	5, 6	000	0
1,250–2,500	3.0	6	00	0, 1
2,500–3,000	3.0, 3.5	6, 8	0	1
>3000	3.0, 3.5, 4.0	8	0	1

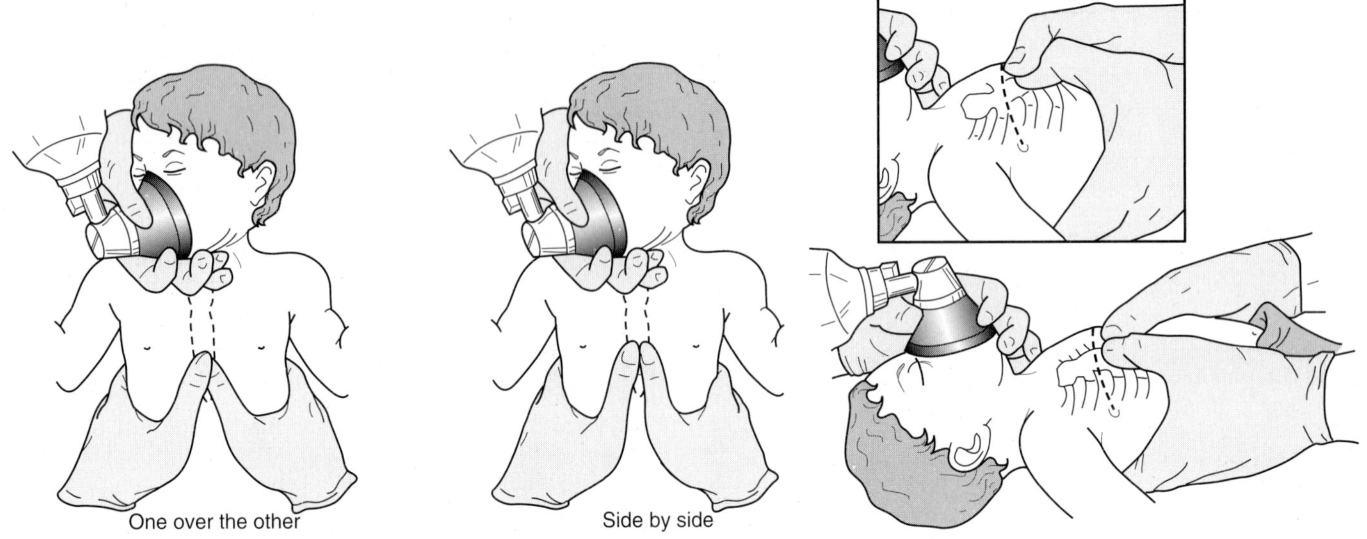

Figure 2.1. **A**: Thumb method of chest compressions. Infant receiving chest compressions with thumb one fingerbreadth below the nipple line and hands encircling chest. **B**: Hand position for chest encirclement technique for external chest compressions in neonates. Thumbs are side by side over the midsternum. In the small newborn, thumbs may need to be superimposed (inset). Gloves should be worn during resuscitation.

volemia such as fetal hemorrhage or maternal hypotension from placental abruption, require volume expansion.

Several methods of vascular access may be used in the newborn. The umbilical vein is often considered a preferred site for vascular access during neonatal resuscitation because it is easily located and cannulated. A skilled resuscitator may elect to cannulate the umbilical artery to obtain arterial blood gases as well as to monitor arterial pressures in a significantly ill infant. Vascular access may also be obtained by placing peripheral catheters in the extremities or scalp.

MEDICATIONS AND VOLUME EXPANDERS

Epinephrine

Epinephrine is the most commonly needed medication for neonatal resuscitation. Because asystole and bradycardia are usually the result of respiratory failure and tissue acidosis, epinephrine therapy is indicated when the newborn's heart rate remains less than 80 beats per minute despite effective ventilation with 100% oxygen and chest compressions for approximately 30 seconds. Epinephrine works because of its α-adrenergic effects. Swine models have demonstrated that α-vasoconstriction in infants increases the diastolic and mean arterial pressures and thus increases the perfusion pressure to the coronary arteries, enhancing oxygen delivery to the heart. The β-adrenergic effects of increased myocardial contractility and stimulation of spontaneous contractions appear less important.

The dose of epinephrine therapy in neonates is 0.01 to 0.03 mg per kg of a 1:10,000 concentration, or 0.1 to 0.3 mL per kg (Table 2.8). It may be administered via an umbilical catheter, a peripheral i.v., an intraosseous line, or the ET tube. The dose should be repeated every 3 to 5 minutes as needed throughout the resuscitation. The safety and efficacy of high-dose epinephrine (0.1 to 0.2 mg per kg) has not been studied in neonates. A concern that large doses of epinephrine may lead to prolonged

TABLE 2.8. Medications for Neonatal Resuscitation

Medication	Concentration	Dosage	Route	Comment
Epinephrine	1:10,000	0.1–0.3 mL/kg	IV, ET	Rapid push, dilute with 2-mL saline via ET tube
Sodium bicarbonate	0.5 mEq/mL (4.2% solution)	2 mEq/kg	IV	Slowly over 2 minutes with effective ventilation
Naloxone	0.4 mg/mL	0.1 mg/kg	IV, ET IM, SC	Rapid push IV, ET preferred
	1.0 mg/mL	0.1 mg/kg	IV, ET IM, SC	Rapid push IV, ET preferred
Dextrose	10%	2–5 mL/kg	IV	Correction of hypoglycemia

ET, endotracheal; IM, intramuscular; IV, intravenous; SC, subcutaneous.

hypertension and subsequent intracranial hemorrhage in neonates has precluded changing dosing recommendations. In addition, the AHA continues to recommend that the dose of endotracheally administered epinephrine remain at 0.01 to 0.03 mg per kg. This is because of the findings by Lindemann in 1984 that ten infants unresponsive to PPV and chest compressions were successfully resuscitated using regularly recommended doses of epinephrine. If the neonate has no vascular access and fails to respond to PPV with 100% oxygen, and a standard dose of epinephrine by the ET route, administration of a larger epinephrine dose (0.1 mg per kg) by the ET route may be considered.

Sodium Bicarbonate

Bicarbonate therapy is indicated in neonatal resuscitation, after establishment of adequate ventilation, for documented metabolic acidosis or presumed metabolic acidosis when other resuscitative measures have failed. The dose is 1 to 2 mEq per kg administered intravenously and slowly over 2 minutes to decrease adverse effects associated with its hypertonicity. For the same reason, only the 0.5 mEq per kg (4.2%) solution should be administered to neonates. If only the 1 mEq per kg solution is available, it should be diluted 1:1 with sterile water before intravenous delivery.

Recommendations for bicarbonate therapy have changed recently. In animal studies performed over the last 40 years, acidosis has been shown to reduce cardiac contractility, blood pressure, and heart rate responses to catecholamines. Subsequently, sodium bicarbonate therapy was recommended before administration of epinephrine. Correction of metabolic acidosis is very dependent on carbon dioxide removal by pulmonary gas exchange. This in turn is reliant on minute ventilation and pulmonary blood flow.

Recently, investigators have discovered that in a resuscitation scenario, both minute ventilation and pulmonary blood flow are decreased. As a result, hypercarbia ensues and exacerbates intracellular acidosis. Therefore, bicarbonate should be administered only to the well-ventilated infant with a documented metabolic acidosis.

Naloxone Hydrochloride

Naloxone is a narcotic antagonist that reverses respiratory depression induced by narcotics. Naloxone is indicated for infants displaying signs of respiratory depression whose mothers have received narcotics within 4 hours before delivery. Prompt and effective oxygenation and ventilation must be provided before administration of naloxone. The current dosing recommendation for naloxone is 0.1 mg per kg, which may be given as 0.1 mL per kg of the 1 mg per mL concentration or 0.25 mg per mL of the 0.4 mg per mL concentration (Table 2.8). This increased dosage from previously published statements has been found more effective in opiate reversal. Naloxone is best administered via the intravenous, intraosseous, or ET routes. Sporadic and delayed absorption may occur if the medication is given intramuscularly or subcutaneously, particularly in an infant with poor perfusion. Furthermore, the resuscitator must remember that repetitive doses of naloxone may be required because the duration of action of narcotics may exceed that of naloxone.

Atropine

Atropine is a parasympatholytic drug that reduces vagal tone and accelerates sinus or atrial pacemakers and atrioventricular conduction. Because vagal stimulation does not cause bradycardia in neonatal resuscitation, atropine is not indicated. Furthermore, many investigators believe that the bradycardic vagally mediated response to hypoxia is a valuable reflex to guide resuscitative efforts and should not be pharmacologically abolished by atropine.

The usual dose of atropine is 0.02 mg per kg with a minimum dose of 0.1 mg and a maximum dose of 2 mg. Because most newborns weigh less than 5 kg, their dose would require the 0.1 mg minimum. If smaller doses are given, paradoxical bradycardia and slowed atrioventricular conduction will likely occur. In conclusion, the efficacy of atropine in newborn resuscitation is unproven and anecdotal and could have deleterious consequences.

Volume Expanders

Volume expanders are indicated for the treatment of hypovolemia. Both historical and physical examination findings suggest the need for volume expansion. Historical factors include fetal hemorrhage from an avulsed cord or trauma, or maternal hypotension from placenta previa, placental abruption, or trauma. Umbilical cord prolapse may cause hypovolemia in the newborn. Physical examination findings include pallor that persists despite oxygenation, weak peripheral pulses with a good heart rate, and a poor response to resuscitation, including effective ventilation.

Volume expanders (Table 2.9) are given intravenously in 10 mL per kg aliquots; after each infusion, the infant is reassessed for improvements in perfusion, blood pressure, and oxygenation. It is appropriate to begin with a bolus of normal saline or Ringer's lactate and proceed to albumin or packed red blood cells based on the infant's clinical response. Volume replacement should be given over 10 minutes to decrease the risk of intracranial hemorrhage from delicate vascular beds.

Postresuscitation Stabilization

After appropriate resuscitative efforts, continuous monitoring and anticipation of complications must occur until the patient is safely transported to a neonatal facility. Priority must be given to thermoregulation by providing the infant with a warm environment and repetitively monitoring the temperature.

SPECIAL SITUATIONS

Meconium

Meconium staining of the amniotic fluid complicates between 10% and 20% of all pregnancies. The risk of meconium at delivery increases to nearly 30% in infants born after 42 weeks' gestation. Approximately 2% to 5% of infants born with meconium in the amniotic fluid will experience some degree of aspiration syndrome, ranging from mild tachypnea to very severe pneumonitis with persistent pulmonary hypertension. The management of an infant born through meconium differs from that previously discussed for other depressed infants. Efforts to remove meconium from the oropharynx and trachea must precede other interventions because of the risk of its aspiration into the lungs with the infant's first breath.

TABLE 2.9. Volume Expanders for Neonatal Resuscitation

Fluid	Dosage	Route
5% albumin	10 mL/kg	IV
Normal saline	10 mL/kg	IV
Ringer's lactate	10 mL/kg	IV
Packed red blood cells	10 mL/kg	IV

IV, intravenous.

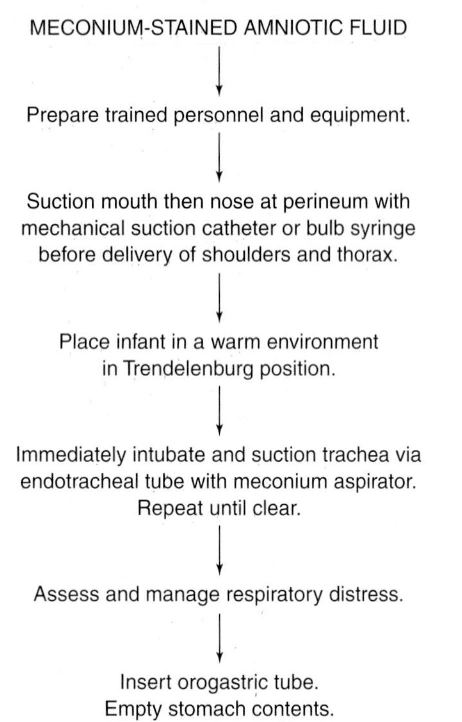

Figure 2.2. Diagram of management of an infant born with meconium-stained amniotic fluid.

When meconium staining is detected during delivery, a sequence of events to prevent aspiration must occur (Fig. 2.2). As soon as the infant's head is delivered, suctioning of the mouth, nose, and posterior pharynx must occur with a 12- or 14-Fr suction catheter or bulb syringe at the perineum. Suctioning must be performed before delivery of the shoulders and thorax to decrease the risk of aspiration. After delivery, the infant is placed in a warm environment in a slight Trendelenburg position, and before other usual resuscitative efforts, meconium suctioning is completed. First, the oropharynx is visualized with a laryngoscope, and any remaining meconium is removed with a suction catheter. Next, the trachea is intubated, and suctioning of the lower airway occurs. Because the ET tube itself is the largest diameter item placed in the trachea, it is the most effective means of suctioning viscous meconium. Thus, a meconium aspirator directly attached between the ET tube and mechanical suction is the preferred method of removing meconium from the lower airway. Negative pressure is applied by occluding the opening on the side of the aspirator with a finger. Mechanical suctioning should not exceed −100 mm Hg. It may be necessary to repeat intubation and suctioning with another ET tube until the aspirated material is clear. Upon completion of tracheal suctioning, orogastric suctioning is performed to empty meconium from the newborn's stomach, which could potentially be aspirated later.

Prematurity

Prematurity greatly increases the likelihood of needing newborn resuscitation. Early involvement of neonatologists and neonatal centers adept in the management of low–birth weight infants is crucial to improve outcome. Only 15% of hospitals have specialized neonatal units. Hospitals without neonatal units need easily available guidelines and established relationships for accessing neonatal consultation and transport. Several factors have added importance in the resuscitation of the preterm infant. These include greater risk for heat loss, greater mechanical ventilation needs, and greater risk of intraventricular hemorrhage.

Premature infants are at greatest risk for heat loss because of their higher ratio of body surface area to body mass. Premature infants require strictest attention to maintenance of normal body temperature.

Premature infants are more likely to develop respiratory distress than term infants are. As a result, assisted ventilation must be provided effectively but gently. ET intubation is usually necessary for surfactant administration and transport to a neonatal facility. Too much ventilatory pressure may result in barotrauma to the lungs and decreased cardiac output as a result of decreased venous return. Good clinical judgment should be used by watching for adequate chest wall rise and listening for good breath sounds. Then, the physician should use the lowest pressure necessary to achieve these clinical end points, which can be confirmed by blood gas analysis. Hyperoxia may lead to complications such as retinopathy of prematurity in low–birth weight infants. Once the infant is stabilized after initial resuscitative care, the fraction of inspired oxygen can be decreased while monitoring pulse oximetry.

Pneumothorax

Pneumothorax is a potentially lethal problem in the neonate because it can rapidly progress to a tension pneumothorax and thereby decrease cardiac output. It is often the result of PPV, positive end-expiratory pressure, or resuscitation.

Pneumothorax is also more common in premature infants with surfactant deficiency and in infants with meconium aspiration. Signs and symptoms include grunting respirations; intercostal, sternal, and substernal retractions; elevated respiratory rate; and tachycardia followed by bradycardia and hypotension. The physical examination findings may include decreased breath sounds and distant heart tones. However, it often may not be possible to diagnose or localize a pneumothorax by auscultation. Transillumination by a high-intensity light in a dark room will reveal increased light transmission on the side of the pneumothorax.

If significant respiratory distress is present and pneumothorax is suspected, rapid decompression may be achieved with a large syringe, 20-gauge needle or catheter over needle, and three-way stopcock. The chest is cleansed with antiseptic solution, and the needle is advanced at the fourth intercostal space in the anterior axillary line or the second interspace in the midclavicular line. This will relieve the tension and decompress the pleural space. Subsequently, a chest tube (8 Fr) may be placed using a standard technique. If the infant is stable, an expedient portable anteroposterior (AP) chest radiograph may be taken to confirm the diagnosis.

Diaphragmatic Hernia

Diaphragmatic hernia is a true neonatal emergency and may be suspected by tachypnea, asymmetric chest wall motion, and a scaphoid abdomen. The diagnosis is confirmed by a chest radiograph showing bowel gas within the thorax. The patient should be given oxygen and a nasogastric tube placed to decompress the stomach. Intubation and PPV are often necessary. The infant must be rapidly evaluated by a pediatric surgeon after ventilation is stabilized and venous access is achieved.

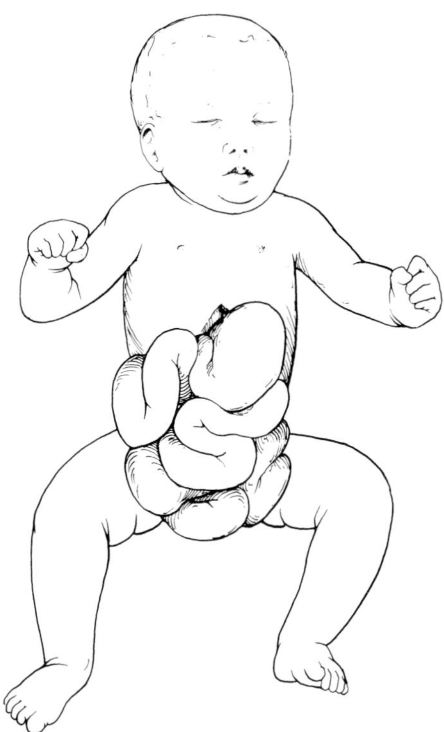

Figure 2.3. Gastroschisis.

Omphalocele/Gastroschisis

Omphalocele and gastroschisis are defects of the umbilical ring that allow herniation of the abdominal contents outside of the abdominal wall. An omphalocele is covered by a thin layer of amnion that may be intact or broken. The abdominal contents are free-floating in the amniotic fluid in gastroschisis (Fig. 2.3). Cardiovascular malformations are commonly associated with omphalocele. The infant must be kept dry and warm, and the eviscerated bowel covered by warm saline-soaked gauze and placed in a plastic bag. If a sac covers the omphalocele and the sac is intact, it should be covered with saline-soaked gauze. A nasogastric tube must be placed and oxygen and i.v. fluids given. The infant may be hypovolemic from peritoneal fluid loss. The physician should maintain good peripheral perfusion and a urine output of 1 to 2 mL per kg per hour. The infant must be evaluated promptly by a pediatric surgeon who can repair these defects.

Spina Bifida

Spina bifida (meningocele, meningomyelocele, and lipomeningocele) involves a wide array of defects. It can range from the least significant form (spina bifida occulta, nonfusion of vertebral laminar arches) to the severe form with meninges and neural tissue protruding, with poorly organized cord tissue exposed to the surface. Neurologic deficit ranges from none to severe impairment and associated hydrocephalus. The child should receive proper supportive care, oxygen and fluid (as needed), sterile moist dressings to the exposed sac or tissues, and prompt referral to a pediatric neurosurgeon.

CHAPTER 3
Shock

Louis M. Bell, M.D.

All physicians who care for ill children will be faced with managing the clinical syndrome of shock. Many common childhood illnesses, such as trauma, gastroenteritis, infection, and accidental drug ingestions, can lead to shock. Ultimately, without timely medical intervention, the child in shock will follow a common pathway to multiorgan system failure and death. Early recognition and appropriate therapy are vital if we hope to reduce the morbidity and mortality associated with this serious syndrome.

DEFINITION OF SHOCK

Shock is defined as an acute syndrome that occurs because of cardiovascular dysfunction and the inability of the circulatory system to provide adequate oxygen and nutrients to meet the metabolic demands of vital organs. Note that this definition recognizes that shock can and does exist without hypotension.

PATHOPHYSIOLOGY

Microcirculatory Dysfunction

The clinical manifestations of shock can be directly related to the abnormalities seen on the tissue, cellular, and biochemical levels. Microcirculatory dysfunction, common to all etiologic types of shock, is characterized by maldistribution of capillary blood flow. Local sympathetic, vasoconstrictor nerve activity and circulatory vasoactive substances (Table 3.1) cause smooth muscle contraction in the precapillary sphincters and arterioles. As shock continues, mechanical obstruction of capillary beds occurs by blockage with cellular debris. Normally, polymorphonuclear leukocytes undergo extensive deformation as they squeeze through the capillaries. Hydrostatic pressure within the capillary makes this possible. However, hydrostatic pressures fall by 30% to 40% during shock states. As a result, capillary beds are blocked and endothelial damage occurs. Subsequent complement activation causes still further aggregation of platelets and granulocytes. During septic shock, exposure to endotoxin directly damages vascular endothelium. Once damaged, endothelial cells can generate procoagulant activity, which may explain the mechanism by which fibrin is deposited in the microcirculation. Superoxide radicals, lysosomal metabolites, and cytokines produced by macrophages and neutrophils for bacterial killing can result in further tissue damage, especially to endothelium, adding to the vicious cycle of damage to the microcirculation.

Tissue Ischemia

Tissue ischemia is also basic to all forms of shock. The consequences of poor tissue perfusion sustain the cascade of events that occur during shock. When there is a lack of oxygen, energy production at the cellular level becomes inefficient, producing only 2 moles of adenosine triphosphate (ATP) per mole of glucose, instead of the normal 38 moles of ATP produced by aerobic metabolism.

TABLE 3.1. Endogenous (Host-Derived) Vasoactive Mediators in Shock

Mediator	Stimulus	Major sources	Major actions
Norepinephrine	Hypovolemia	Sympathetic nervous system	Vasoconstriction
	Head trauma	Adrenal medullae	β_1, β_2 stimulation
Epinephrine	Hypovolemia Hypercapnia	Adrenal medullae	Vasoconstriction α, β_1 stimulation
Angiotensin II	Hypovolemia	Kidneys, brain, blood	Vasoconstriction
Arachidonic acid metabolites			
Leukotrienes	Tumor necrosis factor	Macrophages	Capillary permeability
	Bacterial antigens		Vasoconstriction, release of lysomal hydrolases
Thromboxane A_2	Hypoxia	Platelets	Vasoconstriction, platelet aggregation
Prostaglandins F_2	Hypoxia	Platelets Vascular smooth muscle	Vasoconstriction
Prostaglandins I_2	Hypoxia	Healthy vascular endothelium	Vasodilator counterbalances thromboxane A_2
Myocardial depressant factor	Ischemia Tissue damage	Pancreas	Direct negative inotropic effects
Opiates (B-endorphins)	Hypoxia	Pituitary	Decreased myocardial contractility Decreased sympathetic tone hypotension

In addition, anaerobic metabolism depletes glycogen stores with an accumulation of lactate and associated acidosis. The decreasing energy and acidosis lead to an efflux of potassium and an influx of sodium and calcium with an obligate influx of water into the cell. Cellular swelling and further cellular dysfunction occur, which is seen clinically as edema.

Release of Biochemical Mediators

Biochemical mediators play an important role in the development and continuation of all types of shock. These vasoactive and inflammatory mediators are endogenous (host-derived) products primarily from cells of the nervous system and are hematopoietic in origin. Although in septic shock these mediators are stimulated after exposure to microbial products (e.g., endotoxin) and play a primary role in initiating shock, in hypovolemic and cardiogenic shock, they are released secondarily in response to ischemic cellular injury as just described.

VASOACTIVE MEDIATORS

The vasoactive mediators exert their effect primarily by induction of severe vasoconstriction and vasospasm, induction of platelet aggregation and thrombus formation, increased capillary permeability, and redistribution of blood flow away from vital tissues (Table 3.1).

INFLAMMATORY MEDIATORS

In the past, it was believed that invasive microbial agents were directly responsible for the cellular damage and microcirculatory dysfunction seen in septic shock. However, within the last decade, it has become clear that endogenous inflammation mediators are the real culprits in the pathogenesis of septic shock and that lethal tissue injury occurs when production of these mediators escalates out of control.

Septic shock starts with exposure to microbial products. Perhaps the most potent stimulator of the inflammatory cascade is the outer cell membrane of Gram-negative bacteria, a lipopolysaccharide (LPS) coat, also called endotoxin. Once in the bloodstream, the LPS attaches to a plasma protein called LPS binding protein, or LBP. This complex (LPS-LBP) binds to the CD14 receptor on the surface of the monocyte/macrophage, which leads to stimulation of tumor necrosis factor (TNF) and interleukin-1 (IL-1) and ultimately to the entire cascade of inflammatory mediators.

As a group, these newly described protein mediators are called cytokines (Table 3.2). TNF plays the pivotal role in triggering the production of not only other cytokines but also other inflammatory mediators. TNF is one known endogenous factor that is capable of inducing a broad range of vasoactive and inflammatory mediators. Because of this, treatment of shock with anti-TNF antibodies has been attempted with mixed results (see "Initial Therapy," following). In physiologic amounts, TNF has beneficial effects in tissues and promotes wound healing, tissue remodeling, and neovascularization. In pathogenic amounts, TNF and other inflammatory mediators (Table 3.2) cause severe septic shock in animal models and act primarily by inducing fever, increasing the white blood cell counts, inducing production of procoagulant and cell adhesion molecules by endothelial cells, causing aggregates of hematopoietic cells, and increasing vascular permeability.

NITRIC OXIDE

In 1990, several groups noted that circulatory shock appears to be intimately associated with an increased production of nitric

TABLE 3.2. Endogenous (Host-Derived) Inflammatory Mediators in Shock

Mediator	Stimulus	Major sources	Major action
Platelet-activating factor	TNF Bacterial antigens	Platelets Neutrophils	Thrombosis Vascular permeability
Cytokines			
Tumor necrosis factor (TNF)	Bacterial antigens Severe trauma	Macrophages, Monocytes	Induces other mediators Adhesion to endothelium
Interleukin-1 (IL-1)	TNF Bacterial antigens	Mononuclear Phagocytes	Fever Leukocytosis Acute phase reactants Adhesion to endothelium
Interleukin-6	TNF IL-1	Monocytes Endothelial cells	Fever Leukocytosis Thrombosis
Interleukin-8	Endotoxin TNF	Monocytes Endothelial cells	Neutrophil activation
Complement fragments	TNF Bacterial antigens	Alternate pathway	Chemotache activity
Toxic oxygen species	TNF Bacterial antigens	Neutrophils	Cellular damage

oxide by a variety of different cells. After exposure to TNF-α and IL-1 a variety of cells, including macrophages, vascular endothelium, vascular smooth muscle, hepatocytes, and cardiac myocytes, are induced to increase nitric oxide production. In pathologic amounts, nitric oxide causes vasodilation, vascular hyporesponsiveness, and hypotension. Although nitric oxide has beneficial effects that make it important in host defense against infection, in excessive amounts, nitric oxide leads to hypotension, worsening the shock state. Studies are ongoing to determine whether drugs that inhibit nitric oxide production may be useful in controlling shock.

COMPLEMENT ACTIVATION

The complement system is activated by circulating bacteria and bacterial products. The low–molecular-weight peptides that are released as a result induce both vasoactive and inflammatory effects. Vasoactive effects are seen with C3 and C5 fragments, which promote the release of histamine and other vasoactive mediators, producing increased permeability and vasodilation. Complement fragments also stimulate an inflammatory response by promoting the activation and aggregation of platelets and granulocytes.

MYOCARDIAL DEPRESSANT FACTOR

Myocardial depression occurs in all types of shock. Recent investigation suggests that myocardial depression may occur as a result of mediators that act directly on myocardial tissue. Discovered in 1970, a small peptide called myocardial depressant factor is produced when the pancreas is ischemic and hypoperfused. Myocardial depressant factor has been shown to have negative inotropic effects in isolated heart muscle and causes constriction of the splanchnic vascular bed. In 1985, Parker, using isolated heart muscle preparation, found altered inotropic responsiveness within 1 to 2 hours of endotoxin treatment, demonstrating *in vitro* what is apparent in patients with shock syndrome.

CLINICAL MANIFESTATIONS

Early or Compensated Shock

Regardless of the etiology, shock begins when there is absolute or functional hypovolemia. Absolute hypovolemia exists in cases of severe emesis and diarrhea, trauma with blood loss, peritonitis, and "third-spacing" of fluids or increased capillary permeability, as in sepsis. Functional hypovolemia exists when vascular capacity increases, as in septic shock, spinal cord injury, anaphylaxis, and barbiturate overdose.

The signs of early shock include tachycardia, mild tachypnea, slightly delayed capillary refill (more than 2 to 3 seconds), orthostatic changes in blood pressure or pulse, and mild irritability. These earliest symptoms result from an effort to compensate for shock and increase cardiac output and maintain perfusion of vital organs (brain, heart, kidneys). Unexplained tachycardia without other signs may be one of the earliest signs of shock. Tachycardia occurs to compensate for a diminished stroke volume (Fig. 3.1). Delayed capillary refill occurs as increases in sympathetic tone by endogenous catecholamines cause peripheral vasoconstriction. In some cases of early septic shock, the skin may be warm and dry without a decrease in capillary refill, reflecting cutaneous vasodilation in a state of increased cardiac output and increased venous capacitance—so-called warm distributive shock. As systemic vascular resistance falls, cardiac output must increase to maintain normal arterial pressure. Often, in this form of distributive (septic) shock, the pulse will be bounding and the pulse pressure widened.

Late or Uncompensated Shock

As shock continues, these early compensatory mechanisms are not enough to meet the metabolic demands of the tissue, and uncompensated shock follows (Fig. 3.1). In uncompensated shock, the effects of cellular ischemia with the associated release of vasoactive and inflammatory mediators begin to affect the microcirculation, and the child shows signs of brain, kidney, and cardiovascular compromise.

Tachycardia and tachypnea continue. Tachypnea becomes more severe because an increasing acidosis elicits a compen-

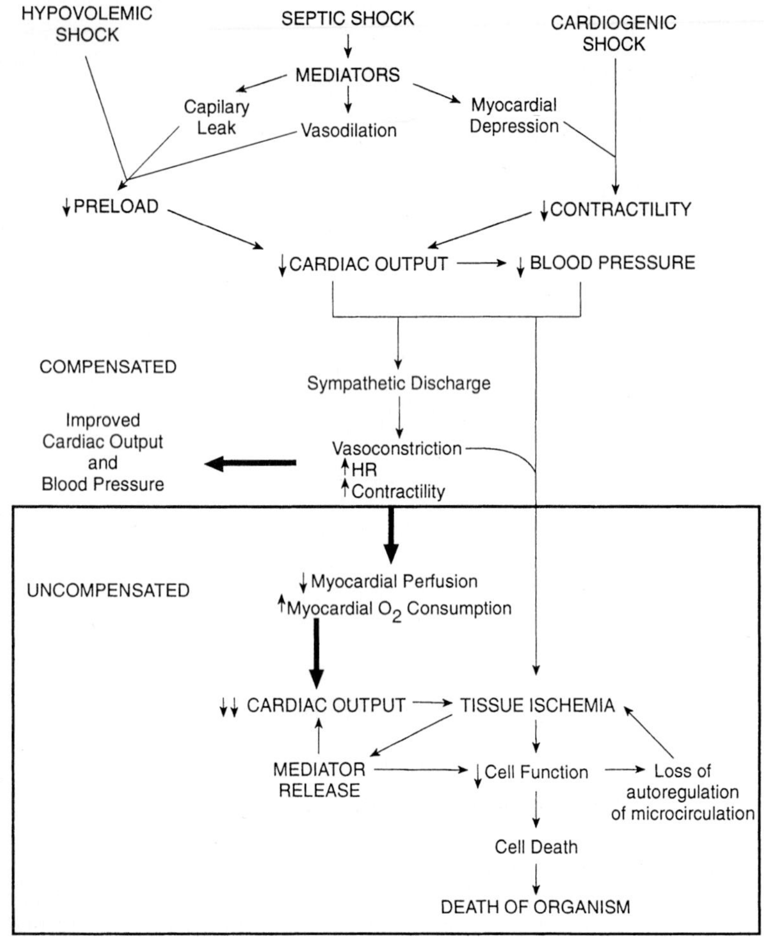

Figure 3.1. Sequence of pathophysiologic events in clinical shock states. (From Witte MK, Hill JH, Blumer JL. Shock in the pediatric patient. *Adv Pediatr* 1987;34:139–174, with permission.)

satory increase in the minute ventilation, resulting in a fall in $PaCO_2$ and a compensatory respiratory alkalosis. The skin may be mottled or pale and extremities cool as vasoconstriction and diminished blood flow to the skin occur. Capillary refill becomes markedly delayed (more than 4 seconds). Hypotension is noted. Decreased cardiac output and vasoconstriction cause renal perfusion, and oliguria is observed. The gastrointestinal tract is also underperfused and may become ischemic. Under these conditions, decreased motility, distension, release of vasoactive and inflammatory mediators, and fluid accumulation may occur. In patients with septic shock, fever (greater than 38.3°C rectally) or hypothermia (less than 35.6°C rectally) may be present.

As perfusion of the brain occurs, irritability progresses to agitation, confusion, hallucinations, alternating periods of agitation and stupor, and finally coma. The multiorgan dysfunction secondary to ongoing shock and exaggerated inflammatory responses has been termed systemic inflammatory response syndrome (SIRS).

The effects of a dysfunctional microcirculation, tissue ischemia, and release of vasoactive and inflammatory mediators obviously affect all tissues, including the pulmonary tissues and vasculature. Damage to the capillary endothelium in the lung allows fluid to fill the interstitium of the intraalveolar septum. If the shock syndrome progresses, fluid accumulation will eventually lead to fluid leakage into the alveolar spaces, which prevents adequate gas exchange. As the damage to the lungs continues, the child demonstrates dyspnea, tachypnea, cyanosis refractory to oxygen therapy, decreased lung compliance, and diffuse alveolar infiltrates. These signs, when grouped together, have been termed the adult respiratory distress syndrome (ARDS), which, despite the name, has been seen in infants as early as 2 weeks after birth. For example, Carcillo found that 11 (32%) of 34 children with septic shock develop ARDS.

TYPES OF SHOCK

Hypovolemia

Hypovolemia (decreased circulating blood volume) is the most common cause of shock in children. The most common cause of hypovolemic shock occurs from water losses associated with diarrhea and vomiting (see Chapter 15). Other causes of hypovolemic shock include blood losses (trauma, gastrointestinal, intracranial hemorrhage), plasma losses (burns, hypoproteinemia, peritonitis), and water losses (glycosuric diuresis, sunstroke).

Distributive Shock

Distributive shock occurs primarily because of vasodilation and pooling of blood in the peripheral vasculature. Causes include anaphylaxis, central nervous system (CNS) or spinal injuries, drug ingestions, and most commonly in children, sepsis. The bacterial etiology of septic shock (and meningitis) is listed in Table 3.3. *Haemophilus influenzae* type b was once the most com-

TABLE 3.3. Bacterial Etiology of Invasive Disease in Infants and Children[a]

Organism
Streptococcus pneumoniae
Neisseria meningitidis
Group B *Streptococcus*
Listeria monocytogenes
Haemophilus influenzae type b
Gram-negative bacilli[b]
Staphylococcus aureus
Pseudomonas aeruginosa
Salmonella enteritidis

[a] Listed in order of most to least frequently isolated from blood or cerebrospinal fluid. Based on data from Schuchat A, et al. *N Engl J Med* 1997;337:970–976.
[b] Includes *Escherichia coli* and *Enterobacter* species.

mon bacterium associated with septic shock in infants and children, but has been virtually eliminated through vaccination.

In 1990, Jacobs and colleagues retrospectively analyzed more than 2,000 admissions to their pediatric intensive care unit over 3 years. They found that 27% (564 cases) of admissions met criteria of sepsis syndrome, which included: (1) clinical manifestations of sepsis; (2) fever (greater than 38.3°C) or hypothermia (less than 35.6°C); (3) tachycardia; (4) tachypnea; and (5) signs of inadequate tissue perfusion (e.g., decreased capillary refill, hypoxemia, oliguria, acidosis, altered mental status). Inotropic support was required to maintain an adequate blood pressure in 268 of 564 patients that met these criteria. However, an etiology for septic shock was found in only 143 (25%) of cases. Meningitis was found in half of these children (71 of 143), and mortality was 10% (14 of 143).

Cardiogenic Shock

Cardiogenic shock can usually be distinguished from other forms of shock because of associated signs of congestive heart failure, including rales auscultated throughout the lungs, a gallop cardiac rhythm, enlarged liver, and jugular venous distension.

Regardless of the etiology, cardiogenic shock leads to decreased cardiac output, in most cases as a result of a decrease in myocardial contractility. As we have seen, direct myocardial damage occurs in all types of shock as a late manifestation. Other common etiologies of cardiogenic shock in children include viral myocarditis, arrhythmia, drug ingestions, postoperative complications of cardiac surgery, metabolic derangements (hypoglycemia), and congenital heart disease.

TREATMENT

Initial Therapy

To determine proper therapy, we should recall the definition and pathophysiology of shock. *Shock* is defined as an acute syndrome that occurs because of cardiovascular dysfunction and the inability of the circulatory system to provide adequate oxygen and nutrients to meet the metabolic demands of vital organs. Therefore, initial therapy in the emergency department can be applied universally, regardless of the etiology of shock, and is directed to reverse or halt further tissue injury. To underscore this, in 1989, Carcillo compared hemodynamic and oxygen use in children with either cardiogenic shock or septic shock. These data suggested that there was little difference physiologically, and therefore, initial treatment should be similar.

Oxygenate/Ventilate
- O_2 by bag-valve-mask
- Intubation (consider early)
- Maintain PaO_2 >65

Vascular Access
- Peripheral vein
- Femoral vein
- Internal jugular
- External jugular
- Subclavian vein
- Intraosseous infusion (consider early in those with hypotension)
- Peripheral venous cutdown

Administer Fluids
- Saline 20 mL/kg initially
- HCT <33% blood; saline
- HCT >33% saline
  - 5% albumin

Drug Therapy
- Positive inotropic agents
- Treat acidosis
- Vasodilator agents
- Hypoglycemia

Specific Therapy
- Control hemorrhage
- Antibiotics (?)
- Immunotherapies (?)

Figure 3.2. Management of shock—overview.

With this pathophysiology in mind, the first steps of therapy are to (1) establish an adequate airway; (2) determine whether breathing is adequate; (3) provide oxygen at 100% FiO_2; (4) establish vascular access and obtain laboratory samples; and (5) provide aggressive fluid resuscitation, beginning with 20 mL per kg of crystalloid 0.9% sodium chloride or Ringer's lactate given intravenously as rapidly as possible (minutes). Reassessment after each therapeutic maneuver is vital (Fig. 3.2). After the initial therapy, the following questions should be addressed: (1) Is tracheal intubation needed? (2) Should additional intravenous therapy be given? If so, blood, crystalloid, or colloid? (3) Are positive inotropic drugs needed? If so, which one initially? (4) What is the urine output? (5) What other drugs are needed (antibiotics)? (6) Should arrangements for admission to the intensive care unit be initiated?

Decision and Monitoring in the Emergency Department

OXYGENATION

Oxygen delivery to the tissues remains our primary focus in children with shock. While the airway and ventilatory effort is assessed, 100% oxygen should be provided via a bag-valve-mask apparatus. Assisted bag-valve-mask may be indicated. If there is any question that the airway is obstructed or that ventilatory effort is inadequate, the insertion of an artificial airway is indicated. We suggest the orotracheal intubation route initially. Measurements of the PaO_2 by an arterial blood sample or pulse oximetry should be performed throughout the decision-making process. The goal is to maintain the arterial oxygen tension above 65 mm Hg; therefore, 100% oxygen should be continued until that is achieved.

VASCULAR ACCESS

Vascular access is vital in treatment. If possible, a large-bore intravenous catheter should be inserted in a peripheral vein. Use of the femoral vein is preferred in infants and younger children. In older children and adolescents, cannulation of the internal jugular, external jugular, and subclavian veins can also be considered. If there is any delay in accomplishing prompt placement of a central venous catheter, an intraosseous line should be placed.

FLUID ADMINISTRATION

After venous access is established, 20 mL per kg of 0.9% normal saline or Ringer's lactate is infused as rapidly as possible. Then reassessment should occur. The decision to give additional intravenous fluids can be based on arterial pressures, heart rate, and oxygenation. If blood pressure is normal, additional fluids will depend on urine output, heart rate, capillary refill, and mental status. If the child remains hypotensive after the initial fluid challenge, an additional 20 mL per kg should be infused and, if possible, titrated against central venous or right atrial pressures because they correlate better with intravascular volume than does systemic arterial pressure. If there is a delay in transfer to the intensive care area, central venous pressure monitoring can be accomplished in the emergency department.

If there is delay in transfer to the intensive care area, fluid management may be directed by right heart filling pressures (central venous pressures). This can be accomplished by using a modification of Weil's "4 and 2 rule" (Fig. 3.3). Central venous pressure (CVP) is observed for 10 minutes. If that pressure is less than 6 mm Hg, 4 mL per kg is infused over 10 minutes, discontinuing the infusion if CVP rises at any time more than 4 mm Hg. If, after the infusion, CVP has risen by less than 4 mm Hg but more than 2 mm Hg, the patient should be observed for 10 minutes. If CVP remains above 2 mm Hg of the starting value, the patient should be monitored without administering additional fluid. If CVP declines to within 2 mm Hg of the initial value, again 4 mL per kg should be infused over 10 minutes. We repeat these maneuvers until the systemic arterial pressure reaches a normal value, the patient manifests other signs of restored circulation integrity, or the "4 and 2 rule" is violated. If the initial CVP lies between 6 and 10 mm Hg, we administer 2 mL per kg over the 10-minute period and look for the same CVP

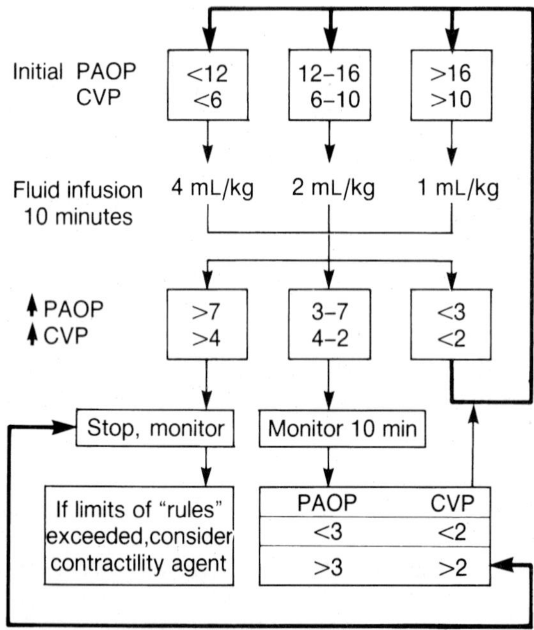

Figure 3.3. "7-3, 4-2 Rules" of Weil. *CVP,* central venous pressure; *PAOP,* pulmonary artery occluded pressure. (Adapted from Weil MH. The "VIP" approach to the bedside management of shock. *JAMA* 1969;207: 337–340.)

changes. If the initial CVP exceeds 10 mm Hg, we infuse 1 mL per kg fluid over 10 minutes and again observe the CVP change.

Two points should be emphasized. First, we examine the change in CVP measurement in response to the fluid infusion, rather than look for an absolute value. Second, because the veins are very distensible vessels and act as a reservoir for fluid, a threefold increase in the volume of fluid contained in the venous system may be necessary before we see changes in CVP. When the pulmonary artery occluded pressure (PAOP) is used, 7 and 3 mm Hg should be substituted for 4 and 2 mm Hg CVP measurements (Fig. 3.3).

CHOICE OF FLUIDS AND BLOOD PRODUCTS

The initial choice of fluid should be 0.9% saline or Ringer's lactate given as described earlier, beginning with 20 mL per kg over minutes. Packed red blood cells should be given at 10 mL per kg over 1 to 2 hours to maintain a hematocrit of 33%. Children with cyanotic heart disease and neonates may require higher hematocrit percentages to ensure adequate tissue delivery.

If the hematocrit is over 30% or if blood is not available, 5% albumin in 0.9% sodium chloride can be used in combination with crystalloid fluids. Initially, albumin can be given in 10 mL per kg doses. When colloids (albumin) are used, appropriate intravascular monitoring should be considered when possible to guard against circulatory overload.

IMPROVING MYOCARDIAL FUNCTION

Catecholamines (adrenergic agents) are the drugs of choice for improving myocardial contractility in patients with shock because of their very short half-life (2 to 3 minutes) and potency (Table 3.4). A brief review of adrenergic receptor physiology is important if we are to have a rational approach to their use.

There are at least three broad populations of adrenergic receptors, termed alpha (α), beta (β), and dopaminergic (DA) receptors. Although all have been subdivided further, in general, β_1-receptors mediate inotropic (contractility), chronotropic (rate), and dromotropic (increased conduction velocity) activity. Beta-$_2$-receptors mediate vasodilation and bronchial smooth muscle relaxation. Alpha-receptors mediate arteriole constriction systemically and bronchial muscle constriction. Dopaminergic receptors, termed DA_1 and DA_2, mediate smooth muscle relaxation and increase renal blood flow and sodium excretion.

Catecholamines may stimulate some adrenergic receptors more strongly than others, providing some rationale for selection. In general, the mechanism of action for most positive inotropic agents seems to be an increased concentration of or sensitivity to intracellular calcium during systole. If the desired effect is not achieved with one agent, combinations of several agents together may be necessary. It is important to note that there may be decreased responsiveness to adrenergic stimulation in patients with congenital heart disease, after heart transplantation, or in those with bronchopulmonary dysplasia.

Currently, dopamine is the first choice to improve cardiac function and improve splanchnic and renal circulation if the patient is relatively stable but remains hypotensive after initial fluid resuscitation. At low dosages (2 μg per kg per minute), dopamine increases renal blood flow up to 50% and sodium excretion up to 100%. Cardiac output is increased with dosages of 5 to 10 μg per kg per minute. Improvement in perfusion as measured by increased urine output, blood pressure, and warming of the extremities can be seen early.

In some cases of profound septic shock and hypotension, epinephrine should be considered initially. A low dose (less than 0.2 μg per kg per minute) of epinephrine stimulates both β_1 cardiac effects and β_2 peripheral vascular effects, which results in an increase in skeletal muscle blood flow and a decrease in di-

TABLE 3.4. Positive Inotropic Agents

Agent	Dose Range (μg/kg/min)	Mechanism[a]	Considerations
Dopamine	2–20	β_1, β_2, DA stimulation	Increases renal flow 1–2 μg/kg/min, cardiac output 5–10 μg/kg/min
Epinephrine	0.1–1.0	β_1, β_2, α stimulation	Dose over 0.3 μg/kg/min associated or α effects
Dobutamine	2.5–15	β_1, β_2 stimulation	Increase cardiac output with no increase in heart rate, not as effective in those <12 months (see text)
Amrinone	1–10	Phosphodiesterase F^{111} inhibition	Positive inotrope with smooth muscle relaxation
Isoproterenol	0.1–1.0	β_1, β_2 stimulation	Increases myocardial oxygen consumption
Norepinephrine	0.1–1.0	α, β_1 stimulation	Infrequent use due to renal vasoconstriction

[a]Adrenergic receptors: Beta (β_1) receptors mediate inotropic, chronotropic, and dromotropic activity; intestinal relaxation. Beta (β_2) receptors mediate vasodilation and bronchial smooth muscle relaxation. Alpha receptors mediate arteriole constriction systemically; bronchial muscle constriction. Dopaminergic receptors (DA) mediate smooth muscle relaxation and increases in renal blood flow and sodium excretion.

astolic blood pressure. Dosages higher than 0.3 μg per kg per minute are associated with increased α-adrenergic effects and increases in blood pressure. If the child is unresponsive to dopamine, epinephrine may be useful in maintaining blood pressure and cardiac output.

When epinephrine is being used, one may need to consider vasodilator therapy. Nutrient flow may be improved, left ventricular stroke work enhanced, and myocardial oxygen consumption decreased by lowering impedance to left ventricular ejections. A short-acting vasodilating drug such as sodium nitroprusside, beginning with 0.1 μg per kg per minute, is preferred. The infusion can be increased until evidence of decreased peripheral vascular resistance exists or until the generally accepted safe maximum of between 8 and 10 μg per kg per minute is reached. Toxicity results from the accumulation of cyanide, which should be monitored. The use of this therapy in the emergency department is rarely needed, although in cases in which transfer to the intensive care unit is delayed, it may be indicated.

Dobutamine should be considered initially in patients with cardiogenic shock because it is a very selective stimulant of β_1 receptors. In patients with cardiogenic shock, dobutamine tends to increase cardiac output without increasing the heart rate. Starting doses should be 2 to 5 μg per kg per minute. However, Perkins found that infants with cardiogenic or septic shock who were less than 12 months of age derived little benefit from dobutamine, demonstrating insignificant increases in cardiac index and stroke index. If dobutamine fails, epinephrine should be used.

Finally, amrinone represents a class of inotropic agents distinct from the catecholamines. Although the mechanism of action is not fully understood, data favor inhibition of phosphodiesterase F^{111}. A direct relaxant effect on vascularity and vasodilation that results in smooth muscle causes afterload, and preload reduction contributes to the improved hemodynamic state. Amrinone facilitates atrioventricular conduction, relaxes smooth muscle, and dilates coronary arteries. At this time, there is seldom an indication to start this agent in the emergency department.

ACID-BASE ABNORMALITIES

It is clear that unless perfusion and ventilation are adequate, infusion of sodium bicarbonate rarely maintains arterial pH. Therefore, bicarbonate should be considered as a temporary and immediate therapy to acutely alter arterial pH so that myocardial performance will be optimized. Ultimately, improved blood flow will result in a decrease in acid products of anaerobic metabolism and only then will pH concentration remain normal. We calculate the dose of sodium bicarbonate according to the following formula: bicarbonate administered in milliequivalents (mEq) equals the body weight (kg) times base excess (BE) times 0.6. In the presence of acute hypercapnia, one-half of the calculated dose is administered and pH remeasured. If correction is not achieved, the remainder is infused. The suggested rate of administration should not exceed 2 mEq per minute.

STEROIDS

In a prospective, randomized, double-blind, placebo-controlled study of adults, Bone concluded that high-dose corticosteroids provided no benefit in the treatment of septic shock.

DISSEMINATED INTRAVASCULAR COAGULATION

As we have seen, microcirculatory dysfunction, tissue ischemia, and cardiovascular dysfunction, regardless of etiology, leads to shock and consumption of coagulation factors and platelets. This consumption is characterized by thrombocytopenia, an increase in fibrin split products, a decrease in fibrinogen, and abnormally prolonged prothrombin time and partial thromboplastin times.

ANTIBIOTICS

Antibiotics are given presumptively in most cases of severe shock when the etiology is unclear. Antibiotics are chosen based on age and suspected bacterial pathogens.

IMMUNOTHERAPIES

Over the last several years, the identification of the mediators of septic shock has led to a better understanding of how these mediators cause and contribute to the pathophysiology of shock. Coincidentally, the use of monoclonal antibody techniques has allowed for the production of large quantities of antibody that are free from human infection and are of known isotype and epitope specificity. This new knowledge has led to the development of a number of investigational therapies aimed at different components of the inflammatory cascade. These therapies can

TABLE 3.5. Experimental Therapies[a] for the Treatment of Septis Shock (Selected)

Category	Product and mechanism of action
Antimicrobial	
E5	Murine IgM monoclonal antibody; binds to lipid A of endo toxin
HA-1A	Human IgM monoclonal antibody; binds to lipid A of endo toxin
Soluble CD14	Blocks binding of endotoxin to macrophage
Anti-CD14 antibody	Blocks binding of endotoxin to macrophage
Anticytokine	
Anti-TNF antibody	Blocks inflammatory cascade
TNF soluble receptor	Binds TNF, inhibits inflammatory cascade
IL-1 receptor antagonist	Blocks IL-1 binding
Nitric Oxide (NO) Inhibitors	
L-NMA	L-arginine analogs; inhibits NO synthase and decreases NO production
L-NAA	Same as above

[a] The safety and efficacy studies of these agents in humans and animals have been mixed. In some cases, use of the above products have resulted in an increased mortality as compared to controls.
Further research is needed.
TNF, tumor necrosis factor; IL-1, interleukin-1.

be divided into three broad categories (Table 3.5): agents aimed at blocking the effects of circulating microbial products, agents that block cytokines, and agents that reduce or prevent nitric oxide production.

Although initially there was much optimism that these products would reduce mortality by blunting the detrimental effects of inflammatory mediators, subsequent animal and human studies have revealed mixed results. In fact, some of these studies have been associated with an increased mortality.

LABORATORY INDICATIONS OF IMPROVEMENT IN SHOCK

The initial phase of treatment for shock is directed to improve oxygen delivery to the tissues by ensuring adequate ventilation, correcting hypovolemia, and improving cardiac function.

The success of the initial resuscitation is usually reflected in signs of improved perfusion (skin, kidneys, brain, heart rate) and indications of normal CVP if invasive monitoring is required. However, other laboratory parameters may be useful, if monitored sequentially, in determining if the shock syndrome is persisting despite early clinical improvement. Sequential measurements of serum lactate levels, and expired CO_2 gas (end-tidal CO_2) may indicate that continued aggressive resuscitation is needed despite signs of improvement.

It has been documented that a 5% reduction in serum lactate in the first hour is a good prognostic sign for patients presenting in circulatory shock. Lactate should fall over time as perfusion and oxygen delivery to the tissue improves. High serum lactate levels (approximately 4 mm per L) or serum lactate levels that continue to rise despite therapy are indications of severe shock. Aggressive therapeutic maneuvers to reverse the shock should be redoubled in this setting.

In addition, end-tidal CO_2 is a noninvasive laboratory value that may indicate continued hypovolemia. In hypovolemia and poor perfusion of the peripheral tissues and pulmonary tissues, CO_2 is not excreted in the lungs. Subsequently, there is a reduction of expired CO_2 gas, which is measured as a decreased end-tidal CO_2. As perfusion improves, end-tidal CO_2 increases. Investigators hope to correlate whether sequential end-tidal CO_2 measurements can be used to titrate the amount of intravenous fluid needed during resuscitation of the patient in shock. These measurements are noninvasive and may be a valuable adjunct in accessing improvements in perfusion in children with severe hypovolemia in the emergency department.

CHAPTER 4
Sedation and Analgesia

Steven M. Selbst, M.D.

One of the most common reasons for seeking care in an emergency department (ED) is to relieve pain and suffering. Injuries and painful medical conditions are common among children, and ED physicians are expected to manage this pain appropriately. Unfortunately, pain control is not often addressed satisfactorily. In 1990, Selbst and Clark found that in the ED setting, 60% of adult patients received adequate analgesia for painful conditions, but only 28% of pediatric patients received adequate analgesia for similar painful conditions. Emergency physicians and pediatricians were equally unlikely to give analgesics to children. There have been great advances in recognition, assessment, and management of pain in children over the last 10 years. The care of infants and children who undergo painful procedures in the ED has improved considerably. However, two recent studies show that children still often fail to receive analgesia for painful conditions. Inadequate dosing of medications for children upon discharge from the ED is a significant problem.

Many theories try to explain why pediatric pain is not successfully managed in the ED. Physicians expect babies to cry, so this nonspecific response to pain often is tolerated instead of controlled. Moreover, because young children and infants cannot describe or localize their pain, it is often ignored or presumed not to exist. Adult patients who clearly indicate that they are in pain generally get a direct response from a physician, whereas a young child who is crying or whimpering may not. In addition, some ED physicians avoid giving adequate analgesics to children because they fear it will lead to drug addiction. This is fear unfounded, however, because narcotic addiction is extremely rare when medications are used appropriately to manage acute pain. Hypotension and respiratory depression are other feared consequences of narcotic use with children, and although these fears may be legitimate, respiratory depression and hypotension are unlikely to occur if proper protocols are adhered to. These un-

TABLE 4.1. Possible Reasons for Inadequate Pain Control in the Emergency Department

Inability of young children to talk
Misconception that infants cannot feel pain
Misconception that children will not remember pain
Misconception that children will get addicted to narcotics
Fear of respiratory depression and hypotension
Unfamiliarity with analgesics and dosages
Other conditions taking priority

likely occurrences should be manageable in the ED, and they should not inhibit the attempt to control pain. Furthermore, it is likely that ED physicians often are forced to concentrate on other aspects of resuscitation and care before managing pain. Plans for pain control, therefore, may be forgotten because of other priorities. Also, in some cases, pain is ignored because it is inconvenient to wait for analgesics to take effect. Thus, some physicians may convince a young child that a painful procedure or repositioning of an extremity will hurt only for a minute. Brute force (instead of medication) is then used, and more pain is inflicted on an already uncomfortable child. Table 4.1 summarizes some reasons for inadequate pain control with children.

MINOR PAIN

Conditions such as headache, myalgia, chest pain, pharyngitis, otitis media, arthralgia, sunburn, strains, and sprains often produce minor pain in children. For treatment of this mild pain, aspirin, acetaminophen, ibuprofen (nonnarcotics), and codeine (narcotic) are excellent oral analgesic medications. *Aspirin* is one of the oldest analgesic medications, but its use has recently declined. It has the advantage of being inexpensive, and it has antiinflammatory effects. Sustained high dosages are needed, however, for the antiinflammatory effect. Thus, in most instances, aspirin is not much better than non-antiinflammatory drugs. Aspirin may be given every 4 hours at a dosage of 10 to 15 mg per kg per dose. Higher dosages increase only the antiinflammatory effect—not the analgesic effect. Buffered aspirin may be tolerated better and absorbed faster, but there is no evidence to show that it acts more rapidly or lasts longer than the nonbuffered variety. Likewise, enteric-coated aspirin is better tolerated but has variable absorption.

There are some definite disadvantages to using aspirin for pain management. It has many side effects, particularly gastrointestinal irritation in some patients, which can lead to nausea and vomiting. Aspirin also inhibits platelet function, which can lead to bleeding with overdosage, and it may cause reversible liver toxicity and central nervous system (CNS) problems (tinnitus, dizziness). Moreover, it may induce bronchospasm in asthmatic patients. Reye syndrome has been associated with the use of aspirin for varicella and flulike illness, but not for control of pain from trauma.

Acetaminophen acts centrally on nonopioid receptors in the brain to inhibit prostaglandin synthetase. Acetaminophen is more expensive than aspirin but is probably a better choice for pain associated with minor trauma or otitis media because it is tolerated better and it comes in liquid form, making it easier to give to young children. In some studies, acetaminophen has been shown to be a less potent analgesic than aspirin, but most claim it is equipotent. One study shows that 1,000 mg of acetaminophen is equal to 60 mg of codeine for postpartum pain. In addition, acetaminophen does not cause bleeding and is less likely than aspirin to cause bronchospasm in asthmatics. Its dosage is 15 mg per kg per dose every 4 hours and takes effect in 20 to 40 minutes, with a peak effect in 2 hours. High dosages are usually well tolerated, but therapy should not exceed 4 to 6 g per day. Acetaminophen has no antiinflammatory effects, and therapeutic doses rarely are associated with side effects; overdose, however, can cause liver toxicity.

Nonsteroidal antiinflammatory drugs (NSAIDs) (e.g., ibuprofen) are excellent choices for treating minor pain such as headache, dysmenorrhea, or musculoskeletal injuries. NSAIDs are thought to be more potent drugs than aspirin, and they have a longer half-life. Like aspirin, NSAIDs act on the peripheral nervous system to block formation of prostaglandins. The dosage is 8 to 10 mg per kg given every 6 hours. The recommended dosage for ibuprofen in older children is 400 mg every 4 to 6 hours for mild to moderate pain. Ibuprofen is available in liquid form, making it suitable for use in very young children. It is nonaddictive and does not cause respiratory or cardiac depression. Although NSAIDs may cause gastrointestinal bleeding, this risk is small. Like aspirin, these agents also cause renal and hepatic dysfunction and should be used with caution in children with renal or hepatic disease. Unlike aspirin, however, their effect on platelets (acetylation) is reversible. They can cause sodium retention, and they have crossreactivity with aspirin, so they should not be used with patients who have aspirin sensitivity.

Finally, *codeine* is a narcotic analgesic that can be given orally (even to young children) to control minor pain. Codeine usually is given orally because it maintains two-thirds of its effectiveness in oral form compared with parenteral use. It is thought to be more potent than aspirin but less potent than meperidine; thus, it is valuable for moderate pain (dental abscess, severe otitis media, or stomatitis) and has a low addiction potential. The dosage is 0.8 to 1.5 mg per kg per dose every 4 to 6 hours. Codeine can be changed into a liquid form for use in young children, and it can be combined with acetaminophen or aspirin to produce an even greater analgesic effect than when either is used alone. Codeine can cause respiratory depression, but this occurs very rarely. It has no renal or hepatic toxicity and does not alter platelet function, but it can cause the same gastrointestinal side effects (e.g., nausea and vomiting) as noted for other narcotics.

Table 4.2 summarizes the advantages and disadvantages of these analgesics for treating minor pain in children.

TABLE 4.2. Analgesics for Mild Pain

Analgesic	Advantages	Disadvantages
Acetaminophen	Well tolerated, safe	Liver toxicity if overdosed
Aspirin	Inexpensive	Gastrointestinal irritation
Ibuprofen	Long duration of action	Gastrointestinal irritation
Codeine	Potent opioid analgesia	Nausea, constipation

MODERATE AND SEVERE PAIN

Opioid medications are extremely important for treating patients in the ED with moderate to severe pain (burns, fractures, sickle cell vasoocclusive crises). Most opioids can cause important adverse effects (respiratory depression and hypotension), but these often are dose-related and may be reversed with naloxone, making opioids safe in the ED setting. Because of pharmacokinetic differences in young infants that may predispose them to respiratory depression, these drugs should be used with caution in infants less than 6 months of age who are not ventilated. Such infants should receive one-fourth to one-third of the initial calculated dosage recommended for older children, and they should be closely monitored. Opioid analgesics can be given by various routes. In general, the intramuscular route should be avoided because the injection itself is painful, it causes delayed drug absorption, and the dosage of drug given cannot be titrated. The intravenous route is more advantageous because titration is possible, although some pain is involved in starting the intravenous line. Some physicians choose to deliver the opioids with a patient-controlled analgesia (PCA) device that allows the patient to self-administer the drug at a safe dosage as it is needed. This allows patients to have some control over their own pain while relieving the ED nurse of time needed to administer the drugs.

For severe pain from a significant burn, sickle cell crisis, fracture, or other injury, *morphine* is an excellent choice. The usual dosage of morphine is 0.1 to 0.15 mg per kg per dose given intravenously over a few minutes. The maximum dose is 10 mg for opioid-naive subjects, which is repeated every 3 or 4 hours. The higher dosage, and a dosing interval of every 1 to 2 hours, is suggested for those who get narcotics often (e.g., those with sickle cell disease or cancer) because they may have some tolerance to the drug. If needed, a subsequent dose is reduced to 0.05 mg per kg if the patient is moderately sedated. Morphine can also be given as a continuous infusion at 0.07 to 0.10 mg per kg per hour, and it can be titrated, if needed (increase 25% every 3 hours). When given intravenously, its effect is almost immediate, with the peak effect occurring in 20 minutes. Morphine can cause pooling of blood by decreasing peripheral vascular resistance, which may result in hypotension. However, this is a concern only in the patient with a severe injury who may be hypovolemic. Certainly, the fluid status of an injured child requires careful attention from the ED staff, but morphine should not be withheld after intravenous fluids have corrected volume depletion. If the child is awake, alert, and screaming in pain, morphine can be given safely as long as the patient is monitored carefully.

Meperidine is another opioid agent that can be used to treat moderate to severe pain. It can be given intravenously or intramuscularly at a dose of 0.5 to 1 mg per kg, given every 2 to 3 hours. The maximum recommended dose for opioid-naive patients is 125 mg. Meperidine is more effective than morphine when given orally, and it reaches peak effectiveness more quickly than morphine when given by the intramuscular route (about 90 minutes). Otherwise, it has no significant advantages over morphine, but there can be problems with it use. For example, it may cause nervousness, tremors, disorientation, and even seizures when used intravenously. Morphine therefore may be a better opioid for severe pain unless a patient indicates that meperidine works best.

Fentanyl is a synthetic opioid that should be given slowly at a dose of 2 to 3 μg per kg intravenously over 3 to 5 minutes. It has a rapid onset of action (a few minutes) and a short duration of action (30 to 40 minutes), which makes it useful in the ED. It is an excellent agent for severe pain from fractures. Fentanyl also has several other advantages. It is a relatively safe drug and rarely causes hypotension, making it an excellent choice for injured children in severe pain.

A study of adult patients found that fentanyl caused hypotension in only 0.4% of patients, and alcohol intoxication may have been responsible for some cases of hypotension. It is thought that hypotension is unusual because histamine is not released when the drug is given. Respiratory depression can occur within minutes of fentanyl administration, but this is reported in only 0.7% of adult patients, some of whom were intoxicated with alcohol. There is a greater risk of respiratory depression when coadministered with other sedatives and in infants younger than 3 months of age. Apnea occurs even less often, and this may be related to the rate of infusion of fentanyl rather than the dosage. Although these adverse effects are serious, they can be reversed with naloxone and reduced if the dosage guidelines are followed and the drug is given slowly. Individualized dosing titrated to effect may reduce these side effects. Also, proper equipment and personnel who can manage an obstructed airway should be nearby when fentanyl is used.

An uncommon event caused by fentanyl is neuromuscular blockade, with severe thoracic and abdominal muscle rigidity. However, this is expected only when high dosages (greater than 15 μg per kg) are used and especially when fentanyl is administered rapidly. Most often, this side effect is reversible with naloxone, but succinylcholine may be required. Despite the problems already noted, fentanyl remains a valuable analgesic that should be used liberally in the ED when a child has severe pain.

Ketorolac tromethamine is a parenteral NSAID that has been used to treat moderate to severe pain. This drug is relatively new, and few data are available regarding its use with children. However, studies with adult patients show intramuscular ketorolac is comparable to narcotic agents and oral ibuprofen for treatment of musculoskeletal pain, headaches, sickle cell crises, and orthopedic injuries with less sedation and fewer side effects. It does not cause respiratory depression or nausea or vomiting. Intravenous ketorolac has been found to be as effective as morphine for postoperative pain in children with fewer side effects. It may have an opioid sparing effect, but this is not well proven. The drug is not yet approved by the Food and Drug Administration for intravenous use, although studies have demonstrated this route to be safe and efficacious in adults and children. Many pediatric centers use ketorolac with a loading dose of 1 mg per kg intravenously to a maximum of 60 mg followed by 0.5 mg per kg intravenously (maximum 30 mg) every 6 hours.

Other Agents

Another semisynthetic agent used occasionally with children in the ED is hydromorphone (Dilaudid), which can substitute for morphine and codeine. This is often given orally, rectally, or parenterally, and the analgesic effects last 4 to 5 hours. Also, hydrocodone (Hycodan) is an oral analgesic that is more potent than codeine with less associated nausea and vomiting. Likewise, oxycodone is 10 times more potent than codeine and about equal to the strength of morphine. Like codeine, it retains about 50% of its efficacy when given orally. It is often combined with aspirin (Percodan) or acetaminophen (Percocet, Tylox). The agents described next are not used in the ED for children. Propoxyphene (Darvon) has been shown to be inferior to aspirin, and in some studies, it was no better than placebo. It has significant addiction potential. Pentazocine (Talwin) is a narcotic agonist–antagonist that is better than placebo but not much better than aspirin. It is expensive and causes dizziness and hallucinations, as well as sedation and gastrointestinal dis-

TABLE 4.3. Analgesics for Severe Pain

Analgesic	Advantages	Disadvantages
Morphine	Rapid onset, potent analgesia	Respiratory depression, hypotension
Meperidine	Potent analgesia	Respiratory depression, seizure
Fentanyl	Potent analgesia, less hypotension	Respiratory depression, apnea
Ketorolac tromethamine	Nonnarcotic	Not well studied in children

comfort. Methadone is an excellent analgesic with actions similar to those of morphine. It is well absorbed from the gastrointestinal tract and reaches peak concentration 4 hours after ingestion. This is a useful drug for treating chronic pain because it has few gastrointestinal side effects, less sedation, and less euphoria. Heroin is not available in the United States for pain control.

Table 4.3 summarizes the advantages and disadvantages of several analgesics used to treat moderate to severe pain.

PROCEDURAL PAIN/CONSCIOUS SEDATION

Children often undergo painful procedures in the ED, including fracture reduction, laceration repair, incision and drainage, burn debridement, gynecologic examination, and foreign body removal. The pain involved with these procedures can be alleviated largely with the appropriate use of analgesics. Because a child's anxiety may further exacerbate the feeling of pain, it is often useful to give the child a combination of an anxiolytic with an analgesic medication before a painful procedure is performed.

The narcotics mentioned earlier commonly are given intravenously just before and during a painful procedure. Some emergency physicians combine opioids with phenothiazines. Morphine and hydroxyzine, combined in an intramuscular injection, are used by some physicians. For years, the combination of meperidine 2 mg per kg, promethazine 1 mg per kg, and chlorpromazine 1 mg per kg has been used for sedation and analgesia ("lytic cocktail," or "DPT"). Because this combination can produce deep and prolonged sedation with respiratory depression, its use is undesirable in the ED. It also requires a painful intramuscular injection and can result in dystonic reactions. Therefore, the use of the lytic cocktail, or DPT, is not recommended.

Sedatives

Sedatives should be used for painless procedures or in combination with analgesics when pain is anticipated.

Diazepam has been used as a sedative in doses of 0.1 to 0.2 mg per kg intravenously or orally. It can also be administered rectally, but the intramuscular route is discouraged because of pain and poor absorption. One retrospective study of children undergoing orthopedic procedures found the combination of fentanyl and diazepam to be safe.

Midazolam has become more popular and may be given at a dose of 0.05 to 0.2 mg per kg slowly, intravenously every 15 minutes as needed. Intranasal midazolam (dose of 0.2 to 0.4 mg per kg) and oral midazolam (dose of 0.2 to 0.5 mg per kg) have also been used with narcotic analgesics before painful procedures are performed. The intranasal route is irritating to the nasal mucosa and may not be tolerated well by the pediatric patient. Midazolam may be preferable over diazepam because it has a shorter onset of action (about 5 minutes) and a more rapid recovery (about 1 to 4 hours). The combination of a benzodiazepine and a narcotic analgesic produces amnesia, sedation, and muscle relaxation, which is preferred for orthopedic procedures and laceration repair. The likelihood of respiratory depression increases when a sedative is added to a narcotic, so proper precautions must be taken to protect the airway.

Propofol is an intravenous anesthetic used for sedation during short procedures, gynecologic examinations, and cardioversion. Propofol does not have analgesic properties of its own. This agent has been used rarely in the ED, but one report found it to be effective when used in combination with fentanyl for fracture reduction, abscess drainage, and chest tube placement in 20 adult patients. There were few side effects in that study, and propofol is advantageous because it has a rapid onset of action, a rapid recovery phase, and amnesic properties. It is a potent sedative, associated with significant respiratory depression, so great caution should be exercised with its use.

Pentobarbital is another sedative that is useful for pediatric procedures. Pentobarbital has no analgesic properties of its own and may increase pain perception, so it is not ideal for painful procedures. Its greatest use is for nonpainful procedures such as sedation of children for imaging studies. Narcotics can also be combined with 4 to 5 mg per kg pentobarbital, but this may result in prolonged sedation, making the combination less convenient to use in a busy ED. Sedation occurs rapidly after intravenous administration, and the effect dissipates in 15 to 20 minutes.

Chloral hydrate is a pure sedative hypnotic. It has no analgesic properties but may be useful for painless procedures such as imaging studies. Unfortunately, the sedation effect is variable and sometimes long lasting, making it less desirable for use in the ED. The peak effect may take 40 to 60 minutes or longer to accomplish. It is usually given orally in a dose of 20 to 75 mg per kg. Vomiting and paradoxic hyperactivity may occur with its use, but it is a relatively safe drug. Cardiac arrhythmia is a rare event associated with large doses, and respiratory depression may be a risk if the patient has obstructive sleep apnea.

In one study of 95 children who received 25 to 30 mg of chloral hydrate orally, there were no adverse cardiovascular, respiratory, or gastrointestinal effects. All sedated children recovered promptly in less than 60 minutes.

Nitrous Oxide

Nitrous oxide gas has been used for analgesia in an emergency setting since 1969. A few studies on children have shown that it is an effective agent for reducing pain when performing painful procedures, and it can be delivered painlessly.

Nitrous oxide has a short duration of action and a sedative, dissociative effect on the patient. The patient may complain of pain but does not seem to experience it (dissociative effect) and does not remember it later (amnesic effect). Patients who receive this gas feel as if they are floating, drowsy, or euphoric. It takes about 4 minutes to induce these effects with a nitrous oxide–oxygen mixture and about 4 to 5 minutes for them to wear off. When used in a 50/50 mixture with oxygen, nitrous oxide provides

TABLE 4.4. Nitrous Oxide–Oxygen Analgesia

Advantages	Disadvantages
Has rapid onset, short duration of action	Fail-safe system required
Causes sedation, dissociation, and amnesia	Expensive equipment
Is useful when local anesthesia is impractical	Scavenger device needed
May be used for young children	Not all patients benefit
Is safe when mixed with oxygen	More personnel required

analgesia, not anesthesia. That is, the patient remains awake during a procedure and is able to follow instructions. These properties make it useful in the emergency setting.

When used properly in a mixture with more than 20% oxygen, nitrous oxide does not produce serious side effects. Nitrous oxide affects the cerebral cortex (not the brainstem), so circulatory and respiratory depression do not occur and there is little relaxation of skeletal muscle. The gas is nonallergenic and not flammable or explosive, but it must be used with oxygen, and it will support combustion if a fire develops. It must be used with a fail-safe system that shuts off the flow of nitrous oxide when oxygen flow stops. The child can hold the mask on his or her face so that it will fall off if the child becomes unresponsive. Nitrous oxide also can be given with a nasal mask, enabling the patient to breathe through the mouth during the procedure. These precautions will avoid possible anoxia, which could be catastrophic. Some patients have experienced vomiting with this mixture of nitrous oxide, but this usually is an inconvenience rather than a danger because the patients maintain their cough and gag reflexes.

Table 4.4 reviews the advantages and disadvantages of nitrous oxide–oxygen analgesia.

Ketamine

Ketamine hydrochloride is another anesthetic agent used when performing wound debridement, foreign body removal, laceration repair, and other painful procedures. It can provide intense analgesia at subanesthetic doses. It causes dissociative amnesia and a trancelike state in which the child can follow commands but cannot respond verbally. The drug can be given intramuscularly (at a dosage of 3 to 4 mg per kg), and it also can be given intravenously (at a dosage of 0.5 to 2 mg per kg). This can be followed by an infusion of 0.01 to 0.2 mg per kg per minute if anesthesia is needed for more than 20 minutes. Ketamine has the advantage of rapid onset of action (1 minute if given intravenously, 5 to 10 minutes if given intramuscularly). It does not cause prolonged sedation and a single intravenous dose has an effect for about 15 minutes. With repeated doses or continuous infusion, the effect of ketamine depends on its elimination half-life and is considerably prolonged (1 to 2 hours). Ketamine can also be given orally (10 mg per kg), in which case sedation occurs in 30 to 45 minutes with duration of effect about 2 hours.

Ketamine does have disadvantages, however, in addition to the pain of injection. Rarely, ketamine causes unusual, unpleasant sensations and dreams with subsequent flashbacks, but benzodiazepines may decrease this reaction if given with ketamine. In a recent prospective study, no children experienced nightmares. Ketamine also can cause increased production of saliva in 11%, and vomiting upon awakening in about 6 % of those who receive this medication. Excess salivation can be effectively prevented by prior administration of atropine (0.01 mg per kg) or glycopyrrolate (0.005 mg per kg). Ketamine does not generally impair pharyngeal or laryngeal function or protective airway reflexes such as cough or swallowing. Thus, the risk of airway compromise is less with ketamine than with some other agents. However, a rare adverse effect is laryngospasm, so precautions should be taken to manage the airway if this develops. Neonates and those with upper respiratory infection are more likely to have laryngospasm, and they should not receive ketamine. Ketamine also can elevate blood pressure, intracranial pressure, and pulmonary artery pressure, so patients with head trauma, CNS malformations, and cardiovascular or respiratory disease should not receive this drug.

Local Anesthetic Agents

LIDOCAINE

Lidocaine is an excellent local anesthetic that has been used frequently in the ED for wound repair, foreign body removal, insertion of intravenous infusion lines or lumbar puncture needles, drainage of abscesses, and arterial puncture. Lidocaine has been shown to reduce pain of lumbar puncture in neonates without decreasing the success of the procedure.

Lidocaine usually is administered as a 1% solution (10 mg per mL) at a dosage of 3 to 5 mg per kg. A 0.5% solution is used for infiltration when large volumes are needed or in smaller patients when it is desirable to limit the total number of milligrams per kilograms given. When vasoconstriction is desired for suturing, lidocaine can be used in combination with epinephrine, at a dosage of (lidocaine) 7 mg per kg. Lidocaine should not be combined with epinephrine for use in areas supplied by end arteries such as the digits, penis, or pinna of the ear. Lidocaine is advantageous because it provides excellent local anesthesia and takes effect quickly (within a few minutes). The effect lasts long enough to complete most procedures (about 1 to 2 hours). It is a safe drug, as few people have a true allergy to it. Serious toxicity, such as seizures and cardiac arrest, can occur, but only when large amounts are injected inadvertently or when the drug is injected directly into a blood vessel.

The major disadvantage of using lidocaine as a local anesthetic is that a painful injection is required for administration. This pain can be reduced, however, if a long, small (27- or 30-gauge) needle is used to produce a "fanning" effect of the anesthetic. When injecting deep into tissue, a larger needle is needed to aspirate blood so that inadvertent injection into a vessel is avoided. Otherwise, the small needle is recommended, and only a small amount of lidocaine should be injected to avoid tissue distortion.

OTHER INJECTABLE LOCAL ANESTHETICS

Bupivacaine 0.25% is similar to lidocaine but may have a longer duration of action and may help reduce pain for 6 hours after a wound is repaired. Diphenhydramine, 0.5% and 1%, has been used and studied as a local anesthetic in adult patients. However, it seems to cause more pain on infiltration than does lidocaine and may cause tissue necrosis. In addition, a recent study shows that saline with 0.9% benzyl alcohol additive (the bacteriostatic compound in multidose vials of physiologic saline solution) provides anesthesia when injected into the skin of children just before placement of an intravenous line. With injection of 1 mL, anesthesia lasts about 2 minutes and there is minimal pain of injection and no side effects.

Topical Anesthetic Agents

LET

Wound repair can often be done painlessly with the use of a topical anesthetic such as LET. LET is a solution of 4% lidocaine,

TABLE 4.5. Suggested Protocol for Use of LET for Wound Repair

1. Apply LET gel directly to the wound.
2. Apply LET for 10–20 min.
3. Alternatively, apply 3–5 mL of LET solution for 3-cm wound.
4. Use cotton-tipped swab to paint solution onto wound.
5. Drip some LET into wound directly.
6. Tape cotton saturated with LET onto wound.
7. Avoid eyes, digits, and mucous membranes.

0.1% epinephrine, and 0.5% tetracaine. It can be made in gel form with hydroxyethyl cellulose. LET has been used successfully and safely for repair of uncomplicated facial and scalp lacerations in children. The major advantage of using LET for suturing is that the anesthetic can be applied painlessly, without the use of a needle. This should reduce the fear and anxiety involved in wound repair and may help the suturing go more smoothly. Even in the small number of children who have inadequate anesthesia from LET, the application of this topical anesthetic will reduce the pain of subsequent administration of lidocaine by injection. The gel can be applied directly to the wound for 15 to 20 minutes, or the solution can be "painted" on to the wound with a cotton-tipped swab, or a saturated cotton ball can be applied to the wound and held in place manually or with tape. Subsequently, the surrounding skin will be well blanched, indicating adequate local anesthesia. Like lidocaine, LET should not be applied to body parts where vasoconstriction is contraindicated.

Table 4.5 suggests a protocol for the use of LET for wound repair.

EMLA CREAM

Some physicians have used topical EMLA cream, which is a eutectic mixture of lidocaine and prilocaine with an occlusive dressing to supply local anesthesia. EMLA has been found helpful in relieving pain associated with intravenous catheter placement, lumbar puncture, and venipuncture in children. This cream may also be useful for draining perirectal abscesses or paronychias, draining arthrocentesis, or accessing subcutaneous drug reservoirs. The EMLA cream must be applied directly to the skin for 60 minutes before it is effective, so it is not practical for many situations in the ED. (Lidocaine does not penetrate well through intact skin.) If preparing for intravenous line placement, one should prepare multiple sites in case the first attempt is unsuccessful. Also, young children may become agitated, perspire, and have difficulty keeping the anesthetic on the skin. This could then mandate additional nursing time for a procedure. The cream works best for procedures where the child is unlikely to view the procedure needle and become agitated (e.g., lumbar puncture, bone marrow aspiration).

Despite these disadvantages, EMLA cream has been gaining popularity in the ED setting when time permits. In one recent study, EMLA was compared with TAC in a controlled, blinded fashion during wound repair in children. It was found to be superior to TAC in that patients treated with EMLA required less supplemental anesthesia than those who received TAC.

NONPHARMACOLOGIC METHODS FOR PAIN CONTROL

Hypnosis

Hypnosis has been used to treat pain in children for several years, and it has been successful in children as young as 2 years of age. Some physicians believe that the technique better serves children than adults because children have vivid imaginations and can more easily intertwine fantasy and reality. Also, it is thought that patients who present to the ED are already in a hypersuggestible state and thus may be more receptive to hypnosis.

This technique involves creating visual images for the child in an effort to reduce pain. For example, one could ask the child to think of the funniest movie he or she has ever seen and to imagine the pain getting less intense with each laugh. Or, the child could be asked to imagine the pain as a color that is fading away and is painted over with the child's favorite color.

Hypnosis is of value for chronic pain syndromes such as migraine headaches or long-term illnesses. It has also been used to treat children with sickle cell disease and painful crises. Such children have been taught self-hypnosis to reduce the frequency and intensity of painful crises, but some required a few outpatient sessions before it became effective.

Hypnosis has also been recommended for the acute management of burns, fractures, and other injuries. In fact, it is thought to be more useful for those entities than when emotional problems are triggers for pain. However, hypnosis may again be less practical than analgesics in this setting in the ED. It may have a role in conjunction with analgesics, but hypnosis cannot completely replace the need for medications in the acute situation. The use of hypnosis for many painful procedures in a busy emergency department has not been well studied.

TABLE 4.6. Summary of Some Choices Useful for Painful Procedures

Agent	Advantages	Disadvantages
Narcotics	Easy administration, may be titrated	Respiratory depression
Nitrous oxide	Painless administration, rapid onset, short duration, dissociative state	Requires more personnel, not always effective
Ketamine	Rapid onset, dissociative state	Hypersalivation, bad dreams (rare), laryngospasm (rare)
LET	Painless administration, low toxicity	Delays procedure slightly
TAC	Painless administration	Seizures, death (if ingested)
Lidocaine	Rapid onset, long duration, safe drug	Painful injection
Hypnosis	No side effects	Time-consuming, not always effective
Restraint	Rarely dangerous, increases success of procedure	May increase child's fear

Distraction and Relaxation Techniques

Distracting a child (e.g., with counting or squeezing a parent's hand) during a painful procedure may help reduce pain. One study shows that asking children to "blow out" air as if they were blowing bubbles was helpful in reducing pain from needle sticks for immunizations. Singing a song or telling a story to a child is also helpful. Children become very involved when listening to their favorite story, and parents can help with this. Paintings on the walls or ceiling of a procedure room may also distract a young child. However, distracting a child may have short-lived success because of a child's limited attention span, and it is less effective than involving the child in a detailed imaginary story. Another study shows that allowing adult patients to listen to music during suture repair provides a safe, inexpensive, and effective adjunct for pain management. It is possible that music or television might provide helpful distraction to older children undergoing painful procedures.

Restraint and Reassurance

Properly restraining a child for a painful procedure can be useful in reducing pain. Although this does not reduce fear or anxiety (in fact, it may heighten them), it allows the physician to perform the task better. This indirectly reduces pain because fewer attempts may be necessary to accomplish the task. The child should be warned honestly about the possible pain, but it is best to allow for the possibility that it may not hurt as much as he or she expects. Table 4.6 summarizes possible means of reducing pain from procedures.

CHAPTER 5

Emergency Airway Management—Rapid Sequence Intubation

Loren G. Yamamoto, M.D., M.P.H., M.B.A.

Management of the airway is a critical initial step in the stabilization of patients who present to the emergency department (ED) with a life-threatening emergency. Tracheal intubation often is the most reliable means of maintaining airway control. Indications for tracheal intubation include cardiopulmonary arrest, apnea, respiratory insufficiency, actual or potential airway obstruction, respiratory depression, severe burns, severe multiple trauma, severe head injury, increased intracranial pressure (ICP), a depressed sensorium, and a loss of the normal protective airway reflexes.

The equipment necessary for tracheal intubation should be readily available at the bedside for immediate access and use during the management of any critically ill patient in the ED (Table 5.1).

TABLE 5.1. Equipment Needed for Rapid Sequence Intubation

Pulse oximeter
End-tidal CO_2 monitor or detector
Electrocardiogram monitor
Uncuffed endotracheal tubes, sizes 2.5 to 6.0
Cuffed endotracheal tubes, sizes 6.0 to 8.5
Endotracheal tube stylets
Laryngoscopes (straight blade sizes 0 to 3, curved blade sizes 2 to 4)
Oral airways
Oxygen masks, preferably a nonrebreather
Ventilation masks in all sizes for bag-valve-mask ventilation
Large and small self-inflating ventilation bag with oxygen reservoir tail and positive end-expiratory pressure (PEEP) valve attachment
Laryngeal mask airways (LMA) in all sizes
Oxygen source
Suctioning source
Large-bore stiff suction tips
Flexible suction catheters
Nasogastric tubes
Tracheostomy tubes
Tracheostomy surgical instrument set
12- and 14-gauge needle catheters for needle cricothyrotomy
Preassembled transtracheal ventilation setup

Rapid sequence intubation (RSI) is not necessarily indicated in cardiac arrest. In cardiac arrest, for example, intubation without RSI would generally be preferable unless cardiopulmonary resuscitation (CPR), brain perfusion, muscle tone, and/or some degree of consciousness were maintained, in which case RSI may be of benefit.

A typical RSI consists of providing atropine to block vagal stimulation, a sedative to induce unconsciousness, and a muscle relaxant to induce paralysis. This typical sequence can become rather complicated when more considerations are added. It should be noted that the drugs for pediatric RSI have been recommended in their most basic forms as (1) atropine, (2) sedative, and (3) muscle relaxant. This chapter addresses the following controversies surrounding RSI: sedative selection, muscle relaxant selection, priming or defasciculation, and adjunctive medications such as lidocaine and fentanyl.

RAPID SEQUENCE INTUBATION SEDATIVES

The most common sedatives used in RSI include thiopental, midazolam (and other benzodiazepines), ketamine, and etomidate. Narcotic analgesics such as fentanyl can also be used, but this is less common. The use of propofol has increased in frequency, but its use is mostly for brief sedation for procedures rather than for RSI. Each of these drugs has beneficial and detrimental properties that must be understood to select the best sedative for RSI in the patient at hand. The advantages and disadvantages of each drug are summarized in Table 5.2.

Thiopental (an ultra–short-acting barbiturate) was initially one of the most commonly used sedatives for RSI. Its advantages are reliable and rapid onset (10 to 20 seconds), short duration, and a cerebral protective effect accomplished by reducing ICP, cerebral metabolism, and oxygen demand. Its main disadvantages are vasodilation and myocardial depression, which may result in hypotension. Thiopental should be avoided or used in lower dosages in hypotensive or hypovolemic patients. These effects can be minimized by slowing the rate of injection. Thiopental causes respiratory depression and may result in coughing, laryngospasm, and bronchospasm. Thiopental is contraindicated in porphyria and status asthmaticus.

Midazolam (and other benzodiazepines such as diazepam) has a slower onset than thiopental does. It is more commonly used for conscious sedation or as an adjunctive agent in general anesthesia. Midazolam is capable of anesthesia induction at higher dosages. Cardiovascular and respiratory depression occur less often than with barbiturates. Lack of recall or anterograde amnesia results from benzodiazepines used for anesthesia. Benzodiazepines should not be used in patients with

TABLE 5.2. Significant Properties of Rapid Sequence Intubation Sedatives

Drug	Onset	Duration	Cerebroprotective effect	Cardiovascular effect	Bronchial effect	Other disadvantages
Thiopental	Rapid	Brief	Good	Significant depression	Bronchospasm	N/A
Midazolam	Less rapid	Brief	Modest	Neutral	Neutral	Titration recommended is not feasible in RSI
Ketamine	Rapid	Brief	Adverse	Stimulatory	Bronchodilatory	Psychic reactions and excessive airway secretions
Etomidate	Rapid	Brief	Good	Neutral	Neutral	Myoclonus, cortisol suppression
Fentanyl	Less rapid	Brief	Modest	Neutral	Neutral	Seizurelike activity and chest wall rigidity
Propofol	Rapid	Brief	Good	Significant depression	Neutral	Less experience with agent in ED RSI

RSI, rapid sequence intubation; ED, emergency department.

glaucoma. Midazolam has many properties that suggest its use for RSI in the ED. Many reports in the literature have advocated its use despite the lack of data to document its efficacy and safety. The dosing range is suggested at 0.1 to 0.3 mg per kg. The lower dosage is probably insufficient to reliably induce unconsciousness. Because these drugs also result in amnesia, studies may never be able to retrospectively assess the degree of unconsciousness attained during RSI.

Although attractive, benzodiazepines have a slower onset than thiopental and have an excessively wide dosing range during which titration is recommended. In RSI, however, titration is undesirable because a rapid induction of unconsciousness and paralysis is the goal, and paralysis makes it impossible to assess consciousness. The use of midazolam in RSI has grown in popularity, largely because it can be used in nearly all clinical situations. Despite this, there appear to be drugs that have advantages over benzodiazepines in specific clinical situations.

Ketamine produces rapid sedation, amnesia, and analgesia. It is described as a dissociative agent that induces a trancelike state in which the patient is unaware, but not necessarily asleep. In combination with a paralyzing agent as in RSI, this difference is not noticeable. Ketamine results in sympathetic stimulation and an increase in systemic blood pressure (BP); however, reduced doses or no sedative are still recommended in potentially hypovolemic patients. Adverse effects, which include ICP elevation, intraocular pressure elevation, hallucinations, excessive airway secretions, and laryngospasm, limit its use to ED patients who have hypotension, hypovolemia, or status asthmaticus. Ketamine increases airway secretions, so routine atropine premedication is recommended. Ketamine has a bronchodilating effect in addition to its sympathetic effect, making it useful for RSI of patients with severe bronchospasm that requires intubation. Ketamine is contraindicated in patients with hypertension, head injury, psychiatric problems, glaucoma, or an open globe injury.

Fentanyl is a short-acting narcotic analgesic that results in rapid analgesia and unconsciousness at higher dosages. Adverse effects associated with fentanyl are less than those of morphine. The doses of narcotics required to produce complete anesthesia are much higher than the doses required for analgesia alone and may vary extensively. Chest wall rigidity may occur with rapid injection of fentanyl, but this is reversible with a muscle relaxant or with naloxone. Fentanyl use has been associated with seizurelike activity. Fentanyl is used most often in cardiovascular surgery in combination with other anesthetics. Although it has some properties useful for RSI done in the ED, literature sources to support fentanyl use for RSI in the ED are lacking. Fentanyl should not be used with monoamine oxidase (MAO) inhibitors.

Propofol use in the ED is a new occurrence. Largely used by anesthesiologists for short-term sedation and general anesthesia, propofol is gaining wider acceptance as an agent for short-term sedation for procedures in the intensive care unit (ICU) and ED. It can be used as a sedative in RSI, but its degree of experience here is limited and it does not have substantial advantages over other sedatives. Propofol shares many features with thiopental. Propofol decreases ICP and cerebral metabolism. The onset of propofol is rapid and brief, but it has significant cardiovascular depression. Although propofol can be used in instances when thiopental could be used, there is more experience with thiopental.

Although myocardial depression is most pronounced with thiopental, all sedatives cause some degree of cardiovascular depression, especially in hypotensive or hypovolemic patients. Because no sedative is entirely free of cardiovascular depression in the hypovolemic or hypotensive patient, such patients should receive reduced dosages or no sedative at all, depending on their cardiovascular status.

SEDATIVE SELECTION

Sedative selection remains one of the most controversial aspects of RSI. The addition of etomidate as a sedative for RSI has extended the sedative selection options. Etomidate appears to have the broadest applicability, but each agent should be well understood so that individual practitioners can make the best decisions about which agent would be most optimal in each clinical situation. No sedative is universally superior. The clinical situation determines the optimal sedative selection. Table 5.3 summarizes sedative selections in different clinical categories.

MUSCLE RELAXANTS

Muscle relaxants result in total muscle paralysis, yet the patient may be fully conscious.

Succinylcholine is a depolarizing muscle relaxant with a rapid onset (30 to 60 seconds) and short duration (3 to 12 minutes). Even though it has been the most common muscle relaxant used in RSI, it has numerous disadvantages. Although not contraindi-

TABLE 5.3. Rapid Sequence Intubation Drugs and Doses (in milligrams)

Age Average weight	Dose (mg/kg)	2 mo 5 kg	6 mo 8 kg	1 yr 10 kg	3 yr 15 kg	5 yr 19 kg	7 yr 23 kg	9 yr 29 kg
1. Preoxygenation: Positive-pressure ventilation with cricoid pressure only if hypoventilating or hypoxic.								
2. Adjunctive agents:								
Atropine: Optional in adults not requiring ketamine (1 mg maximum dose):	0.01–0.02	0.1	0.15	0.2	0.3	0.3	0.4	0.5
Lidocaine: Use when intracranial pressure elevation is suspected (otherwise, it is optional—see text):	1.5–3.0	7–15	12–24	15–30	22–45	30–55	35–70	45–85
3. Assess ability to establish mask ventilation should intubation fail. Do not proceed if inability to mask ventilate is anticipated.								
4. Sellick maneuver (cricoid pressure): Do not release until intubation is confirmed.								
5. Sedation agent: problem specific:								
No hypotension/hypovolemia (excluding status asthmaticus):								
Thiopental:	4–5	20–25	35–40	40–50	60–75	75–95	90–115	120–145
Etomidate:	0.2–0.4	1–2	1.5–3	2–4	3–6	4–7	5–9	6–11
Midazolam:	0.1–0.3	0.5–1.5	0.8–2.4	1–3	1.5–4	2–6	2.5–7	3–9
Mild hypotension/hypovolemia with head injury:								
Thiopental:	2–4	10–20	15–30	20–40	30–60	40–75	50–90	60–110
Etomidate:	0.2–0.3	1–1.5	1.5–2	2–3	3–4	4–5	5–7	6–8
Mild hypotension/hypovolemia without head injury:								
Ketamine:	1–2	5–10	8–16	10–20	15–30	19–38	23–46	29–58
Etomidate:	0.2–0.3	1–1.5	1.5–2	2–3	3–4	4–5	5–7	6–8
Severe hypotension/hypovolemia: Consider the risk of sedatives. Use NO sedative if risk is great.								
Ketamine:	0.35–0.7	1.5–3.5	2.8–5.6	3–7	5–11	7–13	8–16	10–20
Status asthmaticus:								
Ketamine:	1–2	5–10	8–16	10–20	15–30	19–38	23–46	29–58
6. Rocuronium:	0.6–1.0	3–5	5–8	6–10	9–15	12–19	14–23	18–29
7. Intubate (ET tube size):		3.5	3.5	4.0	4.5	5.0	5.5	6.0
ET tube depth at lip:		11 cm	12 cm	13 cm	14 cm	15 cm	16 cm	18 cm
Laryngoscope blade size:		1	1	1	2	2	2	2
8. Optional NG/OG tube:		8 Fr	10 Fr	10 Fr	12 Fr	12 Fr	12 Fr	14 Fr
9. Longer-acting sedation and/or paralysis as needed.								
10. If reversal of rocuronium is needed (see text):								
Atropine:	0.01–0.02	0.1	0.15	0.2	0.3	0.3	0.4	0.5
Edrophonium:	0.5–1.0	2.5–5.0	4–8	5–10	8–15	10–19	12–23	15–29

ET, endotracheal; NG, nasogastric; OG, orogastric.

cated in head injuries, it causes elevated ICP. Intraocular and intragastric pressure elevations may occur. Muscle fasciculations that may result in muscle pain, rhabdomyolysis, and myoglobinuria also may occur. These are more severe in muscular patients and can be prevented by a defasciculating dose of vecuronium before succinylcholine (this is not necessary in children under 5 years of age). Atropine premedication can prevent the bradycardia and excessive bronchial secretions associated with succinylcholine. Other less preventable adverse effects include negative inotropic and chronotropic effects, an association with malignant hyperthermia, hyperkalemia, hypertension, and arrhythmias. Succinylcholine is contraindicated in patients with glaucoma, penetrating eye injuries, significant neuromuscular disease, history or family history of malignant hyperthermia, and pseudocholinesterase deficiency. At 3 to 60 days after trauma or burns (in other words, day 3 or later following trauma or burns), succinylcholine results in an increased frequency of the risks described here and should not be used. Patients with severe burns or large crush injuries may already be acutely hyperkalemic; thus, the decision to use succinylcholine should consider this as well.

Of the nondepolarizing muscle relaxants, rocuronium currently has the fastest onset and shortest duration. Vecuronium is still commonly used because it was the most popular agent before rocuronium. Both agents have minimal cardiovascular effects. Onset times for rocuronium and vecuronium are 30 to 90 seconds and 90 to 120 seconds, respectively. Duration for both drugs is 25 to 60 minutes. Rocuronium comes in a premixed vial ready to use, whereas vecuronium comes in a powder that must be reconstituted. This factor gives rocuronium another advantage when the time to intubation may be prolonged because of medication preparation.

Other nondepolarizing muscle relaxants include pancuronium and atracurium. Pancuronium has a slower onset and more cardiovascular side effects. Atracurium has an onset time similar to that of vecuronium; however, it is associated with histamine release and cardiovascular side effects. Rocuronium is currently the nondepolarizing muscle relaxant of choice, but there is less experience with this drug compared to vecuronium. Other nondepolarizing agents should be eliminated from consideration.

MUSCLE RELAXANT SELECTION

In comparing rocuronium and succinylcholine, rocuronium has fewer adverse effects, whereas succinylcholine has a shorter duration. The onset times are similar. Some view rocuronium as preferable because it is safer. The contrary view is that because of its shorter duration (which allows restoration of spontaneous ventilation within 3 to 12 minutes compared with 25 to 60 minutes for rocuronium), succinylcholine is better if intubation fails. Rocuronium can be reversed pharmacologically with edrophonium and other similar agents; however, this is not clinically routinely useful because reversal cannot be achieved immediately. Reversal must wait for some degree of spontaneous recovery to occur, which happens later than the duration of succinylcholine.

Defasciculation and Priming

Defasciculation refers only to the use of succinylcholine, which may cause fasciculations, muscle pain, rhabdomyolysis, and myoglobinuria. This effect is most pronounced in muscular individuals. Fasciculations may increase muscle tone and increase the risk of gastric regurgitation during RSI. To prevent fasciculations, "defasciculation" is recommended, where one-tenth the paralyzing dose of a nondepolarizing muscle relaxant (e.g., vecuronium 0.01 mg per kg) is administered 1 to 3 minutes before succinylcholine administration. This "defasciculating" dose of vecuronium will prevent fasciculations caused by succinylcholine. Defasciculation is most beneficial in muscular individuals. It is not necessary in children 5 years of age or younger. Note that this defasciculating step delays the time to intubation and adds complexity to RSI.

Priming in RSI refers to nondepolarizing muscle relaxants only. Its purpose is to shorten the onset time of nondepolarizing muscle relaxants. A priming dose is one-tenth the paralyzing dose of a nondepolarizing muscle relaxant. Using vecuronium as an example, a priming dose of 0.01 mg per kg is administered. Five minutes should elapse for the "priming" to take effect. The paralyzing dose of 0.1 mg per kg is now administered. The full paralyzing onset time of vecuronium is about 100 seconds without priming, 50 seconds with priming. Unfortunately, priming adds an additional 5-minute delay to intubation while saving 50 seconds in accelerating the onset of the full dose of vecuronium. Because the onset time of rocuronium is considerably faster, the advantage of priming is minimal. Although some experts still recommend priming, it appears to have little benefit in the ED when immediate intubation is required.

Defasciculation and priming are often confused because they both require one-tenth of the paralyzing dose of a nondepolarizing muscle relaxant. However, the two principles are different even though they have similar characteristics in that they both are optional and they both delay the time to intubation and they both add complexity to the drug administrations in RSI.

ADJUNCTIVE AGENTS

The RSI sequence shown in Table 5.3 considers the use of atropine and lidocaine. Atropine use is considered routine in children to prevent bradycardia, but it is optional in adults unless ketamine is used as a sedative. In this case atropine is recommended in adults as well.

Lidocaine is more controversial. It has been shown to reduce ICP and airway reactivity under certain conditions when given 2 minutes before intubation. If ICP elevation is suspected, a cerebroprotective sedative (thiopental or etomidate) is generally preferred in RSI. Lidocaine is cerebroprotective in isolation, but it is unclear whether lidocaine results in additional benefit when added to a cerebroprotective RSI regimen that includes thiopental or etomidate. Despite this controversy, most practicing academic centers and consensus reports recommend the use of intravenous lidocaine if ICP elevation is suspected. In addition to intravenous lidocaine, topical lidocaine has been recommended to blunt the adverse reaction to tracheal intubation. This adds considerable complexity to the laryngoscopy procedure, especially in patients in whom neck immobilization is critical and/or airway visualization may be less than optimal. The recommendation that lidocaine be used in intubating asthmatics stems from its beneficial effect in attenuating bronchospasm. If one truly believes that lidocaine has such a benefit, then if possible, it should be administered long before the patient requires intubation, as opposed to administering it during RSI.

RAPID SEQUENCE INTUBATION PROTOCOL

After patient assessment, immediate stabilization, and intravenous access, patients should be assessed for any contraindications to RSI or its agents. The major contraindication to RSI is a likelihood that intubation or ventilation might not be possible, as in cases of limited cervical mobility, a receding mandible, limited jaw opening, major facial or laryngeal trauma, upper airway obstruction, or distorted facial or airway anatomy.

To simplify RSI, a table such as Table 5.3 should be adapted and modified to your preferences. This table should be taped to the wall in the critical care area of your ED. This table is not a substitute for thoroughly understanding the characteristics of each agent and the critical thinking necessary to select the agents. What follows explains the protocol given in Table 5.3.

Nasal Intubation Compared with Oral Intubation in the Trauma Patient

Trauma victims who arrive in the ED have suspected cervical spine (C-spine) injuries in addition to other injuries. When it is not possible to rule out a C-spine injury before RSI, the head and neck should be immobilized during intubation.

Unless contraindicated, emergency intubation of pediatric patients should always be done orally. In spontaneously breathing patients, older literature sources have recommended blind nasal tracheal intubation, whereas newer recommendations prefer oral tracheal intubation using RSI. If the need for intubation is emergent, nasal tracheal intubation may not be as reliable as oral tracheal intubation. Nasal tracheal intubation is noxious, and it may cause the conscious patient to gag or become agitated, resulting in more neck movement, an increase in ICP, and possible vomiting. Nasal tracheal intubation is more difficult in children. Epistaxis, sinusitis, and cribriform fracture complications are other concerns with nasal tracheal intubation. Studies have not been able to show that nasal tracheal intubation results in less C-spine movement than oral tracheal intubation.

There is concern that laryngoscopy during oral tracheal intubation may displace a C-spine fracture. When using RSI, however, laryngoscopy manipulation and neck movement are minimized under these more ideal conditions. The concern that the loss of cervical muscle tone on an unstable C-spine will reduce its splinting effect and increase its instability has not been supported by evidence.

ALTERNATIVE INTUBATION AND AIRWAY TECHNIQUES

Because the experience level of most ED physicians is greatest with oral tracheal intubation, it is unwise to deviate from this in managing a critically ill child who requires intubation.

Alternative procedures should be reserved for instances in which conventional airway techniques prove unsuccessful.

Flexible fiberoptic scopes, lighted stylets to guide nasal tracheal intubation, retrograde intubations, and surgical airways all require high skill and experience levels to be done optimally. These procedures have a minimal degree of documented experience in children. Directly visualizing the airway through a fiberoptic scope is appealing; however, it requires extensive practice, and it may be especially difficult in critical intubations or in agitated patients. Intubation aided by bronchoscopy, lighted stylets, and the retrograde wire technique are not recommended in ED RSI because of the lack of spontaneous breathing during RSI and the time required for these procedures.

The Combitube (Sheridan Catheter Corporation, Argyle, NY) is a double-lumen airway that is blindly inserted through the mouth. One lumen exits through the distal end of the Combitube. The other lumen exits through multiple side-holes proximal to the distal end. An inflatable (distal) balloon separates these two (the distal end-hole and the more proximal side-holes). Because the Combitube is inserted blindly, it will enter either the trachea or the esophagus. If it enters the trachea, the distal balloon is inflated and the distal end-hole lumen is used to ventilate the patient just as if this were a conventional endotracheal tube. If the Combitube enters the esophagus, the inflation of the distal balloon occludes the esophagus and the lumen ending in the more proximal side-holes is used to ventilate the patient. The esophageal position of this tube is similar to an esophageal obturator airway. Use of the Combitube requires familiarity with its function and method of insertion. It has been demonstrated to be effective in providing an airway during resuscitation, but failures occur as well. Widespread experience with the Combitube in pediatric patients is lacking.

The laryngeal mask airway (LMA) is a newer airway device. The LMA is not disposable and must be sterilized between uses. LMAs come in several different sizes, and their use in pediatric patients has been demonstrated. Experience with LMAs is growing. The correct insertion and placement position of the LMA is critical. The LMA is inserted blindly, taking about 15 to 20 seconds. LMA insertion methods are best taught using video or hands-on instruction. In-depth understanding of the LMA and previous hands-on experience are required to consider it as an airway management option. The LMA does not prevent aspiration.

Surgical airways may be considered. Complications, including incorrect tube placement, subcutaneous emphysema, pneumomediastinum, pneumothorax, bleeding, tracheal stenosis, subglottic stenosis, arterial injury, blood aspiration, and persistent tracheocutaneous fistulae, are more common when the procedure is performed on an emergency basis in children. Cricothyrotomy is faster and easier to perform than tracheostomy and also has a lower complication rate. However, in small children, the cricothyroid membrane is not readily palpable, and it may be too small for an airway. It is not recommended in children less than 10 years of age.

HEAD TRAUMA

Children with head injuries who have a depressed sensorium may be hypoxic, hypovolemic, hypotensive, or acidotic. Although intracranial hemorrhage alone cannot account for significant hypovolemia that results in shock in an older child or adult, this is possible in an infant.

Unconscious patients should be intubated using RSI and should be hyperventilated. Patients responsive only to painful stimuli may need to be intubated as well. Some patients with lesser degrees of sensorium depression also may need intubation using RSI and hyperventilation, depending on the degree of head injury and the rate of deterioration. Patients at risk of ICP elevation should be given thiopental or etomidate in addition to lidocaine pretreatment as part of RSI unless hypovolemia or hypotension exist, in which case the dose should be reduced or eliminated, depending on the clinical circumstances. Thiopental and etomidate lower ICP and cerebral metabolic oxygen demand.

In patients with evidence of ICP elevation, cerebral dehydration may reduce ICP and prevent impending herniation. This can be done using diuretics (furosemide 1 mg per kg) or osmotic diuretics (mannitol 0.25 to 1.0 mg per kg).

Patients with head injuries may develop posttraumatic seizures related to cerebral contusions, cerebral edema, or intracranial hemorrhage. Under RSI, these seizures are not visible because of pharmacologic paralysis. It is prudent in most instances to give a loading dose of phenytoin (10 to 20 mg per kg) after intubation is confirmed to treat prophylactically any undiagnosed posttraumatic seizure focus.

BURNS

Children with severe burns represent a special form of multiple trauma. Burn patients may also sustain blunt trauma, and ABCs are still the priority. Early intubation using RSI is advocated for patients at risk of airway injury because airway edema is expected to worsen rapidly. These cases include children with evidence of soot in sputum or vomitus, burns of the face, singed nasal hairs, lip burns, wheezing, stridor, or severe burns. The possibility of carbon monoxide poisoning should be considered. It may be preferable to avoid succinylcholine in patients with severe burns for fear of worsening hyperkalemia.

Pulmonary compromise may result from smoke inhalation, burn injury, bronchial edema, bronchospasm, blunt trauma, or adult respiratory distress syndrome (ARDS). Initial chest radiographs may fail to show some of these injuries.

Circumferential burns around an extremity may result in additional swelling and venous and arterial occlusion. Infarction of the extremity distal to this injury can be prevented by early recognition of this fact and surgical release of the constriction. Similarly, circumferential burns about the chest may result in chest wall constriction and respiratory difficulties.

STATUS EPILEPTICUS

In patients presenting to the ED with prolonged seizures, the standard approach of ABC support and immediate administration of benzodiazepines is generally initiated. Loading with i.v. phenytoin and/or phenobarbital may also be considered if seizures continue. This process of administering anticonvulsants and waiting to assess its effect occurs in 5- to 15-minute cycles. If seizures fail to respond to several doses of anticonvulsants, the child could be continuously seizing for an additional 30 to 60 minutes.

Prolonged seizures result in hypoxia and respiratory acidosis due to poor ventilation. The brain is simultaneously hypermetabolic with greater oxygen demand. RSI using thiopental effectively reverses this process. Skeletal muscle activity stops. Oxygenation and ventilation are restored. The brain may still be hypermetabolic because it may still be epileptogenic, but at least the patient is no longer hypoxic and acidotic. Thiopental has potent cerebroprotective and anticonvulsant activity. Simultaneous administration of high dosages of benzodiazepines, phenytoin, and phenobarbital can potently reduce the seizure potential of the brain while maintaining oxygenation and ventilation. The major adverse effect of most anticonvulsants is respiratory depression. Following RSI, this is no longer a concern and maximum doses of anticonvulsants can be administered to provide maximum anticonvulsant activity.

In refractory status epilepticus, the duration of seizures, hypoxia, and acidosis is likely to contribute to cerebral injury. At some point in the management of status epilepticus (e.g., 60 minutes), the failure of conventional anticonvulsants should be recognized and RSI followed by maximum anticonvulsant administration should be considered. Because potentially injurious seizure durations of 40 minutes or more can occur in the management of such patients, it has been my preference to initiate RSI earlier rather than later. The concern that seizures can no longer be visibly appreciated after RSI should be tempered by the clinical benefits of RSI as described. Electroencephalogram monitoring in the ED is often recommended, but it is not feasible in most hospitals.

AGITATED PATIENTS WHO REQUIRE PROCEDURES OR TRANSPORT

Agitated or combative patients with head injuries or possible intracranial lesions that require computed tomography (CT) scanning cannot be scanned in such a condition. Sedation alone can be considered for such patients. In patients who fail to respond to standard sedation measures or in patients who may benefit from tracheal intubation, RSI provides an effective means of immediately securing airway control, breathing, and movement so that imaging can be completed with minimal trauma to the patient. Patients who require transport to another facility and who are agitated and hard to control may be difficult to manage during transport. After the clinical situation has been assessed, RSI may be indicated if its benefits outweigh its risks. Patients are more difficult to monitor during procedures and transports. The immediate detection of unrecognized extubation or hypoxemia is crucial. Portable pulse oximeters and $ETCO_2$ monitors can monitor oxygenation and confirm intubation continuously.

SECTION II

Signs and Symptoms

CHAPTER 6

Abdominal Distension

Joseph E. Simon, M.D.

Abdominal distension is defined as an increase in the volume of the abdominal cavity. Apparent abdominal distension secondary to poor posture, the natural lordosis of childhood, abdominal wall weakness, obesity, and pulmonary hyperinflation may be mistaken for true abdominal distension.

DIFFERENTIAL DIAGNOSIS

Abdominal distension is a nonspecific sign (Table 6.1); common causes are listed in Table 6.2 and life-threatening etiologies in Table 6.3. Bowel distension occurs secondary to mechanical or functional intestinal obstruction, aerophagia, malabsorption, or obstipation. Mechanical obstruction most commonly occurs in infants secondary to congenital malformations (atresias, volvulus, incarcerated hernia) and intussusception and in all ages secondary to previous abdominal surgery with resulting adhesions. Functional obstruction, or ileus, is suggested by tympanitic distension in the absence of bowel sounds. Peritoneal irritation secondary to infection, pancreatic enzymes, bile, or blood is suggested by signs such as involuntary guarding and pain with movement. Fever without peritoneal signs suggests intestinal inflammation, systemic infection, or anticholinergic poisoning. Various poisonings (atroponics), toxins (botulism), and electrolyte disturbances (hypokalemia) may result in an ileus. These will most likely occur in the patient who has no abdominal findings other than tympanitic distension. In particular, the abdomen will be nontender. Finally, posttraumatic gastric distension is an extremely important entity that may result in significant respiratory embarrassment secondary to upward pressure on the diaphragm. It probably is secondary to a combination of aerophagia and ileus.

Free peritoneal air results from intestinal perforation secondary to trauma or inflammation. The child will be toxic, and peritoneal signs will be present.

Extraluminal fluid accumulates in the abdominal cavity because of a decreased serum albumin, inflammation, bleeding, intraperitoneal chyle, and/or increased venous and lymphatic resistance through the portal and hepatic veins. A low serum albumin level is suggested by peripheral edema. It occurs as a result of protein loss secondary to nephrotic syndrome or protein-losing enteropathy, or decreased protein synthesis like that which occurs in cirrhosis and malnutrition. Obstruction of blood flow through the liver is suggested by distended abdominal wall veins, a history of hemoptysis, and an enlarged spleen. The obstruction may occur at the prehepatic level (portal venous thrombosis), within the liver parenchyma (end-stage cirrhosis), at the hepatic veins (Budd-Chiari syndrome), or at the intrathoracic level (congestive heart failure [CHF], pericarditis). Obstruction at the portahepatis usually is idiopathic, although a history of umbilical venous catheterization or omphalitis in the newborn period should suggest this possibility. Although cirrhosis evolves gradually, its clinical presentation may be abrupt. It results from Wilson disease, α_1-antitrypsin disease, biliary atresia, and other congenital problems, or occasionally, from chronic active hepatitis. Obstruction of flow at the hepatic veins or above occurs as a result of Budd-Chiari syndrome, CHF, or constrictive pericarditis. The liver is engorged, resulting in hepatomegaly and right upper quadrant tenderness in each of these entities.

A history of recent trauma and signs of shock point to intraperitoneal bleeding, usually secondary to a splenic or hepatic laceration. An ileus secondary to both peritoneal inflammation and shock likely contributes to the abdominal distension. Trauma in the recent past suggests chylous ascites. Finally, a diffusely tender abdomen suggests infectious peritonitis, pancreatitis, or bile peritonitis.

Extreme hepatomegaly that develops acutely occurs secondary to inflammation, engorgement, or trauma. There will be marked right upper quadrant tenderness and generally systemic toxicity. Causes include hepatitis, CHF, constrictive pericarditis, and congenital enzyme deficiencies. Other causes of extreme hepatomegaly include neoplastic disease, storage diseases, and congenital hemolytic anemias. Generally, hepatomegaly develops gradually in these conditions and is accompanied by many other signs of chronic illness. If neoplastic disease is suspected because of suspicious lymphadenopathy or other masses or if trauma is a consideration, an abdominal tomographic scan should be considered.

Extreme splenomegaly without marked hepatomegaly in the toxic-appearing child suggests intraparenchymal bleeding with an intact capsule, sickle cell sequestration crisis, or malaria. In the nontoxic child, portal hypertension, neoplastic disease, and chronic hemolysis should be suspected. Neoplastic disease often results in a spleen with an irregular surface. Abdominal computed tomography (CT) scan is useful in identifying this possibility. Chronic hemolysis secondary to sickle cell disease, β-thalassemia, and hereditary spherocytosis may result in a very large spleen. In the case of hemoglobin SS disease, but not hemoglobin SC disease or sickle-thalassemia, splenic enlargement is followed by splenic atrophy beyond 5 years of age. A peripheral blood smear generally identifies this group of causes of massive splenomegaly.

Other causes of abdominal distension include cysts, tumors, uterine enlargement, obstructive uropathy, bowel duplication, and inflammation. Cystic lesions include ovarian cysts; mesenteric, omental, or peritoneal cysts; choledochal cysts; and polycystic kidneys. These conditions generally present with a subacute history and physical examination. The exception is torsion

TABLE 6.1. Differential Diagnosis of Abdominal Distension

Spurious
- Poor posture
- Obesity
- Pulmonary hyperinflation
- Lordotic posture of childhood
- Abdominal muscle weakness/hypotonia

Bowel Distension
- Aerophagia
  - Postprandial
  - Post–positive-pressure ventilation (PPV) with bag-mask-valve device
  - TE fistula
- Intestinal obstruction (mechanical)
  - Volvulus
  - Incarcerated hernia
  - Intussusception
  - Adhesive bands
  - Duplications and other masses
  - Meconium ileus
- Ileus
  - Infection
  - Abscess
  - Appendicitis
  - Peritonitis
  - Botulism
  - Gastroenteritis
  - Pneumonia
  - Sepsis
  - Necrotizing enterocolitis
- Intraperitoneal blood (trauma, ruptured ectopic pregnancy)
  - Electrolyte abnormalities
  - Hypokalemia
  - Hypercalcemia
  - Poisoning
  - Anticholinergics
  - Methyldopa
  - Trauma
  - Shock
  - Severe pain secondary to:
  - Biliary colic
  - Renal colic
- Malabsorption
  - Congenital causes
  - Bacterial overgrowth
  - Parasites
  - Formula enteropathy
- Obstipation
  - Functional
  - Hirchsprung's
  - Hypothyroidism

Free Peritoneal Air

Extraluminal Fluid
- Hypoproteinemia
  - Malnutrition
  - Nephrotic syndrome
  - Renal failure
  - Cirrhosis
  - Protein-losing enteropathy
  - Congenital syphilis and TORCH infections
- Blood
  - Hepatic laceration
  - Splenic laceration
- Peritoneal inflammation
  - Bile peritonitis
  - Peritonitis
  - Leukemia
  - Tuberculosis
  - Pancreatitis
- Cirrhosis
  - Biliary atresia
  - Chronic active hepatitis
  - Wilson's disease
  - α_1-Antitrypsin disease
  - Tyrosinemia
  - Galactosemia (late)
  - Chylous ascites
  - Congestive heart failure/pericarditis
  - Budd-Chiari syndrome
  - Portal hypertension

Hepatomegaly
- Congestive heart failure/constrictive pericarditis (chronic)
- Budd-Chiari syndrome
- Biliary atresia
- Inflammation
  - Abscess
  - Acquired immunodeficiency syndrome (AIDS)
  - Hepatitis
  - Tyrosinemia
  - Galactosemia
  - Wilson's disease
  - Congenital syphilis and TORCH infections
- Neoplastic disease
  - Hodgkin's disease
  - Neuroblastoma
  - Leukemia
  - Lymphoma (non-Hodgkin's)
  - Hepatoblastoma
- Storage disease
- Hemolytic anemia
  - Sickle cell
  - β-Thalassemia
  - Malaria
- Hepatic laceration (subcapsular hematoma)

Splenomegaly
- Portal hypertension
- Neoplastic disease
  - Hodgkin's disease
  - Neuroblastoma
  - Leukemia
  - Lymphoma (non-Hodgkin's)
- Hemolytic anemia
  - Sickle cell
  - Spherocytosis
  - β-Thalassemia
  - Malaria
- Inflammation
  - AIDS
- Storage diseases
- Hemorrhage
  - Trauma (subcapsular hematoma)
  - Sequestration (sickle cell)

Mass
- Cysts
  - Choledochal cyst
  - Ovarian cyst
  - Mesenteric cyst
  - Peritoneal cyst
  - Omental cyst
  - Polycystic kidneys
- Obstructive uropathy
- Uterine enlargement
  - Pregnancy
  - Hematocolpos
- Neoplastic disease
  - Wilms' tumor
  - Ovarian tumor
  - Teratoma
- Inflammatory masses
  - Regional enteritis

TE, tracheoesophageal; TORCH, *t*oxoplasmosis, *o*ther infections, *r*ubella, *c*ytomegalovirus infection, and *h*erpes simplex.

TABLE 6.2. Common Causes of Abdominal Distension[a]

Aerophagia (crying, feeding)	Pneumonia/sepsis
Gastroenteritis	Peritonitis
Obstipation	Intra-abdominal bleeding
Pregnancy	Hemolytic disease
Traumatic ileus	Congestive heart failure
Intestinal obstruction (mechanical)	Hepatitis
Obstructive uropathy (infants)	

[a]Listed in approximate order of frequency.

TABLE 6.3. Life-Threatening Causes of Abdominal Distension

Infectious	*Other*
Peritonitis	Intestinal obstruction (mechanical)
Sepsis/pneumonia	Electrolyte abnormality
Botulism	Renal failure
Pancreatitis	Poisoning
Congenital syphilis	Necrotizing enterocolitis
Hepatitis	Intestinal perforation
Tuberculosis	Shock
Congenital	Budd-Chiari syndrome
Tyrosinemia	Congestive heart failure
Galactosemia	Pericarditis
Hemolytic disease	Portal hypertension
Traumatic	Acquired immunodeficiency syndrome
Intra-abdominal bleeding	
Neoplastic	
Leukemia and other malignancies	

of the large ovarian cyst, which produces vomiting and marked abdominal pain. Obstructive uropathy is probably the most common cause of abdominal distension in early infancy. Tumors such as Wilms tumor, an ovarian tumor, and a teratoma generally can be palpated easily as firm, discrete abdominal masses by the time they are causing frank abdominal distension. Bowel duplication can be a subtle diagnosis until a complication such as mechanical bowel obstruction or hematochezia develops. Regional enteritis with sufficient inflammatory mass to cause abdominal distension is preceded by a long history of ob-

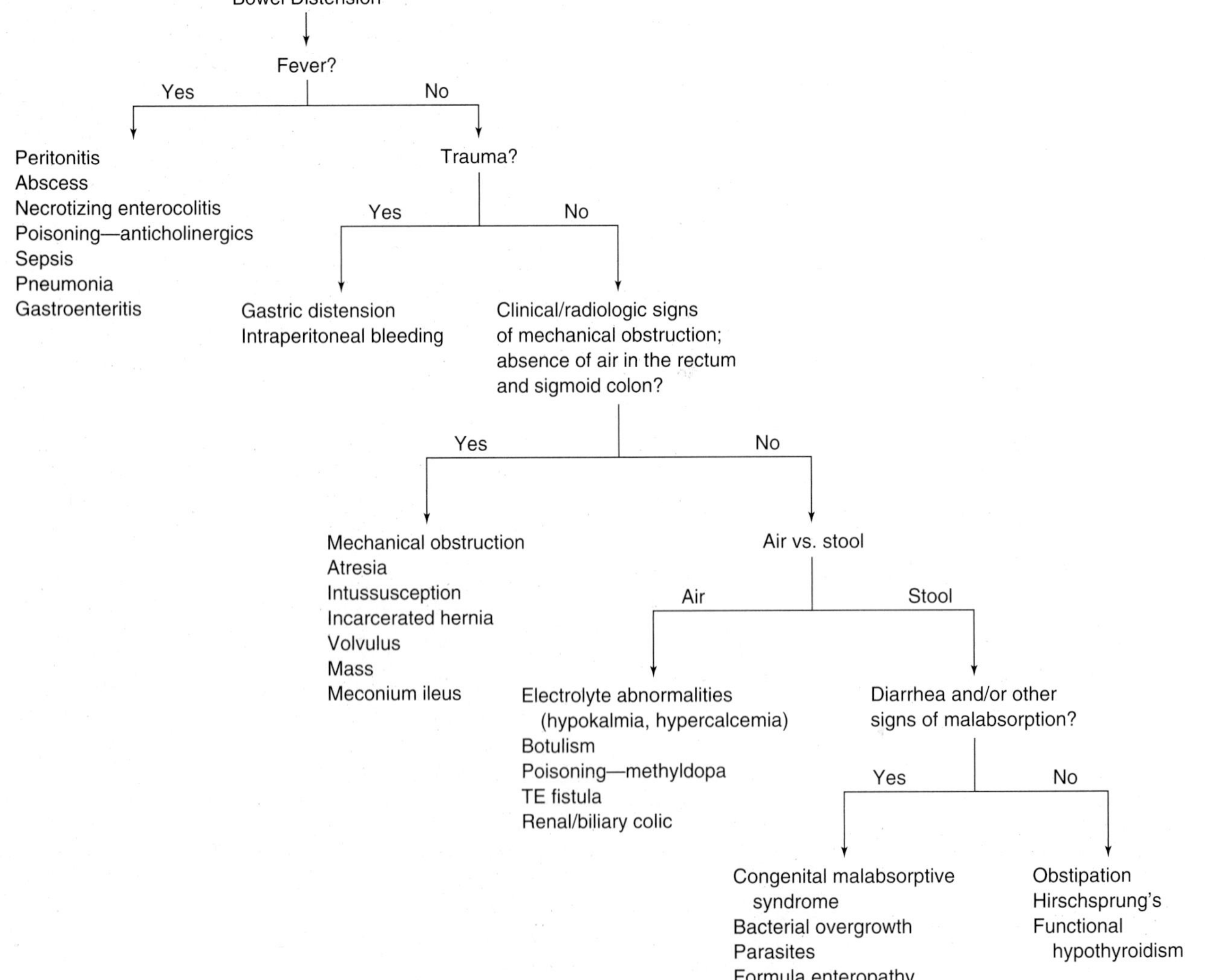

Figure 6.1. Bowel distension.

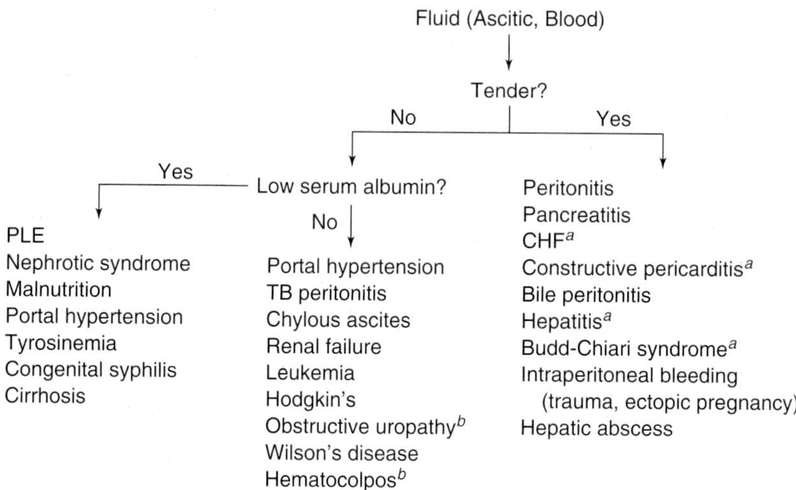

Figure 6.2. Fluid (ascitic, blood).

structive and malabsorptive symptoms. Finally, a midline pelvic mass should suggest pregnancy or hematocolpos.

EVALUATION AND DECISION

History

The history should attempt first to differentiate acute from chronic symptomatology, focusing on rate of progression, recent trauma, weight loss, or weight gain. Next, systemic signs such as fever, anorexia, edema, and lethargy further define the acuteness of the problem and, to some degree, narrow the diagnostic possibilities. Next, symptoms relative to specific organs, including the gastrointestinal (GI), renal, cardiac, and gynecologic systems, should be pursued. These symptoms include vomiting (bilious or nonbilious), abdominal pain, stool history, shortness of breath, cough, hemoptysis, urine output (including strength of stream and any abnormality of urinary color or foamy urine), and menstrual history. Finally, a family history of anemia, early infant death among relatives or metabolic disease, a travel history, and a careful newborn history may be revealing.

Physical Examination

After ruling out life-threatening respiratory embarrassment and shock, the physical examination should focus on determining whether the generic cause of the abdominal distension is bowel (air or stool) (Fig. 6.1), free fluid (Fig. 6.2), massive hepatomegaly (Fig. 6.3), massive splenomegaly (Fig. 6.4), inspissated stool, or a discrete mass (Fig. 6.5). A tympanitic abdomen with intestinal outlines on the anterior abdominal wall suggests bowel distension as the cause of the abdominal enlargement. Tympani in a toxic child without intestinal outlines suggests free air. A fluid wave and dullness suggest ascites. Palpable loops of bowel or a palpable descending colon suggests stool.

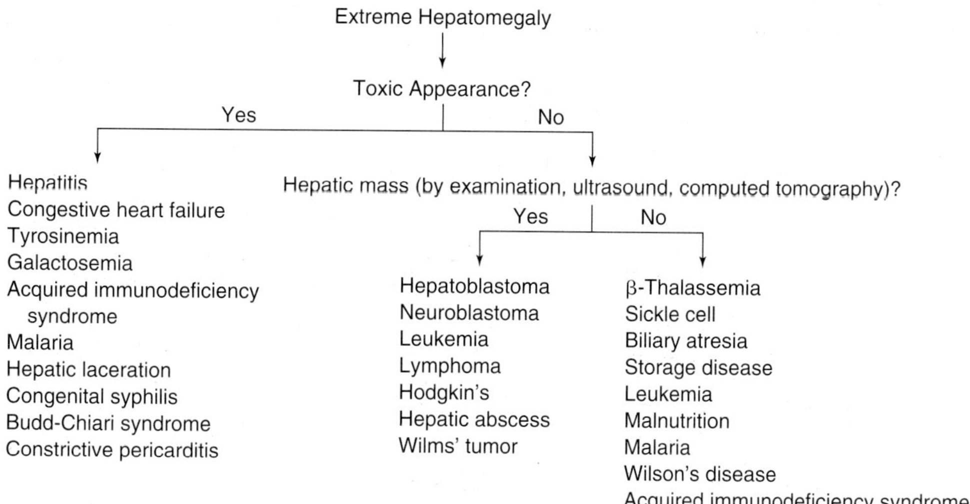

Figure 6.3. Extreme hepatomegaly.

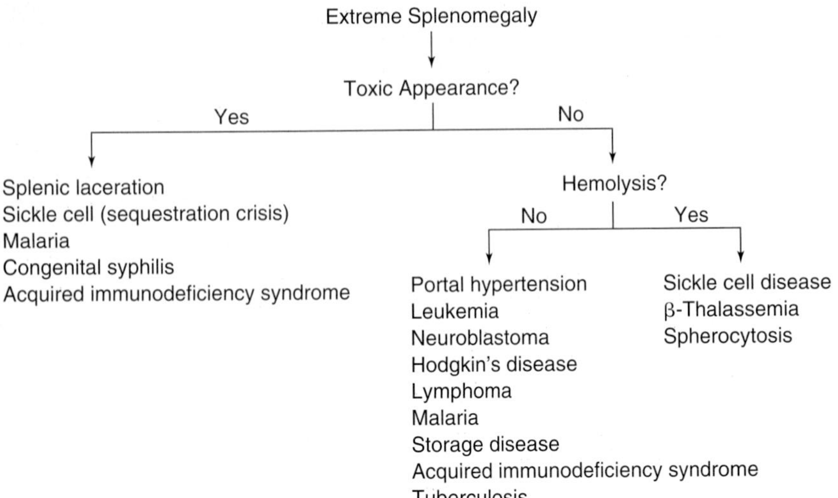

Figure 6.4. Extreme splenomegaly.

Massive hepatomegaly and splenomegaly generally are defined easily by palpation. The examiner must be cautious, however, because other masses may mimic hepatomegaly and, in particular, splenomegaly. Other key physical findings include signs of CHF, abdominal tenderness, edema, signs of trauma or easy bruising, lymphadenopathy, pallor, and jaundice. A rectal examination for a mass, tenderness, and the presence or absence of stool is also helpful. More specific findings may be pursued once an initial hypothesis is made based on the algorithms in this chapter.

Laboratory

The initial laboratory evaluation of abdominal distension is determined by the clinical findings and may include complete blood count with smear, erythrocyte sedimentation rate, reticulocyte count; liver function tests, including serum albumin and clotting studies; electrolytes with blood, urea, nitrogen, creatinine, and amylase; a urinalysis with reducing substances; and a chest radiograph and a two-view abdomen plain radiograph. If intestinal obstruction is suspected, one of the plain radiographs should be a prone cross-table lateral to determine the presence or absence of air in the rectum and sigmoid colon. It is preferable that this study be performed before a rectal examination is done.

Often, after the initial history, physical examination and laboratory evaluation imaging studies will be necessary. Ultrasound, if available, is an excellent first step because it does not involve radiation and often produces a definitive answer. If intestinal obstruction is suspected, an upper GI series is the preferred study (or an air-contrast or barium enema if intussusception is suspected). An abdominal CT scan is the preferred study to evaluate abdominal distension thought to be secondary to trauma.

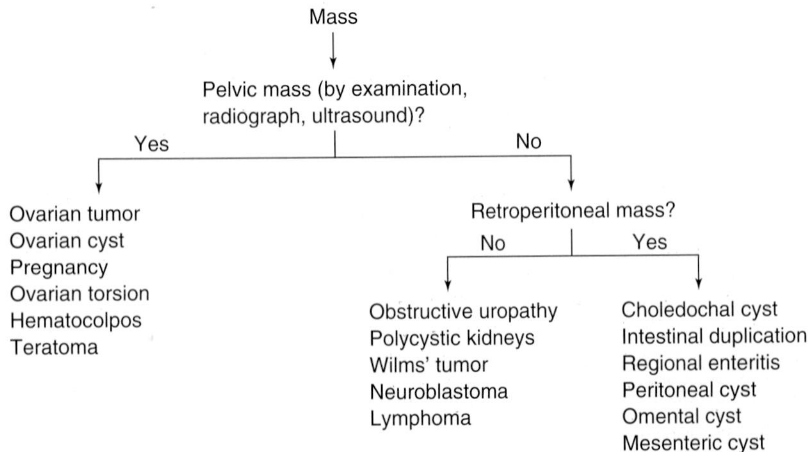

Figure 6.5. Mass.

CHAPTER 7
Apnea

Susan B. Torrey, M.D.

Apnea is the final manifestation of many pathophysiologic processes seen among patients of all ages, but neonates and infants can experience apneic episodes in response to a variety of physiologic and pathophysiologic processes not seen in later life. Differences in maturity of the central nervous system (CNS), respiratory reserve, and susceptibility to infectious agents are among the factors that interact to make the very young patient unique. The causes of apnea in older children are similar to those in adults although the susceptibility and reserve of the child, again, are different. In this chapter, the neonate and young infant are emphasized, but for completeness, the older child also is considered.

Apnea is defined as a respiratory pause of greater than 15 seconds or of any duration if there is associated pallor or cyanosis and/or bradycardia. Apnea must be distinguished from periodic breathing, which is a common respiratory pattern in young infants and is characterized by cycles of short respiratory pause followed by an increase in respiratory rate. Normal newborn infants display respiratory patterns that vary by sex and by conceptual age as well as by sleep state. Premature infants have more apneic episodes, defined for research purposes as respiratory pauses of greater than 2 seconds, than term infants. Normal-term infants experience significantly more episodes of nonperiodic apnea during active sleep than during quiet sleep, although respiratory failure occurs more often during quiet sleep. Severe apnea may be accompanied by change in color, muscle tone, or mental status, or by choking. Such an episode is described as an acute life-threatening event (ALTE).

The differential diagnosis of apnea is extensive (Table 7.1), and several categories are unique to newborns and young infants. For example, apnea may be the only clinical manifestation of seizure activity. This may be particularly difficult for emergency physicians to identify however, because they did not witness the episode, and neurologic examination may be normal in the postictal period. Several infectious processes can cause apnea. Meningitis, in particular, even in the absence of fever, must be included in the differential diagnosis. Respiratory syncytial virus is the predominant cause of bronchiolitis, which may cause apnea in children who were premature or have preexisting lung disease or congenital heart disease. Infant botulism is a diagnosis that will be made, it is hoped, before apnea occurs and must be suspected on the basis of age, symptoms, and clinical findings, such as constipation and decreased muscle tone. Recent data suggest that gastroesophageal reflux often occurs in infants with an ALTE despite the absence of a history of vomiting. Several systemic disease processes, including metabolic abnormalities that result in hypoglycemia, and sepsis, will become evident because the child develops apnea. The presence of congenital abnormalities always must be considered in newborns and in young infants. Finally, there have been well-substantiated reports of life-threatening child abuse as the etiology of ALTE.

Of great concern to both parents and physician is the risk of sudden infant death syndrome (SIDS) for an infant who has an unexplained ALTE. Although any of the diagnoses previously described can result in an ALTE, no cause is identified in about half of patients. No clear relationship exists between an "idiopathic" ALTE and SIDS. Since 1992, the American Academy of Pediatrics has recommended that infants be placed supine or on the side during sleep; a coincident decline in the incidence of SIDS has been observed since that time.

EVALUATION AND DECISION

Initial Stabilization

The first priority of the emergency physician, after immediate resuscitation of the patient, is to identify a life-threatening condition—persistent or recurrent apnea (Fig. 7.1), hypoxia, septic shock, and hypoglycemia, among others. In addition to assessment of the vital signs, including a rectal temperature and blood pressure (BP), the general appearance and mental status should be noted. As apnea is always potentially life threatening, even in the

TABLE 7.1. Differential Diagnosis of Apnea

	Neonate, infant	Older child
Central nervous system	Infection (meningitis, encephalitis) Seizure Prematurity Intraventricular hemorrhage Increased intracranial pressure (ICP) Congenital anomaly (e.g., Arnold-Chiari) Breath-holding spell	Infection Toxin Tumor Seizure Increased ICP (trauma, hydrocephalus) Idiopathic hypoventilation ("Ondine's curse")
Upper airway	Laryngospasm (e.g., gastroesophageal reflux) Infection (e.g., croup) Congenital anomaly (e.g., Down syndrome)	Obstructive sleep apnea Infection (epiglottitis, croup) Foreign body
Lower airway	Infection (pneumonia, bronchiolitis) Congenital anomaly	Infection Asthma
Other	Infant botulism Hypocalcemia, hypoglycemia Anemia Sepsis Arrhythmia Sudden infant death syndrome (SIDS)	Guillain-Barré syndrome Spinal cord injury Flail chest Arrhythmia

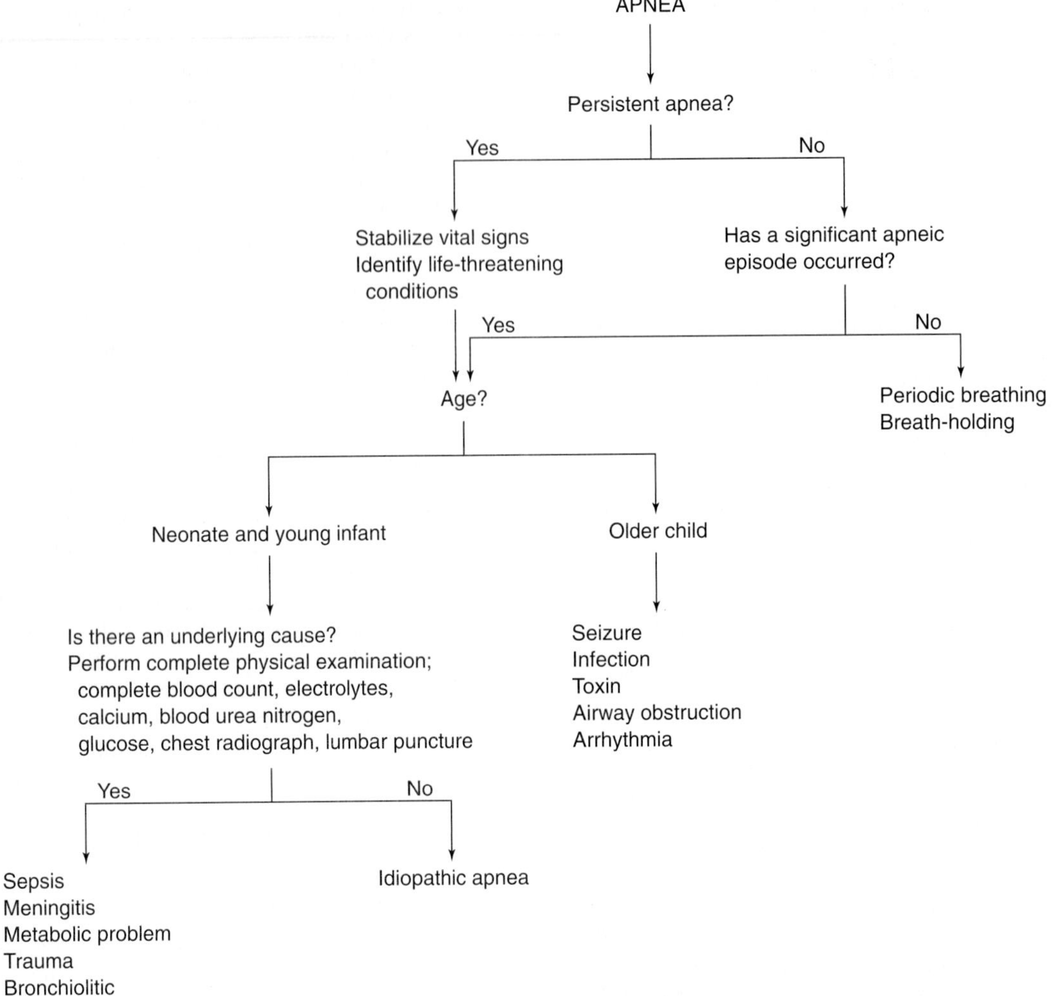

Figure 7.1. Approach to the diagnosis and management of apnea.

absence of abnormal physical findings, appropriate diagnostic studies should be performed to evaluate the child for several common etiologies (Table 7.2). The next phase of evaluation addresses two key questions: Is this episode of clinical significance? and What is the risk of recurrence? Factors to consider include signs of another acute illness, the age of the child, and other possible risk factors for clinically significant or recurrent apnea (Table 7.3).

TABLE 7.2. Common Life-Threatening Conditions That Cause Apnea

Pneumonia	Seizures
Sepsis/meningitis	Intracranial hypertension
Hypoglycemia	Shock

Has a Significant Apneic Episode Occurred?

The key to answering the questions previously outlined is invariably in the history (Table 7.3). The following details should be included: (1) where the event took place; (2) how long the event lasted; (3) whether the infant was awake or asleep; (4) whether there was an associated color change and, if so, to what colors and in what order; (5) description of associated movements, posture, or changes in tone; (6) what resuscitative efforts were made and the infant's response to them; and (7) when was the infant last fed? Attention to the response to these questions may provide the physician with a diagnosis. For example, if an 8-month-old infant was interrupted in a favorite activity, began to cry, turned red and blue, and finally had several seconds of tonic-clonic motor activity, the diagnosis of a breath-holding spell would be straightforward. In contrast, a story of 40 minutes of cyanosis and apnea in a now well-appearing child suggests that parts of the history are unreliable. Other recent events that should be documented are symptoms of other illnesses, including changes in behavior, activity, and appetite, as well as recent trauma and immunizations.

TABLE 7.3. Historical Features of Apnea

History	Significant apnea
Duration of event	Greater than 10 sec
Was child asleep or awake?	Either, but apnea during sleep is more worrisome
Color change	Pallor or cyanosis
Associated movements, posture, or change in tone	Seizure activity Hypotonia "He looked dead"
Resuscitative efforts and response	Color change or hypotonia requiring cardiopulmonary resuscitation to improve
Interval since last feeding	If shortly after feeding, consider gastroesophageal reflux
Where event occurred	Association with sleep, trauma

In many cases an absolute determination of significant apnea cannot be made in the emergency department (ED). Nevertheless, the description of the event may clearly suggest that significant apnea did occur, and hospitalization for further workup, as outlined next, is warranted. A typical case might be the previously well 2-month-old child who was noted by the parents to be apneic during a nap. The infant was described as limp and blue and "looked like he was dead." There was no response to tactile or verbal stimulation for 5 to 10 seconds, but after 15 to 20 seconds of mouth-to-mouth breathing, the child coughed, gagged, and began to breathe. His color improved over the next 30 seconds, and the parents rushed him to the ED. Such a baby may look entirely normal on examination in the ED but be at grave risk for experiencing an ALTE.

The medical history also may provide important information regarding infants at risk for significant or recurrent apnea. The physician should ask specifically about previous similar episodes. Information about perinatal events, including gestational age (birth weight), labor and delivery, maternal health, and nursery course, is helpful. A family history with specific reference to seizures, infant deaths, and serious illnesses in young family members also should be included. Finally, information regarding poisons available in the household may be important in treating an older child.

Is There an Underlying Cause?

A careful physical examination identifies many treatable acute illnesses that can cause apnea; however, the likelihood of an underlying illness varies by age. One clue to serious systemic disease is fever or hypothermia. Tachypnea suggests either a respiratory or metabolic problem, and shock may be secondary to sepsis or hypovolemia from occult trauma. Evaluation of the nervous system should include notation of mental status, palpation of the fontanelles, and funduscopic examination. Dysmorphic features might suggest an underlying congenital abnormality; however, an entirely normal physical examination provides no reassurance that the described event was clinically insignificant and will not recur.

Laboratory evaluation should be guided by the history and physical examination. Tests to consider in the ED include a measurement of blood glucose and serum electrolytes. Any indication that the infant could have a serious infection should be pursued with cultures of blood and urine and by examination of cerebrospinal fluid. Urine and blood for toxologic analysis should be obtained on patients who may have been poisoned. In the child who has no pulmonary findings, an arterial blood gas serves primarily to indicate a persistent abnormality such as hypoxia or a metabolic derangement. For instance, in carbon monoxide poisoning, the PaO_2 may be normal, but metabolic acidosis will be apparent. A significant apneic episode can occur, followed by recovery and a completely normal arterial blood gas determination. Therefore, the arterial or venous blood gas examination does not serve as a screening test for a serious event and should be obtained based on specific indications. Radiologic studies during the initial evaluation might include lateral neck, chest, abdomen, or skull films—again, as indicated by the history and physical examination.

The tasks of the emergency physician faced with a young patient who has had an apneic episode are to identify whether he or she should be hospitalized and to treat underlying conditions. If a careful history and physical examination suggest that a significant apneic episode has not occurred, the diagnosis of periodic breathing or breath holding can be made, and the patient can be discharged after appropriate counseling of the parents and arrangements for follow-up. The evaluation of a young child with apnea, however, rarely will be so straightforward. If historical information indicates that significant apnea has occurred, the infant is at risk for a recurrence of this life-threatening event. An aggressive search for an underlying cause is necessary and often includes laboratory studies, lumbar puncture, chest radiograph, and electrocardiogram (ECG). Hospital admission should be arranged for observation and further diagnostic evaluation.

A significant apneic episode in the absence of systemic disease suggests a diagnosis of primary apnea. In a recent survey of pediatricians in varying types of practices, most reported that they would refer such children to a teaching hospital or to an established infant apnea study program for evaluation. There were considerable differences in opinion regarding the relationship between apnea and SIDS. This is not surprising considering that there is no single etiology for SIDS and little is known about how associated factors relate to the cause of death. This leaves the emergency physician in a quandary. There may not be an explanation for the event that satisfies the physician or the anxious parents. Thus, it is judicious to refer the family to an available specialist or center.

The standard evaluation that usually is pursued is designed to identify known causes of primary apnea. It generally includes in-hospital observation with monitoring as well as an evaluation of the CNS with an electroencephalogram, some type of sleep study, a chest radiograph, and an ECG. Respiratory function is evaluated with a pneumogram, and a barium swallow and esophageal pH study might identify gastroesophageal reflux. An ultrasound or computed tomogram of the head would be indicated if a CNS cause for apnea is suspected. The decision to recommend home cardiorespiratory monitoring is beyond the scope of emergency practice because it necessitates a level of continuity of care and follow-up that cannot be provided by the emergency physician.

In many instances, a thorough history and careful physical examination with appropriate laboratory studies will suggest that a significant apneic event has not occurred and that there is no serious underlying illness. In this situation, the emergency physician should reassure and educate the family before discharging the patient. Good medical practice dictates that the parents also should be given specific instructions regarding indications for another ED visit and a follow-up visit to a primary care provider.

CHAPTER 8
Ataxia

Janet H. Friday, M.D.

Ataxia is defined as a disturbance in coordination of movements and may manifest as an unsteady gait. True ataxia may be difficult to differentiate from clumsiness in toddlers. In older children, ataxia may be confused with weakness or vertigo.

DIFFERENTIAL DIAGNOSIS

Ataxia as a presenting sign invokes a broad differential diagnosis (Table 8.1). Distinguishing among acute, intermittent, and chronic progressive and chronic nonprogressive ataxia may be helpful, although some diagnoses have overlap in their time course at presentation.

TABLE 8.1. Differential Diagnosis

Acute Ataxia	*Chronic, Progressive*
Acute cerebellar ataxia (postinfectious)	Hydrocephalus
Drug intoxication	Posterior fossa tumors
Labyrinthitis	Urea cycle defects
Vasculitis or Kawasaki disease	Multiple carboxylase deficiency
Meningitis	Vitamin E deficiency
Viral encephalitis	Abetalipoproteinemia
Intracranial hemorrhage	Refsum disease
Post-concussion syndrome	Hartnup disease
Benign paroxysmal vertigo	Familial periodic ataxia
Conversion reaction	Freidrich's ataxia
Intermittent	Ataxia telangiectasia
Migraine	Olivopontocerebellar atrophy
Epilepsy	*Chronic, Nonprogressive*
Transient ischemic attacks	Familial
Hartnup disease	Chiari I malformation
Wilson disease	Dandy-Walker malformation
Hereditary paroxysmal ataxia	Joubert syndrome
Maple syrup urine disease	Spastic cerebral palsy
Pyruvate decarboxylase deficiency	Cerebellar agenesis

TABLE 8.2. Common Causes of Acute Ataxia

Acute cerebellar ataxia
Drug ingestion
Guillain-Barré syndrome

TABLE 8.3. Life-Threatening Causes of Ataxia

Meningitis	Neuroblastoma
Drug intoxication	Cerebrovascular accident
Brain tumor	Intracranial hemorrhage

TABLE 8-4. Drugs and Toxins That May Cause Ataxia

Phenytoin	Dextromethorphan
Alcohol	Lead
Carbamazepine	5-Fluorouracil
Benzodiazepines	Ethylene glycol
Tricyclic antidepressants	Primidone
Antihistamines	Phenothiazines

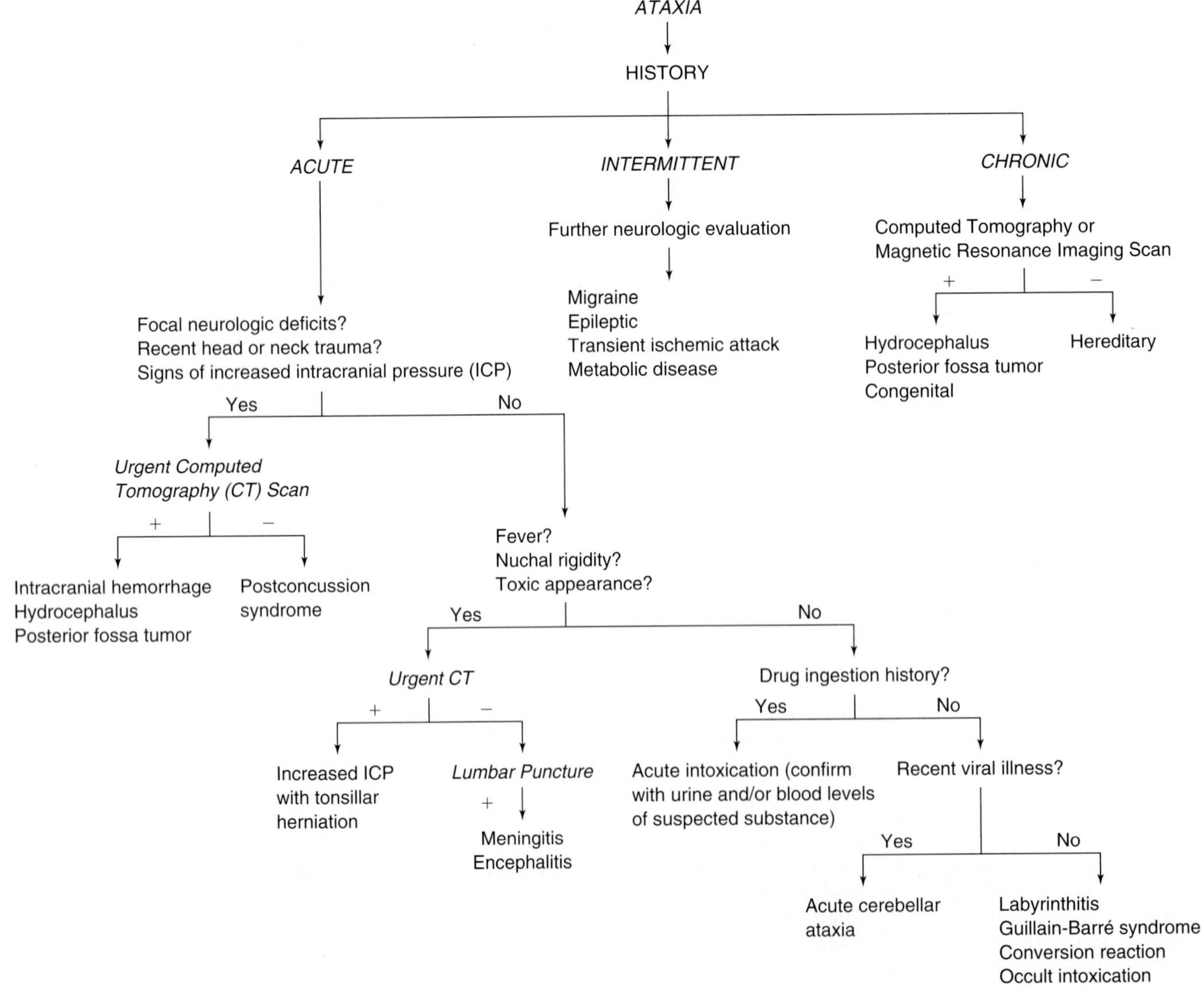

Figure 8.1. The diagnostic approach to the child with ataxia.

Fortunately, common causes of pure ataxia (Table 8.2) are not rapidly progressive. Acute cerebellar ataxia or postinfectious cerebellitis is truncal in nature and occurs 2 to 3 weeks after a viral illness Children ages 1 to 3 years are most commonly affected. Varicella is the classically identified culprit. This self-limiting illness is most severe at its onset, but complete recovery may not occur for several months. Cerebrospinal fluid (CSF) may show mild lymphocytosis and increased protein. Imaging studies are normal.

Toxic ingestions of anticonvulsants, alcohol, and sedative-hypnotics cause ataxia but always in association with depressed mental status However, with other substances (phenytoin, carbamazepine, primidone), ataxia may be the most remarkable feature of intoxication.

When an ataxic patient presents with weakness and areflexia, Guillain-Barré syndrome may be present. If ophthalmoplegia and areflexia are prominent, the Miller-Fisher variant can be suspected. Neuroimaging is normal, and the CSF may show a mild leukocytosis and elevated protein.

Ataxia may be an early prominent sign of posterior fossa tumors (especially medulloblastoma) and other conditions associated with increased intracranial pressure, including hydrocephalus and supratentorial tumors. Labyrinthitis and benign paroxysmal vertigo are rarely seen in young children but are occasionally encountered in adolescents. The sensation of loss of balance generally produces a classic wide-based gait. Conversion disorder should be suspected in a patient who walks with a narrow gait and has elaborate "near falls."

Life-threatening causes of ataxia (Table 8.3) rarely present as ataxia alone. In a few cases, bacterial meningitis has been reported with ataxia as the first symptom. Viral cerebellitis may occur as a result of enteroviral disease. Neuroblastoma may present with titubations, myoclonic ataxia, and chaotic eye movements. The syndrome is immune-mediated. It should be suspected in patients with acute ataxia that waxes and wanes over several days. One should consider vertebrobasilar occlusion in a patient with neck trauma and ataxia, cerebellar hemorrhage with ataxia and headache, and vasculitis in a child with features of Kawasaki disease.

Migraine, seizure, transient ischemic attack, and metabolic disease are the most common causes for intermittent ataxia. Chronic progressive ataxias may have a basis in metabolic defects, some of which are treatable. When a progressive ataxia acutely worsens, this may signify severe hydrocephalus or hemorrhage into a posterior fossa tumor. A variety of familial, metabolic, and congenital causes exist for chronic nonprogressive ataxias.

EVALUATION AND DECISION

The duration and progression of the illness can be established and will help define the ataxia as acute, intermittent, or chronic. Chronic ataxia should be further divided into progressive or nonprogressive. Key historical points to cover include recent illnesses such as varicella or other viral diseases and access to medications or alcohol (Table 8.4). Family history may be helpful in recurrent or genetic causes. Physical examination should focus on signs of increased intracranial pressure (bulging fontanelle, papilledema, bradycardia, hypertension, abnormal respirations), meningeal irritation (nuchal rigidity, Kernig or Brudzinski sign), fever, rash, and evidence of middle ear disease

The decision to pursue specific laboratory testing is outlined in the algorithm shown in Fig. 8.1. Patients with an acute presentation, focal neurologic deficits, recent head trauma, or signs of increased intracranial pressure warrant urgent evaluation via cranial computed tomography scan. Evidence of intracranial hemorrhage, hydrocephalus, or posterior fossa tumor provides an etiology for the ataxia. If the imaging study is normal, the diagnosis may be postconcussion syndrome for patients with head trauma.

If the patient appears "toxic" with fever or nuchal rigidity, emergent imaging of the head is indicated because cerebellar tonsil herniation may cause neck stiffness. If imaging results are negative, a lumbar puncture can be performed safely. When bacterial meningitis is strongly suspected, appropriate antibiotics may be administered before the testing is done.

When other causes have been eliminated, it is prudent to suspect drug or alcohol ingestion (Table 8.4). With the exception of benzodiazepines and tricyclics, the routine toxicologic screen of urine will not detect these drugs. Thus, specific blood levels are indicated when intoxication is suspected.

CHAPTER 9
Coma and Altered Level of Consciousness

Douglas S. Nelson, M.D.

Consciousness refers to the state of being awake and aware of oneself and one's surroundings. It is a basic cerebral function that is not easily compromised; impairment of this faculty may therefore signal the presence of a life-threatening condition. An altered level of consciousness (ALOC) is not in itself a disease. It is a state caused by an underlying disease process, which must be addressed quickly to maximize a patient's chance of recovery. *Coma* refers to a state of complete unawareness and unresponsiveness (e.g., unconsciousness) from which a patient cannot be roused; this represents the most extreme form of ALOC.

DIFFERENTIAL DIAGNOSIS

A differential diagnosis for children presenting in or near coma is shown in Table 9.1. Conditions arising from trauma or disease within the central nervous system (CNS) are separated from those affecting the brain diffusely due to extracranial problems. The more commonly encountered causes of coma are listed in Table 9.2. Life-threatening causes of ALOC must always be considered initially.

Primary Central Nervous System Disorders

TRAUMA

Coma-producing brain lesions that result from trauma include subdural and epidural hematomas, intraparenchymal and subarachnoid hemorrhage, penetrating injuries, cerebral contusion, and diffuse cerebral edema. Patients may present in a comatose state or may be alert for variable periods after impact.

SEIZURES

Level of consciousness (LOC) is greatly diminished both during and after periods of seizure activity. Although generalized seizure activity is readily recognizable by the rhythmic motor activity accompanying an ALOC, partial or absent seizure activ-

TABLE 9.1. Etiology of Acute-Onset Coma/Altered Level of Consciousness

I. Conditions arising from head trauma or primary central nervous system (CNS) disease
  A. Trauma
    1. Intracranial hematoma (subdural, epidural, intraparenchymal)
    2. Cerebral contusion
    3. Cerebral edema
    4. Concussion
  B. Seizures
    1. Status epilepticus
    2. Postictal state
  C. Infection
    1. Meningitis
    2. Encephalitis
    3. Focal infections (brain abscess, subdural empyema, epidural abscess)
  D. Neoplasms
    1. Tumor (± edema, hemorrhage)
  E. Vascular disease
    1. Cerebral infarct (thrombotic, hemorrhagic, embolic)
    2. Central venous thrombosis
    3. Subarachnoid hemorrhage
  F. Hydrocephalus
    1. Obstructive (from tumor or other cause)
    2. Cerebrospinal fluid shunt malfunction

II. Conditions affecting the brain diffusely
  A. Vital sign abnormalities
    1. Hypotension, hypertension
    2. Hypothermia, hyperthermia
  B. Hypoxia
    1. Pulmonary disease
    2. Severe anemia
    3. Methemoglobinemia
    4. Carbon monoxide
    5. Posthypoxic encephalopathy
  C. Intoxications
    1. Sedative drugs: antihistamines, barbiturates, benzodiazepines, ethanol, narcotics, phenothiazines
    2. Tricyclic antidepressants
    3. Anticonvulsants
    4. Salicylates
  D. Metabolic abnormalities
    1. Hypoglycemia (sepsis, insulin overdose, ethanol intoxication)
    2. Hyperglycemia (diabetic ketoacidosis)
    3. Metabolic acidosis
    4. Metabolic alkalosis
    5. Hyponatremia, hypernatremia
    6. Hypocalcemia, hypercalcemia
    7. Hypomagnesemia, hypermagnesemia
    8. Hypophosphatemia
    9. Uremia (kidney failure)
    10. Liver failure
    11. Acute toxic encephalopathy (Reye syndrome)
    12. Inherited metabolic disorders
  E. Other
    1. Intussusception
    2. Dehydration
    3. Sepsis
    4. Psychiatric conditions

TABLE 9.2. Common Causes of Coma/Altered Level of Consciousness

Subdural hematoma	Posthypoxia
Epidural hematoma	Hypoglycemia
Cerebral edema	Toxic ingestions
Postictal state	Meningitis
Hypotension	

ity may present more subtly with staring, tremors, eye blinking, rhythmic nodding, or other inappropriate repetitive motor activity. Seizures of all types except petit mal may be followed by a postictal period, during which obtunded patients gradually regain responsiveness to and awareness of their surroundings.

INFECTION

Coma-inducing infections of the CNS may involve large areas of the brain and surrounding structures, as in meningitis or encephalitis, or they may be confined to a smaller region, as in the case of cerebral abscess or empyema. Bacterial meningitis remains the most common infection severe enough to produce profoundly diminished LOC; despite the overall decrease in total number of cases since the introduction of vaccines effective against *Haemophilus influenzae* and *Streptococcus pneumoniae*. Herpes simplex is the most important agent to consider with encephalitis, as it is treatable with acyclovir. Focal CNS infections include brain abscesses, subdural empyemas, and epidural abscesses.

NEOPLASMS

Alterations in consciousness as a result of intracranial neoplasms may be caused by seizure, hemorrhage, increases in intracranial pressure (ICP) caused by interruption of cerebrospinal fluid (CSF) flow, or direct invasion of the reticular activating system by the malignancy (which is unlikely to cause coma of rapid onset). The location of the tumor determines additional symptoms: ataxia and vomiting for infratentorial lesions versus seizures, hemiparesis, and speech or intellectual difficulties resulting from supratentorial neoplasms. Acute hydrocephalus secondary to tumor growth most commonly presents with headache, lethargy, and vomiting.

VASCULAR

Coma of cerebrovascular origin is caused by interruption of cerebral blood flow (stroke) as a result of hemorrhage, thrombosis, or embolism. Hemorrhage is often nontraumatic, stemming from an abnormal vascular structure such as an arteriovenous malformation (AVM), aneurysm, or cavernous hemangioma. Rupture of an AVM is the most common cause of spontaneous intracranial bleeding among pediatric patients. Aneurysm rupture is less common and is unusual in that repetitive episodes of bleeding may occur ("sentinel bleeds"), with rising morbidity and mortality from each subsequent episode of bleeding. Subarachnoid blood may be present in either case, although more commonly with aneurysm rupture.

Stroke may also occur from thrombosis or embolism of a normal vessel. Cerebral infarction caused by occlusion of the anterior, middle, or posterior cerebral artery usually produces focal neurologic deficit, not coma. Acute occlusion of the carotid artery, however, may produce sufficient unilateral hemispheric swelling that herniation and coma may ensue; infarction may lead to hemorrhage as well. Central venous thrombosis is most commonly seen as a sequela of infections of the ear or sinus or hypercoagulable states.

Swelling or hemorrhage from infarcted brain can cause increased ICP, leading to coma. Less severe, often focal symptoms vary based on the size and location of brain denied adequate blood supply. Vascular accidents in the cerebellum present with combinations of ataxia, vertigo, nausea, occipital headache, and resistance to neck flexion. Coma is an unusual early sign of infarction of cerebral structures but becomes more common as lower anatomic centers are affected. Occlusion of the basilar artery may result in upper brainstem infarction, resulting in rapid onset of coma, as does hemorrhage or infarction of the pons.

CEREBROSPINAL FLUID SHUNT PROBLEMS

Children with congenital or acquired hydrocephalus as a result of prematurity, neoplasm, or trauma depend on the continued function of a neurosurgical shunt to drain CSF and prevent rises in ICP. CSF shunts may malfunction for many reasons, including tubing rupture, valve malfunction, tubing blockage, tubing disconnection, and shunt infection. The risk of failure is greatest during the first 6 months after shunt placement or revision.

Systemic Abnormalities

The second major category of disorders causing coma listed in Table 9.1 arises in organs other than the CNS and affects the brain diffusely. These abnormalities alter neuronal activity by a variety of means, including decreasing metabolic substrates required for normal function (e.g., hypoxia, hypotension, hypoglycemia, other electrolyte abnormalities), altering the rate of intracellular chemical reactions (e.g., hypothermia, hyperthermia), and introducing extraneous toxins into the CNS.

HYPOXIA

Oxygen delivery to the brain may be adversely affected by disorders that compromise a patient's airway, breathing, or circulation. Neurons are the cells most sensitive to oxygen deprivation, and they will cease to function within seconds after being deprived of adequate levels of oxygen

CARDIOVASCULAR ABNORMALITIES

Hypotension may be the product of numerous causes, including hemorrhage, dehydration, sepsis, arrhythmia, and intoxication, but the result is poor cerebral perfusion, which produces diminished mental status. Hypertensive encephalopathy is distinguished by headache, nausea, vomiting, visual disturbance, altered mental status, or coma in the presence of a blood pressure above the ninety-fifth percentile. The acute onset of severe hypertension may reflect ongoing renal (e.g., unilateral renal artery stenosis, acute glomerulonephritis), endocrine (e.g., pheochromocytoma), or cardiac (e.g., aortic coarctation) pathology, or it may be the result of a toxic ingestion (e.g., cocaine). Cerebral hemorrhage may result. Hypertension accompanied by bradycardia may indicate increased ICP.

DISORDERS OF THERMOREGULATION

Hypothermia or hyperthermia in the pediatric patient is usually caused by prolonged environmental exposure to temperature extremes such as those found in cold water or in a closed car in sunlight. The child made comatose as a result of abnormal core temperature will have multiple organ system abnormalities in addition to CNS dysfunction.

TOXIC INGESTIONS

Pediatric toxic ingestions are often not witnessed, may involve a large dose on a milligram per kilogram basis, are rarely intentionally inflicted, and are usually complicated by the young patient's inability to provide information regarding the quantity or identity of the substance ingested. Table 9.1 lists many drug classes that cause coma when an overdose is taken.

METABOLIC ALTERATIONS

Abnormal serum concentrations of any substrate or product involved in neuronal metabolism can produce obtundation, leading to coma. Hypoglycemia is the most common disorder in this category, especially in infants and young children, whose capacity for hepatic gluconeogenesis is limited.

Metabolic acidosis or alkalosis of sufficient degree produces altered mental status. Severe dehydration that leads to significant metabolic acidosis is the most common disorder of this type seen in children. Abnormal concentrations of any serum cation, including sodium, calcium, magnesium, and phosphorus, can produce altered mental status as well. The degree of resulting neurologic compromise will be affected by the duration of the problem and concurrent disorders. Severe dehydration alone, from any cause without significant electrolyte abnormalities, may produce profound lethargy in infants and children as well.

Other causes of metabolic coma in the pediatric age group include kidney or hepatic failure, both of which may result in progressive apathy, confusion, and lethargy. Urea cycle defects may present with coma and hyperammonemia in young infants. Acute toxic encephalopathy (Reye syndrome) is a rare but devastating illness caused by mitochondrial injury of unknown origin that affects all organs of the body, particularly the brain and liver.

MISCELLANEOUS CONDITIONS

Other causes of coma or depressed LOC in children are less easily categorized. Children with intussusception, the most common cause of bowel obstruction in childhood, may have significant apathy and lethargy in addition to vomiting, intermittent abdominal pain, and bloody stools. As a result, they are often treated for dehydration, sepsis, or meningitis before the appropriate diagnosis is discovered. The presence of "currant jelly" stools or a palpable abdominal mass suggests this condition.

Psychiatric disorders may produce a true stuporous state. More commonly, neurologically intact patients attempt to feign unresponsiveness for reasons known only to them, and they may be remarkably successful at remaining immobile despite painful stimuli. The nature of their "impairment" may be discovered by a detailed neurologic examination. Conscious patients will usually avoid hitting their face with a dropped arm, may resist eyelid opening, will raise their heart rate to auditory or painful stimuli, and will have intact deep tendon, oculovestibular, and oculocephalic reflexes.

A useful acronym incorporating the common causes of coma in children has been proposed by Schunk and is listed in Table 9.3; the acronym is based on the names of childhood immunizations: DPT (for *d*ehydration, *p*oisoning, *t*rauma), OPV (*o*ccult trauma, *p*ostictal or *p*ostanoxia, *v*entriculoperitoneal shunt problem), HIB (*h*ypoxia or *h*yperthermia, *i*ntussusception, *b*rain masses), and MMR (*m*eningitis or encephalitis, *m*etabolic, *R*eye syndrome, other *r*arities).

TABLE 9.3. Mnemonic for Causes of Coma

DPT
- *D*ehydration
- *P*oisoning
- *T*rauma

OPV
- *O*ccult trauma
- *P*ostictal or postanoxia
- *V*entriculoperitoneal shunt problem

HIB
- *H*ypoxia or *h*yperthermia
- *I*ntussusception
- *B*rain masses

MMR
- *M*eningitis or encephalitis
- *M*etabolic
- *R*eye syndrome, other *r*arities

(Modified from Schunk JE. The pediatric patient with altered level of consciousness: remember your "immunizations." *J Emerg Nurs* 1992;18:419–421, with permission.)

EVALUATION AND DECISION

An approach for the evaluation of pediatric patients presenting with coma is summarized in Fig. 9.1. All patients need rapid assessment of their airway, breathing, and circulation, followed by a focused history, physical examination, and consideration of laboratory and imaging studies. This approach is based on the selective use of the following critical clinical and laboratory findings: (1) vital signs; (2) a history of recent head trauma, seizure activity, or ingestion; (3) signs of increased ICP or focal neuro-

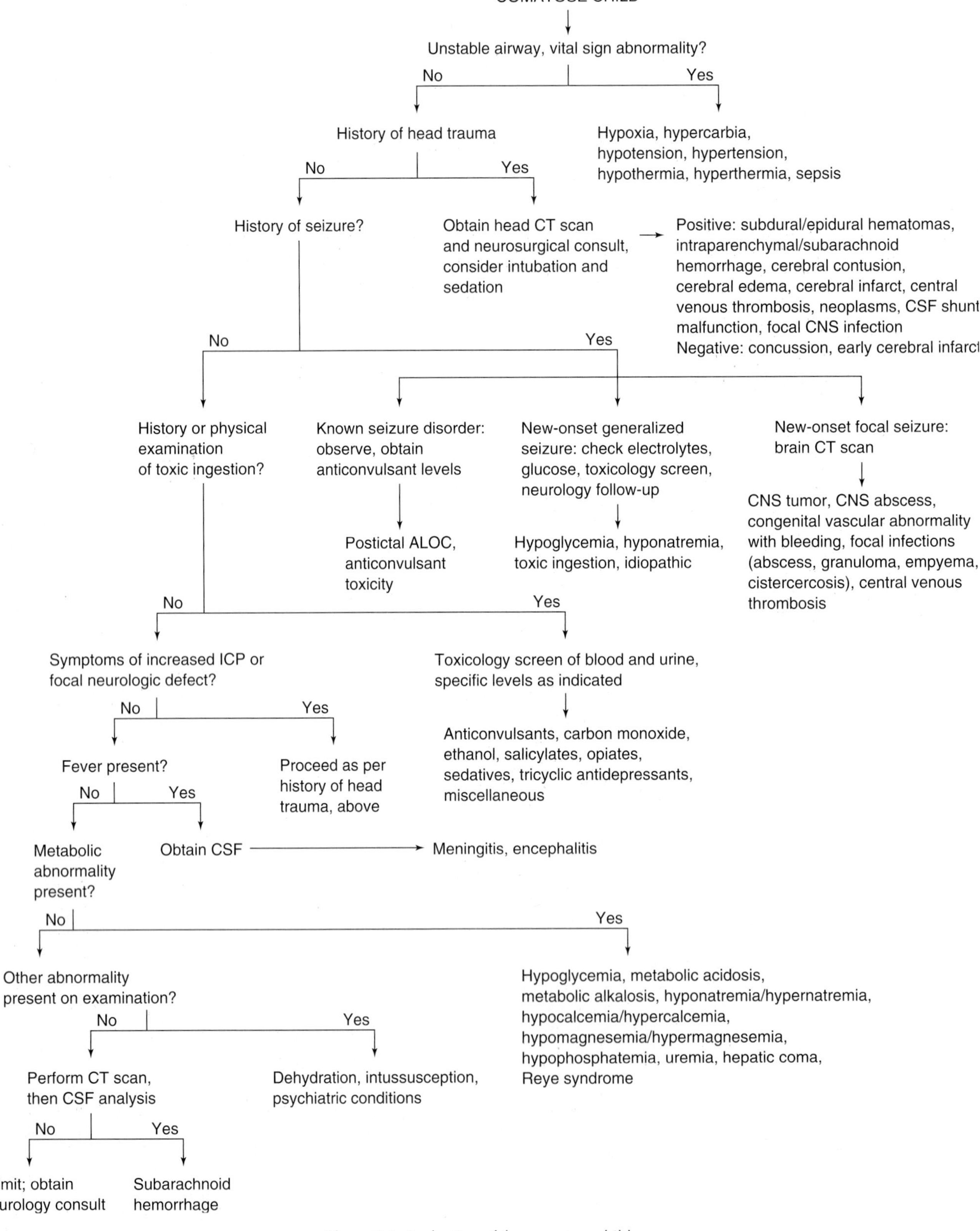

Figure 9.1. Evaluation of the comatose child.

logic abnormality; (4) fever; (5) laboratory results; (6) brain computed tomography (CT) scan results; and (7) CSF analysis. The evaluation of the comatose patient should follow an orderly series of steps, addressing the more life-threatening problems of hypoxia, hypotension, and increased ICP before progressing to the investigation of less urgent disorders. If one or more of the former are present, immediate resuscitative efforts are begun.

Vital Sign Abnormalities

Evaluation and treatment of airway, breathing, and circulatory compromise always take precedence over neurologic problems in the child with ALOC. Airway patency and respiratory effort are both compromised by decreased mental status and may result in hypoxia and/or hypercarbia. The former may be readily measured using pulse oximetry, although values will be inaccurate if a toxic hemoglobinopathy, such as methemoglobinemia or carboxyhemoglobinemia, is present. Hypoxia is usually evident by cyanosis of the lips and nail beds and pulse oximetry values below 90 (see Chapter 12). Arterial blood gas analysis is useful in some cases to quantify respiratory status and to identify altered hemoglobin states. The treatment of hypoxia, regardless of the cause, always begins with supplemental oxygen administered via an appropriate route.

The numeric definition of hypotension varies with age, but pallor and evidence of poor peripheral perfusion, with capillary refill time greater than 4 seconds, is recognizable even before placement of a sphygmomanometer cuff. Immediate administration of intravenous (i.v.) crystalloid therapy starting with 20 mL per kg of normal saline or lactated Ringer's solution is indicated, followed by additional boluses and pressors if needed (see Chapter 3). Efforts should be made during i.v. placement to draw blood for laboratory tests. Of the empiric antidotal therapies often used in adults, only glucose 0.25 to 0.5 g per kg is routinely administered to children; an empiric trial of naloxone (1 to 2 mg) is often justified, whereas flumazenil and thiamine are given only when specific indications for their use exist (see Chapter 78).

Severe hypertension is less easily discerned on physical examination. If confirmed in more than one extremity, antihypertensives should be administered via the i.v. or sublingual route (see Chapters 28 and 76). Mental status should improve after blood pressure is lowered to high normal levels. Patients in hypertensive crises are at risk for hemorrhagic stroke and should be evaluated with a head CT scan if they are neurologically abnormal after blood pressure lowering. Note that hypertension in the comatose patient with increased ICP may represent a physiologic response to maintain cerebral perfusion pressure (by raising mean arterial pressure) and in this context should not be treated with antihypertensives.

Hypothermia and hyperthermia are readily recognized once a core (rectal) temperature less than 35°C or greater than 41°C is obtained. The mental status of these patients should begin to improve as body temperature approaches the normal range. A significant percentage of patients with abnormal core temperatures have drowned, fallen through ice, or were engaged in sporting activities in extreme environments. Head trauma, hypoxia, and/or cervical spine injury may be present in these patients.

History of Head Trauma

The patient with deeply depressed consciousness (GCS score less than 9) after head trauma is presumed to have increased ICP until proven otherwise. Rapid sequence intubation with 1 mg per kg of lidocaine added to standard paralytics and sedatives to blunt rises in ICP caused by laryngeal manipulation is indicated. Cervical spine injury should be assumed and cervical immobilization maintained at all times. An emergent noncontrast brain CT scan should be obtained and neurosurgery consulted.

History of Seizures

The patient with ALOC in the absence of trauma should be evaluated for recent seizure activity with current postictal state (see Chapters 61 and 73). A history of previous seizures, witnessed convulsive activity, and ALOC consistent with previous postictal periods are valuable clues to this etiology of coma. Ongoing seizure activity may be revealed by the presence of muscular twitching, nystagmus, or fluttering of the eyelids. Subtle forms of status epilepticus may require an electroencephalogram (EEG), to diagnose usually performed somewhat later in the evaluation. The mental status examination of the postictal patient should gradually improve over several hours. Although temporary focal neurologic deficits may follow seizures of any cause, they must be presumed to indicate the presence of focal CNS lesions until proven otherwise or resolved.

The evaluation of neurologically depressed patients with seizures varies based on the patient's history, type of seizure, and presence or absence of fever. Patients with a history of seizures should have serum anticonvulsant concentrations measured and be observed until they approach their neurologic baseline. Children who have had a simple febrile seizure (see Chapter 61) should return to their baseline state soon, usually within 1 hour. Those who remain lethargic or irritable past this point (especially after antipyretics have been administered) should be suspected of having meningitis and are candidates for lumbar puncture. Patients with new-onset generalized seizures who do not meet criteria for simple febrile seizures (see Chapters 21, 61, and 73) require more extensive evaluation, which may include measurements of electrolytes (especially sodium, glucose, and calcium), toxicologic screening, examination of CSF, and neurology consultation.

The new onset of focal seizures, with or without the presence of fever, should be evaluated with a head CT scan (using contrast when indicated) to determine the presence of a focal lesion such as a tumor, abscess, or hemorrhage. Only after the results of this study are known should a lumbar puncture be performed. If neuroimaging is unavailable and meningitis or encephalitis is a concern, empiric treatment for bacterial meningitis or herpetic encephalitis may be administered and lumbar puncture deferred (see Chapter 74).

History of Toxic Ingestions

If no history or physical examination findings suggestive of head trauma or seizures are present, a toxic ingestion should be considered, especially in toddlers and adolescents. The availability in the home of any substances capable of depressing CNS function should be thoroughly explored. In general, coma from toxic ingestions is of slower onset than that from trauma and may be preceded by delirium or other abnormal behaviors.

Chapter 78 lists major toxidromes that result from ingestions that produce CNS depression. The pupils of a poisoned comatose patient are a particularly valuable source of information. Miosis occurs with ingestions of narcotics, clonidine, organophosphates, phencyclidine, phenothiazines, and occasionally, barbiturates and ethanol. Mydriasis is produced by ingestions of anticholinergic agents (e.g., atropine, antihistamines, and tricyclic antidepressants) and sympathomimetic compounds (e.g., amphetamines, caffeine, cocaine, LSD, and nicotine). Nystagmus may indicate the ingestion of barbiturates, ketamine, phencyclidine, or phenytoin. Pupillary responses are more likely to be preserved in toxic

TABLE 9.4. Poisons Undetected by Drug Screening That Cause Coma

Miosis present
Clonidine
Chloral hydrate
Organophosphates
Tetrahydrozoline
Bromide
Mydriasis present
Carbon monoxide
Cyanide
Methemoglobinemia
LSD

or metabolic comas. Systemic toxins do not cause unequal pupils; anisocoria should be pursued with neuroimaging.

A toxicologic screen of blood and urine should be considered in all children with coma of unknown origin. Specific assays for other chemicals may be ordered as suspected. A serum acetaminophen level should be ordered in all children with significant ingestions. Table 9.4 lists compounds capable of causing coma that are not typically detected by drug screening; the compounds are grouped by pupillary effects.

The poisoned patient with depressed consciousness should be intubated with a cuffed endotracheal tube for airway protection before decontamination efforts are made. Ipecac-induced emesis is never indicated in the patient with depressed consciousness. Naloxone may be administered as empiric antidotal therapy for coma-producing toxic ingestions involving unknown medications. Flumazenil should not be given to these patients because seizures may result. Its use is limited to pure benzodiazepine overdoses in patients with no history of seizures.

Increased Intracranial Pressure or Focal Neurologic Defect

Nontraumatic causes of increased ICP or focal neurologic deficits include neoplasms, CSF shunt malfunction, and hemorrhage secondary to cerebrovascular disease (see Chapter 73). These patients may present with a history of headache, vomiting, confusion, lethargy, meningism, focal neurologic dysfunction, seizure activity, or deep coma. Initial physical signs of increased ICP include a bulging fontanelle in infants and sluggishly reactive pupils. More severe and prolonged increases in ICP produce a unilaterally enlarged pupil, other cranial nerve palsies (III, IV, VI), papilledema, and Cushing's triad of hypertension, bradycardia, and periodic breathing. All may signal impending or progressive herniation. From the standpoint of the emergency physician, which type of herniation is present is unimportant; all are life threatening, and the initial treatment is identical for all. Endotracheal intubation using rapid sequence induction (with cervical immobilization) is performed to minimize increases in ICP while gaining airway control. Evaluation should parallel that of the patient with a traumatic head injury, with the only change being the increased desirability of using i.v. contrast during CT scan. Urgent neurosurgical consultation is recommended for all patients in this category regardless of the focality of findings on CT scan. Comatose patients with a CSF shunt may need their shunt reservoir or ventricle tapped to decrease ICP.

Fever

Coma accompanied by fever indicates that CNS infection may be present (see Chapters 21 and 74). Resistance to neck flexion is the most important physical finding in meningitis, the most common infection of this type, although children less than 2 years of age may lack this finding. Historical data may also include a steadily increasing headache, irritability, vomiting, and worsening oral intake. Kernig and Brudzinski signs may be present. Other useful physical clues to CNS infection are the rashes that accompany meningococcemia, varicella, and Rocky Mountain spotted fever. The historical and physical findings in encephalitis are similar to those in meningitis; meningism may be absent, however. Seizures are particularly common if herpes simplex is the causative agent.

A history of localized CNS dysfunction or seizures before the onset of febrile coma or the presence of concomitant focal neurologic signs may indicate the presence of a focal cerebral infection such as an abscess, granuloma, or subdural empyema. In addition, either diffuse or focal infections may present with signs of increased ICP secondary to abscess formation, cerebral edema, or blockage of CSF flow. If this is the case, a head CT scan should be obtained before lumbar puncture is performed. A contrast-enhanced study is desirable if concern about focal infection is present. The patient who appears ill should receive antibiotics before neuroimaging is performed.

CSF analysis remains the key to establishing the diagnosis of CNS infection. Abnormalities of CSF white blood cell count (pleocytosis), glucose, and protein occur in roughly predicable patterns with bacterial or viral meningitis, and pathogens may be visible using Gram and other stains (see Chapter 74). CSF pleocytosis in encephalitis is variable and, if present, is usually mild (less than 500 cells per mm^3), with normal levels of glucose and protein being common. CSF in herpes simplex encephalitis contains red blood cells in 50% of cases. Bloody or xanthochromic CSF under increased pressure in the absence of signs of infection indicates subarachnoid hemorrhage.

Metabolic Abnormalities

The presence of a metabolic disorder leading to coma is usually apparent once the results of routine laboratory tests are available. These values for glucose, sodium, potassium, bicarbonate, calcium, magnesium, and phosphorus make any deficiency or excess of these serum components readily apparent and treatable. Blood gas analysis for evaluation of acidosis or alkalosis from metabolic or respiratory causes may be indicated as well. Decreased LOC caused by diabetic ketoacidosis may initially worsen because of a paradoxic temporary decrease in CSF pH and/or cerebral edema complicating therapy.

Renal and hepatic function should be quantified with analysis of blood urea nitrogen, creatinine, and ammonia. Markedly elevated serum blood urea nitrogen and creatinine, oliguria, hypertension, anemia, acidosis, and hypocalcemia indicate the presence of uremic coma as a result of renal failure. Hyperammonemia with decreased mental status is most commonly caused by hepatic failure, acetaminophen ingestion with resultant hepatotoxicity, and Reye syndrome. The hyperammonemia of Reye syndrome is accompanied by a history of antecedent viral illness (possibly varicella), resolving within the past week, and likely treated with aspirin (see Chapter 73). Encephalopathy begins soon after unremitting vomiting; jaundice, scleral icterus, focal neurologic signs, and meningeal irritation are absent. Hyperammonemia without accompanying liver failure in the young infant may indicate the presence of a congenital urea cycle defect.

Coma of Unknown Origin

Patients with coma of unknown origin not falling into any of the diagnostic categories discussed previously usually benefit from a noncontrast brain CT scan, CSF analysis, and neurologic consultation, in that order. Patients presenting in a comatose state usually need admission for continuing treatment, observation, and specialized care, except when there is an easily recognized and reversible cause, such as hypoglycemia in a known diabetic.

TABLE 10.2. Common Causes of Constipation

Functional	Viral illness with ileus
Anal fissure	Dietary

CHAPTER 10
Constipation

Jonathan Markowitz, M.D. and
Stephen Ludwig, M.D.

Constipation is an important problem in the pediatric emergency department for many reasons. It is one of the most common pediatric complaints, accounting for 3% of primary care visits. There are many causes for constipation (Table 10.1), some rare and some very common (Table 10.2). Occasionally, the presentation of constipation is atypical, with chief complaints that on the surface might seem unrelated to the gastrointestinal tract (Table 10.3). Although they are relatively rare, some causes of constipation are potentially life threatening and need to be recognized promptly by the emergency physician (Table 10.4). In addition, constipation can produce symptoms that mimic other serious illnesses, such as appendicitis.

TABLE 10.1. Etiology of Constipation

- I. Functional
  - A. Fecal retention
  - B. Depression
  - C. Harsh toilet training
  - D. Toilet phobia
  - E. Avoidance of school bathrooms
  - F. Fecal soiling
  - G. Anorexia nervosa
- II. Pain on defecation
  - A. Anal fissure
  - B. Foreign body
  - C. Sexual abuse
  - D. Laxative overuse
  - E. Proctitis
  - F. Rectal prolapse
  - G. Rectal polyps
- III. Mechanical obstruction
  - A. Hirschsprung's disease
  - B. Pelvic mass
  - C. Upper bowel obstruction
  - D. Rectal stenosis
  - E. Anal atresia (newborn)
  - F. Meconium ileus (newborn)
- IV. Decreased sensation/motility
  - A. Drug-induced
  - B. Viral "ileus"
  - C. Neuromuscular disease
    - 1. Hypotonia
    - 2. Werdnig–Hoffmann disease
    - 3. Cerebral palsy
    - 4. Down syndrome
  - D. Endocrine abnormalities
    - 1. Hypothyroidism
    - 2. Hyperparathyroidism
    - 3. Hypercalcemia
    - 4. Diabetes insipidus
    - 5. Renal tubular acidosis
  - E. Infant botulism
  - F. Spinal cord tumor
  - G. "Prune belly" syndrome
- V. Stool abnormalities
  - A. Dietary
  - B. Dehydration
  - C. Malnutrition
- VI. Pseudoconstipation
  - A. Breast-fed infant
  - B. Normal variation in stool frequency

EVALUATION AND DECISION

The evaluation of the child presumed to have constipation should begin with a thorough history and physical examination, with special attention given to changes in frequency and consistency of stool for the individual patient in question. A complaint of constipation is not sufficient. A decrease in stool frequency or the appearance of straining often is interpreted as constipation. The physician should be aware of the "grunting baby syndrome": The infant grunts, turns red, strains, and may cry while passing a soft stool. This syndrome is the result of poor coordination between Valsalva and relaxation of the voluntary sphincter muscles. Examination reveals the absence of palpable stool in the rectum or abdomen. Complaints of constipation not supported by history or physical examination are called *pseudoconstipation* (Fig. 10.1).

ACUTE CONSTIPATION

The patient's age and the duration of the constipation are important when determining the cause and significance of the problem. The infant aged younger than 1 year with true constipation is of particularly concern.

Constipation of less than 1 month's duration is termed *acute*. In such cases, history will identify many of the problems responsible for the constipation. A recent viral illness is a common cause of short-lived constipation in the infant. Excessive water loss through vomiting, diarrhea, fever, and increased respiratory rate may cause hard stools. Adynamic ileus or decreased intake after gastroenteritis may cause slower transit time through the colon, and anal fissures after a bout of diarrhea may precipitate painful defecation, resulting in stool retention. The infant may be noted to assume a retentive posture consisting of extension of the body with contraction of the gluteal and anal muscles.

TABLE 10.3. Some Atypical Presentations of Constipation

Anorexia	Refusal to walk
Headaches	Seizure-like activity (shaking, staring spells)
Lethargy	Urinary retention
Limp	Urinary tract infection

TABLE 10.4. Life-Threatening Causes of Constipation

Acute constipation	Chronic constipation
Mechanical obstruction	Hirschsprung's disease
Dehydration	
Infantile botulism	

TABLE 10.5. Some Medications Associated with Constipation

Aluminum	Iron
Amiodarone	Mesalamine
Amitriptyline	Omeprazole
Anticholinergic agents (benztropine, glycopyrrolate, promethazine)	Ondansetron
Antineoplastic agents (procarbazine, vincristine)	Opioids
Benzodiazepines	Phenobarbitol
β-Blockers	Phenothiazines and derivatives (prochlorperazine, promethazine, haloperidol)
Calcium salts	Phenytoin
Calcium-channel blockers	Ranitidine
Cholestyramine	Sucralfate
Diazoxide	Ursodiol

Excessive intake of cow's milk, inadequate fluid intake, and malnutrition should be revealed by a complete diet history. Recent courses of medication cannot be overlooked because many medications can cause constipation (Table 10.5). Ingestion of lead is also a potential and serious reason for constipation.

Acute constipation can be caused by bowel obstruction, but it is normally a less prominent feature than other symptoms. Infantile botulism commonly presents with constipation, weak cry, poor feeding, and decreasing muscle tone.

Simple constipation in an infant should be treated initially with dietary changes. Decreasing consumption of cow's milk and increasing fluid intake when appropriate may be enough to alleviate the symptoms. If the infants does not show improve-

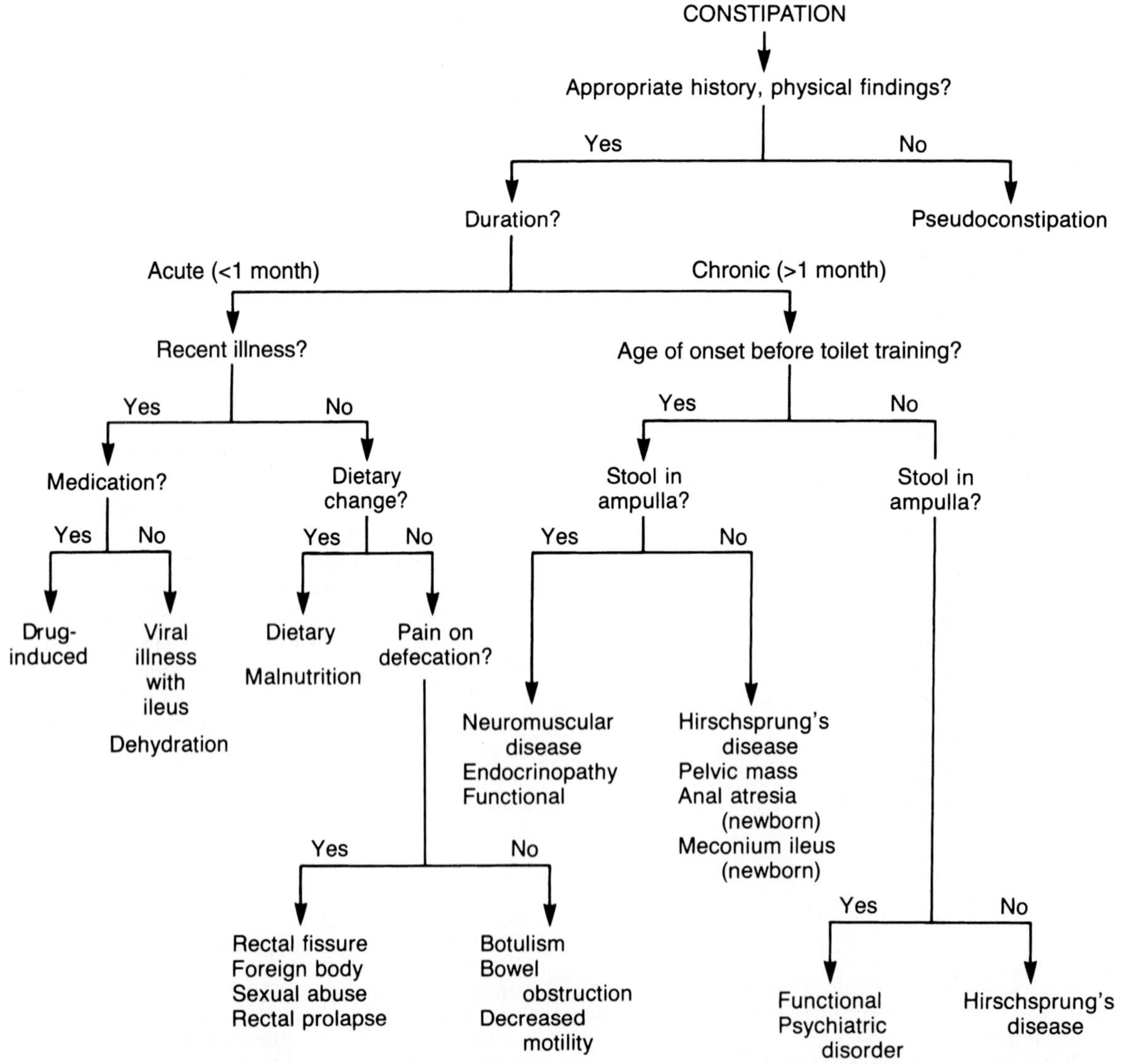

Figure 10.1. Approach to constipation.

ment, constipation can be treated by supplementing the diet with barley malt (Maltsupex) or Karo syrup. Stool lubricants, such as mineral oil, can be administered orally when aspiration is not a concern.

Acute constipation in the child older than 1 year occurs for many of the same reasons as in the infant. History may reveal recent viral illness or use of medication as well as the presence of underlying illness, such as neuromuscular disease. Physical examination suffices to rule out anal malformations and other physical problems that could result in trouble defecating.

CHRONIC CONSTIPATION

Constipation of more than 1 month's duration in an infant is of special concern. Spinal muscular atrophy, amyotonia, congenital absence of abdominal muscles, dystonic states, and spinal dysraphism, which cause problems with defecation, can be readily diagnosed through the history and physical examination.

Anorectal anomalies occur in approximately 1 in 2,500 live births. Anal stenosis causes the passage of ribbon-like stools with intense effort. Diagnosis is made by anal examination, which demonstrates a tight, constricted canal. The condition is treated by repeated anal dilatations, sometimes over several months. The anus can be covered by a flap of skin, leaving only a portion open for passage of stool. This "covered anus" may require anoplasty with dilatation. Anterior displacement of the anus is thought to cause constipation by creating a pouch at the posterior portion of the distal rectum that catches the stool and allows only overflow to be expelled after great straining. The treatment may be medical or surgical.

Hirschsprung disease, or congenital intestinal aganglionosis, is rare but must be considered in the constipated infant because it has the potential to cause life-threatening complications (Table 10.6). The absence of ganglion cells leaves the affected segment tonically contracted, blocking the passage of stool. The segment proximal to the blockage dilates as the buildup of stool progresses. In most cases, the child never feels the urge to defecate because the blockage is proximal to the internal sphincter and anal canal.

In Hirschsprung disease, abdominal examination often yields a suprapubic mass of stool that may extend throughout the abdomen. Rectal examination reveals a constricted anal canal with the absence of stool in the rectal vault, commonly followed by expulsion of stool when the finger is removed. The combination of palpable abdominal feces and an empty rectal vault is abnormal and must be investigated further.

Megacolon in Hirschsprung disease can lead to enterocolitis characterized by abdominal distension; explosive stools, which are sometimes bloody; and fever progressing to sepsis and hypovolemic shock. Enterocolitis represents a major cause of mortality in this condition. Of infants with Hirschsprung disease, 80% are diagnosed within the first year of life. A history of late passage of meconium is often found; if, however, the involved segment is relatively short, the diagnosis may be delayed. If Hirschsprung disease is suspected, the diagnosis is supported by unprepared barium enema, which typically demonstrates narrow bowel rapidly expanding to a dilated area. This transition zone represents the location where the aganglionic, tonically contracted bowel meets the dilated, innervated bowel. In disease where only a short segment of bowel is involved, barium enema may miss the transition zone and anal manometry aids in diagnosis. Confirmation is achieved by demonstration of aganglionosis on biopsy.

Hypothyroidism in the infant may manifest with constipation. Water-losing disorders such as diabetes insipidus and renal tubular acidosis also can contribute to this condition. Particularly among white infants, cystic fibrosis merits consideration because it may lead to an inspissated meconium or stool that is presenting as constipation.

Chronic constipation in the older child is overwhelmingly likely to be functional constipation. Typically, a cycle of stool withholding starts when the child disregards the signal to defecate and strikes a retentive posture, that is, rising on the toes and stiffening the legs and buttocks. Over time, in functional constipation, the rectum dilates and sensation diminishes. Watery stool from higher in the gastrointestinal tract can leak around the large fecal mass, causing involuntary soiling, or *encopresis*. Painful defecation from streptococcal perianal disease or sexual abuse must be remembered as potential precipitants of stool withholding.

A history supportive of functional constipation includes retentive posturing, infrequent passage of very large stools, and involuntary soiling during the peak ages. Physical examination normally reveals palpable stool in the abdomen. The back should be inspected for skin changes over the sacral area suggestive of spinal dysraphism. Normal deep tendon reflexes and strength in the lower extremities in conjunction with a normal anal-wink reflex virtually excludes neurologic impairment. The anus should be normal in placement and appearance. Rectal examination typically yields a dilated vault filled with stool. Abdominal flat plate can be helpful but is not necessary. Failure to thrive is not associated with functional constipation and, if present, should prompt further investigation.

The patient with functional constipation needs no further evaluation before induction of therapy. Treatment begins with evacuation of the stool remaining in the bowel, which can be accomplished most readily with the use of hypertonic phosphate (Fleet) enemas. A mineral oil enema administered the night before the first phosphate enema may soften the existing stool, allowing less painful passage. The phosphate enemas should be given in doses of 3 mL per kilogram of body weight and administered as pairs 1 hour apart every 12 hours until clear. If there is no response after 2 days, more aggressive disimpaction under physician supervision is indicated. Phosphate enemas should be used with caution in patients with renal impairment. Tap water and soapsuds enemas should be avoided because of the possibility of water intoxication.

A lubricant such as mineral oil should be given orally in a dose adequate to overcome stool retention. Fat-soluble vitamins need to be supplemented during this phase of treatment. Reeducation of bowel habits is vital.

Although functional constipation encompasses most cases of chronic constipation in the child more than 1 year old, the less common causes must always be considered. As in the infant, endocrine abnormalities can cause and present as constipation.

TABLE 10.6. Findings in Hirschsprung's Disease and Functional Constipation

	Hirschsprung disease	Functional constipation
Onset in infancy	Common	Rare
Delayed passage of meconium	Common	Rare
Painful defecation	Rare	Common
Stool-withholding behavior	Rare	Common
Soiling	Rare	Common
Stool in rectal vault	Rare	Common
Failure to thrive	Common	Rare

Hypothyroidism is often associated with constipation as well as with sluggishness, somnolence, hypothermia, weight gain, and peripheral edema. Increased serum calcium causes constipation through decreased peristalsis. Causes include hyperparathyroidism and hypervitaminosis D. Diabetes mellitus produces increased urinary water loss, possibly leading to harder stool.

Rarely, an abdominal or pelvic mass may present with chronic constipation. Careful abdominal examination will demonstrate the mass. Rectal masses may present similarly. Follow-up again is emphasized because a mass that does not resolve after clearance of impaction needs further evaluation. Hydrometrocolpos can present with constipation and urinary frequency; therefore, in girls, a genital examination is indicated to document a perforated hymen. One must also remember that intrauterine pregnancy is a common cause of pelvic mass and constipation in adolescent girls.

Children with neuromuscular disorders often develop constipation. Myasthenia gravis, the muscular dystrophies, and other dystonic states can predispose children to constipation through a number of mechanisms. A detailed history and physical examination should recognize most neuromuscular problems, allowing symptomatic treatment to be provided.

Psychiatric problems must not be forgotten in the evaluation of constipation. Depression can be associated with constipation secondary to decreased intake, irregular diet, and decreased activity. Many psychotropic drugs can cause constipation. Anorexia nervosa may present with constipation because of decreased intake or metabolic abnormalities, and laxative abuse can cause paradoxical constipation.

CHAPTER 11
Cough

Richard Bachur, M.D.

Cough is a common pediatric complaint that has a variety of causes. Although cough usually is a self-limited symptom associated with upper respiratory illnesses, it occasionally indicates a more serious process. Under most circumstances, history and physical examination can accurately determine the cause.

DIFFERENTIAL DIAGNOSIS

The causes of cough differ in the type of stimulus and the site of involvement in the respiratory tract (Table 11.1). The common causes of cough are listed in Table 11.2. Potentially life-threatening causes are listed in Table 11.3.

TABLE 11.1. Causes of Cough in Children

Infection	Inhaled particulates
Upper respiratory infection	Smoking
Sinusitis	*Neoplasm*
Tonsillitis	Pharyngeal or nasal polyp
Laryngitis	Hemangioma
Laryngotracheitis (croup)	Papilloma
Tracheitis/tracheobronchitis	Lymphoma
Bronchiolitis	Mediastinal tumors
Acute bronchitis	*Congenital anomalies*
Pneumonia	Cleft palate
Pleuritis	Laryngotracheomalacia
Bronchiectasis/pulmonary abscess	Laryngeal or tracheal webs
Inflammation/allergy	Tracheoesophageal fistula
Allergic rhinitis	Vascular ring
Asthma	Pulmonary sequestration
Laryngeal edema	*Miscellaneous*
Reactive airway disease	Gastroesophageal reflux
Chronic bronchitis	Congestive heart failure
Cystic fibrosis	Swallowing dysfunction
Mechanical or hemical irritation	Granulomatous diseases
Foreign body aspiration	Psychogenic cough
Neck/chest trauma	Foreign body in otic canal
Chemical fumes	

EVALUATION AND DECISION

The history and physical examination are the keys to establishing a diagnosis for cough. The first priority is to recognize and treat any life-threatening conditions: Patients with significant respiratory distress should receive supplemental oxygen and rapid assessment of their airway and breathing (Fig. 11.1).

History

Cough can occur as an acute or chronic symptom, depending on the underlying process. Most common and serious causes of cough have an acute onset (Fig. 11.1). Certain conditions, such as asthma, may manifest as an acute or a chronic history of cough.

The relationship of the cough to other factors is helpful. Cough in the neonate must raise the possibility of congenital anomalies, gastroesophageal reflux, congestive heart failure, and atypical pneumonia (e.g., *Chlamydia*). If the cough began with other upper respiratory tract symptoms or fever, an infectious cause is likely. A cough that started with a choking episode, especially in an older infant or toddler, suggests a foreign body aspiration. Cough associated with exercise or cold exposure, even in the absence of wheezing, may be a sign of reactive airway disease. A primarily nocturnal cough often stems from allergy, sinusitis, or reactive airway disease. Systemic complaints should also be considered for patients with a cough: headache, fever, facial tenderness or pressure (sinusitis), acute dyspnea (asthma, pneumonia, cardiac disease), chest pain (asthma, pleuritis, pneumonia), dysphagia (esophageal foreign body), dysphonia (laryngeal edema or tracheal mass), or weight loss (malignancy or tuberculosis).

The quality of the cough also may be helpful in localizing the process. A barking, seal-like cough with or without stridor supports the diagnosis of laryngotracheitis. A paroxysmal cough associated with an inspiratory "whoop," cyanosis, or apnea is characteristic of pertussis. Tracheitis gives a deep "brassy" cough, whereas conditions accompanied by wheezing (asthma or bronchiolitis) typically produce a high-pitched "tight" (often termed *bronchospastic*) cough. Determining whether a cough is productive can be difficult in young children who often swallow, rather than expectorate, their sputum. Many parents, however, can convey whether the cough is "dry" or "wet." Although a productive-sounding cough may be seen with uncomplicated upper respiratory infections (URIs), sinusitis and lower respira-

TABLE 11.2. Common Causes of Cough

Upper respiratory infection	Acute bronchitis
Sinusitis	Pneumonia
Laryngotracheitis	Allergic rhinitis
Bronchiolitis	Reactive airway disease

TABLE 11.3. Life-Threatening Causes of Cough

Reactive airway disease	Laryngeal edema
Croup	Pertussis
Bronchiolitis	Toxic inhalation
Foreign body	Congestive heart failure
Pneumonia	

tory tract infections are commonly accompanied by a productive cough.

Typically, the onset of cough with rhinorrhea suggests a viral URI; however, if a child with an apparent URI becomes more ill or has persistent symptoms, secondary bacterial infections should be considered.

Physical Examination

Rhinorrhea, congestion, swollen turbinates, sinus tenderness, and pharyngitis are all signs of upper respiratory tract involvement. Allergic features include boggy nasal mucosa, an allergic nasal crease, and allergic "shiners." An otoscopic examination may reveal a small foreign body (e.g., hair) in the otic canal which may cause chronic cough. Laryngitis or stridor generally implies inflammation or obstruction at the level of the trachea or larynx. Unequal breath sounds, wheezes, rhonchi, and rales are signs of lower respiratory tract disease. A careful cardiac evaluation should be performed, and any clubbing should be noted. Young infants may have respiratory distress with localized upper airway congestion, but older infants and children usually have lower respiratory tract disease if significantly distressed (except in the obvious case of stridor).

Ancillary Studies

In most circumstances of children with a cough, the history and physical examination should be sufficient to make a diagnosis. In patients with unexplained cough or significant or persistent pulmonary signs, a chest radiograph is warranted. In children with an uncomplicated exacerbation of their asthma, a radiograph is unnecessary. If a radiolucent foreign body is suspected, inspiratory and expiratory films or decubitus films should be obtained to detect air trapping (see Chapter 22). Other studies

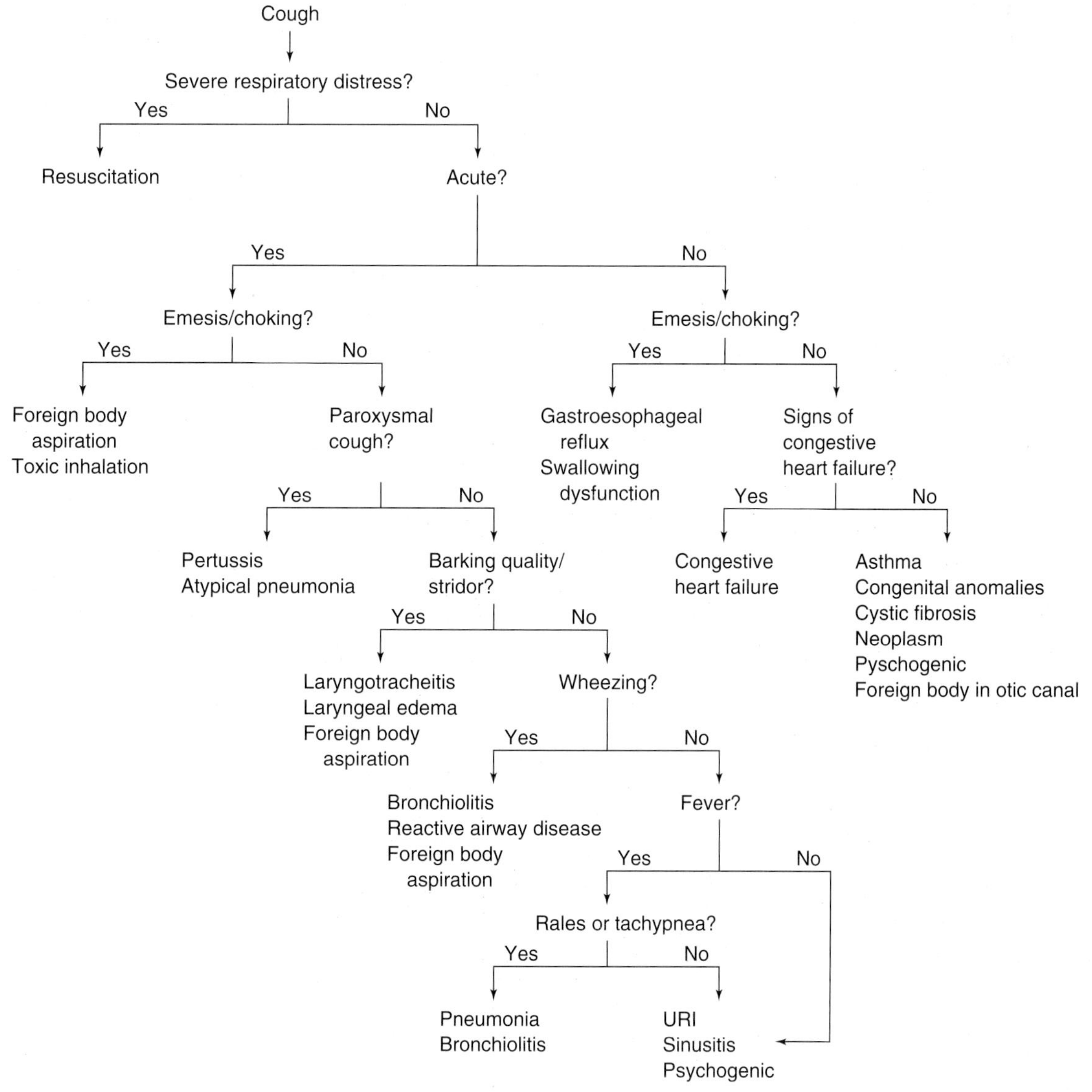

Figure 11.1. Approach to the child with cough.

that could be useful in selected patients include sinus films, lateral neck radiographs, barium swallow, and computed tomography of the sinuses, neck, or chest.

In addition, laboratory tests may be necessary for specific diagnoses. Such tests include a complete blood count and differential, blood culture, tuberculin test, nasopharyngeal swab for rapid assays or culture (commonly for pertussis and respiratory syncytial virus), Wright stain of nasal secretions (eosinophils with allergic rhinitis, neutrophils with sinusitis), and sputum culture and Gram stain (neutrophils and Gram-positive diplococci with pneumococcal pneumonia). Pulmonary function testing can be useful to diagnose or follow obstructive airway disease. In cases of airway masses, airway anomalies, foreign bodies, or atypical pneumonias, bronchoscopy may be necessary.

APPROACH

The major considerations in evaluating a child with cough include the quality of the cough, associated choking or emesis, and the findings of lower respiratory tract signs or fever (Fig. 11.1). Obviously, any child with respiratory distress needs immediate attention to oxygenation and ventilation.

Most patients with cough of acute onset will have a simple URI, asthma, bronchiolitis, or pneumonia. A sudden onset with choking or gagging, especially in the preverbal child, is suspicious for a foreign body aspiration (see Chapter 22). A barky cough, with or without stridor, in a child 3 months to 3 years of age suggests laryngotracheitis. Paroxysms of coughing associated with perioral cyanosis, posttussive emesis, or apnea points to pertussis. Visualizing the posterior pharynx with a tongue blade will elicit an episode of coughing.

Physical examination should include inspection of the nares and oropharynx and auscultation of the chest. Wheezing indicates bronchiolitis, asthma, or, rarely, foreign-body aspiration. Patients with asthma may complain only of cough and deny any wheezing. Careful auscultation during forced exhalation may detect wheezing or a prolonged expiratory phase. In an older child, significant lower airway obstruction can be measured with a handheld peak flow meter. Asymmetric, or focal, wheezing is seen with lower airway masses and foreign bodies. Rales, rhonchi, and decreased breath sounds are characteristic of lower respiratory tract infection.

The remaining patients with a cough of acute onset will have pneumonia or a UTI infection such as viral nasopharyngitis, sinusitis, pharyngitis, or tracheitis. Although rales, decreased breath sounds, or focal wheezing are signs associated with pneumonia, a small proportion of patients with pneumonia may not have any findings by auscultation. Therefore, in cases of significant cough, especially in very young children and those with high fever or elevated white blood cell counts, a chest radiograph is useful to exclude the diagnosis of pneumonia.

Children with chronic cough are likely to have reactive airway disease, allergic rhinitis, or sinusitis. In young children with failure to thrive or recurrent pulmonary infections, cystic fibrosis (see Chapter 85) should be considered. Chronic cough with a history of recurrent pneumonias or chronic bronchitis also can be suggestive of immunodeficiency or anatomic lesions (see Chapter 104). Choking with feeding or emesis followed by cough or wheezing in young infants is typical of gastroesophageal reflux. Newborns who exhibit a cough deserve special consideration for airway anomalies, atypical pneumonias, and congestive heart failure (see Chapter 72). Persistent cough during the day that stops with distraction or sleep is supportive of a psychogenic cause.

CHAPTER 12
Cyanosis

Anne M. Stack, M.D.

Cyanosis, a bluish purple discoloration of the tissues, is a disturbing condition commonly confronted by the pediatric emergency physician. It is most easily appreciated in the lips, nailbeds, earlobes, mucous membranes, and locations where the skin is thin and may be enhanced or obscured by lighting conditions and skin pigmentation. Three factors that ultimately determine the occurrence of cyanosis are the total amount of hemoglobin in the blood, the degree of hemoglobin saturation or qualitative changes in hemoglobin, and the state of the circulation.

DIFFERENTIAL DIAGNOSIS

The most common causes of cyanosis are cardiac and respiratory diseases that lead to a decrease in the arterial paratial pressure of oxygen (P_{O2}), but many other conditions also also can cause a patient to appear blue (Tables 12.1 and 12.2). Life-threatening causes of cyanosis are summarized in Table 12.3.

With regard to the amount of hemoglobin (Hb), polycythemia, as in newborns with twin–twin transfusion, infants of diabetic mothers, children with high erythropoietin states, or other conditions associated with increased red cell mass can give the appearance of cyanosis because of the relative increase in the amount of unsaturated Hb.

The degree of Hb saturation is affected by many factors, which can be grouped conveniently by systems. First is the significant contribution from respiratory conditions. Any circumstance leading to a decrease in the concentration of inspired oxygen, such as a house fire or high altitude, can eventually lead to diminished P_{O2} and cyanosis. Likewise, upper airway obstruction, as with a foreign body, croup, epiglottitis, bacterial tracheitis, tracheal or bronchial disruption, or congenital airway abnormalities, quickly leads to a decrease in the alveolar ventilation and hypoxemia. Cyanosis ensues rapidly when chest wall movement or lung inflation is impeded. This condition is often a result of trauma and includes external chest compression, flail chest, or hemothorax. Tension pneumothorax, whether traumatic or as a result of preexisting lung disease such as asthma or cystic fibrosis, is diagnosed by dyspnea, deviated trachea, and possibly distended neck veins with diminished breath sounds on the affected side. Empyema or pleural effusion caused by infection, malignancy, or large chylothorax may be associated with fever, respiratory distress, dullness to percussion, and an asymmetric examination on auscultation. It is important to keep in mind that any lung dysfunction that directly affects pulmonary gas exchange can lead to cyanosis. The most common conditions in children are asthma, bronchiolitis, pneumonia, cystic fibrosis, pulmonary edema, and hyaline membrane disease. Other causes include bronchopulmonary dysplasia, foreign body or substance aspiration, and congenital pulmonary lesions, to list a few.

Circulatory or vascular conditions leading to diminished arterial P_{O2} are also associated with cyanosis. One of the most common causes of cyanosis in children is congenital heart disease. The causes of cyanotic congenital heart disease are listed in Chapter 26. Cyanosis also can be caused by pulmonary congestion from cardiac failure or left-to-right cardiac lesions leading to increased pulmonary blood flow and diminished diffusion of

TABLE 12.1. Laboratory Evaluation of Cyanosis

I. Respiratory
  A. Decrease in inspired O_2 concentration
  B. Upper airway
    1. Foreign body
    2. Croup
    3. Epiglottitis
    4. Bacterial tracheitis
    5. Traumatic disruption
    6. Congenital anomalies (e.g., vascular malformation,hypoplastic mandible, laryngotracheomalacia)
  C. Chest wall
    1. External compression
    2. Flail chest
  D. Pleura
    1. Pneumothorax
    2. Hemothorax
    3. Empyema/effusion
    4. Diaphragmatic hernia
  E. Lower airway
    1. Asthma
    2. Bronchiolitis
    3. Cystic fibrosis
    4. Pneumonia
    5. Hyaline membrane disease
    6. Adult respiratory distress syndrome
    7. Bronchopulmonary dysplasia
    8. Foreign body/aspiration
    9. Congenital hypoplasia
II. Vascular
  A. Cardiac
    1. Cyanotic congenital defects
      a. Tetralogy of Fallot
      b. Transposition of the great vessels
      c. Truncus arteriosus
      d. Pulmonary atresia
      e. Severe pulmonary stenosis with patent foramen
      f. Tricuspid atresia
      g. Ebstein's anomaly
      h. Total anomalous pulmonary venous drainage
      i. Atrioventricular canal defect
    2. Congestive cardiac failure
    3. Cardiogenic shock
  B. Pulmonary
    1. Pulmonary edema
    2. Primary pulmonary hypertension of the newborn
    3. Pulmonary hypertension
    4. Pulmonary embolism
    5. Pulmonary hemorrhage
  C. Peripheral
    1. Moderate cold exposure
    2. Shock: septic/cardiogenic
    3. Acrocyanosis of the newborn
III. Neurologic
  A. Drug or toxin-induced respiratory depression (e.g., morphine, barbiturates)
  B. CNS lesions (e.g., intracranial hemorrhage, contusion)
  C. Seizure
  D. Breath holding
  E. Neuromuscular disease (e.g., Guillain-Barré, spinal muscular atrophy)
IV. Hematologic
  A. Polycythemia
  B. Methemoglobinemia
V. Dermatologic
  A. Blue dye
  B. Pigmentary lesions
  C. Tattoos

CNS, central nervous system.

O_2 across the gas–blood barrier. (For a detailed discussion of cardiac disease, see Chapter 72.) Several pulmonary vascular abnormalities can lead to cyanosis as well. These include primary pulmonary hypertension of the newborn or pulmonary hypertension from other causes in which, because of high pulmonary pressures, blood is shunted away from the lungs and the child becomes hypoxemic. Pulmonary embolism and pulmonary hemorrhage, although rare in children, also impair lung perfusion and must be considered.

Low perfusion states may lead to local cyanosis, particularly of the hands, feet, and lips. Moderate cold exposure slows transit time for red cells across capillary beds, leading to greater unloading of oxygen to the tissues and local blueness. Patients in septic or cardiogenic shock may have perfusion-related cyanosis with long capillary refill times as a result of vascular collapse of

TABLE 12.2. Common Causes of Cyanosis

I. Local cyanosis
  A. Acrocyanosis of the newborn
  B. Moderate cold exposure
II. Generalized cyanosis
  A. Respiratory dysfunction
  B. Congenital heart disease

TABLE 12.3. Life-Threatening Causes of Cyanosis

I. Respiratory
  A. Decreased inspired O_2 concentration
  B. Upper airway obstruction/disruption
  C. Chest wall immobility
  D. Tension pneumothorax
  E. Massive hemothorax
  F. Lung disease leading to hypoxemia
II. Vascular
  A. Cardiac
    1. Cyanotic congenital defects
    2. Congestive heart failure
    3. Cardiogenic shock
  B. Pulmonary
    1. Pulmonary edema
    2. Primary pulmonary hypertension of the newborn
    3. Pulmonary embolism
    4. Pulmonary hemorrhage
  C. Peripheral
    1. Septic shock
III. Other
  A. Neurologic conditions leading to hypoxemia
  B. Severe methemoglobinemia

sepsis or pump failure. Acrocyanosis, or blueness of the hands and feet with preserved pinkness in the mucous membranes and elsewhere, is seen commonly in newborns and is related to variable perfusion in the extremities. It is seen in well-appearing babies and resolves within the first few days of life.

Neurologic conditions can lead to Hb desaturation and cyanosis as well. Patients who hypoventilate because of central nervous system (CNS) depression, whether from primary CNS lesions or from drugs or toxins that depress the respiratory center, are often centrally cyanotic. Episodic blue spells in infants and young children who are otherwise well may be caused by breath holding, especially when associated with a sudden insult such as fright, pain, frustration, or anger. Vigorous crying is thought to cause cerebral ischemia via vasoconstriction from decreased partial pressure of carbon dioxide (P_{CO2}), decreased cardiac output from Valsalva maneuver, and hypoxemia from apnea. Seizures often are associated with cyanosis from inadequate respiration during the convulsion. A variety of neuromuscular diseases that affect chest wall or diaphragmatic function ultimately may lead to hypoventilation.

With respect to the Hb molecule itself, methemoglobinemia is an unusual but not rare reason for admission to the pediatric emergency department. Young infants with gastroenteritis or oxidant toxin exposure are particularly susceptible to the development of methemoglobinemia as a result of having immature enzyme systems required to reduce Hb. Symptoms caused by decreased blood oxygen content and cellular hypoxia, include headache, dizziness, nausea, dyspnea, confusion, seizure, and coma. Even at low levels, skin discoloration is prominent, often with intense or "slate gray" cyanosis from the presence of methemoglobin as perceived through the skin. (For a more detailed discussion of methemoglobinemia, see Chapter 77.)

Other conditions that can lead to a blue appearance of the skin may be confused with cyanosis. A rare but perplexing presentation is that of the well-appearing child with unusually localized cyanosis, which as the result of head scratching turns out to be related to blue dye of clothing. Certain pigmentary lesions such as mongolian spots can be confused with cyanosis, especially when uncharacteristically large or in unusual locations. Adolescents occasionally "tattoo" areas of the body that may appear as local cyanosis.

EVALUATION AND DECISION

The history and physical examination act as the "jumping-off point" for evaluation of the cyanotic patient. In newborns, congenital cardiac and respiratory diseases are the most common causes. Some older children with cyanosis will have a history of preexisting diseases of the heart or lungs. Exposure to cold, toxins, smoke, or trauma offers a likely explanation in others.

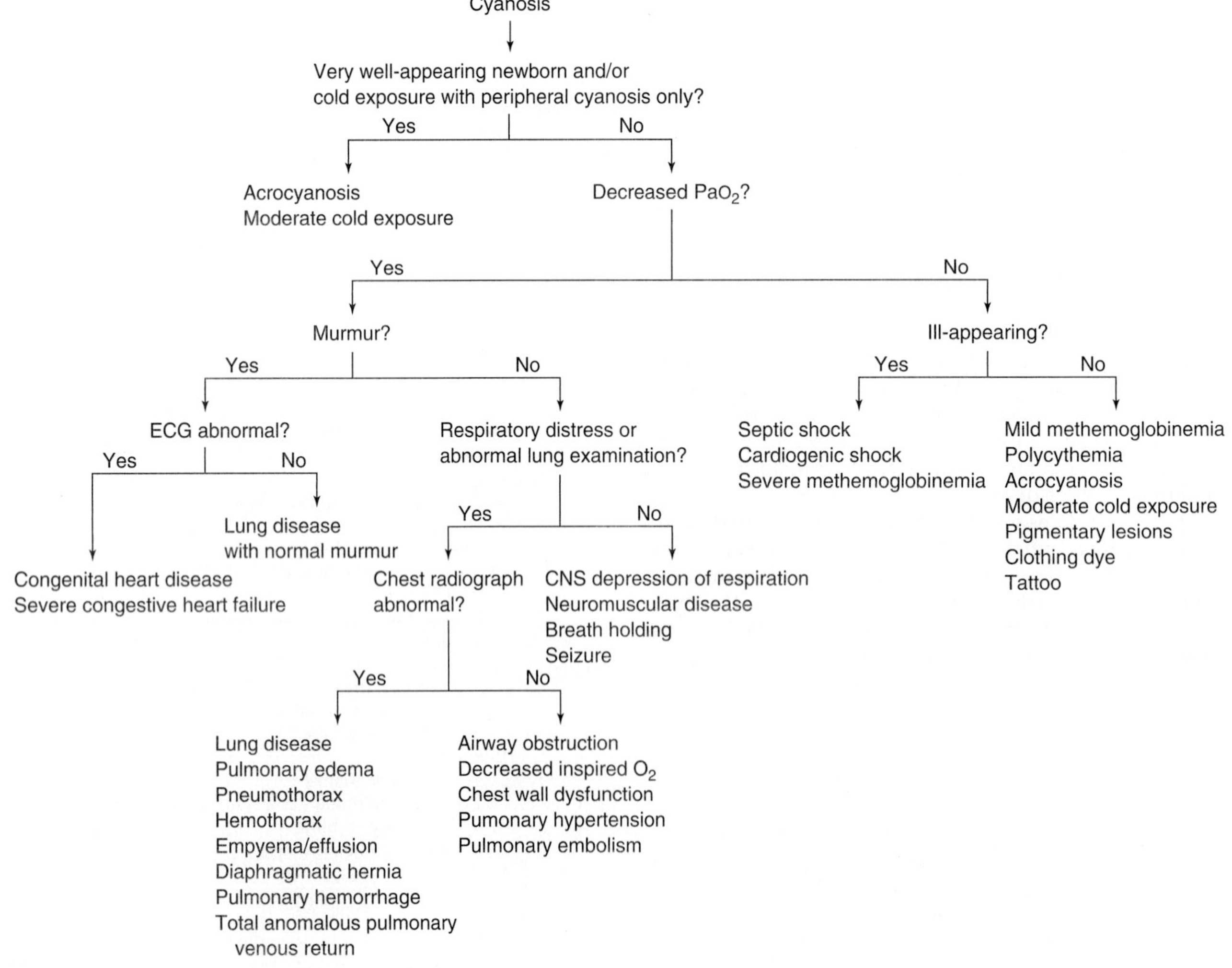

Figure 12.1. Laboratory evaluation of cyanosis.

Physical examination may reveal hypoventilation, shock, pulmonary disease, or a cardiac failure or anomaly.

The path of the laboratory evaluation depends on the historical features and physical findings established on initial encounter (Fig. 12.1). All patients, except well-appearing newborns and well-appearing cold-exposed patients with peripheral cyanosis only, require measurement of arterial P_{O2}. (Oxygen saturation by pulse oximetry may be helpful in determining if hypoxemia is the cause of cyanosis, but it may also be misleading when forms of Hb are present other than oxyhemoglobin and deoxyhemoglobin.) If the P_{O2} is normal, the laboratory evaluation is determined by the degree of ill appearance. Well-appearing oxygenated children with cyanosis usually have less urgent conditions, such as polycythemia, mild methemoglobinemia, cold exposure, newborn acrocyanosis, or dermatologic findings. In this case, laboratory evaluation might include a methemoglobin level and complete blood count, or no further investigation may be warranted. Despite a normal P_{O2}, an ill-appearing cyanotic patient may have a more emergent condition such as severe methemoglobinemia or septic or cardiogenic shock and may require aggressive laboratory investigation, including complete blood count, methemoglobin level, blood cultures, and blood chemistry. Blood with high methemoglobin content may appear very dark or "chocolate brown" and fail to turn red on exposure to air, such as in a drop on filter paper. Treatment then is directed at the underlying cause. Methemoglobinemia may improve with intravenous methylene blue. If the P_{O2} is decreased, oxygen therapy should be instituted. In general, cyanosis caused by decreased alveolar ventilation or diffusional abnormalities often improves with delivery of 100 O_2. Hypoxemia caused by decreased pulmonary perfusion, however, responds little to oxygen therapy. Next, a chest radiograph should be obtained. Abnormalities of the lungs may confirm pulmonary disease as a major contributor to hypoxemia, and changes in the cardiac size or silhouette may suggest cardiac causes. If the chest radiograph is normal, other reasons for diminished arterial P_{O2}, such as CNS or chest wall–related respiratory depression, upper airway obstruction, or pulmonary perfusion abnormalities, must be entertained. If a concomitant murmur or other concern for cardiac disease exists, an electrocardiogram (ECG) is essential. Abnormal electrocardiographic findings suggest cardiac dysfunction, either congenital or acquired (Table 12.1), and the addition of echocardiography will help establish the definitive diagnosis.

CHAPTER 13
Crying and Colic in Early Infancy

Barbara B. Pawel, M.D. and
Fred M. Henretig, M.D.

Crying is the means by which an infant expresses discomfort, ranging from normal hunger and desire for company to severe, life-threatening illness. Many common minor irritations and illnesses can cause crying. Often, however, a normal, thriving infant will develop a chronic pattern of daily paroxysms of irritability and crying known as *colic*. The attacks usually have their onset in the second to third week of life and may last for several hours, more commonly in the late afternoon or evening. Establishing an orderly approach to the infant with unexplained crying is important to rule out the occasional physical illness and to provide preliminary guidance to the family.

EVALUATION AND DECISION

A careful history and physical examination with emphasis on the head, eyes, ears, skin, abdomen, genitalia, and extremities, plus analysis and culture of a urine specimen, usually will enable the physician to diagnose identifiable illnesses or injuries causing severe paroxysms of crying (Table 13.1). Initially, this clinical evaluation must focus on those conditions that are potentially life threatening: meningitis, child abuse, intussusception, incarcerated hernia, severe intoxication, and metabolic disturbance. Other less critical but more common conditions should be sought next; corneal abrasion or foreign body, otitis media, aerophagia, teething, gastroenteritis, and anal fissure are most commonly seen. As noted in Table 13.1, other diagnoses are encountered occasionally.

The history should include special attention to the onset of crying and any associated events—particularly recent immunization ("screaming spells" lasting up to 24 hours have been described after pertussis vaccine), trauma, fever, or use of medications. Physical examination must be thorough, with the infant completely undressed. Vital signs may reveal fever, suggesting infection (although not always present in young infants with serious infections), or hyperpnea, suggesting metabolic acidosis.

The head should be explored for evidence of trauma, and the fontanelle should be palpated. Eyes must be examined with fluorescein to look for corneal abrasion, even in infants with no symptoms referable to the eyes. In addition, eversion of the upper eyelids can exclude a foreign body. Funduscopy should be attempted (retinal hemorrhages are common signs of abuse, especially in "shaken baby" syndrome). Careful otoscopy is required to visualize the tympanic membranes. The heart should be evaluated for signs of congestive failure, arrhythmia, or rare ischemia-producing lesions (Table 13.1). Abdominal and rectal examinations must be done to look for signs of anal fissure or intussusception. The diaper must be removed, and a careful search should be made for incarcerated hernia, testicular torsion, or strangulation of the penis or clitoris by an encircling hair. Because crying may be the primary symptom of an occult urinary infection, a suitable specimen of urine should be obtained for urinalysis and culture. Careful palpation of all long bones despite the absence of obvious signs of trauma can detect fracture sites that otherwise might have been overlooked. Each finger and toe should be inspected closely to rule out strangulation by hair or thread. Further consideration of laboratory evaluation is made in light of the clinical findings.

A low threshold for urine toxicology screening is warranted in the persistently irritable infant, given the escalation in illicit drug use.

Many infants will have a completely negative examination, and the history (or subsequent follow-up) will be suggestive of colic. Over the time in which the crying attacks recur, the infant must demonstrate adequate weight gain (average 5–7 ounces per week in the first months of life) and an absence of physical disorders on several examinations before underlying illnesses can be excluded and colic can be diagnosed confidently (Fig. 13.1). The safest and most effective course of treatment at this time seems to be counseling and empathy.

TABLE 13.1. Conditions Associated with Abrupt Onset of Inconsolable Crying in Young Infants

I. Discomfort caused by identifiable illness
  A. Head and neck
    1. Meningitis
    2. Skull fracture/subdural hematoma
    3. Glaucoma
    4. Foreign body (especially eyelash) in eye
    5. Corneal abrasion
    6. Otitis media
    7. Caffey's disease (infantile cortical hyperostosis)
    8. Child abuse
    9. Prenatal/perinatal cocaine exposure
  B. Gastrointestinal
    1. Excess air (improper feeding/burping technique)
    2. Gastroenteritis[b]
    3. Intussusception[a]
    4. Anal fissure[b]
    5. Cow's milk protein intolerance (CMPI)
    6. Gastroesophageal reflux/esophagitis
  C. Cardiovascular
    1. Congestive heart failure
    2. Supraventricular tachycardia
    3. Coarctation of the aorta
    4. Anomalous origin of left coronary artery from pulmonary artery (ALCAPA)
  D. Genitourinary
    1. Torsion of the testis
    2. Incarcerated hernia
    3. Urinary tract infection
  E. Integumentary
    1. Burn
    2. Strangulated finger, toe, penis (hair tourniquet)
  F. Musculoskeletal
    1. Child abuse
    2. Extremity fracture (following a fall)
  G. Toxic/metabolic
    1. Drugs: antihistamines, atropinics, adrenergics, cocaine (including passive inhalation), aspirin
    2. Metabolic acidosis, hypernatremia, hypocalcemia, hypoglycemia
    3. Pertussis vaccine reactions
II. Colic—recurrent paroxysmal attacks of crying

[a] Life-threatening causes.
[b] Common causes.

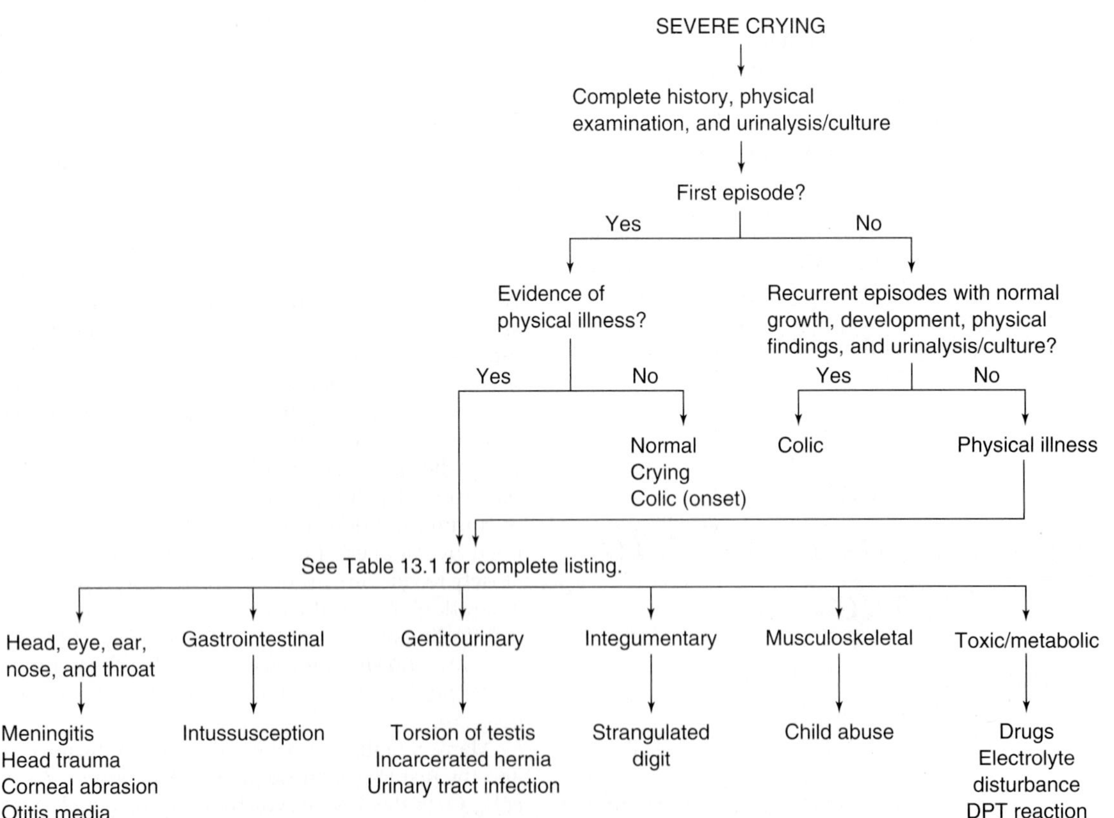

Figure 13.1. Approach to abrupt onset of severe crying in infancy. *DPT,* diphtheria-pertussis-tetanus (vaccine).

CHAPTER 14
Dehydration

Kathy N. Shaw, M.D.

Dehydration is a physiologic disturbance caused by the reduction or translocation of body fluids and is a type of hypovolemic shock. Infants have higher morbidity and mortality rates and are more susceptible to dehydration because of their larger water content, higher metabolic turnover rate of water, renal immaturity, and inability to meet their own needs independently. Because dehydration is not a disease itself, children with various illnesses and circumstances will present to the emergency department with signs of dehydration (Table 14.1).

Dehydration often is categorized by the patient's *osmolarity* (the disturbance of distribution of water among body spaces) and *severity* (degree of fluid deficit), which is helpful in determining fluid therapy. Based on the initial serum sodium, most children have isotonic dehydration (130–150 mEq per liter), whereas others have hypertonic dehydration (> 150 mEq per liter) or hypotonic dehydration (<130 mEq per liter). The terms *isonatremia, hypernatremia*, and *hyponatremia* would be more appropriate. Severity is judged by the amount of body fluid lost or the percentage of weight loss, and the three categories include *mild* (< 50 mL per kilogram of body weight, or <5%), *moderate* (50–100 mL per kilogram of body weight, or 5–10), and *severe* (> 100 mL per kilogram of body weight, or >10).

DIFFERENTIAL DIAGNOSIS

Fluid losses in dehydration result from (1) decreased intake, (2) increased output secondary to insensible, renal, or gastrointestinal losses; or (3) translocation of fluid such as occurs with major burns or ascites (Table 14.1). Diarrhea (see Chapter 15) is the most common cause of dehydration in infants and children and is the leading cause of death worldwide in children less than 4 years of age. In the United States, an average of 300 children under 5 years of age die each year, and an additional 200,000 are hospitalized secondary to diarrheal illnesses with dehydration. Other common causes of dehydration in children include vomiting, stomatitis, or pharyngitis with poor intake secondary to pain, febrile illnesses with increased insensible losses, decreased intake, and diabetic ketoacidosis (Table 14.2). More severe or life-threatening causes are listed in Table 14.3.

TABLE 14.1. Causes of Dehydration

Decreased intake	Mannitol usage
Physical restriction	Nonosmotic
Infant CNS depression	Diabetes insipidus
Anorexia	Sustained hypokalemia/ hypercalcemia
Voluntary or imposed cessation of drinking	Sickle cell disease
Pharyngitis, stomatitis	Chronic renal disease
Respiratory distress	Bartter syndrome
Child abuse	Sodium-losing
Hypothalamic hypodipsia	Congenital adrenal hypoplasia
Increased output	Diuretics
Insensible losses	Sodium-losing nephropathy
Fever	Pseudohypoaldosteronism
Sweating	Gastrointestinal losses
Heat prostration	Diarrhea (see Chapter 15)
High ambient temperature/low humidity	Secretory vs. nonsecretory
	Vomiting (see Chapter 69)
Hyperventilation	Obstructive vs. nonobstructive
Cystic fibrosis	Translocation of fluids
Thyrotoxicosis	Burns
Renal losses	Ascites (e.g., nephrotic syndrome)
Osmotic	
Diabetic ketoacidosis	Intraintestinal
Acute tubular necrosis	Paralytic ileus
High-protein feeds	Postabdominal surgery

CNS, central nervous system.

TABLE 14.2. Common Diagnoses

Gastroenteritis	Febrile illness
Stomatitis/pharyngitis	Diabetic ketoacidosis

EVALUATION AND DECISION

The first step in evaluating a child with dehydration is to assess the severity or degree of dehydration, regardless of the cause (Table 14.4). Most children with clinically significant dehydration will have two of the following four clinical findings: (1) capillary refill greater than 2 seconds, (2) dry mucous membranes, (3) no tears, and (4) ill appearance. Dehydration is a type of hypovolemic shock. *Mild, moderate*, and *severe* dehydration correspond to *impending, compensated*, and *uncompensated* states of shock, respectively (see Chapter 3). If there is severe dehydration or uncompensated shock, the child must be treated immediately with isotonic fluids to restore intravascular volume, as detailed later in this chapter.

History

A thorough history is needed to assess the child with dehydration to determine the cause and degree of dehydration (Fig. 14.1). Particular attention should be paid to the child's output and intake of fluids and minerals. Asking the parents about documented weight loss, amount of urine output, and the presence or absence of tears is helpful in determining the severity of the dehydration.

Physical Examination

Vital signs are important and objective parts of the evaluation of the child with dehydration (Table 14.4). The first sign of mild dehydration is tachycardia, whereas hypotension is a late sign of severe dehydration. Attention should be paid to the overall appearance, mental status, eyes, and skin on physical examination. The mildly dehydrated child usually appears well and may have decreased tearing and a slightly dry mouth. Dry mucous

TABLE 14.3. Life-Threatening Diagnoses

Gastroenteritis (especially infants)	Heat prostration
Diabetic ketoacidosis	Gastrointestinal obstruction
Burns over 25% of body surface area	Cystic fibrosis
Thyrotoxicosis	Diabetes insipidus
Congenital adrenal hyperplasia	Child abuse

TABLE 14.4. Clinical Estimation of Degree of Dehydration[a]

	Mild	Moderate[b]	Severe[b]
Body fluid lost (mL/kg)	<50	50–100	>100
Weight loss (%)	<5	5–10	>10
Stage of shock	Impending	Compensated	Uncompensated
Vital signs			
Heart rate	Slight ↑	↑ (Orthostasis)	↑↑
Respiratory	Normal	Normal	↑ (Hyperpnea)
Blood pressure	Normal	Normal (orthostasis)	↓
Skin			
Capillary refill (finger)	<2 sec	2–3 sec	>3 sec
Elasticity (<2 yr)	Normal	↓	↓↓ (Tenting)
Anterior fontanel	Normal	Depressed	Depressed
Mucous membranes/tongue	Normal/dry	Dry	Dry
CNS			
Mental status	Normal	Altered	Depressed
Thirst	Not thirsty, drinks normally	Thirsty, drinks eagerly	Drinks poorly, not able to drink
Eyes			
Tearing	Normal/absent	Absent	Absent
Appearance	Normal	Sunken	Sunken
Laboratory tests			
Urine			
Volume	Small	Oliguria	Oliguria/anuria
Osmolarity (mOsm/L)	600	800	Maximal
Specific gravity	1.020	1.025	Maximal
Blood			
Blood urea nitrogen	Upper normal	Elevated	High
pH	7.40–7.22	7.30–6.92	7.10–6.80

CNS, central nervous system.
[a] Signs of dehydration may be less evident or appear later in hypernatremic dehydration; conversely, they may be more pronounced or appear sooner in hyponatremic dehydration.
[b] The presence of at least three clinical findings are necessary to predict clinically significant dehydration.

membranes are an early sign of dehydration, but this condition is affected by rapid breathing and ingestion of fluids. Conversely, the severely dehydrated infant classically appears quite ill with lethargy or irritability, a dry mouth, sunken fontanelle, and absent tears. More moderate states of dehydration, however, require more careful evaluation.

Laboratory Tests

Progressive decrease in urine output and increase in specific gravity and osmolarity are expected with increasing severity of dehydration. If the physical examination indicates significant dehydration and there is dilute or copious urine, a renal or adrenal origin is most likely. The presence of glucose or ketones may indicate diabetic ketoacidosis, and a history of disorders of the central nervous system (CNS) suggests diabetes insipidus.

In children who are judged to have moderate to severe dehydration that requires intravenous rehydration, laboratory tests of electrolytes, glucose, blood urea nitrogen, and creatinine usually are obtained to determine osmolarity and renal function. The acid-base status may be assessed further with an arterial or venous blood gas.

DIAGNOSTIC APPROACH

In approaching the patient with presumed dehydration, the initial assessment serves to determine whether shock is present. If the child appears to be in shock, resuscitation is called for immediately and a number of life-threatening disorders need to be considered, as listed in Table 14.3 and discussed in Chapter 3. Patients with obvious burns or diseases that disrupt the integument in the same way (e.g., "scalded skin" syndrome) are presumed to have become dehydrated through transudation of fluids through the skin.

If the patient does not have an obvious cutaneous source for dehydration, gastrointestinal losses provide the most likely explanation. A history of vomiting (see Chapter 69) or diarrhea (see Chapter 15) should be sought. Most children with vomiting or diarrhea have viral gastroenteritis, but many diseases (see Tables 14.1 and Table 69.1 in Chapter 69) produce these symptoms. Additional history serves to establish the adequacy of oral intake. Several common minor infections, such as pharyngitis and stomatitis, as well as more serious disorders of the CNS, cause dehydration as a result of voluntary or involuntary limitation of fluids taken orally.

Next, the history should address the nature and quantity of the urine output. With dehydration, one expects to find oliguria or anuria, as seen with many renal diseases (see Chapter 76). The unexpected discovery of polyuria points to diabetes mellitus or insipidus.

By this point, the physician will have established a diagnosis in most patients. In hot weather or when there is prolonged fever, skin losses must be considered. Patients with cystic fibrosis (see Chapter 85) in particular are prone to dehydration under these conditions because of a high concentration of sodium in the sweat (the finding of hyponatremic dehydration seemingly unexplained by the estimated fluid loss should suggest this diagnosis). Additional considerations are listed in Table 14.1.

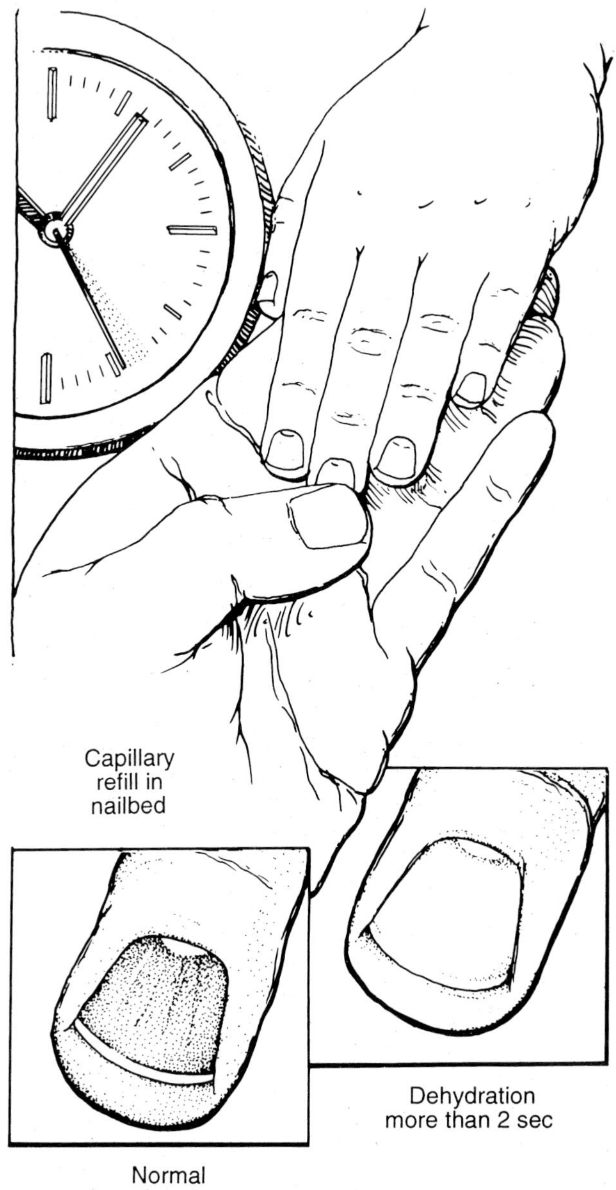

Figure 14.1. Assessing dehydration by capillary refill.

CHAPTER 15
Diarrhea

Gary R. Fleisher, M.D.

Diarrhea refers to a softening in the consistency of the stool with or without an increase in the number of stools. Because of the variability in the frequency and type of stools among children, absolute limits of normalcy are difficult to define. Rather, any deviation from the child's usual pattern should arouse concern, regardless of the actual number of stools or their water content. Some infants, particularly those who are breastfed, often have five or six loose stools daily as their normal routine; other healthy infants may produce only one formed stool every other day.

TABLE 15.1. Common Causes of Diarrhea

Infections
Enteral
Viruses
Bacteria
Nongastrointestinal
Dietary disturbances
Psychogenic disturbances
Miscellaneous
Antibiotic-associated
Secondary lactase deficiency

DIFFERENTIAL DIAGNOSIS

Of the many causes of diarrhea, a few are particularly common: infections with viruses and bacteria, parenteral diarrhea, and diarrhea associated with antibiotic administration (Table 15.1). The single most common disorder seen in the emergency department is viral gastroenteritis. The emergency physician must be vigilant in recognizing the few children who have diseases that are likely to be life threatening from among the majority of children who have self-limiting infections. Particularly urgent are intussusception, pseudomembranous colitis, hemolytic uremic syndrome (HUS), and appendicitis (Table 15.2).

EVALUATION AND DECISION

The initial evaluation of the child with diarrhea should serve the dual purpose of exploring the possible causes and assessing the degree of illness. Preexisting conditions in the child may account for the diarrhea or predispose him or her to unusual causes; in particular, the emergency physician should search for a history of gastrointestinal surgery or chronic illnesses, such as ulcerative colitis or regional enteritis. Immunodeficiency syndromes, neoplasms, and immunosuppressive therapy all can lead to an increased susceptibility to infection. Institutionalized children and those recently returning from underdeveloped countries are more likely to harbor bacterial or parasitic pathogens.

A history of abdominal pain, particularly if severe, raises the index of suspicion for intussusception and appendicitis. Bloody diarrhea points particularly to bacterial enteritis but occasionally occurs with viral infections and may also herald the onset of HUS or pseudomembranous colitis. The combination of episodic abdominal pain and blood in the stool characterizes intussusception. Vomiting in association with diarrhea is very suggestive of viral gastroenteritis, whereas vomiting in isolation (see Chapter 69) is of greater concern.

TABLE 15.2. Life-Threatening Causes of Diarrhea

Intussusception
Hemolytic uremic syndrome
Pseudomembranous colitis
Appendicitis
Salmonella gastroenteritis (with bacteremia in the neonate or compromised host)
Hirschsprung's disease (with toxic megacolon)
Inflammatory bowel disease (with toxic megacolon)

The general physical examination can provide clues to an underlying illness in the child who appears malnourished or small for his or her age. On abdominal examination, the finding of a mass (regional enteritis, intussusception) or evidence of obstruction is important. A rectal examination should be performed in the child who has chronic diarrhea. With overflow stools secondary to prolonged constipation, the rectal ampulla contains a large amount of hard stool, but it often is empty in the patient with Hirschsprung disease. For selected children, laboratory measurements may assist in the evaluation of dehydration, but they often fall in the normal range despite marked loss of fluids.

A diagnostic approach to the pediatric patient with diarrhea is outlined in Fig. 15.1. The physician first should determine whether the child appears seriously ill or has signs of a surgical abdominal process. Once it has been determined that immediate signs of a life-threatening process are absent, more than any other feature, the duration of diarrhea dictates the initial diagnostic considerations. Children with chronic diarrhea (more than 5 days) are likely to have irritable bowel syndrome, infections, inflammatory bowel disease, or various malabsorptive disorders. Such conditions, if uncomplicated, do not require a definitive diagnosis emergently but rather an extensive evaluation over time.

ACUTE DIARRHEA

With the acute onset of diarrhea, most children have an infectious cause for their disorder. Fever, the hallmark of infection, serves as the first branch point in the approach to such patients. Although not all children with infectious enteritis have fevers, the finding of an elevated temperature points strongly in this direction. At the same time, the absence of fever, particularly in the presence of bloody stools, should alert the physician to the possibility of one of several serious noninfectious diseases, particularly intussusception and HUS.

The next question is whether hematochezia (bloody stool) is present. Blood is seen in the stool of approximately 10% of chil-

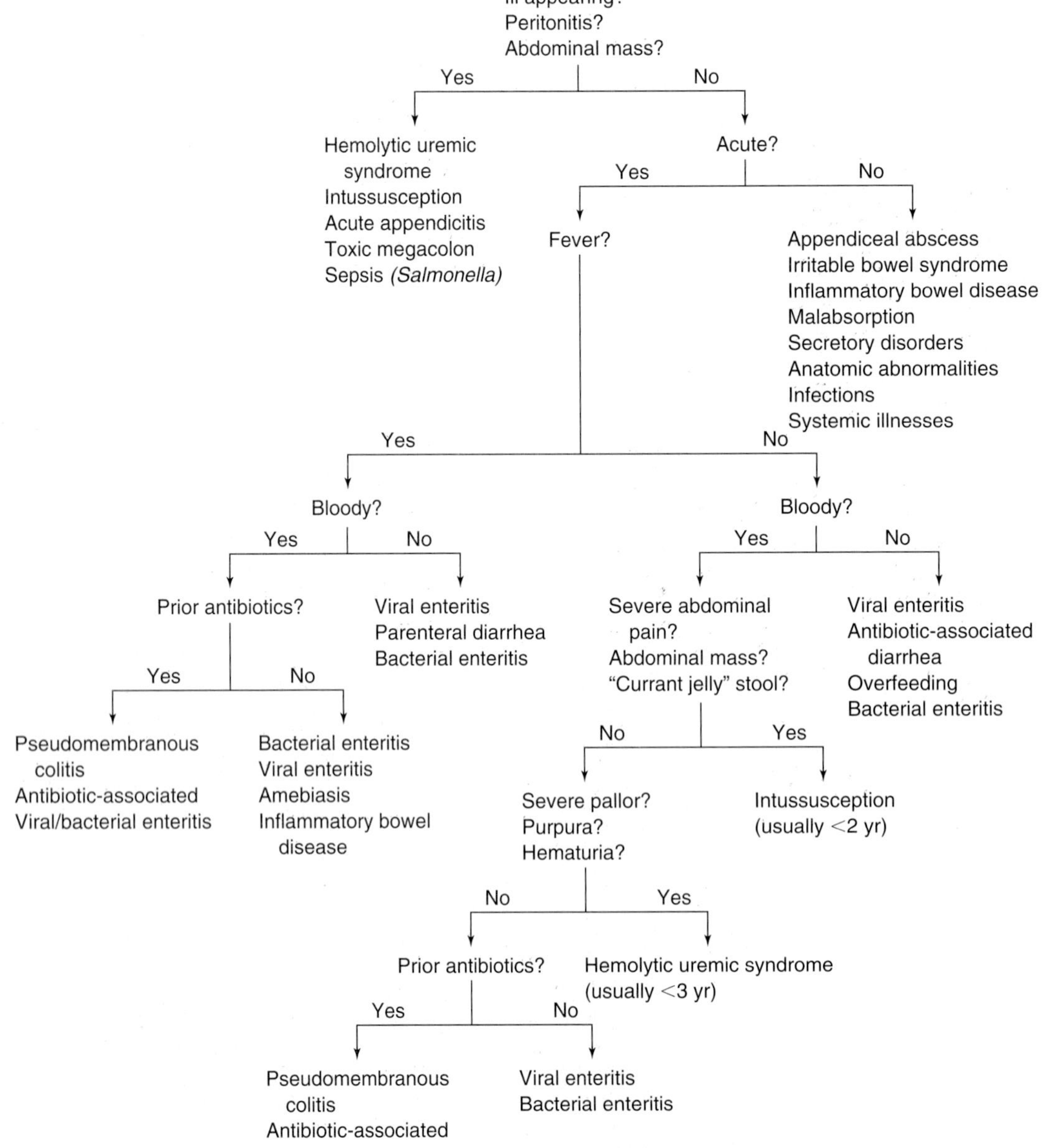

Figure 15.1. Diagnostic approach to the immunocompetent child with diarrhea.

dren with diarrhea. In most cases, the blood appears in small quantities as drops on the surface of the stool and should not be construed as an ominous finding. A small percentage of children with diarrhea, however, have more profuse rectal bleeding. In these patients, one must exclude life-threatening disorders such as intussusception, HUS, and pseudomembranous colitis.

Febrile children with bloody diarrhea (Fig. 15.1) almost invariably have an infectious enteritis. Pseudomembranous colitis should be considered in patients who have received antibiotic therapy, but this diagnosis usually can be discarded on clinical grounds in the absence of systemic toxicity, abdominal distension, and gross blood in the stools. If pseudomembranous colitis is strongly suspected, admission to the hospital and a full diagnostic evaluation should be considered. Bacterial diarrhea should be sought by culture in febrile children with frankly bloody diarrhea but will be found only in 15% to 20% of cases; viral enteritis is much more common. In the first few months of life, in the infant for whom *Salmonella* gastroenteritis represents a more serious illness, a stool smear for polymorphonuclear leukocytes is useful because the finding of sheets of inflammatory cells strongly points to a bacterial origin. Amebiasis merits consideration only in endemic areas and among travelers. Finally, an occasional child with inflammatory bowel disease may present with an initial episode of acute, bloody diarrhea. With most of these children, the physician can elicit a preceding history of weight loss or recurrent abdominal pain; in the remainder, the diagnosis emerges when bloody diarrhea persists in the face of negative cultures.

Most febrile children with nonbloody diarrhea (Fig. 15.1) have viral enteritis. The physician must perform a thorough examination because nonenteric infections, particularly otitis media, may cause "parenteral" diarrhea. For similar reasons, a urine culture is indicated if any historical factors point to an infection of the urinary tract. Although a small percentage of these patients have a bacterial enteritis, routine cultures of stool are not recommended for nonbloody diarrhea of brief duration in otherwise healthy children. Immunocompromised patients, such as those with acquired immunodeficiency syndrome (AIDS) (see Chapter 75), require a more thorough evaluation, including bacterial cultures and examination for ova and parasites.

Afebrile children with bloody diarrhea (Fig. 15.1) represent the most worrisome category because most patients with intussusception, HUS, and pseudomembranous colitis have this constellation of symptoms. In particular, intussusception should be considered carefully in any child less than 1 year of age with bloody diarrhea that does not appear to have an infectious cause. Although the finding of a mass or a currant jelly stool is pathognomonic, a history of severe, colicky abdominal pain in a lethargic child warrants a contrast enema. Obvious pallor, purpura, and hematuria point to HUS, an unusual but potentially life-threatening disease. Once again, prior antibiotic therapy raises the possibility of pseudomembranous colitis. The most common diagnosis, infectious enteritis, should be assigned only after exclusion of the more serious disorders by history, physical examination, and occasionally laboratory or radiographic studies.

Afebrile children with nonbloody diarrhea (Fig. 15.1) usually are judged to have viral enteritis. Those who receive antibiotic agents, such as amoxicillin, may be suffering from a drug-related gastrointestinal disturbance but not usually from pseudomembranous colitis. During the first 6 to 12 months of life, overfeeding may manifest as diarrhea. The clue to this diagnosis is the history of excessive intake in the overweight child. Bacterial enteritis, although a possibility, does not merit a stool culture in the usual clinical circumstances.

CHRONIC DIARRHEA

The evaluation of chronic diarrhea usually requires a period of observation and laboratory evaluation beyond the scope of the emergency department. In the management of these children, the role of the emergency physician is to select those few children who have urgent conditions and refer the remainder to their regular source of care. Particularly in the infant, consideration must be given to Hirschsprung disease and to cystic fibrosis. A history of delayed passage of meconium, constipation since birth, and abdominal distension are compatible with Hirschsprung disease. Malabsorptive stools and respiratory infections suggest cystic fibrosis. Failure to thrive, thrush, and pneumonia occur in association with human immunodeficiency virus (HIV) infection. A stool culture and examination for parasites serve to diagnose the serious infections of the gastrointestinal tract and provide a head start on the evaluation to the physician who subsequently sees the child.

The child who returns to the emergency department with the persistence of an acute diarrheal illness, presumed to be viral in origin and with no evidence of malnutrition or dehydration, often may be managed without an extensive evaluation. Three causes are common: (1) bacterial infections; (2) secondary lactase deficiency from mucosal sloughing; and (3) starvation stools in the child who inadvertently has been continued on a clear liquid diet for several days. A stool culture should be obtained, and testing for clostridial toxin is indicated in the presence of ongoing antibiotic therapy. If the child has remained on a clear liquid diet, gradual refeeding is recommended. Milk and all milk products should be proscribed temporarily when secondary lactase deficiency is suspected.

TREATMENT

Most children, even those with vomiting, will tolerate frequent small feedings, but occasionally delivery of fluids via a nasogastric tube may be helpful. Optimal oral therapy emphasizes the use of appropriate glucose and electrolyte solutions as well as the early reintroduction of feeding. In general, antidiarrheal agents are ineffective and have no role in the treatment of infectious gastroenteritis during childhood; agents that decrease intestinal mobility (i.e., Lomotil) carry an additional risk of toxicity.

CHAPTER 16
Dizziness

Stephen J. Teach, M.D., M.P.H.

"Dizziness" is a common complaint in the pediatric emergency department. *True vertigo* is the perception that the environment is rotating relative to the patient or that the patient is rotating relative to the environment. Preverbal children, unable to articulate the sensation, may merely be irritable, vomit, and prefer to lie still. Unfortunately, most patients who use the term *dizziness* are in fact describing one of numerous nonvertiginous disturbances (*pseudovertigo*), which may be difficult for the practitioner to distinguish from true vertigo. Light-headedness, presyncope, intoxication, ataxia, visual disturbances, unsteadiness, stress, anxiety, and fear from any of numerous causes initially can be described as dizziness. The key element in the history that distinguishes true vertigo is the subjective sense of rotation.

TABLE 16.1. Causes of Vertigo in Children

Peripheral causes	Central causes
Suppurative or serous labyrinthitis	Tumor[a]
External ear impaction	Meningitis[a]
Ramsay Hunt syndrome	Encephalitis[a]
Cholesteatoma	Increased intracranial pressure[a]
Perilymphatic fistula	Multiple sclerosis
Vestibular neuronitis	Trauma[a]
Benign paroxysmal vertigo	Seizure (usually complex partial)
Ingestions[a]	Migraine
Temporal bone fracture[a]	Stroke[a]
Posttraumatic vestibular concussion	Motion sickness
Meniere's disease	Paroxysmal torticollis of infancy

[a] Life-threatening causes of vertigo.

DIFFERENTIAL DIAGNOSIS

Table 16.1 lists the differential diagnosis of true vertigo and highlights the life-threatening causes. Table 16.2 lists the most common causes of vertigo. Table 16.3 lists numerous nonvertiginous conditions that may be described initially as dizziness. Because the spectrum of nonvertiginous conditions is so broad, the following discussion concentrates on true vertigo.

Vertigo follows a dysfunction of the vestibular system and also can be divided into conditions in which hearing is impaired (usually peripheral causes) and conditions in which hearing is spared (usually central causes). Finally, vertigo can be divided into acute (usually infectious, postinfectious, traumatic, or toxic) and chronic recurrent groups (usually caused by seizures, migraine, or benign paroxysmal vertigo of childhood).

INFECTIONS

Both acute and chronic bacterial and viral infections of the middle ear with or without associated mastoiditis can cause both vestibular and auditory impairment (see Chapter 25). Severe untreated, acute suppurative otitis media with effusion may extend directly into the labyrinth. Even without direct invasion of the pathogens, inflammatory toxins can cause a serous labyrinthitis.

Chronic and recurrent otitis media can produce a cholesteatoma of the tympanic membrane, an abnormal collection of keratin caused by repeated cycles of perforation and healing. Cholesteatomas can erode the temporal bone and the labyrinth, producing a draining fistula from the labyrinth that presents as vertigo, nausea, and hearing impairment. Computed axial tomography scans show destruction of the temporal bone.

Viral infections can directly affect the labyrinth or the vestibular nerve; together, these conditions are known as *vestibular neuronitis*. Known pathogens include mumps, measles, and the Epstein-Barr virus. More commonly, a nonspecific upper respiratory tract infection precedes the illness. Onset is usually acute and can be severe. Nystagmus is usually present. Patients prefer to lie motionless with the eyes closed.

TABLE 16.2. Common Causes of Vertigo

Suppurative or serous labyrinthitis	Ingestions
Benign paroxysmal vertigo	Seizure
Migraine	Motion sickness
Vestibular neuronitis	

TABLE 16.3. Common Causes of Pseudovertigo

Depression	Cardiac disease
Anxiety	Anemia
Hyperventilation	Hypoglycemia
Orthostatic hypotension	Pregnancy
Hypertension	Ataxia
Heat stroke	Visual disturbances
Arrhythmia	

MIGRAINE

Vertigo may be a prominent feature of classic migraine or migraine equivalent, in which there is no associated headache (see Chapter 73). Basilar migraine presents as a throbbing occipital headache following the signs and symptoms of brainstem dysfunction (including vertigo, ataxia, tinnitus, and dysarthria). Vertigo from migraine equivalent (without pain) typically is seen in patients with a family history of migraine headache and is associated with other transient neurologic complaints (e.g., weakness, dysarthria). Symptoms may suggest temporal lobe epilepsy. The latter is distinguished by altered consciousness.

The differential diagnosis of headache and vertigo includes a brainstem or cerebellar mass, hemorrhage, and infarction. These uncommon disorders are best assessed by magnetic resonance imaging (MRI).

BENIGN PAROXYSMAL VERTIGO

Considered by many to be a form of migraine, benign paroxysmal vertigo is most common in children between the ages of 1 and 5 years. Patients have recurrent attacks, usually one to four per month, and occasionally in clusters. Onset is sudden—the child often cries out at the start of each episode—and is associated with emesis, pallor, sweating, and nystagmus. Episodes are brief, lasting up to a few minutes, and may be mistaken for seizures. Consciousness and hearing are preserved, and the neurologic examination is otherwise normal. The disorder spontaneously remits after 2 to 3 years.

OTOTOXIC DRUGS

Most agents that disturb vestibular function also will disturb auditory function. Specific agents include aminoglycoside antibiotics, furosemide, ethacrynic acid, streptomycin, minocycline, salicylates, and ethanol. Toxic doses of certain anticonvulsants and neuroleptics can produce measurable disturbances of vestibular function, although associated complaints of vertigo are rare.

POSTTRAUMATIC VERTIGO

Several mechanisms account for posttraumatic vertigo. The most obvious is fracture through the temporal bone with damage to the labyrinth. Presentation includes vertigo, hearing loss, and hemotympanum. Computed tomography (CT) scanning of the temporal bone should be obtained when there is hemotympanum or posttraumatic evidence of vestibular dysfunction.

More subtle causes of posttraumatic vertigo include trauma-induced seizures, migraine, or a postconcussion syndrome. The latter disorder (vestibular concussion) typically follows blows to parieto-occipital or temporoparietal regions and presents with headache, nausea, vertigo, and nystagmus. Hyperextension and flexion ("whiplash") injuries can be associated with vestibular dysfunction, probably caused by basilar artery spasm with subsequent impairment of their labyrinth and cochlear connections. Symptoms may mimic basilar artery migraine.

SEIZURES

Two types of seizures are associated with vertigo: vestibular seizures (seizures causing vertigo) and vestibulogenic seizures ("reflex" seizures brought on by stimulating the semicircular canals or vestibules by sudden rotation or caloric testing). Vestibular seizures, the more common type, consist of sudden onset of vertigo with or without nausea, emesis, and headache and invariably are followed by loss or alteration of consciousness. The electroencephalogram (EEG) is abnormal. Anticonvulsants may be of benefit.

MOTION SICKNESS

Motion sickness is precipitated by a mismatch in information provided to the brain by the visual and vestibular systems during unfamiliar rotations and accelerations. The most common situation occurs when a child travels in a car or airplane and is deprived of visual stimulus that confirms movement. Symptoms include vertigo, nausea, and nystagmus. Attacks can be prevented if the patient watches the environment move in a direction opposite to the direction of body movement. In car travel, encouraging children to "look out the window" is helpful.

MENIERE DISEASE

Uncommon in children younger than 10 years old, Meniere disease is characterized by episodic attacks of vertigo, hearing loss; tinnitus, nystagmus, and autonomic symptoms of pallor, nausea, and emesis. Between episodes, patients complain of impaired balance. The underlying cause is believed to be an overaccumulation of endolymph within the labyrinth, which causes a rupture (endolymphatic hydrops). Typical attacks last from 1 to 3 hours and usually begin with tinnitus, a sense of fullness within the ear, and increasing hearing impairment. Attacks are intermittent and unpredictable, often lasting for years, and at times evolving to permanent hearing loss.

MISCELLANEOUS CAUSES

Vertigo can occur at any point in the clinical course of multiple sclerosis when the central demyelination interferes with the vestibular nuclei in the brainstem or its efferents or afferents. Diagnosis is confirmed by MRI and lumbar puncture. Paroxysmal torticollis of infancy consists of spells of head tilt associated with nausea, emesis, pallor, agitation, and ataxia. Episodes are brief and self-limited and may recur for months or years. The cause is unclear, although some researchers regard it as a prelude to later benign paroxysmal vertigo (considered by some to be a migraine variant). Perilymphatic fistula is an abnormal communication between the labyrinth and the middle ear, with leakage of perilymphatic fluid through the defect. It may be congenital or acquired by trauma, infection, or surgery. Diagnosis is made by exploring the middle ear exploration. Finally, vertigo may be associated with diabetes mellitus and chronic renal failure.

EVALUATION AND DECISION

Differentiation of True Vertigo and Pseudovertigo

Evaluation of children complaining of dizziness begins by separating those with true vertigo from those with pseudovertigo (Tables 16.1 and 16.3). True vertigo always is associated with a subjective sense of rotation of the environment relative to the patient or of the patient relative to the environment. Acute attacks are usually accompanied by nystagmus. Pseudovertigo is suggested by complaints of light-headedness, flushing, weakness, ataxia, unsteadiness, weakness, fatigue, pallor, anxiety, stress, and fear.

TRUE VERTIGO (FIG. 16.1)

History and Physical Examination

Sudden onset of sustained vertigo suggests central or peripheral trauma, infection, central stroke, or ingestion. Chronic recurrent episodes suggest seizures, migraine, or benign paroxysmal vertigo. More persistent episodes suggest brainstem or cerebellar mass lesions. Recurrent, transient, altered mental status suggests seizure or basilar migraine. Episodes of prior head injury suggest concussion syndromes. Recent upper respiratory tract infections may suggest vestibular neuronitis. History of ototoxic drugs or intoxicants is important, as is a family history of migraine. The age of the patient is especially helpful: Benign paroxysmal vertigo is unusual after age 5 years, whereas Meniere disease is unusual before age 10 years.

The physical examination focuses on the middle ear and on neurologic and vestibular testing. Perforation or distortion of the tympanic membrane should be noted. A pneumatic bulb will enable the examiner to determine whether abrupt changes in the middle-ear pressure trigger an episode of vertigo, a suggestion that a perilymphatic fistula may be present (Hennebert's sign).

Both vestibular and cerebellar disorders manifest with an unsteady gait. The two can be distinguished by the presence or absence of nystagmus and, in the verbal child, by the presence or absence of a sense of rotation. In addition, if cerebellar dysfunction is present, there will be a breakdown of rapid alternating movements and finger-to-nose movements.

Nystagmus is a highly specific sign for both central and peripheral vertiginous disorders. A patient complaining of dizziness from vertigo may not have nystagmus at the time he or she is examined. Initially, nystagmus should be sought in all positions of gaze and with changes in head position. Peripheral vestibular disorders are characterized by a "jerk" nystagmus with the slow component toward the affected side. Central lesions are characterized by nystagmus with the fast component toward the affected side and reversal of the fast component when changing from right to left lateral gaze. The Nylen-Barany test is performed by moving a child rapidly from a sitting to a supine position with the head 45 degrees below the edge of the examining table and turned 45 degrees to one side. Nystagmus and a vertiginous sensation may

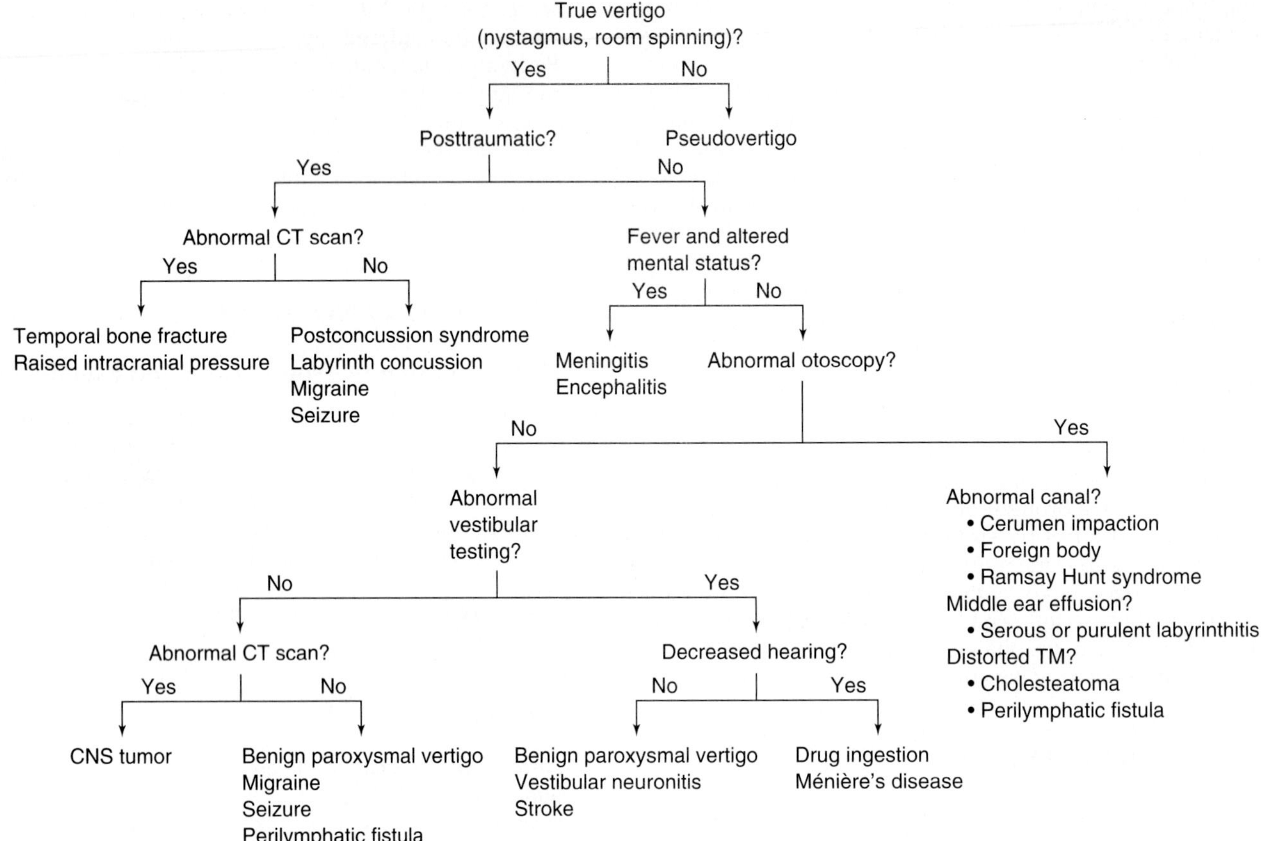

Figure 16.1. Approach to the child with true vertigo.

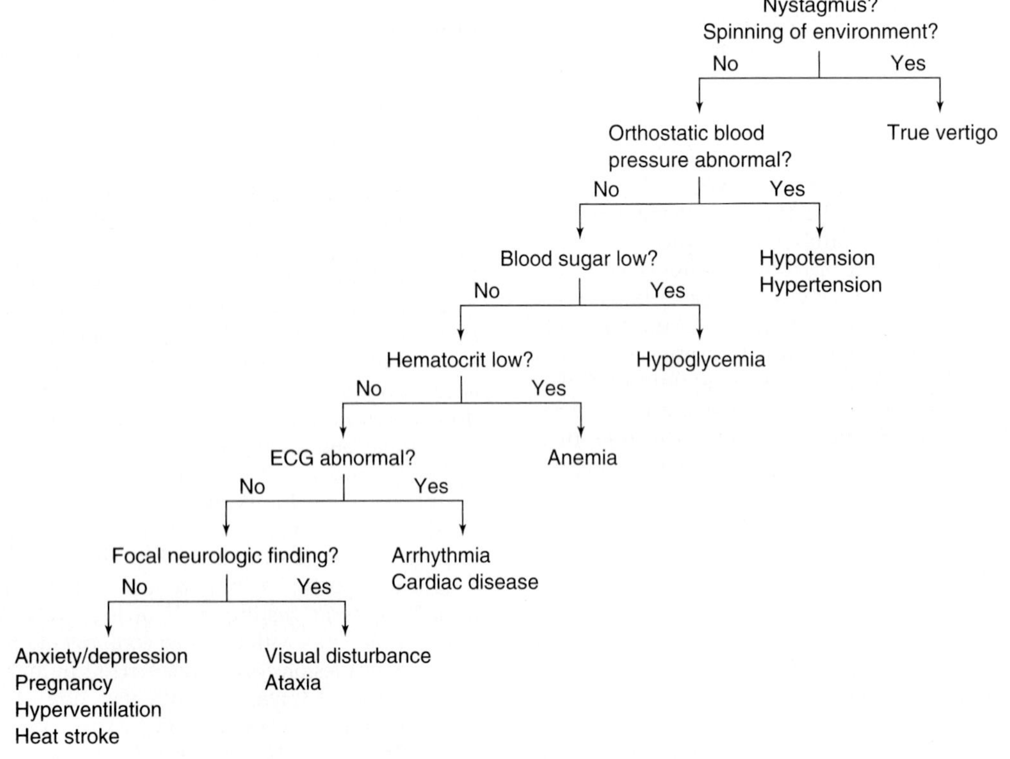

Figure 16.2. Approach to the child with pseudovertigo.

result as the vestibular system is stressed. Certain features of the nystagmus elicited may be helpful in distinguishing central from peripheral vestibular dysfunction. In central dysfunction, for example, onset of nystagmus is immediate; in peripheral vestibular disorders, it is delayed. The cold caloric response tests for integrity of the peripheral vestibular system.

Laboratory Data

Laboratory investigations have a limited role in the evaluation of vertigo. Useful initial tests include a complete blood count, serum glucose measurement, and an electrocardiogram. Together, these tests may help to identify patients with pseudovertiginous conditions caused by anemia, hypoglycemia, and rhythm abnormalities. Further laboratory testing may reveal diabetes or renal failure, both of which have been associated with vertigo. Toxicologic testing, including specific anticonvulsant levels and an ethanol level, if indicated, may be helpful. A lumbar puncture is indicated in cases of suspected meningitis or encephalitis.

Radiologic imaging of the central nervous system is indicated in cases of chronic and recurrent vertigo to exclude mass lesions. Children with vertigo and an underlying bleeding diathesis or a predisposition toward ischemic stroke (i.e., sickle cell disease) also may require an emergent cranial CT or MRI. Posttraumatic vertigo, especially when accompanied by hearing loss or facial nerve paralysis, is best assessed by computed axial tomography, including adequate images of the temporal bone.

PSEUDOVERTIGO (FIG. 16.2)

Pseudovertigo refers to a broad array of diagnoses that present with symptoms such as light-headedness, presyncope, intoxication, ataxia, visual disturbances, unsteadiness, stress, anxiety, and fear. Uniformly absent are a sense of rotation and ocular nystagmus. Underlying causes are numerous; several of the most common causes are listed in Table 16.3. Careful consideration of the patient's age, sex, detailed history, and physical examination, together with a limited number of ancillary tests, may help to establish the specific diagnosis.

CHAPTER 17
Edema

Lydia Ciarallo, M.D.

Edema, the abnormal swelling of tissues from accumulation of fluid in the extravascular space, is a common emergency problem. This fluid characteristically appears either in the dependent portions of the extremities or lower back; in distensible tissues such as the eyelids, scrotum, or labia; or in organs or extremities at the site of tissue damage. The major mechanisms that lead to the formation of edema are decreased intravascular oncotic pressure (clinically indicated by a decreased serum albumin), increased venous or lymphatic pressure, and vasculitis from an allergic or hypersensitivity reaction.

DIFFERENTIAL DIAGNOSIS

Numerous diseases can cause localized or generalized edema on the basis of the three major pathophysiologic mechanisms already discussed (Table 17.1). The most common origin for localized edema in children is an allergic reaction. Idiopathic nephrosis is the most likely source for generalized edema (Table 17.2). Although most children who develop edema will have self-limiting disorders, potentially life-threatening conditions (Table 17.3) may be seen, including allergic reactions that involve the upper airway, bacteremic cases of cellulitis (see Chapter 74), thrombophlebitis, and dysfunction of the kidney, liver, or heart.

TABLE 17-1. Causes of Edema

Decreased oncotic pressure
Protein loss
Protein-losing enteropathy
Nephrotic syndrome
Cystic fibrosis
Reduced albumen synthesis
Liver disease
Malnutrition
Increased hydrostatic pressure
Increased blood volume from Na^+ retention
Congestive heart failure
Primary renal Na^+ retention
Acute glomerulonephritis
Henoch-Schönlein purpura
Premenstrual edema or pregnancy
Venous obstruction
Constrictive pericarditis
Acute pulmonary edema
Portal hypertension
Budd–Chiari syndrome
Local venous obstruction
Thrombophlebitis
Increased capillary permeability
Allergic reaction
Inflammatory reactions
Burns
Cellulitis
Hereditary angioneurotic edema
Pit viper envenomations
Other
Edema of the newborn
Lymphedema

EVALUATION AND DECISION

When evaluating the child with edema, initially the physician must determine whether the patient has a localized or generalized process. Even if the complaint appears to be confined to one anatomic area, a thorough examination is necessary, checking in particular for edema around the eyes, the scrotum, and the feet. If there is any suspicion of generalized swelling, a urinalysis is indicated to rule out proteinuria (renal disease often leads to the formation of edema without other clinical findings). Acquired hypoproteinemia from hepatic or intestinal dis-

TABLE 17.2. Common Causes of Edema

Localized
Allergic reaction
Cellulitis
Trauma
Generalized
Nephrosis

TABLE 17.3. Life-Threatening Causes of Edema

Localized
- Allergic reaction with airway involvement
- Cellulitis
- Group A streptococcus with varicella
- Pit viper envenomations
- Thrombophlebitis

Generalized
- Cardiac disease
  - Congestive heart failure
  - Pericardial effusion
- Renal disease
  - Nephrosis
  - Nephritis
- Hepatic failure

ease is unusual, and congestive heart failure (CHF) produces myriad findings.

LOCALIZED EDEMA

Children seek care more often for localized than for generalized edema (Fig. 17.1). Rarely, an infant will have unexplained, localized swelling of an extremity since birth. In this situation, congenital lymphedema (Milroy disease) should be considered; Turner syndrome may be associated with bilateral leg edema and Noonan syndrome with pedal edema. More commonly, the swelling arises over a few days. Most of these lesions result from minor trauma, infection of the subcutaneous tissues, or allergic (urticarial) reactions. Rapid onset of painful swelling typically follows pit viper envenomation (see Chapter 80). Tenderness to palpation points to trauma or infection, and fever with warmth over the lesion often occurs with the latter (Table 17.4). On the eyelids and over the ankles, insect bites are likely to produce a noticeable swelling, which can be difficult to distinguish from cellulitis. A therapeutic response to an antihistamine (diphenhydramine) or to a subcutaneous dose of epinephrine can aid in the diagnosis of an allergic reaction. When local edema occurs on the face, the physician should evaluate the child carefully for concurrent laryngeal involvement. When facial edema is severe or recurrent or when there is a family history of a similar problem, hereditary angioedema (see Chapter 81) is a consideration. Other causes of facial edema include acute sinusitis, dental abscess, orbital or buccal cellulitis, and cavernous sinus thrombosis. A history of environmental exposure can be helpful in the diagnosis of sunburn, frostbite, and plant-induced dermatitis. Sickle cell anemia can cause painful limb edema, as in the case of toddlers with dactylitis. Thrombophlebitis rarely occurs in the prepubertal child but may affect the adolescent; weightlifting and the use of oral contraceptive pills predispose teenagers to this condition. Finally, pregnant young women may develop edema in the lower extremities.

GENERALIZED EDEMA

Generalized edema, usually an indication of significant underlying disease, occasionally occurs with less serious conditions. Certain drugs (oral contraceptive pills, lithium, nonsteroidal antiinflammatory agents) may cause some people to become edematous; cessation of the drug produces a resolution of the

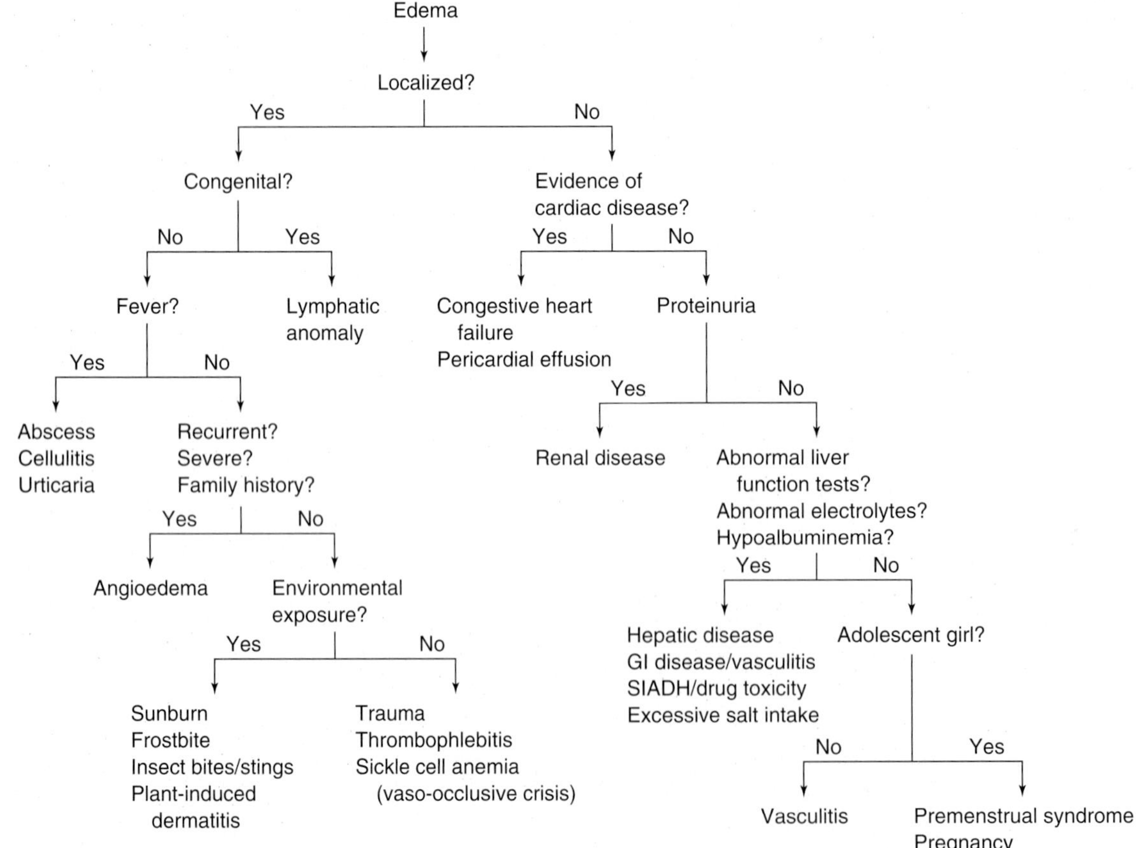

Figure 17.1. Edema in children.

TABLE 17.4. Differentiation among the Common Causes of Localized Edema

	Fever	Local tenderness	Local warmth	Lesion/color
Allergic reaction	No	No	No	Erythematous
Trauma	No	Yes	No	Violaceous
Infection	Usually	Yes	Yes	Erythematous or violaceous

swelling. Just before menstruation, young women may complain of "bloating."

The clinical manifestations of CHF or pericarditis are rarely subtle when these conditions are hemodynamically severe enough to produce edema. Tachycardia, tachypnea, adventitial pulmonary sounds, and hepatomegaly suggest CHF (see Chapter 72). In the child with a pericardial effusion, a pulsus paradoxus greater than 10 to 20 mm Hg, muffled heart tones, and jugular venous distension may occur. A chest radiograph often shows an enlarged cardiac silhouette with both conditions. An electrocardiogram with ST-segment elevation and generalized T-wave inversion on the tracing may suggest pericarditis with a pericardial effusion. Echocardiography is diagnostic.

Generalized edema that is not cardiovascular in origin most often arises secondary to diseases of the kidneys, particularly idiopathic nephrotic syndrome (see Chapter 76). Occasionally, other forms of the nephrotic syndrome, glomerulonephritis, hemolytic uremic syndrome, or Henoch-Schönlein purpura (HSP) are responsible. The detection of significant proteinuria (3+ or 4+) confirms the diagnosis of nephrotic syndrome or nephritis, and affected children require admission to the hospital for evaluation and treatment. In the child with HSP, the edema usually affects the lower extremities predominantly and often is accompanied by a purpuric eruption (despite normal platelet count and coagulation studies).

In the absence of proteinuria or signs of CHF, occult diseases of the gastrointestinal tract or liver remain considerations. An initial laboratory evaluation, including liver function tests, electrolyte levels, and measurement of total protein and albumin, should be performed. Abnormalities in these studies often suggest involvement of a specific organ system or severe vasculitis with protein leak.

By the process of exclusion, the child with normal screening laboratory tests and no abnormal physical findings except generalized edema is likely to have some type of vasculitis. The finding of a normal albumin does not rule out vascular disease. In teenaged girls, otherwise unexplained edema may occur in the premenstrual period and carries a benign prognosis.

CHAPTER 18
Epistaxis

Fran Nadel, M.D. and Fred M. Henretig, M.D.

Epistaxis (nosebleed) is a common symptom in young children and may be alarming to parents, who often overestimate the amount of blood loss. An orderly approach to the history and physical examination is necessary to identify the small minority of patients who require laboratory evaluation or referral for further treatment.

DIFFERENTIAL DIAGNOSIS

Many types of local and systemic disorders can cause epistaxis (Table 18.1). Local factors predominate in etiologic importance (Table 18.2). In addition to minor accidental trauma and habitual picking, any cause of acute inflammation will predispose the nose to bleeding. Acute upper respiratory infections contribute to the onset of epistaxis. Allergic rhinitis also may be a factor. Staphylococcal furuncles, foreign bodies, telangiectasias (Osler-Weber-Rendu disease), hemangiomas, or evidence of other uncommon tumors may be found on inspection. Juvenile nasopharyngeal angiofibroma usually is seen in adolescent boys with nasal obstruction, mucopurulent discharge, and severe epistaxis. These tumors may bulge into the nasal cavity but often re-

TABLE 18.1. Differential Diagnosis of Epistaxis

- Local predisposing factors
  - Trauma, direct and picking
  - Local inflammation
  - Acute viral upper respiratory tract infection (common cold)
  - Bacterial rhinitis
  - Nasal diphtheria (rare)[a]
  - Congenital syphilis
  - Usually a blood-tinged discharge
  - β-Hemolytic streptococcus
  - Foreign body
  - Acute systemic illnesses accompanied by nasal congestion:
  - Measles, infectious mononucleosis, acute rheumatic fever
  - Allergic rhinitis
  - Nasal polyps (cystic fibrosis, allergic, generalized)
  - Staphylococcal furuncle
  - Telangiectasias (Osler–Weber–Rendu disease)
  - Juvenile angiofibroma[a]
  - Other tumors, granulomatosis (rare)[a]
  - Rhinitis sicca
- Systemic predisposing factors
  - Hematologic diseases[a]
    - Platelet disorders
      - Quantitative: idiopathic thrombocytopenic purpura, leukemia, aplastic anemia
      - Qualitative: von Willebrand's disease, Glanzmann's disease, uremia
      - Other primary hemorrhagic diatheses: hemophilias, sickle cell anemia
      - Clotting disorders associated with severe hepatic disease, DIC, vitamin K deficiency
    - Drugs: aspirin, nonsteroidal anti-inflammatory drugs, warfarin, rodenticide
    - Vicarious menstruation
  - Hypertension[a]
    - Arterial (unusual cause of epistaxis in children)
    - Venous: superior vena cava syndrome or with paroxysmal coughing seen in pertussis and cystic fibrosis

DIC, diffuse intravascular coagulopathy.
[a] Life-threatening condition.

TABLE 18.2. Common Causes of Epistaxis

Trauma	Rhinitis sicca
Foreign body	Viral rhinitis
Allergic rhinitis	

quire examination of the nasopharynx to be identified. A rare childhood malignant tumor, nasopharyngeal lymphoepithelioma, may cause a syndrome of epistaxis, torticollis, trismus, and unilateral cervical lymphadenopathy. *Rhinitis sicca* refers to a condition that is common in northern latitudes during the winter, in which low ambient humidity, exacerbated by dry hot-air heating systems, leads to desiccation of the nasal mucosa with concurrent tendency to frequent bleeding. Other rare local causes of epistaxis include nasal diphtheria and Wegener granulomatosis.

Children rarely present with a nosebleed as their only manifestation of a more systemic disease. In children with severe or recurrent nosebleeds, a positive family history, or constitutional signs and symptoms, the physician should consider a systemic process. Von Willebrand disease and platelet dysfunction are two of the more common systemic diseases that cause recurrent or severe nosebleeds. Other less common systemic factors include hematologic diseases such as sickle cell anemia, leukemia, hemophilia, and clotting disorders associated with severe hepatic dysfunction or uremia. Arterial hypertension rarely is a cause of epistaxis in children. Increased

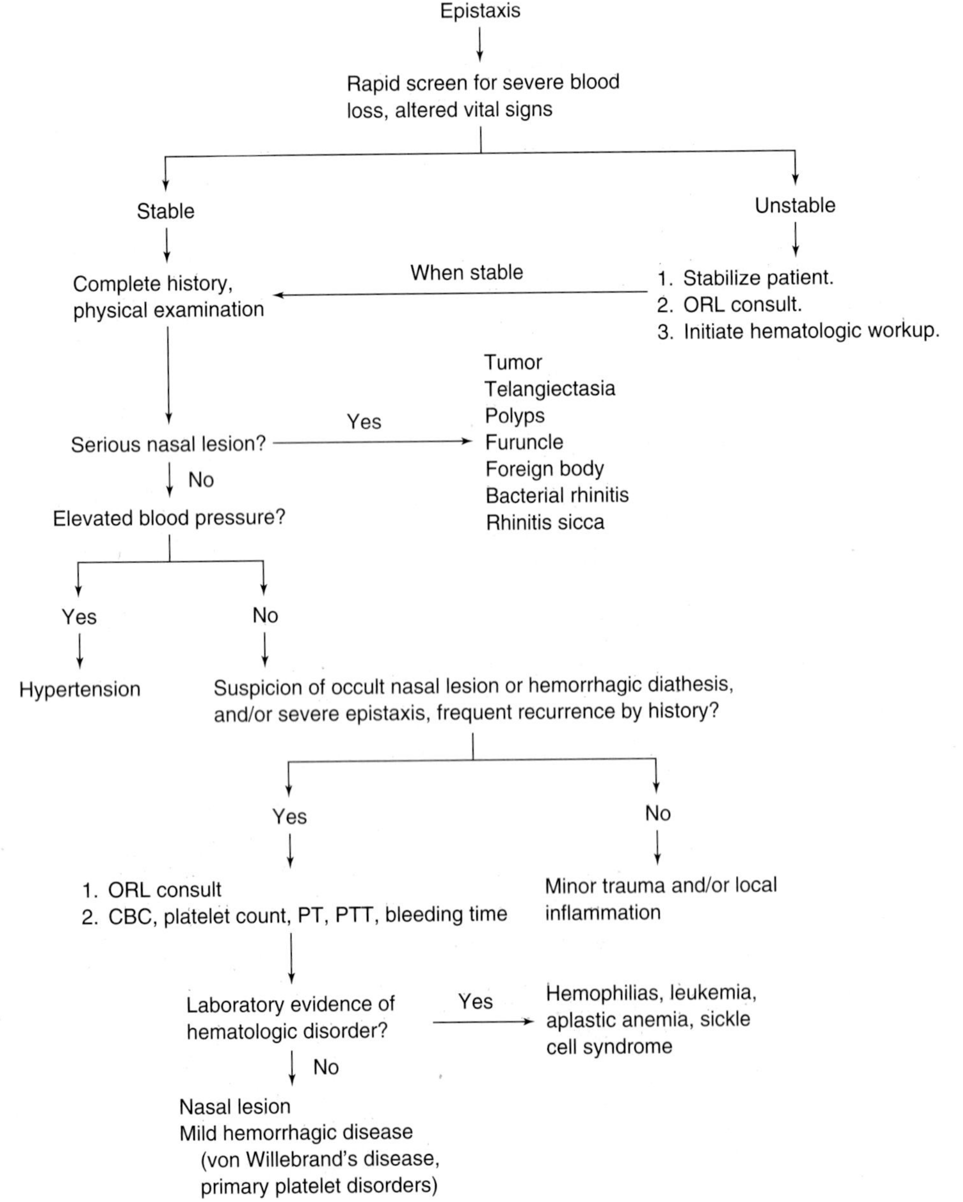

Figure 18.1. Approach to diagnosis of epistaxis. ORL, otorhinolaryngologist; CBC, complete blood count; PT, prothrombin time; PTT, partial thromboplastin time.

nasal venous pressure secondary to paroxysmal coughing, such as that occurring in pertussis or cystic fibrosis, occasionally causes nosebleeds. *Vicarious menstruation* refers to a condition occasionally found in adolescent girls in whom monthly epistaxis related to vascular congestion of the nasal mucosa occurs concordant with menses.

EVALUATION AND DECISION

After treating any emergent problems, the evaluation of the child with epistaxis begins with a thorough history (Fig. 18.1). Specific features to be sought include frequency of occurrence, difficulty in control (and adequacy of simple at-home first aid), a history of trauma, nose picking, frequent upper respiratory infection, allergic and chronic discharge, and obstructive symptoms. Often, asking children which finger they pick their noses with will elicit a more honest answer.

Often, parents will note hematemesis or melena, prompting them to seek urgent medical attention. Specific questions regarding evidence for any systemic hemorrhagic disorder or family history of bleeding are asked. In adolescent girls, relation to menses is noted.

Physical examination must include a complete general examination with special attention to vital signs, including blood pressure, evidence of hematologic disease (enlarged nodes, organomegaly, petechiae, or pallor), and, of course, inspection of the nasal cavity after reasonable efforts to stop the bleeding. On examination, one is looking for the site of bleeding, mucosal color, excoriations, discharge, a foreign body or other mass, and septal hematomas.

All patients discharged from the emergency department after evaluation for significant epistaxis should be given specific instructions on nares compression and indications for repeat evaluation. For patients with specific local abnormalities, such as tumors, polyps, or telangiectasias, referral to an otorhinolaryngologist is necessary. Such a referral also might be considered, even with questionable findings on the emergency department nasal examination, if bleeding was severe, recurrent, or suspected to be posterior in origin.

Finally, evaluation for hemorrhagic diathesis should be done in any child with pertinent positive findings on history, family history, or physical examination. This evaluation usually would include prothrombin time, partial thromboplastin time, complete blood count, and bleeding time. Although the yield would be low in the absence of corroborative clinical features, some children with isolated epistaxis that seems particularly severe or frequently recurrent might also deserve such screening.

CHAPTER 19
Eye—Red

Alex V. Levin, M.D.

When approaching the problem of "red eye," it is important to determine which tissues are involved. This chapter is confined to disorders in which the conjunctiva, episclera, or sclera are inflamed, causing the "white of the eye" to appear red or pink. The term *conjunctivitis* should be reserved for disorders in which the conjunctiva is inflamed. Red eyes may be caused by local factors, intraocular disease, or systemic problems. Tables 19.1, 19.2, and 19.3 list common and life-threatening causes of red eye.

TABLE 19.1. Common Causes of Red Eye[a]

Conjunctivitis
Infectious: viral, bacterial, chlamydial
Allergic or seasonal
Chemical (or other physical agents such as smoke)
Systemic disease (see Table 19.3)
Juvenile rheumatoid arthritis with iritis
Varicella with conjunctival lesion
Trauma
Corneal or conjunctival abrasion
Iritis
Foreign body
Dry-eye syndromes
Abnormalities of the lids and/or lashes
Blepharitis
Trichiasis due to epiblepharon
Sty or chalazion (external or internal hordeolum)
Molloscum of lid margin
Periorbital or orbital cellulitis
Contact lens–related problems
Infectious keratitis (corneal ulcer)
Allergic conjunctivitis
Corneal abrasion
Poor fit
Overwear

[a] Not listed in order of frequency. List not meant to be complete.

Often the cause of a red eye can be identified based on the history alone. Attention must be paid to documenting whether the inflammation is unilateral or bilateral, diffuse or sectional, and acute or chronic. When the inflammation is bilateral, it is helpful to know whether both eyes were involved simultaneously or sequentially.

EVALUATION AND DECISION

The approach to the child who presents in the emergency department with a red eye is outlined in the flowchart shown in Figure 19.1. Any child who wears contact lens regularly, even if the lens is not in the eye at the time of the examination, should be referred to an ophthalmologist within 12 hours if he or she has red eye. Other than removing the contact lens when possible (topical anesthesia may be helpful), further diagnostic or therapeutic interventions by the pediatric emergency physician are not indicated in these patients. It is recommended that empiric antibiotics not be started because the ophthalmologist may want to culture the cornea.

Numerous systemic diseases may be associated with ocular inflammation. A representative sample can be found in Table

TABLE 19.2. Life-Threatening Causes of Red Eye[a]

Systemic disease (see Table 19.3)
Child abuse
Blunt trauma
Instillation of noxious substances (Munchausen syndrome by proxy)
Traumatic intracranial arteriovenous fistula (very rare)

[a] List not meant to be complete.

TABLE 19.3. Systemic Conditions That May Be Associated with Red Eye[a]

Collagen vascular disorders
Juvenile rheumatoid arthritis
Infectious diseases
Varicella, measles, mumps, otitis media
Kawasaki disease
Inflammatory bowel disease
Cystic fibrosis
Vitamin A deficiency
Cystinosis
Leukemia
Ectodermal dysplasia
Trisomy 21
Cornelia de Lange syndrome
Status postradiation therapy including ocular field
Bone marrow transplantation
Stevens–Johnson syndrome

[a] Not a complete list: intended to demonstrate multiorgan system representation.

19.3. In some systemic diseases, the associated ocular abnormality involves intraocular inflammation (iritis, vitreitis), which might cause secondary conjunctival infection. Patients with these diseases also may have coincidental ocular inflammation unrelated to their underlying conditions.

Traumatic injury can result in a red eye because of corneal or conjunctival abrasion, hyphema, iritis, or rarely, traumatic glaucoma (Chapter 97). Very rarely, head injury causes the development of an intracranial arteriovenous fistula that may present with proptosis, chemosis, red eye, corkscrew conjunctival blood vessels, and decreased vision. If there is no fluorescein staining of the conjunctiva or cornea and there is no obvious evidence of severe intraocular injury (e.g., hyphema, ruptured globe), the examiner may need to consider the possibility of noxious material coming in contact with the eyeball at the time of trauma. Both acidic and alkaline substances may cause a red eye (Chapter 105). Likewise, a foreign body may cause ocular pain and inflammation. All the recesses and redundant folds of the conjunctiva must be inspected.

It often is wise to inspect the position of the eyelashes before performing these manipulations. Eyelashes that turn against the ocular surface (*trichiasis*) can cause a red eye that is accompanied by pain or foreign-body sensation. The condition may be so mild that slitlamp biomicroscopy is required to detect it, despite significant symptoms. It is particularly common in patients who have had prior injury or surgery to the eyelid and in patients of Asian background.

In the absence of an abrasion of the cornea or conjunctiva, any foreign body, or trichiasis, the painful red eye caused by trauma may have iritis. This may not present for up to 72 hours after the trauma was sustained. Photophobia and visual blurring also may occur. The pupil may be smaller. Occasionally, one sees a cloudy inferior cornea caused by the deposition of inflammatory cells and debris on the inner surface. Iritis also may occur in association with systemic disease or as an isolated idiopathic ocular finding. Traumatic iritis and nontraumatic iritis often are indistinguishable except by history. Topical steroids should not be prescribed by the primary care physician.

Episcleritis and scleritis also may cause a painful red eye. Although episcleritis usually is an isolated ocular abnormality, scleritis often is associated with an underlying systemic disease, particularly the collagen vascular disorders. Both entities may present with focal or diffuse inflammation. A nodular elevation involving the sclera may be seen. The eye may be tender, and the inflamed area may have a bluish hue. There also may be pain on

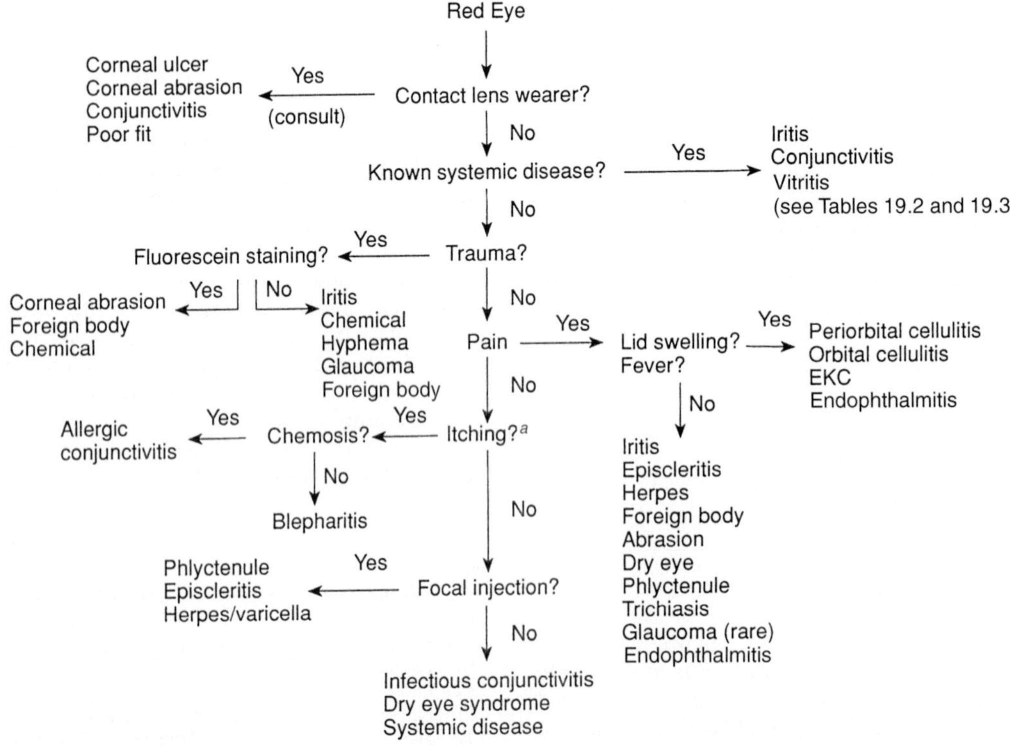

Figure 19.1. Approach to the child with red eye. EKC, epidemic keratoconjunctivitis (adenovirus).

attempted movement of the eye. Diagnosis and treatment require slitlamp examination and ophthalmologic consultation.

Another cause of painful ocular inflammation is herpetic corneal infection, which may be caused by the simplex or varicella-zoster viruses. Usually, there is no concomitant dermatologic manifestation except in association with chickenpox, when a unilateral or bilateral lesion may be seen on the conjunctiva (usually near but not on the cornea) with focal injection. Herpetic corneal ulcers require urgent treatment to prevent corneal scarring and vision loss. Patients with herpetic corneal ulcers may have a history of prior recurrent painful red eye, although herpes occasionally is painless because of induced corneal hypoesthesia. Herpes simplex is virtually always unilateral. Fluorescein staining of the cornea may reveal a linear branching pattern. If the infected area is located eccentrically on the corneal surface, the injection may be localized to the quadrant of conjunctiva adjacent to the lesion.

If eye pain is relieved by a drop of topical anesthetic (Chapter 97), the patient must have a surface problem (e.g., foreign body, abrasion). If the pain is not relieved and periorbital swelling and fever are present, the red eye may be caused by periorbital or orbital cellulitis. These are emergent conditions (Chapter 105). Eye pain and marked lid swelling also may be associated with epidemic keratoconjunctivitis (EKC) secondary to adenovirus. When questioned further, patients may reveal that they actually have a sandy foreign-body sensation rather than true ocular pain. The presence of pseudomembranes is a fairly diagnostic sign. Low-grade fever and tender preauricular adenopathy also may occur, making it difficult to distinguish EKC from periorbital cellulitis; however, EKC usually affects the eyes consecutively and bilaterally. There also may be associated prominent photophobia and tearing, which is not usually seen in cellulitis.

Itching is another important diagnostic symptom. When it is associated with swelling of the conjunctiva, giving it the appearance of a blister-like elevation, allergic conjunctivitis should be suspected. Often there is no known causative agent, and there may be associated periocular swelling. The condition may be unilateral or bilateral and usually has an acute or hyperacute onset. Photophobia, tearing, and lid swelling also may occur. The emergency physician can prescribe topical antihistamines or vasoconstrictors as well as a cool compresses to relieve the symptoms.

Itching also may accompany blepharitis, an idiopathic disorder in which there is suboptimal flow of secretions from the glands normally present in the eyelids. Because these glands participate in the formation of the lubricating tear film that normally covers the eye, the deficiency of flow may result in an abnormal tear film and rapid corneal desiccation. Symptoms are aggravated by activities associated with prolonged staring and a decreased blink rate (reading, television viewing, and video games) or going outside on windy days. Patients may have photophobia and a sandy foreign-body sensation. To compensate for the tear-film deficiency, reflex excess tearing may occur from the lacrimal gland. The most characteristic sign is erythema of all four eyelid margins and flaking and crusting at the base of the eyelashes. Slitlamp examination is helpful in making this diagnosis and is necessary to rule out the presence of corneal involvement.

Although itching and pain may be minor symptoms associated with several types of conjunctivitis, it is usually the absence of these symptoms that should lead to a suspicion of an infectious cause. Conjunctivitis usually causes diffuse inflammation of the conjunctiva, either unilaterally or bilaterally. The differentiation of bacterial, viral, chlamydial, and other types of conjunctivitis sometimes is difficult (Chapter 105). Purulent discharge is particularly characteristic of bacterial infection. Diffuse injection also may be a sign of a previously unrecognized underlying systemic disease.

If the injection is localized, the examiner should consider a specific list of diagnostic possibilities. A phlyctenule appears as a small nodule on the conjunctiva at or near the corneal–conjunctival junction, usually with concomitant blepharitis. It usually represents an immune response to bacteria located on the surface of the eye or eyelid. Episcleritis and scleritis also may manifest with focal involvement, as previously discussed. Localized injection of the conjunctiva may be an indicator of an imbedded foreign body, herpes, chickenpox, or other focal processes that require the attention of an ophthalmologic consultant.

Although much feared, glaucoma in children is very rare. Congenital glaucoma usually is not associated with a red eye or pain. Small children who have glaucoma often have enlarged eyes (*buphthalmos*) with tearing, photophobia, and sometimes heterochromia. Acute acquired glaucoma causes a painful red eye, perhaps associated with corneal clouding and decreased visual acuity. Acquired glaucoma, however, usually is associated with trauma, other anatomic abnormalities, or iritis that would be apparent on examination. Because it is difficult to determine intraocular pressure in children, ophthalmologic consultation is required in all cases.

CHAPTER 20
Eye—Visual Disturbances

Robert A. Felter, M.D.

Sudden loss or deterioration of vision (or *diplopia*) can be caused by numerous diseases and injuries (Tables 20.1–20.3). Although such cases are rare in the pediatric patient, a systematic approach is necessary to reach a correct diagnosis and to minimize permanent visual impairment. The patient's age, underlying disease conditions, visual history, and history of possible injury must be determined. It is important to remember that up to 5% of abused children present with ocular injuries and 40% of abused children will have ocular findings. The recent increase in survival of extremely low–birth weight infants has led to many children with varying degrees of visual disturbances that may not be readily noticed. The extent of the visual impairment and the rapidity of its onset also are vital pieces of information. A careful eye examination, including gross and ophthalmoscopic examination, determination of extraocular movement, and visual acuity, together with the history, leads to correct diagnosis and management of the patient (see Chapter 105).

Few ocular conditions in the pediatric population are truly emergent (Table 20.4), but many are urgent; most can be treated by the emergency physician or can be referred for appropriate follow-up with an ophthalmologist. Many conditions that a pediatric ophthalmologist sees are not discussed here because they rarely are seen in the emergency department. Such conditions include congenital eye disorders and amblyopia. Sudden onset of diplopia may be secondary to many of the conditions listed, as a direct effect of trauma, infection, central nervous system pathology (tumor or shunt malfunction), or hysterical reaction. Likewise, head tilt may represent a visual disturbance and requires a complete ophthalmologic evaluation, although the condition also may be caused by musculoskeletal problems in the neck. Conditions that are more likely

TABLE 20.1. Causes of Acute Visual Disturbances

	Traumatic	Nontraumatic
Periorbital	Eyelid hematoma, edema from trauma	Orbital or periorbital cellulitis, tumor, allergic edema
Cornea and conjunctiva	Chemical burns, thermal burns, ultraviolet or infrared burns, laceration of cornea	Conjunctivitis (bacterial, viral, fungal)
Anterior chamber	Traumatic iritis, hyphema, posttraumatic cataract, dislocation of lens, glaucoma	Acute iritis, glaucoma, uveitis
Posterior chamber	Vitreous hemorrhage	Endophthalmitis
Retina	Severed retinal artery, retinal tears or detachment, commotio retinae	Retinal vein or artery obstruction, spontaneous
Cortex	Head trauma	Optic neuritis, toxins, hysteria, hypoglycemia, leukemia, cerebrovascular accidents, migraine
Other	Carotid artery trauma	Poisoning, shunt malfunction, vitamin A deficiencies, measles

to be seen in the emergency department are emphasized in this chapter.

DIFFERENTIAL DIAGNOSIS

Trauma and infections are the two most common causes of acute visual impairment in otherwise healthy children seen in the emergency department, and these two processes can interfere with any part or all of the visual pathway (Tables 20.1 and 20.2). Children with shunts for hydrocephalus may have a variety of visual disturbances—from complete blindness to transient diplopia. Any child with an acute visual disturbance and a shunt must undergo evaluation of the functioning of the shunt.

Vision may be limited by periorbital diseases such as orbital cellulitis, tumor, or infection or swelling of the eyelids. The history and physical examination usually make these diagnoses obvious. Blunt trauma to the eye may cause a blowout fracture of the orbit. Visual impairment may be limited to double vision when the patient is looking in a certain direction, particularly upward. Testing the extraocular movements reveals the limitation. Careful inspection of the globe also is necessary.

Diseases of the cornea that cause visual impairment are predominantly infectious or traumatic. Infections of the cornea and conjunctiva can be caused by bacteria, viruses, and fungi (see Chapters 19 and 105). All these diseases may present as a unilateral or bilateral process, usually affecting only the conjunctiva and cornea. Onset is variable but usually occurs over 1 or 2 days, and vision is not greatly impaired. With a recent eye injury or foreign-body intrusion, fungal infections are possible. In the United States, the most common corneal infection that causes permanent visual impairment is herpes simplex. A careful ophthalmoscopic or slitlamp examination will reveal the characteristic dendritic ulcers of herpes simplex infection after the eye has been stained with fluorescein.

Traumatic injuries to the cornea include one of the true ophthalmologic emergencies: alkali burns. Alkali burns in general carry a worse prognosis than acid burns. Rapid treatment of this condition is imperative to prevent permanent visual impairment. The cause of the chemical injury usually is obvious from the history. Both ultraviolet and infrared light can cause damage to the cornea, resulting in severe pain and photophobia within 24 hours of exposure. Lacerations with perforation of the cornea usually affect other parts of the eye as well and can lead to significant visual impairment. Careful inspection of the globe with associated lid trauma is mandatory.

The anterior chamber of the eye consists of the aqueous humor, the iris, and the lens. Acute iritis is rare in children, and the cause often is uncertain. There is a sudden onset of pain, redness, and photophobia that usually affects one eye only. The degree of visual impairment varies with the severity of the inflammation. Certain diseases have associated iritis, such as juvenile rheumatoid arthritis. Blunt trauma also can cause iritis, but vision is only slightly impaired unless other structures are involved. Trauma also can cause a hyphema or hemorrhage into the anterior chamber. This can result in little to severe visual impairment in the affected eye, depending on the extent of bleeding and associated trauma. Traumatic injuries

TABLE 20.2. Common Conditions That Cause Acute Visual Disturbances

Trauma
Chemical burns
Hyphema
Rupture of globes
Periorbital infection
Conjunctivitis

TABLE 20.3. Causes of Acute Diplopla

Blowout fractures
Poisoning
Central nervous system pathology (tumor, bleed)
Shunt malfunction
Exercise
Arnold-Chiari malformation
Myasthenia gravis
Head trauma

TABLE 20.4. Emergent Conditions That Cause Visual Disturbances
Alkali or acid burns
Central retinal artery occlusion

can lead to cataract formation, usually within a few days of injury, but onset may be delayed for years. Dislocation of the lens after trauma causes significant visual impairment but can be recognized easily with a careful examination. Glaucoma and a retinal detachment may be late complications of blunt trauma. Congenital glaucoma is a major preventable cause of blindness in children; most cases manifest within the first 6 months of life. Corneal clouding, buphthalmos, or asymmetry in eye size may be the chief complaint. If any one of these is noted as a primary complaint or an incidental finding, immediate referral is required.

Injury or infection that involves the anterior chamber may lead to increased intraocular pressure. Glaucoma may become evident days to years after the initial trauma or infection. Pain around the eye, blurred vision, and, occasionally, nausea and vomiting in a patient with glaucoma or a recent eye injury may represent an acute attack of glaucoma. The diagnosis is made easily with tonometry.

The uvea consists of the iris, ciliary body, and choroid. One or all portions of the uvea may become inflamed, causing uveitis. Iritis and iridocyclitis may be called *anterior uveitis*, whereas inflammation of the choroid is often called *posterior uveitis*. The etiologies may be divided into *infectious* and *noninfectious*. Infectious uveitis may be caused by viruses, bacteria, fungi, or helminths. The most common cause of posterior uveitis in children is toxoplasmosis; *Toxocara canis* is second. Noninfectious causes include sarcoidosis and sympathetic ophthalmia. Measles, mumps, and pertussis may be associated with uveitis that is not the result of invasion by the agent causing the infection. Vogt–Koyanagi–Harada syndrome is a panuveitis with meningeal and cutaneous findings. Prompt treatment of this syndrome is necessary for optimal visual outcome.

In addition to blurred vision in one or both eyes, anterior uveitis also is associated with pain in the affected eye, headache, photophobia, and conjunctival injection. Anterior uveitis may be confused with conjunctivitis or an acute attack of glaucoma. In posterior uveitis, the pain and photophobia may be less pronounced, but there may be a more pronounced visual impairment.

The posterior chamber is composed of the vitreous humor. The vitreous gel usually is clear, and any diseases that affect the clarity will impair vision. Certain chronic conditions such as uveitis can cause deposits in the vitreous humor, but the visual impairment is very gradual. Infections inside the eye (*endophthalmitis*) usually result from a penetrating injury, surgery, or an extension of a more superficial infection. Bacterial infections develop more rapidly than do fungal infections. The child will have severe pain in or around the eye and, with bacterial infections especially, may have fever and leukocytosis. The process usually is unilateral, and vision is severely compromised. Purulent exudate is formed in the vitreous humor, and ophthalmoscopic examination may reveal a greenish color with the details of the retina lost. A *hypopyon*—that is, accumulation of pus in the anterior chamber—usually is present.

Either penetrating or blunt trauma (see Chapter 97) to the eye can lead to vitreous hemorrhage, but this is uncommon in children. Diabetes mellitus, hypertension, sickle cell disease, and leukemia may cause vitreous hemorrhage as well as retinal tears, central retinal vein occlusion, and tumor. There is a sudden loss or deterioration of vision in the affected eye. Findings on examination depend on the degree of hemorrhage. Blood clots may be visible with the ophthalmoscope, or the fundus reflex may be black, obscuring the retina in more severe cases.

Retinal vein and artery obstruction also are uncommon in pediatric patients. With central retinal artery occlusion, there is a sudden, painless, total loss of vision in one eye. If only a branch is occluded, a field loss will result. Ophthalmoscopic examination reveals the cherry-red spot of the fovea, the optic nerve appears pale white, and the arteries are narrowed significantly. A Marcus–Gunn pupil (relative afferent defect) may be present and may be diagnosed by shining a light in one eye, then in the other. When the light is shone in the normal eye, both pupils will constrict. When light is shone in the damaged eye, the pupil will dilate.

The retinal artery may be severed by trauma or obstructed by emboli, as in a patient with endocardial thrombi or arterial obstructions in systemic lupus erythematosus (SLE) and in diseases with hypercoagulability, such as sickle cell disease. The arterial spasm associated with migraine may lead to retinal artery obstruction.

As with retinal artery occlusion, retinal vein occlusion causes a painless loss of vision. Visual loss may be severe, with total occlusion of the central retinal vein, or it may be less pronounced, with branch obstruction. Examination of the retina reveals multiple hemorrhages with a blurred, reddened optic disc. The arteries are narrowed, the veins engorged, and patchy white exudates may be evident. These findings will be limited to one area in branch occlusion. Retinal vein obstruction, although rare, may occur with trauma or diseases such as leukemia, cystic fibrosis, or retinal phlebitis.

As mentioned, a tear in the retina may lead to vitreous hemorrhage, causing decreased vision in the affected eye. If the tear is in the macula, the visual loss will be severe. A tear in the retina may not cause immediate visual impairment. Retinal detachment from a retinal tear may be delayed for years. The visual impairment may go unnoticed if the detachment is peripheral. As the detachment progresses or when it involves more central areas, the patient will complain of cloudy vision with lightning flashes (*photopsia*). This may be followed by a shadow or curtain in the visual field. Visual acuity may remain normal if the macula is not involved. Examination of the eye will reveal a lighter appearing retina in the area of detachment, and it may have folds. Flashing lights or visual-field defects, after trauma, should raise the suspicion of retinal detachment. Retinoschisis, splitting of the layers of the retina, may be seen in the shaken baby syndrome.

Commotio retinae, or Berlin edema—that is, edema of the retina—may follow blunt ocular trauma by 24 hours. The visual loss is variable, and the retina will appear pale gray because of the edema, but the macula usually is spared.

Optic neuritis is involvement of the optic nerve by inflammation or demyelinization. The process usually is acute and may be unilateral or bilateral. Loss of vision may take from hours to days, and visual impairment ranges from mild loss to complete blindness. Patients often complain of disturbance of color vision. Pain may be absent or present on movement of the eye or palpation of the globe. It rarely is an isolated event in children. Causes include meningitis, viral infections, immunizations, encephalomyelitis, Lyme disease, and demyelinating diseases. Exogenous toxins and drugs (e.g., lead poisoning, long-term chloramphenicol treatment) also may cause optic neuritis.

Various toxins are capable of causing impaired vision. The loss may be gradual or sudden, depending on the particular

TABLE 20.5. Causes of Cortical Blindness

Cardiac arrest
Status epilepticus
Hypoxia
Perinatal asphyxia
Cerebral infarction
Meningitis
Encephalitis
Subacute sclerosing leukoencephalitis
Hypoglycemia
Uremia
Hydrocephalus
Shunt malfunction
Head trauma
Cardiac surgery
Cerebral or vertebral angiography
Drugs (steroids)
Carbon monoxide poisoning
Occipital epilepsy
Postictal states

toxin. Toxins usually act on ganglion cells of the retina or on optic nerve fibers, causing contraction of the peripheral field, central visual defect, or a combination. Methyl alcohol, when ingested, may cause bilateral sudden blindness, which may be complete and permanent or may have a more gradual onset. With methyl alcohol ingestion, associated symptoms include nausea, vomiting, abdominal pain, headache, dizziness, delirium, and convulsions. Other toxins include halogenated hydrocarbons, sulfanilamide, quinine, and quinidine. Large doses of salicylates may cause amblyopia. Digitalis may cause transient amblyopia, visual blurring, or the perception of yellow halos around light (*xanthopsia*).

Visual impairment also may result from interference with the visual cortex of the brain. Cortical blindness has many causes (Table 20.5). Head trauma (see Chapters 31 and 92) may cause total loss of vision soon after the event. This has been called *footballer migraine* because of its association with head trauma in soccer. Even trivial head trauma has been known to cause blindness. The apparent hysterical reaction that follows head trauma, especially in young children, may represent complete blindness in a child unable to express the problem or who is too frightened by the experience. The physical examination may be completely normal. There may be a delay of onset, but the entire course is usually brief, lasting minutes to hours. This form of blindness often is confused with hysterical blindness, the latter being a diagnosis of exclusion. Monocular blindness may be caused by trauma to the carotid artery on the affected side.

Migraine headaches are a common cause of bilateral field loss (*hemianopsia*) in adolescents. This field loss usually lasts less than 1 hour. It almost always is misidentified by the patient as loss of vision in only one eye. Headache and nausea after such an episode are the rule but occasionally may be absent.

EVALUATION AND DECISION

The absolute ophthalmologic emergencies are alkali burns, a ruptured globe, and retinal artery occlusion. The diagnosis of the first is by history, and therapy must be initiated promptly to minimize the damage to the eye. If there is any doubt about the actual substance to which the eyes have been exposed, treatment for an alkali burn is always prudent. A ruptured globe must be suspected with any possible penetrating injury to the eye. The injury may be subtle, and the vision may be normal. If a possibility of a ruptured globe exists, the eye should be protected and the patient should have immediate evaluation by an ophthalmologist. Retinal artery thrombosis is rare in children, but it should be suspected when there is sudden, unilateral painless loss of vision and a predisposing condition. Predisposing conditions include those associated with emboli, such as endocardial thrombi or amniotic fluid; conditions with arteritis leading to obstruction, as in SLE; disease states associated with hypercoagulability, such as sickling hemoglobinopathies; and conditions with arterial spasm, such as severe hypertension.

If alkali burns, a ruptured globe, and retinal artery occlusion can be excluded, the patient may be evaluated more carefully before instituting therapy. When visual acuity is being determined, the history may be obtained. Significant historical information includes episodes of recent trauma, unilateral or bilateral nature of the loss, and association of pain in or around the eye (Fig. 20.1). Most children seen in the ED will have a traumatic or infectious process.

SEVERE VISUAL LOSS ASSOCIATED WITH TRAUMA

Severe bilateral visual loss associated with trauma is the result of head trauma, causing cortical blindness. This condition usually is totally reversible in less than a few hours.

Any of the traumatic injuries that cause severe unilateral loss of vision may cause bilateral loss if both eyes are involved. The mechanism of injury should be determined. If there is any possibility of a penetrating injury or rupture of the globe, the involved eye should be protected from further damage by shielding until a careful examination can be performed by a skilled physician. If the globe is intact and no penetration by a foreign body occurred, an ophthalmoscopic or slitlamp examination usually leads to the correct diagnosis. These conditions include chemical burns of the cornea, hyphema, dislocation of the lens, vitreous hemorrhage, detachment or tear of the retina, and commotio retinae.

SEVERE VISUAL LOSS NOT ASSOCIATED WITH TRAUMA

With severe bilateral visual loss not associated with trauma, the possibility of toxins must be explored. Also, cortical blindness may cause a similar picture, but this is rare and generally associated with another problem, such as hypoglycemia, leukemia, and cerebrovascular or anesthetic accidents. If severe visual loss is unilateral and painful, endophthalmitis must be suspected, but once again, such loss usually is the result of a previous penetrating injury or an extension of a local infectious process. If a headache is associated with the visual loss, migraine may be implicated. If the severe loss is unilateral and painless, retinal artery or vein occlusion or retinal detachment may be diagnosed by ophthalmoscopic examination. Optic neuritis will also present this way.

MILD VISUAL LOSS WITH TRAUMA

If the visual loss is unilateral, not severe, and if trauma recently occurred, corneal abrasions, traumatic cataracts, and small hyphemas should be sought. A blowout fracture may cause

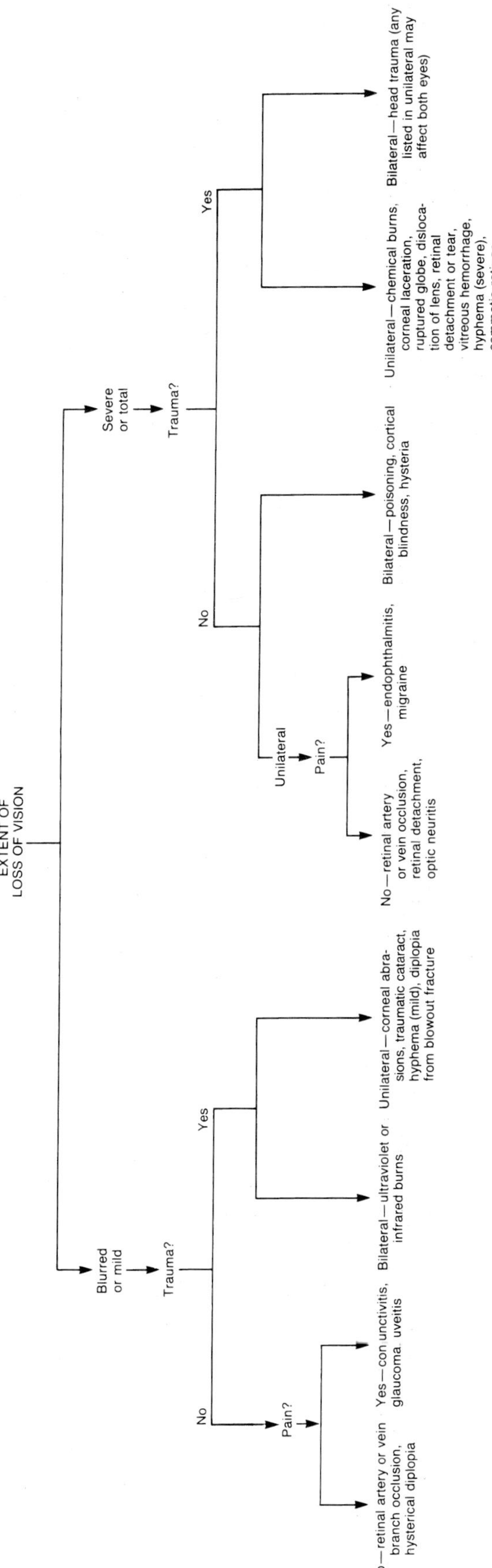

Figure 20.1. Diagnostic approach to visual disturbances.

diplopia, but if each eye is examined individually, the visual acuity should be normal. If the process is bilateral, exposure to ultraviolet or infrared light should be considered.

MILD VISUAL LOSS WITHOUT TRAUMA

When the visual loss is mild and nontraumatic, and if the process is unilateral and painful, conjunctivitis, uveitis, and acute attacks of glaucoma are possible. If the process is painless, retinal vein or artery branch occlusion may be suspected. Any of these processes may be bilateral as well.

CHAPTER 21
Fever

Elizabeth R. Alpern, M.D. and
Fred M. Henretig, M.D.

Fever, the abnormal elevation of body temperature, has been recognized for centuries by physicians as a sign of disease. Furthermore, the problem of the febrile child is one of the most commonly encountered in clinical pediatrics, accounting for as many as 20% of pediatric emergency department (ED) visits. The approach outlined in this chapter helps the physician treat a febrile child in the ED and proceed systematically with the appropriate diagnostic steps and the institution of therapy. The principal causes of fever in children are listed in Table 21.1.

EVALUATION AND DECISION

The physician caring for a febrile child should concentrate on discovering the cause of the fever and treating the underlying illness. Any fever may signify serious infection; however, severe *hyperpyrexia*, defined as a temperature of 41.1°C (106°F) or higher, more often is associated with diagnoses of pneumonia, bacteremia, or meningitis. If no specific treatment for the determined diagnosis is necessary, the physician's goal is then to provide appropriate supportive care and follow-up.

A complete history and physical examination will provide most important clues in determining the diagnosis of children with febrile illnesses. The general impression obtained in the first few moments of an evaluation is extremely important in the recognition of potentially life-threatening causes of fever (Table 21.2). Signs of severe or life-threatening infections heralded by fever should be sought early in the examination. Central nervous system infections may be marked by fever with altered sensorium, convulsion, meningismus, or focal neurologic deficits. Children younger than 2 years of age with meningitis, however, often do not have meningismus, but they may instead have irritability, anorexia, lethargy, vomiting, or a bulging fontanelle. Severe upper airway infections may manifest with stridor, excessive drooling, and tripod positioning. A child with pneumonia, pericarditis, endocarditis, or sepsis syndrome may display dyspnea or tachypnea, cyanosis or pallor, tachycardia, and hypotension, as well as altered mental status. Hemorrhagic rashes may signal bacterial or rickettsial infections such as meningococcemia or Rocky Mountain spotted fever.

Although the index of suspicion for serious febrile illness must be high throughout the evaluation of each child, most

TABLE 21.1. Principal Conditions Associated with Fever in Children

Infections
- Central nervous system
  - Meningitis
  - Encephalitis
  - Brain abscess
- Ocular
  - Periorbital (preseptal) cellulitis
  - Orbital cellulitis/abscess
- Airways and upper respiratory tract
  - Common cold (upper respiratory infection)
  - Pharyngitis/tonsillitis
  - Otitis media
  - Acute cervical adenitis
  - Acute sinusitis
  - Peritonsillar, retropharyngeal, lateral pharyngeal wall abscess
  - Croup
  - Epiglottitis
- Oral cavity and salivary glands
  - Alveolar abscess
  - Viral stomatitis (herpangina, herpetic gingivostomatitis)
  - Parotitis (mumps, acute suppurative parotitis)
- Pulmonary
  - Bronchiolitis
  - Pneumonia bronchitis
  - Pulmonary tuberculosis
  - Lung abscess
- Cardiac
  - Myocarditis
  - Endocarditis
  - Pericarditis
- Gastrointestinal
  - Acute gastroenteritis (viral, salmonella, shigella)
  - Appendicitis
  - Peritonitis
  - Pancreatitis
  - Acute mesenteric adenitis
  - Hepatitis
  - Cholangitis
  - Intra-abdominal abscesses
- Genitourinary
  - Urinary tract infection/pyelonephritis
  - Perinephric abscess
  - Acute salpingitis, tuboovarian abscess
  - Acute prostatitis
  - Epididymitis, orchitis
- Musculoskeletal
  - Septic arthritis
  - Osteomyelitis
  - Myositis
- Cutaneous
  - Cellulitis
  - Necrotizing fasciitis
  - Exanthems (systemic infections usually associated with prominent rashes)
    - Viral: roseola, rubeola, rubella, varicella, hand-foot-mouth disease (coxsackievirus)
    - Bacterial toxin: scarlet fever
  - Syphilis (secondary)
  - Meningococcemia (occasionally other primary septicemia)
  - Rocky Mountain spotted fever
  - Systemic infections
    - Bacterial sepsis (primary–especially meningococcemia)
    - "Occult bacteremia" (especially pneumococcal)
    - Viruses (Epstein–Barr, adenovirus) Lyme disease
    - Rickettsial (Rocky Mountain, spotted fever, ehrlichiosis), chlamydial, fungal, parasitic, and unusual bacterial infections
    - Toxic shock syndrome
    - Miliary tuberculosis

Vasculitis syndromes and hypersensitivity phenomena
- Acute rheumatic fever
- Juvenile rheumatoid arthritis
- Systemic lupus erythematosus
- Polyarteritis nodosa
- Kawasaki disease
- Dermatomyositis/polymyositis
- Mixed connective tissue disease
- Henoch-Schönlein purpura
- Serum sickness
- Stevens–Johnson syndrome
- Drug and immunization reactions

Neoplasms
- Leukemia
- Neuroblastoma
- Lymphoma
- Ewing's sarcoma

Poisonings
- Atropine poisoning
- Salicylate poisoning
- Cocaine poisoning
- Amphetamine poisoning
- LSD poisoning
- Miscellaneous drug (e.g., phenothiazines, antidepressants and others with anticholinergic effect)

Central nervous system (CNS) disorders
- CNS lesions in hypothalamus/brainstem
- Prolonged seizures
- Riley–Day syndrome

Metabolic diseases
- Thyrotoxic crisis
- Etiocholanolone fever
- Acute intermittent porphyria

Miscellaneous conditions
- Dehydration
- Intravascular hemolysis
- Hemorrhage into an enclosed space
- Anhydrotic ectodermal dysplasia
- Extreme environmental heat excess
- Familial Mediterranean fever
- Sarcoidosis
- Chronic inflammatory bowel disease
- Factitious
- Major trauma (crush injuries)
- Other rare causes

CNS, central nervous system.

childhood illnesses with fever are minor and self-limiting. Once the physician has ascertained that the child is not in immediate danger, the examination should focus on sites of common pediatric infections, including the ears, nose, and throat; cervical lymph nodes; respiratory, gastrointestinal, and genitourinary tracts; and skin, joints, and skeletal system. (Table 21.3).

Many febrile exanthems are characteristic enough to be diagnostic (see Chapters 53–56, 58, and 74). Varicella, rubeola, scarlet fever, and Coxsackievirus all can be identified by their pathognomonic rashes. If a child with chickenpox presents several days into the illness with a new fever, the possibility of group A β-hemolytic streptococcal co-infection needs to be fully evaluated. Children with fever and petechiae may have invasive meningococcal disease, disseminated streptococcal infection, or Rocky Mountain spotted fever; however, they also may simply have a less serious viral infection or streptococcal pharyngitis.

TABLE 21.2. Life-Threatening Acute Febrile Illnesses

Infection
- Central nervous system
  - Acute bacterial meningitis
  - Encephalitis
- Upper airway
  - Acute epiglottitis
  - Retropharyngeal abscess
  - Laryngeal diphtheria (rare)
  - Croup (severe)
- Pulmonary
  - Pneumonia (severe)
  - Tuberculosis, miliary
- Cardiac
  - Myocarditis
  - Bacterial endocarditis
  - Suppurative pericarditis
- Gastrointestinal
  - Acute gastroenteritis (fluid/electrolyte losses)
  - Appendicitis
  - Peritonitis (other causes)
- Musculoskeletal
  - Necrotizing myositis (gas gangrene)/fasciitis
- Systemic
  - Meningococcemia
  - Other bacterial sepsis
  - Rocky Mountain spotted fever
  - Toxic shock syndrome

Collagen-vascular
- Acute rheumatic fever
- Kawasaki disease
- Stevens-Johnson syndrome

Miscellaneous
- Thyrotoxicosis
- Heat stroke
- Acute poisoning: atropine, aspirin, amphetamine, cocaine
- Malignancy

Differentiation of these entities is crucial and is based on the clinical appearance of the patient and laboratory evaluation. A child with petechiae only above the nipple line, normal white blood cell (WBC) count, and well appearance is less likely to have invasive disease. Any child who appears ill, has a laboratory abnormality, or has progressive petechial rash needs a full evaluation, including lumbar puncture and antibiotic administration.

Recent public health measures have changed the frequency and risk of certain febrile illness in children. A published report from the Centers for Disease Control and Prevention revealed that the *Haemophilus influenzae* type B vaccine has drastically changed the risk and causative agents for meningitis in children. There has been a 94% reduction in the incidence of *H. influenzae* meningitis and a shift in the median age of those affected from 15 months to 25 years of age. The current rarity of epiglottitis in children is also due to this decline in *H. influenzae* infections. Recognition of this epidemiologic change is crucial in evaluating and treating the febrile child. An analogous, although less complete, reduction in infections due to *Streptococcus pneumoniae* is currently under way following the introduction in the year 2000 of a vaccine effective against seven of the most prevalent pneumococcal serotypes.

Both *H. influenzae* and *S. pneumoniae* historically have caused the great majority of cases of occult bacteremia, defined as the presence of pathogenic bacteria in the blood of a well-appearing febrile child in the absence of an identifiable focus of infection (see Chapter 74). Children most commonly suspected to be at risk for occult bacteremia are those between the ages of 3 and 36 months with a temperature of 39° C (102.2° F) or higher. Traditional estimates of the incidence of bacteremia, in the range of 1.5% to 3% of highly febrile children aged 3 to 36 months, are in the process of being revised downward. Infants younger than 3 months, who are susceptible to infections with gram-negative enteric rods and group B streptococcus, remain at increased risk for invasive disease and therefore necessitate different evaluation and treatment.

Given these general considerations, an algorithmic approach to the child with an acute (< 5 days) febrile illness can be formulated by using the following key features: overall degree of toxicity and presence of signs or symptoms of life-threatening disease, immunocompromised host status, patient's age, degree of fever, and presence of localizing features on history and physical examination (Fig. 21.1). Laboratory studies are indicated

TABLE 21.3. Common Causes of Fever

Infections
- Central nervous system
  - Acute bacterial meningitis
  - Viral meningoencephalitis
- Ocular
  - Periorbital cellulitis
  - Orbital cellulitis
- Upper respiratory tract
  - Common cold
  - Pharyngitis/tonsillitis
  - Cervical adenitis
  - Croup
  - Acute sinusitis
  - Otitis media
- Oral cavity and salivary glands
  - Alveolar abscess
  - Herpangina
  - Herpetic gingivostomatitis
  - Mumps (unimmunized child)
- Pulmonary
  - Acute tracheobronchitis
  - Bronchiolitis
  - Pneumonia
- Gastrointestinal
  - Acute gastroenteritis
  - Appendicitis Tubo-ovarian abscess
- Genitourinary
  - Urinary tract infection
  - Acute salpingitis
- Musculoskeletal
  - Septic arthritis
  - Osteomyelitis
- Cutaneous
  - Cellulitis
  - Viral exanthems (esp. varicella, measles if unimmunized)
  - Scarlet fever
  - Miscellaneous systemic infections associated with prominent rash (e.g., meningococcemia and Rocky Mountain spotted fever)
- Systemic
  - Primary septicemia-especially meningococcemia
  - "Occult" bacteremia-especially pneumococcal
  - Viral syndromes Vector-borne disease-especially Lyme toxic shock syndrome

Miscellaneous
- Drug and vaccine reactions, including serum sickness
- Kawasaki disease
- Salicylate poisoning

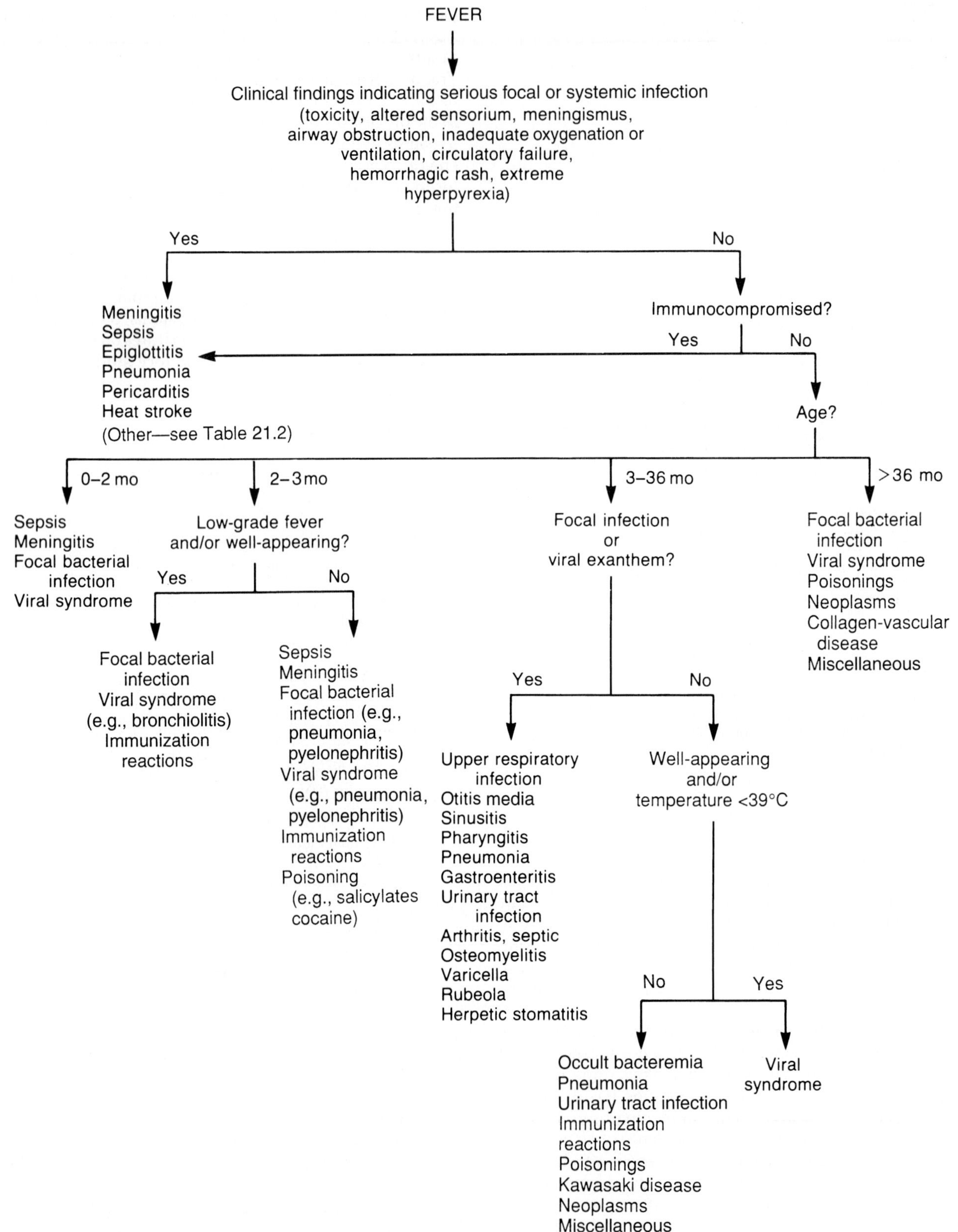

Figure 21.1. Approach to the evaluation of the febrile child.

only for selected situations as defined by these clinical features. Most older febrile children seen in the ED need no ancillary testing.

Infants less than 2 months of age are at increased risk of serious bacterial infections and bacteremia and are more difficult to assess clinically than older children. Thus, all children with temperatures of 38°C (100.4°F) or higher who are less than 2 months of age should receive full laboratory investigation for serious infection ("sepsis workup"), including CBC, blood culture, urine analysis, urine culture, and lumbar puncture with cerebrospinal fluid (CSF) for cell count, glucose, protein, and culture. Infants less than 1 month old are usually admitted to the hospital for observation with presumptive antibiotic therapy. Herpes simplex virus polymerase chain reaction or culture with presumptive antiviral treatment should be considered in neonates with historical concerns or physical findings of skin, eye, or mouth lesions; respiratory distress; seizures; or signs of sepsis. Stool for leukocytes and culture should be obtained if diarrhea is present. A recent meta-analysis showed that respiratory findings are good predictors of clinically significant positive chest radiographs in children less than 3 months of age. Therefore, chest radiographs may be obtained only when there are clinically evident respiratory symptoms. In children 1 to 2 months of age, a standardized observation scale (Yale Observation Scale) is not sensitive enough on its own to identify serious illness. Many recent studies have found that children between 1 and 2 months of age, not pretreated with any antibiotics, and who have a pristine physical examination and completely benign laboratory evaluation may be safely discharged home with careful observation and close follow-up. For such a disposition, parents should be able to watch the infant closely for changes in symptoms, should have ready access to health care, and should be willing to return for evaluation. Other studies have shown that empiric intramuscular ceftriaxone offers a safe and effective management strategy in this age group, particularly when close follow-up is less assured.

An additional dilemma involves the young infant who is described as having either tactile fever alone or fever confirmed by rectal temperature at home but who is afebrile on arrival. Although there is no consensus on the approach to this situation, it seems prudent to consider a careful clinical evaluation in all young infants with a history of fever, including one or more repeat temperature measurements over 1 to 2 hours in the ED after the baby is unbundled. If there is a reliable history of elevated rectal temperature, a sepsis workup should be considered seriously, along with a subsequent disposition based on the evolution of temperature pattern, clinical findings, and laboratory results. The infant with only a history of tactile fever whose repeated temperatures are normal and who has an entirely normal clinical evaluation may be assessed as not requiring laboratory studies.

Children between 2 and 3 months of age are evaluated clinically for the degree of fever and the degree of irritability. Occasionally, an infant at this age may truly "look great," despite having significant fever, and will be judged as requiring symptomatic treatment only without aggressive laboratory investigation or hospitalization. A sepsis workup, however, should be done for infants with high fever and mild to moderate irritability or a full fontanelle. These infants should be hospitalized if signs of a serious bacterial infection (e.g., cellulitis, pneumonia, septic arthritis, osteomyelitis, urinary tract infection, or UTI) are present. If all laboratory results are normal, such a child may be discharged on symptomatic treatment or antibiotics or both if a minor infectious focus (i.e., otitis media) is found. Even with normal laboratory parameters, however, these patients are at risk for bacteremia and subsequent focal infection, including meningitis. Therefore, it has been our tendency to admit infants who are aged 2 to 3 months who have fever and marked irritability, even when CBC and CSF are initially normal.

The febrile child between 3 and 36 months of age with signs of focal infection (e.g., irritability, meningismus, tachypnea, flank tenderness) should be evaluated with the appropriate diagnostic tests and treated for the identified infection. If a child with a temperature of 39°C (102°F) or higher does not have localizing symptoms or laboratory or radiograph results indicative of definitive focal infection, this child should be evaluated with a blood culture for occult bacteremia unless he or she is over 6 months of age and fully immunized against both *H. influenzae* and *S. pneumoniae*.

There has been considerable controversy in the literature about the appropriate initial treatment of children at risk of such occult bacteremia (see Chapter 74). Currently, several options are available to physicians facing this common but challenging situation in the ED (see Chapter 74). One approach is to obtain a blood culture and provide expectant therapy without antibiotics, including antipyretics, close observation for progression of symptoms, and reevaluation for any positive culture. A multivariable model was designed to predict occult pneumococcal bacteremia in children aged 3 to 36 months with temperatures of 39°C or higher and without focal infection. Age less than 24 months, high temperature, and absolute neutrophil count of 10,000/mm^3 or more (WBC 15,000/mm^3 or more) were identified as independent predictors of occult pneumococcal bacteremia and therefore may help delineate patients at highest risk. Others have differed with the published clinical practice guidelines regarding empiric antibiotic therapy, and even to the necessity of obtaining blood cultures in children who do not appear toxic.

An overall prevalence of occult UTI in young children without an identified source of infection has been established to be between 3% and 5%. The risk is highest in febrile white girls less younger than 2 years and in uncircumcised boys younger than 1 year. Laboratory testing is indicated for young febrile children without an identifiable focus of infection. One approach is to obtain a urinalysis and urine culture in febrile boys less than 6 months of age as well as in any age febrile boy who is uncircumcised and not yet toilet trained. Febrile girls less than 2 years of age should undergo urine studies if any two of the following characteristics are present: fever of 39°C (102.2°F) or higher, 1 year of age or younger; white, fever lasting 2 days or longer; or no identifiable source of infection. Aseptic urethral catheterization or suprapubic aspiration is an appropriate method to obtain urine for the diagnosis of UTIs. Positive dipstick urinalysis with microscopic evidence of pyuria (≥5 WBC per high-power field) or any bacteria per high-power field has a sensitivity between 65 and 83; therefore, urinalysis alone is not adequate to diagnose UTI. Urine dipstick and culture should be performed for all children at significant risk for occult UTI (see Chapter 74).

Simple febrile seizures occur in 3% to 5% of all children (see Chapter 61). The dilemma that faces the emergency physician is to decide whether a febrile seizure is truly such or if a child presenting with a fever and seizure requires a lumbar puncture to rule out meningitis. The threshold to perform a lumbar puncture should be extremely low in children younger than 12 months of age (because of the difficulty in recognizing the signs and symptoms of meningitis in very young infants) and in children pretreated with antibiotics (because symptoms of partially treated meningitis may be minimal or absent). Children with atypical febrile seizures should be closely evaluated for CNS infection and a lumbar puncture strongly considered.

Children older than 36 months of age usually can be managed on the basis of degree of irritability, evidence of meningeal signs, and other foci of infection found on history and physical examination. These children need not be screened routinely for occult bacteremia. After excluding meningitis, there are several important infections that may be present in ill-appearing, febrile children in this age group, without obvious initial focus. These include meningococcemia, Rocky Mountain spotted fever, salmonellosis or shigellosis, and pyelonephritis (see Chapter

74). Early institution of presumptive therapy may be lifesaving in some of these situations; so their possibility must be borne in mind with toxic, febrile children of any age. Obviously, if certain high-risk features are missed during the initial triage (or evolve after triage) and are encountered early during the physician's careful clinical assessment (e.g., a significant hemorrhagic rash), the child must be managed with extreme urgency (as befits the reclassification into the high-risk category).

Other causes of acute febrile episodes should be kept in mind, including intoxications, environmental exposure, and immunization reactions. Poisonous exposures to aspirin, atropinic agents, amphetamines, antihistamines, and cocaine present with hyperpyrexia (see Chapter 78). Additional uncommon febrile drug reactions include the serotonin syndrome occurring with the combined use of monoamine oxidase inhibitors and analgesic, antitussive, or psychotropic serotonergic medications (e.g., meperidine, dextromethorphan, fluoxetine), and the neuroleptic malignant syndrome (see Chapter 78). A history of environmental exposure in the face of severe hyperpyrexia may represent heat stroke rather than an infectious cause for the increased temperature (see Chapter 79). The diphtheria–pertussis–tetanus immunization is associated with fever that occurs within 48 hours (occurring less often with DTaP vaccine administration). Fever, at times accompanied by a faint rash, may occur 7 to 10 days after immunization with the live-attenuated measles vaccine or the measles–mumps–rubella vaccine.

Fevers of unknown origin are defined as daily temperatures of 38.5°C (101.3°F) or higher for at least 2 weeks without discernible cause. Infections commonly causing prolonged fever in children include Epstein-Barr virus infections, osteomyelitis, *Bartonella henselae* infections (cat-scratch disease), UTIs, Lyme disease, and human immunodeficiency virus. Noninfectious causes of prolonged fever include neoplasms, collagen vascular diseases, and inflammatory disorders (ulcerative colitis or Crohn disease).

CHAPTER 22

Foreign Body—Ingestion and Aspiration

Jeff E. Schunk, M.D.

Through play, experimentation, and normal daily activities, children are likely to place foreign bodies just about anywhere. Once an object or foodstuff is in a child's mouth, it can lodge in the respiratory tree or be ingested. Young age (6 months to 4 years), a tendency to hold objects in the mouth, easy distractibility, inappropriate-for-age foods, and inappropriate playthings place the child at risk for foreign-body aspiration or ingestion. Often, the "choking episode" completely clears the foreign body; however, the sequelae of an aspirated object can range from an immediate life-threatening event to a slowly evolving pneumonia. The seriousness of the foreign-body ingestion is determined by the nature of the object (e.g., round, long, sharp, corrosive) and the potential level of lodgment in the gastrointestinal (GI) tract. Fortunately, children typically swallow round rather than sharp objects. Generally, most ingested foreign material is well tolerated, and many ingestions go unnoticed by the family as well as by the child.

DIFFERENTIAL DIAGNOSIS

Gastrointestinal Foreign Body

ESOPHAGUS

Impaction in the esophagus is the most common and most serious consequence of ingestion of a foreign body. Most childhood esophageal foreign bodies are round objects. Naturally, children with esophageal strictures are at increased risk for recurrent esophageal impactions, even with foodstuffs. Foreign bodies that remain lodged in the esophagus may lead to potentially serious complications. Therefore, it is imperative that the physician be alert to the possibility of esophageal foreign bodies, especially in the susceptible 6-month- to 4-year-old age group.

STOMACH AND LOWER GASTROINTESTINAL TRACT

Objects that can pass safely into the stomach generally traverse the remainder of the GI tract without complication. This may not be true of some long (> 5 cm) objects that are unable to negotiate the turns of the duodenum and some other tight bends in the lower GI tract. This also may not be true of some very sharp objects (sewing needles are particularly high risk), which may perforate the hollow viscera.

Respiratory Foreign Body

UPPER AIRWAY

Foreign bodies that lodge in the upper airway can be immediately life threatening. Children with foreign bodies in their upper airways present with acute respiratory distress, stridor, increased respiratory effort, or complete obstruction of their upper airway. For patients with complete airway obstruction, emergency treatment depends on proper application of basic life support skills. Back blows and chest compressions are used in infants, and the Heimlich maneuver is used in toddlers, children, and adolescents. If these methods fail to dislodge the foreign body, rapid progression to direct visualization and manual extraction is necessary (see Chapters 1 and 5).

LOWER RESPIRATORY TRACT

Because of the ubiquitous nature of the presenting symptoms, the frequency of the asymptomatic presentation, and the potential for false-negative and false-positive screening radiographs, childhood foreign bodies of the lower tracheobronchial tree present a diagnostic challenge to all who treat children. Foreign bodies of the lower respiratory tract are seen more commonly in children less than 3 years of age. In children, aspirated foreign bodies show only a slight propensity to lodge in the right lung. Organic matter accounts for most aspirations, with nuts and seeds (e.g., sunflower and watermelon) accounting for 30% to 70%, followed by other food products, including apples, carrots, and plants and grasses (Table 22.1). Plastics and metals make up a minority of aspirated objects, and coin aspiration has been reported only rarely.

The diagnosis of foreign body aspiration is often delayed. Symptoms at diagnosis include cough in 75% to 90%, wheezing in 50% to 75%, and respiratory distress in 25% to 60%. The classic clinical triad of an aspirated foreign body (wheeze, cough, and decreased breath sounds) is present in only about one third of all cases of pediatric foreign body aspiration. This triad is more likely to occur the more delayed the evaluation from the aspiration event. Approximately 20% of patients with aspirated foreign bodies are asymptomatic; however, in most surveys of pediatric foreign-body aspiration cases, a history of aspiration, if sought, is present in more than 75% of patients.

TABLE 22.1. Aspirated Foreign Bodies in Children Recovered at Bronchoscopy[a]

Foreign body	Percent
Peanuts	38
Other nuts	10
Other organic (food) material	16
Seeds, weeds, or twigs	7
Plastics	6
Popcorn	6
Pins, screws, tacks, or nails	6
Crayons	2
Rocks or stones	1
Miscellaneous[b]	8

[a] Included a total of 440 foreign bodies removed.
[b] Included cotton/lint, earrings, bullet shell casings, tooth, staple, shirt label, pellet, spring, aluminum foil, seashell, pencil lead, screwdriver, chalk, chain, coin, chicken bone, plaster, Styrofoam cup fragment, and others.
Adapted from Black RE, Johnson DG, Matlak ME. Bronchoscopic removal of aspirated foreign bodies in children. *J Pediatr Surg* 1994;29:682–684, with permission.

EVALUATION AND DECISION

Unknown Location

Generally, the symptom complex and history that surround the event provide the clues necessary to decide whether to evaluate the respiratory tract or GI tract. Symptoms of cough, respiratory distress with tachypnea or retractions, stridor, wheezing, or asymmetric aeration suggest a foreign body in the airway. Although symptoms of gagging, vomiting, drooling, dysphagia, pain, or localization may suggest esophageal impaction, impacted esophageal foreign bodies may induce secondary airway symptoms; either location may induce coughing, vomiting, or gagging initially; and both types may be asymptomatic. If the history and physical examination do not provide the necessary clues, initial evaluation with a chest radiograph (to include the upper abdomen and oropharynx) will suffice as the first screen for a radiopaque esophageal or gastric foreign body. Coupling this with an expiratory chest radiograph (as outlined later) screens for an aspirated foreign body. Alternatively, the combination of a soft-tissue lateral neck and a "wide" chest radiograph that includes oropharynx and abdomen is also used as an initial search for foreign body.

Gastrointestinal Foreign Body

ESOPHAGEAL FOREIGN BODY: DIAGNOSIS

Children with esophageal foreign bodies often have a history of having swallowed the foreign body. Symptoms associated with esophageal impaction include pain with swallowing, refusal to eat, foreign-body sensation or localization, drooling, and vomiting. When these symptoms are associated with a history of foreign-body ingestion, the diagnosis is straightforward. In the absence of an ingestion history, the diagnosis may be more subtle because these same symptoms occur with such common childhood ailments as acute gastroenteritis, pharyngitis, and gingivostomatitis. Any patient with swallowing difficulty requires a thorough examination, including mouth, oropharynx, neck, chest, and abdomen as well as a radiologic evaluation in some cases (see Chapter 45).

The approach to a child who has ingested a foreign body is outlined in Figure 22.1. Children may be asymptomatic with an esophageal foreign body. Studies have demonstrated that 30% to 40% of children who showed coins in the esophagus were asymptomatic in the emergency department. Therefore, it is suggested that all children with a history of ingested foreign bodies undergo radiographic evaluation, with the exception of the asymptomatic patient who has ingested a small (< 1 cm in maximum diameter), nonsharp object (Fig. 22.1). If the foreign body is not radiopaque (and yet is large enough to become impacted) and the patient's symptoms suggest esophageal im-

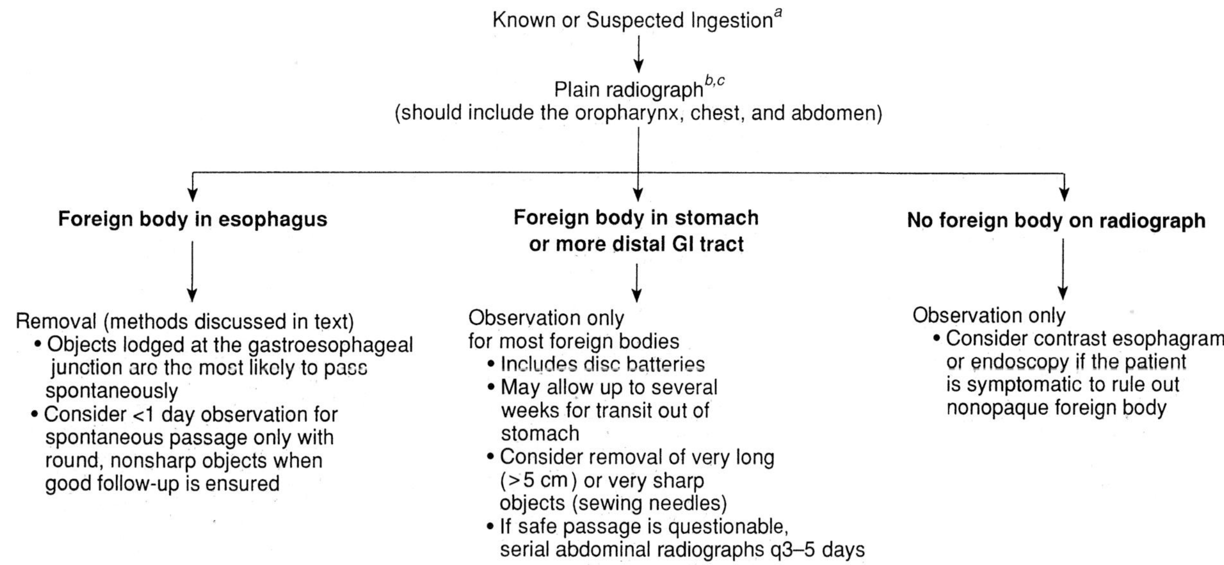

Known or Suspected Ingestion[a]
Plain radiograph[b,c]
(should include the oropharynx, chest, and abdomen)
Foreign body in esophagus
Foreign body in stomach or more distal GI tract
No foreign body on radiograph
Removal (methods discussed in text)
• Objects lodged at the gastroesophageal junction are the most likely to pass spontaneously
• Consider <1 day observation for spontaneous passage only with round, nonsharp objects when good follow-up is ensured
Observation only for most foreign bodies
• Includes disc batteries
• May allow up to several weeks for transit out of stomach
• Consider removal of very long (>5 cm) or very sharp objects (sewing needles)
• If safe passage is questionable, serial abdominal radiographs q3–5 days
Observation only
• Consider contrast esophagram or endoscopy if the patient is symptomatic to rule out nonopaque foreign body
[a] If the suspected foreign body is small (<1 cm), not sharp, and the patient is without symptoms, radiographs are not indicated.
[b] In the patient with a known nonradiopaque foreign body with symptoms of esophageal foreign body, go directly to esophagram or endoscopy.
[c] In the patient with a prior history of esophageal surgery (e.g., TEF repair) or stricture, who presents with symptoms of an esophageal foreign body after eating (especially meats, including chicken and hot dogs), go directly to esophagram.

Figure 22.1. Management of ingested foreign body.

paction, it is necessary to use contrast esophagrams to rule out an esophageal foreign body. Fortunately, childhood esophageal foreign bodies tend to be radiopaque (e.g., coins), and so diagnosis with plain radiographs is not difficult. Children with a predisposing condition who have symptoms of an esophageal foreign body after eating should have contrast esophagrams; plain radiographs are not necessary. Similarly, with nonradiopaque ingestions and symptoms suggestive of impaction in children without underlying conditions, contrast esophagrams, or esophagoscopy should be performed initially.

Handheld metal detectors may provide an alternative to conventional radiography as an initial screen when a coin ingestion is suspected. In study situations, these devices compare favorably with radiography in determining the presence or absence of a coin and determining coin location.

ESOPHAGEAL FOREIGN BODY: REMOVAL

In general, once an esophageal foreign body is detected, it should be removed promptly. It may be prudent to allow a period of less than 1 day for spontaneous passage of round, noncorrosive objects in the asymptomatic patient. Removal methods currently used include rigid esophagoscopy with the patient under general anesthesia, flexible endoscopy (with or without conscious sedation), and for round objects, a balloon-tipped catheter under fluoroscopic guidance or bougienage to advance the object into the stomach. All these methods have a high success rate; provincial opinion and local referral patterns will dictate which method is used. Esophagoscopy with the patient under general anesthesia has been the method of choice for many years. Use of medications (e.g., glucagon, diazepam) to reduce muscular tone, to enhance esophageal motility, or to relax the lower esophageal sphincter has been suggested to facilitate passage from the esophagus. This has not been investigated thoroughly enough to offer guidelines for routine clinical application and dosing.

STOMACH AND LOWER GASTROINTESTINAL TRACT

As mentioned, most foreign bodies of the stomach and lower GI tract can be managed expectantly. Management recommendations for sharp objects are varied but conservative—watchful waiting usually is safe. Sewing needles seem to have increased propensity for perforation, however, and should probably be removed. Long objects (>5 cm) also should be removed from the stomach. If the long or very sharp object has passed out of the stomach at the time of evaluation or, in any instance, to a place where a safe journey through the remainder of the GI tract is questionable, serial abdominal radiographs taken every 3 to 5 days and serial examinations may be necessary to document continued passage. Most round objects (e.g., coins) will traverse the GI tract in 3 to 8 days without any complication.

Respiratory Foreign Body

LOWER RESPIRATORY TRACT: DIAGNOSIS

A high clinical index of suspicion is necessary to diagnose foreign-body aspiration accurately and promptly. Symptoms seen in pediatric foreign body ingestions also are present in other common diseases such as upper respiratory tract infection, bronchiolitis, pneumonia, and asthma. A few radiographic techniques serve as the most important diagnostic aids. Yet, when the clinical suspicion of foreign-body aspiration is high (a good history for aspiration, new onset of symptoms with focal physical findings), the lack of confirmatory radiographic studies should not dissuade the clinician from pursuing bronchoscopy for diagnosis and treatment. In patients diagnosed early, as many as one third have normal chest radiographs. The abnormal findings seen on a chest radiograph include air trapping, atelectasis, and consolidation. The more time that has elapsed since the aspiration event, the more likely the chest radiograph will be abnormal and the greater

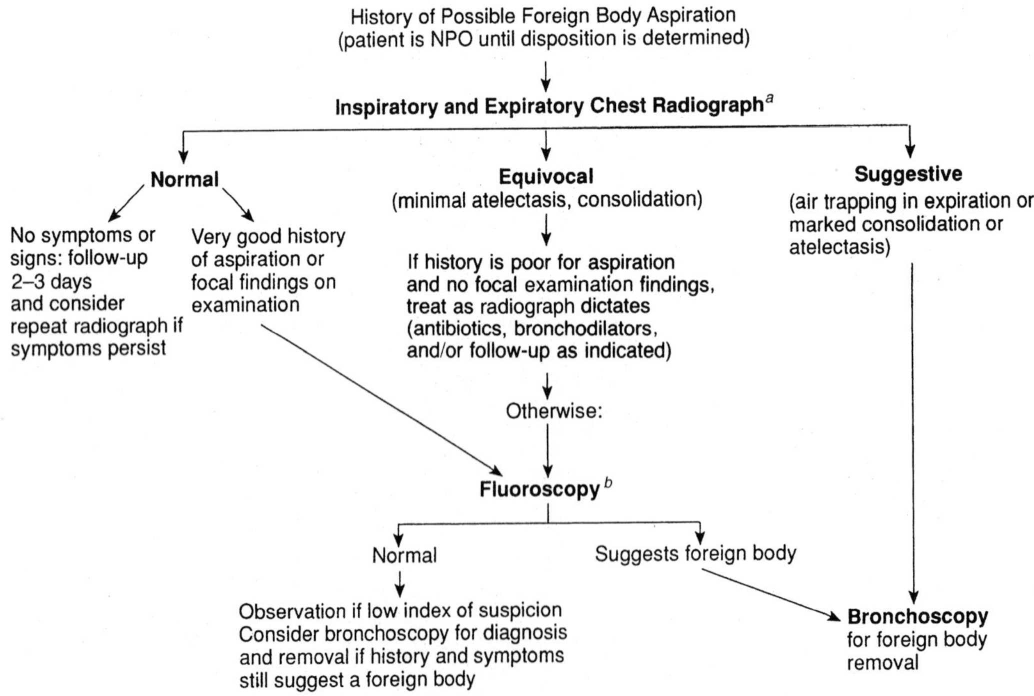

Figure 22.2. Guidelines for management of the child with suspected aspiration of a foreign body.

the percentage of patients who exhibit consolidation and atelectasis.

Inspiratory and expiratory films comparing the relative deflation of the two lungs may demonstrate unilateral air trapping indicative of a foreign body. In some series, up to 80% of the foreign bodies demonstrated abnormalities using inspiratory and expiratory chest radiographs. In the young or uncooperative child, in whom obtaining an adequate expiratory film may be difficult, lateral decubitus chest radiographs (both obtained during inspiration) that compare the relative deflation of the dependent lung may be a useful adjunct. In equivocal cases, chest fluoroscopy may show mediastinal shift during respiration; unfortunately, even this technique does not have 100% sensitivity.

The approach to diagnosing foreign-body aspiration is outlined in Figure 22.2. In instances in which a respiratory foreign body is being considered, the patient should be kept on a nil per os (NPO) basis until the diagnosis is confirmed or the decision for bronchoscopy is made. The first step in the patient suspected of foreign-body aspiration is inspiratory and expiratory chest radiographs. If these studies are normal, the aspiration history is poor, the material uncommonly aspirated, and the patient has mild or no symptoms without focal findings on physical examination, then discharge with follow-up in a few days usually is adequate. If diagnosis is still unclear after plain films and there is a historical or clinical suspicion of aspiration, fluoroscopy may be obtained, looking for air trapping and evidence of mediastinal shift away from the foreign body. In some instances in which there are focal physical findings (unilateral wheeze, decreased aeration) and a good aspiration history, the patient might go directly to bronchoscopy. Similarly, in some cases, despite normal radiographic evaluation (including fluoroscopy), when there is a high clinical index of suspicion, bronchoscopy is necessary to confirm the presence of a pulmonary foreign object.

A history of aspirated foreign body should be sought in all cases of new-onset respiratory distress, wheezing, or cough, with special consideration to the high-risk children from 6 months to 4 years of age. History taking should include questions about recent choking episodes, especially when eating nuts (peanuts), seeds, apples, and carrots. The differential diagnosis of foreign-body aspiration includes many common childhood diseases, including upper respiratory infection, bronchiolitis, viral and bacterial pneumonitis, and reactive airway disease; specific questioning concerning aspiration events should be explored.

LOWER RESPIRATORY TRACT: REMOVAL

Once a foreign body of the lower respiratory tract has been identified, bronchoscopic removal is performed with the patient under general anesthesia. This technique is successful in more than 98% of cases, and only rarely is a thoracotomy required.

CHAPTER 23
Gastrointestinal Bleeding

Sigmund J. Kharasch, M.D.

Gastrointestinal (GI) bleeding is a relatively common problem in pediatrics. Most infants and children who arrive in the emergency department (ED) with what appears to be GI bleeding have an acute, self-limited GI hemorrhage and are hemodynamically stable. In such patients, three important questions must be asked: (1) Is the patient really bleeding? (2) Is the blood coming from the GI tract? and (3) Is there more than a trivial amount of blood? Children with only a few drops or flecks of blood in the vomit or stool should not be considered "GI bleeders" if their history and physical examinations are otherwise unremarkable. Likewise, many substances ingested by children may simulate fresh or chemically altered blood. Red food coloring (as in some cereals, antibiotic and cough syrups, Jell-O, and Kool-Aid), as well as fruit juices and beets, may resemble blood if vomited. Melena may be confused with dark or black stools and results from iron supplementation, dark chocolate, bismuth, spinach, cranberries, blueberries, grapes, or licorice. In these cases, confirmation of the absence of blood with Gastroccult (vomitus) and Hematest or Hemoccult (stool) tests will allay parental anxiety and prevent unnecessary concern and workup. Gastroccult is a specific and sensitive assay, stable in an acid environment, which can detect as little as 300 μg per deciliter of hemoglobin. A careful search for other causes of presumed GI bleeding, such as recent epistaxis, dental work, and sore throat, should be sought.

In most cases of upper and lower GI bleeding, the source of the bleeding is inflamed mucosa (infection, allergy, drug induced, stress related, or idiopathic). The emergency physician must be vigilant in differentiating inflammatory conditions that are often self-limited from causes that may require emergent surgical or endoscopic intervention, such as ischemic bowel (intussusception, volvulus), structural abnormalities (Meckel diverticulum, angiodysplasia), and portal hypertension (esophageal varices).

INITIAL ASSESSMENT

The differential diagnosis of GI bleeding is broad. A systematic approach to all patients includes the following: (1) assessment of the severity of the bleeding and institution of appropriate resuscitative measures; (2) establishing the level of bleeding within the GI tract; (3) pertinent history, physical examination, and laboratory tests based on knowledge of age-related causes; and (4) emergency treatment based on general categories of causes. All patients with a significant bleeding episode should have a nasogastric tube placed for diagnostic purposes (Fig. 23.1). In patients with hematemesis or melena, a positive examination of a nasogastric aspirate confirms an upper source of GI bleeding, whereas a negative result almost always excludes an active upper GI bleed.

UPPER GASTROINTESTINAL BLEEDING

Differential Diagnosis

As seen in Tables 23.1, 23.2, and 23.3, there is considerable overlap between age groups and causes of upper GI bleeding. Mucosal lesions, including esophagitis, gastritis, stress ulcers, peptic ulceration, and Mallory–Weiss tears, are the most common sources of GI bleeding in all age groups (see Chapter 82). Of all cases of upper GI bleeding in children, 95% are related to mucosal lesions and esophageal varices.

Hematemesis in a healthy newborn is most likely to result from swallowed maternal blood either at delivery or during breast-feeding (i.e., cracked nipples). The Apt-Downey test can differentiate neonatal from maternal hemoglobin based on the conversion of oxyhemoglobin to hematin when mixed with alkali. Although rare, hemorrhagic disease of the newborn should be considered with prolongation of the prothrombin time, if vitamin K has not been administered.

Significant and sometimes massive upper GI hemorrhage in a newborn infant may occur with no demonstrative anatomic le-

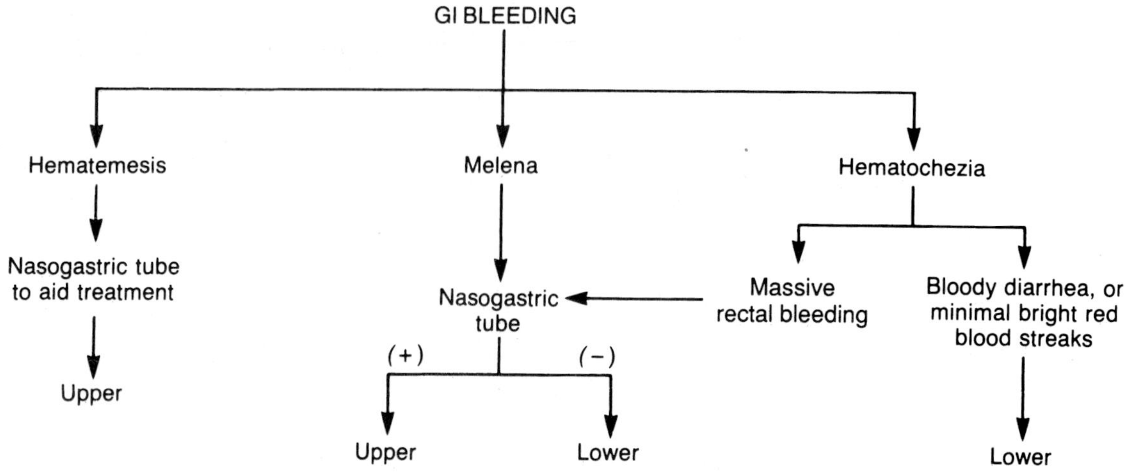

Figure 23.1. Establishing level of gastrointestinal bleeding.

sion or only "hemorrhagic gastritis" at endoscopy. This is usually a single, self-limited event that is benign if treated with appropriate blood replacement and supportive measures.

Critically ill children of any age are at risk for developing stress-related peptic ulcer disease. Such ulcers occur with life-threatening illnesses, including shock, respiratory failure, hypoglycemia, dehydration, burns (Curling ulcer), intracranial lesions or trauma (Cushing ulcer), renal failure, and vasculitis. These ulcers may develop within minutes to hours after the initial insult and primarily result from ischemia. Hematemesis, melena, and perforation of a viscus may accompany stress-associated ulcers. Hematemesis secondary to gastroesophageal reflux and esophagitis is uncommon but should be considered in patients who are severely symptomatic with vomiting or aspiration. Hematemesis following the acute onset of vigorous vomiting or retching at any age suggests a Mallory–Weiss tear.

Idiopathic peptic ulcer disease is a common cause of GI bleeding in preschool and older children. Younger children have less characteristic symptoms, often localize abdominal pain poorly, and may have vomiting as a predominant symptom. Older children and adolescents describe epigastric pain in a pattern typical of adults. *Helicobacter pylori* has emerged as a leading cause of secondary gastritis, particularly in older children. Similar to adults, pediatric patients with evidence of *H. pylori* infection often are treated with antibiotics, bismuth preparations, and H_2 antagonists or omeprazole.

In older children, the possibility of bleeding esophageal varices must be considered in the differential diagnosis of upper GI bleeding. Although variceal bleeding is rare in infancy, esophageal and gastric varices associated with portal hypertension are the most common cause of severe upper GI hemorrhage in older children. One half to two thirds of these children have an extrahepatic presinusoidal obstruction, often resulting from portal vein thrombosis, as the cause of portal hypertension. Omphalitis with or without a history of umbilical vein cannulation, dehydration, and a number of other factors may contribute. Other children with portal hypertension have hepatic parenchymal disorders such as neonatal hepatitis, congenital hepatic fibrosis, cystic fibrosis, or biliary cirrhosis associated with biliary atresia. Two thirds of patients with portal hypertension develop bleeding before 5 years of age, and 85% do so by 10 years of age.

Evaluation and Decision

Once it has been determined that a significant upper GI bleed has occurred and hemodynamic stability is restored, identification of the specific disorder is the next step (Fig. 23.2). If the

TABLE 23.1. Etiology of Upper Gastrointestinal Bleeding Based on Age (in order of frequency of occurrence)

Neonatal period (<4 wk)	Infancy (<2 yr)	Preschool age (2–5 yr)	School age (>5 yr)
Swallowed maternal blood	Gastritis	Epistaxis	Gastritis
Hemorrhagic gastritis	Esophagitis	Gastritis	Mallory–Weiss tear
Stress ulcer	Mallory–Weiss tear	Esophagitis	Peptic ulcer
Idiopathic	Stress ulcer	Mallory–Weiss tear	Stress ulcer
Bleeding diathesis	Pyloric stenosis	Toxic ingestion	Toxic ingestion
Esophagitis	Vascular malformation	Stress ulcer	Esophagitis
Duplication	Toxic ingestion	Foreign body	Inflammatory bowel disease
Vascular malformations	Duplication	Vascular malformation	Esophageal varices
		Esophageal varices	Vascular malformation
		Hemobilia	Hemobilia

TABLE 23.2. Common Causes of Upper Gastrointestinal Bleeding Based on Age

Neonatal period	Preschool age
Swallowed maternal blood	Epistaxis
Infancy	Gastritis
Gastritis	Mallory–Weiss tear
Mallory–Weiss tear	School Age
Esophagitis	Gastritis
	Peptic ulcer
	Mallory–Weiss tear

bleeding is mild and self-limited or the gastric aspirate negative, a minor mucosal lesion is likely. Although mucosal lesions such as esophagitis, gastritis, or peptic ulcer disease can present with severe bleeding, most often bleeding from mucosal lesions is self-limiting and will respond to conservative medical management. For patients with persistent or recurrent hemorrhage, emergent endoscopy may be necessary if the bleeding is considered life threatening (continued transfusion requirement, hemodynamic instability). In a small percentage of patients in whom bleeding is massive, which makes endoscopic visualization impossible, angiography or radionuclide studies (technetium-sulfur colloid/Tc-labeled red blood cells) may be indicated. Treatment of specific mucosal conditions and esophageal varices is discussed in Chapter 82.

Eighty to eighty-five percent of upper GI bleeding stops spontaneously, regardless of the source, before or early in the hospital course. In stable patients who have stopped bleeding, double-contrast barium examination of the upper GI tract and endoscopy provide valuable and often complementary information. In this group of patients, endoscopy need not be performed on an emergent basis and may be done electively in the

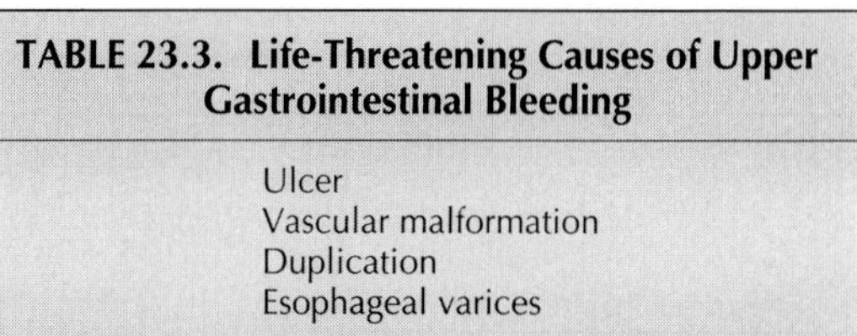

TABLE 23.3. Life-Threatening Causes of Upper Gastrointestinal Bleeding

Ulcer
Vascular malformation
Duplication
Esophageal varices

first 12 to 24 hours after admission. Elective endoscopy should be performed in patients who stop bleeding spontaneously but who have required transfusion or have a history of previously unexplained upper GI bleeding episodes.

LOWER GASTROINTESTINAL BLEEDING

Differential Diagnosis

NEONATAL PERIOD (0–1 MONTH)

As is true for upper GI bleeding, a common cause of blood in the stool in well infants is the passage of maternal blood swallowed either at delivery or during breast-feeding from a fissured maternal breast. Although hemorrhagic disease of the newborn is uncommon after prophylactic administration of vitamin K at delivery, maternal drugs that cross the placenta, including aspirin, phenytoin, cephalothin, and phenobarbital, may interfere with clotting factors and cause hemorrhage. Infectious diarrhea can occur in very young infants, and stools may contain blood or mucus. Common bacterial pathogens in this age group include *Campylobacter jejuni* and *Salmonella.*

In ill-appearing infants with lower GI bleeding, midgut volvulus, necrotizing enterocolitis, and Hirschsprung disease should be considered (Table 23.4). Malrotation with midgut volvulus is most common during this period. Initially, bilious

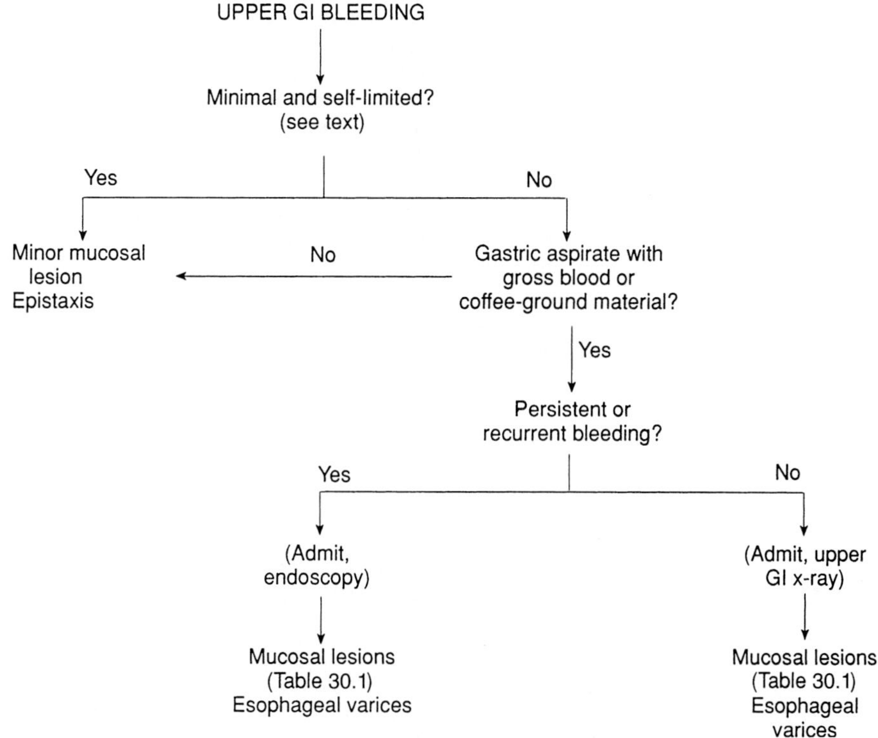

Figure 23.2. Diagnostic approach to upper gastrointestinal bleeding.

TABLE 23.4. Etiology of Lower Gastrointestinal Bleeding Based on Age[a]

Neonatal period	Infancy (1 mo–2 yr)	Preschool age (2–5 yr)	School age (>5 yr)
Well infant			
Swallowed maternal blood	Anal fissure	Anal fissure	Infectious colitis
Infectious colitis	Infectious colitis	Infectious colitis	Polyps
Milk allergy	Milk allergy	Juvenile polyps	Inflammatory bowel disease
Hemorrhagic disease	Nonspecific colitis	Intussusception	Hemorrhoids
Duplication of bowel	Juvenile polyps	Henoch-Schonlein purpura	Meckel's diverticulum
Meckel's diverticulum	Intussusception	Meckel's diverticulum	Hemolytic uremic syndrome
Sick infant			
Infectious colitis	Meckel's diverticulum	Hemolytic uremic syndrome	Pseudomembranous colitis
Midgut volvulus	Duplication	Inflammatory bowel disease	Ischemic colitis
Hirschsprung's disease	Hemolytic uremic syndrome	Peptic ulcer	Peptic ulcer
Disseminated coagulopathy	Inflammatory bowel disease	Pseudomembranous enterocolitis	Angiodysplasia
Necrotizing enterocolitis	Pseudomembranous enterocolitis	Ischemic colitis	
Intussusception	Ischemic colitis	Angiodysplasia	
Congestive heart failure	Lymphonodular hyperplasia		

[a] Listed in the order of frequency of occurrence.

vomiting, abdominal distension, and pain are present. Melena is seen in 10% to 20% of patients and signifies vascular compromise. Of all cases of necrotizing enterocolitis, 10% occur in term infants. These patients can present with nonspecific signs of sepsis (temperature instability or apnea and bradycardia) as well as with specific GI tract findings, such as abdominal distension, pain, and abdominal wall erythema. GI bleeding can be in the form of guaiac-positive or grossly bloody stools. Hirschsprung disease with enterocolitis may present with GI bleeding in the newborn period. Enterocolitis occurs in up to 25% of children with Hirschsprung disease. The risk of enterocolitis remains high until about 6 months of age. The diagnosis should be considered in any newborn who does not pass meconium in the first 24 to 48 hours of life.

Other common causes of lower GI bleeding are listed in Table 23.5. Life-threatening causes are listed in Table 23.6.

INFANCY (1 MONTH TO 2 YEARS)

In the first 2 years of life, anal fissures are the most common cause of rectal bleeding and usually are associated with hard stools or constipation. Milk or soy enterocolitis usually occurs during the first month of life or shortly thereafter. These infants can present with chronic diarrhea, stools containing blood or mucus, or less commonly, fulminant colitis and shock. Breast-fed infants whose mothers drink cow's milk may develop an allergic colitis that responds to removal of cow's milk from the mother's diet. Infectious enterocolitis as a cause of bloody diarrhea is common in all age groups. Bacterial causes (*Salmonella*, *Shigella*, *Campylobacter*, pathogenic *Escherichia coli*, and *Yersinia enterocolitica*) should be identified with stool cultures. In symptomatic infants and children, the presence of leukocytes in a stool smear for white cells may aid in preliminary diagnosis. Pseudomembranous colitis should be considered in any infant or child with bloody stools and a history of recent antibiotic therapy. "Nonspecific colitis" has been demonstrated to be a common cause of hematochezia in infants less than 6 months of age. Although the cause of nonspecific colitis is unknown, it may represent a variation in the colonic response to viral invasion.

Meckel diverticulum should be suspected in infants or young children who pass bright or dark red blood per rectum. Intermittent painless bleeding or massive GI hemorrhage can occur. Sixty percent of complications from Meckel diverticulum (hemorrhage and intestinal obstruction) occur in patients less than 2 years of age.

Idiopathic intussusception may occur in children 3 months to 1 year of age, with 80% occurring before 2 years of age. In children older than 3 years, a lead point (polyp, Meckel diverticulum, or hypertrophied lymphoid patch) is often found. Paroxysmal pain may be associated with guaiac-positive stools or hematochezia. Lethargy alone (without pain) has been in-

TABLE 23.5. Common Causes of Lower Gastrointestinal Bleeding Based on Age

Neonatal period	Preschool age
Swallowed maternal blood	Anal fissure
Infectious colitis	Infectious colitis
Milk allergy	School age
Infancy	Infectious colitis
Anal fissure	
Infectious colitis	
Milk allergy	

TABLE 23.6. Life-Threatening Causes of Gastrointestinal Bleeding

Midgut volvulus	Pseudomembranous colitis
Intussusception	Ischemic colitis
Meckel's diverticulum	Peptic ulcer
Hemolytic uremic syndrome	

creasingly recognized as a presenting symptom of intussusception in young children. Lymphonodular hyperplasia is a common cause of rectal bleeding in this age group and may cause mild, painless hematochezia. The nodular lymphoid response is self-limited and does not require any specific therapy. Intestinal duplications are an uncommon cause of lower GI bleeding and, when diagnosed, usually are found in children less than 2 years of age. Duplications can be found anywhere in the GI tract but are most common in the distal ileum. These usually present with obstruction and lower GI bleeding.

PRESCHOOL (2–5 YEARS)

The two conditions most likely to cause bleeding in children 2 to 5 years of age are juvenile polyps and infectious enterocolitis. Polyps may cause painless rectal bleeding in this age group. Significant bleeding is unusual. Infectious causes of colitis are similar to those discussed in younger age groups. Hematochezia is often a manifestation of systemic disease in infancy and throughout childhood. Hemolytic uremic syndrome is the most prevalent of these conditions reported in infants and children up to 3 years of age. Bloody diarrhea may precede the development of renal and hematologic abnormalities. GI manifestations of Henoch-Schönlein purpura (HSP) occur in 50% of patients and include colicky abdominal pain, melena, and bloody diarrhea. These symptoms precede the characteristic rash in 20% of patients. GI complications of HSP include hemorrhage, intussusception, and rarely intestinal perforation.

Angiodysplasia is a rare cause of GI bleeding but can be associated with massive hemorrhage. Vascular lesions of the GI tract probably have a congenital basis. Several recognized syndromes, including Rendu–Osler–Weber syndrome, blue rubber bleb syndrome, and Turner syndrome may be associated with intestinal telangiectasia.

SCHOOL AGE (5 YEARS THROUGH ADOLESCENCE)

For the most part, the diagnostic considerations relevant to the preschool child apply to school-aged and adolescent children with the addition of inflammatory bowel disease. Toxic megacolon is a life-threatening presentation of both ulcerative colitis and Crohn disease.

Evaluation and Decision

Rectal bleeding is a common complaint in the pediatric age group (Fig. 23.3). The causes of lower GI bleeding vary significantly with age and often are transient and benign. Occasionally, lower GI bleeding reflects a life-threatening pathologic condition, and establishment of a specific diagnosis becomes urgent.

The priority of the emergency physician in evaluating the patient with lower GI bleeding is to identify lower tract bleeding associated with intestinal obstruction. Intussusception and a late presentation of midgut volvulus secondary to malrotation are the major types of intestinal obstruction associated with lower GI hemorrhage. All causes of abdominal obstruction (e.g., adhesions, incarcerated hernia, appendicitis) eventually cause bleeding, however, if diagnosis is delayed and vascular compromise occurs.

Severe lower GI bleeding leading to hemodynamic instability or requiring transfusion is rare in pediatrics, and gastric lavage is essential in these cases to rule out a possible source in upper GI tract. Meckel diverticulum is the most common cause of severe lower GI bleeding in all age groups. Following Meckel's diverticulum, Crohn disease and arteriovenous malformation are prominent causes of massive lower GI bleeding in adolescents.

The urgency and extent of evaluation of patients with lower GI bleeding will depend on the amount of bleeding, the patient's age, and associated physical findings. In a healthy infant with a few streaks of blood in the stool and a normal examination, stool culture and observation are reasonable. If hematochezia is found and nasogastric aspirate is negative, significant pathology must be sought. Flat and upright abdominal radiographs should be performed if an obstructive process (e.g., intussusception, volvulus) is suspected by history or physical examina-

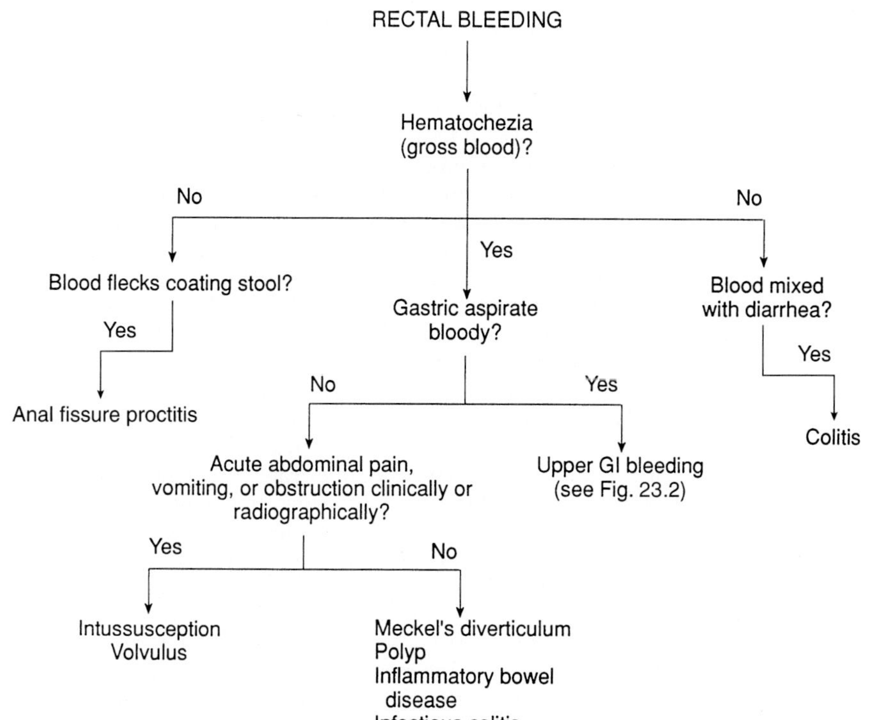

Figure 23.3. Diagnostic approach to lower gastrointestinal bleeding.

tion. The absence of radiographic findings should not, however, deter the physician from pursuing further diagnostic evaluation. A barium or air enema examination is diagnostic and often therapeutic in children with intussusception. If obstruction is not considered likely, the decision to perform contrast enema examination or colonoscopy will depend on the diagnosis that is suspected. Air-contrast barium enema is extremely valuable in the detection of polyps or inflammatory bowel disease. Indications for colonoscopy include severe bleeding, moderate but persistent bleeding with a negative double-contrast barium enema, or a lesion of unknown nature seen on barium enema. If undefined bleeding persists, radionuclide studies or angiography should be considered. A technetium scan may detect ectopic gastric mucosa as seen in Meckel diverticulum, whereas angiography will help to identify bleeding vascular malformations in the GI tract. Ongoing, undiagnosed GI hemorrhage accounts for fewer than 10% of cases in infants and children. Exploratory laparotomy may be necessary and lifesaving in these circumstances.

CHAPTER 24
Groin Masses

Bruce L. Klein, M.D. and
Daniel W. Ochsenschlager, M.D.

Children occasionally present to the emergency department with an inguinal mass. There are many different causes, ranging from inconsequential to serious (Table 24.1). One generally can ascertain the correct diagnosis based on the age and sex of the child, the location of the mass, how painful it is, how rapidly it has evolved, and whether there are any associated symptoms or signs (Fig. 24.1). Lymph node enlargement and retractile, undescended, and traumatically dislocated testes are discussed in this section. Hernia and hydrocele (as well as scrotal masses) are addressed in Chapters 50 and 103.

DIFFERENTIAL DIAGNOSIS

Lymphadenopathy and Lymphadenitis

A healthy child can have a few small nodes normally. These tend to be less than half a centimeter long, and they are oval, firm, slightly moveable, and nontender. If the nodes are enlarged (especially unilaterally) or tender, erythematous, or suppurating, further evaluation is necessary (see Chapter 37).

TABLE 24.1. Causes of Inguinal Masses

Painful
Torsion of an undescended testicle[a]
Trauma (e.g., dislocated testicle)[a]
Incarceration or strangulation of an indirect inguinal hernia[a]
Lymphadenitis
Usually or comparatively painless
Hernia
Hydrocele
Lymphadenopathy
Retractile or undescended testicle

[a] Urgent or emergent condition.

Inguinal adenopathy—nodes that are enlarged but nontender—often is part of a more generalized lymphadenopathy. The list of causes of generalized lymphadenopathy is extensive and includes collagen vascular diseases (e.g., juvenile rheumatoid arthritis, serum sickness), immunologic disorders (e.g., chronic granulomatous disease), metabolic diseases (e.g., Gaucher disease, Niemann–Pick disease), and certain anemias (e.g., sickle cell disease, thalassemia). Inguinal nodes may be enlarged because of malignancy (e.g., acute lymphocytic leukemia), but this is rarely the sole presentation of a malignant tumor. Of note, some local tumors, such as testicular tumors, metastasize to the inguinal nodes. Although many infections, particularly viral ones (e.g., human immunodeficiency virus, Epstein–Barr virus), produce inguinal adenopathy, these usually cause generalized lymphadenopathy as well as hepatosplenomegaly and other abnormalities.

Inflammation or infection of the gluteal region, perineum, genitalia, or ipsilateral lower extremity is the most common cause of isolated inguinal adenopathy or adenitis. These areas must be examined carefully. Chronic eczema, tinea cruris, or an innocuous inflammation (an insect bite or diaper rash) may produce lymphadenopathy. In such cases, treatment of the underlying condition suffices. If lymphadenitis—enlargement with tenderness, erythema, or suppuration—is detected, the node itself is probably infected. Group A β-hemolytic streptococcus, *Staphylococcus aureus,* or an enteric organism is the usual pathogen, depending on the site of the primary infection. A culture from the primary site or node aspirate helps identify the organism. Most children can be treated as outpatients with oral antibiotics (e.g., cephalexin or amoxicillin–clavulanate), but children with severe symptoms should be admitted and treated with intravenous antibiotics (e.g., oxacillin, cefazolin). Abscesses caused by these pathogens should be incised and drained (see Chapter 74).

Venereal diseases can result in inguinal adenopathy or adenitis in adolescents (see Chapter 74). Herpes is a common cause of genital ulcerations and bilaterally enlarged, painful lymph nodes. Enlarged lymph glands occasionally precede the appearance of vesicles. Oral acyclovir shortens the duration of symptoms and viral shedding in primary disease but is less effective in recurrences.

The chancre of primary syphilis is painless and indurated and has raised, firm borders, a shallow, smooth base, and no exudate. Bilateral (70%) and unilateral, nontender inguinal adenopathy is common.

Chancroid is more common in developing countries than in the United States. It is caused by *Haemophilus ducreyi,* which is hard to isolate and requires selective media. Unlike syphilis, the chancroid ulcer is painful and soft and has ragged edges and a deep, friable base covered with a dirty yellow exudate. About half of patients develop painful adenitis, usually unilaterally. The node or nodes often suppurate and drain spontaneously.

Lymphogranuloma venereum, which occurs mostly in tropical and subtropical countries, is caused by *Chlamydia trachomatis.* The genital papule, vesicle, or ulcer often is missed because it is painless, inconspicuous, and transitory. One or more unilaterally enlarged, moderately tender, fluctuant nodes are characteristic. If left untreated, these nodes drain and form fistulae.

Granuloma inguinale is caused by the gram-negative bacillus *Calymmatobacterium granulomatis.* Granuloma inguinale is rare in the United States but untreated will result in extensive subcutaneous granulomas (pseudobuboes), which mimic suppurative lymph glands. The initial small, relatively painful, red nodule or vesicle progresses to a red mass of granulomatous tissue, which ulcerates and coalesces.

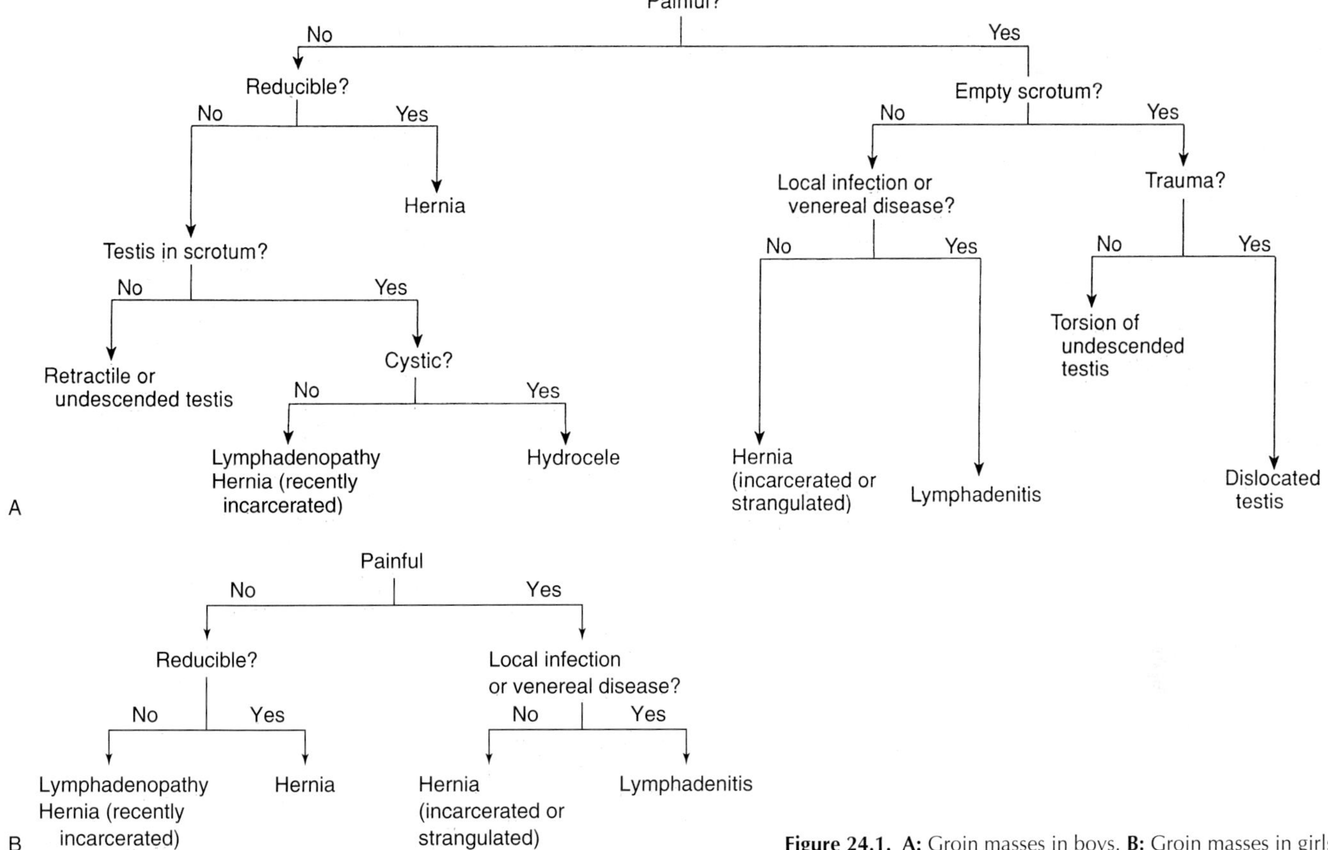

Figure 24.1. **A:** Groin masses in boys. **B:** Groin masses in girls.

An enlarged, tender inguinal node can be caused by plague, brucellosis, tularemia, or cat-scratch disease if the portal of entry for the infective organism is the lower extremity. *Yersinia pestis,* which causes plague, is extremely rare in the United States and is commonly transmitted by flea bites. The buboes are firm and nonfluctuant but extremely tender. The overlying skin is often warm and edematous. Tularemia is caused by a tick bite. Enlarged tender lymph nodes precede the appearance of a small papule that later ulcerates. Infection with *Bartonella henselae* (cat-scratch disease) results in regional lymphadenopathy that is usually red, indurated, and warm.

Filariasis, which is found in the tropics, can produce adenopathy or adenitis associated with lower extremity lymphedema and scrotal pathology.

RETRACTILE, UNDESCENDED, OR TRAUMATICALLY DISLOCATED TESTES

If the inguinal mass is firm, oval, and nontender and is associated with an empty scrotum, it probably is a retractile or undescended testis. A retractile testis, in contrast to a truly undescended one, is pulled into its abnormally high position by a hyperactive cremasteric reflex and can be milked back into the scrotum by the examiner. The scrotum appears fully developed when the testicle is retractile. Although it may retract again, ultimately it will assume a normal position; therefore, no treatment is needed. An undescended testicle is found in 2% to 4% of term boys. The testis can lodge anywhere along its natural line of descent, for example, intraabdominally, in the inguinal canal, or just outside the external inguinal ring. It also may be discovered in an ectopic location, for example, in a superficial pouch near the external ring or, less commonly, in the abdominal, suprapubic, perineal, or femoral areas.

Although intraabdominal testes are most at risk, cancer also occurs more often in the contralateral descended testis. An undescended testicle is particularly prone to torsion and more likely to be injured from trauma. In such cases, if it is located in the inguinal region, it presents as a painful groin mass. Finally, 90% of undescended testicles are associated with a patent processus vaginalis, increasing the chance that a hernia will develop.

Finally, a traumatically dislocated testicle may be discovered in the groin. Testicular dislocation occurs primarily in the older adolescent and young adult but is uncommon even then. It usually follows major trauma, in particular, a motor-vehicle accident. An associated injury, such as a pelvis or femur fracture, often is found. Despite swelling, ecchymosis, and tenderness, the scrotum feels empty. As mentioned, sometimes the testis is palpated in an abnormal location, most often in the groin in the superficial pouch anterior to the external oblique aponeurosis.

EVALUATION AND DECISION

In evaluating groin masses, one should consider the sex of the child, the presence or absence of pain, status of the testes (in boys), response to attempted reduction, history of trauma, and findings of local infection.

Boys (Fig. 24.1A)

In boys, pain often heralds a potentially emergent condition, including torsion of an undescended testis, an incarcerated or strangulated hernia, or a significant injury. One begins the evaluation by carefully palpating the scrotum. An empty scrotum points to a dislocated testis after trauma or spontaneous torsion of an undescended testis. In a boy with bilaterally descended testes, an isolated, painful groin mass may represent an incarcerated or strangulated inguinal hernia. The finding of penile lesions, such as those of herpes or syphilis, or obvious signs of inflammation (erythema, fluctuance) suggests inguinal lymphadenitis.

Painless groin masses in boys are usually not urgent. If the mass is reducible, it is an inguinal hernia, which calls for elective surgical repair. The absence of a testis in the scrotum on the side of the mass suggests a retractile or undescended testis. A retractile testis is more likely in the boy presenting with new-onset swelling; the diagnosis can be confirmed in most cases by "milking" the testis into the scrotum. When both testes are descended, a painless mass is likely to be either a hydrocele or an enlarged lymph node. One must keep in mind that a recently incarcerated hernia may be painless and is easily confused with a solitary, enlarged lymph node.

Girls (Fig. 24.1B)

As for girls, one can approach the diagnosis of groin masses by first ascertaining the presence or absence of pain. The highest priority in girls with painful masses is to identify an incarcerated or strangulated hernia. Local lesions or signs of inflammation point to lymphadenitis.

Although hernias occur less often in girls than in boys, they are still relatively common. The ability to reduce a mass with gentle pressure confirms this diagnosis. When a painless mass is irreducible, a recently incarcerated hernia (particularly involving an ovary) or an enlarged lymph node represents the most likely causes.

CHAPTER 25
Hearing Loss

Robert J. Vinci, M.D.

Acute hearing loss is of two main types: conductive and sensorineural. Several serious—even life-threatening—disorders can accompany acute hearing loss. Therefore, prompt clinical evaluation is mandated when hearing loss is suspected.

Hearing loss can occur as an isolated symptom or in association with auditory or central nervous system (CNS) dysfunction. The differential diagnosis of hearing loss includes congenital and acquired causes. It may be produced by the abnormal transmission of sound waves to the inner ear (*conductive hearing loss*) or by the defective processing of sound waves (*sensorineural hearing loss*) in the inner ear (Table 25.1). In young children, the possibility of acute hearing loss may be suspected by parents when the child does not respond to noise or to simple commands. Abnormal or delayed language development may be a sign of a more chronic process. Older children and adolescents may complain directly of hearing difficulty.

TABLE 25.1. Differential Diagnosis of Hearing Loss

Conductive hearing loss
Middle-ear effusion
Acute or chronic
Impacted cerumen
Foreign-body of external ear
Canal
Ossicle dysfunction (ossification)
Cholesteatoma
Acute trauma
Hemotympanum
Rupture of the tympanic membrane
Disruption of the inner ear
Ossicles
Malformation of the external ear canal
Sensorineural hearing loss
Congenital or neonatal
Anatomic abnormalities
Aplasia of the inner ear (Michel's aplasia)
Abnormal cochlea development
Mondini's aplasia
Scheibe's aplasia
Alexander's aplasia
Syndromes (more than 70 described with hearing loss)
Waardenburg syndrome
Jervell and Lange-Nielsen syndrome (prolonged Q-T syndrome)
Usher's syndrome
Alport's syndrome
Chromosomal abnormalities
Trisomy 13–15
Trisomy 18
Trisomy 21
Infections
TORCH
Congenital syphilis
Metabolic
Hypothyroidism
Storage disorders
Neonatal
Birth asphyxia
Kernicterus
Use of ototoxic drugs
Acquired infection
Bacterial meningitis
Viral labyrinthitis
Acute otitis media
Vascular insufficiency
Sickle cell disease
Diabetes mellitus
Polycythemia
Anatomic defect
Perilymphatic fistula
Trauma
Temporal bone fracture
Noise-induced injury
Barotrauma
Lightning
Tumor
Acoustic neuroma
CNS tumors
Leukemic infiltrates
Neurofibromatosis
Autoimmune disease
Miscellaneous
Kawasaki disease
Hypothyroidism
Hypoparathyroidism
Idiopathic

TORCH, toxoplasmosis, rubella, cytomegalovirus, and herpes simplex; CNS, central nervous system.

DIFFERENTIAL DIAGNOSIS

Conductive Hearing Loss

In children, conductive hearing loss occurs when there is a decrease in the transmission of sound waves to the cochlea from an external source. Commonly, middle ear effusion (acute or chronic), impacted cerumen, foreign body in the external ear canal, and ossification of the middle-ear ossicles produce conductive hearing loss (Table 25.1). In children with chronic recurrent otitis media (OM), a cholesteatoma—an epidermal inclusion cyst of the middle ear—may develop and cause a slowly progressive conductive hearing loss. Acute head injury, especially in association with a basilar skull fracture, may produce a conductive hearing loss secondary to hemotympanum, rupture of the tympanic membrane, or disruption of the inner ear ossicles. Rarely, the conductive hearing loss may be secondary to malformations of the external or middle ears, such as absence of the external ear canal.

Congenital Sensorineural Hearing Loss

Approximately 1 of every 750 infants is born with congenital hearing loss. Diagnostic possibilities include genetic disorders, chromosomal abnormalities, metabolic and storage diseases, and abnormal development of the auditory apparatus (Table 25.1). Congenital hearing loss secondary to aplasia of the inner ear (Michel aplasia) and abnormal cochlear development (Mondini aplasia) or absence of parts of the cochlear apparatus (Scheibe aplasia, Alexander aplasia) are reported in children. Sensorineural hearing loss has been described in more than 70 syndromes, including Waardenburg syndrome (facial dysmorphism, white forelock), Jervell and Lange-Nielsen syndrome (prolonged Q-T syndrome), Usher syndrome (retinitis pigmentosa and sensorineural hearing loss), and Alport syndrome (nephritis, optic abnormalities, and hearing loss). The chromosomal disorders caused by trisomies (especially trisomies 13, 14, 15, 18, and 21) are associated with defects in hearing. Many of these patients are diagnosed because of anatomic features associated with each of these disorders, although the hearing loss that occurs may be present at birth or develop over time. Individual patients with presumed idiopathic sensorineural hearing loss have a recurrence rate in siblings of 10%, much closer to the 25% to 50% rate of an inherited disorder than the overall risk of 1 in 750 for the general population. These data support the theory that the etiology of presumed isolated causes of sensorineural hearing loss may be genetic in origin.

Acquired Sensorineural Hearing Loss

Although acquired sensorineural hearing loss occurs less commonly than congenital hearing loss, the absence of associated symptoms may make it a more difficult diagnosis. An array of clinical problems can produce sensorineural hearing loss during childhood.

Acute Infection

Hearing loss secondary to bacterial meningitis is the most common cause of acquired sensorineural hearing loss. Untreated congenital syphilis is another infection associated with acquired sensorineural hearing loss. Hearing loss also has been described with congenital infections caused by rubella, toxoplasmosis, cytomegalovirus (CMV), and perinatally acquired herpes simplex infections.

Viral infection of the labyrinth (also called *viral cochleitis*) secondary to mumps, parainfluenzae, adenovirus, herpes simplex, CMV, and rubeola have been described and confirmed by serologic studies. Labyrinthitis usually has symptoms related to inflammation of the inner ear and involvement of the vestibular apparatus, and patients may complain of vomiting, tinnitus, and vertigo.

Vascular Insufficiency

Sudden hearing loss secondary to vascular insufficiency has been described in pediatric patients. Vascular insufficiency may compromise blood flow to the cochlea, producing a hypoxic insult to the sensitive nerve cells in the organ of Corti. Once injured, these nerve cells may not regenerate and profound sensorineural hearing loss can develop. In children, sickle cell disease, long-standing diabetes mellitus, and hyperviscosity states associated with polycythemia can compromise cochlear blood flow and produce sudden hearing loss.

Perilymphatic Fistula

Anatomic defects in the bony or membranous enclosure that normally surrounds the perilymphatic space can produce a perilymphatic fistula. These defects may produce an anomalous communication between the middle and inner ear compartment and should be considered in the differential diagnosis of the pediatric patient with acute sensorineural hearing loss. A perilymphatic fistula can occur at any age. The sudden ingress of air into the inner ear is thought to produce the symptom complex of hearing loss, tinnitus, vertigo, dizziness, and nystagmus. Trauma usually underlies the development of a fistula. This is especially true in any patient who has a recent history of vigorous exercise or changes in barometric pressure associated with airplane travel or scuba diving. Although unilateral hearing loss is most common, bilateral hearing deficits have been described. Occasionally, a perilymphatic fistula will develop in a child with previously abnormal hearing. Therefore, this diagnosis needs to be considered in any patient who has sudden onset of hearing loss, fluctuation in hearing, or complaints of progressive hearing loss, regardless of baseline hearing function. Patients with a perilymphatic fistula generally have a normal otoscopic examination. If a tympanogram is performed, middle-ear effusion is usually absent. Emergent referral to an otolaryngologist is warranted because surgery may be required for closure of the anatomic defect.

Head Trauma

Both the vestibular and cochlear nerves can be injured with fractures of the temporal bone. Assessment of audiologic function should be considered in any child with major head trauma; computed tomography (CT) scan may be required to diagnose these injuries.

Acoustic Trauma

Immediate, severe, and permanent hearing loss can follow even a short period of exposure to sounds greater than 140 dB. Exposure to sounds in the 80- to 100-dB range can produce hearing loss with chronic exposure and most commonly is diagnosed in adolescents. Rock concerts, stereo headphones, machinery, and explosive devices are capable of producing sound at the intensity required to produce this condition.

Chronic or Recurrent Otitis Media

A history of chronic or recurrent OM may predispose patients to the development of sensorineural hearing loss. This hearing loss is thought to be related to inflammatory changes in the inner ear that are produced by the diapedesis of toxins through the round window membrane. Such involvement of the inner ear has been confirmed pathologically by the presence of labyrinthitis in patients with acute OM. Because middle-ear effusions produce a

TABLE 25.2. Common Causes of Acute Hearing Loss

Conductive hearing loss	Sensorineural hearing loss
Middle-ear effusion	TORCH infections
Impacted cerumen	Birth asphyxia
Foreign body of external ear canal	Acute otitis media
	Viral labyrinthitis
	Bacterial meningitis
	Perilymphatic fistula
	Trauma
	Acoustic neuroma

TORCH, toxoplasmosis, rubella, cytomegalovirus, and herpes simplex.

conductive hearing loss, the clinician must be aware of the possibility of OM producing a mixed picture.

Miscellaneous

Acoustic neuroma, CNS tumors, and leukemic infiltrates also are associated with sensorineural hearing loss. Other considerations in pediatric patients include Kawasaki disease, hypothyroidism, lightning injury, hyperlipidemia, and the use of ototoxic drugs in the neonatal period. Finally, some children will have no demonstrable cause for their hearing loss.

EVALUATION AND DECISION

Any complaint of hearing loss requires prompt evaluation. Common causes of acute hearing loss are listed in Table 25.2.

TABLE 25.3. Life-Threatening Causes of Acute Hearing Loss

Acute head injury
Brain tumor
Leukemic infiltrate
Vascular insufficiency

Life-threatening causes of acute hearing loss are rare in pediatric patients (Table 25.3). The initial step in evaluation is to confirm the presence of acute hearing loss (Fig. 25.1). Although sophisticated hearing tests are best performed by an audiologist, the emergency physician should attempt bedside testing of gross hearing function.

Once hearing loss is established, the next step in the emergency department (ED) is to differentiate conductive from sensorineural hearing loss with the use of tuning fork tests (Fig. 25.1). Conductive hearing loss can be confirmed by the Weber test. In the Weber test, a vibrating, 512-Hz tuning fork is placed in the midline of the patient's forehead. The patient will describe the sound as being more prominent on the side of the conductive hearing loss or the side opposite the sensorineural hearing loss. For the Rinne test, the vibrating tuning fork is placed against the mastoid process. When the patient signals that the vibration has ceased, the tuning fork is placed adjacent to that ear to determine whether the patient can hear the sound of the still-vibrating tuning fork. Patients with conductive hearing loss will not be able to hear the tuning fork. This is a negative Rinne test (bone conduction greater than air conduction). Sensorineural hearing loss shows up as a positive Rinne test (air conduction

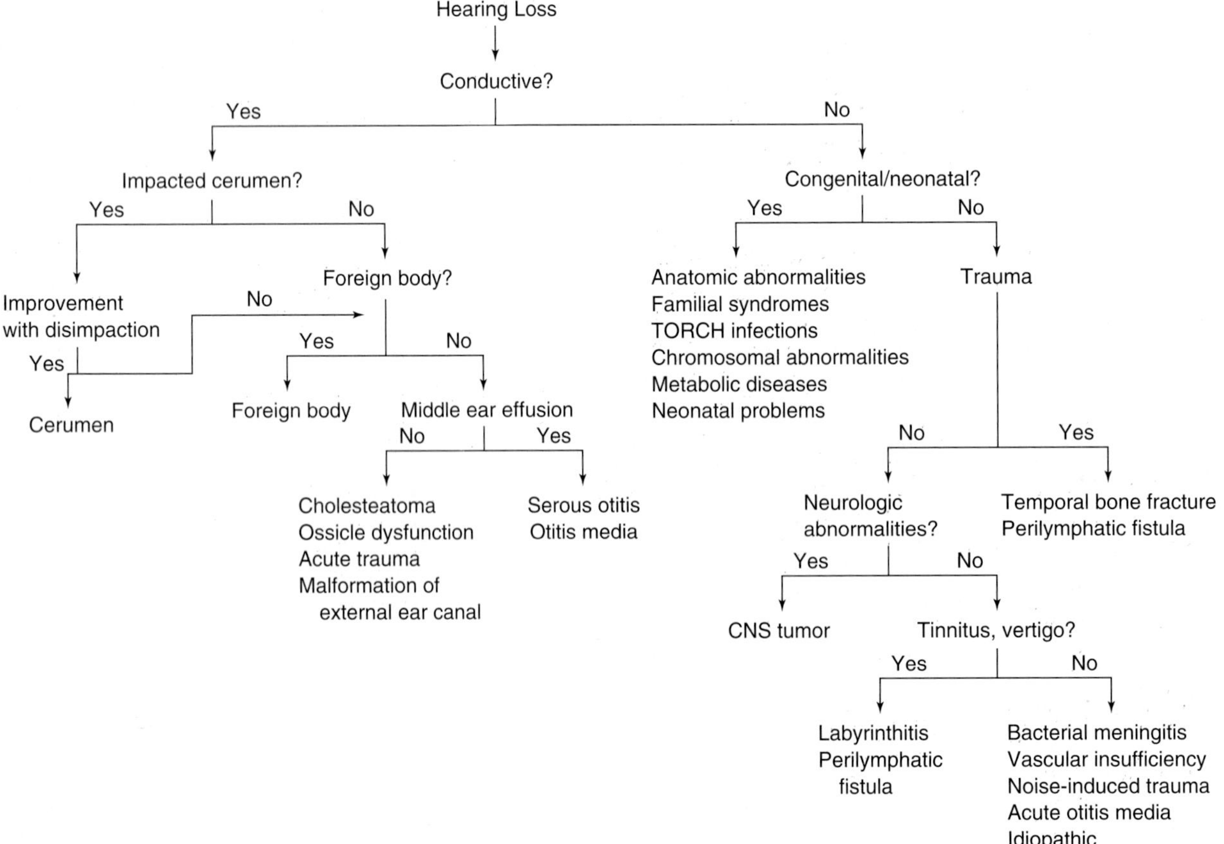

Figure 25.1. Evaluation of hearing loss.

greater than bone conduction). Finally, a test by confrontation is done by placing a tuning fork at a point equidistant from both ears. Regardless of the type of hearing loss, the patient will report the sound to be higher on the side with normal hearing.

Laboratory evaluation is seldom necessary in the ED; when needed, it should focus on diagnosis that may be contemplated after obtaining a detailed history and physical examination. Complete blood count and peripheral blood smear, renal function tests, serologic tests for syphilis, TORCH (toxoplasmosis, rubella, cytomegalovirus, and herpes simplex) titers, and bacteriologic cultures should be performed only if the history and physical suggest an associated diagnosis. Thyroid function tests, lipid profile, and serum calcium levels should be individualized in the context of clinical findings.

In children with the clinical suspicion of intracranial pathology, a radiologic evaluation assists in the diagnosis. Patients with known or suspected congenital malformation of the middle and inner ears should be evaluated with a CT scan because bony detail is essential for diagnosis. Inner-ear abnormalities have been demonstrated in 8% to 20% of patients with sensorineural hearing loss. A CT scan also should be performed in patients with suspected fracture of the temporal bone. Magnetic resonance imaging (MRI) is replacing the CT scan for the diagnosis of acoustic neuroma. With the addition of paramagnetic contrast, high-resolution scanning, and thin-section techniques, excellent detail of the internal auditory canal can be achieved.

Most children with decreased hearing in the ED have a conductive hearing loss. If impacted cerumen is seen on examination, it must be removed because it may be the cause of the decreased hearing and it prevents further evaluation. Children whose hearing improves after disimpaction and who have a normal otoscopic examination need no further treatment. Patients without impacted cerumen and those who fail to improve after removal of cerumen may have a foreign body in the ear canal. Only large objects that completely obstruct the external auditory canal should impair hearing; thus, this diagnosis is easily established during otoscopic examination.

The next step in the evaluation is a careful examination of the tympanic membrane, including pneumatic otoscopy. Many patients will show evidence of a middle-ear effusion, the most common cause of hearing loss seen in the ED. Rarely, a cholesteatoma may been seen through the translucent tympanic membrane. Sensorineural hearing loss is seen less often in the ED. Most children with sensorineural hearing loss have congenital problems that are diagnosed during the course of routine care, although occasional cases will be brought to the attention of the emergency physician. Among the acquired causes, those that must be diagnosed urgently include CNS tumors, vascular accidents, and perilymphatic fistula. In cases of acquired sensorineural hearing loss, a history of trauma should be sought. Direct blows to the head may cause temporal bone fractures or a perilymphatic fistula, and sudden changes in pressure may injure the cochlea. If there is no preceding trauma, a careful neurologic examination should be performed, looking for evidence of CNS tumors. A CT scan is indicated if these lesions are suspected. The most common cause of acquired sensorineural hearing loss seen in children in the ED without a history of trauma is viral labyrinthitis. These patients usually have associated tinnitus, vertigo, and vomiting but no focal neurologic abnormalities. Most of the remaining causes of hearing loss are idiopathic. Vascular insufficiency merits consideration in children with sickle cell anemia, diabetes mellitus, and collagen vascular disease. If the cause of the hearing loss remains uncertain, otolaryngologic consult and evaluation should be considered.

CHAPTER 26
Patients with Heart Murmurs

Benjamin K. Silverman, M.D.

In a "first-encounter" examination of a child, the emergency physician often hears a cardiac murmur—one previously known to the family or one freshly discovered—and then he or she must determine how to fit this finding into the sometimes complicated evaluation of the patient's current illness. Is the murmur an incidental finding of no relevance? Is it suggestive of heart disease? If so, are there cardiac-related symptoms? Is it related to life-threatening illness, not necessarily of cardiac origin?

Certain priorities prevail that should precede the further definition of the murmur per se. It is not important to pinpoint a primary cardiac diagnosis immediately, but it is essential to determine whether the patient is in cardiac decompensation, whether the patient's life is at risk, and whether there is incipient need for evaluation by a cardiologist or cardiac surgeon.

The ultimate goal of the chapter is to provide criteria for determining whether a patient's murmur is irrelevant or associated with life-threatening illness of cardiac or extracardiac origin and whether the patient needs cardiac consultation immediately, eventually, or not at all.

EVALUATION AND DECISION

Neonates and older infants usually have clinical presentations that differ from those in older children. Therefore, in our first-encounter evaluation, we divide murmur patients by two age groupings: from birth to 3 years of age (Fig. 26.1) and over 3 years of age (Fig. 26.2). Table 26.1 lists conditions that may be associated with murmurs.

Infants Less Than 3 Years of Age

Neonates or children less than 3 years of age in whom a murmur is heard require extremely careful assessment but are not necessarily in serious difficulty. The lead point in the evaluation is the presence or absence of cyanosis, preferably confirmed by pulse oximetry.

Infants Less Than 3 Years of Age Who Are Cyanotic (Fig. 26.1A)

Any infant who has a murmur and appears cyanotic should have a thorough physical examination and also should have an electrocardiogram (ECG), chest film, pulse oximetry, and possibly arterial gases. If the physical examination is normal, except for the cyanosis and the murmur, and the ECG, film, and pulse oximetry are normal, the infant probably has a normal murmur and a noncardiac cause of only apparent cyanosis (peripheral acrocyanosis, polycythemia)

A cyanotic infant who appears well but has an abnormal ECG and chest film and has diminished arterial saturation by oximetry or blood gas evaluation probably has cyanotic heart disease of a type not likely to cause early trouble. This could include tetralogy of Fallot, transposition of the great vessels with single ventricle, truncus arteriosus, Ebstein anomaly, tricuspid atresia, anomalous pulmonary venous drainage, or moderately severe pulmonary stenosis with shunting through an atrial or ventricular septal defect.

If the cyanotic infant appears acutely ill, the likelihood is that the chest film and the ECG and pulse oximetry will be abnormal. If the findings on physical examination suggest congestive heart failure (CHF), the infant probably has severe cyanotic congenital heart disease or an extremely severe acyanotic defect with the cyanosis related to poor perfusion and failure. Defects in the neonate could include extreme aortic or pulmonary stenosis, pulmonary atresia with intact ventricular septum, and hypoplastic left heart. In the somewhat older infant, considerations include tricuspid atresia, Ebstein anomaly, large arteriovenous malformation, atrioventricular canal defect, large ventricular septal defect, and total anomalous pulmonary venous drainage. Early echocardiography (ECHO) is indicated.

If the evaluation of the sick cyanotic infant does not suggest CHF and the saturation improves somewhat with crying and in oxygen, the infant probably has primary lung disease caused by infection, hypoperfusion, or pulmonary arteriolar hypertension. If the saturation by oximetry of an infant without heart disease does not improve with oxygen, the patient may have methemoglobinemia (see Chapter 78).

Infants Less Than 3 Years of Age Who Are Not Cyanotic (Fig. 26.1B)

If the infant's physical examination is negative and the infant appears well, except for the murmur, the murmur may represent a congenital cardiac defect that is physiologically insignificant at the time (e.g., small patent ductus, atrial or ventricular septal defect, mild aortic or pulmonary stenosis, partial anomalous pulmonary venous drainage), or it may represent a normal murmur. These children can have follow-up by their primary care physician. If doubt exists about the infant's status because of the intensity or transmission of the murmur, an ECG and chest film should be ordered; if normal, they confirm the above impression. Peripheral pulmonary stenosis, related to angulation of the distal pulmonary arteries, is a common cause of normal murmurs in neonates; this murmur transmits

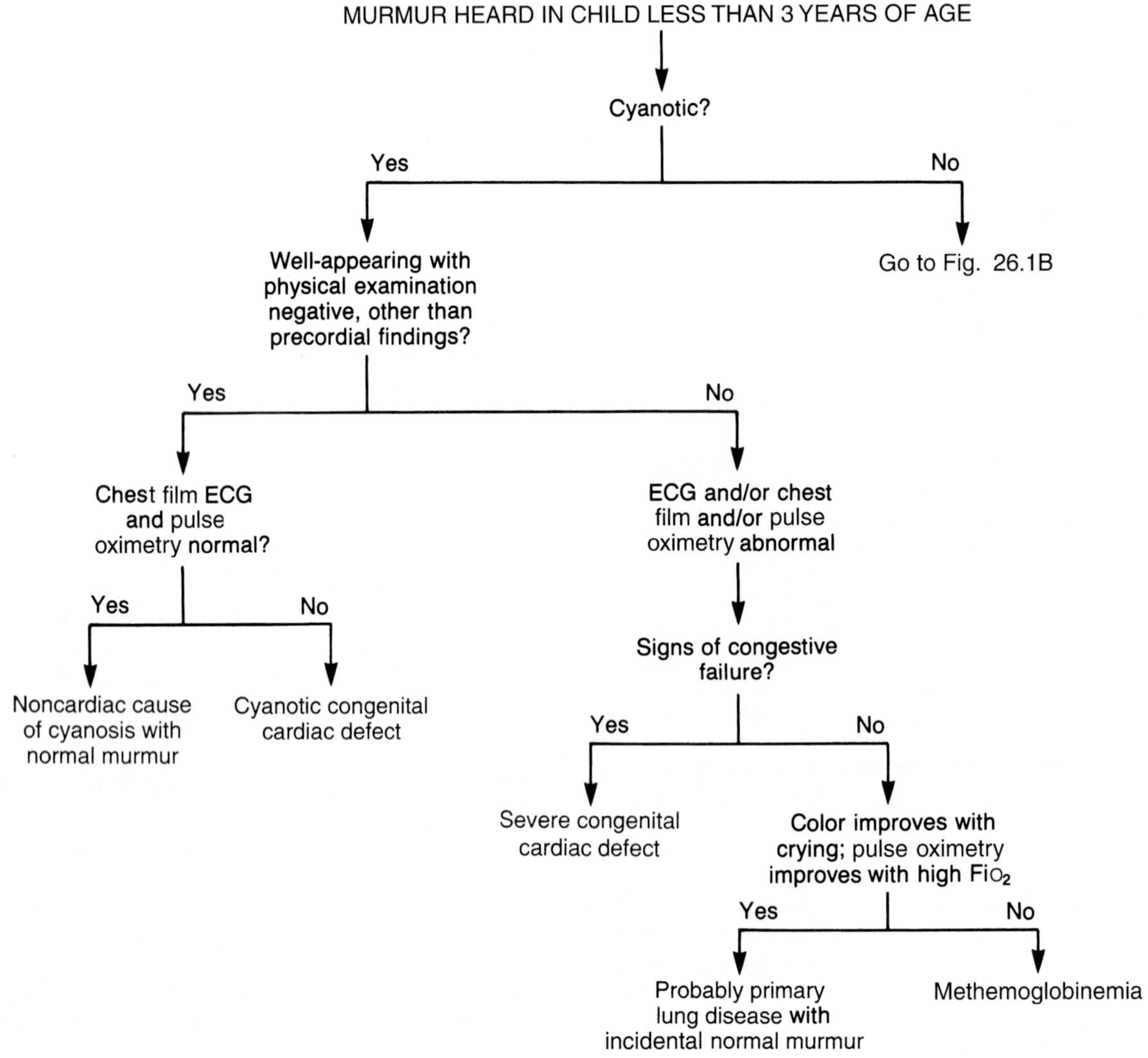

Figure 26.1. A: Assessment of a cyanotic infant less than 3 years of age in whom a murmur is heard. **B:** Assessment of an acyanotic child less than 3 years of age in whom a murmur is heard. VH, ventricular hypertrophy.

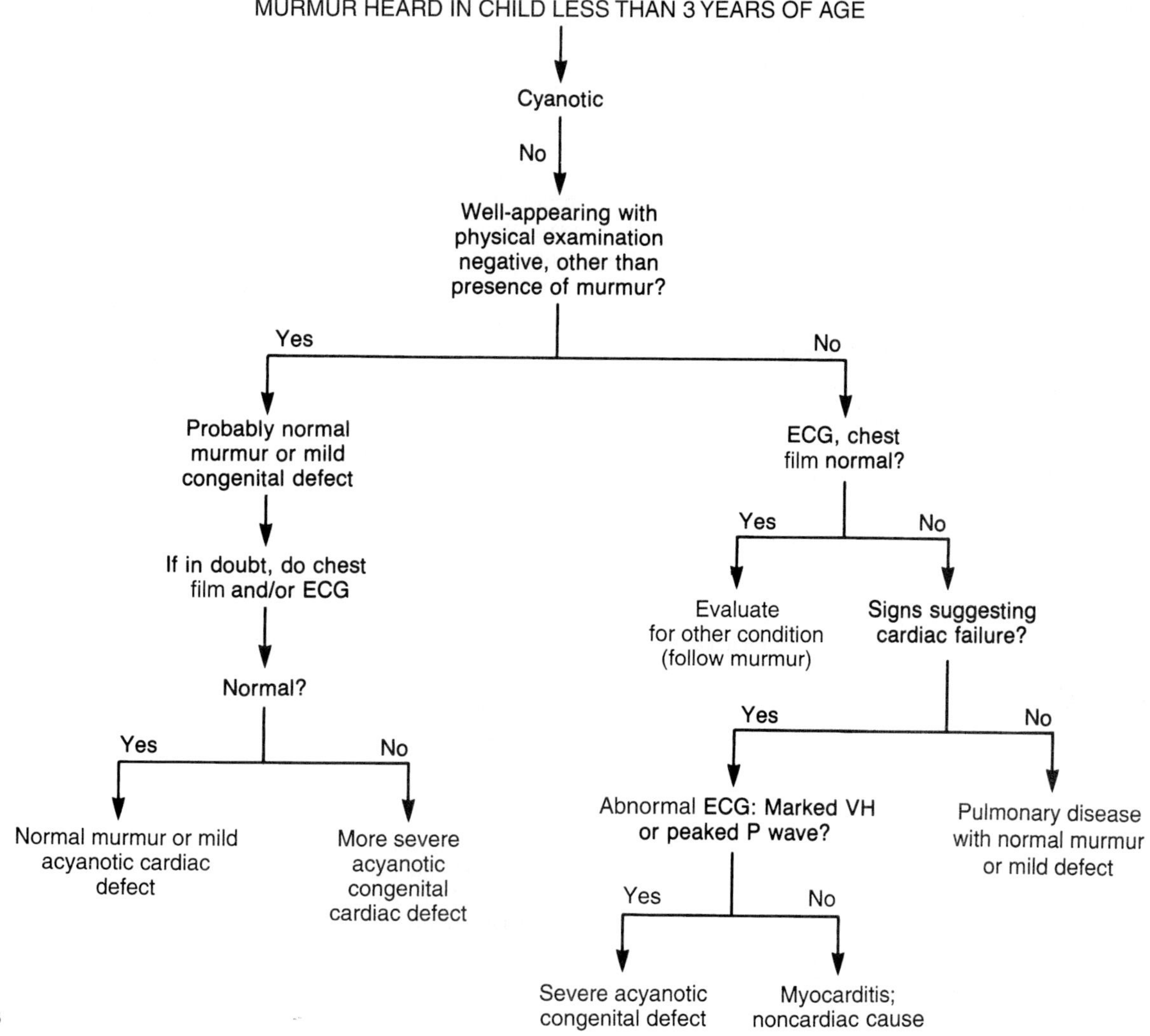

Figure 26.1. *(Continued)*

well to the back, may be quite loud, and in time will not be discernible.

If the ECG shows abnormal atrial or ventricular hypertrophy and the chest film shows cardiac enlargement or abnormal pulmonary vasculature, a more serious degree of the same acyanotic defects, or possibly an acyanotic tetralogy of Fallot, is likely, and nonemergent referral to a cardiologist is warranted.

If the acyanotic infant with a murmur appears ill, an ECG and chest film should be obtained. If these are normal, the murmur is most likely inconsequential, and the infant should be evaluated for an underlying medical or surgical illness related to the presenting complaints at this visit. It is important to think of noncardiac conditions, such as severe anemia or hyperpyrexia, as causes of the murmur.

If the infant has signs suggesting cardiac failure, ECG findings of marked ventricular hypertrophy or tall and pointed P waves might be indicative of a severe acyanotic congenital cardiac defect (e.g., large ventricular septal defect, large patent ductus, severe aortic or pulmonary stenosis).

An infant in failure with only T-wave or ST-segment changes on ECG may have viral myocarditis, primary myocardial disease, or an extracardiac problem that causes high cardiac output (severe anemia, large arteriovenous malformation). Some of these infants, although not cyanotic on the basis of their underlying lesion, may show a degree of cyanosis with diminished saturation on pulse oximetry because of the hypoperfusion related to cardiac failure.

If the chest film or ECG is not normal and the infant appears ill but does not have signs that suggest CHF, a primary pulmonary disease should be considered, with the murmur being either a normal one or representing a milder acyanotic defect.

Children 3 Years and Older

By the time children who live in geographic areas in which modern medical care is available reach 3 years of age, most congenital lesions have been discovered and many have been surgically repaired. Acquired cardiac and noncardiac illnesses, therefore, play a more prominent role in assessment. Still, some congenital lesions go unrecognized, some do not require surgery, and others that require surgery have not had access because of economic or social reasons.

Normal murmurs are by far the most common ones discovered at a first encounter with an older child. Table 26.2 describes the characteristics generally associated with a normal murmur. If the examining physician is satisfied that the murmur is a normal one and the child has no other symptoms referable to the cardiovascular system, cardiac consultation is neither necessary nor advisable. Still, it often is difficult to distinguish a normal murmur from the murmur of such intracardiac lesions as small atrial or ventricular defects or mild aortic or pulmonic stenosis; the management guidelines outlined in this chapter obviate the need for the emergency physician to be concerned about such a differential. For the purposes of the ED evaluation, it is important to determine only whether the patient is in difficulty or needs further evaluation. Again, the presence or absence of cyanosis is the lead finding.

Children 3 Years of Age and Older Who Are Not Cyanotic (Figs. 26.2A and 26.2B)

The acyanotic child with a murmur who seems most likely to have a normal murmur may have a mild acyanotic congenital defect, a healed rheumatic carditis, or a mitral valve prolapse. The femoral artery pulsations always should be palpated for the possibility of coarctation of the distal aorta. In mitral valve prolapse, a midsystolic "click" is a more constant finding than the murmur, which follows the click and is quite variable. These children should have follow-up by their primary care physician. If doubt exists because of the intensity or transmission of the murmur, an ECG and chest film should be ordered. If these are normal, one has further assurance that primary care follow-up is all that is necessary. If these are abnormal, there is concern about the possibility of a more severe acyanotic defect or moderately severe healed rheumatic carditis.

In evaluating the acyanotic child who appears acutely ill and has a murmur, a careful history should be taken regarding prior or recent antecedent illness, including a significant sore throat or "viral" illness. If there is such a history, the possibility of swollen, red, and tender joints should be sought. If these are present, the child is febrile, and an ECG is abnormal, the child should be hospitalized to be evaluated for the possibility of acute rheumatic fever (see Chapter 72). On the other hand, the acyanotic ill child with objective joint findings but a normal ECG is more likely to have a normal murmur with a concurrent

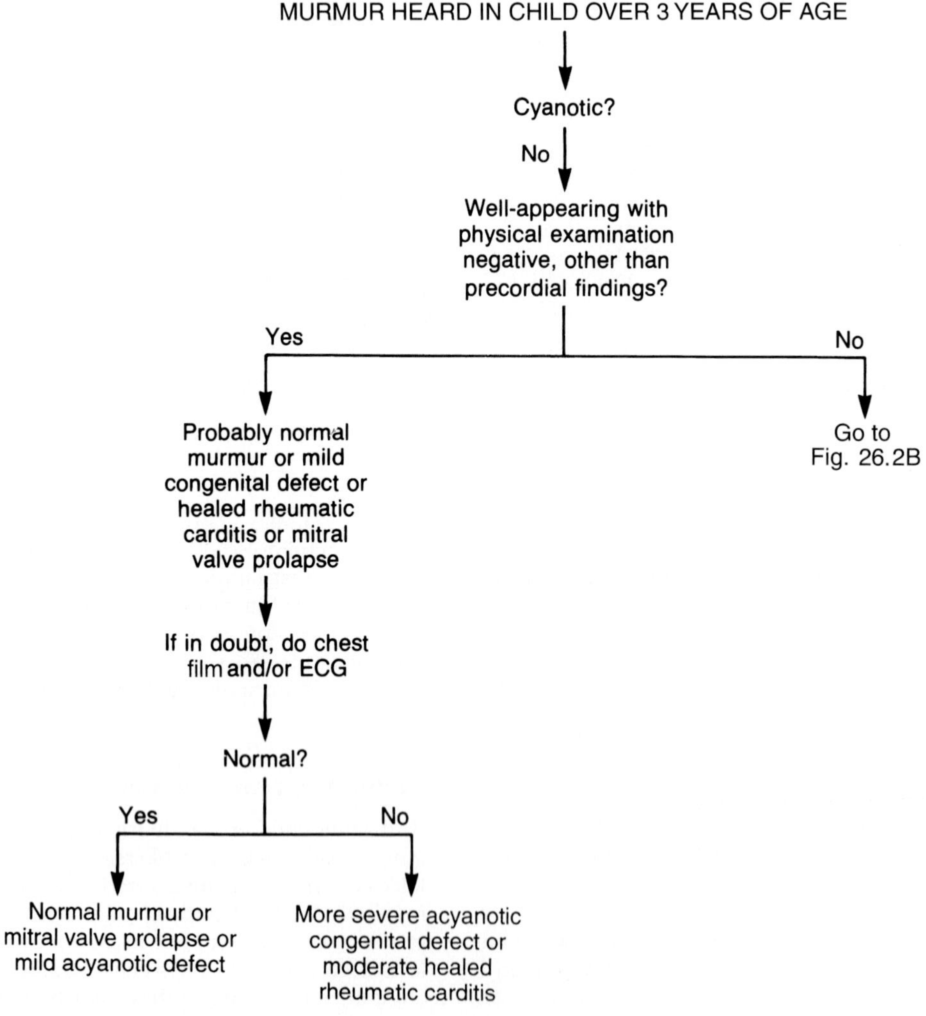

Figure 26.2. **A:** Assessment of an acyanotic, well-appearing child 3 years of age or older in whom a murmur is heard. **B:** Assessment of an acyanotic, sick child 3 years or older in whom a murmur is heard. **C:** Assessment of a cyanotic child 3 years of age or older.

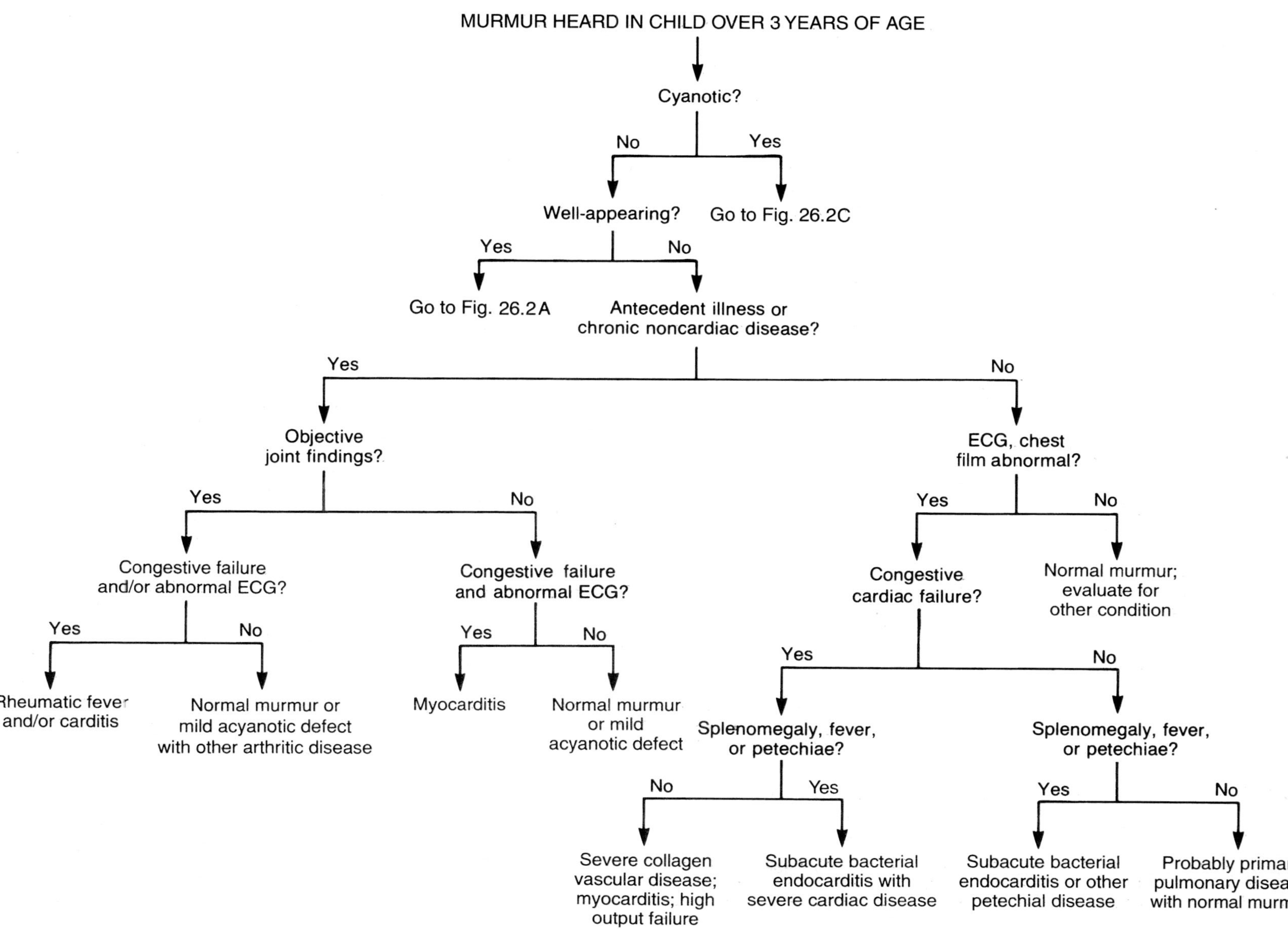

Figure 26.2. *(Continued)*

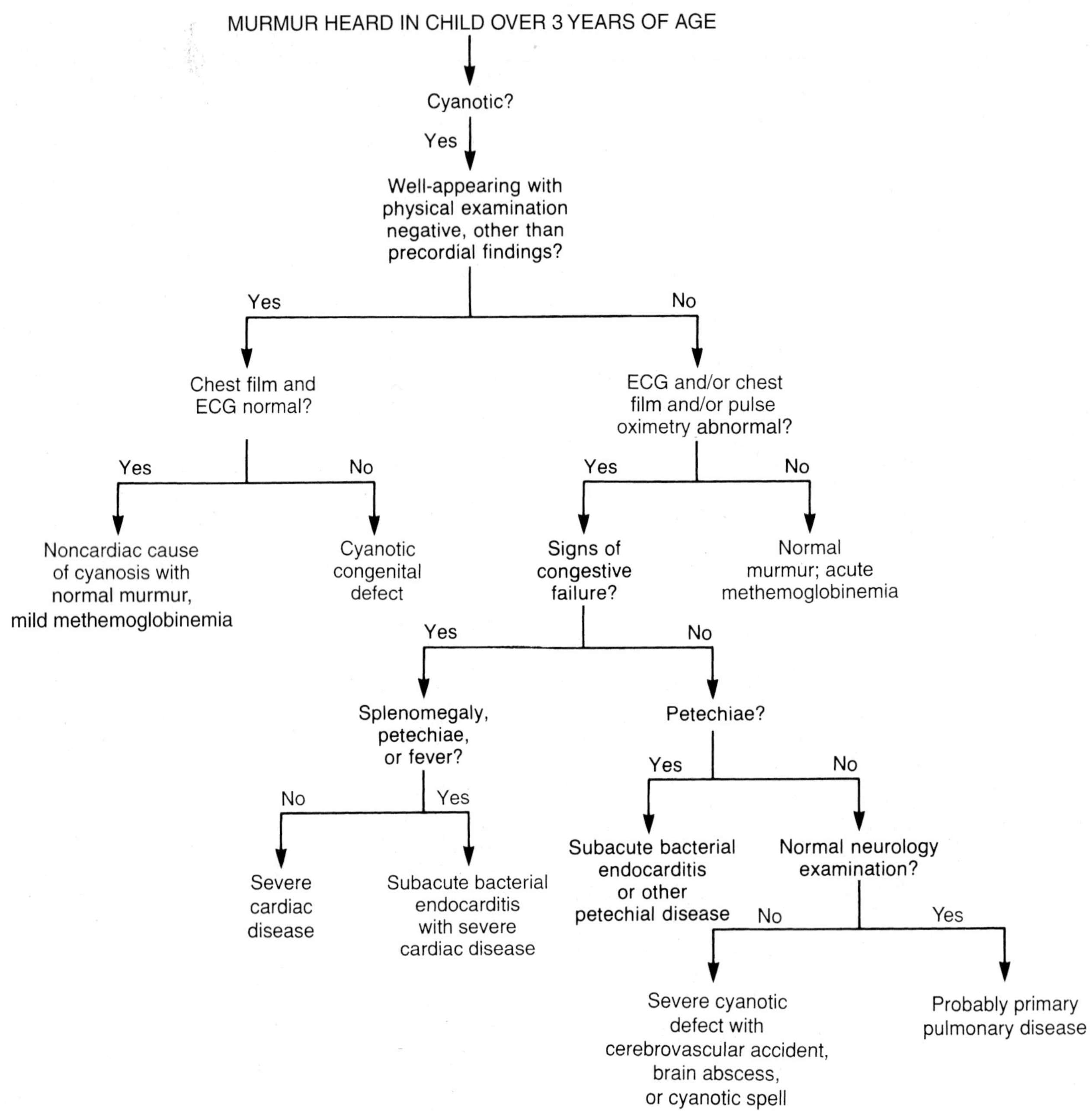

Figure 26.2. *(Continued)*

arthritic-like illness, such as Henoch-Schzönlein purpura (HSP), juvenile rheumatoid arthritis, or septic arthritis. These children need diagnostic evaluation of their acute illness and follow-up of the murmur.

The ill-appearing acyanotic child who has a murmur and a history of known chronic or recent antecedent illness but has no objective joint findings should have an ECG and a chest film taken. If the ECG shows ST-segment and T-wave abnormality and if the heart is enlarged, the patient probably has myocarditis, with the murmur resulting from turbulence created by ventricular dilation and atrioventricular valve insufficiency. The cause could be viral, collagen vascular, toxic, or endocrine (see Chapters 72 and 86). These children must be admitted for evaluation and therapy.

The ill-appearing acyanotic child who has a murmur but no chronic or recent antecedent illness and who shows signs of CHF may have severe acyanotic heart disease, myocarditis, or high-output failure secondary to severe anemia, large arteriovenous malformation, or thyrotoxicosis. Early ECHO is indicated.

Whether in congestive failure or not, the ill-appearing child with a murmur and fever should be examined carefully for splenomegaly and petechiae on the skin surface, on the conjunctivae, and under the nailbeds. If these are found, although the murmur could represent the entire list of cardiac diseases, the important immediate concern is that of infectious endocarditis (see Chapter 72).

If the patient with a murmur and petechiae is not showing signs of failure, the murmur may be normal or represent a mild acyanotic defect. In addition to infectious endocarditis, consideration must be given to other conditions that manifest with petechiae, such as meningococcemia, idiopathic thrombocytopenic purpura (ITP), HSP, and rickettsial infection. Blood

TABLE 26.1. Conditions That May Be Associated with Presence of a Cardiac Murmur[a]

Infancy
- Cardiac
  - Noncyanotic
    - Normal murmur ("innocent" murmur)
    - Congenital defects
      - Patent ductus arteriosus
      - Atrial septal defect
      - Ventricular septal defect
      - Aortic stenosis
      - Coarctation of aorta
      - Pulmonary stenosis
      - Partial anomalous pulmonary venous drainage
    - Myocarditis
    - Primary myocardial disease
  - Cyanotic
    - Congenital defects
      - Tetralogy of Fallot
      - Transposition of the great vessels
      - Truncus arteriosus
      - Pulmonary atresia
      - Severe pulmonary stenosis with patent foramen
      - Tricuspid atresia
      - Ebstein's anomaly
      - Total anomalous pulmonary venous drainage
      - Atrioventricular canal defect
      - Hypoplastic left heart
  - Congestive cardiac failure
    - Secondary to any of the above, as well as noncardiac causes listed below
- Extracardiac
  - Severe anemia
  - Arteriovenous malformation
  - Pulmonary insufficiency (including infection, hypoperfusion, pulmonary arterial hypertension)
  - Hyperpyrexia

Older child
- Cardiac
  - Normal murmur
  - Congenital defect
  - (Same list as for infancy-both cyanotic and noncyanotic)
  - Mitral valve prolapse
  - Myocarditis (viral, collagen, toxic, endocrine, genetic)
  - Acute rheumatic fever
  - Healed rheumatic carditis
  - Subacute bacterial endocarditis
  - Congestive cardiac failure (associated with any of above or the below noncardiac diseases)
- Extracardiac
  - Severe anemia
  - Arteriovenous malformation
  - Pulmonary insufficiency
  - Thyrotoxicosis
  - Hyperpyrexia

[a] It should be kept in mind that *any* pediatric problem may be coincidentally associated with the presence of a normal cardiac murmur or with one of the other conditions in the above list. The algorithms and chapter text are constructed to help sort out the significance of the murmur in the context of patient management.

cultures should be drawn, appropriate emergency treatment initiated, and the child admitted for further evaluation and treatment.

If the acyanotic ill-appearing child with a murmur is not in failure, has no splenomegaly or petechiae, and had a normal ECG, the murmur is most likely normal or associated with the high cardiac output of hyperpyrexia or anemia. These children should be evaluated for their underlying condition.

TABLE 26.2. Characteristics Usually Associated with A "Normal" Murmur

Timing: midsystole
Intensity: grades I through IV
Location of maximal intensity: midsternal border
Radiation: possibly to the precordium and neck, but not the back
Quality: "twangy" or "vibratory"
Heart sounds: readily definable, including splitting of S2

Children 3 Years and Older Who Are Cyanotic (Fig. 26.2C)

As with infants, cyanotic older children with murmurs should have an ECG, chest film, pulse oximetry, and possibly arterial gases after a careful history and complete physical examination. If a patient is tested with these and the results are normal, except for the cyanosis and murmur, the child probably has a noncardiac cause of the cyanosis (polycythemia). The murmur may be normal or associated with a coincidental acyanotic congenital defect. The primary condition should be investigated. The cyanotic child who is not acutely ill but has an abnormal ECG, chest film, and pulse oximetry has cyanotic heart disease that possibly could be improved surgically.

If the cyanotic child appears acutely ill and has signs of CHF, severe cardiac disease is present. The causes could include a decompensating congenital cyanotic cardiac defect, in which case the cyanosis would be intense (Table 26.1), or failure secondary to acquired disease, in which the cyanosis is related to hypoperfusion and usually less intense.

Whether or not there are signs of congestive failure in the cyanotic child with a murmur, if there is fever, splenomegaly, or petechiae on the skin, on the conjunctivae, or under the nailbeds, blood cultures should be drawn for the likelihood of infective endocarditis. If the child is not in failure and petechiae are found, infective endocarditis is still a possibility, but other noncardiac causes of petechial presentations must be considered (e.g., meningococcemia, Valsalva maneuvers, ITP, HSP). Blood cultures should be drawn and the child admitted.

A careful neurologic examination should be part of the evaluation of every ill child with cyanotic heart disease. If findings are abnormal, consideration must be given to the complications of hypoxemic "spells," cerebrovascular accident, or, if the patient is febrile, brain abscess.

If the ill cyanotic child with a murmur and abnormal chest film shows significant improvement of oxygen saturation with supplemental oxygen, the child most likely has primary pulmonary disease. The ECG abnormality, if one is found, most likely would consist of tall, pointed P waves and evidence of right ventricular hypertrophy.

In the cyanotic child with a murmur who has a normal ECG and chest film, abnormal pulse oximetry, but normal arterial partial pressure of oxygen (P_{O2}), the possibility of acute toxin-induced methemoglobinemia must be considered, with the murmur being normal or representing a mild acyanotic condition.

CHAPTER 27
Hematuria

Erica L. Liebelt, M.D.

Hematuria, the presence of red blood cells (RBCs) in the urine, is a common presenting complaint in the emergency department (ED). The presence of 5 to 10 or more RBCs per high-power field (HPF) is abnormal and warrants further workup.

DIFFERENTIAL DIAGNOSIS

The differential diagnosis of hematuria is vast and can be categorized based on whether the site of bleeding is within the urinary system (glomerular, extraglomerular) or secondary to a systemic process (Table 27.1). The most common causes of hematuria (Table 27.2) are UTI (either cystitis or pyelonephritis), acute poststreptococcal glomerulonephritis, and trauma, the latter two also being the most common of the potentially life-threatening causes. Other potentially serious causes of hematuria (Table 27.3) include hematologic disorders, renal stones with obstruction, tumors, and hemolytic uremic syndrome (HUS). Other glomerular causes of hematuria that are primary renal diseases include nonstreptococcal postinfectious glomerulonephritides, membranous glomerulonephritis, immunoglobulin A (IgA) nephropathy, and Alport syndrome (hereditary nephritis). Hematuria as a manifestation of a systemic condition is most commonly seen in children with vasculitides, such as in Henoch-Schönlein purpura (HSP), systemic lupus erythematosus (SLE), and polyarteritis nodosa.

Extraglomerular causes of hematuria include congenital anomalies such as diverticula of the urethra and bladder; hemangiomas in the bladder; cysts of the kidneys, as in polycystic or multicystic kidney; and obstruction of the ureteropelvic junction. In addition to congenital anomalies, renal vein thrombosis secondary to a coagulation disorder or to placement of an umbilical catheter is a cause of hematuria in the neonate. Wilms tumor is a common childhood solid tumor associated with hematuria in 12% to 25% of cases. Nephrolithiasis should be considered if there is a family history or a predisposing condition such as recurrent infection, bladder dysfunction (seen in myelomeningocele), or chronic diuretic therapy (as seen in infants with bronchopulmonary dysplasia). Hypercalciuria and cystinuria are metabolic diseases that also predispose patients to renal stones and hematuria. Finally, urethral prolapse, seen most commonly in girls 2 to 4 years of age, may present with vaginal bleeding that can contaminate a collected urine specimen and be misinterpreted as hematuria.

TABLE 27.1. Principal Causes of Hematuria in Children

- Renal
  - Extraglomerular
    - Trauma
    - Urinary tract infection (cystitis, pyelonephritis)
    - Hemorrhagic cystitis (bacterial, viral, drugs)
    - Stones
    - Hypercalciuria
    - Interstitial nephritis
    - Polycystic kidney disease
    - Renal vein thrombosis
    - Papillary necrosis
    - Wilms' tumor
    - Posterior urethral valves
    - Hydronephrosis
    - Ureteropelvic junction obstruction
    - Urethritis
    - Urethral diverticula
    - Urethral prolapse
    - Foreign body
    - Hemangiomas
  - Glomerular
    - Acute poststreptococcal glomerulonephritis
    - Other postinfectious glomerulonephritis
    - IgA nephropathy
    - Alport's syndrome (hereditary nephritis)
    - Exercise
    - Familial benign hematuria
    - Other chronic nephritides (membranoproliferative, membranous)
- Extrarenal
  - Coagulation disorders–hemophilia, platelet disorders
  - Sickle cell disease or trait
  - Anticoagulant therapy
  - Drugs–aspirin, nonsteroidal anti-inflammatory drugs, phenacetin, penicillins, cephalosporins, cyclophosphamide
- Systemic diseases
  - Leukemia
  - Serum sickness
  - Henoch–Schönlein purpura
  - Hemolytic uremic syndrome
  - Systemic lupus erythematosus
  - Polyarteritis nodosa
  - Subacute bacterial endocarditis
  - Shunt nephritis
  - Tuberculosis
  - Hepatitis

IgA, immunoglobulin A.

EVALUATION AND DECISION

The initial evaluation of hematuria must begin with confirmation of blood in the urine. The most important role for the emergency physician in evaluating a child with hematuria is to identify serious, treatable, and progressive conditions such as trauma, nephritis associated with hypertension, bleeding disorders, and infection.

Blood in the urine may come from sources outside the urinary tract. Vaginal hemorrhage in the female secondary to infection, foreign body, or trauma (sometimes secondary to abuse) may contaminate the urine. In addition, parents may report finding blood in the urine when, in fact, a rectal fissure has caused a small hemorrhage, producing a mixture of blood and urine in the diaper or underwear. In prepubertal girls, urethral prolapse may present with vaginal bleeding, which may be confused with hematuria.

Urine dipsticks positive for blood require microscopic examination of the urine. Hemoglobinuria from hemolysis and myoglobinuria from rhabdomyolysis will cause a positive dipstick reaction for blood and an absence of RBCs on urine microscopy. Many dyes, drugs, and pigments will change the urine color to

TABLE 27.2. Common Causes of Hematuria

- Urinary tract infection–cystitis, pyelonephritis
- Trauma (kidney, bladder, urethra)
- Acute poststreptococcal glomerulonephritis
- Sickle cell disease or trait
- Interstitial nephritis
- Benign hematuria
- Urethritis

TABLE 27.3. Life-Threatening Causes of Hematuria

Trauma (kidney, bladder)
Acute glomerulonephritis
Hemolytic uremic syndrome
Renal stones with obstruction
Tumor
Hematologic disorders
Toxins

pink, red, brown, or black but will not result in a positive dipstick test for blood. A partial list includes beets, blackberries, urates, aniline dyes, bile pigments, porphyrin, diphenylhydantoin, phenazopyridine (Pyridium), rifampin, deferoxamine, phenolphthalein, ibuprofen, methyldopa, chloroquine, homogentisic acid, and *Serratia marcescens* infection.

The history taking for infants and neonates with hematuria should include questions about umbilical vessel catheters (renal venous or arterial thrombosis), passage of clots on voiding (hemorrhagic disorders), abdominal swelling or palpable mass (tumor, polycystic disease, ureteropelvic junction obstruction, posterior urethral valves), and significant birth asphyxia (corticomedullary necrosis). Dysuria or frequency in children and adolescents suggests cystitis, whereas flank, abdominal, or back pain suggests trauma, genitourinary infection, or stones as the cause. Sore throat, upper respiratory infection, or pyoderma (preceding or appearing concurrently with the onset of hematuria) points to acute postinfectious glomerulonephritis. A history of gross hematuria with a concomitant viral upper respiratory or gastrointestinal infection also may suggest IgA nephropathy. Hematuria associated with systemic disorders may be uncovered by eliciting a history of skin rashes and arthralgia or arthritis as seen in HSP and SLE. Both sickle cell anemia and sickle cell trait are associated with chronic, asymptomatic gross hematuria. Finally, a history of drug use, especially the use of penicillins and cephalosporins, may point to interstitial nephritis as the cause. Antibiotic-associated tubulointerstitial nephritis is associated with high-dose, long-term antibiotic therapy and is characterized clinically by fever, rash, eosinophilia with pyuria, eosinophiluria, hematuria, proteinuria, and nonoliguric renal failure. Family history of renal stones, deafness, nephritis, renal anomalies, or hematologic disease may suggest a diagnosis in the child such as Alport syndrome (hereditary nephritis), sickle cell anemia, or hemophilia.

Physical examination of a child with hematuria should always include measurement of blood pressure. Hypertension may accompany glomerulonephritis, obstructive uropathy, Wilms tumor, polycystic kidney, or vascular disease. Periorbital edema and facial swelling may be the first physical signs of nephritis. Urethral prolapse presents as a doughnut-shaped mass at the site of the urethral meatus, which is usually hyperemic and friable with scant bloody drainage.

Bruising of the abdomen, flank, or back should raise the s uspicion of trauma, including child abuse, as a cause of hematuria. Tenderness of the flank or lower abdomen may signal pyelonephritis, obstructed kidney, or lower UTI. Flank or abdominal masses suggest Wilms tumor or hydronephrosis, hydroureter, or polycystic kidney. Petechial or purpuric lesions on the skin and arthritis may accompany hematuria seen in vasculitic syndromes such as HPS, HUS, and SLE. Pallor may be a sign of anemia from chronic renal insufficiency, HUS, hemoglobinopathy, leukemia, or tumors.

Glomerular bleeding is indicated by RBC casts, cellular casts, tubular cells, tea-colored or smoky brown urine, and proteinuria 2+ or greater by dipstick. In addition, the presence of dysmorphic RBCs or acanthocytes (ring-formed RBCs with one or more protrusions of different shapes and sizes) as well as measurement of the mean volume of urine erythrocytes using a Coulter counter have been used as markers of glomerular bleeding (erythrocyte volume <50 m^3). In contrast, nonglomerular bleeding is suggested by red or pink urine, blood clots, no proteinuria (or less than 2+ in the absence of gross hematuria), and normal morphology of erythrocytes. Calcium oxalate crystals may be seen in the urine of patients with renal stones.

EVALUATION AND DECISION

A clinical algorithm for evaluating hematuria in the ED is shown in Figure 27.1. The first step is to confirm the presence of true hematuria. If a traumatic cause for the hematuria is suspected based on the history or physical findings, emergent evaluation for serious anatomic lesions must be initiated. Parenchymal contusions, lacerations, renal transections, and pedicle disruptions are possible injuries. Hematuria is the cardinal marker of renal injury, with the severity paralleling the magnitude of the injury (except for renal pedicle injuries, which may have no associated hematuria). Microscopic hematuria greater than 20 to 50 RBC per HPF, gross hematuria, or a history of significant mechanism of injury to the flank or abdomen necessitates emergent imaging. Hematuria disproportionate to the injury may indicate a congenital renal anomaly or tumor.

If there is no history of trauma, coagulopathies should be considered as a cause; however, the medical history alone usually will point to this cause because the sudden occurrence of isolated hematuria in a previously healthy child is unlikely with either a congenital or acquired bleeding disorder. Hematuria in a child known to have hemophilia or a related disorder often requires minimal investigation and is managed in accordance with standard protocols. If an acquired coagulopathy is suspected, a complete blood count (CBC) with platelet count, prothrombin time, and partial thromboplastin time is warranted.

If trauma and coagulopathies are considered unlikely, identifying the site of bleeding as either glomerular or nonglomerular (based on urinalysis and other signs or symptoms) can direct further evaluation and diagnosis. Acute glomerulonephritis characterized by hypertension, edema, RBC casts, proteinuria, and tea-colored urine most often follows a streptococcal infection and merits serious consideration in the ED because it may cause significant hypertension and pulmonary edema requiring immediate intervention. HUS is a serious disorder that may present with glomerular-induced hematuria and proteinuria as well as a characteristic microangiopathic hemolytic anemia, thrombocytopenia, and renal failure. Laboratory studies useful in children suspected of having nephritis include a CBC and measurement of the erythrocyte sedimentation rate, blood urea nitrogen, serum creatinine, complement levels, and antistreptococcal antibodies. Other nephritides may be associated with vasculitis (HSP, SLE, periarteritis nodosa, Wegener granulomatosis) and may require further diagnostic evaluation before a specific diagnosis is made.

Most children without a history of trauma who are evaluated for gross or microscopic hematuria in the ED have a UTI. The findings of pyuria and bacteriuria on urinalysis suggest an infectious cause, although their absence does not exclude either pyelonephritis or cystitis; thus, a urine culture is essential if no other cause has been uncovered.

Severe flank pain radiating to the groin is characteristic of renal colic from calculi, which may present with either gross or microscopic hematuria. Stones may occur in children with metabolic abnormalities or stasis secondary to obstruction and

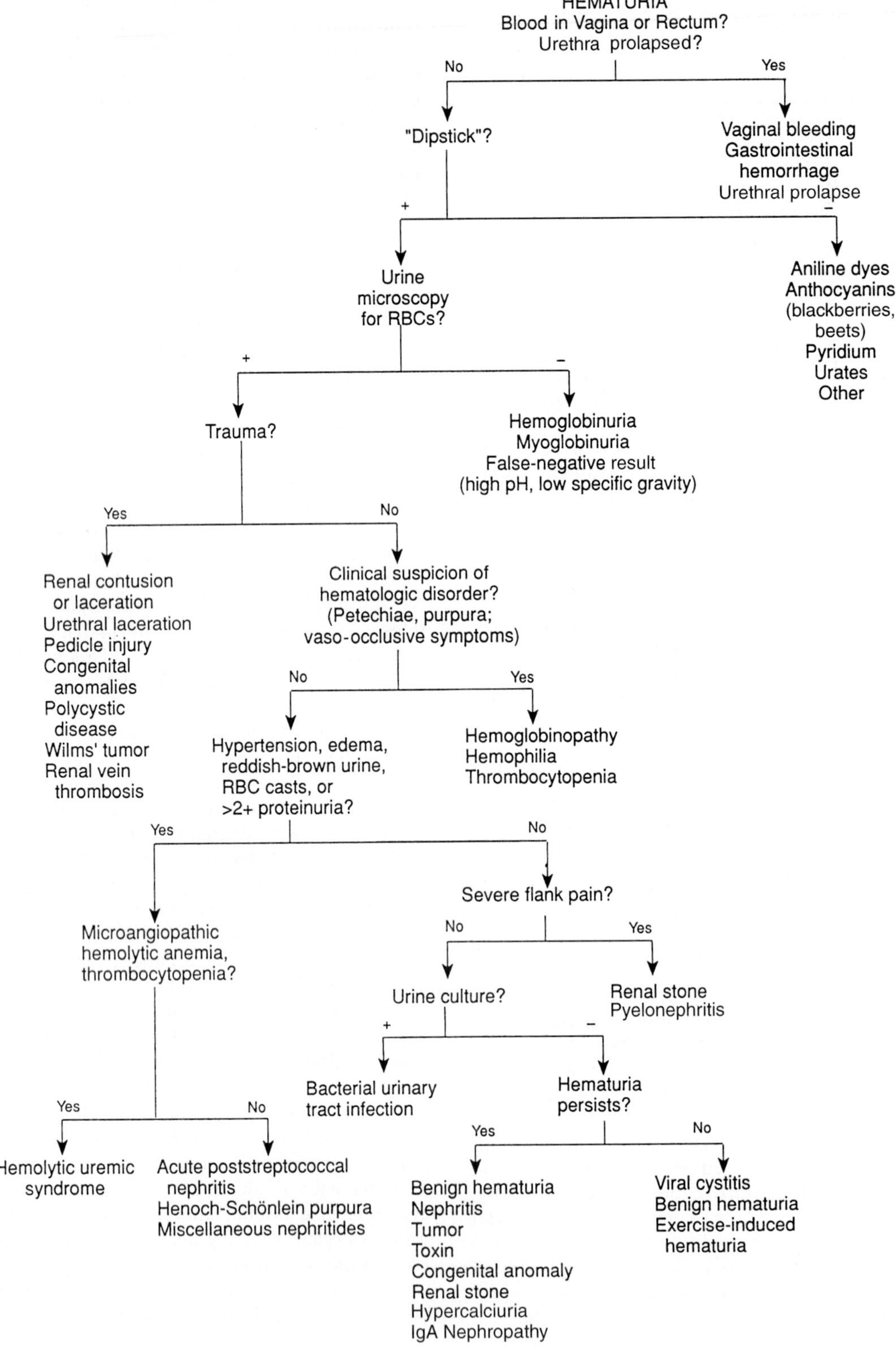

Figure 27.1. Approach to hematuria in the emergency department.

in premature infants taking furosemide, especially those with bronchopulmonary dysplasia. Crystals may be seen on urinalysis; further investigation with intravenous pyelography, renal ultrasound, or spiral computed tomography (CT) usually confirms stones if a plain abdominal radiograph does not reveal the presence of radiopaque material.

Hematuria that persists after the previously mentioned causes have been ruled out or deemed unlikely based on history and physical examination usually does not require further evaluation in the ED and should be pursued by the primary health care provider, possibly in collaboration with a pediatric nephrologist.

CHAPTER 28
Hypertension

James G. Linakis, M.D., Ph.D.

Until recently, hypertension was considered predominantly a disorder of adulthood; however, a wide variety of diseases (Table 28.1) have now been described that elevate the blood pressure in young children and adolescents, and these groups may suffer from essential hypertension. Various etiologies for hypertension have a predilection for infants or children of various ages (Table 28.2). Those entities that lead to extreme elevations in blood pressure are life threatening (Table 28.3).

The Second Task Force on Blood Pressure Control in Children divided hypertension into two distinct classes: *Significant (moderate) hypertension* was defined as blood pressure measurements persistently between the 95th and 99th percentiles for age and sex, and *severe hypertension* was defined as blood pressure measurements persistently at or above the 99th percentile for age and sex (Table 28.4). For the sake of the present discussion, the classification system of The Second Task Force can be expanded to include two additional terms. *Hypertensive urgency* is a severely elevated blood pressure that may be potentially harmful but is without evidence of end-organ damage or dysfunction. For the purposes of evaluation and treatment, blood pressure measurements at or above "severe" levels should be considered a hypertensive urgency even in the absence of symptoms. *Hypertensive emergency* describes a situation in which elevated blood pressure is associated with evidence of secondary organ damage such as hypertensive encephalopathy or acute left ventricular failure.

TABLE 28.1. Complete Differential Diagnosis of Hypertension

Essential hypertension	Neurologic
Obesity	Increased intracranial pressure
Pain	Familial dysautonomia
Anxiety	Guillain-Barré syndrome
Renal	Poliomyelitis
Glomerular disease	Drug-induced/toxicologic
Parenchymal disease	Amphetamines
Obstructive uropathy	Epinephrine
Renal vascular disease	Phenylpropanolamine
Pyelonephritis	Methylphenidate
Hemolytic uremic syndrome	Ephedrine
Henoch–Schönlein purpura	Pseudoephedrine
Renal trauma	Anticholinergics
Renal stones	Cocaine
Hypoplastic kidney	Phencyclidine
Nephrotic syndrome	Methysergide
Polycystic disease	Reserpine overdose
Tumors	Monoamine oxidase inhibitors
Fibrosis	Clonidine overdose
Acute renal failure	Ocular phenylephrine
Endocrine	Anabolic steroids
Pheochromocytoma	Oral contraceptives
Congenital adrenal hyperplasia	Corticosteroids
Primary aldosteronism	Heavy metal poisoning
Primary hyperparathyroidism	Miscellaneous
Cushing's syndrome	Hypercalcemia
Hyperthyroidism	Hypernatremia
Cardiovascular	Acute intermittent porphyria
Coarctation of aorta	Neurofibromatosis
Patent ductus arteriosus	Tuberous sclerosis
Arteriovenous fistula	Malignant hyperthermia
Bacterial endocarditis	
Valvular insufficiency	
Vasculitis	

EVALUATION AND DECISION

In the emergency department (ED), the extent of assessment of the child with hypertension depends on the level of blood pressure and the clinical signs and symptoms of the child at presentation. The asymptomatic child with incidental, newly diagnosed mild or moderate hypertension ("significant" in Table 28.4) generally requires a brief but thorough history and physical examination with emphasis on detecting pathophysiologic risk factors for hypertension and signs and symptoms of the complications of chronic hypertension. Barring the discovery of any of these, the child should be referred for follow-up and further evaluation with his or her primary care physician.

The workup of a child with severe hypertension requires careful evaluation for the presence of clinical findings that may represent either the primary cause of the elevated blood pressure or the secondary, systemic effects. Relevant history includes frequent urinary tract infections, unexplained fevers, hematuria, dysuria, frequency, and edema—all suggestive of possible renal disease. A history of umbilical artery catheterization as a neonate may indicate risk of renal artery stenosis. Ingestion of prescription, over-the-counter, or illicit drugs may support the diagnosis of drug-induced hypertension. Alternatively, a history of sweating, flushing, palpitations, fever, and weight loss may indicate a pheochromocytoma.

Physical examination should concentrate on identifying involved organ systems. Thus, the cardiac examination should inspect for evidence of congestive heart failure (CHF) and pulmonary edema. Femoral pulses should be palpated because their absence suggests aortic coarctation. Neurologic evaluation should include funduscopic examination for such hypertensive changes as hemorrhages, infarcts, and disc edema. In addition, testing of the pupillary light reflex and visual acuity and observation for sensorimotor symmetry should be included. Abdominal examination may reveal the presence of a bruit or palpable kidneys, implicating a renovascular or renal cause for the hypertension.

Ancillary investigations depend on the severity of the child's hypertension. In the child with severe hypertension, a number of laboratory studies are appropriate. Complete blood count, electrolytes, blood urea nitrogen, serum creatinine, and uric acid and urinalysis are warranted in the asymptomatic child with severe hypertension. In addition, urine culture should be obtained in all girls and in boys with known renal pathologic conditions. In the child with hypertensive emergency, early intravenous access also should be established.

In symptomatic children with hypertension, further evaluation includes an electrocardiogram and chest radiograph. These tests help evaluate myocardial function and the extent of damage from hypertension as well as the presence of CHF. Although several additional sophisticated and invasive studies exist for the evaluation of hypertension, these are rarely part of the routine ED assessment.

In some instances, the cause of hypertension is already known, as in a child with end-stage renal disease, or it is immediately apparent, as in an adolescent who has used cocaine. When the cause is not readily identified, a systematic approach is indicated (Fig. 28.1). Because diseases of the genitourinary tract are among the more common sources for hypertension in children, a logical starting point is to ascertain whether the his-

TABLE 28.2. Common Causes of Hypertension

Age group	Cause
Newborn infants	Renal artery thrombosis, renal artery stenosis, congenital renal malformations, coarctation of the aorta, bronchopulmonary dysplasia
Infancy to 6 yr	Renal parenchymal diseases,[a] coarctation of the aorta, renal artery stenosis
6–10 yr	Essential hypertension (including obesity), renal artery stenosis, renal parenchymal diseases
Adolescence	Essential hypertension (including obesity), renal parenchymal diseases

[a] Includes renal structural and inflammatory lesions as well as tumors.
Adapted from the Task Force on Blood Pressure Control in Children. Report of the second task force on blood pressure control in children—1987. *Pediatrics* 1987;79:1–25, with permission.

TABLE 28.3. Selected Life-Threatening Causes of Hypertension[a]

Age group	Cause
Infancy	Coarctation of the aorta, valvular insufficiency, congenital adrenal hyperplasia, renal vascular disease, renal parenchymal disease
Childhood	Renal parenchymal disease, renal vascular disease, coarctation of the aorta, pheochromocytoma, increased intracranial pressure, bacterial endocarditis, drug-induced/toxicolrogic
Adolescence	Renal parenchymal disease, pheochromocytoma, toxemia of pregnancy, drug-induced/toxicologic

[a] Any increase in blood pressure that is sufficiently acute or elevated to cause systemic symptoms should be considered life-threatening.

TABLE 28.4. Classification of Hypertension by Age Group

Age group	Significant hypertension (mm Hg)[a]	Severe hypertension (mm Hg)[b]
Newborn-7 days	Systolic BP ≥96	Systolic BP ≥106
8–30 days	Systolic BP ≥104	Systolic BP ≥110
Infant (<2 yr)	Systolic BP ≥110	Systolic BP ≥118
	Diastolic BP ≥63	Diastolic BP ≥82
Children (3–5 yr)	Systolic BP ≥116	Systolic BP ≥124
	Diastolic BP ≥74	Diastolic BP ≥84
Children (6–9 yr)	Systolic BP ≥121	Systolic BP ≥130
	Diastolic BP ≥81	Diastolic BP ≥86
Children (10–12 yr)	Systolic BP ≥127	Systolic BP ≥134
	Diastolic BP ≥83	Diastolic BP ≥90
Adolescents (13–15 yr)	Systolic BP ≥135	Systolic BP ≥144
	Diastolic BP ≥86	Diastolic BP ≥92
Adolescents (16–18 yr)	Systolic BP ≥142	Systolic BP ≥150
	Diastolic BP ≥92	Diastolic BP ≥98

[a] The values in this table are based on boys of larger than average height for age, and on the older age of the range given. Values for girls, children of ages in the lower end of the ranges given, and children smaller than 95th percentile for age will have values that are slightly lower. For a more comprehensive listing of values, see Task Force on Blood Pressure Control in Children. Report of the second task force on blood pressure in children—1987. *Pediatrics* 1996; 98:649–658. Adapted with permission from the Task Force on Blood Pressure Control in Children. Report of the second task force on blood pressure control in children—1987. *Pediatrics* 1987;79:1–25.
BP, blood pressure.

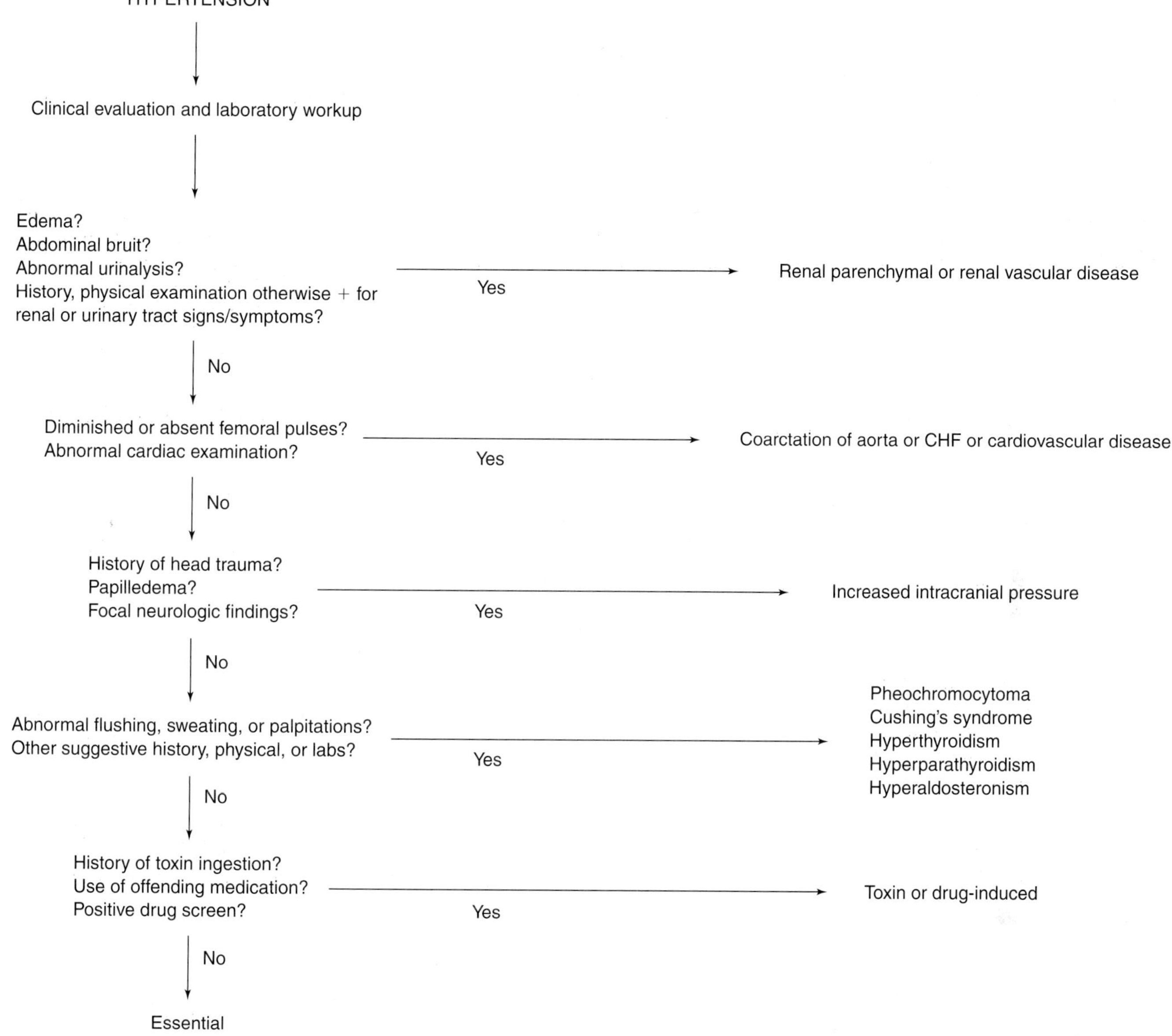

Figure 28.1. Diagnostic approach to acute hypertension in a previously healthy child. (See Fig. 28.2 for initial triage and stabilization for significant or severe hypertension.)

tory suggests prior urinary infection, whether the physical examination identifies signs of renal disease (e.g., edema or an abdominal bruit of renal artery stenosis), or whether the urinalysis is abnormal. Of the cardiovascular causes, coarctation of the aorta is the most likely to manifest in a toddler or older child with previously undiagnosed hypertension. Physical examination of patients with this lesion is notable for femoral pulses that are absent or diminished compared with those in the upper extremities. When a careful evaluation of the renal and cardiovascular systems is not revealing, a detailed neurologic examination is in order because any condition accompanied by increased intracranial pressure may elevate the systemic blood pressure. The history and signs of head trauma (see Chapter 92) are usually obvious but may be occult when injuries in young children are not witnessed or are intentionally inflicted. The emergency physician should specifically examine the fundi for papilledema and ascertain the presence of ataxia or other focal neurologic findings. Although the endocrine disorders are relatively rare, careful history taking and a directed physical examination may identify temperature sensitivity, obesity, a goiter, abdominal striae, or abnormal pigmentation suggestive of hyperthyroidism or Cushing syndrome. Intermittent headaches and flushing occur with pheochromocytoma. Finally, specific questioning about the ingestion of illicit drugs or other medications and a toxicologic screen are appropriate when no other cause for hypertension is apparent. A negative evaluation for a source of an elevation of blood pressure in the ED is compatible with, but not sufficient for, the diagnosis of essential hypertension. Follow-up is always indicated, usually accompanied by further testing in patients under the age of 10 years.

MANAGEMENT

The decision to treat a child with hypertension in the ED setting depends on the acuteness of the rise in blood pressure, the presence of symptoms, preexisting medical problems, and the extent of end-organ damage (Fig. 28.2).

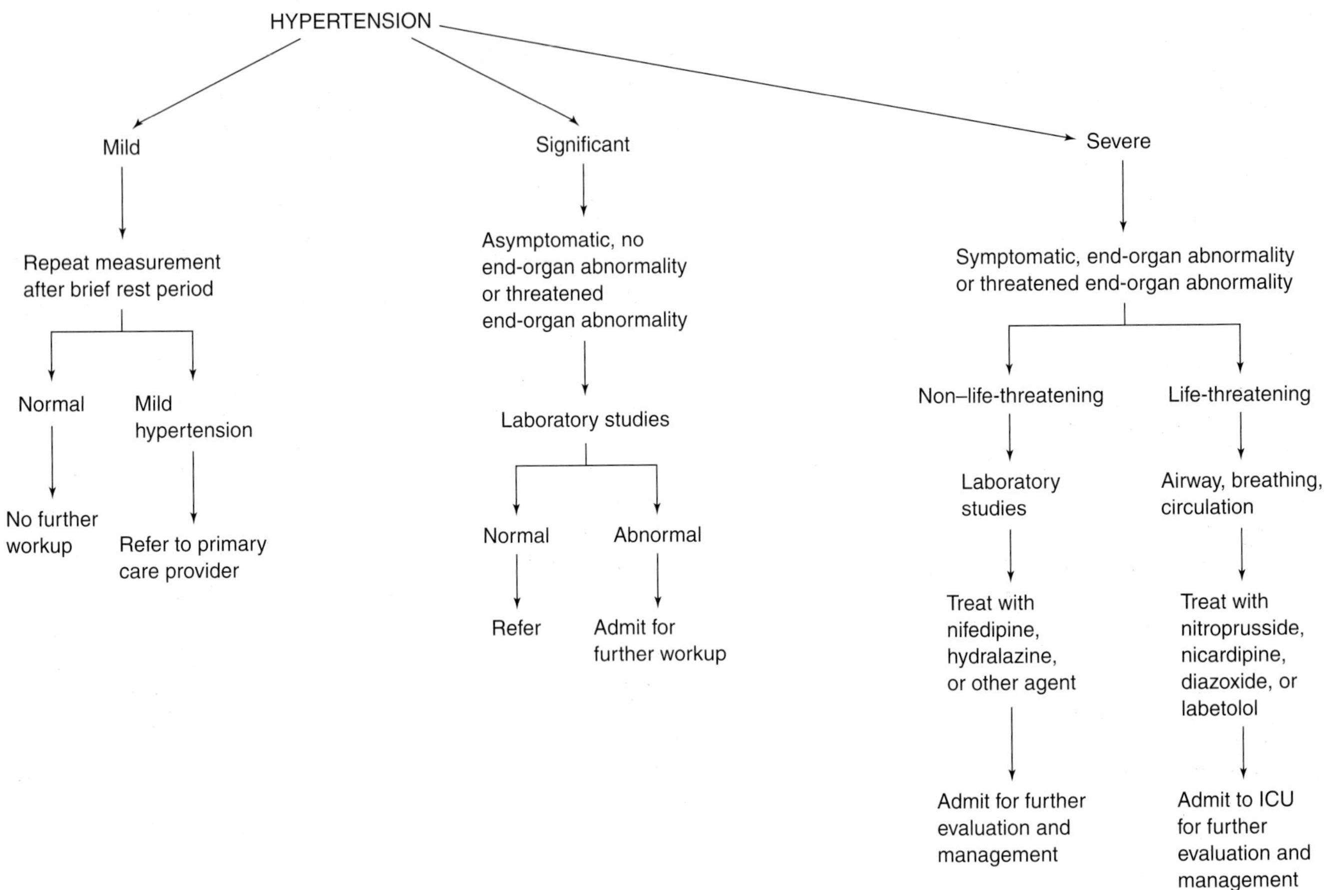

Figure 28.2. Approach to the initial emergency department triage and stabilization of the hypertensive child.

TABLE 28.5. Drugs Commonly Used for the Treatment of Hypertensive Emergencies in Children

Drug	Dosage	Onset of action	Duration of action	Mechanism of action	Side effects/comments
Sodium Nitroprusside	0.5–8.0 μg/kg/min i.v. infusion	Seconds	During infusion only	Vasodilation of arterioles and veins	Very potent—must be given in ICU setting. May cause headache, abdominal pain, chest pain
Nicardipine	1.0–10.0 μg/kg/min i.v. infusion	2–5 min	30 min–4 hr (depends on duration of infusion)	Vasodilation of arteries	Limited experience in pediatrics; headache is common; tachycardia, dizziness, nausea vomiting, abdominal pain can occur. Relatively contraindicated with increased ICP
Labetalol	0.5–3.0 mg/kg/hr i.v. infusion *or* 0.5 mg/kg initial bolus, then 0.5–1.5 mg/kg/hr infusion	2–5 min	12–24 hr	β and α-adrenergic blockade	Fatigue, dizziness GI upset, headache. Contraindicated in asthma, heart failure, heart block, pheochromocytoma
Diazoxide	1–2 mg/kg i.v. infusion push every 10–15 min until desired blood pressure obtained	3–5 min	4–12 hr	Vasodilation of arterioles	Increases heart rate and cardiac output; hypotension has caused coma and renal failure; hyperglycemia, hyperuricemia, salt and water retention
Hydralazine	0.1–0.5 mg/kg	10–20 min mg/kg	3–6 hr	Direct relaxation of smooth muscle, arteries, veins	Less potent than other agents; headaches, tachycardia, dizziness, palpitations, flushing
Nifedipine	0.25–0.50 mg/kg sublingually or p.o. (bite and swallow)	5–15 min	6 hr	Calcium channel blocker—decreases peripheral vascular resistance	Dizziness, flushing; difficult to administer exact dosages

ICU, intensive care unit; IV, intravenous; ICP, intracranial pressure; GI, gastrointestinal; p.o., orally.

For children with hypertensive emergencies (i.e., blood pressure associated with evidence of end-organ damage or dysfunction), treatment must be rapid and, at the same time, cautious. In most emergent cases, it is recommended that blood pressure be reduced gradually—generally by about 25 over several minutes to several hours, depending on the severity of the emergency (Chapter 76).

The choice of which drug to use in the ED treatment of a child with hypertensive crisis depends on the severity of the patient's hypertension, the patient's current medications, the suspected cause of the hypertension, and the organs involved. Thus, hypertension caused by a catecholamine-secreting tumor (pheochromocytoma) might best be controlled with an a β-blocking agent such as phentolamine. On the other hand, if hypertension is associated with an intracerebral bleed, medications that cause an increase in cerebral blood flow, such as nifedipine and nicardipine, are best avoided.

In addition to treating the elevation in blood pressure, the child with complications of hypertension also may require treatment for the specific complications. Thus, the child with seizures or CHF often requires the standard treatment for those problems in addition to antihypertensive therapy. When other complications are thought to be secondary to severe hypertension, however, treatment of the hypertension should take precedence. Of course, attention to airway, breathing, and circulation are to be given priority over all other therapeutic interventions.

Specific Therapy

Generally, only children presenting with hypertension that falls into the categories of hypertensive emergency or hypertensive urgency require pharmacologic intercession in the ED. As mentioned, the medication used depends on a number of factors, including the treating physician's familiarity with the antihypertensive agents.

Hypertensive Emergencies

Children with hypertension and major end-organ abnormalities such as CHF, encephalopathy, or seizures require immediate blood pressure reduction. Careful attention to airway, breathing, and circulation is followed by establishment of vascular access and treatment with one of the following parenteral medications (Table 28.5).

Hypertensive Urgencies

Drugs that are lower in potency or slower in onset are more appropriate for hypertensive crises not accompanied by life-threatening manifestations. These include, in particular, nifedipine and hydralazine (Table 28.5).

CHAPTER 29
Immobile Arm

Sara A. Schutzman, M.D.

An infant or child brought for evaluation of an "immobile arm" is not moving the limb because of pain or weakness. These children can be considered as having an upper extremity equivalent of "limp"; by using historical information, physical findings, selective radiologic studies, and laboratory tests, the physician can evaluate and treat children with this complaint.

DIFFERENTIAL DIAGNOSIS

Table 29.1 lists most conditions that cause decreased use of the arm. Trauma is the most common cause of decreased arm movement in children. Any injury from the clavicle to the fingertips can cause pain in a child and lead to diminished use of the limb; these injuries range from serious (fracture or dislocation with neurovascular compromise) to a simple contusion. Most young children with diminished arm use have a radial head subluxation ("nursemaid's elbow"), fracture, or soft-tissue injury. Although one can often elicit a history of trauma, the diagnosis must be considered even in its absence because of unwitnessed events in preverbal children or, less commonly, intentional injuries inflicted by caretakers who are not forthcoming. With musculoskeletal injuries, the child may have an obvious abnormality such as a deformity or a contusion or more subtle findings of localized tenderness or decreased arm movement. Children with hemophilia may have hemarthrosis or hematoma with minimal trauma. Radiographs are useful for demonstrating most fractures or dislocations but may appear normal with Salter type I fractures and nursemaid's elbow as well as with contusions and other minor soft-tissue injuries.

Although much less common than trauma, infection also may cause decreased use of an arm. There may be a history of fever, and onset of arm disuse often is less abrupt than with trauma. The infection can be located at any point from the shoulder to finger and may be superficial (e.g., cellulitis, paronychia) or deep.

Other inflammatory causes of arm pain include noninfectious arthritis and myositis. In addition to a swollen, tender joint, children with arthritis caused by postinfectious, Lyme, and rheumatologic diseases may have multiple joint involvement, rash, fever, adenopathy, heart murmur, hematuria, or bloody stools.

Tumors are an uncommon cause of diminished arm use. With leukemia or neuroblastoma, fever, abdominal mass, hepatosplenomegaly, or pathologic adenopathy also may be found.

Children with neurologic abnormalities may have diminished use of an arm because of weakness, with or without pain.

TABLE 29.1. Differential Diagnosis of the Immobile Arm

Trauma	Inflammation
Fracture	Arthritis
Dislocation/subluxation	Juvenile rheumatoid
Hemarthrosis (hemophilia)	Other collagen vascular
Soft-tissue injury	Postinfectious
Nerve injury	Lyme
Splinter/hair tourniquet	Myositis
Infection	Infarction
Septic arthritis	Hemoglobinopathy
Osteomyelitis	Hand-foot syndrome
Soft-tissue infection	Acute pain crisis
Cellulitis	Avascular necrosis
Abscess	Avascular necrosis
Lymphangitis	Neurologic
Paronychia/felon/tenosynovitis	Radiculopathy
Tumor	Plexopathy
Primary musculoskeletal	Neuropathy
Bone	Injury
Cartilage	Traction
Soft tissue	Pressure
Bone marrow infiltration	Laceration
Leukemia	Miscellaneous
Neuroblastoma	Reflex sympathetic dystrophy
Lymphoma	

TABLE 29.2. Common Causes of Diminished Arm Use

Newborn/infant
Fractured clavicle
Brachial plexus injury
Septic arthritis/osteomyelitis
Infant/preschool
Nursemaid's elbow
Fracture
Soft-tissue injury

An isolated monoplegia may be caused by a radiculopathy, plexopathy, or neuropathy that results from compression, inflammation, or injury. Trauma, particularly traction on the arm, commonly leads to neurologic abnormalities (e.g., brachial plexus injury from birth); however, nontraumatic conditions may have an abrupt onset with no apparent antecedent illness. The child will have diminished arm movement and weakness, and he or she may even experience pain; unlike the previously discussed causes of arm disuse, however, the pain (if present) usually is not reproducible with palpation and is not accompanied by swelling or redness.

Children with hemoglobinopathies (most commonly sickle cell disease) may present with decreased arm use because of vasoocclusive crisis, causing ischemia or infarction of bone marrow with acute bone pain. Long bones are commonly affected; however, young children often have involvement of the small bones of the hands and feet (*dactylitis*). Usually, no precipitating events are identified.

TABLE 29.3. Life- and Limb-Threatening Causes of Diminished Arm Use

Septic arthritis/osteomyelitis
Leukemia/other malignancy
Fracture with neurovascular compromise

Several other, much less common, processes can cause decreased upper limb use. These include avascular necrosis of the humeral head or capitellum in otherwise healthy children and reflex sympathetic dystrophy. Table 29.2 lists common causes of diminished arm use. Table 29.3 lists life- and limb-threatening causes of diminished arm use.

Evaluation and Decision

When a child is brought for evaluation of diminished arm use, the physician first should determine whether this decrease in mobility resulted from a specific traumatic event (Fig. 29.1). If the history is classic for radial head subluxation, the patient is

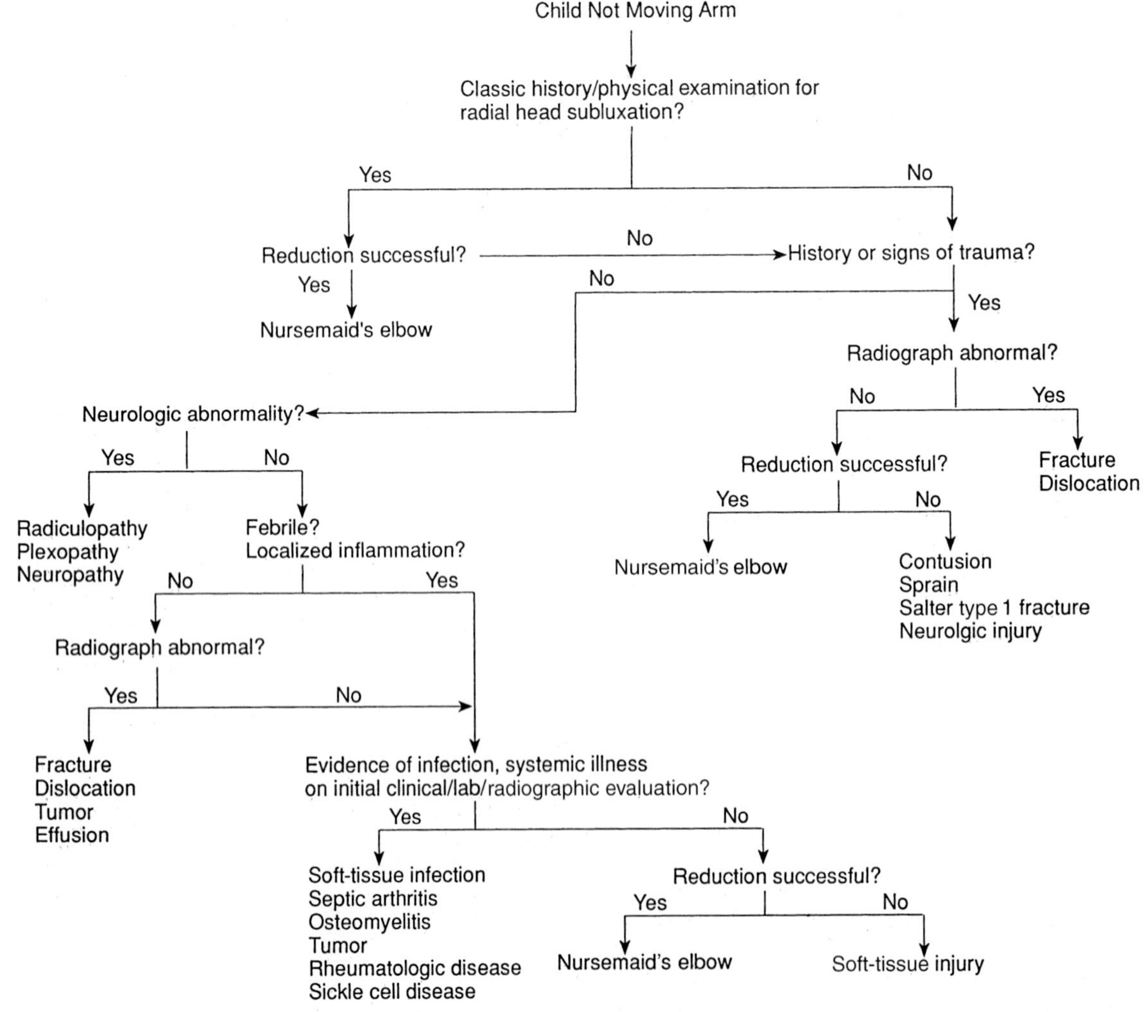

Figure 29.1. Approach to the child with diminished arm use.

holding the arm pronated and slightly flexed, and there is no localized tenderness or swelling, the physician may attempt reduction. If the child does not regain full use of the arm quickly, as in most other cases of trauma, radiographs should be obtained. For many conditions, the radiographic studies make the diagnosis (e.g., fracture, dislocation). Normal radiographs in the setting of acute trauma usually imply soft-tissue injury, and the patient should be treated symptomatically with close follow-up, provided neurovascular integrity is established. If radiographs appear normal but the child has reproducible tenderness localized to the epiphyseal plate, the patient should be treated for a Salter type I fracture. Occasionally, a child with a nursemaid's elbow may have an atypical history (e.g., "fell onto the arm"); if radiographs exclude a fracture but the patient is holding the arm in a characteristic position, a reduction should be attempted.

Children with neurologic abnormalities should be evaluated urgently to localize the site and cause of the impairment; the appropriate subspecialist (neurologist, neurosurgeon) should be involved.

If the child has no clear history of trauma but is afebrile and has no obvious localizing findings of infection, the limb should be evaluated radiographically. Abnormalities revealed might include fracture, dislocation, tumor, or effusion. If radiographs are normal in these children, one could consider obtaining a complete blood count (CBC), erythrocyte sedimentation rate (ESR), or CRP, blood culture, or hemoglobin electrophoresis to evaluate for occult infectious or inflammatory processes.

Children who are febrile, have signs of localized inflammation (e.g., warm, swollen joint), or have evidence of systemic illness should have CBC, ESR or CRP, and blood culture obtained in addition to radiographs. Based on specific findings, further evaluation might include arthrocentesis, bone scan, or rheumatologic tests. When the initial history, physical examination, laboratory tests, and radiographs localize site and cause of the pathology, the physician can begin specific treatment.

A few children with no history of trauma in whom a thorough initial evaluation is unrevealing will have a nursemaid's elbow. Therefore, an attempt at reduction is warranted in selected cases. Children with persistently diminished arm movement who are afebrile and nontoxic and who have no localizing findings, normal neurovascular function, and normal laboratory tests likely have an occult soft-tissue injury and can be treated as outpatients. A few of these children may have indolent pathologic processes or occult fractures; therefore, close follow-up must be ensured. These patients should be reevaluated every few days until normal arm use is regained or until evidence of a pathologic process develops. If arm disuse persists, a more extensive evaluation to diagnose or exclude occult fracture, infection, tumor, or collagen vascular disease is in order.

CHAPTER 30
Injury—Ankle

Angela C. Anderson, M.D.

Young children with ankle injuries may complain of pain anywhere from their midcalf to their toes because it is often difficult for children to localize pain. Conversely, disease in the lower leg and foot can cause referred pain to the ankle.

TABLE 30.1. Differential Diagnosis of Traumatic Injuries That Cause Ankle Pain

Leg	Sprains
Tibial fractures	Contusions
(toddler's fracture)	Osteochondritis dissecans
Fibular fractures	Hemarthrosis
Contusions	Foot
Compartment syndrome	Fractures
of the calf	Talar
Ankle	Navicular
Fractures	Fifth metatarsal (Jones fracture)
Distal tibial	Calcaneal
Distal fibular	Sprains
Physeal	Contusions

DIFFERENTIAL DIAGNOSIS

A number of traumatic injuries can cause ankle pain (Table 30.1). Although trauma is the most common cause of ankle pain in children, infectious, rheumatologic, inflammatory, neoplastic, and hematologic abnormalities also should be considered (Table 30.2). Again, a complaint of ankle pain may result from a lesion anywhere between the knee and the toe, particularly in the preverbal child. The most common injuries vary according to age (Table 30.3).

Ankle Fractures

Fractures of the ankle account for 5.5% of all fractures in pediatrics. The system used to classify ankle fractures in children differs from the one used in adults because of the presence of growth plates and the possible implications of physeal injuries. The Salter-Harris classification is most commonly applied, as described in Chapter 101.

Inversion ankle injuries in the preadolescent most commonly cause a Salter type I fracture of the distal. Clinically, the patient has swelling about the lateral malleolus and tenderness at the distal fibular physis. Fractures confined to the physes may not be visible on a routine radiograph.

As skeletal maturity (and physeal closure) progresses, the relative strengths of various parts of the tibia change. As a re-

TABLE 30.2. Differential Diagnosis of Ankle Pain

Trauma	Brodie's abscess (subacute osteomyelitis of the distal tibia)
Fractures	Rheumatologic
Sprains	Juvenile rheumatoid arthritis
Contusions	Rheumatic fever
Osteochondritis dissecans	Reiter's syndrome
Hemarthrosis	Hematologic
Inflammatory	Sickle cell disease (pain crisis)
Tendonitis	Hemophilia (hemarthrosis)
Synovitis	Osteochondroses (avascular necrosis)
Periostitis	Kohler's disease (navicular)
Sever's disease (calcaneal apophysitis)	Freiberg's disease (second metatarsal)
Infectious	Tumors
Osteomyelitis	Ewing's sarcoma
Soft-tissue abscess	Osteoid osteoma
Septic joint	

TABLE 30.3. Common Injuries Associated with Ankle Pain According to Age

Toddler	Child	Adolescent
Spiral fracture of tibia	Salter I fracture of distal fibula	Ankle sprain
Soft-tissue contusion	Soft-tissue contusion	Soft-tissue contusion

sult, the same mechanism of injury may cause very different fracture patterns, depending on the patient's age.

Diagnosis of these fractures may be difficult because routine radiographs may not show the fracture line well. If displacement is minimal, the only radiographic sign may be a slight widening of the lateral tibial physis or a faint vertical fracture line through the epiphysis on anteroposterior or oblique views. In some cases, the only finding may be local tenderness in the area of the lateral tibial physis.

Ankle Sprains

Ankle sprains in the child or preadolescent are less common than fractures because the ligaments in this age group are much stronger than growth plates or even bone. If a ligamentous injury occurs in a child with an open growth plate, an associated avulsion fracture is almost always present. Once skeletal maturity is reached, however, ankle sprains become the most common of sports injuries.

Inversion injuries cause 85% of ankle sprains. The most commonly injured structures are the lateral ligaments. Three lateral ligaments support the ankle joint: the anterior talofibular, the calcaneofibular, and the posterior talofibular. The anterior talofibular is the weakest and most commonly injured of the three.

Eversion injuries account for 15% of ankle sprains. The deltoid ligament, which supports the medial aspect of the ankle, is most commonly affected by this mechanism. It is made up of deep and superficial fibers. Eversion also may cause disruption of the tibiofibular syndesmosis, which connects the distal tibia and fibula.

EVALUATION AND DECISION

The approach (Fig. 30.1) to the evaluation and diagnosis of traumatic ankle injuries relies primarily on physical findings and the results of radiographic evaluation. Initially, pulses and sensation are assessed. Loss of pulses or sensation suggests a fracture or dislocation and the need for a rapid reduction; when available without delay, orthopedic consultation is advisable. After immobilization to prevent further compromise and the provision of analgesia, a radiograph should be obtained immediately. If neurovascular status is adequate and the general inspection reveals no obvious abnormalities, the remainder of the physical examination should be continued as described previously.

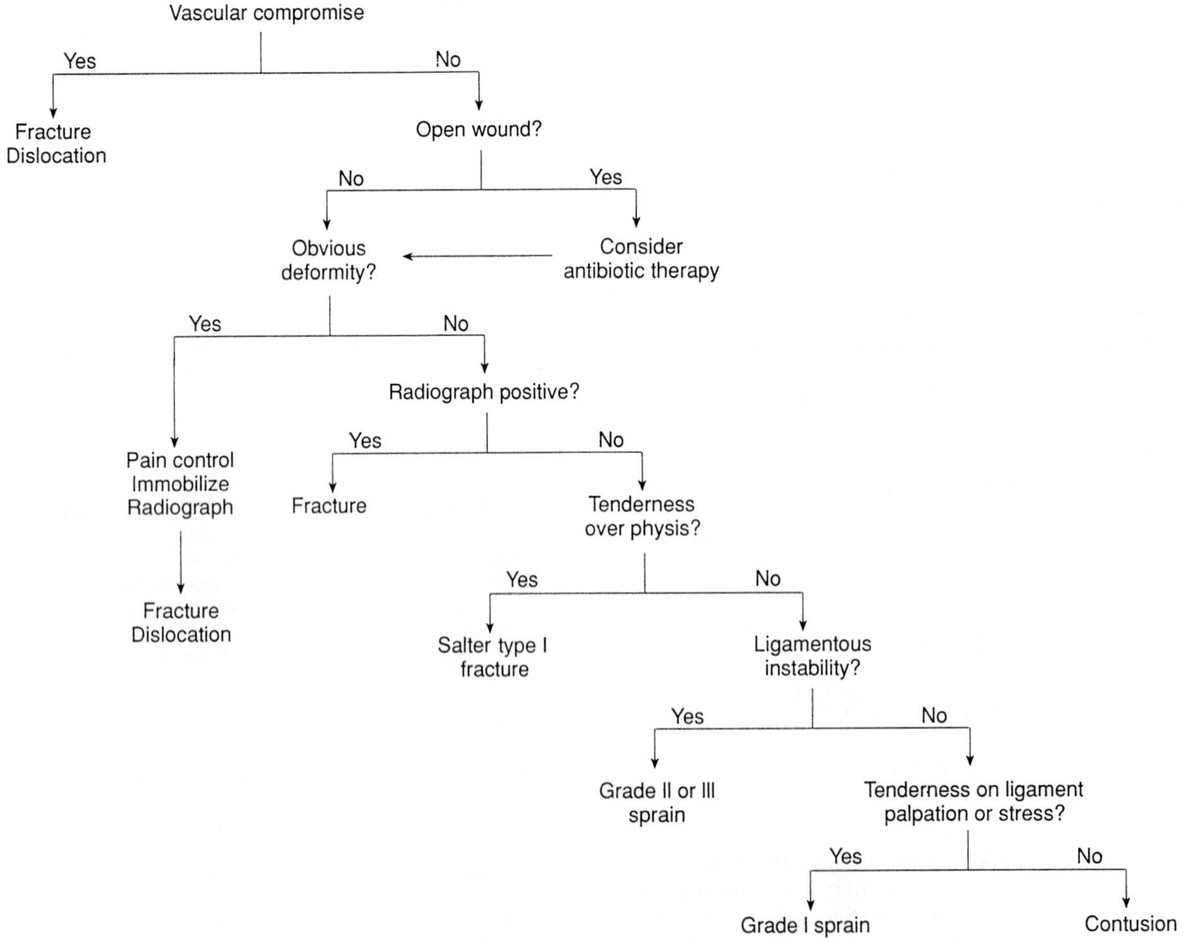

Figure 30.1. Evaluation and diagnosis of traumatic ankle injuries.

Next, the area should be examined for open wounds. If open wounds are present, the physician should fashion a sterile saline dressing and immobilize the extremity before obtaining a radiograph. In addition, the administration of intravenous antibiotic therapy and tetanus prophylaxis should be considered.

If radiographic studies indicate a fracture or dislocation, the specific injury should be treated (see Chapter 101). Analgesia should be administered as needed.

If no fracture is evident on radiography but tenderness is elicited over a physis, the diagnosis of a Salter type I injury is made and appropriate immobilization performed. A negative radiograph in the absence of bony tenderness suggests the diagnosis of contusion or ligamentous injury. The diagnosis of a grade II or III sprain is rendered in the patient with joint instability. If the ankle is stable but pain is elicited with ligamentous stress or palpation, a grade I sprain is diagnosed.

TREATMENT

Fractures

Fracture reduction usually can be accomplished by reversing the mechanism of injury. Closed reduction and a short leg cast are usually adequate for Salter-Harris type I and type II fractures of the distal tibia and fibula. Often, younger children require placement of a long leg cast, even for minor fractures, because of their ability to slip out of short leg casts, whether accidentally or intentionally.

One study recommends the use of a tubular bandage (Tubigrip, Seton Health Care PLC) and crutches—in lieu of a short leg plaster cast—in patients with clinically suspected but nonradiographically evident Salter-Harris type I fractures of the distal fibula. The group treated with the tubular bandage had a shorter time to recovery; however, further study is required to determine whether this method is adequate.

Sprains

A common approach to the treatment of ankle sprains is described by the mnemonic *RICE* (rest, ice, compression, elevation). This treatment approach should be initiated within 36 hours of the injury.

Splinting

If swelling or pain is severe, a stirrup or posterior splint should be applied to the ankle. Air splints also can be used; they allow dorsiflexion and plantar flexion while maintaining medial and lateral stability.

CHAPTER 31
Injury—Head

Sara A. Schutzman, M.D.

PEDIATRIC HEAD TRAUMA

Head injuries in children are common, accounting for 600,000 emergency department (ED) visits annually. The most common mechanisms of injury for the entire pediatric group are falls (37%), motor vehicle (18%) and pedestrian (17%) accidents, and bicycle injuries (10%); most fatal injuries occur because of motor vehicle-related injuries. The mechanism of pediatric head injury varies with age; younger children are more likely to fall or be abused, whereas older children often are injured in sporting or motor vehicle accidents (in addition to falls).

Many of the serious neurologic complications of head injury are evident soon after the traumatic event; however, some life-threatening injuries can appear initially as trivial head trauma. To manage head injuries best, the physician must approach the child in a systematic manner to address all injuries (because global resuscitation is the first priority of cerebral resuscitation), identify and treat any neurologic complications, and prevent ongoing cerebral insult.

DIFFERENTIAL DIAGNOSIS

Head trauma may cause injuries of the scalp, skull, and intracranial contents. Although each is discussed here separately, the clinician must remember that these injuries may occur alone or in combination, and all potential injuries must be kept in mind when dealing with each.

Scalp

The scalp consists of five layers of soft tissue that cover the skull; contusions and lacerations of this structure are common results of head trauma. Subgaleal hematomas may result from more forceful blows if vessels in the fourth layer bleed and dissect the galea from the periosteum, or they may be signs of an underlying skull fracture. In subperiosteal hematomas, or cephalohematomas, the swelling is localized to the underlying cranial bone and most often occurs with birth trauma. Scalp lacerations may occur with or without underlying contusions or fractures and often require suturing.

Skull

Linear, diastatic, depressed, compound, and basilar skull fractures may result from head trauma. Linear fractures account for 75% to 90% of skull fractures in children and often manifest with localized swelling and tenderness. Their presence reflects the degree of traumatic impact. Because the force required to fracture a child's skull is significant, risk of an intracranial injury (ICI) is significantly more likely (as much as 10 to 20 times) with a fracture. The second feature important in linear skull fractures derives from their location; those that cross the path of a major vascular structure (middle meningeal artery, large dural sinuses) signal potential for intracranial hemorrhage from these vessels.

Diastatic fractures are traumatic separations of cranial bones at one or more suture sites. A depressed skull fracture is present when the inner table of the skull is displaced by more than the thickness of the entire bone. Compound fractures are those that communicate with lacerations.

Basilar skull fractures often are difficult to detect on routine radiographs or computed tomography (CT) scans; however, their location produces clinical signs that lead to the diagnosis. Fractures of the petrous portion of the temporal bone may cause hemotympanum, hemorrhagic or cerebrospinal fluid (CSF) otorrhea, or Battle's sign (bleeding into mastoid air cells with postauricular swelling and ecchymosis). Fracture of the anterior skull base may cause a dural laceration with subsequent drainage of CSF into paranasal sinuses and rhinorrhea. Anterior venous sinus drainage may cause blood leakage into the periorbital tissues ("raccoon's eyes"). Given the location of basilar skull fractures, associated CN palsies may occur. CT scan is indicated to try to localize the area of fracture and to identify any associated intracranial pathology (which occurs in approximately 20% of children with basilar skull fractures who have a Glasgow Coma Scale [GCS] score of 15 and a nonfocal neurologic examination).

Intracranial Injury

CONCUSSION

Concussion is the most minor brain injury and is characterized by posttraumatic alteration in mental status that may or may not involve loss of consciousness. The child may have a depressed level of consciousness, pallor, vomiting, amnesia, and confusion; however, the clinical picture usually normalizes within several hours without specific therapy.

POSTTRAUMATIC SEIZURES

Posttraumatic seizures can be divided temporally into immediate, early, and late, and they occur in 5% to 10% of children hospitalized for head trauma. Immediate seizures occur within seconds of the trauma and probably represent traumatic depolarization of the cortex. They usually are generalized and rarely recur. Early seizures occur within 1 week of the trauma (most occur within 24 hours) and often are the result of focal injuries (contusion, laceration, ischemia, edema). Late seizures occur more than 1 week after the traumatic event and may be attributed to scarring associated with local vascular compromise, distortion, and mechanical irritation of the brain. These seizures are more likely to occur in children with severe head injuries, dural lacerations, and intracranial hemorrhages. A substantial number of the latter will have subsequent seizures.

CEREBRAL CONTUSION

Cerebral contusion is a bruising or crushing of brain and often results from blunt head trauma. Children with cerebral contusion may have had loss of consciousness (not imperative), may show a depressed level of consciousness or symptoms of vomiting or headache, and may have focal neurologic signs or seizures.

EPIDURAL HEMATOMA

Epidural hematoma (EDH) is a collection of blood between the skull and dura. An overlying fracture is present in 60% to 80% of cases. Depending on the location and vascular structure involved, the hemorrhage may be of arterial or venous origin; injury to the middle meningeal artery often is responsible for temporal EDH. The classic pattern of a lucid interval between initial loss of consciousness and subsequent neurologic deterioration occurs in only a minority of children with EDH. Furthermore, patients occasionally may develop EDH after relatively minor trauma with no history of loss of consciousness. Although many children present with significant lethargy, focal neurologic signs, or a clinical pattern consistent with temporal lobe herniation as the hematoma expands, some children with EDH are alert, have a nonfocal neurologic examination, and have only symptoms of headache or persistent vomiting; nevertheless, rapid deterioration can ensue.

SUBDURAL HEMATOMA

Subdural hematoma (SDH) occurs as a result of bleeding between the dura and the arachnoid membranes covering the brain parenchyma. An SDH may result from direct trauma or from shaking injuries that can cause tearing of the cortical bridging veins or bleeding from the cortex itself. An SDH may be bilateral, and often, there is an associated underlying brain injury. Skull fractures occur in only a minority of cases. Children with SDH often have seizures, may present with evidence of acutely elevated intracranial pressure (ICP), or may have more nonspecific signs of vomiting, irritability, or low-grade fever. Physical examination often reveals an irritable or lethargic infant or child with a bulging fontanel who may or may not have neurologic abnormalities. CT scan commonly demonstrates crescent-shaped subdural collections.

INTRACEREBRAL HEMATOMA

Posttraumatic intracerebral hematomas are unusual in children. Blood within the parenchyma usually is the result of severe focal injury or penetrating trauma, usually manifests with severe neurologic compromise, and often portends a poor prognosis.

SUBARACHNOID HEMORRHAGE

Subarachnoid hemorrhage may occur after head trauma (including shaking injuries in infants) and may cause headache, neck stiffness, and lethargy in the child.

ACUTE BRAIN SWELLING

The most common diagnosis in children with severe head injury (GCS score of less than 8) is diffuse cerebral swelling. In one study, this occurred in 50% of cases, whereas intracranial hemorrhages were less common (reported in 20% of cases). These children have a depressed level of consciousness and may have focal neurologic signs or symptoms of herniation.

PENETRATING INJURIES

Penetrating head injuries are uncommon in children and may be caused by bullets, teeth (e.g., dog bites), or other objects (e.g., dart, pencil, pellet) penetrating the skull. These injuries have obvious potential for extensive damage to the brain and intracranial vessels.

EVALUATION AND DECISION

The general approach is essentially the same as with any child who presents with trauma, paying particular attention to potential CNS damage. Following the ABCs (airway, breathing, and circulation) of resuscitation, the physician must systematically evaluate and stabilize the child with head trauma. The goals of management are to define specific anatomic lesions (e.g., skull fracture) and to prevent secondary brain injury. One approach (Fig. 31.1) to diagnosing complications of head trauma involves determining whether a penetrating injury has occurred. If so, brain or vascular injury is likely, and emergent CT scanning and neurosurgical consultation are mandated in addition to stabilization.

If the head injury has resulted from blunt trauma, it must be determined whether an intra-cranial injury (ICI) is present. Suggestive history includes loss of consciousness (especially if more than brief); prolonged, focal, or early seizure; and definite bony abnormality or underlying condition that predisposes to ICI (e.g., coagulopathy). Physical findings indicative of possible intracranial abnormalities include a GCS score of less than 15, focal neurologic abnormalities, a definite palpable bony depression, and signs of a basilar skull fracture. If any of these findings are present, then, in addition to supportive therapy, CT scan and possible neurosurgical consultation are indicated. Abnormalities on the CT scan might include intracranial hemorrhage, diffuse cerebral swelling, or skull fracture; if the CT scan is normal, concussion or extracranial injury has likely occurred.

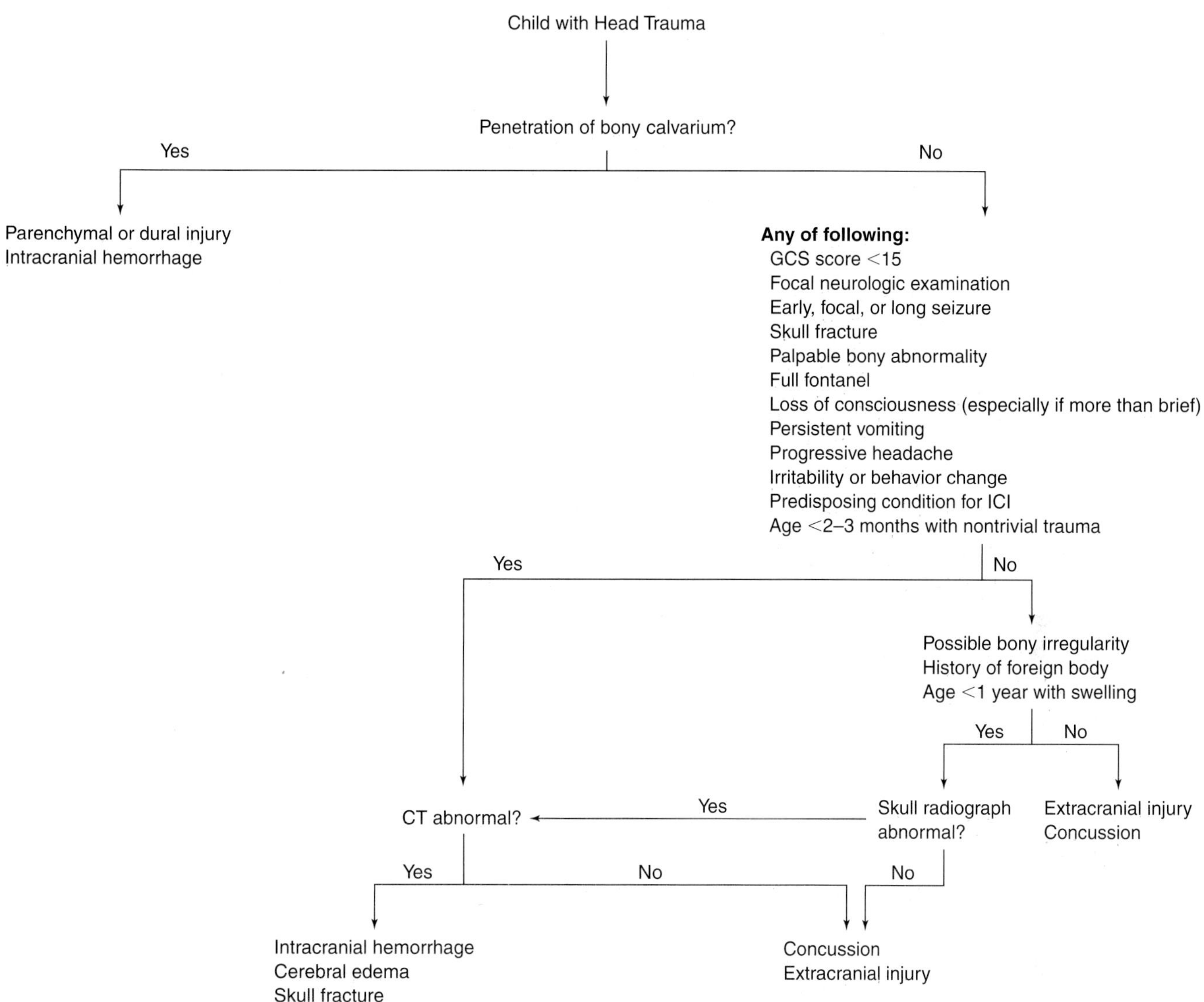

Figure 31.1. Approach to the child with head trauma. *GCS,* Glasgow Coma Scale; *ICI,* intracranial injury; *CT,* computed tomography.

If these findings are not present, the child will be alert with a nonfocal neurologic examination. The drowsy child who quickly becomes alert or the child with a history of momentary loss of consciousness who is alert with a nonfocal examination may show no evidence of intracranial complications; however, the child may have had more than a trivial head injury. If these patients do not undergo a CT scan, they should be observed in the ED for at least 4 to 6 hours after the injury for signs and symptoms of complications, including neurologic abnormalities, mental status depression, persistent vomiting, and progressively severe headache. A CT scan should be obtained if these signs or symptoms develop. As previously stated, discrete abnormalities may be identified on CT scan; however, if the scan is normal, the child has experienced a concussion or extracranial injury.

Children likely to display abnormalities on skull radiographs but in whom immediate imaging of intracranial contents is not indicated include those who are awake and alert but in whom there is a history of a foreign body, possible penetration of the bony calvaria, or question of a palpable bony irregularity. Another relative indication for skull radiographs is a significant subgaleal hematoma, especially if it overlies the middle meningeal groove. One should also consider obtaining skull radiographs in infants under the age of 1 year with a history of a fall of more than 3 feet onto a hard surface or with a palpable hematoma (if they have not undergone CT) because an infant's skull has limited ability to withstand trauma.

Skull radiographs may show an extracranial or intracranial foreign body, may reveal a fracture, or may be normal. Obviously, immediate CT scan (with neurosurgical consultation) is mandated for patients with an intracranial foreign body because neuronal or vascular damage is likely. CT is also indicated if skull radiographs demonstrate a skull fracture because this significantly increases the likelihood of an associated ICI. The child with normal skull radiographs and examination who is alert has likely experienced an extracranial injury or a concussion.

The remaining children who sustained impact of minimal force, had no loss of consciousness, and are alert and asymptomatic with normal examinations likely have only minor head trauma with or without extracranial injuries, including contusions and lacerations. Home observation is appropriate management for most of these patients. Rarely, intracranial compli-

TABLE 31.1. Criteria for Discharge with Home Observation

Traumatic force not life threatening	No intracranial abnormalities on CT (if obtained)
Glasgow Coma Scale score of 15	Reliable caretakers who are able to return if necessary
Nonfocal neurologic examination	No suspicion of abuse or neglect
No significant symptoms	
No history of prolonged loss of consciousness (or normal CT if it did occur)	

CT, computed tomography.

cations develop in these children, causing symptoms hours after the traumatic event; therefore, caretakers should be given a printed list of signs and symptoms indicative of increased ICP with instructions to check the child at regular intervals and to return to the ED if symptoms occur. The caretakers must be reliable and able to return with the child if necessary, and there must be no suspicion of abuse or neglect; otherwise, admission for observation in the hospital should be considered (Table 31.1).

CHAPTER 32
Injury—Knee

Marc N. Baskin, M.D.

Acute pain or injury to the knee is a common complaint in the emergency department (ED). The emergency physician can provide appropriate therapy or determine the need for consultation, based on a comprehensive history, physical examination, and an appropriate radiographic evaluation.

DIFFERENTIAL DIAGNOSIS

Differential diagnoses for the injured knee are given in Table 32.1.

Acute Injuries

FRACTURES

A separation fracture of the distal femoral epiphysis (wagon-wheel injury) occurs most commonly during contact sports or in car accidents. It is classified by the Salter-Harris. The patient has severe pain, refuses to bear weight, and experiences joint and soft-tissue swelling and possibly deformity.

Separations of the proximal tibial epiphysis are more rare than those of the distal femoral epiphysis and also are likely to involve vascular compromise because of the proximity of the popliteal artery to the posterior aspect of the tibial epiphysis. The patient will have severe pain, limited range of motion (ROM), and commonly, a hemarthrosis. If displaced, the knee will be deformed.

Acute traumatic avulsion of the tibial tubercle is caused by acute stress on the knee's extensor mechanism. The patient will have tenderness and swelling over the tibial tubercle and is unable to extend the knee fully. A lateral radiograph is diagnostic.

Fractures of the patella are more common in adults because the child's patella is surrounded by cartilage, protecting it from

TABLE 32.1. Differential Diagnosis of the Injured Knee

Acute injuries	Dislocations and subluxations
Fractures	Patellar[b]
Distal femoral epiphysis[a]	Knee joint[a]
Proximal tibial epiphysis[a]	Subacute injuries
Tibial tubercle avulsion	Osgood-Schlatter disease[b]
Patella	Patellofemoral pain syndrome[b]
Tibial spine avulsion	Patellar tendon tendinitis ("jumper's knee")
Osteochondral fractures	Prepatellar bursitis
Soft-tissue injuries	Osteochondritis dissecans
Collateral ligament sprain or rupture	Baker's cyst
Anterior cruciate ligament sprain or rupture	Iliotibial band friction syndrome
Posterior cruciate ligament sprain or rupture	Other
Meniscal tears	Pathologic fractures[a]
Quadriceps tendon rupture	Hip disease
Patellar tendon rupture	Slipped capital femoral epiphysis
Hamstring strain[b]	Aseptic necrosis of the femoral head
Posttraumatic infections	
Septic arthritis[a]	
Osteomyelitis[a]	
Cellulitis	
Septic prepatellar bursitis	

[a] Life- or limb-threatening causes of the injured knee.
[b] Common causes of the injured knee.

direct trauma. A medial avulsion fracture suggests that the mechanism was a patellar dislocation that spontaneously reduced.

Analogous to an adolescent who ruptures the anterior cruciate ligament, children sustain avulsion fractures of the tibial spine at the point where the anterior cruciate ligament inserts. The patient will have a hemarthrosis and will be unable to bear weight. If the patient tolerates an examination, the Lachman test may be positive because the injury is similar mechanically to an anterior cruciate ligament tear. Anteroposterior (AP), lateral, and intercondylar or tunnel view radiographs will show the avulsed fragment. The visible ossified fragment may be small because the tibial spine is mostly radiolucent cartilage.

Osteochondral fractures are fractures of articular cartilage and underlying bone not associated with ligamentous attachments. These fractures usually involve the patella and occur during patellar dislocations or may involve the femoral condyle. Occasionally, a patient sustains a direct blow to the knee, but more commonly, the knee is injured during a twisting injury. The patient has severe pain, holds the knee flexed, and refuses to bear weight. Often, the patient has immediate swelling of the knee consistent with a hemarthrosis.

DISLOCATIONS

Patellar dislocation occurs as the quadriceps muscles pull along the patellar tendon to extend the knee. This often recurrent injury rarely occurs from direct force but rather happens more often during dancing or gymnastics. The patient may feel or hear a ripping or popping sensation or sound. The patient complains of intense pain and holds the knee flexed. The patella is visible more laterally than normal. The dislocation may be reduced before radiographs are taken.

In a child, the knee joint itself rarely dislocates; usually, the distal femoral or proximal tibial epiphysis separates first. Dislocation occurs only with trauma that involves significant force, such as a high-speed motor vehicle accident.

SOFT-TISSUE INJURIES

Medial or lateral collateral ligament injuries are rare when the epiphysis is open because the involved ligaments are stronger than the growth plate. In older patients, the medial collateral ligament may be damaged by a blow to the lateral side of the knee during contact sports or stress during a skiing accident, when the athlete "catches an edge" and falls forward with the leg rotated externally. Severe collateral ligament injury may be associated with anterior cruciate ligament (ACL) or meniscal damage.

ACL injuries occur in many scenarios but usually involve rotational forces on a fixed foot. The patient often reports the sensation of a "pop." The joint usually swells rapidly as a result of hemarthrosis and has a marked decrease in ROM. The Lachman test is sensitive in detecting ACL injuries but may be falsely negative soon after the injury when the knee is swollen and painful. ACL injuries are rare before adolescence because ACL's insertion point in a child, the tibial spine, is incompletely ossified. Therefore, the same force that would produce an ACL injury in an adolescent will cause an avulsion fracture of the tibial spine in a child.

Posterior cruciate ligament injuries are extremely rare and usually result from direct force on the tibial tubercle, pushing the tibia posteriorly on the femur. The posterior drawer sign will be present in most cases.

The menisci can be injured when the knee is twisted during weight bearing. The patient may report a popping sensation and the feeling of the knee "giving out." More chronically, the patient may report that the knee suddenly refuses to extend fully, "locking up," and then suddenly "unlocking." Joint-line tenderness is almost always present but must be differentiated from the tenderness associated with collateral ligament injuries. An effusion is commonly detected. Acutely, the injury may be difficult to diagnose because the patient has significantly reduced ROM, making the classic McMurray sign difficult to elicit. The Apley compression test requires less knee flexion and may be easier for the patient to tolerate. Radiographs generally are normal. A subluxating patella, ACL injury, or osteochondral fracture also may cause a popping sensation, and the patellofemoral pain syndrome may be associated with "giving way" of the knee.

The quadriceps or patellar tendon can rupture acutely, especially in an older athlete who jumps or falls a great distance. The tendon will be tender directly over the rupture, and the patella may be positioned abnormally. A hemarthrosis may be present, and radiographs may show the abnormally positioned patella.

The three hamstring muscles (semitendinosus, semimembranosus, and the biceps femoris) flex the knee and may be strained in young athletes. The semitendinosus and semimembranosus insert along the medial popliteal space, and the biceps femoris tendon runs laterally. The patient may describe an acute pain or even a pop in the back of the thigh. Often, this injury presents subacutely with posterior thigh and popliteal knee pain when the hamstrings are strained by repetitive use.

POSTTRAUMATIC INFECTION

Although not considered injuries, acute infections may present after a vague history of trauma. Physical findings of acute infection are present. The most common disorders are septic arthritis, osteomyelitis, cellulitis, and septic prepatellar bursitis.

Subacute Injuries

Many subacute knee problems manifest acutely in the ED. Osgood-Schlatter disease of the tibial tubercle may lead to similar symptoms as a traumatic avulsion of the tubercle; however, with Osgood-Schlatter disease, the symptoms have been noted for days or weeks. The symptoms of Osgood-Schlatter disease are exacerbated by squatting or jumping, but they do not cause the same disability as an acute avulsion. The disease is usually seen in patients between 10 and 15 years of age. The patients have localized tenderness and occasionally swelling over the tibial tubercle. The patient will refuse to extend the knee against force (e.g., perform a deep-knee bend) and have difficulty going up or down stairs, although they may have a normal gait on a level surface.

Patellofemoral pain syndrome (PFPS) or chondromalacia patella may be caused by malalignment of the extensor mechanism of the knee. The patient with PFPS has patellar pain with running and especially going down inclines or stairs. The patient also may have the sensation of the knee giving out when descending, although an actual fall usually does not occur. The patient has pain when sitting for a prolonged time with the knee flexed at 90 degrees. The pain disappears once the patient is ambulatory. This is called the movie sign. On examination, the patient may have the malalignment just mentioned, tenderness of the articular surface of the patella, and a positive patellar stress test. This test is performed with the patient in the supine position with the knee fully extended. The patient is asked to relax the quadriceps so that the physician can move the patella. With the patella pulled inferiorly, the physician should gently press down on it and ask the patient to tighten the quadriceps. (A younger patient should be asked to "push the knee into the examination table.") This will move the patella superiorly as the physician continues to press down. A patient with PFPS will have acute pain with this maneuver; radiographs, however, are normal.

Patellar tendon tendonitis, or "jumper's knee," occurs in patients during their growth spurt, especially those involved in

TABLE 32.2. Summary of Diagnostic Maneuvers for the Injured Knee

Maneuver	Diagnosis
Collateral laxity test	Collateral ligament injury
Lachman test	Anterior cruciate ligament injury
Posterior drawer test	Posterior cruciate ligament injury
McMurray test	Meniscal injury
Apley compression test	Meniscal injury
Patellar apprehension test	Patellar subluxation
Patellar stress test	Patellofemoral pain syndrome

jumping (knee extension) sports. The knee is tender on the inferior pole of the patella and the adjacent patellar tendon, but not on the tibial tubercle; radiographs generally are normal.

Prepatellar bursitis occurs after acute or chronic trauma to this bursa, which overlies the patella. The patient will have swelling over the anterior aspect of the knee, especially over the patella. A septic bursitis may need to be ruled out by needle aspiration.

Osteochondritis dissecans is the separation of a small portion of the femoral condyle with the overlying cartilage. The patient usually is an adolescent with a 1- to 4-week history of nonspecific knee pain. The physical examination may be normal or the femoral condyle may be tender. Because AP and lateral radiographs may not show the lesion, a tunnel or intercondylar view should be obtained.

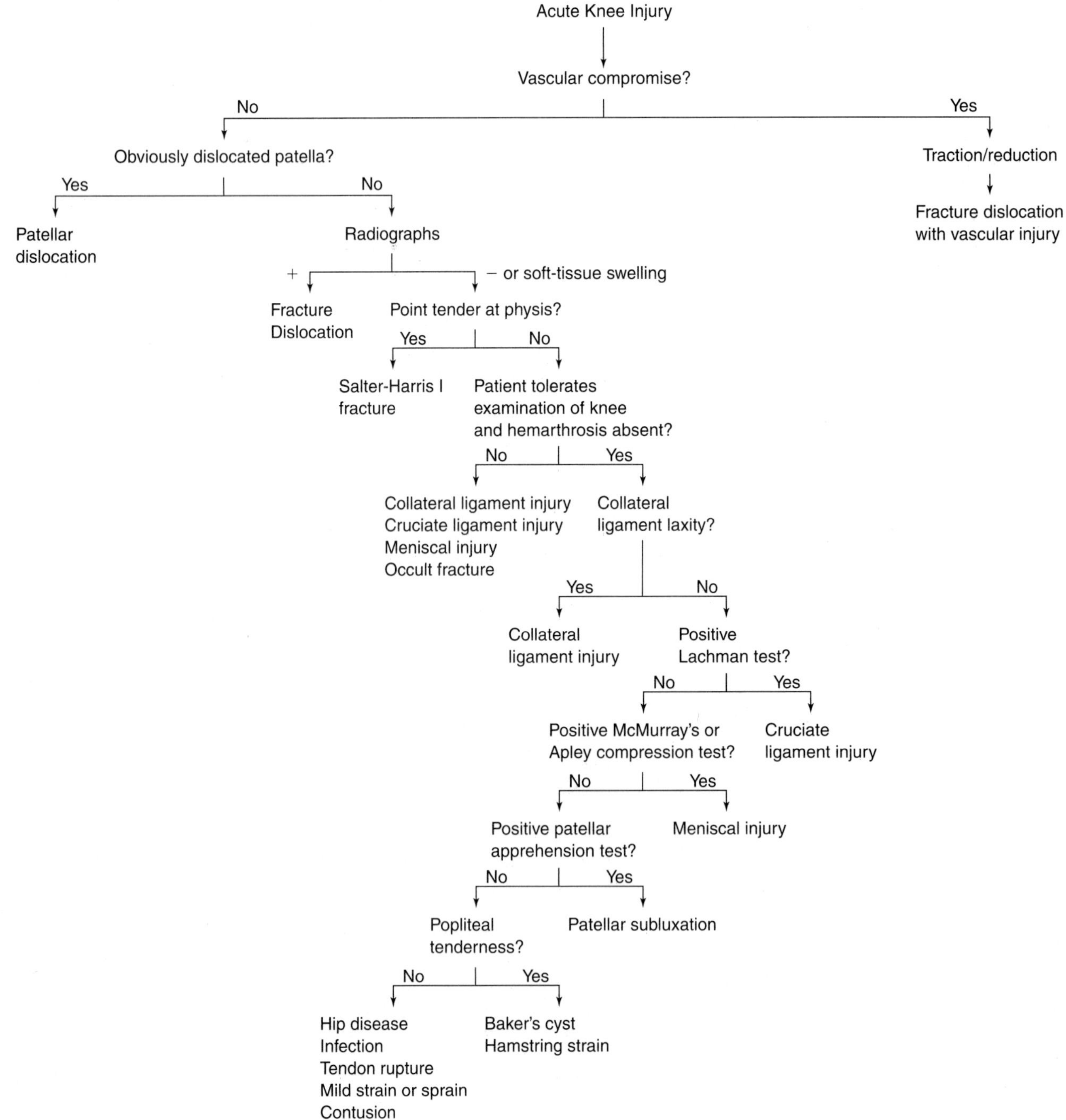

Figure 32.1. Approach to the patient with an acute knee injury.

Iliotibial band syndrome usually occurs in older runners who complain of pain over the lateral aspect of the knee. The iliotibial band moves in an anterior or posterior direction across the lateral femoral condyle as the knee flexes and extends. This repetitive movement may cause the pain. When examined, the patient is tender over the lateral femoral epicondyle, palpable 2 cm above the joint line. Radiographs are normal.

Baker's cyst is a herniation of the synovium of the knee joint or a separate synovial cyst located in the popliteal fossa. The patient complains of popliteal pain and swelling only if the cyst enlarges. The sac can be palpated in the posterior medial aspect of the popliteal space and may be transilluminated. For the most part, radiographs will be normal or show soft-tissue swelling.

In any patient with knee pain, with or without a history of trauma, benign (e.g., osteochondroma and nonossifying fibroma) and malignant tumors (e.g., osteosarcoma or Ewing sarcoma), the various causes of monoarticular arthritis (see Chapter 49), and hip disease that may present with knee pain (e.g., slipped capital femoral epiphysis or aseptic necrosis of the femoral head) must be considered.

EVALUATION AND DECISION

Four points are critical in the patient's history: (1) the activity and forces that led to the injury (e.g., direct or indirect force, direction of the force, and whether the foot was planted); (2) any sensations or noises (e.g., "locking," "pops," "snaps," "rips," or "tears"); (3) the initial location of the pain; and (4) the timing of any swelling. The physician should test for collateral and cruciate ligament damage, meniscal injuries, patellar subluxation, and PFPS, using the appropriate maneuvers (Table 32.2). Each test is described in the appropriate differential diagnosis section. All patients with acute knee injuries should have AP and

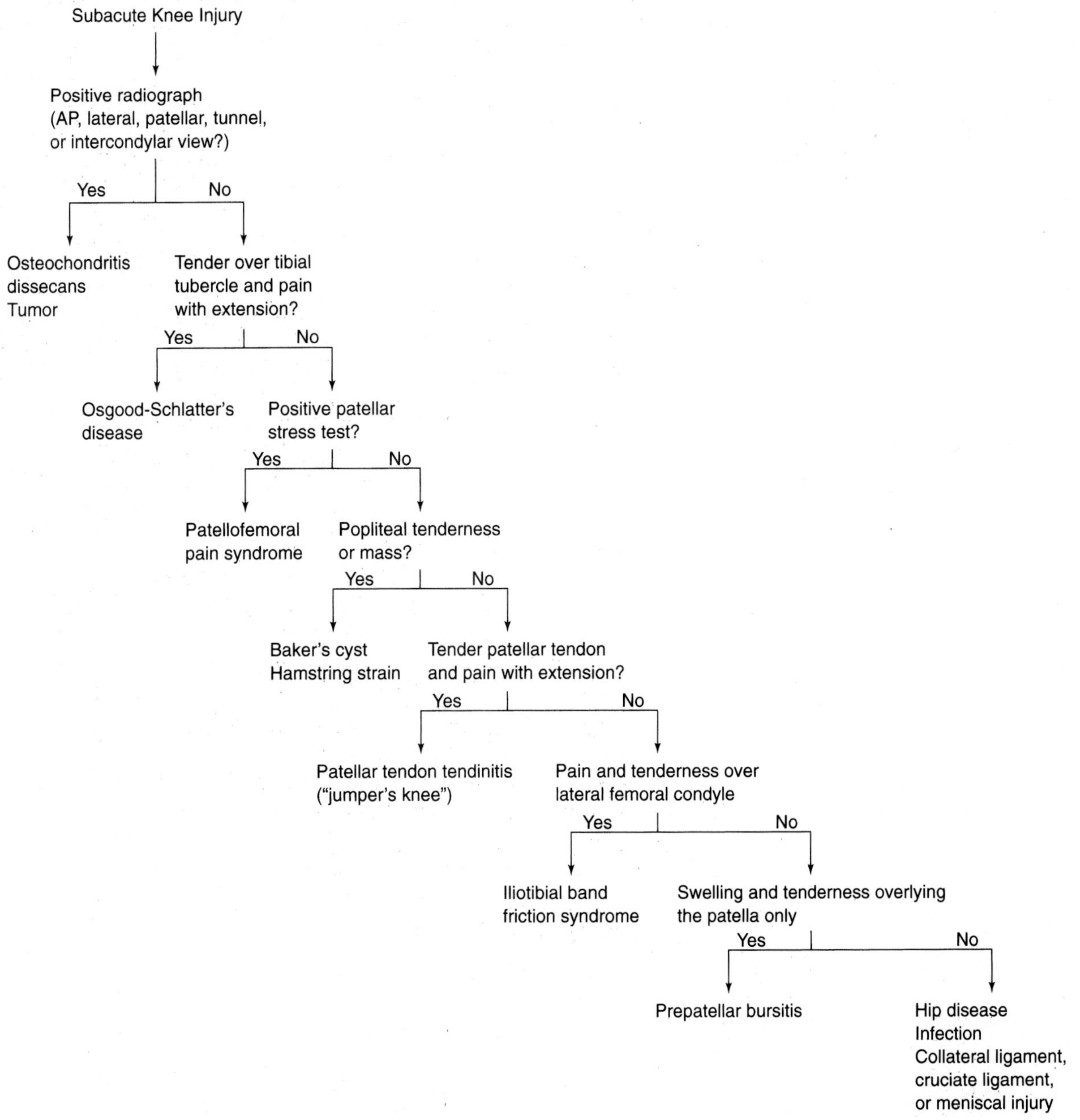

Figure 32.2. Approach to the patient with a subacute knee injury.

lateral radiographs, and if indicated, a patellar (or skyline view) radiograph should be taken. If the injury is more chronic, an intercondylar or tunnel view should also be taken to evaluate for osteochondritis dissecans.

The possibility of abuse in young children must always be considered, especially if the injury is unexplained, the history is implausible, or the seeking of medical care was unreasonably delayed.

Figure 32.1 summarizes an approach to the child with an acutely injured knee. If the initial evaluation suggests vascular compromise, traction and reduction of the knee should be attempted and an emergency orthopedics consultation should be obtained. If the patella is obviously dislocated, it may be reduced before obtaining radiographs. Postreduction radiographs and a careful examination for physeal tenderness then can exclude the diagnosis of a fracture. If the patient's knee is too painful or swollen to allow a complete examination or if the patient has a hemarthrosis, ligament or meniscal damage should be suspected, and the knee should be immobilized for a maximum of 3 days until seen by an orthopedic surgeon.

If the patient tolerates an examination, a series of maneuvers may suggest collateral ligament injury, cruciate ligament injury, meniscal injury, or patellar subluxation as the diagnosis (Table 32.2 summarizes the diagnostic maneuvers for the knee). Next an assessment for popliteal tenderness to exclude a Baker's cyst or hamstring strain is performed. Finally, if no signs of infection or hip disease exist, the patient may have a tendon rupture or a mild sprain, strain, or contusion.

Often, a patient may come to the ED with a history of trauma and knee pain that has been present for more than 1 or 2 days (Fig. 32.2). In addition to the standard AP, lateral, and patellar views, a tunnel or intercondylar view should be taken to exclude a fracture, tumor, and osteochondritis dissecans. If the initial knee and hip examinations do not suggest a diagnosis and no signs of infection exist, the diagnostic maneuvers in Table 32.2 should be completed. The patient may have an old collateral ligament, cruciate ligament, or meniscal injury and may require an orthopedic referral.

CHAPTER 33
Injury—Shoulder

Marc N. Baskin, M.D.

This chapter focuses on the diagnosis of the child with an overtly painful, injured shoulder. Children have different causes for their shoulder injuries than do adults because of their open growth plates, and young patients may be more difficult to examine because of anxiety and limited verbal skills.

DIFFERENTIAL DIAGNOSIS

The differential diagnosis depends mainly on exactly where the patient has pain. In this chapter, injuries are described anatomically, from the sternoclavicular joint to the humeral shaft (Tables 33.1 and 33.2).

Physeal (growth plate) separations of the medial clavicle are caused by indirect trauma that forces the shoulder medially and separates the growth plate. This injury mimics the sternoclavicular dislocations seen in adults. Most separations are anterior,

TABLE 33.1. Differential Diagnosis of the Injured Shoulder

Sternoclavicular joint	Rotator cuff
Dislocation[a]	Impingement
Sprain	Tear
Clavicle	Humerus
Physeal separation of medial end of the clavicle	Fracture of proximal humeral physis
Fracture	Stress fracture of proximal humeral physis ("Little League shoulder")
Contusion ("shoulder pointer")	Fracture of shaft
Osteolysis	Biceps tendon tendinitis
Acromioclavicular joint dislocation or sprain ("shoulder separation")	Pathologic fracture[a]
Scapula fracture	Referred pain (from)
Glenohumeral joint	Myocardium[a]
Dislocation ("shoulder dislocation")	Diaphragm[a]
	Neck
	Thoracic outlet syndrome

[a] Potentially life-threatening conditions.

and the patient has swelling and tenderness over the sternoclavicular joint. If the dislocation is posterior, the aorta or trachea may be injured; the child may remain asymptomatic or complain of choking or difficulty breathing. If the growth plate and ligaments are not disrupted by the injury, a simple sprain has occurred.

The clavicle is a commonly fractured bone in children, with fractures occurring most often in the middle or lateral third of the bone. A neonate's birthing injury or an infant's greenstick fracture of the clavicle may go unnoticed until the focal swelling of the developing callus is noted. In the older child, the arm droops down and forward, and the head may be tilted toward the affected side because of sternocleidomastoid muscle spasm. Localized swelling, tenderness, and crepitations may be noted.

Older children with a clavicular contusion or "shoulder pointer" may have swelling and tenderness over the distal clavicle. Osteolysis of the distal clavicle with resorption of the bone may develop after minor injuries to the clavicle. Patients experience chronic pain and mild swelling 2 to 3 weeks after the initial injury.

AC joint injuries usually cause fractures of the distal clavicle in patients less than 13 years of age. Older children may injure the AC joint ("shoulder separations") either by a direct blow to the shoulder or by transmitted force from a fall on an outstretched hand. The child will have pain with any motion of the shoulder and tenderness over the AC joint. In a first-degree sprain, the clavicle is not elevated above the acromion. In second- and third-degree sprains, swelling and elevation should be present. Bilateral "stress view" radiographs of the AC joint may be obtained to compare the separation on the normal and affected sides. Scapula fractures are rare in pediatrics and usually

TABLE 33.2. Common Causes of the Injured Shoulder

Clavicle fracture	Humerus
Glenohumeral joint	Fracture of proximal humeral physis
Dislocation ("shoulder dislocation")	Fracture of shaft
Subluxation	

occur only after major direct trauma such as a motor vehicle accident or a fall from a height.

Shoulder or glenohumeral joint dislocations are rare in children less than 12 years old. The trauma can damage the axillary nerve or fracture the humeral head. More than 95% of all dislocations are anterior, and less than 5% are posterior. The patient will be in severe pain, supporting the affected arm internally rotated and slightly abducted (i.e., the patient cannot bring the elbow to his or her side). The shoulder contour is sharp, unlike the smooth contour of the opposite shoulder, and the acromion is prominent. Sensation over the shoulder, especially laterally (axillary nerve distribution), and distal pulses should be documented. If the patient has a history consistent with dislocation but has more range of motion than expected and the radiograph is normal, the patient may have spontaneously reduced a dislocated shoulder or only sprained the ligaments overlying the glenoid fossa and subluxated the glenohumeral joint.

Actual tears of the rotator cuff are rare before 21 years of age. However, if the rotator cuff muscles are weak, the humeral head is displaced upward during overhead motion and may impinge the tendon of the supraspinatus muscle as it runs below the acromion. Impingement symptoms usually occur with repetitive overhead motions (e.g., throwing a ball). The pain is poorly localized. The patient may have mild tenderness under the acromion when the arm is abducted and may have increasing pain when the arm is abducted passively between 80 and 120 degrees.

Because the ligamentous attachments are stronger than the growth plate, fracture separations of proximal humeral epiphysis occur until the patient's epiphysis closes between 16 and 19 years of age. The injury occurs because of direct or indirect trauma, such as a backward fall or an attempt to break a fall with a hand. The patient usually has mild swelling and local tenderness. Stress fractures of the proximal humeral epiphysis, or "Little League shoulder," are caused by repetitive internal rotation of an abducted, externally rotated shoulder during the throwing motion. The child has diffuse shoulder pain that worsens after throwing. The proximal humerus may be tender, and radiographs show widening of the proximal humeral epiphysis.

Transverse or comminuted fractures of the humeral shaft may occur from direct trauma, whereas spiral fractures usually occur from indirect trauma (e.g., a fall on a hand). If the history is implausible, inconsistent from one caretaker to another, or the patient is less than 2 years of age, the child should be evaluated for physical abuse. The patient will have obvious pain, tenderness, and local deformity. Care must be taken not to miss an associated neurovascular injury because the radial nerve runs along the humeral shaft. Radial nerve damage results in weakness of wrist extension and anesthesia of the skin between the first and second metacarpals.

Shoulder pain is rarely related to tendonitis of the tendon of the long head of the biceps. This tendon runs through the bicipital groove just anterior and medial to the greater humeral tuberosity. The patient often has chronic pain and tenderness over the bicipital groove.

A painful shoulder or fracture that follows minimal trauma may be caused by a benign or malignant tumor or by nonneoplastic bone lesions. Osteochondromas (exostoses) are outgrowths of benign cartilage from the bone adjacent to the epiphysis and present with a mass adjacent to a joint. The nonossifying fibromas (called fibrous cortical defects if smaller than 0.5 cm) are common asymptomatic lesions that may lead to pathologic fractures.

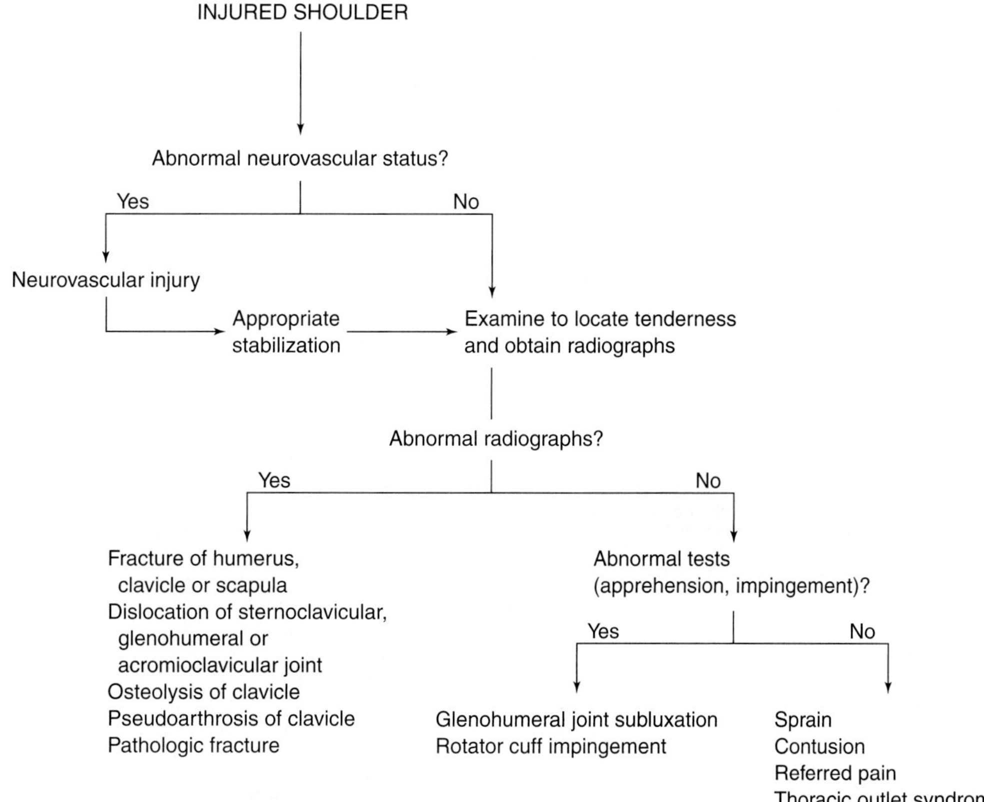

Figure 33.1. Approach to the patient with an injured shoulder.

The malignant chondroblastoma is a rare tumor, but its most common location is the proximal humerus. The patient often has joint pain from effusion associated with this tumor. Osteogenic sarcomas and Ewing sarcoma are more common but involve the humerus in only 10% of cases.

Unicameral and aneurysmal bone cysts are asymptomatic until the bone fractures, but they are not neoplastic lesions. Unicameral cysts are more likely to affect the humerus.

Shoulder pain also may be referred from the neck (e.g., cervical disc herniation), myocardium, or diaphragm (e.g., a splenic hematoma) after trauma to those areas.

Thoracic outlet syndrome, with compression of the medial cord of the brachial plexus (C8–T1) may rarely present as shoulder pain. The pain and anesthesia most commonly follow the dermatome of the ulnar nerve. The pain may be reproduced by 180 degrees of forward flexion; radiographs should include the neck to exclude a cervical rib.

EVALUATION AND DECISION

Initially, the patient's neurovascular status is assessed and fracture stabilization provided, if necessary (Fig. 33.1).

If the child seems anxious, the uninjured side is examined first. The examiner carefully palpates the entire shoulder from sternoclavicular joint to the shaft of the humerus. Swelling and tenderness at the sternoclavicular joint suggests a physeal separation or dislocation at this site. The clavicle is covered only by a thin platysma muscle and a fracture is easily seen and palpated. Just lateral to the clavicle is the AC joint. Elevation of the clavicle above the acromion or tenderness of the articulation suggests AC joint dislocation ("shoulder separation") or contusion. With the shoulder in external rotation, palpation just lateral to the acromion will locate the greater tuberosity of the humerus. Just in front of the greater tuberosity is the tendon of the long head of the biceps within the bicipital groove. Pressure may produce exquisite tenderness in this area, so palpation should be gentle; if uncertainty about a finding of tenderness exists, a comparison with the examination of the uninjured side is helpful. Finally, the proximal humeral shaft and the scapula are palpated.

Once the pain has been localized, appropriate radiographs are obtained, and when indicated, two additional specific tests are performed: the apprehension test for shoulder subluxation and the impingement test for rotator cuff impingement.

As previously discussed, patients with normal radiographs and negative maneuvers are most likely to have sprains or contusions, but occasionally, they may be experiencing referred pain.

CHAPTER 34

Jaundice—Unconjugated Hyperbilirubinemia

Kenneth D. Mandl, M.D., M.P.H.

Jaundice—a yellowish discoloration of the skin, tissues, and bodily fluids—indicates an elevated serum bilirubin concentration. Hyperbilirubinemia results from increased production or impaired excretion of bilirubin. Both physiologic and pathologic etiologies may give rise to unconjugated (or indirect) hyperbilirubinemia; to distinguish, the clinician must consider the patient's age, the rate of increase and peak level of serum bilirubin, and the historical features of the case. Prompt evaluation and therapy for unconjugated hyperbilirubinemia are particularly important for infants less than 1 week old. If bilirubin levels rise too high, these young infants risk developing neurodevelopmental deficits as well as kernicterus.

DIFFERENTIAL DIAGNOSIS

For patients with primarily unconjugated hyperbilirubinemia who are beyond the neonatal period, the most common causes are hemolytic processes resulting in overproduction of bilirubin (Table 34.1). Extravascular blood in a concealed hemorrhage may also be metabolized into supraphysiologic concentrations of bilirubin. Infants and children with jaundice may have enzyme deficiencies or other conditions that impair the hepatic uptake or conjugation of bilirubin. Upper gastrointestinal (GI) obstruction generally causes conjugated hyperbilirubinemia but may occasionally be associated with an unconjugated hyperbilirubinemia. In the neonatal period, physiologic and breast milk jaundice are common. The potential for maternal–fetal blood group incompatibility is critical to recognize.

TABLE 34.1. Causes of Primarily Unconjugated Hyperbilirubinemia

Excess bilirubin production
- Intravascular hemolysis
  - Intracorpuscular
    - Glucose-6-phosphate dehydrogenase deficiency
    - Sickle cell disease
    - Thalassemia
    - Hereditary spherocytosis, hereditary elliptocytosis
  - Extracorpuscular
    - Autoimmune hemolytic anemia
    - Microangiopathic hemolytic anemia
    - Drug-induced hemolytic anemia
- Extravascular hemolysis
  - Concealed hematomas
  - Hyperspleni sm

Infection
  - Bacterial sepsis
  - Malaria (causes hemolysis)

Inherited disorders of bilirubin metabolism
- Gilbert syndrome
- Crigler-Najjar syndrome type II

Neonatal only
- Physiologic hyperbilirubinemia
- Nonphysiologic hyperbilirubinemia
- Jaundice related to breast-feeding
- Hemolysis
  - Intravascular
    - Maternal–fetal blood group incompatibility (ABO, Rh, other)
    - Polycythemia
  - Extravascular
    - Cephalohematoma
    - Neonatal intracranial hemorrhage
    - Swallowed blood during birth
  - Upper gastrointestinal obstruction
    - Pyloric stenosis
    - Meconium ileus
    - Hirschsprung disease
    - Duodenal atresia
  - Endocrine
    - Congenital hypothyroidism
    - Infant of a diabetic mother
  - Inherited disorders of bilirubin metabolism
    - Crigler-Najjar syndrome type I
    - Galactosemia (early)
    - Lucey-Driscoll syndrome

Excess Bilirubin Production

The numerous causes of hemolysis may be classified as intravascular or extravascular. Intravascular hemolysis may be further divided into intracorpuscular and extracorpuscular defects (Table 34.1). Inborn errors of metabolism, such as glucose-6-phosphate dehydrogenase (G6PD) deficiency, may result in destruction of RBCs. Hemoglobinopathies, including sickle cell disease, can result in hemolysis, as can the impairments in hemoglobin chain synthesis that occur in the thalassemias. Defects in the RBC membrane found in hereditary spherocytosis and hereditary elliptocytosis increase the fragility of the corpuscles. Extracorpuscular causes of RBC destruction include the autoimmune, microangiopathic, and drug-induced hemolytic anemias.

Hematomas, pulmonary hemorrhages, and other collections of extravasated blood undergo hemolysis and, if sufficiently large, can elevate serum levels of unconjugated bilirubin. Various hypersplenic states, including splenic sequestration crisis in sickle cell disease, may result in anemia with accompanying hemolysis and hyperbilirubinemia.

Infection

Jaundice may be a harbinger of serious infection. Bacterial endotoxins reduce bile flow and can cause hyperbilirubinemia. The neonate with jaundice as well as poor feeding, lethargy, or fever should be evaluated for sepsis and urinary tract infection. However, sepsis is exceedingly rare among well-appearing jaundiced neonates who have no additional signs or symptoms, occurring at a rate considerably below 1%. Malaria, caused by *Plasmodium* species, is endemic in tropical regions. In patients with malaria, a high degree of parasitemia may result in massive hemolysis presenting with jaundice.

Inherited Disorders of Bilirubin Metabolism

Gilbert syndrome is a common cause of mild, intermittent, unconjugated hyperbilirubinemia that occurs in as many as 6% of the population. Patients generally do not present until late childhood or early adolescence, when they may develop nonspecific abdominal pain, nausea, and mild jaundice during an intercurrent illness. Other liver function studies are normal, and there is no evidence of hemolysis or hepatosplenomegaly. The serum bilirubin rarely exceeds 5 mg/dL.

Crigler-Najjar syndrome is characterized by the absence or deficiency of the enzyme bilirubin glucuronyl transferase. Type I, the more severe form, manifests soon after birth and is associated with high morbidity and mortality. Type II, the milder form, caused by an incomplete enzyme deficiency, typically presents in infancy or later in childhood but has been reported to first appear as late as adolescence.

SPECIAL CONSIDERATIONS IN THE NEONATE

Physiologic Neonatal Hyperbilirubinemia

Most newborns develop a mild hyperbilirubinemia; approximately 60% manifest clinical signs of physiologic jaundice. Physiologic jaundice peaks between 3 and 5 days of life in the term infant and requires no treatment. Because at high levels bilirubin may be associated with neurotoxic effects, careful attention should be paid to distinguishing physiologic from nonphysiologic jaundice.

Nonphysiologic Neonatal Hyperbilirubinemia

One to two percent of newborns require readmission within the first week of life, and up to 85 of these readmissions are for nonphysiologic neonatal hyperbilirubinemia. Jaundice in the term newborn is nonphysiologic if it is conjugated or appears within the first 24 hours of life. Other indications that jaundice is not physiologic are a peak serum total bilirubin concentration of 17 mg per dL or higher in the breast-fed infant and 15 mg per dL or higher in the formula-fed infant. Also, infants with persistence of jaundice beyond the first week of life, or whose serum bilirubin level increases more than 5 mg per dL per day, should be followed closely for nonphysiologic jaundice. Risk factors for nonphysiologic neonatal hyperbilirubinemia include history of a sibling with hyperbilirubinemia, breast-feeding, lower gestational age, maternal diabetes, bruising (from birth trauma), and Asian race. Dehydrated neonates may develop unconjugated hyperbilirubinemia.

Breast-Feeding and Jaundice

Breast-fed newborns develop a greater degree of hyperbilirubinemia more often than do formula-fed newborns. Breast-milk jaundice, occurring in 1% of newborns, is associated with the breast milk itself and may be hormonally mediated or related to intestinal excretion and resorption of bile. Many cases of jaundice in breast-fed infants are caused by nonoptimal breast-feeding practices that result in dehydration.

Hemolysis

Birth trauma, when associated with a cephalohematoma, extensive bruising, or swallowed maternal blood, can result in hyperbilirubinemia. Intracranial, pulmonary, or other concealed hemorrhage also can lead to extravascular hemolysis. Similarly, polycythemia, caused by delayed clamping of the cord or maternal–fetal or fetal–fetal transfusion (in multiple gestations), increases the RBC mass and causes jaundice in neonates.

When maternal antibodies are produced against fetal red cell antigens, the neonate can develop a Coombs' positive isoimmune hemolytic anemia. The risk of kernicterus in infants with hyperbilirubinemia as a result of isoimmune hemolytic anemia is much greater than the risk in infants with nonhemolytic causes of jaundice. Fetal Rh and A and B blood group antigens are most commonly etiologic in the hemolysis syndrome, although dozens of antigens have been implicated.

Upper Gastrointestinal Obstruction

Pyloric stenosis, meconium ileus, Hirschsprung disease, duodenal atresia, and other causes of upper GI obstruction may present with jaundice and clinical signs of obstruction. In neonates, obstruction can increase enterohepatic circulation or decrease the enzyme activity responsible for bilirubin uptake, resulting in unconjugated hyperbilirubinemia. In contrast, older children and adults with upper GI obstruction and jaundice generally have a conjugated hyperbilirubinemia.

Endocrine Disorders

Unconjugated hyperbilirubinemia may be the presenting sign of congenital hypothyroidism, preceding other manifestations by several weeks. The mechanism probably relates to reduced bile flow. Other signs that may be present include persistent poor feeding, prolonged jaundice, constipation, and hypotonia. Infants of diabetic mothers are also at increased risk of jaundice, with as many as 19 developing nonphysiologic hyperbilirubinemia.

Inherited Disorders of Bilirubin Metabolism

Very high, rapidly rising levels of bilirubin not responsive to phototherapy raise concern for Crigler-Najjar syndrome type I or Lucey-Driscoll syndrome. Lucey-Driscoll syndrome is probably caused by an inhibition of glucuronyl transferase. Infants with galactosemia may exhibit an unconjugated hyperbilirubinemia during the first week of life. Older infants with galactosemia tend to have a conjugated hyperbilirubinemia. Infants with galactosemia usually also present with vomiting, failure to thrive, poor feeding, abdominal distension, and hypoglycemia.

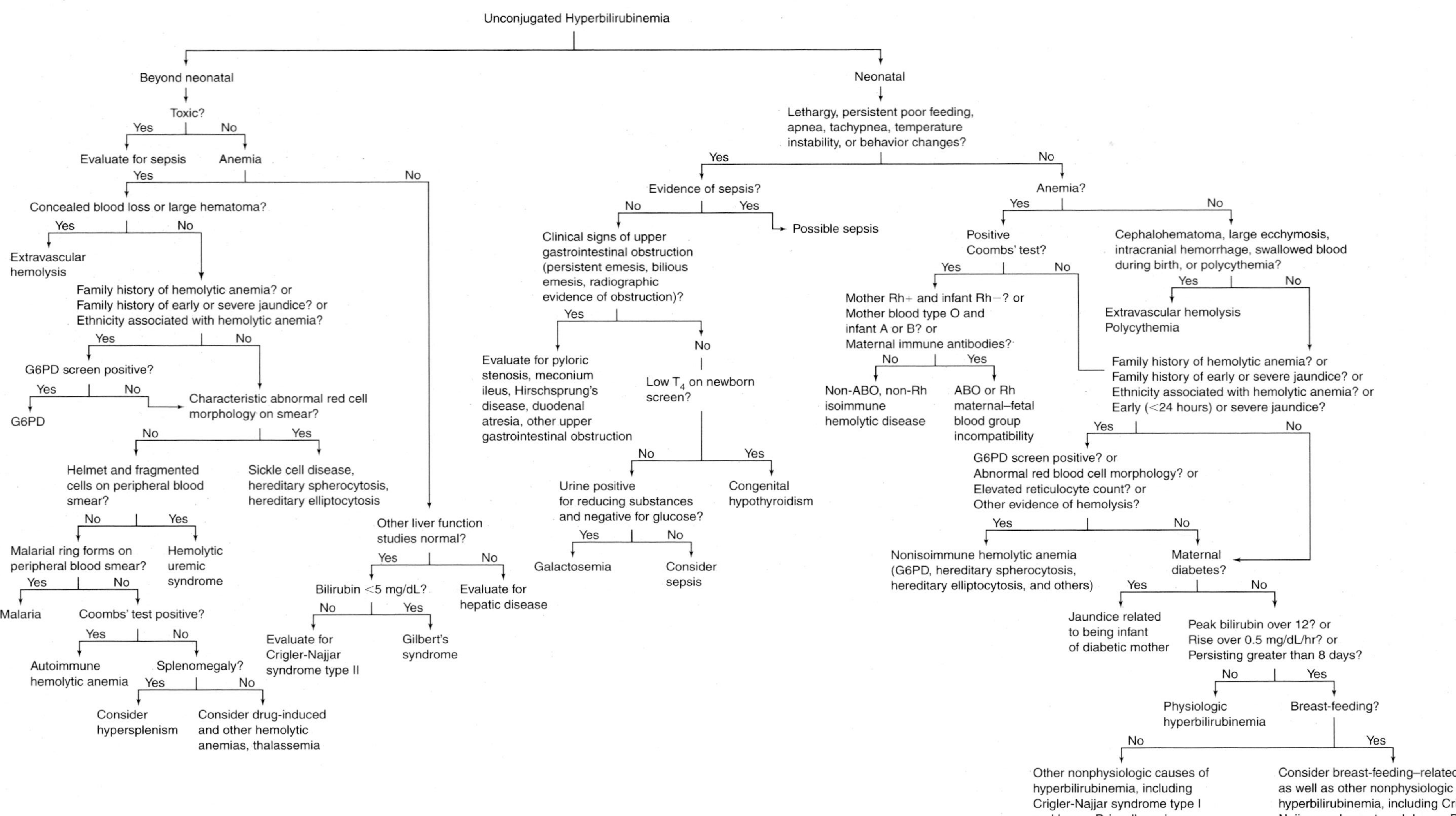

Figure 34.1. Evaluation of the pediatric patient with unconjugated hyperbilirubinemia.

EVALUATION AND DECISION

An approach to the patient with unconjugated hyperbilirubinemia is outlined in Fig. 34.1. Hemolysis and Gilbert syndrome are the most common cause of jaundice in the patient beyond the neonatal period (Table 34.2). During the neonatal period, physiologic jaundice and breast-feeding–related jaundice are the most likely causes. The differential diagnosis is broad, and evaluation should always begin with a detailed history and physical examination. A general clinical history may help guide the workup. An infant who has been lethargic or apneic or a child who has been ill and febrile may require evaluation for serious bacterial infections (Table 34.3). A neonate with persistent or bilious emesis may have an upper GI obstruction. In the neonate, poor feeding, lethargy, apnea, tachypnea, and temperature instability are highly concerning.

Laboratory Testing

The serum bilirubin level should always be determined. Jaundiced patients beyond the neonatal period should be evaluated for anemia with a complete blood count (CBC) and reticulocyte count. Those with evidence of anemia and/or hemolysis should have a peripheral blood smear examined microscopically. Testing for G6PD should be performed if the patient has risk factors or a consistent clinical presentation. Hemoglobin electrophoresis may be used to diagnose hemoglobinopathies such as sickle cell disease and thalassemia. If hepatomegaly is present or if there is no evidence of anemia, liver function studies should be performed. Patients with no laboratory abnormalities other than serum unconjugated bilirubin below 5 mg per dL have Gilbert syndrome, a benign condition.

SPECIAL LABORATORY CONSIDERATIONS IN THE NEONATE

In neonates, it may be important to determine the rate of rise of serum bilirubin with serial measurements. The clinician must know whether a newborn has a set-up for maternal–fetal isoimmune anemia. Therefore, either the mother's blood and Rh type and antibody status should be obtained, or the infant's blood type should be determined and Coombs testing performed. A neonate with probable physiologic jaundice does not need to undergo an anemia or hemolysis workup if he or she has no family history of hemolytic disease, no maternal–fetal blood group incompatibility, and no physical stigmata of anemia.

If clinical signs of obstruction are present, the patient should undergo appropriate laboratory testing such as abdominal radiographs, ultrasound, or upper GI series with contrast. The neonate with fever or ill appearance should be evaluated for serious bacterial infection, with peripheral white blood cell count, urine analysis, and cerebrospinal fluid analysis as well as blood, urine, and cerebrospinal fluid cultures. Results of the newborn screen for congenital hypothyroidism may be available. The newborn with symptoms of congenital hypothyroidism needs to have a determination of T_4 level. A newborn with poor feeding, vomiting, or failure to gain weight should be evaluated for galactosemia. If the newborn with galactosemia has already started feeds, the urine will contain reducing substances (Clinitest positive) but no glucose.

TABLE 34.2. Common Causes of Primarily Unconjugated Hyperbilirubinemia

Excess bilirubin production
- Glucose-6-phosphate dehydrogenase deficiency
- Sickle cell disease

Infection
- Malaria (causes hemolysis)

Inherited disorders of bilirubin metabolism
- Gilbert syndrome

Neonatal only
- Physiologic hyperbilirubinemia
- Nonphysiologic hyperbilirubinemia
- Jaundice related to breast-feeding
- Overproduction of hemoglobin
  - Hemolysis
    - Maternal–fetal blood group incompatibility (ABO, Rh, other)
    - Cephalohematoma

TABLE 34.3. Life-Threatening Causes of Primarily Unconjugated Hyperbilirubinemia

Acute hemolysis

Infection
- Bacterial sepsis
- Malaria (causes hemolysis)

Neonatal only
- Nonphysiologic hyperbilirubinemia
- Hemolysis
  - Maternal–fetal blood group incompatibility (Rh, ABO, other)
  - Polycythemia
- Upper gastrointestinal obstruction
- Endocrine
  - Congenital hypothyroidism
- Inherited disorders of bilirubin metabolism
  - Crigler-Najjar syndrome type I
  - Galactosemia (early)
  - Lucey-Driscoll syndrome

Approach

BEYOND THE NEONATAL PERIOD

In all children with jaundice, a total bilirubin level with fractionation and CBC should be performed. If a patient appears acutely ill, the physician should proceed with the appropriate evaluation and treatment for sepsis. Among well-appearing patients, the hematocrit determines the likely diagnostic possibilities and appropriate studies.

Anemia

Anemic children are suspect for having hemolytic processes, including autoimmune hemolytic anemia, hemoglobinopathies (e.g., thalassemia or sickle cell anemia), enzyme deficiencies (e.g., G6PD), red cell membrane defects (e.g., spherocytosis), hypersplenism, drug reactions, hemolytic uremic syndrome, and malaria. Extravascular hemolysis and resultant jaundice occur occasionally in children with concealed blood loss or large hematomas. A family history of hemolytic anemia and severe jaundice, particularly among children of Mediterranean descent, suggests G6PD deficiency, whereas abnormal RBC morphology points to sickle cell anemia, hereditary spherocytosis, or heredity elliptocytosis. Additional clues on the peripheral smear include helmet and fragmented cells in hemolytic uremic syndrome and ring forms in malaria.

A positive Coombs test is seen with autoimmune hemolytic anemia. In patients with splenomegaly, hemolysis may lead to jaundice. Finally, drug reactions and unusual hemolytic anemias should be considered.

Normal Hematocrit

When unconjugated hyperbilirubinemia occurs without anemia, abnormal liver function studies (transaminases, prothrombin time, and partial thromboplastin time) differentiate hepatic disease from inherited disorders of bilirubin metabolism.

Among these latter disorders, only Gilbert syndrome, which produces a mild elevation in the serum bilirubin level, is at all common.

NEONATAL PERIOD

As for older children, an ill appearance and/or fever suggest sepsis. Other disorders likely to cause lethargy include bowel obstruction, hypothyroidism, and inborn errors of metabolism, such as galactosemia. Among well-appearing neonates, the presence of anemia serves as an important point in the differential diagnosis.

Anemia

The foremost consideration in the infant with indirect hyperbilirubinemia and anemia is isoimmune hemolytic disease, caused by blood group incompatibility, because this disorder may lead to kernicterus. The diagnosis can be established by determining the blood group and Rh status of the maternal–infant dyad in combination with a Coombs test in the infant. Other disorders that produce jaundice include enzymatic and structural disorders of the red cells (e.g., G6PD, hereditary spherocytosis) and the poorly understood occurrence of jaundice in infants of diabetic mothers.

Normal Hematocrit

In the absence of anemia, extravascular hemolysis is a common cause of jaundice in the newborn, with the breakdown of hemoglobin occurring in a cephalohematoma, large ecchymosis, or from swallowed blood. In addition, polycythemic infants are prone to jaundice. Also, hemolysis of even small amounts of hemoglobin may markedly elevate the serum bilirubin level in the infant with an immature liver. Thus, the same disorders that are diagnosed in anemic infants may occur in the jaundiced neonate with a normal hematocrit.

Most infants with indirect hyperbilirubinemia will have a negative evaluation for the disorders previously listed. If the bilirubin level is less than 12 mg per dL, rises slowly, and resolves before 8 days of age, one can diagnose physiologic hyperbilirubinemia without further laboratory studies. When these conditions are not met, the most likely cause for the jaundice is the hormonal impairment of bilirubin conjugation. Other possibilities, either alone or in combination with breast milk, include Crigler-Najjar and Lucey-Driscoll syndromes.

MANAGEMENT

For patients beyond the neonatal period, the management of hyperbilirubinemia is primarily directed at identification and treatment of the underlying cause. In contrast, newborns with jaundice require careful monitoring and sometimes specific therapies for hyperbilirubinemia because the neonatal central nervous system is susceptible to the toxic effects of bilirubin. The emergency physician may initiate the management of term newborn infants with jaundice and arrange hospitalization or subsequent follow-up after discharge. The management of premature infants with hyperbilirubinemia is highly specialized and not discussed here.

The goal of neonatal hyperbilirubinemia management is to prevent neurotoxicity, encephalopathy, and kernicterus. The jaundiced newborn needs to be kept well hydrated, and enteral feeding should be encouraged to promote bilirubin excretion. When bilirubin levels rise significantly, phototherapy and exchange transfusion may be indicated.

Phototherapy can be initiated with either an overhead bank of lights or a fiberoptic light source in a blanket. Indications for phototherapy and exchange transfusion vary according to the age of neonate. For the term neonate who develops jaundice after the first day of life and has no evidence of hemolysis, indications for phototherapy and exchange transfusion are shown in Table 34.4. When there is evidence of isoimmune hemolysis, phototherapy should be started immediately and a neonatologist should be consulted regardless of bilirubin level. Phototherapy is relatively contraindicated in patients with conjugated hyperbilirubinemia because it can cause the "bronze baby syndrome." When bilirubin levels are toxic, exchange transfusion may be necessary.

For jaundiced, breast-fed infants, the interruption or discontinuation of breast-feeding should be discouraged. Any of several management strategies, however, are accepted: (1) the infant may be observed while normal breast-feeding continues; (2) if bilirubin levels are high (Table 34.4), the infant may continue to breast-feed while receiving phototherapy; (3) breast-feeding may be supplemented with or without administration of phototherapy; and (4) breast-feeding may be interrupted and formula may be substituted with or without administration of phototherapy.

TABLE 34.4. Management of Hyperbilirubinemia in the Healthy Term Newborn[a]

	Total serum bilirubin level (mg/dL)			
Age (h)	Consider phototherapy[b]	Phototherapy	Exchange transfusion if intensive phototherapy[c] fails	Exchange transfusion an tensive phototherapy
<24				
24–48	≥12	≥15	≥20	≥25
49–72	≥15	≥18	≥25	≥30
>72	≥17	≥20	≥25	≥30

[a] Term infants who are clinically jaundiced at ≤24 hours old are not considered healthy and require further evaluation.
[b] Phototherapy at these total serum bilirubin levels is a clinical option, meaning that the intervention is available and may be used *on the basis of individual clinical judgment.*
[c] Intensive phototherapy should produce a decline of total serum bilirubin of 1 to 2 mg/dL within 4 to 6 hours and the total serum bilirubin level should continue to fall and remain below the threshold level for exchange transfusion. If this does not occur, it is considered a failure of phototherapy.
Adapted with permission from the American Academy of Pediatrics practice parameter for management of hyperbilirubinemia in the healthy term newborn.

CHAPTER 35

Jaundice—Conjugated Hyperbilirubinemia

Jonathan I. Singer, M.D.

The presence of jaundice in a child can be a useful indicator of occult pathology. The finding of icterus should set in motion a careful diagnostic search to elucidate the cause. The ultimate goal, to identify precisely the cause of the clinical syndrome, may rest in some cases with the longitudinal caretaker. In all cases, however, the emergency physician at first visit must separate patients whose admission can be temporized from those who require urgent intervention and/or immediate hospitalization.

DIFFERENTIAL DIAGNOSIS

Conjugated hyperbilirubinemia, defined as an elevated total bilirubin with greater than 30% direct reacting, always is pathologic. The differential diagnosis includes a variety of structural defects, infections, hepatotoxins, inborn errors of metabolism, and familial syndromes (Table 35.1). Although only a few diseases commonly cause conjugated hyperbilirubinemia (Table 35.2), all are serious. In addition, several less common conditions are important considerations because they are life threatening (Table 35.3).

EVALUATION AND DECISION

The approach to the patient with conjugated hyperbilirubinemia is shown in Fig. 35.1.

TABLE 35.2. Common Causes of Conjugated Hyperbilirubinemia

Infancy	Childhood
Idiopathic cholestasis	Viral hepatitis
Biliary atresia	Hepatotoxins
Perinatal infections (TORCH)	
Sepsis/urinary tract infection	

TORCH, toxoplasmosis, other infections, rubella, cytomegalovirus infection, and herpes simplex.

Infants Less Than 8 Weeks Old

The onset of conjugated hyperbilirubinemia in the first 2 months of life may be abrupt or insidious. Infants with generalized viral infections acquired in utero and during the birthing process are more likely to present shortly after birth. Perinatal cytomegalovirus (CMV) infection, rubella, toxoplasmosis, herpes simplex, and syphilis may account for irritability, jitteriness, seizures, microcephaly, hepatomegaly, icterus, and petechiae.

The diagnosis of sepsis or urinary tract infection should be considered in any infant who abruptly develops icterus. Hyperbilirubinemia may occur antecedent to blood cultures becoming positive and may precede findings of anorexia, vomiting, abdominal distension, fever, hepatomegaly, or alterations in respiratory pattern or sensorium.

Infants with intrahepatic and extrahepatic biliary atresia have a failure of bile secretion associated with a significant hyperbilirubinemia. Although symptoms vary in onset, they usually are less acute than those seen in the infectious states. Infants affected with atresia generally appear well, with the exception of jaundice and hepatomegaly. Infants with complete obstruction pass clay-colored stools.

The characteristic clinical pattern with idiopathic cholestasis consists of onset of jaundice in the second or third week of life.

TABLE 35.1. Causes of Conjugated Hyperbilirubinemia in Infants and Children

First 8 Weeks of life	*Childhood*
Hepatic disorders	Hepatic disorders
Biliary atresia	Hepatotoxins (drugs, chemicals)
Intrahepatic biliary hypoplasia	Byler disease
Idiopathic hepatocellular cholestasis or neonatal hepatitis syndrome	Dubin-Johnson syndrome
Ischemic hepatitis	Rotor syndrome
Perinatal infections	Infections
Toxoplasmosis	Viral hepatitides (A through E)
Rubella	Epstein-Barr virus, coxsackievirus, echovirus
Cytomegalovirus	Liver abscess (usually anicteric)
Varicella-zoster	Myocarditis
Herpes simplex	Urinary tract infection
Coxsackievirus	Suppurative cholangitis
Bacterial sepsis	Peritonitis
Leptospirosis	Pneumonia
Urinary tract infection	Metabolic disorders
Metabolic disorder	Wolman disease
Galactosemia	Zellweger syndrome
Galactokinase deficiency	Glycogen storage (III, IV)
Hereditary fructose intolerance	Wilson disease
Hereditary tyrosinemia	Biliary tree disorders
α_1-antitrypsin deficiency	Choledocholithiasis
Cystic fibrosis	Pancreatic disease
Biliary tree disorders	Miscellaneous
Spontaneous perforation of the bile duct	Abdominal crisis, sickle hemoglobinopathy
Choledochal cyst	Hepatorenal syndrome

TABLE 35.3. Life-Threatening Causes of Conjugated Hyperbilirubinemia

Fulminant hepatic failure	Abdominal crisis, sickle hemoglobinopathy
Septicemia	Hepatorenal syndrome
Intraabdominal sepsis	Reye syndrome (usually anicteric)
Pyogenic liver abscess	
Suppurative cholangitis	
Peritonitis	

Initially, stool color is normal, but the stools may become acholic after several weeks. The presence of acholic stools may make it difficult to differentiate between obstructive jaundice caused by hepatocellular disease and that caused by obstruction of the biliary tree.

The inherited and metabolic conditions (e.g., galactosemia, tyrosinemia, cystic fibrosis, α_1-antitrypsin deficiency) associated with conjugated hyperbilirubinemia are typically insidious in onset. Although of a diverse nature, these diseases largely are characterized by inconstant jaundice, failure to thrive, developmental delay, and metabolic derangements. Unexplained fatality in the sibship or unexplained pulmonary, gastrointestinal, neurologic, or psychiatric disturbance in other family members may provoke diagnostic consideration.

The priorities for the emergency physician are to diagnose medically treatable infections, to identify metabolic disorders for which effective therapy is available, and to detect extrahepatic obstructive lesions that are amenable to surgical correction. The evaluation begins with cultures of cerebrospinal fluid, blood, urine, and stool. Infants also should have complete blood and platelet counts and should be tested for prothrombin time, hepatic enzymes (AST, ALT, and GGT), ammonia, albumin, total protein and protein electrophoresis, alkaline phosphatase, electrolytes, blood urea nitrogen, creatinine, and blood sugar. Urine should be tested for reducing substances. Additional studies useful for the longitudinal care physician include sweat iontophoresis, α_1-antitrypsin, TORCH (toxoplasmosis, other infections, rubella, CMV infection and herpes simplex) and hepatitis B virus serology, immunoglobulin M (IgM), urine examination for CMV, red blood cell galactose1-phosphate uridyltransferase activity, stool examinations, abdominal ultrasonography, and hepatobiliary scintigraphy.

Inpatient observation is appropriate in this age group because the diagnosis rarely can be established in the emergency department (ED). Empiric therapy for sepsis or urinary infection often is warranted, pending culture results.

Children More Than 8 Weeks Old

In the evaluation of conjugated hyperbilirubinemia beyond infancy, it is necessary to know whether there has been exposure to contagion or a potential for sexual or vertical transmission of infections such as hepatitis or human immunodeficiency virus (HIV). Other risk factors for hepatitis (e.g., needle sticks, hemodialysis, transplant, transfusion of blood products or factor use) need to be excluded. The physician should pursue possible exposure to industrial toxins or foods previously implicated in hepatic injury (e.g., carbon tetrachloride, yellow phosphorus, tannic acid, alcohol, mushrooms of the Amanita species). The emergency physician must inquire about use of acetaminophen, salicylates, erythromycin estolate, ceftriaxone,

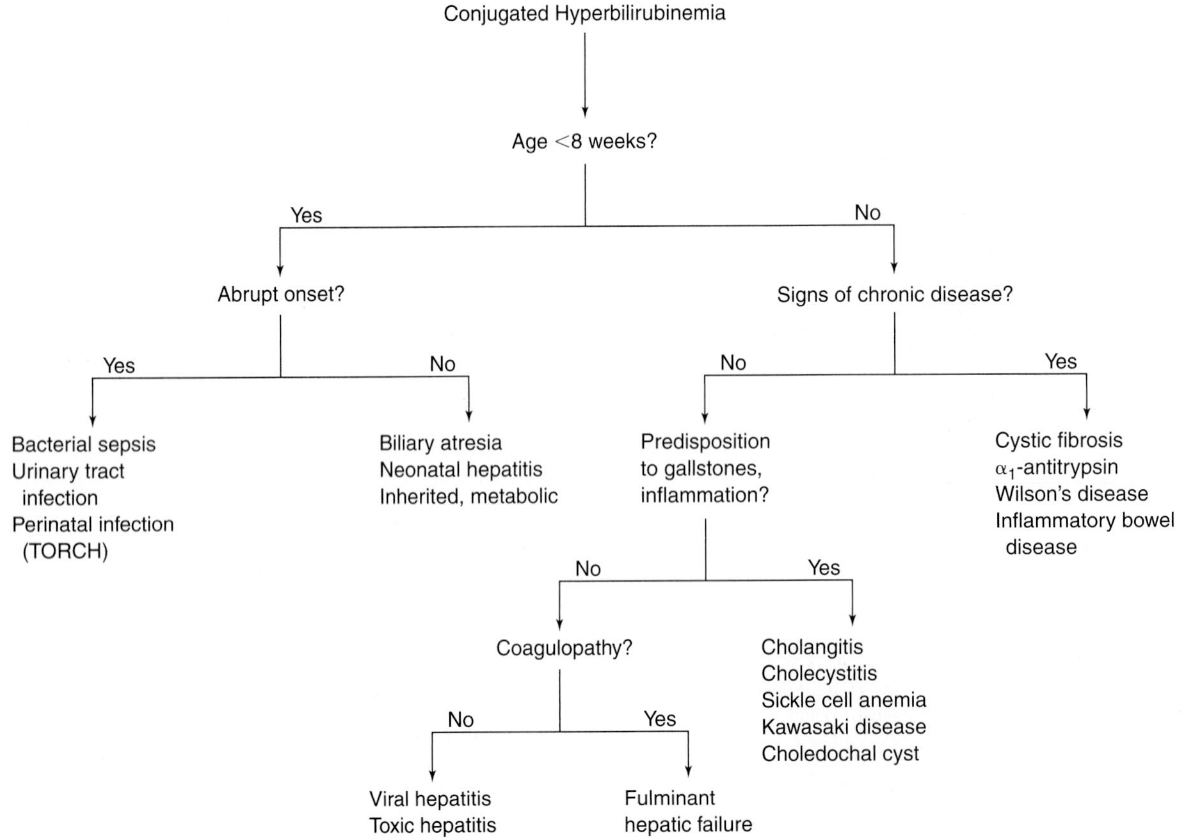

Figure 35.1. Approach to the patient with conjugated hyperbilirubinemia.

rifampin, iron salts, nitrofurantoin, oxacillin, methimazole, tetracycline, trimethoprim–sulfamethoxazole, diphenylhydantoin, isoniazid, and paraaminosalicylic acid (PAS). The presence of prior episodes of jaundice, acholic stools, and/or abdominal pain may suggest an underlying disorder, predisposing the patient to obstruction of the biliary tree. Other historical points include the presence of fever, arthralgia, arthritis, conjunctivitis, rash, pruritus, vomiting, diarrhea, weight loss, color of the urine, abnormal bruising or spontaneous bleeding, and changes in mental status.

An examination that focuses on ongoing physical signs of liver disease may result in greater accuracy in clinical evaluation of the older jaundiced patient. These signs include skin changes (spider angioma, excoriations, palmar erythema) and peripheral edema. The abdominal examination should include observations of the venous pattern, presence of ascites, mass, or peritoneal irritation. There should be an estimation of liver size, contour, and tenderness, as well as an estimate of spleen size. The clinician should exclude cardiovascular dysfunctions such as hypoxemia, systemic venous congestion, and low cardiac output. Observations should be made of mental status and neuromuscular changes.

Patients with cystic fibrosis, α_1-antitrypsin deficiency, Wilson disease, or inflammatory bowel disease tend to have symptoms that remit and relax. However, slow progression is the rule. Patients with α_1-antitrypsin deficiency may have onset of respiratory or hepatic complaints at any age. Similarly, infants who have failure to thrive from cystic fibrosis may develop obstruction at any age in the extrahepatic or intrahepatic ducts and, transiently or persistently, may exhibit jaundice. Patients with ulcerative colitis and Crohn disease may become symptomatic intermittently with episodes of cholestasis. The degree of hepatic derangement and expression of neurologic abnormality is variable with Wilson disease. Patients typically exhibit dysarthria, tremors, rigidity, or psychic disturbances before the diagnosis is entertained. Rarely, patients at a younger age without prodromal events have acute jaundice and hepatomegaly and progress to hepatic failure.

Biliary calculi and acute inflammation of the gallbladder are uncommon causes of conjugated hyperbilirubinemia in the pediatric population. However, a subset of patients is predisposed to these complications. Cholelithiasis may complicate any of the hemolytic anemias, particularly in patients with sickle hemoglobinopathies. Cholecystitis may accompany a variety of acute focal infections, such as pneumonia or peritonitis, and may occur in the course of bacterial sepsis. Right upper quadrant abdominal mass, pain, and jaundice constitute the classic triad in the diagnosis of choledochal cyst. The clinical recognition may be delayed until there is a complication, such as cholangitis. An acute, painful right upper quadrant mass associated with jaundice also may occur in the course of acute hydrops of the gallbladder from Kawasaki disease or systemic streptococcal infection.

In the previously healthy child, the most common cause of conjugated hyperbilirubinemia is acute hepatitis. The illness may be abrupt in onset, with fever, urticaria, and arthralgia as primary manifestations. More often, the illness is insidious. Viral hepatitis is characterized by low-grade fever and gastrointestinal complaints such as anorexia, malaise, nausea, vomiting, and abdominal pain before the jaundice. Liver enlargement with hepatitis (A, B, C, and non-A, non-B, non-C), varicella, herpesvirus, coxsackievirus, echovirus, Epstein-Barr virus, and adenovirus infection is inconstant. Hepatic tenderness is a more reliable finding. Rarely, ascites can accompany hepatitis virus infection. Splenomegaly is the rule with Epstein-Barr virus but is unusual with the other agents. On occasion, hepatitis may be associated with a distinctive erythematous papular eruption localized to the limbs (Gianotti disease).

Toxic hepatitis, unlike viral hepatitis, does not have a prolonged prodrome. Acute nausea, vomiting, and malaise are followed in 1 to 2 days by alterations in mental status and deterioration of liver function. Most patients with toxic hepatitis will have an identifiable exogenous precipitant. Children with fulminant hepatic failure typically experience anorexia, nausea, vomiting, malaise, and fatigue—all symptoms indistinguishable from those expected with viral hepatitis. The patient's jaundice becomes more profound, and vomiting becomes protracted. Hyperexcitability, mania, and subtle psychomotor abnormalities may be seen. Coagulopathy, ascites, and sudden decrease in liver size are often the prelude to the development of frank neuromuscular signs.

The objectives of the emergency physician are to render supportive care to those icteric patients with infectious and metabolic derangements and to identify those cases in which jaundice is caused by mechanical obstruction or hepatic failure. The impression based on a targeted history, physical examination, and clinical algorithms can be bolstered with the following laboratory examinations: complete blood count, platelet count, prothrombin time, total and direct bilirubin, transaminase, alkaline phosphatase, electrolytes, blood urea nitrogen, and creatinine. Urinalysis, culture, and toxicologic screen should be considered. Chest and abdominal radiographs are indicated when there are pulmonary parenchymal complaints or significant abdominal findings. Other laboratory tests that are often available immediately and that may provide useful information in specific circumstances are serum ammonia, albumin, total protein, cholesterol, pH, and carbon dioxide. If available, abdominal sonography or computed tomography may occasionally be helpful. Results of several important blood and urine tests may not be of immediate use. Such studies, which are appropriate, include serum for bile acids, ceruloplasmin, protein electrophoretic pattern, serologic evidence of recent infection (e.g., Epstein-Barr virus, mycoplasmal or hepatitis profiles), polymerase chain reaction assays, and enzyme-linked immunosorbent assay and autoantibody test. Urinary analysis includes assessment of organic acids and copper. These investigations may be helpful, however, to the longitudinal caretaker who must maintain a vigilant watch over the jaundiced patient.

Children more than 8 weeks old with conjugated hyperbilirubinemia should be admitted to the hospital at the time of their presentation in all cases in which life-threatening conditions may exist (Table 35.3). Inpatient treatment also is suggested when intravenous fluids are necessary to treat symptomatic hypoglycemia or electrolyte imbalance and when operative intervention may prove necessary. Icteric patients who have been diagnosed previously with confidence and who have exacerbation of their symptoms may require admission to reappraise their status. The physician also may be influenced to admit the patient when poor parenting or geographic barriers inhibit consistent observations. Admission also is indicated for patients who require further diagnostic intervention, such as liver biopsy or scintigraphy, to arrive at a definitive diagnosis.

CHAPTER 36
Limp

Susanne Kost, M.D.

Limping is a common complaint in the pediatric acute-care setting. A *limp* is defined as an alteration in the normal walking pattern for the child's age. The causes of limping are numerous, ranging from trivial to life threatening, but most children who limp do so as a result of pain, weakness, or deformity. The evaluation of a child with a limp demands a thorough history and physical examination, using an age-based approach.

DIFFERENTIAL DIAGNOSIS

The extensive differential diagnosis of the child with a limp may be approached from several angles: by disease category, location of pathology, or age of the child. Table 36.1 presents the differential diagnosis by disease category; Table 36.2 organizes the differential diagnosis by age and location of pathology. The most common causes of limp are outlined in Table 36.3, and potentially life- or limb-threatening conditions are listed in Table 36.4. This section reviews the differential diagnosis within the framework of an algorithmic approach (Fig. 36.1).

The most common cause of limping in all ages is trauma, either acute or repetitive microtrauma (stress fractures). Older children who limp as a result of trauma can generally describe the mechanism of injury and localize pain well. The toddler and preschool-age groups, with their limited verbal ability and cooperation skills, often provide a diagnostic challenge. A common type of injury in this population (often not witnessed) is the aptly named "toddler's fracture," a nondisplaced spiral fracture of the tibial shaft that occurs as a result of torsion of the foot relative to the tibia. Occult fractures of the bones in the foot also occur in young children. Initial plain radiographic findings may be subtle, or at times nonexistent, but will become apparent in 1 to 2 weeks. Bone scans will identify these lesions sooner. Another fracture often lacking initial radiographic confirmation is a Salter-Harris type I fracture, which presents as tenderness over a physis after trauma to a joint area. Stress fractures may also lack overt radiographic findings. Common sites for overuse injury include the tibial tubercle (Osgood-Schlatter disease), the anterior tibia ("shin splints"), and the calcaneus at the insertion of the Achilles tendon (Sever disease). More information on the subject of fractures is found in Chapter 101.

TABLE 36.1. Differential Diagnosis of Limp by Disease Category

Trauma or overuse	*Congenital*
Fracture	Vertical talus
Stress fracture	Tarsal coalition
Soft-tissue injury	Other congenital limb abnormalities
Spondylolisthesis	Spinal dysraphism
Herniated nucleus pulposus	Inguinal hernia
Infectious	*Neurologic*
Septic arthritis	Muscular dystrophy
Osteomyelitis	Peripheral neuropathy
Lyme arthritis	Reflex sympathetic dystrophy
Discitis	*Neoplasia*
Pelvic inflammatory disease	Benign bone tumors
Inflammatory	Malignant bone tumors
Transient synovitis	Leukemia
Reactive arthritis	Intraabdominal tumors
Rheumatic disease	Sacral tumors
Appendicitis	Spinal cord tumors
Developmental or acquired	*Metabolic*
Developmental dysplasia of the hip	Rickets
Blount disease	Hyperparathyroidism
Limb length discrepancy	*Hematologic*
Torsional deformities	Sickle cell disease
Avascular necrosis	Hemophilia
Slipped capital femoral epiphysis	
Testicular torsion	

Trauma may also induce limping as a result of soft-tissue injury. Joint swelling and pain out of proportion to the history of injury raises the possibility of a hemarthrosis as the initial presentation of a bleeding disorder (see Chapter 77). Severe soft-tissue pain and swelling in the setting of a contusion or crush injury suggests compartment syndrome. With compartment syndrome, pain is exacerbated by passive extension of the affected part; pallor and pulselessness are late findings. Severe pain of an entire limb out of proportion to the history of injury suggests reflex sympathetic dystrophy (RSD). RSD is most common in young adolescent girls. It may be accompanied by mottling and coolness of the extremity, presumably as a result of abnormalities in the peripheral sympathetic nervous system.

A limp that is accompanied by a history of fever or recent systemic illness is likely to be infectious or inflammatory in origin. However, the absence of fever does not preclude the possibility of a bacterial bone or joint infection, and many infections are preceded by a history of minor trauma. Septic arthritis is the most serious infectious cause of joint pain and limp. Exquisite pain with attempts to flex or extend the joint is characteristic of septic arthritis, and the degree of pain with motion serves as a helpful clinical sign in distinguishing bacterial joint infection from inflammatory conditions (see Chapters 74 and 108).

Rheumatic conditions that may result in limp are numerous; many are accompanied by systemic symptoms and characteristic skin rashes. Examples include Lyme disease, Henoch-Schönlein purpura, erythema multiforme, acute rheumatic fever, juvenile rheumatoid arthritis, and systemic lupus erythematosus. Occasionally, limping from arthralgia will precede the development of the arthritis and systemic involvement. An approach to the child with joint pain is found in Chapter 49.

In the absence of obvious trauma, fever, or systemic symptoms, the next step in the approach to the differential diagnosis of a limp is to determine the locality of the findings and the degree of pain. Localized pain suggests repetitive microtrauma, bone tumor, or an acquired skeletal deformity. Repetitive microtrauma may be responsible for avascular necrosis of the foot bones in two locations: the tarsal navicular bone (Kohler disease) in younger children and the metatarsal heads (Freiberg disease) in adolescents. Both benign and malignant bone tumors may present with a painful limp. Benign lesions include bone cysts (unicameral or aneurysmal), fibrous dysplasia, and eosinophilic granulomas. Osteoid osteoma, caused by a painful nidus of vascular osteoid tissue, is another benign lesion unique to young people. The most common malignant pediatric bone tumors are osteogenic sarcoma and Ewing sarcoma. Bone tumor pain may be acute or chronic, with acute pain usually related to a pathologic fracture. Examples of acquired skeletal abnormalities causing painful limp include tarsal coalition and osteochondritis dissecans. Tarsal coalition occurs as a result of gradual calcification of a congenital cartilaginous bar between tarsal bones;

TABLE 36.2. Differential Diagnosis of Limp by Age and Location of Pathology

	Long bone	Skin/soft tissue	Any joint	Hip	Knee	Ankle/foot	Spine
Toddler	Fracture Toddler's Salter type I Periostitis Osteomyelitis Vasoocclusive crisis Congenital anomaly	Contusion Strain Foreign body Immunization Infection	Septic arthritis Reactive arthritis Rheumatic disease Systemic JRA Hemarthrosis	Transient synovitis DDH	Occult trauma Blount disease Referred hip pain	Poor shoe fit Occult trauma Vertical talus Kohler disease	Dysraphism Infection Tumor
School age	Fracture Salter type I Discrepant limb length Osteomyelitis Tumor Vasoocclusive crisis	Contusion Strain Myositis Growing pains Infection	Sprain Reactive arthritis Rheumatic disease EM, HSP, ARF Septic arthritis Lyme arthritis	Transient synovitis AVN	Baker's cyst Referred hip pain	Poor shoe fit Salter type I fracture Tarsal coalition Kohler disease	Dysraphism Infection Tumor
Adolescent	Fracture Tumor Osteomyelitis	Contusion Strain Tendonitis RSD	Sprain Reactive arthritis Rheumatic disease IBD, SLE Septic arthritis Gonococcal Lyme arthritis	SCFE	Osgood-Schlatter disease Osteochondritis dissecans Chondromalacia Baker's cyst Referred hip pain	Poor shoe fit Salter type I fracture Bunion Freiberg disease Sever disease	Scoliosis Spondylolisthesis Herniated disc Infection Tumor

JRA, juvenile rheumatoid arthritis; DDH, developmental dysplasia of the hip; EM, erythema multiforme; HSP, Henoch-Schönlein purpura; ARF, acute rheumatic fever; AVN, avascular necrosis; RSD, reflex sympathetic dystrophy; IBD, inflammatory bowel disease; SLE, systemic lupus erythematosus; SCFE, slipped capital femoral epiphysis.

it presents most commonly as a painful flatfoot in school-aged children. Osteochondritis dissecans is related to separation of articular cartilage from underlying bone; it most commonly affects the knees of adolescent boys.

Localized findings without pain suggest congenital or slowly developing acquired limb abnormalities. Three disorders of the hip fit into this category, each of which is characteristic of a specific age group. Developmental dysplasia of the hip (DDH) includes a spectrum of abnormalities ranging from mild dysplasia to frank dislocation. Most affected children with access to primary care are diagnosed with abnormal hip abduction on routine examination in infancy. Occasionally, the diagnosis will be missed, and the child then presents at the onset of walking with a painless short-leg limp, or waddling gait if bilateral, with weakness of the abductor musculature. Legg-Calvé-Perthes (LCP) disease, an avascular necrosis of the capital femoral epiphysis, presents in young school-aged children as an insidious limp with mild, activity-related pain. Slipped capital femoral epiphysis (SCFE) presents in young, typically obese, adolescents with an externally rotated limp. The amount of pain experienced is related to the rate of displacement of the epiphysis, ranging from none to severe. LCP and SCFE are more common in boys. Other acquired skeletal deformities that may cause painless limp include limb length inequality, Blount disease (with marked bowing of the proximal tibias), and torsional deformities. Baker's cyst of the popliteal tendon may cause limping with minimal local discomfort.

Limping in the absence of localized limb findings suggests a systemic (or nonlimb) source such as the spine or abdomen. A painful limp without localization or with migratory bone pain suggests a hematologic or oncologic cause such as sickle cell disease or leukemia. Limping with bilateral leg pain localized to the muscles, especially the calves, suggests myositis. Benign acute childhood myositis is common during influenza epidemics. Recurrent diffuse aches after periods of vigorous activity, usually worse at night, suggest benign hypermobility syndrome or "growing pains." A painless, poorly localized limp may occur with metabolic bone disease (e.g., rickets). Spinal problems that can cause leg pain, weakness, or limp include dysraphism, vertebral infection, spondylolisthesis, and herniated disc. Spinal dysraphism refers to a spectrum of abnormalities in the development of the spinal cord and vertebrae ranging from obvious (myelomeningocele) to occult (tethered cord). Associated neurologic and musculoskeletal

TABLE 36.3. Common Causes of Limp

Trauma Fracture Soft-tissue injury Overuse injuries *Transient synovitis* *Infection* Septic arthritis Osteomyelitis	*Rheumatic Disease* *Other Hip Disorders* Developmental dysplasia Legg-Calvé-Perthes disease Slipped capital femoral epiphysis

TABLE 36.4. Life- or Limb-Threatening Causes of Limp

Septic arthritis Osteomyelitis Tumor Developmental dysplasia of the hip	Slipped capital femoral epiphysis Epidural abscess Appendicitis

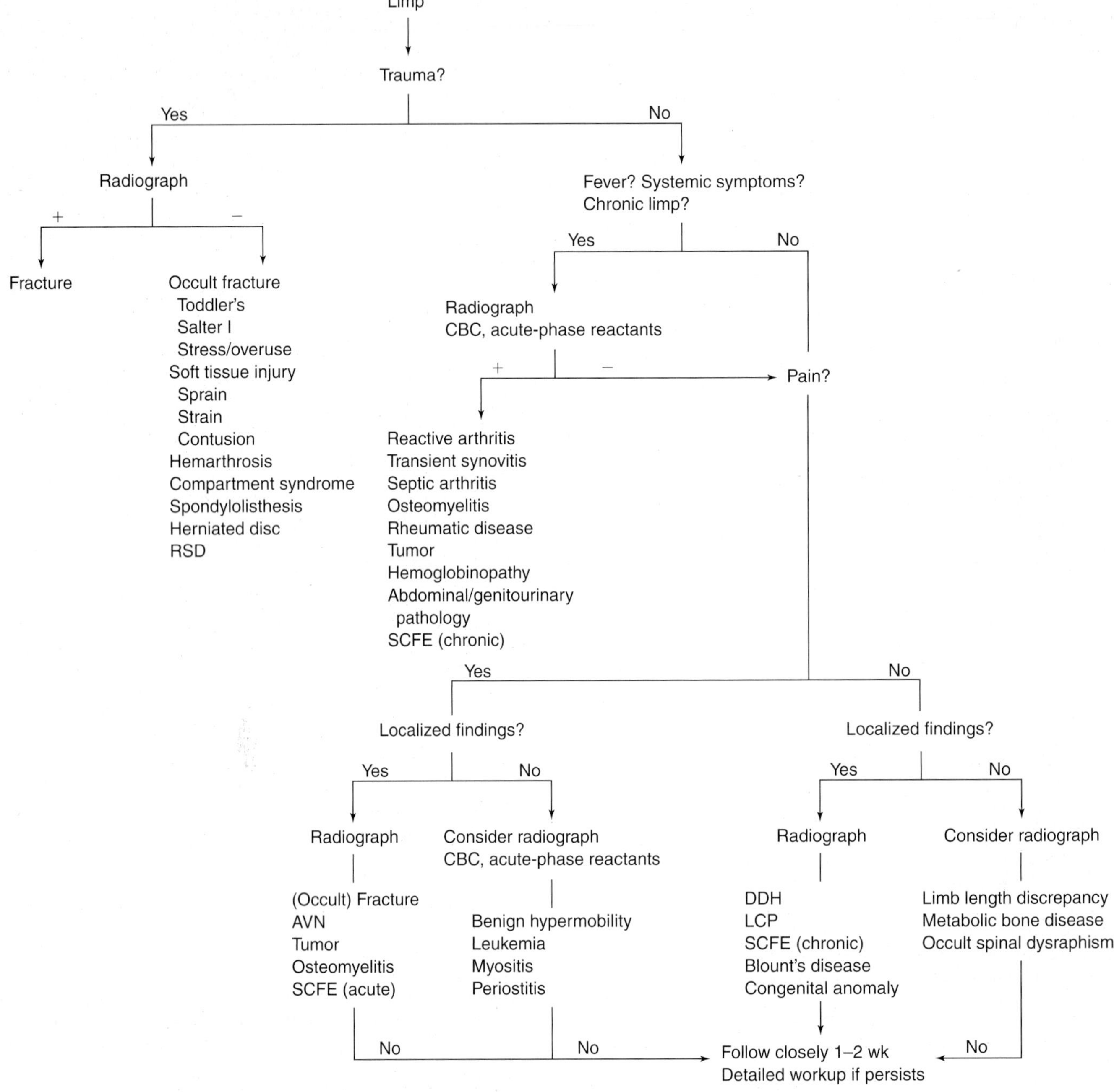

Figure 36.1. Algorithmic approach to the child with a limp. *RSD,* reflex sympathetic dystrophy; *CBC,* complete blood count; *SCFE,* slipped capital femoral epiphysis; *AVN,* avascular necrosis; *DDH,* developmental dysplasia of the hip; *LCP,* Legg-Calvé-Perthes disease.

findings, including pain, atrophy, high arches, and tight heel cords, may develop in early childhood. Vertebral infection typically presents with fever and back pain. Spondylolisthesis and herniated disc are rare in young children but may be seen in adolescents who complain of back pain or radicular pain. Intraabdominal pathology that can result in limp includes appendicitis, pelvic or psoas abscess, and renal disease. Solid tumors, most commonly neuroblastoma, can cause limp through retroperitoneal irritation or extension into the spinal canal. Likewise, a sacral teratoma may affect the nerves of the cauda equina or sacral plexus. Testicular pain may present with limping in a boy who is reluctant or embarrassed to admit the true source of his discomfort.

EVALUATION AND DECISION

Evaluation and decision are presented in Fig. 36.1.

History

A history of trauma should be addressed, keeping in mind the inherent difficulty in obtaining an accurate trauma history in very young children. Conversely, obvious trauma in the absence of a consistent history raises the question of inflicted injury. In more chronic presentations, any cyclical or recurrent patterns should be noted. Stiffness and limp primarily in the morning suggest rheumatic disease, whereas evening symptoms suggest weakness or overuse injury.

Physical Examination

The physical examination in a limping child should begin with observation of the child's gait, along with a complete examination with attention to the musculoskeletal and neurologic systems. The musculoskeletal examination begins with inspection of the limbs and feet for swelling or deformity. The spine should be inspected for curvature, both standing and bending forward, and the soles of feet and toes should be checked for foreign bodies and calluses. The bones, muscles, and joints should be palpated for areas of tenderness; range of motion of all joints should be checked; and limb lengths (from anterior superior iliac spine to medial malleolus) and thigh and calf circumference should be measured for asymmetry. The neurologic examination should include inspection of the spine for lumbosacral hair or dimple (indicating possible spinal dysraphism), and testing of strength, sensation, and reflexes. The abdomen and external genitalia should be examined for tenderness or masses, and the skin for rashes. A rectal examination may be indicated if sacral pathology is suspected. Finally, wear patterns on the child's shoes may provide clues to the nature and duration of the limp.

Laboratory and Imaging

Plain radiographs remain a mainstay of the workup of a limping child. They provide an excellent means of screening for fracture, effusion, lytic lesions, periosteal reaction, and avascular necrosis. In a child with an obvious focus of pain, the radiographs may be obtained with views specific to that area, noting that children with knee pain may have hip pathology. In a young child or a child lacking obvious focus for the limp, anteroposterior (AP) and lateral views of both lower extremities (including the feet) should be ordered as an initial screen. In toddlers lacking a focus of pain and in older children in whom hip pathology is suspected, AP and frog-leg lateral views of the pelvis are required. Radiographs of the spine are necessary if the child has neurologic signs or symptoms.

In children whose limp is associated with fever or systemic illness, laboratory studies, including a complete blood count (CBC) and an erythrocyte sedimentation rate (ESR), are indicated. In some institutions, a C-reactive protein (CRP) is obtained as a sensitive acute-phase reactant. These studies serve as screens for infection, inflammation, malignancy, and hemoglobinopathy. Laboratory studies are also indicated in the absence of fever if the child has been limping for several days without evidence of trauma on plain films. Children with evidence of infection or inflammation with a joint effusion may require arthrocentesis for definitive diagnosis. In areas of endemic Lyme disease, a Lyme titer is a reasonable initial screening test in a patient with arthritis. A creatine phosphokinase (CPK) level may be helpful if muscle inflammation is suspected.

When the initial history, physical examination, imaging, and laboratory evaluation indicate the cause of the limp, specific treatment can be initiated. Abnormalities in the initial workup without a definitive diagnosis should prompt further imaging or laboratory studies. Bone scintigraphy is more sensitive than plain radiographs for occult fracture, infection, avascular necrosis, and tumor; however, it is not specific for a given pathologic process. Computed tomography (CT) is an excellent imaging modality for cortical bone; it serves as a useful diagnostic adjunct in certain fractures, bony coalitions, and bone tumors. Ultrasound (US) is the preferred modality for diagnosing hip effusions; it is also useful for guiding needle aspirations of the hip joint. Magnetic resonance imaging (MRI) is useful in imaging the spinal cord, avascular necrosis, and bone marrow disease.

If the initial workup in a limping child is completely normal, including screening radiographs and laboratory studies, the child may be followed closely as an outpatient. These children should be examined every few days until improvement is noted or a cause is determined. If the limp persists beyond 1 to 2 weeks without a diagnosis, further workup or consultation with a specialist is indicated.

CHAPTER 37
Lymphadenopathy

Richard Malley, M.D.

Lymphadenopathy is defined as swelling of the lymph nodes. Because the differential diagnosis of lymphadenopathy is extensive, it is helpful to distinguish localized from generalized lymphadenopathy. *Localized, or regional, adenopathy* generally occurs in response to a focal infectious process, although rarely other causes may need to be considered. *Generalized lymphadenopathy* is defined as enlargement of more than two noncontiguous lymph node regions. The most common causes of generalized adenopathy are systemic infections (bacterial or viral), autoimmune diseases, and neoplastic processes.

DIFFERENTIAL DIAGNOSIS

Acute Regional Adenopathy

The clinician caring for a child with acute regional adenopathy will benefit from knowledge of the anatomic distribution of nodes in the area and their drainage areas, as described in Table 37.1. The location of lymphadenopathy is often suggestive of a possible cause. For instance, in the head and neck region, swollen nodes are often a response to focal infectious processes occurring in areas that drain in the region of the nodes. Occipital nodes most commonly enlarge in response to bacterial or fungal scalp infections or to chronic inflammation such as occurs in seborrheic dermatitis. Because preauricular nodes drain the conjunctiva and lateral eyelids, these often enlarge in viral conjunctivitis. Epidemic keratoconjunctivitis caused by adenoviruses often presents with an enlarged preauricular node. Similarly, the presence of submaxillary and submental nodes points to the possibility of an infectious process in the oral cavity.

The differential diagnosis of cervical adenopathy is more extensive, mainly because the anatomy of the region is more complex. As can be seen in Table 37.1, nodes in the cervical region can be divided into three areas: the superior deep nodes below the angle of the mandible, the superficial cervical nodes found anteriorly and posteriorly along the sternocleidomastoid muscle, and the inferior deep nodes at the base of the neck. Enlargement of superior deep or superficial nodes raises the possibility of a lingual, external ear, or parotid gland process. In contrast, the inferior deep nodes have a much wider drainage area, including the head and neck, upper extremities, and the thoracic and abdominal regions. Swelling of these nodes, in particular scalene and supraclavicular nodes, can be the first sign of occult thoracic or abdominal pathology, such as malignancy. Therefore, nodes found in these regions must be investigated

TABLE 37.1. Regional Adenopathy

Site	Drainage area	Common causes	Less common causes
Occipital	Posterior scalp/neck	Tinea, seborrhea pediculosis	Rubella
Preauricular	Conjunctiva Lateral eyelids Temporal skin	Viral conjunctivitis *Chlamydia* conjunctivitis	Pannaud syndrome of cat-scratch disease Trachoma Tularemia
Submaxillary	Lip, gums, teeth, buccal mucosa	Chronically cracked lips, dental caries/infection, herpetic gingivostomatitis	
Submental			*Acute less common* Kawasaki syndrome
Cervical Superior (deep) Superficial Anterior Posterior Inferior (deep) Scalene Supraclavicular	Tongue External ear Parotid gland Entire head/neck Larynx, trachea Thyroid gland Arms/superficial thorax Lungs/mediastinum Abdomen	*Acute common* Viral upper respiratory infection Bacterial infection head/neck Primary bacterial adenitis Epstein-Barr virus *Chronic common* Cat-scratch disease Atypical mycobacterium Mycobacterium tuberculosis	*Chronic less common* Anaerobic infection Epstein-Barr virus Cytomegalovirus Toxoplasmosis Tularemia Histoplasmosis Leptospirosis Brucellosis Sarcoid Sinus histiocytosis Hodgkin disease Non-Hodgkin lymphoma Lymphosarcoma Rhabdomyosarcoma
Axillary	Upper extremity Chest wall Upper lateral abdominal wall Breast	Upper extremity inflammation Cat-scratch disease	Rheumatologic disesae hand/wrist Rat-bite fever Toxoplasmosis
Epitrochlear	Ulnar side hand/forearm	Chronically inflamed hand Local infection	Secondary syphilis Rheumatologic disease hand/wrist Tularemia Cat-scratch disease
Inguinal	Scrotum/penis Vulva/vaginal mucosa Skin/lower abdomen Perineum/gluteal region Lower anal canal Lower extremities	Lower extremity inflammation Genital herpes Primary syphilis	Chancroid Lymphogranuloma-venereum
Iliac Palpable deeply over inguinal ligament	Lower extremities Abdominal viscera Urinary tract	Lower extremity inflammation Trauma Appendicitis Urinary tract infection	
Popliteal	Knee joint Skin of lower leg/foot	Severe local infection	

carefully, with thorough physical examinations and, if necessary, radiographic examinations.

By far, the most common cause of acute cervical adenopathy is a viral upper respiratory tract infection. In these cases, lymph nodes are generally symmetrically enlarged and are soft and minimally tender, if tender at all. Bacterial cervical adenitis is also a common cause of cervical lymphadenopathy in children, particularly in preschool-age children. It is usually caused by group A β-hemolytic *Streptococcus* or *Staphylococcus aureus*, although anaerobes (usually penicillin-sensitive) may also be involved, particularly in oral infections. If left untreated, these nodes may become erythematous and eventually fluctuant (see Chapter 74).

Epstein-Barr virus (EBV), the agent of infectious mononucleosis, commonly causes posterior cervical lymphadenopathy in older children and adolescents. The classic presentation of a child with EBV. The diagnosis is made most easily with the detection of a positive heterophile agglutinating antibody (monospot), although it is important to remember that this test may be falsely negative in children under the age of 7 years.

A rarer, but important, cause of acute cervical lymphadenopathy is Kawasaki disease, a systemic febrile syndrome of as yet undefined cause. Kawasaki disease, also called mucocutaneous lymph node syndrome, occurs most often in children less than 4 years of age and is rare after 8 years of age. The presence of a large node in the cervical area, in association with fever of greater than 5 days' duration, bilateral conjunctival injection with limbal sparing, mucous membrane involvement, peripheral edema or erythema, and a polymorphous truncal rash, should alert the physician to the possibility of this disorder.

Axillary adenopathy is commonly present with any infection or inflammation of the upper extremities. Most commonly, injuries to the hand, such as occur after falling or with puncture wounds or bites, may present with concomitant axillary adenopathy. Similarly, epitrochlear nodes, which are not normally palpable in children, may become inflamed after infections of the third, fourth, or fifth finger; medial portion of the hand; or ulnar portion of the forearm.

Inguinal adenopathy most often results from lower extremity infection, although sexually transmitted diseases may also be responsible. For example, acute genital infection with herpes simplex virus (HSV)-2 often presents with tender inguinal adenopathy, occasionally as the only sign. Similarly, chancroid, lymphogranuloma venereum, and syphilis may present with inguinal nodal swelling and tenderness. Enlarged iliac nodes are palpable deeply over the inguinal ligament and become inflamed with lower extremity infection, urinary tract infection, abdominal trauma, and appendicitis. Of note, iliac adenitis, which can present with fever, limp, and inability to fully extend the leg, may mimic the signs and symptoms of septic hip arthritis. Iliac adenitis may also be confused with appendicitis, but the pain initially occurs in the thigh and hip rather than in the periumbilical region or right lower quadrant.

Chronic Regional Adenopathy

Organisms such as *Bartonella* (the etiologic agent of cat-scratch disease), mycobacteria, and atypical mycobacteria are most commonly responsible for chronic adenopathy. Cat-scratch disease, caused by *Bartonella henselae*, is a relatively common cause of chronic axillary or cervical adenopathy (see Chapter 74). Tuberculous cervical lymphadenitis, otherwise known as scrofula, most commonly involves the posterior cervical nodes. Atypical mycobacterial adenitis usually involves young children, less than 5 years of age, and is generally unilateral. The node is rarely more than 3 cm in size. Overlying skin may turn a deep purple and gradually thins, developing a parchment-paper appearance. Fluctuation and ulceration occur commonly. Infected patients generally appear well, with a notable absence of any systemic symptoms.

Other less common causes of chronic adenopathy deserve mention. A prolonged heterophile-negative adenopathy unresponsive to a trial of antibiotics should raise suspicion for one of these possibilities. Cytomegalovirus (CMV) infection, which is characterized by cervical adenopathy, pharyngitis, and atypical lymphocytosis, may cause prolonged adenopathy in younger children. Toxoplasmosis typically presents as a single, nontender posterior cervical node. Brucellosis, associated generally with axillary and cervical lymphadenopathy, and tularemia with cervical adenopathy, are rare infectious causes of chronic adenopathy in children.

Noninfectious etiologies may also cause chronic regional adenopathy. Various malignancies, such as Hodgkin disease, lymphosarcoma, neuroblastoma, and rhabdomyosarcoma, may all present with chronic cervical lymphadenopathy (see Chapter 89). For example, Hodgkin disease usually presents as a slowly growing, painless firm node in the upper third of the neck. Lymphosarcoma also presents as a firm painless node, but it occurs in younger children than those with Hodgkin disease and more commonly involves extranodal sites such as tonsils. Rhabdomyosarcoma, the most common solid tumor of the head and neck in children, often involves the nasopharynx, middle ear, mastoid, or orbit, but it can also occur as a painless mass anywhere in the head and neck.

Particularly in African-American children, sarcoidosis must be entertained with bilateral chronic cervical adenopathy. Scalene nodes are involved in more than 80% of cases. An abnormal chest film, with hilar adenopathy and peribronchial fibrosis, suggests sarcoidosis. Sinus histiocytosis, a benign form of histiocytosis, can present as a large painless cervical adenopathy. The clinical presentation often includes fever, anemia, leukocytosis, and elevated erythrocyte sedimentation rate.

Generalized Lymphadenopathy

Various systemic illnesses are associated with generalized lymphadenopathy (Table 37.2). The most common causes of generalized lymphadenopathy include bacterial or viral illnesses that disseminate systemically. As an example, the high incidence of vomiting and abdominal pain in streptococcal pharyngitis has been attributed to abdominal node inflammation and swelling, suggesting a more systemic pattern of adenopathy in streptococcal disease. Rarer bacterial causes of generalized lymphadenopathy include bacterial illnesses such as brucellosis and leptospirosis, diagnoses that may be suggested by occupational or dietary history. Common viral causes of generalized adenopathy include EBV or CMV mononucleosis, rubella, and measles in parts of the world where the disease is endemic. Another cause of generalized adenopathy includes human immunodeficiency virus (HIV) infection. HIV infection in children can present with persistent generalized adenopathy, hepatosplenomegaly, and failure to thrive. Generalized lymphadenopathy may occasionally be the only presenting symptom in a child with vertical HIV infection.

Noninfectious systemic disease may also present with generalized adenopathy. Approximately 70% of patients with systemic lupus erythematosus (SLE) or juvenile rheumatoid arthritis (JRA) manifest generalized adenopathy during the acute

TABLE 37.2. Generalized Adenopathy

Systemic infection	*Autoimmune disease*
Bacterial	Juvenile rheumatoid arthritis
Bacteremia	Systemic lupus erythematosus
Scarlet fever	Serum sickness
Subacute bacterial endocarditis	Autoimmune hemolytic anemia
Syphilis	*Primary lymphoid neoplasm*
Tuberculosis	Hodgkin disease
Brucellosis	Non-Hodgkin lymphoma
Viral	*Metastatic neoplasm*
Varicella	Acute lymphocytic leukemia
Rubella	Acute myelogenous leukemia
Rubeola	Neuroblastoma
Epstein-Barr virus	*Histiocytosis*
Cytomegalovirus	Letterer-Siwe
Human immunodeficiency virus	Histiocytic medullary reticulosis
Fungal	*Storage disease*
Histoplasmosis	Gaucher disease
Coccidioidomycosis	Niemann-Pick disease
Parasitic	*Drugs*
Toxoplasmosis	Phenytoin
Malaria	Isoniazid
	Miscellaneous
	Hyperthyroidism

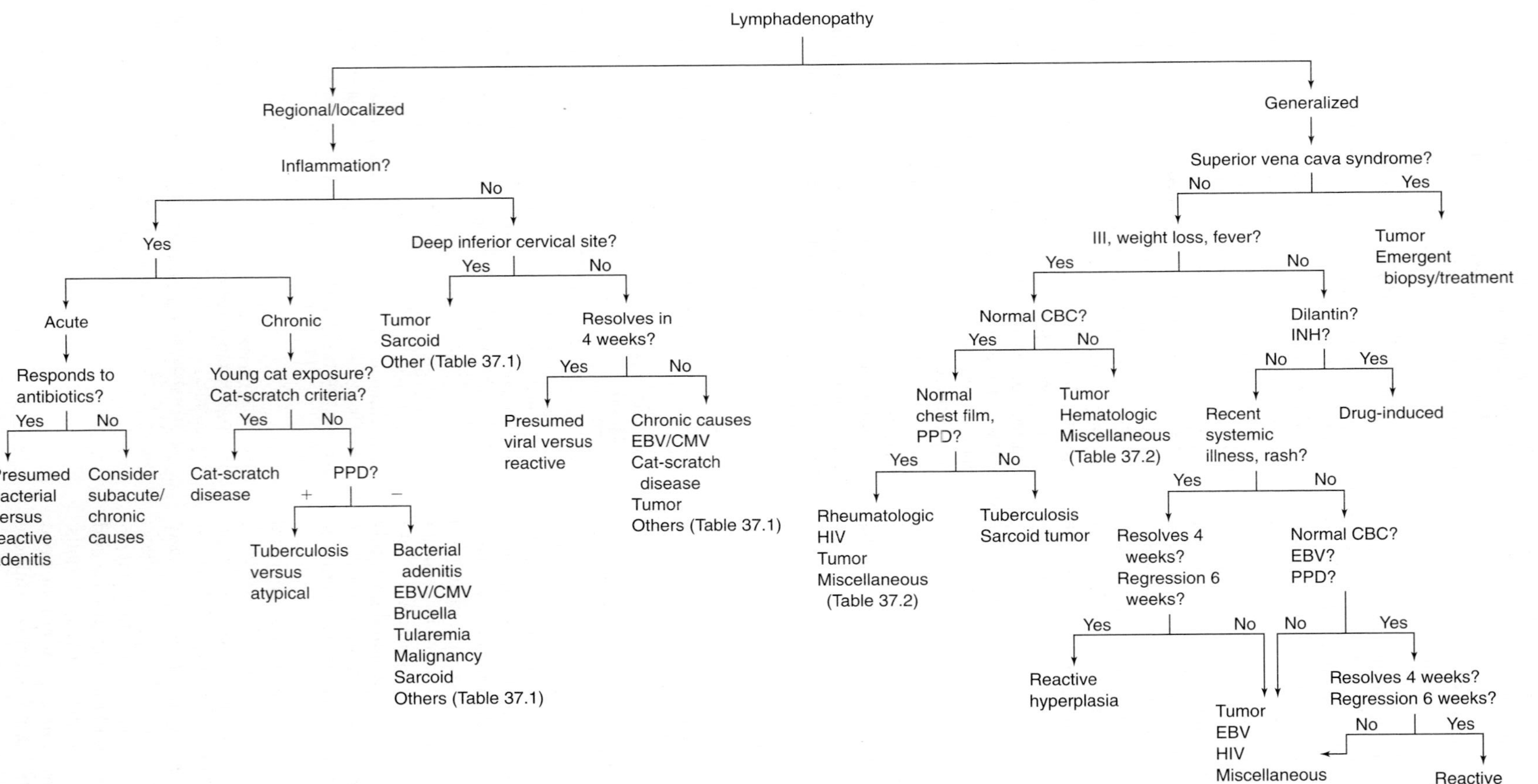

Figure 37.1. The diagnostic approach to the child with lymphadenopathy. *PPD,* purified protein derivative; *EBV,* Epstein-Barr virus; *CMV,* cytomegalovirus; *CBC,* complete blood count; *HIV,* human immunodeficiency virus.

phase of illness. The lymphadenopathy of serum sickness often occurs in the presence of the exanthem but may be seen without rash.

Neoplastic disease that causes generalized adenopathy may be primary to the lymph node as in Hodgkin and non-Hodgkin lymphoma, or it may be metastatic to the node with invasion of the node by extrinsic malignant cells as in leukemia or neuroblastoma (see Chapter 89). Hodgkin disease, as discussed previously under "Chronic Regional Adenopathy," usually manifests as cervical adenopathy. In contrast, non-Hodgkin lymphoma may present with rapidly enlarging, diffuse adenopathy, often accompanied by abdominal pain, vomiting, and diarrhea secondary to abdominal node involvement. Another neoplastic condition that can present with generalized adenopathy includes leukemia.

Histiocytosis presents as a spectrum of disease, ranging from a benign, isolated eosinophilic granuloma found in a long bone of an older child to the malignant multiorgan histiocytic infiltration found in infants with Letterer-Siwe disease (see Chapter 89). Lymphadenopathy often occurs in histiocytosis and can be an isolated finding; however, it usually occurs in association with other manifestations of disease.

Rarer causes of systemic adenopathy include lipid storage diseases (Gaucher disease and Niemann-Pick disease), which can cause diffuse adenopathy and are almost always associated with hepatosplenomegaly. Bone marrow biopsy, showing lipid-laden histiocytes, is diagnostic.

Certain drugs, most notably phenytoin (Dilantin), are associated with generalized adenopathy, appearing 1 to 2 weeks after drug initiation and disappearing 3 to 4 weeks after the drug is discontinued. This generalized adenopathy may or may not be associated with other systemic signs (hepatosplenomegaly, pruritic rash, fever, anemia, and leukopenia).

Finally, hyperthyroidism can be associated with a nonspecific lymph node hyperplasia, but one should see other signs and symptoms of the illness, such as tachycardia, hypertension, diaphoresis, weight loss, goiter, lid lag, and hyperreflexia, on physical examination.

Life-Threatening Lymphadenopathy

Several disorders associated with lymphadenopathy, primarily but not exclusively oncologic, can be life threatening (Table 37.3). The superior vena cava (SVC) syndrome is an example of life-threatening adenopathy. Superior mediastinal syndrome is a variant of SVC syndrome, with additional respiratory symptoms caused by trachea or bronchus compression.

EVALUATION AND DECISION

The approach to the patient with lymphadenopathy focuses initially on the history and examination findings, with emphasis on the distribution of enlarged nodes: regional or generalized (Fig. 37.1). Regional lymphadenopathy should be categorized as acute or subacute/chronic.

The most common causes of acute regional lymphadenopathy include reactive hyperplasia, acute bacterial adenitis, and EBV infection (infectious mononucleosis). Findings of acute inflammation, such as erythema and tenderness, point to bacterial adenitis (see Chapter 74).

The presence of systemic symptoms may suggest other causes of acute regional adenopathy. For example, the presence of pharyngitis, hepatosplenomegaly, and periorbital edema should suggest EBV infection. Several days of high fever, rash, and swelling of the extremities in the presence of a large node should alert the physician to the possibility of Kawasaki disease.

The evaluation of subacute or chronic regional adenopathy includes consideration of various infectious and noninfectious causes. Exposure to cats should alert the physician to the possibility of cat-scratch disease. The possibility of tuberculosis or atypical mycobacteria can be evaluated by placing a positive purified protein derivative (PPD) test on the patient or can be elicited by a history of exposure to a patient with active tuberculosis. Malignancies and chronic systemic disorders (sarcoid) are less common causes of subacute or chronic regional adenopathy. Either the location (e.g., supraclavicular) or persistence of the node points to a neoplastic disease or to another serious process.

The evaluation of generalized lymphadenopathy involves consideration of systemic diseases that may be associated with adenopathy. The presence of systemic signs of illness, such as weight loss and fever, may be seen in subacute bacterial endocarditis, HIV, tuberculosis, brucellosis, and syphilis. A recent, brief febrile illness, at times with a rash, is characteristic of EBV, tuberculosis, mononucleosis, or acute HIV infection. Signs of toxicity suggest less commonly encountered causes (tumors, collagen vascular disease, sarcoid). In the absence of toxicity, and particularly if the adenopathy begins to resolve within 4 weeks of presentation, the diagnosis of reactive hyperplasia is most likely.

TABLE 37.3. Life-Threatening Conditions Associated with Lymphadenopathy

Superior vena cava syndrome	Acute myelogenous leukemia
Hodgkin disease	Neuroblastoma
Non-Hodgkin lymphoma	Letterer-Siwe disease
Neuroblastoma	Coronary artery aneurysm
Bone marrow failure/multiorgan infiltration	Kawasaki disease
Acute lymphocytic leukemia	

CHAPTER 38
Neck Mass

Constance M. McAneney, M.D. and Richard M. Ruddy, M.D.

Neck masses include any visible swelling that disturbs the normal contour of the neck between the shoulder and the angle of the jaw. In the pediatric population, the four basic classifications of neck lesions are congenital, inflammatory, traumatic, and neoplastic. Congenital anatomic defects of the neck are often inapparent or minimally recognizable at birth but develop into significant cystic masses later. Included in this category are cystic hygromas, branchial cleft cysts, hemangiomas, thyroglossal duct cysts, and dermoids. Inflammatory masses are the most common and usually represent structures normally present, such as lymph nodes that are undergoing changes from the infectious causes. Traumatic neck masses are usually caused by hematoma surrounding vital structures and may lead to significant distress. Malignant lesions of the head and neck must be ruled out, but fortunately, they are fairly uncommon.

TABLE 38.1. Life-Threatening Causes of Neck Mass

Hematoma secondary to trauma
- Cervical spine injury
- Vascular compromise or acute bleeding
- Late arteriovenous fistula

Subcutaneous emphysema with associated airway or pulmonary injury
Local hypersensitivity reaction (sting/bite) with airway edema
Airway compromise with epiglottitis, tonsillar abscess, or infection of floor of mouth or retropharyngeal space (with adenopathy)
Bacteremia/sepsis associated with local infection of a cyst (cystic hygroma, thyroglossal, or branchial cleft cyst)
Non-Hodgkin lymphoma with mediastinal mass and airway compromise
Thyroid storm
Mucocutaneous lymph node syndrome with coronary vasculitis
Tumor—leukemia, lymphoma, rhabdomyosarcoma, histiocytosis X

True medical emergencies arise if neck masses compromise adjacent vital structures, including the airway, carotid blood vessels, and cervical spinal cord. In rare cases, the principal threat to life is from systemic toxicity. Infection that leads to septicemia or the effects of excess hormone secretion in thyroid storm can lead to uncompensated shock.

This chapter first emphasizes recognition of masses that represent true emergencies (Table 38.1). Then, the approach to nonemergent, but commonly seen, lesions is described (Table 38.2). Table 38.3 lists causes of neck masses of children by origin.

EVALUATION AND DECISION

The initial history and physical examination should screen rapidly for airway or vascular compromise with consideration of integrity of the cervical spine. The presence of stridor, hoarseness, dysphagia, and drooling indicates respiratory compromise. The quality of breathing, level of consciousness, and integrity of the cervical spine should also be assessed. Appropriate resuscitative measures should be taken if respiratory or vascular compromise is evident. The cervical spine should be immobilized if there is history of trauma or the initial evaluation leads to suspicion. Table 38.1 lists disorders that constitute true emergencies because of local pressure on vital structures or because of systemic toxicity.

Child with Neck Mass and Respiratory Distress or Systemic Toxicity

Trauma may cause bleeding or hematoma formation near vital structures such as the carotid artery or trachea. If the trauma involves the cervical spine, a hematoma may occur over fractured vertebrae. Symptomatic arteriovenous fistulas may appear weeks after neck trauma. The progression of a pneumomediastinum to pneumothorax can be rapid and requires close observation of the tachypneic child with a "crepitant" neck mass. Acutely, this may be caused by trauma to the chest and rib cage or by severe airway obstruction caused by asthma or a foreign body. In children with obstructive lung diseases, such as asthma and cystic fibrosis, high transpulmonary pressure generated in these diseases forces air through small alveolar leaks into the mediastinum or pleural space. This may produce a pneumomediastinum that dissects into the neck. Anaphylactic reaction with neck swelling may precipitate an acute emergency if the swelling compromises the airway. Severe, local reactions to bee stings or to other sensitizing allergens may cause enough tissue edema to obstruct the trachea.

Infections associated with life-threatening processes include retropharyngeal, lateral pharyngeal, and peritonsillar abscesses. Rarely, epiglottitis may present with associated cervical adenitis or the appearance of submandibular mass from ballooning of the hypopharynx. Occasionally, branchial cleft cysts or cystic hygromas become infected and progress to mediastinitis, or laryngoceles may become acutely infected and obstruct air flow.

TABLE 38.2. Common Causes of Neck Mass

Lymphadenopathy secondary to viral or bacterial infection
Cervical adenitis (bacterial)
Hematoma
Benign tumors—lipoma, keloid
Congenital cyst (squamous epithelial cysts)

TABLE 38.3. Differential Diagnosis of Neck Mass by Etiology

Congenital
- Squamous epithelial cyst (congenital or posttraumatic)
- Pilomatrixoma (Malherbe's calcifying epithelioma)
- Hemangioma and cystic hygroma (lymphangioma)
- Branchial cleft cyst
- Thyroglossal duct cyst
- Laryngocele
- Dermoid cyst
- Cervical rib

Inflammatory
- Infection
  - Cervical adenitis—streptococcal, staphylococcal, fungal, mycobacterial; cat-scratch disease, tularemia
  - Adenopathy—secondary to local head and neck infection
  - Secondary to systemic "infection"—infectious mononucleosis, cytomegalovirus, toxoplasmosis, others
  - Focal myositis—inflammatory muscular pseudotumor
- "Antigen"-mediated
  - Local hypersensitivity reaction (sting/bite)
  - Serum sickness, autoimmune disease
  - Pseudolymphoma (secondary to phenytoin)
  - Kawasaki disease
  - Sarcoidosis
  - Caffey-Silverman syndrome

Trauma
- Hematoma
  - Sternocleidomastoid tumor of infancy (fibromatosis colli)
  - Subcutaneous emphysema
  - Acute bleeding
  - Arteriovenous fistula
  - Foreign body
- Cervical spine fracture

Neoplasms
- Benign
  - Epidermoid
  - Lipoma, fibroma, neurofibroma
  - Keloid
  - Goiter (with or without thyroid hormone disturbance)
  - Osteochondroma
  - Teratoma (may be malignant)
  - "Normal" anatomy or variant
- Malignant
- Lymphoma—Hodgkin disease, non-Hodgkin lymphoma
- Leukemia
- Other—rhabdomyosarcoma, neuroblastoma, histiocytosis X, nasopharyngeal squamous cell carcinoma, thyroid or salivary gland tumor

Massive tonsillar hypertrophy with infectious mononucleosis or dental infection that spreads to the floor of the mouth (Ludwig angina) and neck may cause neck masses and airway compression. Children with human immunodeficiency virus (HIV) infection (see Chapter 75) may have parotitis or generalized lymphadenopathy, particularly visible in the neck as a presenting complaint. Hyperthyroid symptoms may accompany masses originating from the thyroid gland. Similarly, patients with the mucocutaneous lymph node syndrome often have cervical lymphadenopathy and, on rare occasions, have active life-threatening vasculitis of the coronary vessels.

Neck tumors in children may become large enough to encroach on vital structures. Cystic hygromas and hemangiomas occasionally enlarge sufficiently enough to interfere with feeding or to obstruct the airway. Lymphoma, an uncommon but important cause of neck mass, is suggested especially by painless enlargement (often of supraclavicular nodes) that occurs over several weeks in the older school-age child. When mediastinal nodes are involved, the patient may rapidly develop a blockage of the intrathoracic trachea that is accentuated on lying down. Other tumors, such as rhabdomyosarcoma, leukemia, neuroblastoma, and histiocytosis X, are life threatening because of local invasion and metabolic and hematologic effects.

Child with Neck Mass and No Distress

Most children in the emergency department with a neck mass are not in distress; the leading diagnoses are reactive adenopathy and acute lymphadenitis from viral or bacterial infection. A common concern, however, is which neck mass bears the diagnosis of malignancy and requires biopsy or further evaluation. Figure 38.1 describes a pathway to facilitate some of the differential diagnoses by category, and Figure 38.2 diagrams the locations of many of the causes of neck mass.

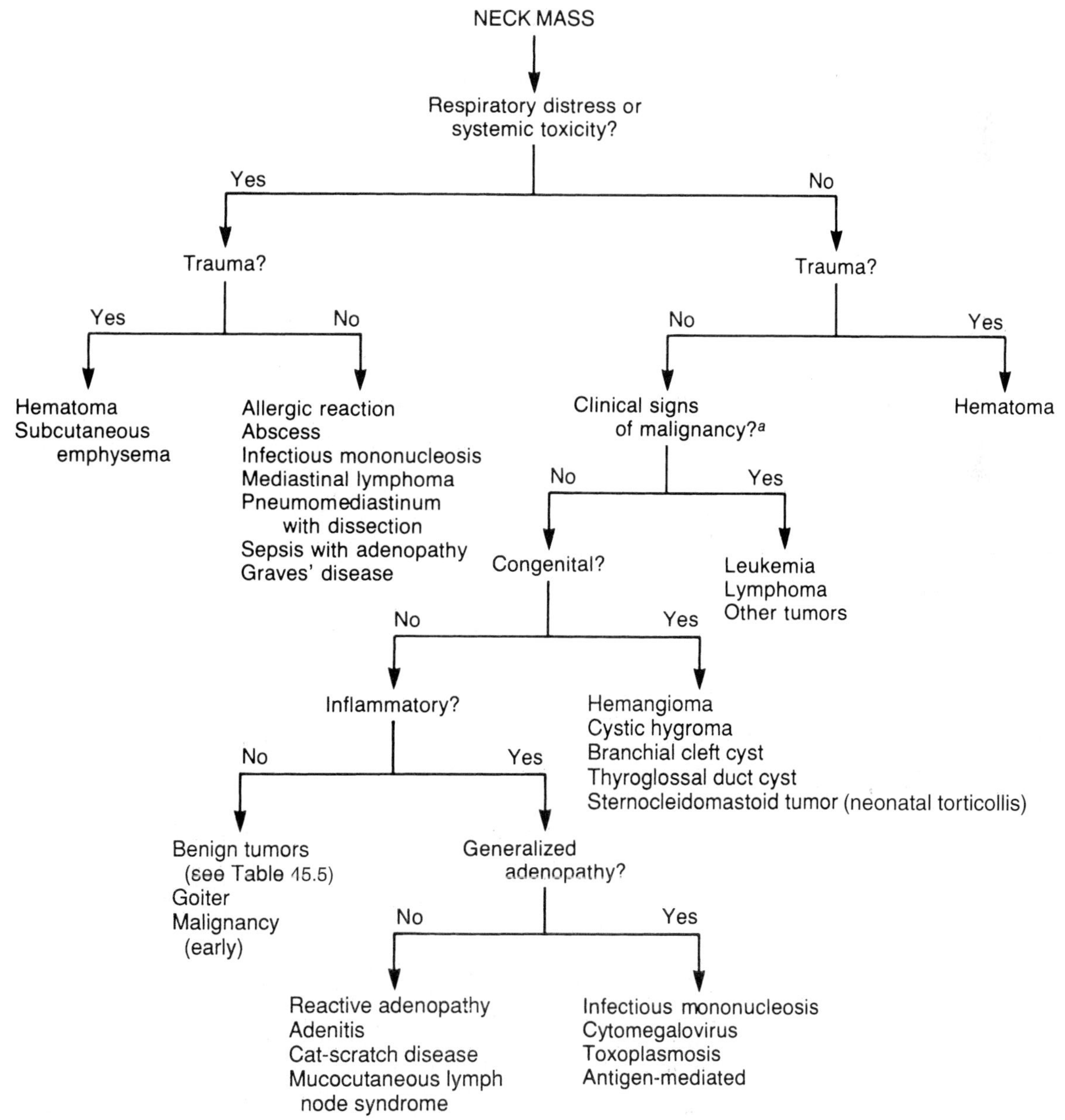

[a]Malignancy: nontender, >3-cm diameter (and firm), enlarging mass of several weeks' duration, ulceration, location deep to superficial fascia or fixed to tissue; supraclavicular mass; systemic lymphadenopathy and bruising; superior vena cava syndrome.

Figure 38.1. Evaluation of the child with a neck mass.

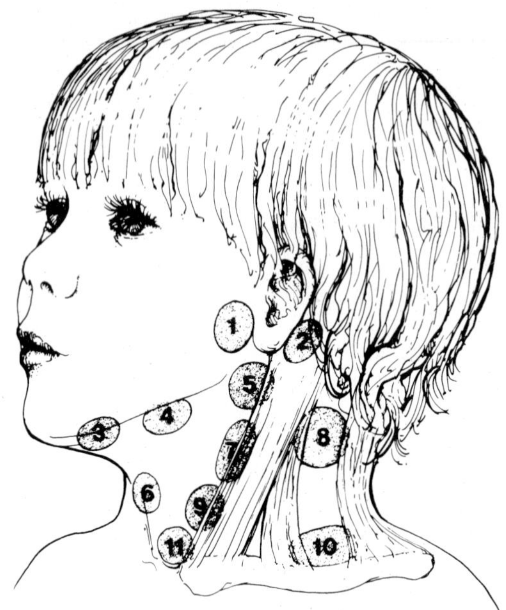

Figure 38.2. Differential diagnosis of neck mass by location.
Area 1. Parotid: Cystic hygroma, hemangioma, lymphadenitis, parotitis, Sjögren and Caffey-Silverman syndrome, lymphoma.
Area 2. Postauricular: Lymphadenitis, branchial cleft cyst (first), squamous epithelial cyst.
Area 3. Submental: Lymphadenitis, cystic hygroma, sialadenitis, tumor, cystic fibrosis.
Area 4. Submandibular: Lymphadenitis, cystic hygroma, sialadenitis, tumor, cystic fibrosis.
Area 5. Jugulodigastric: Lymphadenitis, squamous epithelial cyst, branchial cleft cyst (first), parotid tumor, *normal*—transverse process C2, styloid process.
Area 6. Midline neck: Lymphadenitis, thyroglossal duct cyst, dermoid, laryngocele, *normal*—hyoid, thyroid.
Area 7. Sternomastoid (anterior): Lymphadenitis, branchial cleft cyst (second, third), pilomatrixoma, rare tumors.
Area 8. Spinal accessory: Lymphadenitis, lymphoma, metastasis (from nasopharynx).
Area 9. Paratracheal: Thyroid, parathyroid, esophageal diverticulum.
Area 10. Supraclavicular: Cystic hygroma, lipoma, lymphoma, metastasis, *normal*—fat pad, pneumatocele of upper lobe.
Area 11. Suprasternal: Thyroid, lipoma, dermoid, thymus, mediastinal mass.
(Modified with permission from May M. Neck masses in children: diagnosis and treatment. *Clin Pediatr* 1976;5:17.)

Details of chronicity, size, and progression and evidence of inflammation help distinguish between infection and neoplasm. Characteristics that some authors have found associated with malignancy include masses that are firm and larger than 3 cm in diameter, nonpainful, progressively enlarging, ulcerating, deep to fascia or fixed to tissue, or discovered in a newborn. These criteria are sensitive but not specific for cancer. Even with these characteristics, most lesions are benign congenital cysts or inflammatory masses. The length of time the "node" is present is not discriminating in that, often, inflammatory nodes that are biopsied have been present for longer than 3 to 6 months. The general appearance and color of the child is important, as is the presence of hepatosplenomegaly or an abdominal mass, indicating a high suspicion for a malignancy.

Congenital Masses

Thyroglossal duct cysts are the most common congenital cyst of the neck. They develop in the midline along the line of descent of the thyroid gland in the neck anywhere from the base of the tongue to the sternal notch. *Cystic hygromas* are cystic lymphatic malformations occurring in the posterior triangle of the neck. Most are identified at birth, but some may be recognized after injury or upper respiratory infection when "herniation" has occurred after crying, coughing, or other forceful Valsalva maneuvers. Cystic hygromas appear discrete, soft, mobile, nontender, and vary greatly in size. *Branchial cleft anomalies* are lesions most commonly occurring from defects in the development of the second branchial arch, giving rise to firm masses along the anterior border of the sternocleidomastoid muscle. Branchial cleft sinuses are painless and present with drainage at the junction of the middle and lower thirds of the sternocleidomastoid muscle. Cysts that are usually fluctuant, mobile, and nontender may occur if the sinus tract becomes blocked. Probing or injecting the tract may lead to infection. *Hemangiomas* are common head and neck lesions identified in infancy. These soft, mobile, nontender, bluish or reddish lesions tend to get larger in the first year of life and then involute over the next several years. *Neonatal torticollis* results from sternocleidomastoid fibrosis and shortening of the muscle. Presenting symptoms of torticollis occur in the first 3 weeks of life, with the infant holding his or her face and chin away from the affected side and the head tilted toward the fibrous mass. The mass is firm and seems attached to the muscle.

Inflammatory Masses

Cervical lymphadenopathy is the most common reason for neck masses in children. Up to 90% of children between the ages of 4 and 8 years can have cervical adenopathy without obvious associated infection or systemic illness. Lymphadenopathy in newborns and young infants is rare and warrants investigation. Supraclavicular lymphadenopathy is considered pathologic and should be biopsied. Etiology for cervical adenopathy includes bacterial or viral infection either from local, regional, or systemic illness.

Cervical lymphadenitis occurs when acute infection is present within the lymph node (see Chapter 74). Bacteria are the most common causes and include penicillin-resistant *Staphylococcus aureus* and group A β-hemolytic streptococci. Common presentation is usually one or more cervical lymph nodes that become acutely enlarged, tender, warm, and erythematous after an upper respiratory illness, pharyngitis, tonsillitis, or otitis media. Systemic symptoms of fever and malaise may be present. If fluctuation is present, needle aspiration is indicated. The purulent fluid should be sent for Gram stain and culture with antibiotic selection based on test results. If resolution of the lymphadenitis does not occur after needle aspiration and antibiotics, incision and drainage should be performed.

Cat-scratch disease is another common cause of lymph node enlargement in children. Typically, regional lymph nodes enlarge 2 to 4 weeks after a cat scratch (usually a kitten). Fever and malaise may have been present initially and usually a single node is involved. The area around the lymph node is warm, tender, indurated, and erythematous.

Mycobacterial infection of the cervical lymph nodes is most often caused by the atypical strains of *Mycobacterium avium-intracellulare and M. scrofulaceum*. The enlarged lymph nodes are generally submandibular in region and red, rubbery, and minimally tender to palpation. If systemic manifestations are present, an immune deficiency should be considered. On the other hand, clinical systemic signs of tuberculosis accompany cervical lymphadenopathy caused by *M. tuberculosis*.

Cervical lymphadenitis can be the result of viral infections, most commonly mononucleosis. Classically, the patient has diffuse lymphadenopathy with prominent cervical lymphadenopathy and large, hypertrophied tonsils. *Epstein-Barr virus* is the most common cause of mononucleosis. Systemic symptoms of fever, malaise, and the presence of hepatosplenomegaly are common.

Kawasaki disease (mucocutaneous lymph node syndrome) is associated with a single enlarged cervical lymph node, conjunctival injection without drainage, erythematous mouth, cracked lips, strawberry tongue, erythematous rash, induration of the palms of hands and soles of the feet, and fever of at least 3 days' duration.

Neoplasms

Presentation is usually a painless, firm, fixed cervical mass. Systemic symptoms may not be present. Differentiating between a benign and malignant lesion can be difficult. Cervical lymphadenopathy that does not resolve with standard therapy should raise suspicion for a malignancy. Neoplastic etiologies for neck mass in children include Hodgkin and non-Hodgkin lymphoma, rhabdomyosarcoma, neuroblastoma, thyroid carcinoma, and nasopharyngeal carcinoma.

CHAPTER 39

Neck Stiffness

Nathan Kuppermann, M.D., M.P.H.

Commonly, neck stiffness is accompanied by neck pain. However, certain clinical conditions may lead a child to hold the neck in an abnormal posture without neck pain. Torticollis is a variation of neck stiffness. The child holds the head tilted to one side and the chin rotated in the opposite direction, reflecting unilateral neck muscle contraction. This chapter reviews the differential diagnosis of neck stiffness or malposition, including torticollis, both with and without neck pain, in children.

DIFFERENTIAL DIAGNOSIS

The differential diagnosis of neck stiffness is best organized around a few important historical/clinical questions: (1) Is there a history of trauma? (2) Is there evidence of an infectious or inflammatory process (e.g., history or presence of fever)? and (3) Is there evidence of spinal cord involvement? Table 39.1 lists most causes of neck stiffness in children, Table 39.2 lists the common causes, and Table 39.3 lists the life-threatening causes. The following description categorizes the causes of neck stiffness in children by underlying mechanism and severity.

Neck Stiffness Associated with Trauma

LIFE-THREATENING CAUSES

Fractures of the cervical spine in children are uncommon, occurring in 1% to 2% of hospitalized pediatric trauma patients. Although some children with fractures of the cervical spine are unresponsive at the time of evaluation, most are alert and verbal, complain of neck pain, and have no demonstrable neurologic deficit. Subluxations of the cervical spine are more common than fractures and may result from minor trauma (e.g., falls from low heights) as well as more severe trauma (see Chapter 93). The most commonly occurring of these is rotary atlantoaxial subluxation, which generally does not compromise the spinal canal because the transverse ligament of the atlas remains intact. Rotary subluxation typically causes neck pain and torticollis. With rotary atlantoaxial subluxation, an anteroposterior open-mouth radiograph typically shows the rotation of C1 on C2, with the odontoid in an eccentric position relative to C1. Computed tomography (CT) scans of the neck can confirm equivocal cases. Most patients with rotary subluxation can be treated with a soft collar and antiinflammatory medications. Atlantoaxial subluxation with compromise of the spinal canal results from ligamentous laxity or rupture and resultant anterior movement of the atlas on the axis. Children with Down syndrome are susceptible to atlantoaxial subluxation because of laxity of the transverse ligament of the atlas. Radiographic findings of atlantoaxial subluxation may include a widened predental space and prevertebral soft-tissue swelling. Treatment involves immobilization and cervical traction.

The ligamentous laxity and hypermobility of the pediatric cervical spine predispose children to spinal cord injuries without radiographic abnormality (SCIWORA syndrome). Children younger than 8 years of age are most susceptible. Children with SCIWORA syndrome generally experience significant or progressive paralysis within 48 hours of a traumatic injury. Some children, however, may have transient neurologic symptoms that remit, then recur within the next day with worsening neurologic abnormalities.

Epidural hematomas of the cervical spine are uncommon but may occur even after apparently minor trauma. These may compress the spinal cord, leading to progressive neurologic symptoms and signs. Subarachnoid hemorrhage after trauma may lead to neck stiffness but is accompanied by headache and/or other physical findings of head trauma.

NONLIFE-THREATENING CAUSES

Fracture of the clavicle in children is common and may cause torticollis because of sternocleidomastoid (SCM) muscle spasm. However, the diagnosis is usually clear because pain is localized to the clavicle and not to the neck. Blunt trauma to the neck may result in neck pain as a result of muscular contusion and/or spasm. This is a diagnosis of exclusion, however, and should not be entertained until a detailed physical (neurologic) examination and radiographs of the cervical spine exclude the possibility of a more serious injury.

Neck Stiffness Associated with Infectious/Inflammatory Conditions

LIFE-THREATENING CAUSES

Bacterial meningitis is the most important infectious cause of neck stiffness and is almost always accompanied by fever. Children with meningitis typically have findings of neck stiffness on physical examination, although this may not be apparent in young infants and in children with meningeal infection who lack an inflammatory response.

Several other important infectious processes may have neck stiffness and usually fever as presenting signs. Retropharyngeal abscess is an infection that occupies the potential space between the posterior pharyngeal wall and the anterior border of the cervical vertebrae. Most commonly caused by group A streptococcus, oral anaerobic organisms, and *Staphylococcus aureus,* these infections cause clinical toxicity, drooling, and stridor. Lateral radiographs of the neck reveal soft-tissue swelling anterior to the upper cervical vertebral bodies.

Infectious processes involving the spine (osteomyelitis, epidural abscess, discitis) in children can involve the cervical

TABLE 39.1. Causes of Neck Stiffness or Malposition

Trauma Fracture of the cervical spine Subluxation of the cervical spine SCIWORA syndrome Epidural hematoma of the cervical spine Subarachnoid hemorrhage Clavicular fracture Muscular contusions/spasm of the neck *Infectious/inflammatory conditions* Bacterial meningitis Retropharyngeal abscess Infections of the spine (osteomyelitis, epidural abscesses, discitis) Rotary atlantoaxial subluxation as a result of local inflammation and/or otolaryngologic procedures (Grisel syndrome) Cervical lymphadenitis Intervertebral disc calcification Collagen vascular diseases (juvenile rheumatoid arthritis, ankylosing spondylitis, psoriatic arthritis, and other spondyloarthropathies) Pharyngotonsillitis Upper respiratory tract infection Upper lobe pneumonia Otitis media and mastoiditis Viral myositis	*Tumors and other space-occupying lesions of the central nervous system* Brain tumor Spinal cord tumor Other tumors of the head and neck (osteoid osteoma, eosinophilic granuloma, orbital tumor, acoustic neuroma, osteoblastoma, metastatic tumor to the spine, nasopharyngeal carcinoma, bone cyst) Other space-occupying lesions of the head and neck (Arnold-Chiari malformation) Other space-occupying lesions of the spinal cord (neurenteric cyst, arteriovenous malformation, syringomyelia) *Congenital conditions* Congenital muscular torticollis Skeletal malformations (Klippel-Feil syndrome, Sprengel deformity, hemiatlas, basilar impression, occipitocervical synostosis) Atlantoaxial instability secondary to congenital conditions (Down syndrome, Klippel-Feil syndromes, os odontoideum, Morquio syndrome) Benign paroxysmal torticollis *Miscellaneous* Ophthalmologic, neurologic, and/or vestibular causes (strabismus, cranial nerve palsies, extraocular muscle palsies, refractive errors, myasthenia gravis, migraine headaches) Sandifer syndrome Spontaneous pneumomediastinum Spasmus nutans Dystonic reaction Psychogenic

SCIWORA, spinal cord injuries without radiographic abnormality.

region, although they occur most commonly in the thoracic and lumbar areas. Localized pain, fever, and elevation of erythrocyte sedimentation rate (ESR) generally accompany all of these. Epidural abscesses may occur in the cervical spine, although lower spine involvement is much more common. When these abscesses arise in the cervical region, severe neurologic deficits may occur. Infectious discitis is uncommon in children. Most children with infectious discitis are younger than 3 years of age. Disease is usually in the lumbar or thoracic vertebrae rather than in the cervical region, with lower back pain and limp being the most common presenting complaints (see Chapter 43).

TABLE 39.2. Common Causes of Neck Stiffness or Malposition

Trauma Minor trauma (cervical muscular contusions, strains, and spasm) Clavicular fracture Rotary atlantoaxial subluxation *Infectious/inflammatory conditions* Bacterial meningitis Cervical lymphadenitis	Pharyngotonsillitis and other upper respiratory tract infections Viral myositis Muscle spasm Rotary atlantoaxial subluxation *Congenital conditions* Congenital muscular torticollis *Miscellaneous* Dystonic reaction

NONLIFE-THREATENING CAUSES

Atlantoaxial subluxation rarely may occur as a result of inflammatory processes in the head and neck region (e.g., rheumatoid arthritis, systemic lupus erythematosus, tonsillitis, pharyngitis) or after otolaryngologic procedures (e.g., tonsillectomy, ade-

TABLE 39.3. Life-Threatening Causes of Neck Stiffness or Malposition

Trauma Injuries to the cervical spine (fractures, subluxation, SCIWORA, epidural hematoma) Subarachnoid hemorrhage *Infection* Bacterial meningitis Retropharyngeal abscess Infections of the spine (osteomyelitis, epidural abscesses, discitis) Atlantoaxial subluxation with anterior displacement of the atlas as a result of local inflammation	*Tumors and other space-occupying lesions of the central nervous system* Brain tumor Spinal cord tumor Other tumors and space-occupying lesions of the head, neck, and spinal cord *Congenital conditions* Atlantoaxial instability secondary to congenital conditions

SCIWORA, spinal cord injuries without radiographic abnormality.

noidectomy). This condition, also called Grisel syndrome, is believed to occur as a result of ligamentous laxity after an infectious or inflammatory process. Most children with Grisel syndrome have torticollis and neck pain, often localized to the SCM muscle. Fever and dysphagia are common as well.

Cervical lymphadenitis, either acute or chronic, is a common cause of neck stiffness. The child with this condition typically has tender swelling over the lateral aspect of the neck, with or without fever.

Intervertebral disc calcification (IDC) in children is an uncommon, generally self-limited condition in which the nucleus pulposus of one or more intervertebral discs calcifies. Both the underlying cause of the condition and the cause of acute symptoms are unknown. It is generally thought that acute symptoms are secondary to some inciting event (e.g., mild trauma, viral infection) that results in an inflammatory response, possibly because of the release of calcium crystals. Children typically present with 24 to 48 hours of neck pain associated with neck stiffness or torticollis; fever is often present as well.

Collagen vascular disease in children may involve the cervical spine and lead to neck stiffness and/or pain. Children with juvenile rheumatoid arthritis may have either insidious or acute onset of symptoms, which commonly include neck stiffness. However, isolated cervical disease is unusual. Cervical involvement in ankylosing spondylitis is a late finding, as it is in other spondyloarthropathies. Girls with psoriatic arthritis, however, may have cervical involvement preceding sacroiliac and lumbar involvement.

Pharyngotonsillitis and upper respiratory tract infections may cause neck pain, although this is generally localized to tender cervical lymph nodes. Another common cause is viral myositis. Otitis media and mastoiditis have also been reported as causes of torticollis. Upper lobe pneumonia may cause pain referred to the neck. Muscle spasm as a cause of torticollis is a diagnosis of exclusion after eliminating the possibility of more serious underlying causes.

Neck Stiffness Associated with Space-Occupying Lesions of the Central Nervous System

LIFE-THREATENING CAUSES

Children with tumors of the posterior fossa, the most common location for pediatric brain tumors, may present with head tilt or torticollis. Posterior fossa tumors may cause any of a number of other symptoms and signs (vomiting, headache, ataxia, disturbances in vision including diplopia, papilledema, cranial nerve deficits, corticospinal or corticobulbar signs). Head tilt may result from attempts to compensate for diplopia. However, neck stiffness is thought to result from irritation of the accessory nerve by the cerebellar tonsils trapped in the occipital foramen or by tonsillar herniation.

Typically, spinal cord tumors cause pain at the site of the tumor and neurologic defects (sensory and motor defects, impaired bowel and bladder function), but symptoms may be very slow to develop, often leading to delays in diagnosis. Spinal cord tumors may also cause torticollis. Patients with these tumors may also hold their heads in a forward flexed position ("hanging head sign").

Other tumors of the head and neck, including orbital tumors, acoustic neuromas, nasopharyngeal carcinomas, osteoblastomas, and metastatic tumors to the spine, may cause torticollis. Arnold-Chiari malformations may also cause torticollis. Uncommon space-occupying lesions of the cervical spine such as neurenteric cysts, arteriovenous malformations, and syringomyelia may also cause neck pain and stiffness, generally accompanied by neurologic findings.

NONLIFE-THREATENING CAUSES

Osteoid osteoma is a benign bone tumor that typically affects older children and adolescents. If the osteoma is in the cervical spine, neck pain results. Eosinophilic granulomas and bone cysts are other benign (and rare) lesions of the spine that may cause neck pain. Congenital muscular torticollis is the most common cause of torticollis in infancy. Klippel-Feil syndrome is characterized by congenital fusion of a variable number of cervical vertebrae, which may result in atlantoaxial instability. Limitation in range of motion of the neck is the most common physical sign. In addition to limited neck motion, the classic triad also includes a low hairline and a short neck; the triad, however, is seen in fewer than half of patients. Sprengel deformity is characterized by congenital failure of the scapula to descend to its correct position. The scapula rests in a high position in relation to the neck and thorax. In its most severe form, the scapula may be connected by bone to the cervical spine and limit neck movement. Hemiatlas is a malformation of the first cervical vertebra, which may cause severe, progressive torticollis. Basilar impression is a condition resulting from anomalies at the base of the skull and vertebrae, which lead to a short neck, headache, neck pain, and cranial nerve palsies due to compression of the cranial nerves. Many congenital conditions, including Klippel-Feil syndrome, achondroplasia, and neurofibromatosis, may cause basilar impression. Commonly associated with basilar impression is occipitocervical synostosis, a condition in which fibrous or bony connections between the base of the skull and the atlas cause neck pain, torticollis, high scapula, and several neurologic symptoms.

Several congenital conditions may be associated with atlantoaxial instability and predispose the patient to cervical subluxation. In addition to Down and Klippel-Feil syndromes, these include other skeletal dysplasias and os odontoideum (aplasia or hypoplasia of the odontoid). Children with these conditions should be screened for atlantoaxial instability. Morquio syndrome is a mucopolysaccharidosis resulting in flattening of the vertebrae and multiple skeletal dysplasias. The odontoid process of the axis is underdeveloped and may lead to atlantoaxial subluxation.

Benign paroxysmal torticollis of infancy presents as recurrent episodes of torticollis in association with pallor, agitation, and vomiting. Typical onset is between 2 and 8 months of age, and the condition tends to remit by 2 to 3 years.

Miscellaneous Causes of Neck Stiffness

Head tilt or neck malposition may result from abnormalities of vision (strabismus, cranial nerve palsies, extraocular muscle palsies, refractive errors) or the vestibular apparatus. The child attempts to correct for the disturbance through changes in neck position. Careful ophthalmologic and neurologic examinations of the child with head tilt are necessary to exclude these possibilities. Torticollis has also been reported in patients with migraine headaches. Patients with myasthenia gravis may develop torticollis, but ptosis, impairment of extraocular muscular movement, and other cranial nerve palsies are generally earlier signs. Sandifer syndrome is the constellation of torticollis, gastroesophageal reflux, and hiatal hernia. Spontaneous pneumomediastinum may present with neck pain and torticollis: crepitus is generally palpated along the neck. Spasmus nutans is an acquired condition of childhood, characterized by nystagmus, head nodding, and torticollis. Children with these findings typically become symptomatic in the first 2 years of life. Certain drugs with dopamine-2 receptor antagonists can cause acute dystonic reactions with torticollis. These include many neuroleptic and antiemetic agents, such as haloperidol, prochlorperazine, and metoclopramide. Hysterical patients may present with torticollis. This diagnosis can be made only after excluding other more serious causes.

EVALUATION AND DECISION

The approach to the child with a stiff or malpositioned neck should focus initially on whether there is spinal cord involvement, as detailed in Fig. 39.1. If secondary to trauma, one should suspect cervical spine fracture or subluxation, spinal epidural hematoma, or SCIWORA syndrome. In the setting of fever, a spinal epidural abscess should be considered. Atlantoaxial subluxation secondary to otolaryngologic diseases or procedures should be considered in children with spinal cord involvement and consistent histories. Finally, spinal cord tumors and other space-occupying lesions should be considered if the development of symptoms is gradual and not associated with trauma or fever.

The next issue that should be considered is whether the neck stiffness is the result of an acute traumatic event. Fractures and subluxations/dislocations will generally be identified on plain radiography of the cervical spine. Other modalities (e.g., flexion–extension views, CT, MRI) may be useful to detect ligamentous injury, rotary subluxation, or spinal epidural hematomas. Muscle strain and/or contusion is a diagnosis of exclusion. If other symptoms in addition to the neck stiffness are present, appropriate studies should be obtained. For example, the patient with neck stiffness and headache may have a subarachnoid hemorrhage for which a head CT scan would be indicated. The patient with clavicle fracture may have spasm of the SCM muscle and torticollis.

Fever in the setting of neck stiffness suggests the presence of an infectious, inflammatory, or neoplastic process. The presence of meningitis must be excluded either clinically or with a lumbar puncture (see Chapter 74).

After the presence of meningitis has been excluded in the febrile patient with neck stiffness, the examination should focus on the presence or absence of a cervical mass. If a cervical mass is identified, a history of contact with cats and constitutional symptoms suggestive of malignancy should be elicited. If the cervical mass is tender, a trial of antibiotics directed at the most common bacterial pathogens and the placement of a purified protein derivative skin test to screen for tuberculosis may be all that is necessary. If the cervical mass does not respond to an appropriate trial of antibiotics, cat-scratch disease, atypical mycobacterial infection, or malignancy may be the cause.

If no palpable cervical mass is present, a more in-depth evaluation may be necessary, based on the history and physical ex-

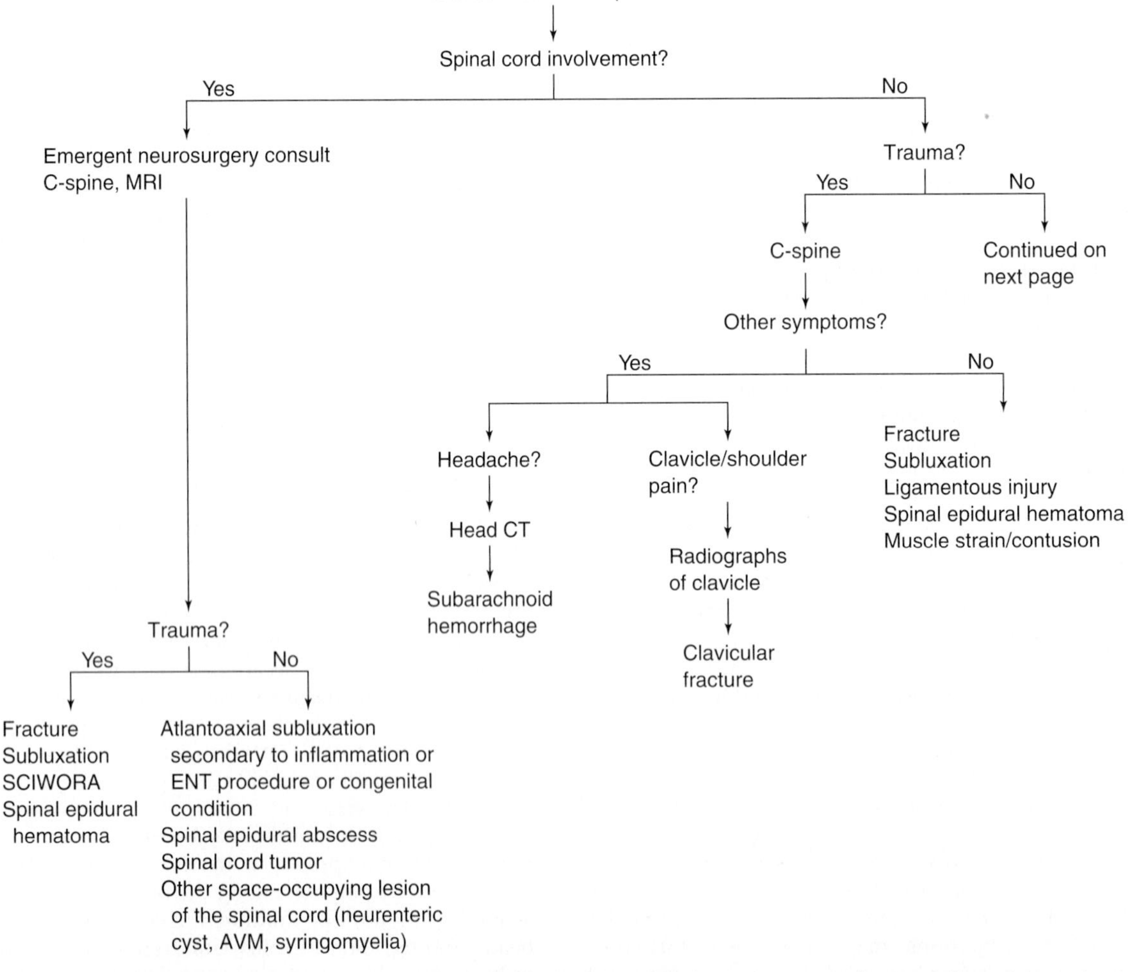

Figure 39.1. Approach to the child with stiff or malpositioned neck. *C-spine,* cervical spine radiograph; *MRI,* magnetic resonance imaging; *ENT,* ear, nose, throat; *AVM,* arteriovenous malformation; *CT,* computed tomography; *CBC,* complete blood count; *ESR,* erythrocyte sedimentation rate; *TB,* tuberculosis; *SCM,* sternocleidomastoid.

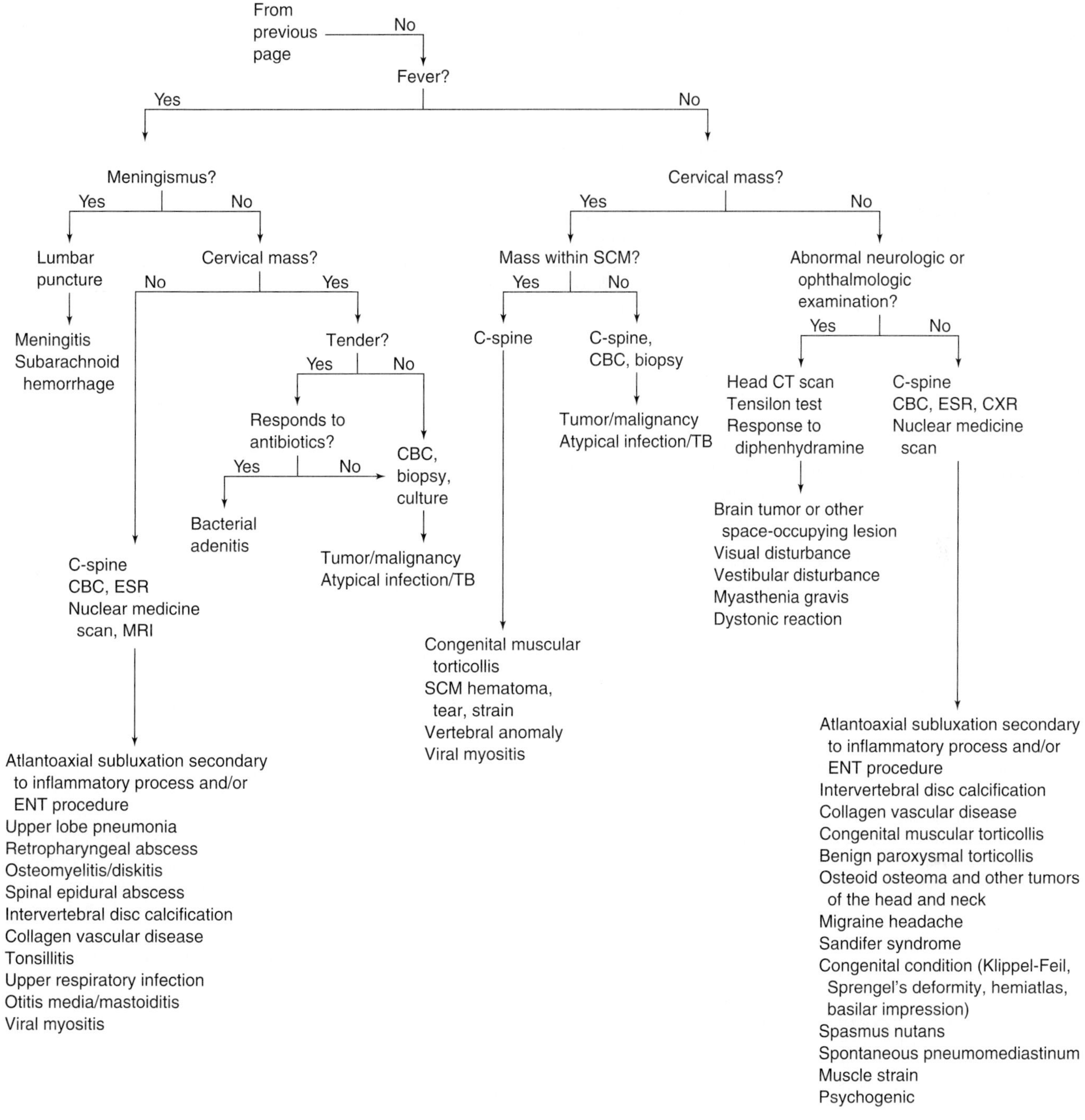

Figure 39.1. *(Continued)*

amination of the child. Radiographs of the cervical spine will diagnose retropharyngeal abscess in the febrile child with stridor, drooling, and neck stiffness and may detect atlantoaxial subluxation in the child with otolaryngologic disease or who has recently had an otolaryngologic procedure. Radiographs of the cervical spine may also be useful in detecting other diseases involving the cervical spine, including vertebral osteomyelitis, infectious discitis, intervertebral disc calcification, and neck stiffness from collagen vascular disease. White blood count or ESR will be elevated in most children with these conditions, as well as those with spinal epidural abscesses and infections of the head and neck (e.g., tonsillitis, mastoiditis). If plain radiography is not diagnostic, technetium scans will identify vertebral osteomyelitis or discitis. CT or MRI of the spine will identify spinal epidural abscesses and can be helpful if routine radiographs are equivocal in several of the previously described conditions. Finally, an upper lobe pneumonia identified on chest film may be the cause of neck stiffness in the febrile child.

In the afebrile child with neck stiffness, the presence of a cervical mass within the SCM suggests congenital muscular torticollis (in an infant) or a SCM hematoma or tear. Radiographs of the cervical spine should be obtained to exclude more serious conditions. If the cervical mass is not within the SCM, a malignancy or atypical infection may be the cause and a complete blood count and biopsy of the mass should be considered.

For the afebrile child with neck stiffness and/or malposition of the neck and no cervical mass, a careful ophthalmologic and neurologic examination should be performed to exclude the possibility of a brain tumor, other space-occupying lesions of the brain, visual disturbances, and vestibular disturbance causing the abnormal neck posture. Often, the patient does not have true neck pain but is attempting to correct for these disturbances through changes in head position. A head CT scan is necessary to exclude the possibility of a space-occupying lesion of the brain, including brain tumor. The child with myasthenia gravis generally has ptosis and weakness of extraocular muscles and may develop torticollis. A trial of intravenous edrophonium chloride (Tensilon) is diagnostic because symptoms will improve immediately; however, edrophonium chloride should not be given to young infants, who are especially prone to this agent's ability to cause cardiac arrhythmias. Children with torticollis after taking neuroleptic or antiemetic medications will usually respond to intravenous diphenhydramine.

Finally, the child with neck stiffness without fever, cervical mass, or abnormal ophthalmologic or neurologic examination may have any of a number of conditions. Many of the disorders mentioned as typically being associated with fever are commonly seen without fever as well (atlantoaxial subluxation in the child with otolaryngologic diseases or after otolaryngologic procedures, intervertebral disc calcification, collagen vascular disease). Furthermore, infants with congenital muscular torticollis may not have SCM masses that are detectable on physical examination. Some children with neck stiffness may have dysmorphic features, suggesting specific skeletal malformation syndromes or cervical subluxation in a child with Down syndrome. Chronic symptoms may suggest a congenital syndrome, collagen vascular disease, or a neoplastic process, but children with these conditions may also present with acute onset of symptoms. Osteoid osteoma and other benign tumors of the head and neck may be detected by plain radiography of the cervical spine. A chest radiograph is indicated for the child with neck stiffness in association with a history of severe coughing and/or retching because an upper lobe pneumonia or spontaneous pneumomediastinum may be the cause. Finally, if no cause can be identified after a complete history, detailed examination, and careful radiographic and laboratory evaluation, muscle spasm or hysteria may be the cause of torticollis.

CHAPTER 40
Oligomenorrhea

Jan E. Paradise, M.D.

Oligomenorrhea can be defined as an interval of more than 6 weeks between two menstrual periods. If menstrual cycles do not resume within 3 to 6 months, the term *secondary amenorrhea* is applied. Oligomenorrhea should be distinguished from hypomenorrhea, a nonpathologic pattern of light but regular menstrual periods. The differential diagnosis of oligomenorrhea is given in Table 40.1.

TABLE 40.1. Differential Diagnosis of Oligomenorrhea Organized by Pathophysiology of Disorder or Condition

- Hypothalamic–Pituitary axis disorders
  - Disorders of weight and/or energy expenditure
  - Anorexia nervosa
  - Strenuous exercise
  - Marked thinness or weight loss
  - Chronic illness
  - Delayed maturation
  - Psychological stress
  - Central nervous system tumors
  - Pseudocyesis
- *Ovarian disorders*
  - Ovarian failure
    - Gonadal dysgenesis
    - Cancer chemotherapeutic agents
    - Pelvic irradiation
    - Autoimmune diseases
  - Hormone-secreting tumors
- *Uterine disorders*
  - Endometrial destruction
    - Surgical
    - Tuberculous
- *Hyperprolactinemia*
  - Lactation
  - Drugs (see Table 40.2)
  - Pituitary adenoma
  - Hypothyroidism
- *Hyperandrogenism*
  - Polycystic ovary syndrome
  - Adrenal disease
- *Miscellaneous conditions*
  - Pregnancy
  - Hormonal contraception
    - Hypothyroidism or hyperthyroidism

EVALUATION AND DECISION

Diagnosis of Pregnancy

"Is she pregnant?" is always the first question to answer in evaluating an adolescent with one or several missed menstrual periods (Fig. 40.1). If she is pregnant prompt diagnosis and referral are important for the teenager who intends to seek a therapeutic abortion, as well as for the one who plans to continue her pregnancy.

Early pregnancy is not always easy to recognize. Symptoms of fatigue, nausea, vomiting (not necessarily in the morning), urinary frequency, and breast growth or tenderness are common, but by no means are they universal or specific. On pelvic examination, the first indications of pregnancy are softening of the lower uterine segment (Hegar sign) and of the cervix (Goodell sign) at 4 to 6 weeks after the last menstrual period. By 6 weeks' gestation, the uterus changes from pear-shaped to globular, and by about 8 weeks, the vagina and cervix acquire a bluish hue (Chadwick sign). These changes occur in ectopic as well as in intrauterine pregnancies. After 12 weeks, the uterine fundus is palpable above the symphysis pubis on abdominal examination. Fetal movement can be discerned after about 16 weeks.

To determine pregnancy, β-human chorionic gonadotropin (hCG) tests, are specific and sensitive, identifying total levels of hCG as low as 5 mIU per mL in serum and 25 mIU per mL in urine. Because the serum concentration of hCG in pregnant patients reaches 100 mIU/mL by about the time of the next anticipated menstrual period, the clinician can detect pregnancy in nearly all patients within about 9 days after conception (before the menstrual period has been missed) and in essentially all patients who have missed a period, including those with ectopic pregnancies that produce abnormally low levels of hCG. If a patient with one or several missed menstrual periods also complains of abdominal pain or abnormal vaginal bleeding, the diagnosis of *ectopic pregnancy* must be entertained (see Chapter 67). Three-fourths of women with ectopic pregnancies experience 1 to 12 weeks of amenorrhea before abnormal bleeding or pain eventually prompts them to seek medical attention.

Pseudocyesis is a rare cause of amenorrhea in women who believe they are pregnant and who exhibit many presumptive symptoms and signs of pregnancy, including nausea, vomiting, hyperpigmented areolae, galactorrhea, and abdominal distension. The diagnosis is made when a patient who insists that she is pregnant nevertheless has no true uterine enlargement, no demonstrable fetal parts or heart sounds, and a negative pregnancy test.

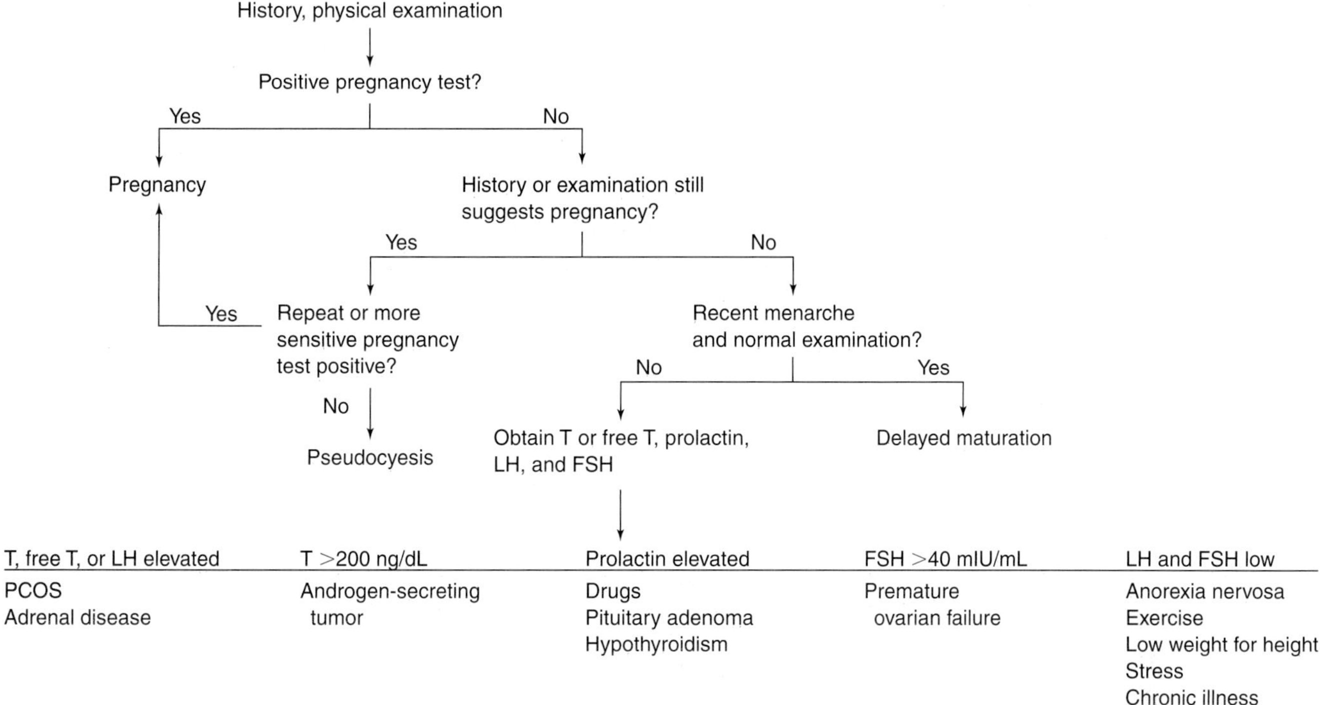

Figure 40.1. Differential diagnosis of oligomenorrhea. *T,* testosterone; *LH,* luteinizing hormone; *FSH,* follicle-stimulating hormone; *PCOS,* polycystic ovary syndrome.

Evaluation of Nonpregnant Patients

During the first 2 years after menarche, irregular menstrual cycles are common. As a rule, if an adolescent who complains of oligomenorrhea is fewer than 2 years past menarche, is not sexually active, and has no signs suggestive of any specific cause of oligomenorrhea (hirsutism, obesity, galactorrhea, extreme thinness), further investigation is not warranted. Adolescents with a pattern of oligomenorrhea that has continued for longer than 2 years after menarche or that began after a regular menstrual pattern had already been established need further evaluation.

HIRSUTE OR OBESE PATIENTS

Classically, hirsutism, obesity, ovarian enlargement, and amenorrhea or infertility constitute the clinical features of *polycystic ovary syndrome* (PCOS, previously the Stein-Leventhal syndrome). However, patients with PCOS are a heterogeneous group with varying combinations of these features. In some cases, clinically evident hyperandrogenism is accompanied by peripheral insulin resistance, hyperinsulinemia, and acanthosis nigricans (HAIR-AN syndrome).

Partial or late onset *congenital adrenal hyperplasia* is a rare cause of oligomenorrhea associated with hyperandrogenism that is usually indistinguishable clinically from PCOS. Other rare causes, including *Cushing disease* and *ovarian and adrenal tumors,* should be suspected in patients with hirsutism accompanied by signs of glucocorticoid excess or virilization (marked acne, deepening of the voice, or clitoromegaly), and in those with testosterone levels above 200 ng per dL.

GALACTORRHEA

Hyperprolactinemia occurs in approximately 25% of adult women with secondary amenorrhea but is a much less common cause of oligomenorrhea in adolescents. Nevertheless, the possibility of hyperprolactinemia must be considered in all adolescents with oligomenorrhea because only 40% to 50% of hyperprolactinemic patients have spontaneous or expressible galactorrhea. The constellation of oligomenorrhea, galactorrhea, and hyperprolactinemia can be produced by drugs (Table 40.2) that block pituitary dopamine receptors or interfere in other ways with dopaminergic or serotoninergic central nervous system pathways, by the discontinuation of birth control pills, by cutaneous or neurogenic stimulation of the breasts, and by excessive secretion of prolactin itself (e.g., primary hypothyroidism, pituitary adenoma). Rarely, in hypothyroid patients, hypothalamic thyroid-releasing hormone acts as a prolactin-releasing factor, resulting in galactorrhea. Breast-feeding is an obvious physiologic cause of prolactin secretion and oligomenorrhea. The occasional patient with galac-

TABLE 40.2. Partial List of Drugs That Can Cause Hyperprolactinemia and/or Galactorrhea

Antipsychotic and antidepressant agents	*Drugs Used to Treat Gastrointestinal Disorders*
Amoxapine (Asendin), clomipramine (Anafranil), chlorpromazine (Thorazine), thioridazine (Mellaril), prochlorperazine (Compazine), fluphenazine (Prolixin), other phenothiazines	Cimetidine (Tagamet)
Haloperidol (Haldol)	Metoclopramide (Reglan)
Pimozide (Orap)	*Antihypertensive agents*
Risperidone (Risperdal)	Methyldopa (Aldomet)
Thiothixene (Navane)	Reserpine (Hydromox, Serpasil, others)
	Verapamil (Calan, Isoptin)
	Opiates
	Codeine
	Morphine

torrhea but a normal prolactin level should be reevaluated periodically in an effort to identify a treatable cause of the problem.

NORMAL AND THIN PATIENTS

Among adolescents who do not have hirsutism, obesity, or galactorrhea, suppression of the hypothalamic–pituitary axis is the most common cause of oligomenorrhea that occurs or persists for at least 2 years after menarche. *Abnormalities of body weight* are probably the most common sources of this central disturbance. This is in accordance with the clinical observation that many patients with serious chronic illnesses, malnutrition, or rapid weight loss develop amenorrhea. The observations that amenorrhea often precedes substantial weight loss in patients with anorexia nervosa and that amenorrheic ballet dancers experience menarche and resume menses during intervals of rest unaccompanied by weight gain give credence to the hypothesis that psychological stress and energy expenditure deficits may have additional, independent effects on the hypothalamic–pituitary axis.

Other diagnostic possibilities for oligomenorrheic patients with no abnormal physical findings include a wide variety of conditions. About half of women using contraceptive *medroxyprogesterone* injections for 12 months have amenorrhea; after 2 years of use, the proportion with amenorrhea is 68%. Amenorrhea also occurs in about 2% of menstrual cycles among patients taking *birth control pills* that contain 50 µg or less of estrogen. However, amenorrhea persisting 12 months after the last injection of medroxyprogesterone or 6 months after birth control pills have been stopped should be evaluated in the standard fashion. The diagnoses uncovered among patients with "postpill amenorrhea" are nearly as heterogeneous as those seen in amenorrheic patients who have never taken birth control pills.

Hypothyroidism and, less commonly, *hyperthyroidism* can produce menstrual irregularities. Many patients with hyperprolactinemia and oligomenorrhea do not have concomitant galactorrhea that would otherwise prompt a medical investigation. Similarly, although hirsutism and obesity are classic features of PCOS, many adolescent patients with oligomenorrhea and the endocrinologic abnormalities of PCOS lack one or both of these signs. A history of hot flashes, antineoplastic chemotherapy, pelvic irradiation, or autoimmune disease suggests the diagnosis of *premature ovarian failure*. *Endometrial destruction* that results from overly vigorous curettage or pelvic tuberculosis is a rare cause of oligomenorrhea.

DIAGNOSTIC PROCEDURES

Patients with oligomenorrhea but few other symptoms or signs of disease require laboratory evaluation to differentiate among the many potential causes of oligomenorrhea after pregnancy has been excluded (Fig. 40.1). Determinations of serum levels of follicle-stimulating hormone (FSH), testosterone (T) or free testosterone (free T), and prolactin are needed in order to corroborate the suspected diagnosis or to categorize the patient whose history and physical examination have provided few diagnostic clues. Prepubertal levels of luteinizing hormone (LH) and FSH indicate hypothalamic–pituitary suppression in a postmenarchal patient; this pattern is commonly found. An elevated LH:FSH ratio of greater than 2.5 can be found in about one-third of patients with PCOS. The finding of a mildly elevated total or free T level constitutes strong evidence for a diagnosis of PCOS. FSH values over 40 mIU per mL suggest ovarian failure as the cause for oligomenorrhea. An elevated prolactin level is likely to indicate a pituitary microadenoma in patients who are not using any of the drugs known to cause hyperprolactinemia and galactorrhea (Table 40.2).

CHAPTER 41
Oral Lesions

Mark G. Roback, M.D.

Oral lesions commonly occur in infancy and childhood and may represent a wide range of illnesses—from benign lesions that completely resolve without intervention to those associated with life-threatening diseases. The differential diagnosis includes a large number of localized congenital and acquired causes; however, lesions associated with systemic disease must also be considered (Fig. 41.1 and Table 41.1). Most often, patients with isolated complaints (e.g., a mouth sore or mass, drooling, pain, fever) represent common, self-limited conditions (Table 41.2). Systemic and potentially life-threatening diseases (Table 41.3) may present initially with isolated mouth findings, necessitating a complete history and physical examination in all patients with oral lesions.

DIFFERENTIAL DIAGNOSIS

Congenital Oral Lesions

Epstein's pearls occur in more than 60% of newborns as small, white milia in the midline of the hard palate. These epithelial inclusion cysts are often found in clusters and resolve over the first few months of life. Epithelial pearls are similar to Epstein's pearls and appear as shiny, small, white, self-limited lesions that occur on the gums. Bohn's nodules are also self-limited cysts that appear on the mandibular or maxillary dental ridges. Dental lamina cysts occur on the alveolar ridge of newborns and represent trapped remnants of the dental lamina. Natal teeth represent the premature eruption of primary teeth. Epulis is a congenital fibrous, sarcomatous tumor that arises from the periosteum of the mandible or maxilla. Lymphangioma is a benign congenital tumor of lymphatic vessels appearing on the tongue, lips, or buccal mucosa at birth or in early infancy. Hemangiomas are benign vascular malformations present at birth that may become more apparent as the patient grows.

Infectious Oral Lesions

Candidiasis, or thrush, is white plaques on the buccal mucosa, gingivae, and palate that will not "rub off" with a tongue blade. When thrush occurs after infancy, the immune status of the patient must be considered.

Herpes gingivostomatitis, most commonly caused by herpes simplex virus type 1 (HSV-1), represents primary infection that typically occurs in young children and infants. These patients have pain, fever, and drooling. *Herpes labialis* manifests as recurrent painful lesions that occur on the lips, most often the lower lip. Hand–foot–mouth disease is characterized by discreet shallow erosions in the mouth, especially on the soft palate, accompanied by erythematous papulovesicular lesions on the hands and feet. High fever may be associated with this enteroviral-mediated disease (typically coxsackievirus) that is self-limited in nature. Herpangina is also a group A coxsackievirus infection that causes vesicles or ulcers on the pharynx of patients with fever, muscle aches, and malaise.

The characteristic "strawberry tongue" seen in streptococcal scarlet fever is the result of hypertrophic red papillae on a thick white coat. Palatal petechiae are often present as is the typical "sandpaper" papular rash on an erythematous base that

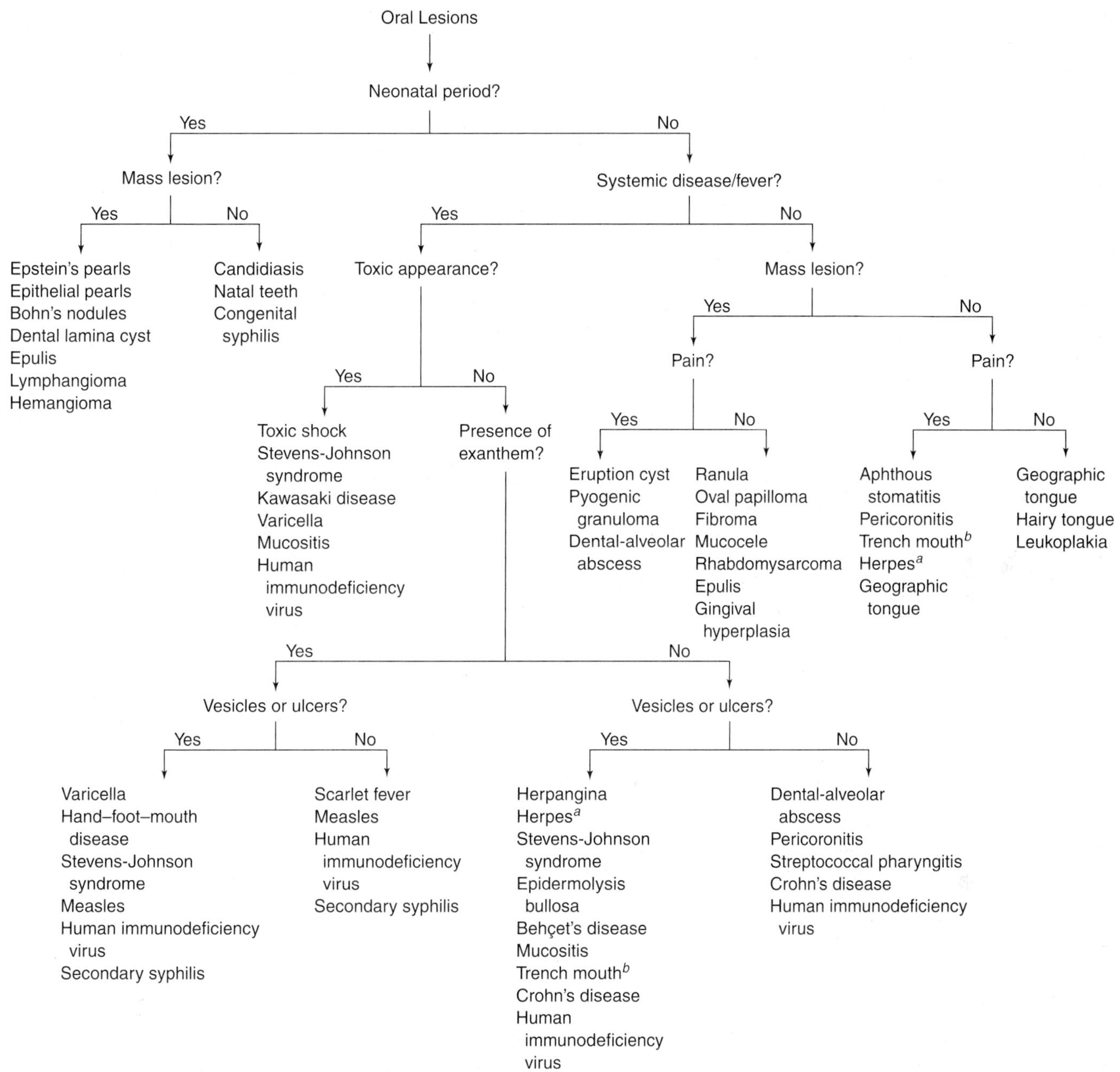

Figure 41.1. Oral lesions.

blanches on palpation, involving the trunk and back. Streptococcal pharyngitis without exanthem often presents with strawberry tongue and palatal petechiae.

Koplik's spots are pinpoint white macules on markedly erythematous mucous membranes and occur during the prodrome of measles, which includes cough, coryza, conjunctivitis, and fever. Varicella lesions occurring in the mouth result in painful vesicles, which may become unroofed on an erythematous base.

Oral lesions commonly associated with human immunodeficiency virus (HIV)-infected patients include candidiasis, hairy leukoplakia, herpes simplex, aphthous ulcers, and necrotizing ulcerative gingivitis. Blue, purple, or red macules, papules, or nodules on the palate suggest oral Kaposi sarcoma, whereas diffuse swelling, discrete nodules, or ulcers of any oral mucosal surface may indicate non-Hodgkin lymphoma.

The pain, erythema, and swelling of the gingiva seen with dental-alveolar abscesses may be associated with fever and loosening or extrusion of the associated tooth. Significant lymphadenopathy and facial cellulitis may develop. Pericoronitis is local infection of the gingiva surrounding an erupting tooth. Acute necrotizing ulcerative gingivitis, also called trench mouth or Vincent angina, is a spirochetal infection of the gingiva that

TABLE 41.1. Differential Diagnosis of Oral Lesions

Congenital oral lesions	Syphilis
Epstein's pearls	Acquired (secondary)
Epithelial pearls	Congenital
Bohn's nodules	Hairy tongue
Dental lamina cysts	*Tumorous oral lesions*
Natal teeth	Eruption cyst
Epulis (gum boil)	Oral papilloma
Lymphangioma	Fibroma
Hemangioma	Mucocele
Infectious oral lesions	Ranula
Candidiasis	Pyogenic granuloma
Herpes simplex virus (HSV)	Rhabdomyosarcoma
Gingivostomatitis—primary	*Oral lesions associated with systemic disease*
Labialis—recurrent (cold scores)	Stevens-Johnson syndrome
Hand–foot–mouth disease	Toxic shock syndrome
Herpangina	Mucositis
Scarlet fever	Kawasaki disease
Streptococcal pharyngitis	Crohn disease
Measles	Behçet syndrome
Varicella	Epidermolysis bullosa
Human immunodeficiency virus (HIV)	*Miscellaneous oral lesions*
Dental-alveolar abscess	Aphthous stomatitis
Pericoronitis	Geographic tongue
Acute necrotizing ulcerative gingivitis (trench mouth)	Gingival hyperplasia
	Leukoplakia

occurs in adolescents. Patients report tender, bleeding gums and breath that has a fetid odor. Gums are hyperemic and appear "punched-out" secondary to tissue loss between the teeth.

Although infection is present at birth, the oral lesions of congenital syphilis may not become obvious until several months of age. Erythematous papules are seen in the mouth and other mucocutaneous sites. *Hutchinson teeth*, peg-shaped, superior, central incisors, are not present until later in life. The secondary stage of acquired syphilis is characterized by patches of ulcers or raised lesions in the mouth and is seen in association with generalized rash, fever, malaise, and adenopathy.

Patients receiving long-term antibiotic therapy may develop elongation of filiform papillae of the dorsum of the tongue and a "hairy" appearance from fungal overgrowth called hairy tongue. Hairy leukoplakia of the lateral aspects of the tongue is found in HIV-infected patients in association with intraepithelial proliferation of Epstein-Barr virus infection.

Tumorous Oral Lesions

Eruption cysts are associated with the eruption of teeth and appear on the alveolar ridge and may contain blood. Oral papillomas are typically benign, although a small percentage of papillomas may become malignant. They are fingerlike extensions from the epithelium of the tongue, gums, lips, or buccal mucosa. Fibroma is found on the tongue, lips, buccal mucosa, or palate

TABLE 41.2. Common Causes of Oral Lesions

Candidiasis	Hand–foot–mouth disease
Aphthous stomatitis	Herpangina
Herpes simplex virus	
Gingivostomatitis—primary	
Labialis—recurrent	

TABLE 41.3. Life-Threatening Causes of Oral Lesions

Stevens-Johnson syndrome	Toxic shock syndrome
Kawasaki disease	Human immunodeficiency virus

and is a benign, smooth mass with a sessile base. Ranula is a retention cyst or mucocele of the submaxillary or sublingual ducts. Ranulas are typically seen on the underside of the tongue or on either side of the frenulum on the floor of the mouth.

Mucoceles arise secondary to obstruction of salivary glands. Mucoceles are soft, well-demarcated masses. Patients are typically asymptomatic. Pyogenic granuloma represents granulation tissue that develops in response to an irritant such as trauma or foreign body. Most commonly found on the gingiva, pyogenic granulomas are also found on the tongue, lips, and buccal mucosa. Rhabdomyosarcoma is a rare malignant tumor of the oral cavity. These lesions are characterized by rapid growth. They are ulcerative in nature and may present with bleeding.

Oral Lesions Associated with Systemic Disease

Stevens-Johnson syndrome, a severe form of erythema multiforme, consists of an inflammatory process that typically involves the skin and mucous membranes. Oral lesions are erythematous plaques on the mucosa of the oral cavity and lips that develop into vesicles or bullae and may become hemorrhagic. Toxic shock syndrome may manifest erythema of the oropharynx and a strawberry tongue in patients with a diffuse erythematous macular exanthem, hyperemic mucous membranes, fever, and signs of shock. Toxin-mediated disease associated with streptococci also presents with diffuse erythema of the skin and oropharynx and may progress to septic shock. Mucositis presents as ulcers, exudate, and pseudomembranes on the gingivae and buccal mucosa of patients with neutropenia oftentimes secondary to chemotherapy. Kawasaki disease is a potentially life-threatening disorder that typically presents with an array of findings, including prolonged fever, rash, lymphadenopathy, nonpurulent conjunctivitis, and edema of the hands and feet. Oral changes of Kawasaki disease include red, dry, cracked lips; erythematous oropharynx; and strawberry tongue.

The inflammatory lesions of Crohn disease may occur in any portion of the gastrointestinal tract. Oral lesions, seen most often in adolescents and young adults, consist of ulcers, polypoid papulous hyperplastic mucosa, and edema found on the lips, gingiva, vestibular sulci, and buccal mucosa. Chronic, recurrent ulcers surrounded by erythema and gray exudate are found anywhere in the oral cavity in patients with Behçet syndrome. Similar lesions occur on the skin, and the genitourinary tract may also be involved. More than 15 types of hereditary epidermolysis bullosa have been described. This rare, vesiculobullous condition affects mucous membranes and teeth as well as the skin. Scarring may lead to restriction of mouth opening.

Miscellaneous Oral Lesions

Aphthous stomatitis is ulceration of the oral epidermis of unknown cause. These recurrent lesions typically present as 5- to 10-mm ulcerations with a rim of erythema on the buccal mucosa, lips, and lateral aspect of the tongue. The lesions are painful, but patients do not experience fever. Geographic tongue represents a benign inflammatory disorder that results in migratory smooth annular patches on the tongue. Although typically asymptomatic, patients may complain of pain. Gingival hyperplasia is seen in patients receiving long-term anticonvulsant therapy with phenytoin. Leukoplakia of the oral mucosa develops secondary to chronic smokeless tobacco use. These painless, leathery, white patches or plaques occur in areas of greatest tobacco exposure, typically on the mucosa of the buccal sulcus.

EVALUATION AND DECISION

Neonates with oral lesions can be divided into two groups based on the morphology of the lesions. Discrete masses usually represent congenital disorders, most of which are self-limited. Candidiasis, which involves the oral cavity more diffusely, is also common.

Among older children, toxic-appearing patients require immediate evaluation for potentially life-threatening disease. Patients with conditions listed in Table 41.3 have associated findings such as diffuse cutaneous rash, hyperemia of other mucous membranes, or poor perfusion indicative of shock. However, Stevens-Johnson syndrome may cause isolated oral lesions initially and then rapidly progress to systemic involvement. Once life-threatening causes have been considered, additional history and physical examination may lead to diagnosis of other systemic diseases. Weight loss, abdominal pain, and diarrhea with or without blood suggest Crohn disease, whereas genital ulceration in an adolescent boy points to Behçet syndrome or secondary syphilis.

The presence of rash and fever makes disorders of infectious etiology more likely. Measles, varicella, scarlet fever, and hand–foot–mouth disease are generally diagnosed by history and physical examination alone. Infectious causes of oral lesions without exanthem may display obvious findings such as cachexia and alopecia in the neutropenic patient with mucositis, or they may be relatively localized to the oropharynx as in herpangina, herpes gingivostomatitis or labialis, and dental infections, which may or may not have fever and lymphadenopathy.

Oral lesions without overt signs of systemic disease are mostly congenital or tumorous in nature. Lesions found in the newborn and during infancy are largely self-limited, and most will resolve spontaneously.

Children and adolescents experience an array of oral lesions not associated with obvious signs of systemic disease that are typically further delineated by considering the type of lesion (i.e., mass, vesicle, ulcer) and whether they are painful. Most of these processes require little or no therapy. Rhabdomyosarcoma is an obvious exception to this observation.

CHAPTER 42
Pain—Abdomen

Richard M. Ruddy, M.D.

Abdominal pain is a common complaint of children who come to the emergency department. Although most children with acute abdominal pain have self-limiting conditions, the pain may herald a serious medical or surgical emergency. The principal causes of abdominal pain in children and adolescents are summarized in Table 42.1. Table 42.2 highlights those disorders that are life threatening. Clearly, the most difficult challenge continues to be making a timely diagnosis of appendicitis and other causes of an acute condition in the abdomen early enough to reduce the rate of complications.

EVALUATION AND DECISION

The assessment of the patient with abdominal pain hinges on any history of trauma, the patient's age, the onset and chronicity of the pain, the related symptoms and pertinent history, and the physical findings (Fig. 42.1).

Abdominal Pain with Trauma

The physician should perform a rapid, gentle physical examination to separate superficial injury (e.g., muscle contusion) from significant intraabdominal trauma (e.g., splenic rupture or hepatic hematoma). In children who are unstable at presentation and have obvious serious or multiple injuries or a severe mechanism of injury, a rapid, aggressive workup is indicated. Children with localized and acute pain after blunt trauma may appear surprisingly well but have significant solid organ or hollow viscus trauma. When an intraabdominal injury is suspected in a stable patient, an urgent computed tomographic (CT) scan should be obtained to assist in pinning down a diagnosis. Abdominal pain with trauma is also reviewed in Chapters 90, 91, and 95.

Abdominal Pain without Trauma

After stabilization, when required, the next priority is to identify the child who requires immediate or potential surgical intervention, whether for appendicitis, intussusception, or other congenital or acquired lesions. Next, an effort is directed to diagnose any of the medical illnesses from among a large group of acute and chronic abdominal and extraabdominal inflammatory disorders that require emergency nonsurgical management. Table 42.2 lists life-threatening causes of abdominal pain by age groups. Finally, the physician is left to deal with a host of self-limiting or nonspecific causes of abdominal pain, including nonorganic etiologies. The algorithm presented in this chapter for the approach to abdominal pain without trauma has been designed on the basis of three branch points: age; chronicity; and the presence of obstruction, peritonitis, or a mass.

Infant Less Than 2 Years Old

ACUTE PAIN

In evaluating the uncomfortable infant, as described in the algorithm, the clinician looks first at the onset of "pain," separating acute from recurrent. Then, an evaluation is made of additional symptoms as they occurred chronologically. Obstruction may present with isolated vomiting, and a low-grade fever suggests an inflammatory process, including peritonitis. Diarrhea as an early feature often heralds gastroenteritis. Cough (sometimes with posttussive emesis) may suggest pneumonia, bronchiolitis, or asthma. The story of episodic colicky pain with interposed quiet intervals, even in the absence of a "currant jelly" stool, makes one suspicious of intussusception or, occasionally, mid-gut volvulus.

An ileus, manifesting clinically with distension and absent bowel sounds, often accompanies surgical conditions, sepsis, and infectious enterocolitis. Ileus may be seen with pneumonia or a urinary tract infection (UTI). If an abdominal mass is palpable, intussusception, abscess, or neoplasm (commonly of renal origin) is likely. An incarcerated hernia and intussusception are the most common causes of obstruction in this age range. Signs of partial or complete obstruction with peritonitis indicate a per-

TABLE 42.1. Causes of Acute Abdominal Pain

Infancy (<2 yr)	Preschool age (2–5 yr)	School age (>5 yr)	Adolescent
		Common	
Colic (age <3 mo) Acute gastroenteritis "Viral syndromes"	Acute gastroenteritis Urinary tract infection Trauma Appendicitis Pneumonia, asthma Sickling syndromes "Viral syndromes" Constipation	Acute gastroenteritis Trauma Appendicitis Urinary tract infection Functional abdominal pain Sickling syndromes Constipation "Viral syndromes"	Acute gastroenteritis Gastritis (primary or alcohol-induced) Colitis (food intolerance) Trauma Constipation Appendicitis Pelvic inflammatory disease Urinary tract infection Pneumonia, bronchitis, asthma "Viral syndromes" Dysmenorrhea Epididymitis Lactose intolerance Sickling syndromes Mittelschmerz
		Relatively uncommon	
Trauma (possible child abuse) Intussusception Intestinal anomalies Incarcerated hernia Sickling syndromes	Meckel's diverticulum Henoch-Schönlein purpura (anaphylactoid purpura) Toxin Cystic fibrosis Intussusception Nephrotic syndrome	Pneumonia, asthma, cystic fibrosis Inflammatory bowel disease Peptic ulcer disease Cholecystitis, pancreatic disease Diabetes mellitus Collagen vascular disease Testicular torsion	Ectopic pregnancy Testicular torsion Ovarian torsion Renal calculi Peptic ulcer disease Cholecystitis or pancreatic disease Meconium-ileus equivalent (cystic fibrosis) Collagen vascular disease Inflammatory bowel disease Toxin
		Rare	
Appendicitis Volvulus Milk allergy Tumors (e.g., Wilms) Toxin (heavy metal) Disaccharidase deficiency Malabsorptive syndromes	Incarcerated hernia Neoplasm Hemolytic uremic syndrome Rheumatic fever, myocarditis, pericarditis Hepatitis Inflammatory bowel disease Choledochal cyst Hemolytic anemia Diabetes mellitus Porphyria	Rheumatic fever Toxin Renal calculi Tumor Ovarian torsion Meconium-ileus equivalent (cystic fibrosis) Intussusception Pyomositis of abdomen	Rheumatic fever Tumor Abdominal abscess

Modified from Liebman W, Thaler M. Pediatric considerations of abdominal pain and the acute abdomen. In: Sleisenger M, Fortran J, eds: *Gastrointestinal disease.* Philadelphia: WB Saunders, 1978.

forated viscus from intussusception, volvulus, or occasionally, appendicitis or Hirschsprung disease.

On auscultation of the chest, locally decreased or tubular breath sounds or adventitious sounds (i.e., crackles) suggest pneumonia. A "silent" pneumonia, particularly in a lower lobe, may present with abdominal pain and normal chest and abdominal examination. Abdominal pain and pallor can occur in neoplasia, as with bleeding into an abdominal Wilms tumor, hepatoma, or neuroblastoma. The presence of pallor and pain also raises the possibility of sickling hemoglobinopathies with the development of either a vasoocclusive crisis or a splenic sequestration. Abdominal pain may be associated with jaundice when rapid hemolysis is related to acute splenic enlargement or with every dysfunction in acute hepatitis. If bruising is noted, hemophilia or leukemia may be the cause of abdominal pain in the ill child. At times, an intraabdominal vasculitis that causes pain may precede the rash of Henoch-Schönlein purpura.

CHRONIC PAIN

When apparent abdominal pain is recurrent or chronic in infants less than 3 months of age and is not accompanied by other findings or symptoms, the physician often makes a diagnosis of "colic" (see Chapter 13). However, one must consider recurrent intussusception; malrotation with intermittent volvulus; milk allergy syndrome; and various malabsorptive diseases such as cystic fibrosis, celiac disease, and lactase deficiency.

LABORATORY TESTING

In most instances, the history and physical examination lead the emergency physician to the diagnosis.

Child 2 to 5 Years Old

ACUTE PAIN

Symptoms such as anorexia and vomiting suggest distension of an intraabdominal viscus; rectal bleeding points to infectious enterocolitis, intussusception, Meckel's diverticulum, or more rarely, inflammatory bowel disease (IBD). Extraabdominal complaints, such as cough, sore throat, and headache, are commonly present; they often indicate a viral syndrome, pharyngitis, or pneumonia. Urinary symptoms may occur with pyelonephritis, and polydipsia with polyuria may herald the onset of diabetes mellitus with abdominal pain from ketoacidosis. Children with known past intraabdominal pathology or surgery may develop complications of their prior illnesses.

The presence of guarding or persistent abdominal tenderness with gentle palpation warns the emergency physician of a serious abdominal emergency. Persistent right lower quadrant pain or tenderness on palpation alone suggests a need for surgical evaluation. This is the most consistent finding in patients discharged to home with early appendicitis. Usually, during a quiet, relaxed examination, the pain from gastroenteritis abates; other "referred" abdominal pains (e.g., from pneumonia or tonsillitis) often seem to disappear when the child is reassessed in a calm fashion. Ill children with abdominal pain occasionally have life-threatening diseases (Table 42.2) or the more uncommon diseases (Table 42.1). The physical examination of such patients may show jaundice (hepatitis, hemolytic anemia), rash or arthritis (Henoch-Schönlein purpura), cardiac murmurs (rheumatic fever), friction rubs (pericarditis), or "acetone" on the breath (diabetes mellitus).

CHRONIC PAIN

A history of recurrent abdominal pain suggests conditions such as sickle cell anemia, IBD, cystic fibrosis, or asthma. Chronic constipation can occur in children between 2 and 5 years of age, but true psychogenic or other nonorganic abdominal pain is fairly uncommon in this preschool age group.

Child 5 to 12 Years Old

ACUTE PAIN

The presence of fever, cough, vomiting, and/or sore throat suggests an infectious cause. Associated diarrhea may be from infectious colitis, IBD, or an appendiceal abscess irritating the bowel. A genitourinary history of discharge or suspicion of sexual abuse may be difficult to elicit in this age range but must be sought. With UTIs, urinary frequency and dysuria usually occur. Finally, pain that begins periumbilically and migrates to the right lower quadrant after several to 24 hours suggests appendicitis, a more common diagnosis in the older child.

Localized tenderness in the right lower quadrant or diffuse tenderness with involuntary guarding raise the suspicion of appendicitis or other diseases that cause peritonitis.

As in younger children, it is critical to assess for an atypical presentation of appendicitis. Careful extraabdominal examina-

TABLE 42.2. Life-Threatening Causes of Acute Abdominal Pain

Infancy (<2 yr)	Preschool age (2–5 yr)	School age (5–12 yr)	Adolescent (>12 yr)
		Abdominal	
Intestinal anomalies (generally <1 mo) Intussusception Trauma (possible child abuse) Severe gastroenteritis (with prostration) Incarcerated hernia Hirschsprung disease Volvulus Appendicitis Tumors (e.g., Wilms)	Trauma Intussusception Appendicitis Incarcerated hernia Meckel's diverticulum Obstruction secondary to prior abdominal surgery Peritonitis (i.e., nephrosis)	Trauma Appendicitis Megacolon (from inflammatory bowel disease) Peptic ulcer disease (with perforation) Peritonitis (primary or secondary) Aortic aneurysm Acute, fulminant hepatitis	Trauma Ectopic pregnancy Appendicitis Intraabdominal abscess secondary to pelvic inflammatory disease, cholecystitis, appendicitis, inflammatory bowel disease Peptic ulcer disease—bleeding or perforation Pancreatitis Megacolon (from inflammatory bowel disease) Aortic aneurysm Acute fulminant hepatitis
		Nonabdominal	
Metabolic acidoses secondary to inborn errors of metabolism, heart disease Toxic overdose Sepsis Hemolytic uremic syndrome	Toxic overdose[a] Hemolytic-uremic syndrome Diabetic ketoacidosis Sepsis Myocarditis, pericarditis	Toxic overdose[a] Sepsis Diabetic ketoacidosis Collagen vascular disease	Collagen vascular disease Diabetes mellitus (infection or ketoacidosis) Drug abuse/overdose

[a] Alcohol, amphetamines, aspirin, insecticide, iron, lead, phencyclidine, plants.

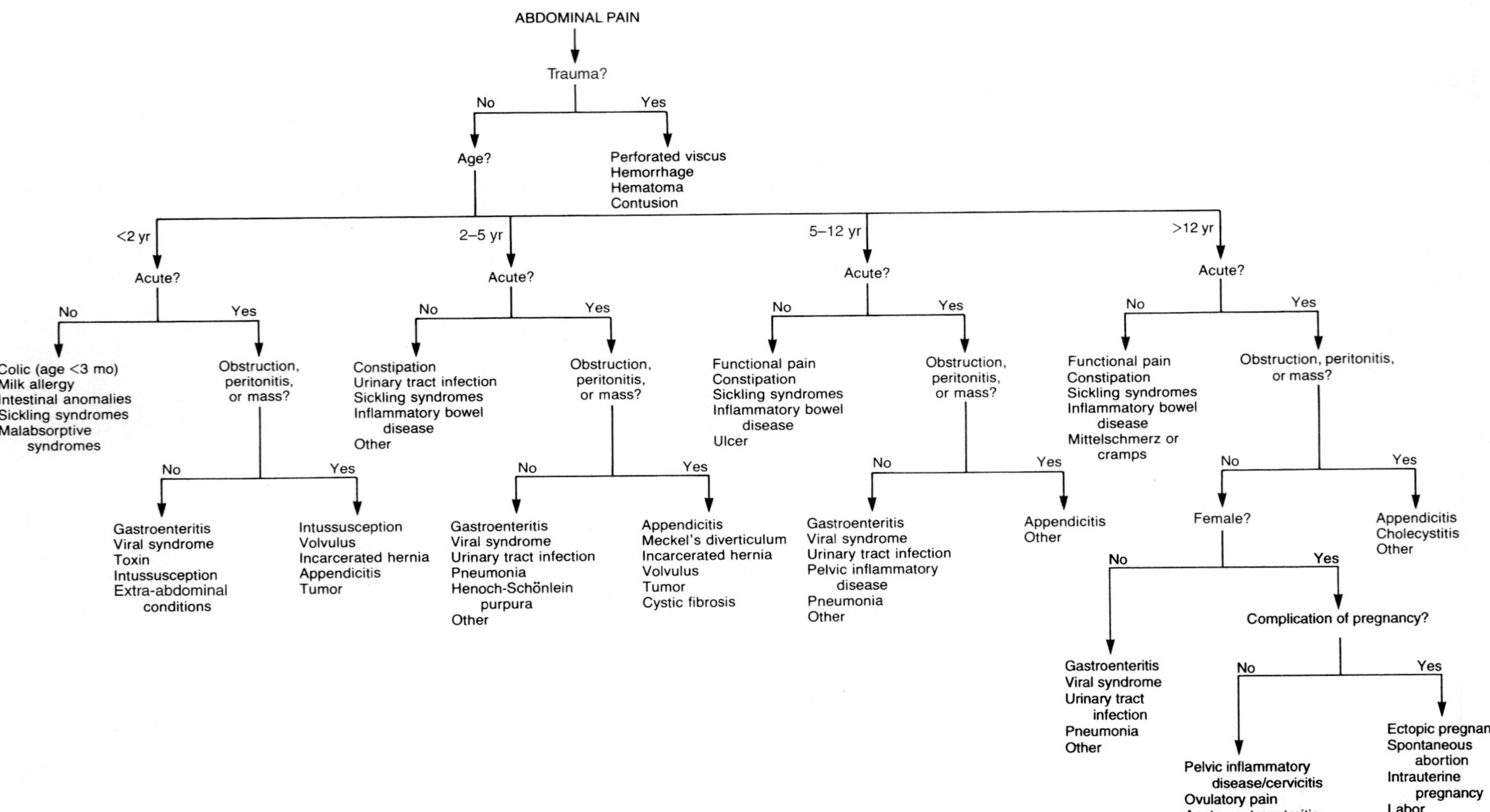

Figure 42.1. Evaluation of the child with abdominal pain.

tion is paramount to discover many of the infectious causes of abdominal pain. Rectal examination should be performed along with visualization of the genitalia in the young girl while in the knee–chest or frog leg position (see Chapter 83).

CHRONIC PAIN

Chronic abdominal pain may occur as a result of many of the conditions listed in Table 42.1. Important considerations are chronic infection with an enteric pathogen and IBD. When the history and physical examination suggest a mild, self-limiting disease or a nonorganic basis for the abdominal pain, however, the emergency physician should refrain from overusing the laboratory or radiography department to allay the parents' fear of organicity. The syndrome of functional abdominal pain precipitates more than 80% of outpatient physician visits by children for abdominal pain. The presentation of such pain is generally episodic, emanating from the umbilicus and, by definition, has no organic cause. The pain rarely occurs during sleep and has no particular associations with eating, exercise, or other activities.

Adolescent More Than 12 Years Old

ACUTE PAIN

Acute pain with peritonitis in the adolescent boy usually results from appendicitis. Assessment also must include that for testicular torsion or epididymitis. The adolescent girl with peritoneal findings may have appendicitis, pelvic inflammatory disease (PID), or less commonly, cholecystitis or ectopic pregnancy.

Boys without peritoneal signs often have gastroenteritis or a viral syndrome. Girls are more prone to UTIs or pyelonephritis; ectopic pregnancy, although uncommon, must be considered because this diagnosis may not produce peritoneal irritation before rupture. Gravid girls may be suffering from a complication of pregnancy or any of the usual disorders that cause abdominal pain as listed in Tables 42.1 and 42.2.

CHRONIC PAIN

Chronic abdominal pain in the adolescent is similar to that in the younger child, with the exception of an increased prevalence of IBD and the need in girls to consider long-standing gynecologic ailments such as dysmenorrhea, endometriosis, and chronic PID. It is particularly difficult to establish the cause of chronic pain when dealing with adolescents on an episodic basis, making appropriate referral essential.

CHAPTER 43
Pain—Back

Howard M. Corneli, M.D.

As a rule, back pain in children is meaningful until proved otherwise. Although back pain is less common in children than in adults, it is also far more likely to signify pathology.

DIFFERENTIAL DIAGNOSIS

A complete list of causes might run for pages, but for our purposes, we can divide the likely childhood causes into a few categories (Table 43.1). Trauma is a major problem in children. Acute injury, especially with axial loading, may cause compression fractures, which are more common in children. Compression fractures present with localized pain over the affected vertebra or vertebrae. The signs of back strain and lumbar disc herniation are similar to those in the adult, but in adolescence, these diagnoses should be made with caution, and in childhood, they are distinctly rare.

TABLE 43.1. Causes of Back Pain

Traumatic, posttraumatic, or stress-induced
Compression fracture
Spondylolysis
Spondylolisthesis
Disc herniation (rare in childhood)
Muscle or ligament strain/overuse
Spinal epidural hematoma (traumatic or spontaneous)
Nontraumatic
Infectious

Injury may be less obvious when it is chronic or recurrent. Especially common among adolescents is spondylolysis. This represents a weakening or discontinuity of the pars interarticularis, which connects the vertebrae at the facet joints. If the vertebra slips forward on the one beneath, the resulting condition is called spondylolisthesis. Either condition can cause back pain, most often in the lower lumbar area or at the L5–S1 level. Another condition linked to overuse, Scheuermann disease, is seen especially in adolescents as anterior wedging of several vertebrae, especially in the thoracic spine.

Rare but dangerous causes of back pain deserve special vigilance in the child. A spinal epidural hematoma may follow a fall or blow, sometimes presenting days later, or it may arise spontaneously, especially in patients with bleeding disorders or those who are receiving anticoagulant therapy. Back pain may only briefly precede symptoms of spinal cord compression. Spinal epidural abscess may present with back pain, low-grade fever, and signs of spinal cord compression. Percussion usually elicits spinal tenderness.

Infectious causes of back pain are many. Vertebral osteomyelitis and discitis present in a similar fashion. A limp or failure to bear weight may be more obvious than back pain in the young child, who is most susceptible to these infections. Paraspinal or psoas abscess and pyomyositis in paraspinal or pelvic muscles may present as back pain. Iliac osteomyelitis and sacroiliac joint infection also may present as back pain. Osteomyelitis of the ribs occurs rarely. The more rare infections include spinal tuberculosis (Pott disease) and brucellosis, in which small vertebral abscesses may accompany lymphadenopathy and hepatosplenomegaly.

Infections outside the musculoskeletal axis that cause back pain include urinary tract infection (UTI), which may cause flank pain with or without upper tract infection; pneumonia; and meningitis. These infections in children may lack the obvious symptoms seen in older patients. Pneumonia can be surprisingly silent. Cough may be minimal. Meningitis occasionally may be identified by parents primarily as back pain. This is especially true in infants who are noted to fuss when moved; a parent may note that it hurts the child to move the back. Myalgias and generalized backache may be seen in influenza, mononucleosis, streptococcal pharyngitis, and other generalized infections. Postinfectious conditions include transverse myelitis, which may follow an upper respiratory infection; back pain may precede weakness by as much as 1 to 2 days.

Abdominal conditions that may present as back pain include pancreatitis, in which the steady, penetrating pain radiates prominently to the back. Gallbladder pain may radiate to the back as well, and appendicitis, especially in a retrocecal location, can cause radiation to the back or pain and tenderness in the flank.

Collagen vascular diseases that cause back pain include ankylosing spondylitis and juvenile rheumatoid arthritis (with sacroiliitis), especially pauciarticular type II disease. Both of these conditions chiefly affect boys over 8 years of age. The back is notably stiff to flexion, especially in the lumbar region. Spondylitis also may be seen in association with Reiter syndrome, regional enteritis, ulcerative colitis, and psoriasis.

A painful, rapidly progressive scoliosis or atypical curvature suggests serious spinal pathology, often with neuromuscular involvement. Idiopathic scoliosis demonstrates back pain only in the most severe cases.

A host of neoplastic causes, both benign and malignant, may present with back pain (Table 43.1). These are not so rare that they can be ignored in any evaluation of back pain. Ewing sarcoma may mimic infection, with fever, leukocytosis, and rarefaction of bone on radiographs. Leukemia, and especially lymphoma, may present as back pain.

Sickle cell disease and other hemoglobinopathies may cause back pain. Dissecting aortic aneurysm has been reported rarely in children, usually with hypertension or with Marfan syndrome and other connective tissue disorders. Table 43.1 lists other miscellaneous causes of back pain.

Psychogenic back pain should be diagnosed with caution in children. Even if suspicion of a psychological component exists, a thorough investigation should be undertaken to exclude organic causes.

EVALUATION AND DECISION

The first task in a child with back pain is to rule out any sign of neurologic involvement. (Fig. 43.1). Conditions that affect the

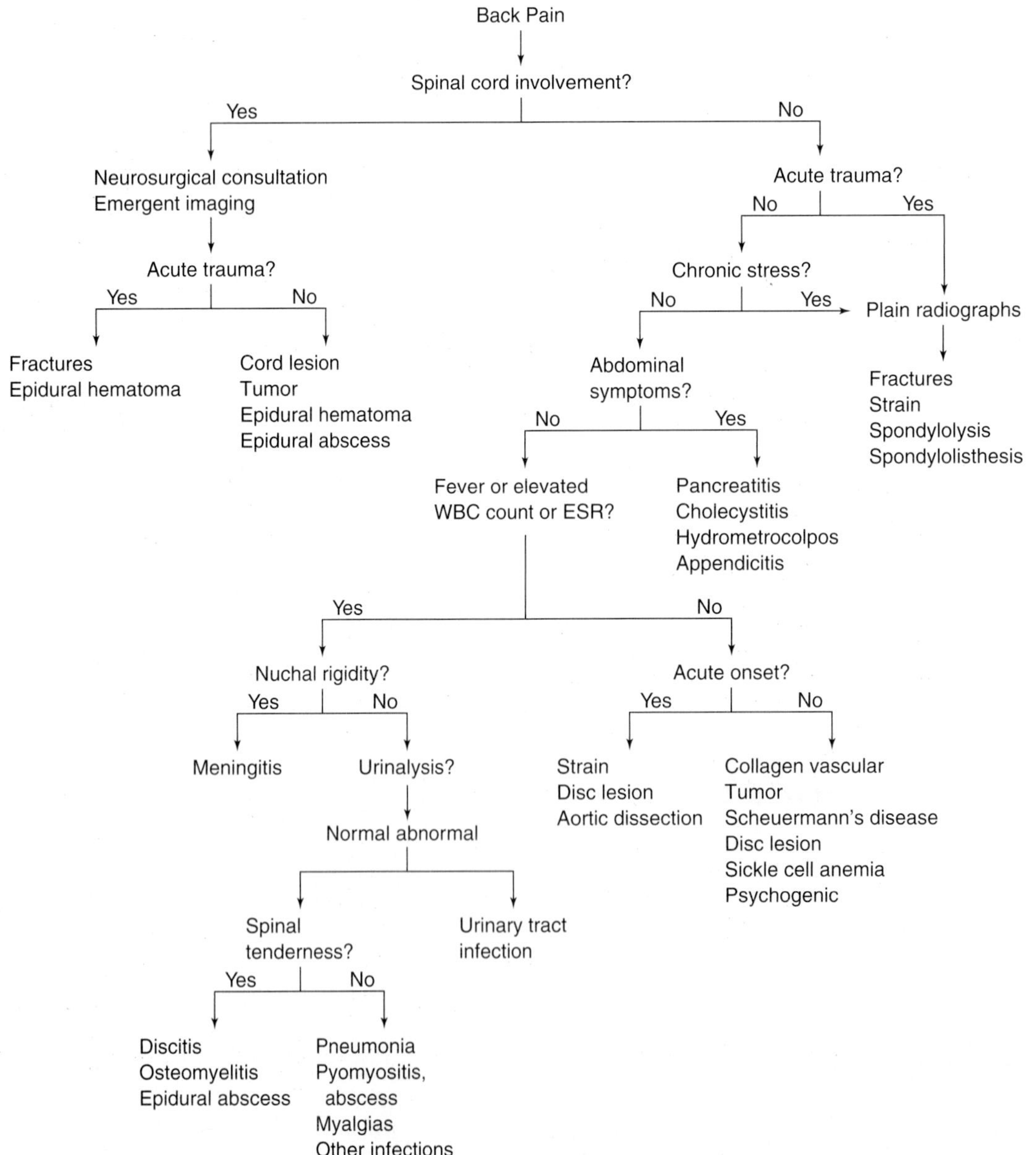

Figure 43.1. Approach to the diagnosis of back pain. *WBC*, white blood cell; *ESR*, erythrocyte sedimentation rate.

spinal cord are seen often enough in children that their gravity should be borne in mind throughout the evaluation.

Systemic symptoms should be carefully reviewed. Fever, fatigue, poor appetite, weight loss, or a decrease in walking or weight bearing usually signify a worrisome illness. Night pain that awakens the patient from sleep is associated with spinal tumor and, if relieved by aspirin or nonsteroidal antiinflammatory drugs, suggests osteoid osteoma or osteoblastoma. Sciatica may signify disc herniation, especially in the adolescent athlete or laborer.

A history of trauma is important in evaluating back pain but may be misleading in the young child whose frequent minor injuries may be seen by the parents as the trigger for a problem that actually is nontraumatic. Adolescents with stress injuries may not identify trauma in connection with back pain. Certain injury histories suggest specific diagnoses; vertical loading of the spine, as when a child lands in a seated position after a fall, often is associated with compression fractures of the vertebrae.

In adolescents with back pain, a history should be sought of sports-related, lifting-related, or work-related exposures to back stress. Weight lifters, gymnasts, football players, and participants in many similar sports have well-known tendencies to hyperextend the back. Unfortunately, not all teenagers who develop stress injuries are engaged in such easily identified activities. As excessive competition in sports is introduced to younger and younger children, such injuries may be seen earlier in childhood.

Fever is likely, of course, to signify infection, and infection both in the back and in adjoining areas is a common cause of back pain. However, fever is sometimes seen with neoplastic and collagen vascular causes of back pain. Even more importantly, children with musculoskeletal infections are afebrile at presentation in a significant proportion of cases.

Age may be suggestive of cause. The preschool-age child is unlikely to have overuse injuries, spondylolysis, or ankylosing spondylitis; however, infectious causes are more likely at this age. Family history may be positive in ankylosing spondylitis and related conditions. History may reveal an underlying disease, chronic inactivity (in the bedridden child), or drug therapy that may cause osteoporosis, which increases the risk of bony injury, especially compression fracture.

Chronicity of back pain may suggest collagen vascular conditions, Scheuermann disease, or perhaps, a developmental defect in the spine, but tumors may progress slowly with chronic back pain being the only noted symptom. Likewise, the acute onset of pain or neurologic symptoms often may be the first signs of a chronic (but expanding) mass lesion.

In many cases, the cause of back pain remains obscure even after a thorough history and physical examination. Here, the physician faces an important decision. In the younger child, it is appropriate to seek consultation or to proceed to imaging studies. Plain films may reveal a narrowed disc space in discitis; bone scan may reveal discitis or vertebral osteomyelitis, even in the absence of fever and bony changes; magnetic resonance imaging (MRI) may reveal a spinal or paraspinal tumor. In the preteen or teenage patient, a history of likely back strain (or the appearance of clues to psychosomatic pain previously mentioned) may warrant a trial of empiric therapy; even here a complete physical examination and screening radiographs and laboratory studies should be documented, and close follow-up should be ensured. (Further treatment of the varying causes of back pain is discussed in specific sections of this book.)

CHAPTER 44
Pain—Chest

Mary D. Patterson, M.D. and
Richard M. Ruddy, M.D.

The complaint of chest pain uncommonly represents a life-threatening emergency in children, in contrast to the same complaint in adults. This chapter first briefly reviews the pathophysiology of chest pain, then outlines the differential diagnosis in children, and finally presents the evaluation, as appropriate in the emergency department.

DIFFERENTIAL DIAGNOSIS

A differential diagnosis of chest pain in children is included in Table 44.1. Most chest pain in children is caused by acute respiratory disease, musculoskeletal injury, anxiety, or inflammation (Table 44.2). Often, the physician does not make a causative diagnosis of the chest pain and calls it idiopathic in origin. This idiopathic chest pain actually may be unrecognized organic disease, such as gastroesophageal reflux. Although much less common, chest pain in association with cardiorespiratory distress demands immediate attention. Table 44.3 lists the life-threatening causes of chest pain by disease and mechanisms for decompensation.

In the case of trauma, cardiac or pulmonary compromise may arise from direct injury to the heart, great vessels, or lung (see Chapter 94). Chest pain in the nontraumatized, yet dyspneic or cyanotic patient, most often stems from a respiratory problem, such as acute pneumonitis, empyema, pleurisy, asthma, or pneumothorax (either spontaneous or associated with cystic fibrosis [CF] or asthma). Rarely, severe chest pain in an acutely ill child results from a myocardial infarction (MI) that comes from aberrant coronary vessels, other underlying cardiac diseases (aortic stenosis), an acute arrhythmia, pericardial disease, or pulmonary embolus. Pediatricians do not often think of pulmonary embolus early on. Usually, this may have associated risk factors, such as recent trauma, particularly spinal injury, or known cardiorespiratory problems. More recently, acute chest pain associated with ischemia, arrhythmia, or myocardiopathy may be secondary to acute or chronic cocaine exposure. Nonorganic chest pain may appear to cause respiratory distress in the hyperventilating teenager, but close examination should distinguish this syndrome from serious problems.

Mild to moderate strain or injury from exercise or trauma may produce a contusion or rib fracture. Inflammation of nerves, muscles, bones, costochondral junctions, the esophagus, or the lower respiratory tract often causes organic chest pain. Both respiratory infection (pneumonia or bronchitis) and allergic respiratory disease (asthma) are important causes to consider. Spontaneous pneumomediastinum and pneumothorax may occur in patients with reactive airway disease, CF, or as a result of barotrauma (e.g., Valsalva maneuver, forceful vomiting or coughing). Aspiration of a foreign body into the trachea or esophagus may occur without such history in a toddler or even in an older child. Unrecognized disease rarely causes isolated chest pain in a child who otherwise appears well, but the physician should consider drug exposure (e.g., cocaine, methamphetamine, nicotine, β-agonist abuse). In addition, attention should be paid to diagnosing the rare patient with progressive obstructive heart disease, angina, mitral valve prolapse, or early

TABLE 44.1. Causes of Chest Pain

Musculoskeletal/neural	Pneumonia
Muscle	Cystic fibrosis
Trauma—contusions, lacerations	Pneumothorax, hemothorax, chylothorax
Infection—myositis	Empyema
Texidor twinge	Subphrenic abscess
Breast	Malignancy
Physiologic (fullness during menses or pregnancy)	Postpericardiotomy syndrome
Mastitis	Pulmonary embolus/infarction
Fibrocystic disease	Vasoocclusive crisis (sickle cell anemia)
Tumor (adenoma, other)	Cholecystitis
Bone	Pneumomediastinum
Trauma—contusions, rib fractures	*Esophageal*
Osteitis, osteomyelitis	Foreign body
Costochondritis	Caustic ingestion
Tumor—eosinophilic granuloma, other	Chalasia (esophagitis)[a]
"Slipping rib" syndrome	Infection–*Candida*
Intercostal nerve	*Cardiac (angina, pericardial, aortic)*
Neuritis—zoster, trauma	Angina—coronary insufficiency, anomalous vessels, pulmonary hypertension[b]
Toxin	Obstructive heart disease
Dorsal root	Aortic stenosis, pulmonary stenosis
Trauma	Asymmetric septal hypertrophy (IHSS)
Radiculitis—viral, postviral	Pericardial defects and effusions, pericarditis
Spinal disease—scoliosis	Acute arrhythmias[b]
Tracheobronchial (proximal bronchi)	Myocarditis[b]
Foreign body	Aortic aneurysm—idiopathic, syphilitic, Marfan syndrome
Infection	*Central*
Tracheitis	Anxiety—hyperventilation
Bronchitis	Idiopathic
Pneumonia	
Cystic fibrosis	
Asthma	
Pleural (parietopleura and diaphragm)	
Trauma—penetrating	
Pleurisy—viral, mycobacterial	

[a] Associated mitral valve prolapse.
[b] Associated drug-induced (especially cocaine).

pericardial or myocardial inflammation (see Chapter 72). A large group of children (up to 50%) will be left whose pain best fits into an anxiety-induced or idiopathic category.

EVALUATION AND DECISION

Child with Thoracic Trauma

If any evidence of trauma to the chest exists (see Chapter 94), the patient requires rapid evaluation and may need immediate resuscitation as well (Fig. 44.1A). Correction of cardiac or respiratory insufficiency may diagnose, as well as treat, the cause of chest pain. Alveolar ventilation should be assessed for adequacy and bilateral symmetry to distinguish acute respiratory failure from hemothorax or pneumothorax. In children with chest trauma, tachycardia with hypotension generally is caused by hypovolemia secondary to a hemothorax, hemopneumothorax, or vascular injury. Reduced cardiac output and perfusion, however, also may be secondary to a rhythm disturbance (from a myocardial contusion, tension pneumothorax) or cardiac tamponade (which causes muffling of the heart sounds and pulsus paradoxus). A discrepancy of the pulse or blood pressure between the extremities points to aortic diseases, such as traumatic avulsion or aneurysm, as the cause of chest pain. Ruptured esophagus and tracheobronchial disruption may result from rapid deceleration injuries and may present with chest pain, respiratory distress, and hypotension.

Many children with thoracic injuries but no respiratory distress also complain of chest pain. Although a careful examination is mandatory in an effort to exclude significant intrathoracic trauma, the cause of the pain usually resides in the chest wall: contusions of the soft tissues or rib fractures. Rib fractures in young infants suggest child abuse. In older children, a predisposing cause for fracture (e.g., bone cyst, tumor) should be sought.

TABLE 44.2. Common Causes of Chest Pain

Functional (anxiety/psychosomatic)
Musculoskeletal contusion/strain
Costochondritis/myositis
Cough or respiratory infections (bronchitis, pneumonia, pleurisy, upper respiratory infections)
Asthma
Gastroesophageal reflux
Idiopathic

Child with No Thoracic Trauma

Initially, the physician needs to assess for cardiorespiratory instability. Next, the physician should inquire about a history suggestive of prior cardiorespiratory disease (Fig. 44.1B). Children with respiratory illnesses such as asthma or CF are at

TABLE 44.3. Life-Threatening Causes of Chest Pain

Category	Disease/injury	Decompensation
Traumatic	Rib fracture	Tension pneumothorax or shock from hemothorax
	Cardiac contusion	Arrhythmia or myocardial infarction
	Laceration—heart or great vessel	Shock
	Contusion—great vessels	Dissecting aneurysm/shock
	Pulmonary contusion	Adult respiratory distress syndrome
Cardiac	Congenital heart disease (precorrection or postcorrection)	Arrhythmia, shock, pulmonary hypertension
	Myocardial infarction (anomalous coronary artery)	Arrhythmia, cardiogenic shock
	Myocarditis	Arrhythmia, cardiogenic shock
	Pericarditis	Tamponade
	Rheumatic heart disease	Arrhythmia, congestive heart failure
	Aortic aneurysm	Rupture-shock, dissection
	Obstructive cardiac disease	Acute hypertension
Pulmonary	Pneumothorax (asthma, cystic fibrosis, spontaneous)	Tension pneumothorax, pulmonary hypertension, shock
	Hemothorax	Shock, hypoxemia
	Pulmonary infection or empyema	Pulmonary hypertension, sepsis
	Aspiration—foreign body	Acute airway obstruction, progressive pulmonary hypertension
	Acute asthma	Tension pneumothorax, pulmonary hypertension
	Pulmonary embolus	Pulmonary infarction, hypertension
	Pulmonary venoocclusive disease	Pulmonary hypertension
	Tumor (chest wall, chest, or mediastinum)	Airway compromise, progression of tumor
Miscellaneous	Drug ingestion/overdose (especially cocaine)	Arrhythmia, cardiomyopathy, shock
	Sickle cell crisis	Pulmonary infarction or hypertension
	Cholecystitis	Sepsis, peritonitis

risk for pneumothorax, acute respiratory failure from mucous plugging or pneumonitis, and acute pulmonary hypertension. Severe hypoxemia may accompany their chest pain. Auscultatory findings, such as rales or wheezing, may be minimal when obstructive pulmonary disease is moderately severe. In the child with a history of cardiac arrhythmias (see Chapter 72), congenital heart disease, cardiac surgery, or pericardial effusions, chest pain may signal an exacerbation of the underlying problem. Although uncommon in children, acute pulmonary embolus should be considered when chest pain

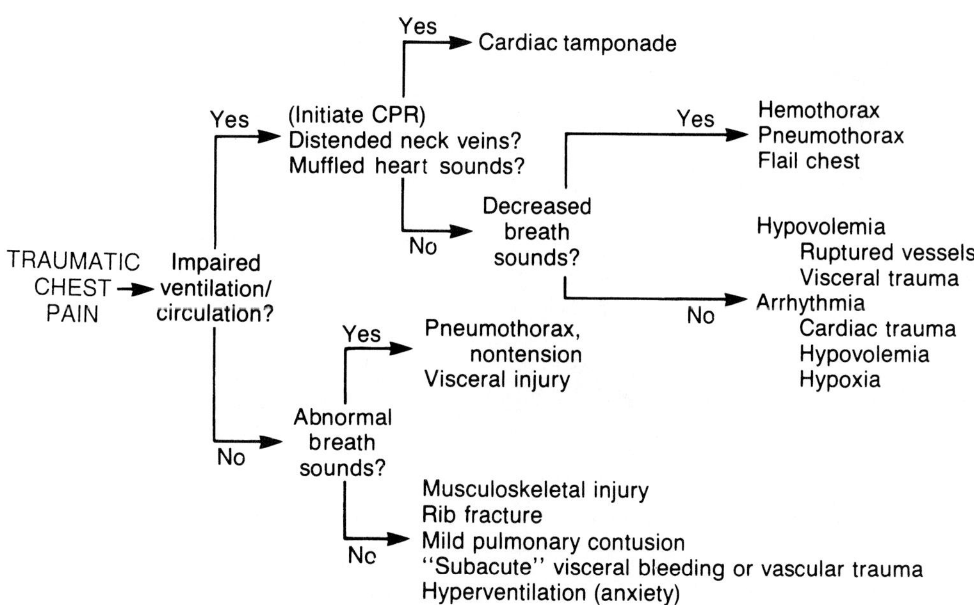

Figure 44.1A. Diagnostic approach to traumatic chest pain. *CPR,* cardiopulmonary resuscitation.

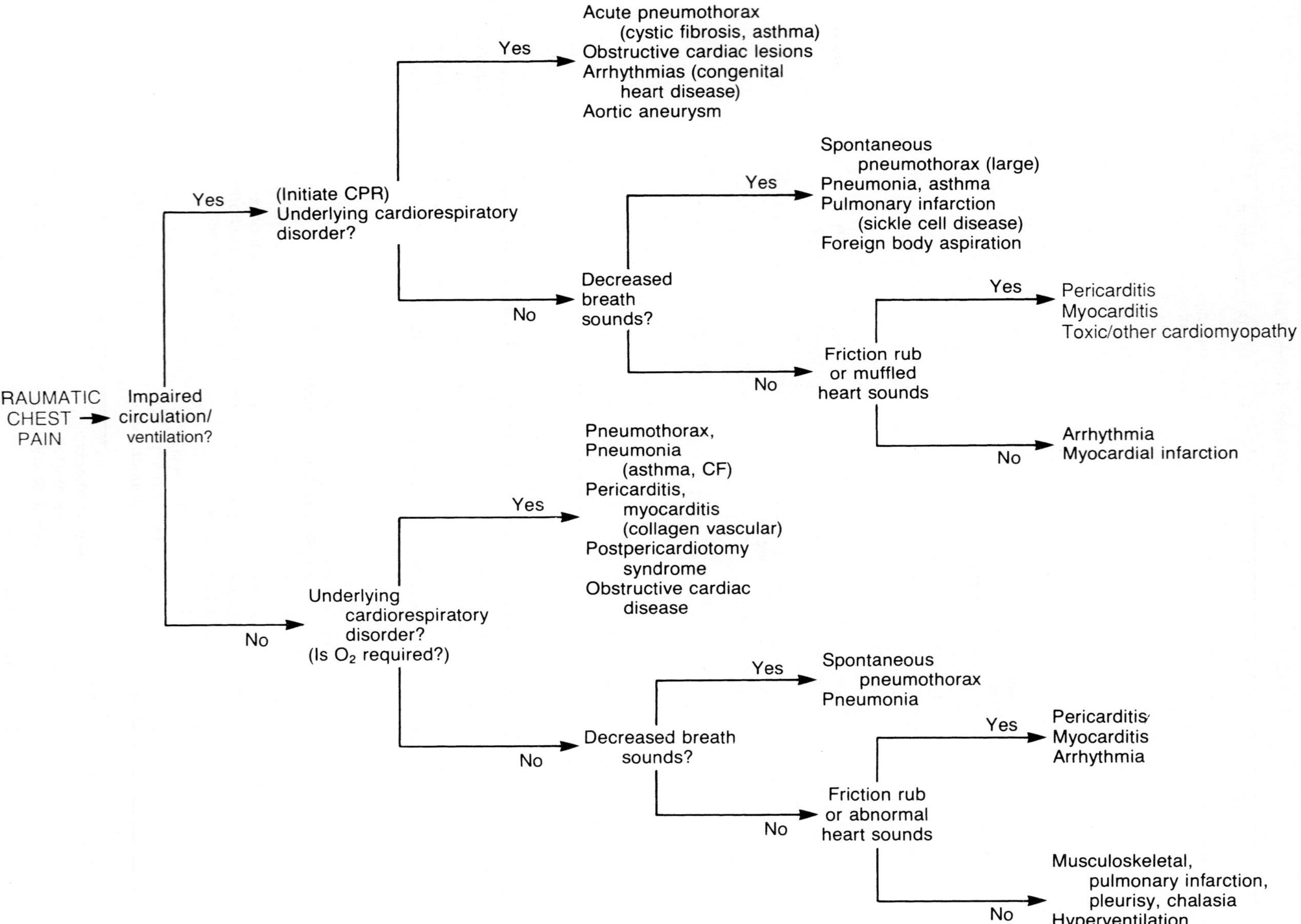

Figure 44.1B. Diagnostic approach to atraumatic chest pain. *CPR*, cardiopulmonary resuscitation; *CF*, cystic fibrosis.

with the sense of impending doom and/or risk factors (e.g., obesity, birth control pills, pregnancy, collagen vascular disease, nephrotic syndrome, cigarette smoking, recent surgery, a positive family history) is present. Pulmonary embolus may occur as a complication of an underlying disease, medical therapy, or surgical repair.

In the absence of prior cardiopulmonary disease or trauma, the approach must be directed toward unmasking evidence for any of the serious cardiorespiratory illnesses listed in Table 44.3. In particular, chest pain associated with exertion, syncope, or palpitations is concerning. A history of untreated Kawasaki disease or hyperlipidemia has been associated with MI at an early age. However, most children with chest pain will be found to have less severe acute inflammatory processes of the respiratory tract or musculoskeletal system or a psychosomatic disturbance.

Infectious diseases of the respiratory tract are associated with fever, malaise, cough, and coryza and may involve several family members simultaneously. A first asthmatic attack should be suspected when an associated night cough, history of wheezing, or family history of atopy is present. The physical examination in asthma shows a prolonged expiratory phase of respiration, variable degrees of chest hyperinflation, and wheezing accentuated by a forced expiratory effort. In musculoskeletal inflammation, one should be able to elicit tenderness of the chest wall and a "trigger point," where palpation reproduces the pain. Reproduction of the pain by a "hooking maneuver" performed over the lower anterior ribs implicates the "slipping rib syndrome." Pain following a dermatome unilaterally suggests intercostal neuritis; children with zoster (shingles) may have pain preceding the development of rash.

When focal, peripheral pain is found without a trigger point, the physician should consider pain referred from areas of sensory nerve overlap. A relationship of the pain to eating or swallowing suggests esophageal disease, and often, the physical examination may appear normal. Some of these patients will have a thin body habitus and/or cardiac findings of mitral valve prolapse. A foreign body (e.g., a coin) in the proximal esophagus commonly manifests with chest discomfort and drooling in the young child. Similarly, an aspirated foreign body may cause dull, aching chest pain associated with cough. Auscultation and plain radiographs of the chest do not always reveal the object or signs of an obstructed upper or lower airway. "Texidor twinge," or pericardial "catch," is a relatively common cause of short duration and sharp pain in healthy teenagers and young adults, often related to exercise and located in the left substernal region. It may be produced by stretching of the supporting ligaments of the heart and is easily distinguishable from angina by its sudden, stabbing onset, a duration of less than 60 seconds, and the absence of referral to other areas. Cigarette smoking has been associated with chest pain in teenagers and adults.

A thorough examination usually uncovers evidence of the cardiac and respiratory causes of chest pain listed in Tables 44.1 through 44.3. In addition to the usual cardiac and pulmonary examination, one should search for trigger points on the chest wall and changes in pain associated with positional changes. Chest pain relieved by leaning forward is consistent with pericarditis; whereas chest pain that is worsened by reclining may represent gastroesophageal reflux or hiatal hernia. Extrathoracic abnormalities, such as a rash or arthritis, may provide clues to collagen disorders or other systemic illness. Marfan syndrome should be suspected in the tall, thin patient whose upper extremity span exceeds his or her height. During examination of the heart and lungs, it is useful to relate normal findings to the child and family because this reassurance often serves as the major "treatment" of self-limiting or functional problems.

A large group of children with chest pain will have no evidence of organic disease and no history of underlying cardiorespiratory disease or trauma. They may have a family history of chest pain. Often, there will be a stressful situation that has precipitated the episode. Complaints of chest pain and other somatic aches often are chronic, with no abnormalities noted on the physical examination. Such children have psychogenic chest pain.

CHAPTER 45
Pain—Dysphagia

Ronald A. Furnival, M.D. and
George A. Woodward, M.D.

Dysphagia is defined as any difficulty or abnormality of swallowing. Dysphagia is not a specific disease entity but is a symptom of other, often clinically occult, conditions and may be life threatening if respiration or nutrition are compromised. Odynophagia (pain on swallowing) or sialorrhea (drooling) may also be present in the dysphagic pediatric patient.

DIFFERENTIAL DIAGNOSIS

The differential diagnostic list for dysphagia is extensive and is commonly divided into preesophageal or esophageal disorders (Table 45.1). Preesophageal causes of dysphagia are further subdivided into anatomic categories, including nasopharyngeal, oropharyngeal, laryngeal, and generalized problems. Infectious and inflammatory disorders of either anatomic region may disrupt swallowing, whereas neuromuscular problems tend to be predominantly preesophageal, given the autonomic function of the esophagus. However, the esophagus can be affected by motility disorders intrinsic to smooth muscle. Finally, the differential diagnosis includes several systemic conditions that may affect the normal swallowing process.

In the adult patient, dysphagia most commonly results from a variety of neuromuscular disorders, whereas the pediatric patient more often has swallowing difficulty from congenital, infectious, inflammatory, or obstructive causes (Table 45.2). In the newborn or infant, swallowing may be disturbed as a result of prematurity, often associated with respiratory and neurologic disabilities. Gastroesophageal reflux is common in infants, although in a small percentage of patients, it may persist into childhood with reflux esophagitis. Ingestion or aspiration of a foreign body must always be considered in the toddler who has either the acute or chronic onset of dysphagia.

Life-threatening causes of dysphagia may involve airway compromise, serious local or systemic infection, and inflammatory disease (Table 45.3). The newborn may have a congenital anatomic abnormality such as tracheoesophageal fistula, with aspiration of swallowed fluid into the lungs, or may have traumatic injury to the upper airway and esophagus from iatrogenic instrumentation in the delivery room. The older child may have a foreign body in the airway or esophagus, with the possibility of complete airway obstruction (see Chapter 22). Numerous infectious processes may present with dysphagia and can threaten airway integrity. These include epiglottitis, retropharyngeal abscess, Stevens-Johnson syndrome, and central nervous system (CNS) infections.

TABLE 45.1. Differential Diagnosis of Dysphagia

Preesophageal (nasopharynx, oropharynx, larynx)

Mechanical/anatomic

- General
  - Congenital syndromes
    - Pierre-Robin
    - Treacher-Collins
    - Crouzon
    - Goldenhar
    - Cornelia de Lange
  - Cysts (tongue, larynx, epiglottis)
  - Tumors (neuroblastoma)
  - Lymphangioma
  - Foreign body aspiration
  - Traumatic (external, endotracheal intubation, endoscopy)
- Nasopharyngeal
  - Choanal stenosis/atresia
  - Nasal septum deflections
- Oropharyngeal
  - Cleft palate/lip
  - Submucosal cleft
  - Macroglossia
    - Down syndrome (trisomy 21)
    - Beckwith-Wiedemann syndrome
  - Micrognathia
  - Lip/teeth defects
  - Tongue/sublingual masses
    - Hemangioma
    - Lymphangioma
    - Lingual thyroid
    - Thyroglossal duct cyst
    - Branchial cleft cyst
  - Hypopharyngeal stenosis
  - Temporomandibular joint ankylosis
  - Pharyngeal diverticula (congenital/traumatic)
  - Adenoidal/tonsillar hypertrophy
- Laryngeal
  - Tracheostomy
  - Tracheoesophageal fistula
  - Cervical vertebral osteophytes
  - Airway obstruction
  - Laryngomalacia

Inflammatory/infectious

- General
  - Tetanus
  - Botulism (especially infant botulism)
  - Poliomyelitis
  - Angioneurotic edema
  - Sydenham chorea
  - Juvenile rheumatoid arthritis
  - Stevens-Johnson syndrome
- Nasopharyngeal
  - Nasal septal abscess
  - Sinusitis
- Oropharyngeal
  - Stomatitis (infectious, allergic)
  - Retropharyngeal abscess
  - Peritonsillar abscess
  - Cervical adenitis
- Laryngeal
  - Epiglottitis
  - Diphtheria
  - Thyroiditis

Neuromuscular

- Prematurity
- Hypoxic injury
- Head trauma
- Neurologic impairment
  - Cerebral palsy
  - Developmental delay
  - Meningitis
  - Cerebral abscess
  - Cerebral cortical atrophy/hypoplasia/agenesis
  - Arnold-Chiari malformation
  - Cerebrovascular disease
- Cranial nerve palsies (V, VII, IX–XII)
  - Palatal paralysis
  - Laryngeal paralysis
- Spinal cord impairment
  - Syringomyelia
  - Cricopharyngeal incoordination/spasm
  - Moebius syndrome
  - Myotonic muscular dystrophy
  - Guillain-Barré syndrome
  - Werdnig-Hoffman
  - Myasthenia gravis
  - Myotonic dystrophy
  - Dermatomyositis

Miscellaneous

- Familial dysautonomia (Riley-Day syndrome)
- Prader-Willi syndrome
- Cerebrohepatorenal syndrome
- Vitamin deficiencies (pellagra, scurvy)
- Acrodynia
- Infantile Gaucher disease
- Psychiatric
  - Globus hystericus ("lump" in throat sensation)
  - Pseudodysphagia
  - Conversion reaction
  - Hyperphagia
  - Munchausen by proxy
- Respiratory distress

Esophageal causes of dysphagia

Mechanical/anatomic

- Tracheoesophageal fistula
- Esophageal atresia/stenosis
- Esophageal diverticula/duplication
- Esophageal strictures
  - Congenital (webs, fibromuscular, tracheobronchial remnants)
  - Acquired (corrosive ingestion, esophagitis, postoperative)
- Foreign body ingestion
- Thermal injury (burn from hot food/drink)
- Esophageal tumors (hamartomas, leiomyoma, rhabdomyoma)
- External esophageal compression
  - Cardiovascular anomalies (aberrant right subclavian artery, vascular rings, double aortic arch)
  - Mediastinal tumors/infiltrations
  - Atopic thyroid
  - Diaphragmatic hernias
  - Paraesophageal hernia
  - Hiatal hernia
- Altered esophageal motility
  - Achalasia
  - Gastroesophageal reflux
  - Esophageal spasm

Inflammatory/infectious

- Infectious esophagitis
  - *Candida albicans*
  - Herpes simplex
  - Cytomegalovirus
  - Human immunodeficiency virus
- Reflux esophagitis
- Allergic esophagitis
- Radiation injury
- Mediastinitis
- Esophageal perforation
- Crohn disease
- Chagas disease (*Trypanosoma cruzi,* a South American parasite)

Miscellaneous

- Connective tissue disease
  - Scleroderma
  - Systemic lupus erythematosus
  - Polymyositis
  - Dermatomyositis
  - Sjögren syndrome
  - Behçet's disease
- Hyperkalemia, hypermagnesemia
- Muscular hypertrophy of esophagus
- Central nervous system tumors
- Demyelinating diseases
- Epidermolysis bullosa congenita
- Lesch-Nyhan syndrome
- Wilson disease
- Dyskeratosis congenita
- Opiz-Frias syndrome
- Lipidosis
- Myxedema
- Thyrotoxicosis
- Alcoholism
- Diabetes
- Amyloidosis
- Posttruncal vagotomy, antireflux surgery

TABLE 45.2. Common Causes of Dysphagia

Newborn/infant	*Child*
Prematurity	Foreign body aspiration/ingestion
Tracheoesophageal fistula	Caustic ingestion
Choanal stenosis/atresia	Infectious
Birth trauma	Neurologic impairment (cerebral palsy, mental retardation, head trauma)
Congenital abnormalities	Inflammatory
Gastroesophageal reflux	
Respiratory illness	
Neurologic/neuromuscular disease	
Infectious (botulism, candidiasis, herpetic esophagitis)	
Inflammatory	

TABLE 45.3. Life-Threatening Causes of Dysphagia

Foreign body aspiration/ingestion	Polio
Tracheoesophageal fistula	Diphtheria
Upper airway obstruction	Central nervous system infection/abscess
Traumatic esophageal perforation	Stevens-Johnson syndrome
Epiglottitis	Corrosive ingestion
Retropharyngeal abscess	Laryngeal paralysis
Botulism	
Tetanus	

EVALUATION AND DECISION

The evaluation of dysphagia in the pediatric patient begins with a detailed history, including pregnancy and delivery, family history, feeding history, growth and development, and a history of other illness (Table 45.4). Evaluation of the stable dysphagic patient may proceed on the basis of age and acute versus chronic onset of symptom development (Fig. 45.1). The neonate and young infant will require evaluation techniques and consideration of the age-related differential diagnoses outlined in Table 45.2, whereas the older child with an acute onset of dysphagia generally requires a more urgent approach.

Prenatal polyhydramnios, maternal infection, maternal drug or medication use, bleeding disorders, thyroid dysfunction, toxemia, or irradiation may lead to swallowing problems in the newborn or infant (Fig. 45.1). Fetal neurologic development may be altered by prenatal difficulties and may result in dysphagia after birth. Maternal myasthenia gravis may also cause temporary feeding problems in the newborn. A history of traumatic delivery may result in neurologic injury or laryngeal paralysis. Newborn intubation may be associated with trauma to the trachea, larynx, or esophagus, as well as hypoxic brain injury. A history of prematurity, developmental delay, failure to thrive, hypotonia, or associated congenital abnormalities may indicate a neuromuscular cause for dysphagia. Anatomic abnormalities of the trachea, larynx, or esophagus commonly present in infancy as respiratory problems during feeding, although vascular lesions that result in extrinsic compression of the esophagus may remain silent until the introduction of solid foods, and occasionally into adulthood. Gastroesophageal reflux in infants may manifest as vomiting shortly after feeding or with a history of nighttime cough or emesis. Intrinsic lesions,

TABLE 45.4. Important Historical Features for Dysphagia

General	*Newborn/infant*
Age of onset	Prematurity
Acute/gradual onset	Pregnancy history
Weight gain	Infections
Growth and development	Medications (especially antihypertensives)
Periodic or constant	Bleeding
Pain (location/quality)	Toxemia
Fever	Thyroid dysfunction
Ingestion history (foreign bodies or caustics)	Polyhydramnios
Difficulty chewing	Fetal irradiation
Difficulty swallowing	Birth history
Change in voice quality	Birth trauma
Altered swallowing sensation (lump, sticking, or foreign body)	Hypoxia
	Endotracheal intubation or resuscitation
Drooling/salivation	Cough/gag/cyanosis/fatigue/stridor/irritability with feeding
Solid/liquid intolerance	
Cough/choking while feeding	Feeding times greater than 30 min
Respiratory symptoms after feeding (stridor, wheezing, or apnea)	Respiratory distress associated with feeding
	Vomiting or regurgitation
Vomiting (gastric contents) vs. regurgitation (food without gastric contents, esophageal disorders)	Level of alertness
	Weight gain or failure to thrive
	Nasal regurgitation
Nasopharyngeal regurgitation	Refusal to eat age-appropriate foods
Gastroesophageal reflux	Recurrent pneumonias
Peptic ulcer disease	Family history of neuromuscular disease
Tobacco or alcohol usage	
Recent esophageal or airway instrumentation	
Arthritis, degenerative joint disease	
Antibiotic use	
Chemotherapy	
Underlying illness, immunodeficiency	

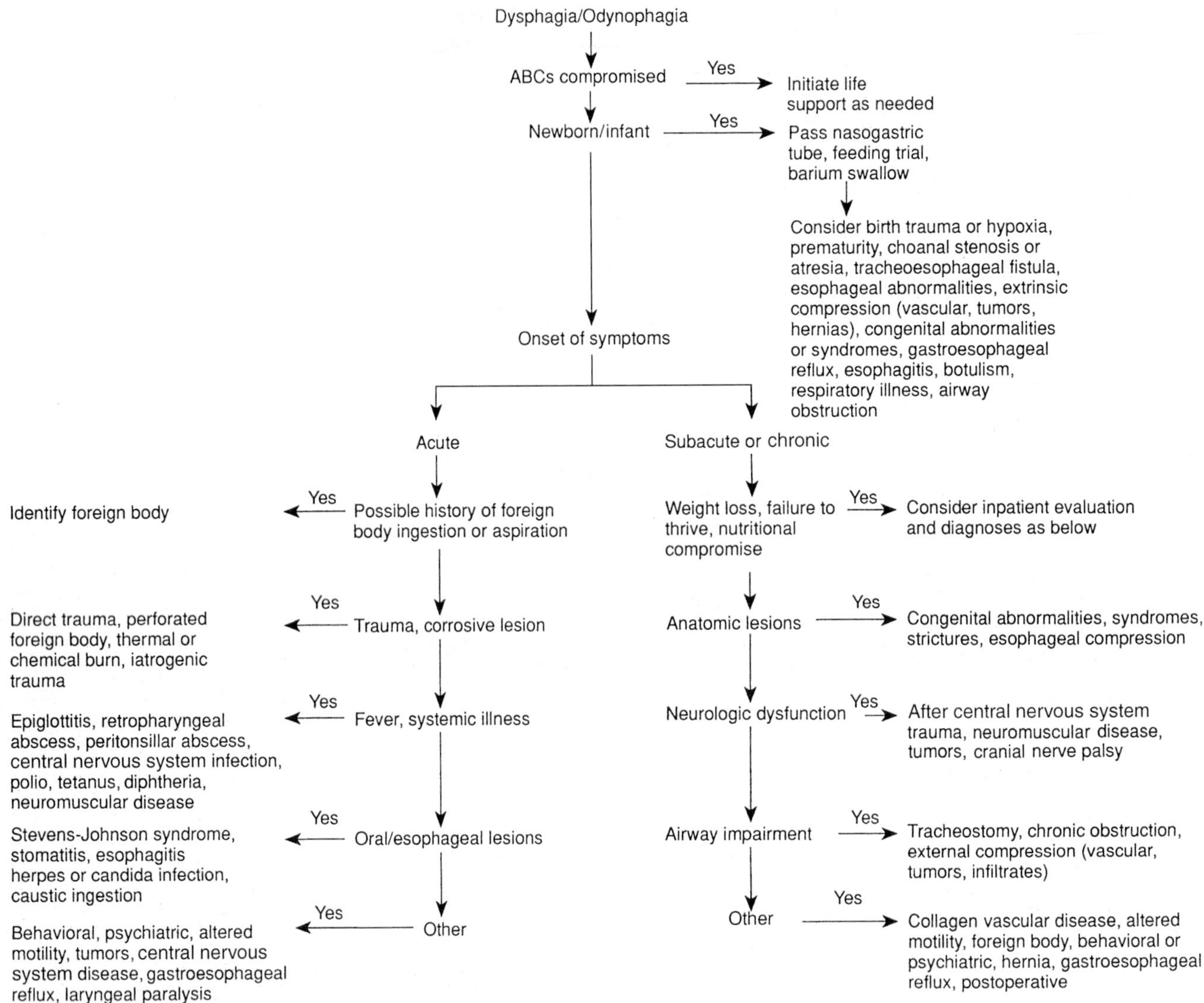

Figure 45.1. Evaluation scheme for the child with dysphagia or odynophagia. *Radiographic options:* neck, chest, abdomen, inspiratory/expiratory films, lateral decubitus films, fluoroscopy, contrast studies, ultrasonography, echocardiography, angiography, computed tomography, magnetic resonance imaging. *Laboratory options:* complete blood count, blood gas, cultures, toxin identifications, nutritional and electrolyte profiles. *Consultant options:* pediatrics, general surgery, otolaryngology, gastroenterology, neurology, infectious disease, cardiology, pulmonology, rheumatology, oncology, nutrition, speech therapy, occupational therapy.

from inflammation, tumor, or foreign body, may create problems with solid food but cause no difficulty with liquids. Infants with previously unrecognized neuromuscular disorders commonly present initially with dysphagia, particularly for liquids; drooling; prolonged feeding time; weak suckle; or nasal reflux of swallowed material. A history of fever may indicate an aspiration pneumonia or other infectious or inflammatory causes of dysphagia.

In the child beyond the neonatal period, witnessed or suspected foreign bodies, either ingested or aspirated, should be investigated with plain radiographs (or contrast studies if a radiolucent object is considered) and, if identified, emergently removed (see Chapter 22). A history of neck trauma or caustic ingestion should lead to the suspicion of aerodigestive tract abnormalities. These patients may present dramatically with neck pain, drooling, and evidence of facial or other trauma, but they may also have a subacute presentation (see Chapters 78, 93, and 98). Presence of fever or signs of systemic illness may result from potentially life-threatening infectious or inflammatory conditions (Table 45.3). Less severe problems (gingivostomatitis or thrush) may present with mouth lesions and can be managed on an outpatient basis after careful assessment of hydration status. Severe problems, including Stevens-Johnson syndrome, herpetic esophagitis, and diphtheria, may be discovered on a detailed examination and may require inpatient management.

Patients with a nonacute history of swallowing difficulty can be evaluated and treated as shown in Fig. 45.1. The initial emphasis with these patients lies more in determination of nutritional status and development issues than in acute emergency department intervention, although prolonged feeding difficulty can develop into a life-threatening problem. The child with obvious anatomic abnormalities, neurologic impairment, specific syndromes, or a tracheostomy may need referral to appropriate subspecialists after initial evaluation. The child without obvious anatomic or neurologic abnormality who has weight loss or failure to thrive may be evaluated as an outpatient.

Radiographic evaluation of the stable dysphagic patient usually begins with an examination of the airway and soft tissues of the neck, looking for evidence of a foreign body, mass, airway impingement, or other abnormality. A chest radiograph may suggest aspiration pneumonia, congenital heart disease, or mediastinal abnormality or, as in the patient with achalasia, demonstrate fluid levels within an enlarged esophagus. Computed tomography (CT) scan, echocardiography, or angiography may further identify problems suspected from initial studies.

Fiberoptic endoscopy under local or general anesthesia may be indicated for suspected mass lesion, stricture, caustic ingestion, inflammatory lesion, or foreign body. In addition, nasopharyngoscopy allows direct visualization of the swallowing process and can document aspiration and functional esophageal disorders.

CHAPTER 46
Dysuria

Gary R. Fleisher, M.D.

Dysuria, or the sensation of pain when voiding, stems from irritation of the bladder, the urethra, or both. In addition, (1) young children may complain of painful urination when they are instead experiencing related symptoms, such as pruritus, and (2) parents may interpret various nonspecific statements or behaviors by their children as indicative of painful urination. Dysuria is a commonly reported symptom that has a number of different causes (Table 46.1), but it usually stems from one of several common disorders of childhood and adolescence (Table 46.2). Most children with dysuria as a chief complaint have disorders of the genitourinary tract. Although patients with urethritis secondary to systemic illnesses may have dysuria as one of their many symptoms, it is only occasionally the principal reason for a visit to an emergency department (ED). Most diseases causing dysuria are self-limited or easily treated; however, the rarely seen systemic causes of urethritis or the spread of some bacterial pathogens beyond the genitourinary tract may be life threatening (Table 46.3).

DIFFERENTIAL DIAGNOSIS

Systemic Conditions

Systemic conditions of dysuria as listed in Table 46.1.

Stevens-Johnson syndrome is a severe manifestation of erythema multiforme, which may affect the mucous membranes throughout the body, producing conjunctivitis, oral ulceration, and urethritis. The rash that occurs in most patients often has the appearance of target lesions. Although usually self-limited, in some cases, pulmonary involvement leads to death. Reiter syndrome is characterized by conjunctivitis, arthritis, and urethritis. Rarely diagnosed, it is more common in males. Also rare, Behçet syndrome is another multisystem disease that may cause urethral ulceration and dysuria.

Localized Conditions

Localized conditions of dysuria are listed in Table 46.1.

Infection of the genitourinary tract is the predominant cause of dysuria. Pyelonephritis is the most serious of these disorders, usually manifesting with fever, often above 39°C (102.2°F), and flank pain or tenderness (older children and adolescents). Patients with cystitis may or may not have fever, which is usually low grade, and suprapubic pain or tenderness. Urethritis is a more localized infection, which often produces a discharge. In adolescents, *Neisseria gonorrhoeae* and *Chlamydia trachomatis* are the most common pathogens. When herpes simplex causes urethritis, vesicles are usually apparent on examination. Younger children may develop a nonspecific bacterial urethritis with involvement of the glans penis (balanitis) or both the glans and the prepuce (balanoposthitis).

In young children, certain drugs taken systemically and topical exposures to a variety of chemicals have been reported to irritate the urethral mucosa; however, these findings have not been well documented. Potential local irritants include detergents, fabric softeners, perfumed soaps, and possibly bubble baths. These patients have either no physical findings or only mild erythema but no discharge.

Minor injury is another relatively common cause of urethral irritation. In older children and adolescents, normal self-exploratory sexual play, masturbation, voluntary sexual activity, or sexual abuse may be the source of the trauma. As for patients with chemical urethritis, the examination is generally unremarkable.

TABLE 46.1. Causes of Dysuria

Systemic conditions	Chemical irritation
Stevens-Johnson syndrome	Detergents
Reiter syndrome	Fabric softeners
Behçet syndrome	Perfumed soaps
Localized conditions	Bubble baths (?)
Infection	Medication
Pyelonephritis	Trauma
Cystitis	Local injury
Viral	Masturbation
Bacterial (*Escherichia coli* and other organisms)	Miscellaneous
Urethritis/balanitis	Hypercalciuria/urinary stones
Neisseria gonorrhoeae	Labial adhesions
Chlamydia species	Psychogenic dysuria
Herpes simplex	*Complaints misinterpreted as dysuria*
Other	Pinworms
	Sexual abuse

TABLE 46.2. Differential Diagnosis of Common Causes for Dysuria

Disorder	Cause	Age	Fever	Tenderness
Pyelonephritis	*Escherichia coli*/other bacteria	All	Common, ≥38.5°C	Flank
Cystitis	Viruses/*E. coli*, other bacteria	All	Occasional, ≤38.5°C	Suprapubic
Infectious urethritis	*Neisseria gonorrhoeae*/ *Chlamydia trachomatis*	Adolescents	None	Prostate/pelvic (occasional)
Chemical/traumatic urethritis	Physical insult	Children	None	None

The passage of a stone is an uncommon cause of dysuria in children. In these cases, the dysuria is usually proceeded by flank pain and is often accompanied by hematuria. Labial adhesions occur relatively often in young girls. Although they are most often asymptomatic, they may cause dysuria on occasion. Throughout childhood and into adolescence, a complaint of dysuria may be psychogenic in origin, occurring in the absence of inflammation in the genitourinary tract.

Complaints Misinterpreted as Dysuria

Complaints misinterpreted as dysuria are listed in Table 46.1.

Enterobius vermicularis (pinworms) infests the perianal area, but occasionally spreads to the vagina in young girls. The pruritus that accompanies this infestation may be expressed as dysuria. Young children who have experienced sexual abuse may complain of pain in their genital area or may exhibit behaviors that are interpreted by adult observers as indicative of genital pain.

EVALUATION AND DECISION

When evaluating a child with dysuria, the physician should ask about trauma and exposure to chemicals such as detergents, fabric softeners, perfumed soaps, bubble baths, and medications that have been reported to irritate the mucosal lining of the urethra or bladder. A negative history for injury may not be accurate because most trauma is not recalled by young patients or, in the case of masturbation or abuse, may be denied. The detection of sexually transmitted diseases, a common cause of dysuria in adolescents, may be facilitated by obtaining a history about the nature and extent of sexual activity.

Some children may have a suggestive constellation of symptoms and signs in addition to dysuria. As examples, the adolescent girl with abdominal and pelvic discomfort probably has pelvic inflammatory disease and the 6-year-old child with fever and flank pain most likely has pyelonephritis. Various systemic disorders (Table 46.1) may cause conjunctivitis, oral ulceration, arthritis, and cutaneous lesions.

TABLE 46.3. Life-Threatening Causes of Dysuria

Stevens-Johnson syndrome
Gonococcal urethritis/vaginitis (when complicated by pelvic inflammatory disease or systemic spread)

In addition to a routine physical examination, special attention should be directed to the genitourinary tract. A swollen or edematous urethral meatus or a discharge from the urethra or vagina will localize the source of the symptoms in an otherwise well child to the genitalia, obviating the need to look extensively for other diseases. In particular, vesicles occur with infections caused by herpes simplex. Labial adhesions are easily recognized on inspection in young girls.

The most important tasks for the emergency physician are to recognize the rare but serious systemic syndromes and to diagnose or exclude infections (Fig. 46.1). If the history and general examination do not suggest a systemic condition, the next step is to examine the genitalia. Lesions in this area, such as vesicles or ulcers, are seen with Stevens-Johnson and Behçet syndromes, but they more likely represent an infection with herpes simplex, even in the preadolescent child.

A urethral or vaginal discharge suggests an infection of the genitalia: urethritis in the boy, and urethritis or vaginitis in the girl. *N. gonorrhoeae* is an organism that commonly causes disease in this area.

If no discharge is seen, the physician should obtain a urinanalysis and urine culture. A positive result on testing by dipstick (leukocyte esterase and/or nitrites) or the finding of pyuria (more than 5 to 10 white blood cells per high-power field) increases the likelihood of bacterial infection (urethritis, cystitis, or pyelonephritis) but does not prove the diagnosis. Inflammatory conditions, such as chemical urethritis, and nonbacterial infections may also evoke a leukocyte response.

In the young child with dysuria in the absence of pyuria, local trauma and chemical irritation are the most likely causes for the pain. Because a few children with urinary tract infections (UTIs) do not have either a positive result on testing by dipstick or pyuria, most physicians obtain a urine sample for culture, particularly from febrile patients. On the other hand, some experts would argue that the likelihood of infection is low enough in the absence of positive indicators on urine analysis that no further testing is needed. Adolescents require cultures of the genital tract to diagnose mild gonococcal or chlamydial infections.

When no other cause for dysuria is found in a prepubertal girl who has adhesions of her labia minora, these adhesions may be responsible for the painful urination. Most girls with labial adhesions, however, are asymptomatic. Thus, infection or another cause for dysuria should be excluded in girls with this finding.

A few patients with a normal examination and negative cultures may complain persistently of dysuria. In this setting, idiopathic hypercalciuria provides a potential diagnosis. If suspected, the diagnosis can be confirmed by measurement of

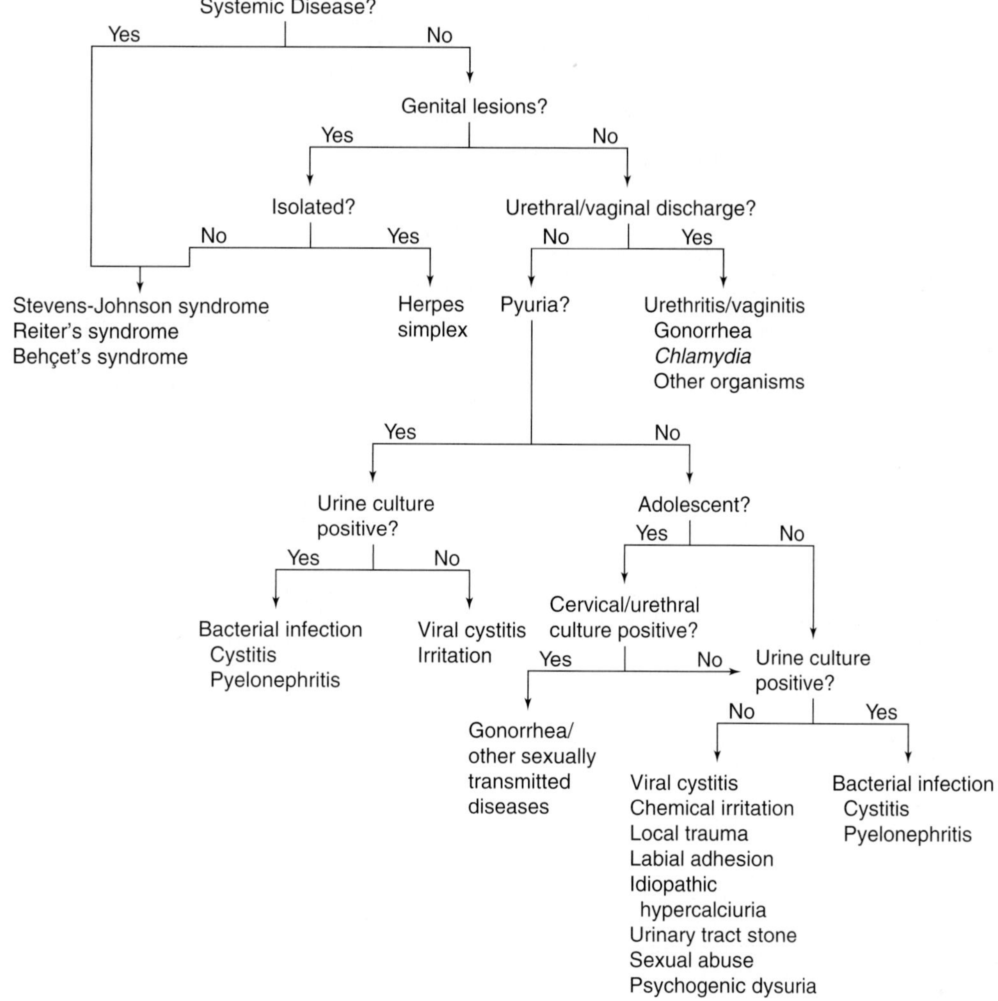

Figure 46.1. Approach to the diagnosis of dysuria.

calcium excretion in the urine. Another possible explanation is that the patient is experiencing vaginal pruritus secondary to pinworms. Confirmation of this diagnosis requires either identification of the larvae or ova or a response to a trial of mebendazole.

Last, the physician should give consideration to both sexual abuse and psychogenic dysuria. In most of these cases, further evaluation outside of the ED will be needed.

CHAPTER 47
Pain—Earache

Amy M. Arnett, M.D.

Ear pain is a common symptom of many different conditions in or around the ear (Tables 47.1 to 47.3). Preverbal children may present with fussiness, crying, or waking intermittently at night. Children may have difficulty differentiating tinnitus from ear pain. Ear pain may be otogenic or nonotogenic in origin. A complete history and physical examination is necessary, focusing not only on the ear but on adjacent areas and those regions innervated by nerves which also innervate the ear. Patients with accompanying central nervous system symptoms, vertigo, or cranial nerve deficits need more extensive evaluation.

DIFFERENTIAL DIAGNOSIS

Otogenic Causes

Trauma is usually evident by physical examination. Hematomas of the pinna resulting from blunt trauma may occur over the cartilaginous portion or upper half of the ear lobe between the perichondrium and the underlying cartilage.

The most common complication of ear piercing is superimposed infection—usually with *Staphylococcus aureus*. Nickel earrings may cause earlobe dermatitis. Preauricular pits are asymptomatic until they become infected. Physical examination reveals a warm, erythematous, tender area anterior to the tragus. Frostbite of the auricle is painful. The ear usually appears pallid secondary to vasoconstriction. With thawing, it becomes hyperemic and edematous, and vesicles may appear. Furunculosis is a Gram-positive, usually staphylococcal infection of a hair follicle at the external auditory meatus that causes marked pain and occasional otorrhea. This generally occurs in the cartilaginous part of the canal and may cause cervical adenopathy. Coalescence of furuncles produces a carbuncle or abscess, which

TABLE 47.1. Causes of Earache

Otogenic	Nonotogenic—referred pain
External	*Trigeminal nerve (V)*
Trauma	Oral cavity—stomatitis, gingivitis, trauma
Ear piercing—infection/dermatoses	Dental—impacted teeth, trauma, caries, abscess
Preauricular pit infection	Temporomandibular joint dysfunction
Frostbite	Sinusitis
Furunculosis	Mastoiditis
Herpes zoster oticus or Ramsay Hunt syndrome	Parotitis
Canal	*Facial nerve (VII)*
Otitis externa—swimmer's ear	Bell palsy
Otomycosis	Herpes zoster infection—Ramsay Hunt syndrome
Foreign body	*Glossopharyngeal nerve (IX)*
Dermatoses—seborrhea or psoriasis	Otopharynx—tonsillitis, posttonsillectomy, retropharyngeal abscess
Impacted cerumen	Nasopharynx
Trauma	*Vagus nerve (X)*
Tympanic membrane/middle ear	Larynx—trauma, foreign body
Acute otitis media	Esophagus—foreign body, burn
Otitis media with effusion/serous otitis media	*C2/C3*
Traumatic perforation	Lymphadenitis
Myringitis	Branchial cleft cysts
Hemotympanum	C-spine—trauma, infection
Aerotitis or acute barotitis	*Psychogenic*
Cholesteatoma	*Drug ingestions (causing tinnitus)*
Inner ear/periauricular structures	Quinine, quinidine, ethacrynic acid, salicylates, nicotine, aminoglycosides
Labyrinthitis	
Subperiosteal abscess/acute mastoid osteitis	
Intracranial infections	
Facial nerve palsy	

requires drainage. Herpes zoster oticus, or Ramsay Hunt syndrome, is a painful viral infection characterized by vesicles on the auricle, the external auditory meatus, and occasionally, the tympanic membrane (TM). Complications include facial paralysis, hearing loss, and vertigo. Other cranial nerves may be affected.

Otitis externa (OE) usually presents in warm, humid weather. Because swimming can predispose the canal to this condition, it is often called swimmer's ear. The initial presenting symptom may be pruritus. Scratching the canal may damage the skin and predispose the area to secondary bacterial infection. Ear pain, itching, and discharge are the primary complaints. Examination reveals a tender auricle, a mildly erythematous canal with edema, and foul-smelling, gray–green discharge. A serious complication of OE is malignant or necrotizing external otitis, which is a fulminant bacterial otitis externa with *Pseudomonas aeruginosa*. This may extend beyond the limits of the external auditory canal, producing cellulitis, chondritis, osteitis, osteomyelitis, and facial nerve paralysis.

Impacted cerumen in the canal is a common cause of ear pain or discomfort. Ear wax removal is often necessary for evaluating ears. Careful immobilization is essential. Removal under direct visualization through an otoscope is ideal. An ear curette or small cotton swab may be used. Hard cerumen may cause bleeding with removal when adherent to the canal. The wax may be softened with a ceruminolytic agent, then irrigated with warm water. A plastic syringe attached to the plastic tubing end cut from a butterfly needle may be used. Foreign bodies can elicit a painful inflammatory reaction. Physical examination visually confirms a foreign body. Otomycosis is a fungal infection of the external canal. It may be acute or chronic, primary or secondary to bacterial infection and prolonged use of antibiotic drops. The primary complaint may be pruritus. On physical examination, the canal contains gray, white, or blackish debris that resembles dirty cotton and has an erythematous and edematous canal wall.

Dermatoses of the ear can cause ear discomfort as well. Seborrheic dermatitis and psoriasis can affect the external auditory canal and produce scaling or drainage. The primary complaint may be itching. Usually, other areas are affected as well, including the retroauricular region and scalp. Removal of crusts can be helpful.

TABLE 47.2. Common Causes of Earache

Otogenic	Nonotogenic
Acute otitis media	Dental caries or abscess
Otitis externa	Pharyngitis
Foreign body	Sinusitis
	Cervical adenopathy

TABLE 47.3. Life-Threatening Causes of Earache

Hemotympanum secondary to basal skull fracture
Local spread of acute otitis media to:
- mastoid cavity—subperiosteal abscess with acute mastoid osteitis
- vascular structures—lateral sinus thrombosis
- intracranial region—meningitis, extradural abscess, subdural empyema, focal encephalitis, brain abscess
- temporal bone—facial nerve paralysis
- inner ear—labyrinthitis

Acute otitis media (AOM) is the most common illness resulting in office visits to physicians who care for children (see also Chapter 74). History often includes recent viral upper respiratory infection followed by deep-seated otalgia, fever, and decreased hearing. The four major criteria when examining the TM for AOM are position, color, translucency, and mobility. AOM may show a hyperemic, opaque, bulging TM with poor mobility. The drum may be bulging with serous fluid or yellow pus in the middle ear space. The auricle is usually normal. A conductive hearing loss may result from accumulation of fluid in the middle ear and impairment of the drum motion. Otitis media with effusion (OME) or serous otitis media is an inflammation of the middle ear in which a collection of liquid is present in the middle ear space, which is usually mucoid or serous without signs or symptoms of infection.

Although rare, dangerous complications of AOM include local spread to the mastoid cavity, soft-tissue and vascular structures of the neck, intracranial region and temporal bone, or inner ear. On examination for subperiosteal abscess with acute mastoid osteitis, the pinna may be displaced inferiorly and anteriorly with obliteration of the postauricular crease as a result of swelling. The eardrum may appear gray, not bulging or perforated. This most commonly occurs in infants 4 to 12 months old.

TM perforation may be caused by pressure from fluid behind the membrane or by external trauma. Trauma often occurs with compressive injuries such as a slap with an open hand or injuries from instruments such as cotton-tipped applicators being placed into the ear canal. Pain may be severe immediately after the injury, but it becomes duller with time. Acute hearing loss, facial paralysis, and severe vertigo associated with the perforation call for ORL evaluation because of possible ossicular damage or direct injury to the facial nerve or labyrinth.

Bullous myringitis is a painful, usually viral but possibly bacterial or mycoplasmal infection of the TM characterized by serous or hemorrhagic vesicles or blebs. Treatment consists of analgesics and possible oral antibiotics.

Hemotympanum secondary to basal skull fracture may be a serious finding on examination of the ear. The TM may appear dark red or purple secondary to the blood behind it. These patients may have other findings consistent with basal skull fractures such as Battle sign—ecchymoses behind the ear, raccoon eyes—periorbital ecchymoses, or cerebrospinal fluid (CSF) drainage from the nose or ears.

Aerotitis, or acute barotitis, is a special type of AOM caused by middle ear barotrauma. A sudden change in altitude in an airplane or the pressure exerted during deep sea diving can cause eustachian tube closure and produce a severe and painful pressure change in the middle ear with extravasation of blood into the middle ear space. The drum may appear blue because of bleeding behind it. The patient has severe pain and hearing loss. Physical examination reveals a hemorrhagic TM.

Cholesteatomas may be visualized in the middle ear. These cystlike structures, which consist of epithelial cells and cholesterol, may be congenital or acquired, often secondary to previous perforation with residual TM epithelial cells in the middle ear.

Nonotogenic Causes

Inflammation, infection, neoplasm, or trauma along the course of any nerves innervating the auricle or the external auditory canal, including cranial nerves V, VII, IX, and X and cervical nerves C2 and C3, can produce pain that the patient may interpret as originating in the region of the ear. Sinusitis, sialadenitis, or lymphadenitis are common reasons for referred ear pain. Early mumps may present as ear pain before obvious parotid swelling. Facial nerve (VII) pain may be a precursor of Bell palsy or herpes zoster oticus. Pharyngitis or tonsillitis, is another common cause of referred earache. Peritonsillar abscess or cellulitis may produce unilateral pain. Earache may also occur after adenotonsillectomy. Nasopharyngeal or oropharyngeal tumors, such as lymphoma or rhabdomyosarcoma, although rare in children, may be associated with ear pain.

Cervical nerves C2 and C3 supply the mastoid and posterior pinna; therefore, ear pain may result from cervical spine injuries, arthritis, or disc disease as well as any generalized neck disorder.

When otologic examination is normal and no pathology is found in the distribution of the cranial or cervical nerves the pain may be psychogenic, especially in a person with anxiety or depression. Also, children may not be able to describe tinnitus and refer to it as pain. Certain drug ingestions such as quinine, quinidine, salicylates, nicotine, ethacrynic acid, and aminoglycosides are possible causes.

EVALUATION AND DECISION

Particularly important components of the examination include the external ear, the auditory canal, the TM, the surrounding structures of the head and neck, and the neurologic evaluation (Fig. 47.1).

EXTERNAL EAR EXAMINATION

External problems are usually obvious on initial examination. Trauma, erythema, or vesicles on the auricle may be easily seen. Palpation of the area around the ear may reveal swelling or tenderness either from nodes, mastoiditis, parotitis, or preauricular pit infection.

Abnormal Otoscopy

Otogenic causes are readily diagnosed by visualization with otoscopy. Inflammation in the canal or middle ear, foreign bodies, abnormal lesions, perforations, or cholesteatomas may be seen. Evaluation of the TM for signs of infection includes describing position, color, degree of translucency, and mobility. Erythema alone is not sensitive as a predictor of infection because it may occur from increased blood flow with crying. Mobility is evaluated by applying pressure to the rubber bulb attached to the otoscope with a good seal in the canal and looking for inward movement with positive pressure and outward movement with negative pressure. Purulent discharge in the canal may be wicked out with cotton to better visualize the TM for a perforation or foreign body. Any patient with accompanying vertigo, facial nerve palsy, hemotympanum, or central nervous system symptoms requires further evaluation with computed tomography scan.

Normal Otoscopy

A normal otoscopic evaluation should prompt a search for referred pain. Evaluation of the cervical spine, oropharynx, and neck should reveal possible sources of inflammation from shared sensory nerves. Radiographs to evaluate dental sources are usually not required emergently. A history of possible drug ingestions should be obtained. If there is a clinical suspicion of disease in the nasopharynx or larynx, an examination with a nasopharyngoscope may be needed. Patients with a completely normal examination and no other accompanying complaints should be referred back to their physician for follow-up before a psychogenic cause is given.

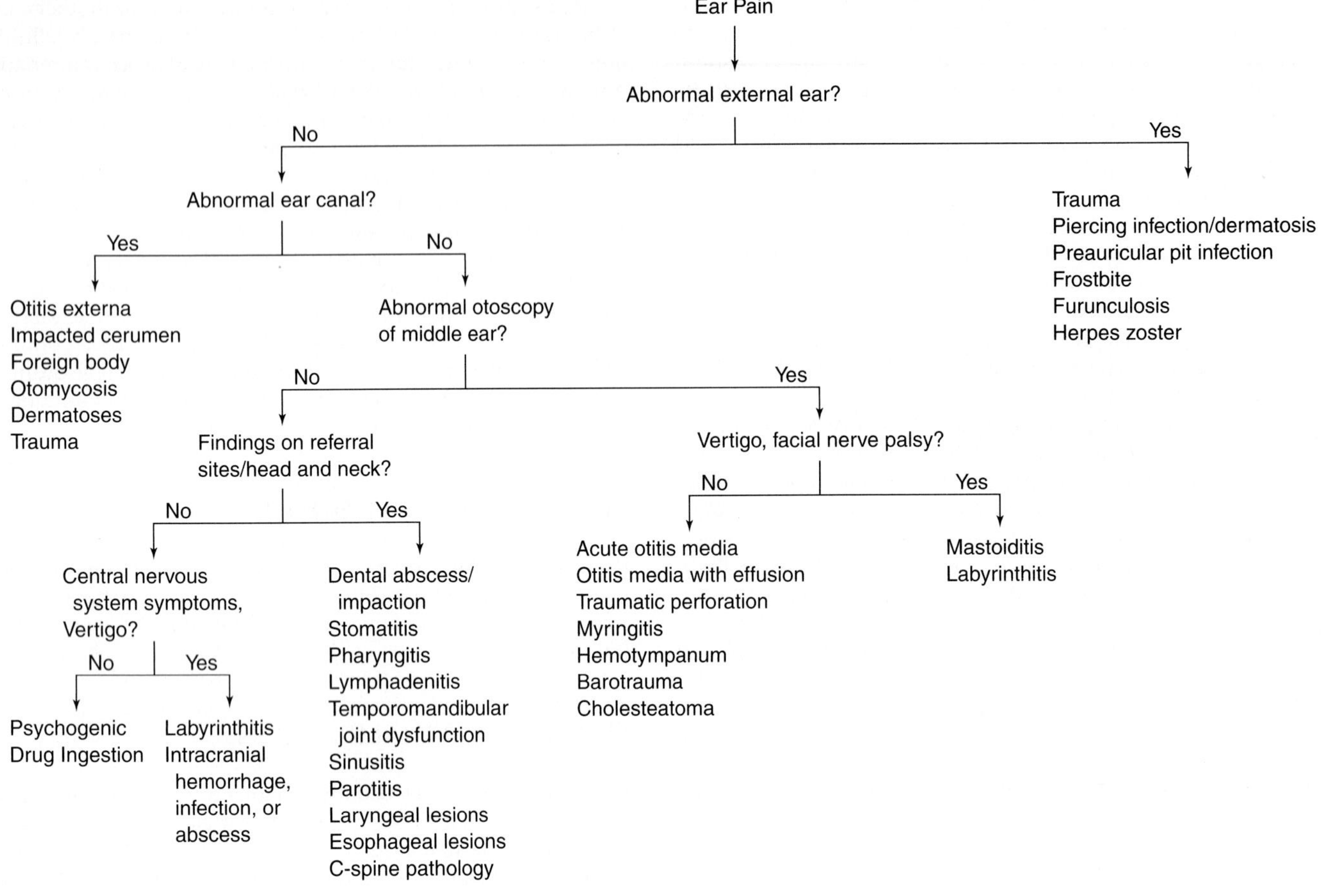

Figure 47.1. Approach to the diagnosis of earache.

CHAPTER 48

Headache

Christopher King, M.D.

Headache occurs with regularity and is almost always benign, but in a small subset of patients, it can portend a potentially life-threatening illness. Distinguishing which child among the many with headache has a serious underlying process can almost always be done successfully after a thorough history and physical examination.

TABLE 48.1. Pathophysiologic Classification of Headaches

Vascular	*Traction/compression*
Febrile illness	Increased intracranial pressure
Migraine	Cerebral edema
Systemic hypertension	Hydrocephalus
Hypoxia	Intracranial hemorrhage or hematoma
Muscle contraction	Brain abscess
Tension	Tumor
Fatigue	Lumbar puncture
Inflammation	*Others*
Intracranial infections	Posttraumatic
Meningitis	Psychogenic
Encephalitis	Ocular
Dental infections	
Sinus infections	

DIFFERENTIAL DIAGNOSIS

A comprehensive discussion of the various causes of headache in pediatric patients (Table 48.1) is beyond the scope of this chapter. The conditions described here are those most likely to be seen in acute- and emergency-care settings (Table 48.2) and those with the greatest potential for imminent morbidity or mortality (Table 48.3).

TABLE 48.2. Common Causes of Headache

Vascular	*Muscle contraction*
Febrile illness	Tension
Migraine	Fatigue
Inflammatory	*Others*
Sinus infections	Psychogenic
Dental infections	Ocular
	Posttraumatic

Vascular

Migraine headaches are typically chronic and remitting, with a characteristic pattern that is easily described by the patient or parents. Often, a strong family history of migraines is present.

TABLE 48.3. Life-Threatening Causes of Headache

Vascular	*Traction/compression*
Hypertension	Increased intracranial pressure
Hypoxia	Tumor
Inflammatory	Hemorrhage/hematoma
Meningitis	
Encephalitis	

For the emergency physician, the main issue with patients with migraines is generally pain control because the diagnosis is already known. However, a significant change in the quality, severity, or timing of headaches in these patients may represent a separate and potentially more serious problem. In such cases, the clinician should not be dissuaded by the existing diagnosis from pursuing an appropriate workup as indicated.

Headaches accompanying fever are also thought to be mediated by vascular effects. Because fever is such a common symptom, this is probably the most common cause of headaches in pediatric patients seen in the emergency department (ED). Hypertension is another possible cause of vascular headaches in children.

Finally, hypoxia is a potent stimulus for cerebral vasodilation and can produce headaches on that basis. Therefore, children with an acute hypoxic insult (e.g., carbon monoxide poisoning) or those with disease states that predispose to hypoxia (e.g., cystic fibrosis, cyanotic heart disease) may present with headaches resulting from an acute process or an exacerbation of an underlying illness.

Muscle Contraction

Headaches can be caused by contraction of the scalp or neck muscles. This is the classic "tension" headache that so often plagues adults. These headaches usually occur when a patient has experienced prolonged periods of mental or emotional stress. The patient can often localize a specific site where the pain is felt, and the involved muscles may be tender to palpation. Although muscle contraction is an unlikely cause of headache in younger children, the stress of life during adolescence will often produce this type of headache. Onset is typically at the end of the day. A headache that is present on arising in the morning or that awakens a patient from sleep would be an unusual manifestation of muscle contraction.

Inflammation

Children with bacterial meningitis or encephalitis may present with headache, although this is usually only one of a constellation of symptoms, such as fever, lethargy, neck pain, confusion, or coma. Headache is unlikely to be the sole complaint in these patients. However, an older child or adolescent who has viral meningitis can present with a severe headache, minimal or mild neck discomfort, and no other signs of significant illness. Rare causes of inflammatory headache include retroorbital cellulitis or abscess and cerebral abscess. Focal findings on neurologic and/or ocular examination will normally provide clues to these unusual diagnoses.

Headaches can also be caused by inflammatory processes affecting other structures of the head and neck. For example, pediatric patients with pharyngitis caused by group A streptococcus will often complain of headaches. In a child who has difficulty localizing pain, otitis media and otitis externa can also present as headache. Pediatric patients with sinusitis will sometimes complain of facial or periorbital pain, although younger children may simply have a persistent nasal discharge. Dental abscess can be overlooked as a cause of headache-type pain because it is a relatively uncommon finding in children. Finally, inflammation of the temporomandibular joint (TMJ syndrome) is a rare cause of unilateral headaches in children. These patients typically report increased pain while chewing and have point tenderness over the mandibular condyle.

Traction/Compression

The most important conditions in this category are intracranial hemorrhage and brain tumor. An intracranial hemorrhage produces displacement of surrounding tissues and, in cases of more significant bleeding, increased intracranial pressure. In the pediatric population, this is most often the result of a severe head injury (see Chapter 92). However, in rare cases, a child can have a nontraumatic intracranial hemorrhage from a ruptured vascular anomaly (e.g., an arteriovenous malformation) that leads to bleeding into the brain parenchyma and ventricles. As with other vascular events, this type of hemorrhage is characterized by the abrupt onset of severe pain. By contrast, headaches resulting from a brain tumor typically have a more insidious onset. The child will often complain of progressively worsening headaches for several weeks or even months. Additional symptoms, such as persistent vomiting or gait abnormalities, may also be present. Unfortunately, the physical examination can be normal during the early phase of the illness, and as mentioned previously, this commonly leads to a delay in diagnosis. Other processes that cause headache as a result of traction and compression include pseudotumor cerebri, hydrocephalus, and persistent spinal fluid leak after lumbar puncture.

Psychogenic

Although less common than in adults, headaches of psychogenic origin are seen in children as well. Possible causes include school avoidance behavior, malingering with secondary gain issues, and a true conversion disorder. These patients often have a history of chronic headaches that have been unresponsive to various treatment methods, and they may have undergone a battery of tests without receiving a diagnosis.

EVALUATION AND DECISION

As stated previously, the diagnosis for pediatric patients presenting with headache will be evident in all but a small minority of cases after a thorough history and physical examination. Laboratory tests and imaging modalities are rarely needed. Even if a definitive diagnosis cannot be established immediately, the identification of a potentially life-threatening cause of headaches will almost always be possible before the child leaves the ED. Concern about the possibility of a more serious cause warrants aggressive use of whatever diagnostic or therapeutic interventions are indicated, such as a computed tomography (CT) scan of the head, lumbar puncture, or intravenous antibiotics. An approach to the diagnostic evaluation of a child with headaches is outlined in Fig. 48.1.

Clinical Assessment

HISTORY

The presence of a high fever, decreased activity, and poor oral intake is suggestive of a serious inflammatory cause such as

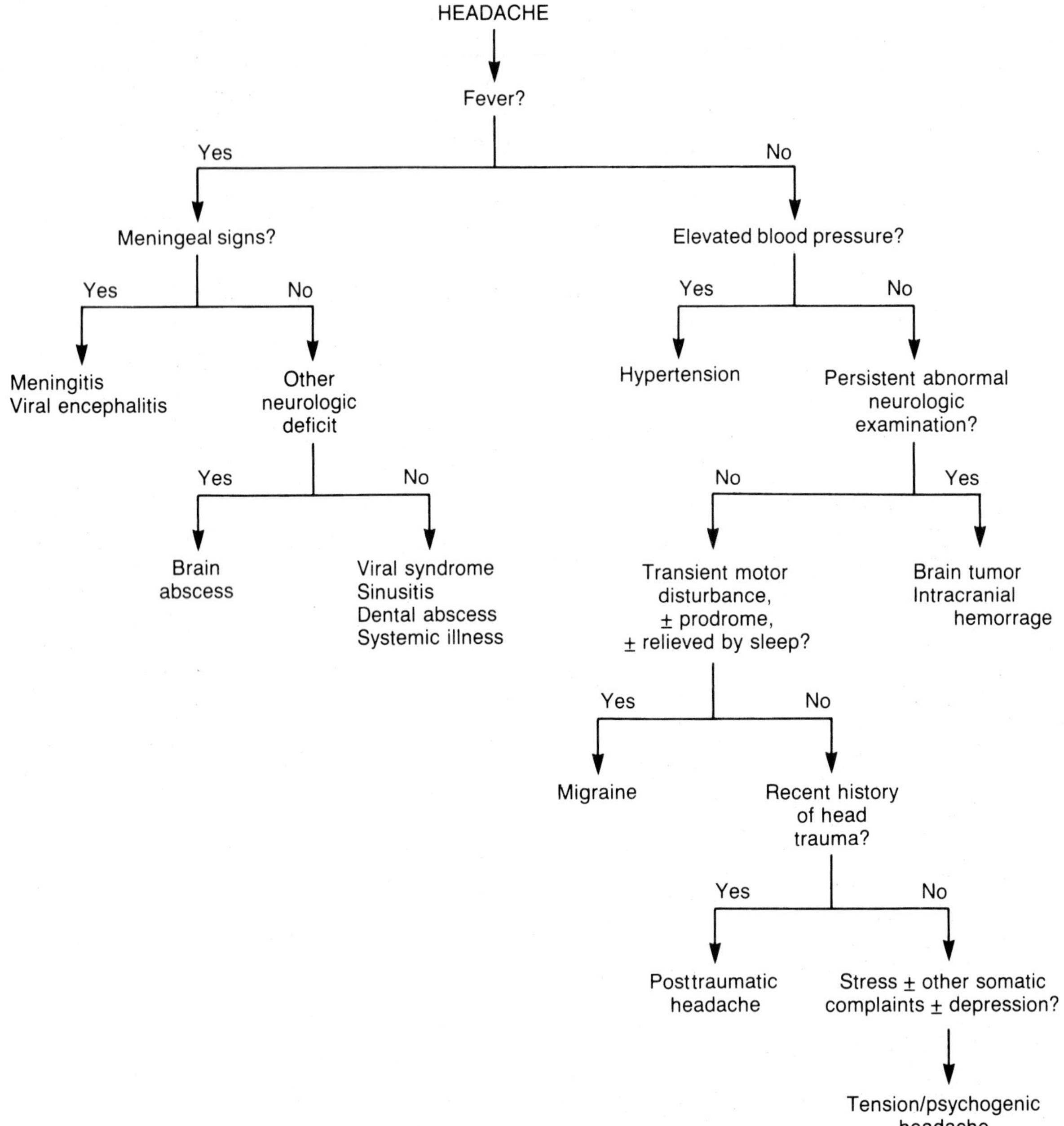

Figure 48.1. Approach to the diagnosis of headache.

meningitis. A patient with these same symptoms who also has an abrupt change in mental status may have encephalitis. If a child has been relatively well but has complained of headache associated with persistent nasal discharge (especially if it is purulent), this may be caused by a sinusitis. A child with tooth pain, ear pain, or sore throat may also have a readily apparent reason for headaches.

One of the more important points to investigate is the mode of onset. A headache that starts abruptly and causes extreme pain may represent a vascular event such as a ruptured arteriovenous malformation, whereas a headache with a more gradual onset would be inconsistent with this diagnosis. The frequency and duration of headaches can also provide valuable clues about the origin of headaches. A child who complains of constant pain for several days without respite (i.e., goes to sleep with it, wakes up with it) will commonly have a tension headache or, perhaps more likely, a psychogenic headache. On the other hand, a patient who presents with headaches that have progressively become more frequent or prolonged may have a more serious underlying condition. Similarly, a child with headaches that have steadily worsened in severity over time warrants careful evaluation, again given the limitations of a child's description of pain.

The time and circumstances of occurrence are also important historical points to ascertain. For example, headaches that are present when a child arises each morning or that awaken a child at night should raise suspicion about a possible brain tumor. In contrast, headaches that occur only later in the day are typically related to stress and result from muscle contraction. In addition, any precipitating events that consistently cause or exacerbate a headache should be identified. If an older child has a headache that is significantly worse when leaning down (e.g., to pick up

TABLE 48.4. Characteristic Historical Findings of Brain Tumor Headaches in Children

Nocturnal headache or pain on arising in the morning
Worsening over time (severity, frequency, and/or duration)
Associated with vomiting (although may also occur with migraine), especially if vomiting gets progressively worse
Behavioral changes
Polydipsia/polyuria (craniopharyngioma)
History of probable neurologic deficits (e.g., ataxia/incoordination/ "clumsiness," blurred vision, or diplopia)

Reprinted with permission from Honig PJ, Charney EB. Children with brain tumor headaches: distinguishing features. *Am J Dis Child* 1982;136:121–141.

something off the floor), this is most likely to be caused by sinusitis, although in rare cases, this history may be present in a child with a brain tumor.

Any relevant details about the patient's medical history and family history should routinely be obtained. As mentioned previously, children with cystic fibrosis or congenital heart disease may have headaches caused by worsening hypoxia. Likewise, a child with renal disease may develop headaches in response to an elevated blood pressure. In general, the most important question regarding family history is whether anyone has had migraine headaches. Abrupt onset of headache in several family members may suggest carbon monoxide poisoning. Sometimes, a constellation of historical findings may suggest a brain tumor (Table 48.4).

PHYSICAL EXAMINATION

The first step of the examination is to assess the patient's appearance. Does the child look sick or well? Does the child appear to be in severe pain, mild pain, or no pain at all? This initial evaluation represents the first important branch point in the decision algorithm for patients with headache (Fig. 48.1). Thus a child who appears ill may have a more serious underlying condition, such as meningitis or an intracranial hemorrhage, requiring a rapid examination and prompt initiation of treatment.

The vital signs should also be assessed, particularly the temperature and blood pressure. Significant hypertension, usually resulting from undiagnosed renal disease, is a rare but potentially dangerous cause of headaches that can affect children of any age. Macrocephaly may be the result of hydrocephalus, and short stature can be associated with a craniopharyngioma that causes impaired pituitary function.

The head and neck examination will sometimes reveal an obvious source of headache in a child. The scalp should be examined for evidence of head injury. Even when no history of trauma exists, the child may have had an unwitnessed event, or the history may be intentionally misleading with a victim of child abuse. Tenderness of the scalp or neck muscles is often present with headaches resulting from stress and muscle contraction. The eyes should be examined to detect any abnormalities in pupillary responses or extraocular movements. A sluggish pupil may be caused by an expanding mass lesion that causes compression of the third cranial nerve, and pain with extraocular movements may be elicited with a retroorbital cellulitis or abscess. The eyegrounds should also be carefully examined for signs of papilledema. The clinician may find an otitis media or otitis externa when the ears are examined. Streptococcal pharyngitis as a cause of headaches may be evident as swelling, erythema, and exudates of the tonsillar pillars. Facial tenderness and erythema are sometimes seen in children with maxillary or frontal sinusitis. The teeth and gingiva should be examined for evidence of inflammation or abscess. Nuchal rigidity can be a sign of meningitis, intracranial hemorrhage, or in rare cases, brain tumor. If a child has a ventricular shunt, assessment of shunt function should be performed when appropriate.

Examining the skin is also important for the child with headaches. Because the skin and central nervous system have a common embryologic origin, cutaneous lesions are sometimes seen with neurologic disorders. For example, a child with numerous hyperpigmented spots scattered over the body (café-au-lait spots) most likely has neurofibromatosis. Similarly, children with tuberous sclerosis will almost always have several small hypopigmented spots (ash leaf spots) that are more apparent when viewed under a Wood ultraviolet lamp.

Every child with a complaint of headaches obviously needs a complete neurologic examination. Any new focal finding suggests the presence of a focal lesion, such as a tumor or hemorrhage. Some children with migraine headaches develop focal neurologic abnormalities as part of their migraine syndrome (e.g., ophthalmoplegia), but parents can normally confirm that this is not a new problem. As mentioned previously, the mental status of a child with headaches must always be carefully assessed. A diminished level of consciousness may be the result of encephalitis, a large intracranial hemorrhage, or significantly elevated intracranial pressure. Cranial nerve abnormalities may result from an elevated intracranial pressure or direct compression by a mass lesion. Any evidence of gait abnormalities or deficits in fine motor coordination points toward cerebellar malfunction.

CHAPTER 49
Joint Pain

Richard J. Scarfone, M.D., M.C.P.

Arthritis is joint inflammation marked by swelling, warmth, and limitation of motion, whereas arthralgia is simply pain without inflammation of the joint space. The diagnostic approach is challenging because the differential diagnosis is lengthy (Table 49.1), clinical and laboratory findings are rarely specific for a particular disease, and the disease pattern for many of the conditions listed is often greatly variable. Among the most common causes of joint pain in children are bacterial infections, trauma, and postinfectious conditions (Table 49.2). Although rare, several life-threatening causes (Table 49.3), including acute rheumatic fever and leukemia, must be considered.

DIFFERENTIAL DIAGNOSIS

The possible causes of joint complaints in children are extensive (Table 49.1), but infectious and traumatic causes are the most common (Table 49.2). Children between 6 to 24 months of age have the highest incidence of nongonococcal bacterial (septic) arthritis, and boys are affected twice as often as girls. Among adolescents, disseminated gonococcal infection with polyarthritis occurs three to five times more often in girls, often during menstruation. Of note, few patients report lower abdominal pain or vaginal discharge concurrently and cultures of blood and synovial fluid are typically negative. The highest yield for

TABLE 49.1. Joint Pain—Differential Diagnosis

Infection	Ligamentous sprain
Nongonococcal bacterial (septic)	Bursitis
Staphylococcus aureus	Tendonitis
Haemophilus influenza	Slipped capital femoral epiphysis
Group B streptococci	Legg-Calvé-Perthes disease
Escherichia coli	Osteochondritis dissecans
Gonococcal	Chondromalacia patellae
Viral	Osgood-Schlatter disease
Mycobacterial	*Immune-mediated/vasculitic*
Fungal	Chronic idiopathic arthritides of childhood
Postinfectious	Serum sickness
Viral: hepatitis B, parvovirus, Epstein-Barr virus (EBV), cytomegalovirus (CMV), varicella-zoster, herpesvirus 6, enterovirus, adenovirus	Kawasaki disease
	Inflammatory bowel disease
	Systemic lupus erythematosus
	Henoch-Schönlein purpura
Bacterial: acute rheumatic fever, Lyme disease, chlamydia (Reiter syndrome), mycoplasma, *Shigella, Campylobacter*	*Other*
	Toxic synovitis of the hip
	Malignancy .
Trauma/overuse	Leukemia
Contusion	Neuroblastoma
Hemarthrosis	Bone tumor
Fracture	Hemophilia
	Metabolic

establishing the diagnosis is by Gram stain of the skin lesions showing Gram-negative intracellular diplococci or by culturing the cervix, rectum, or throat.

In the absence of a clear history of a tick bite, Lyme disease is a challenging clinical diagnosis because only about 40% to 70% of children have the characteristic erythema migrans rash, constitutional symptoms may be mild, and serologic tests have a high incidence of false positivity. The diagnosis relies on the specific Western blot confirmation of a positive serology.

Toxic synovitis is a poorly understood inflammation of the hip joint, usually afflicting children 3 to 6 years of age. The diagnosis is typically made on clinical grounds, and this self-limited disease does not result in joint destruction.

Reactive, or postinfectious, arthritis is probably more common than septic arthritis. Arthritis secondary to various enteric infections is not rare in children and parvovirus B19 is also a common cause of acute arthritis in adolescents and young adults. *Chlamydia trachomatis* infection of the genitourinary tract should be considered in any sexually active adolescent with new onset arthritis. Traumatic injuries to a joint may cause periarticular swelling or an effusion indicative of a hemarthrosis. A host of other conditions may come to light in the setting of minor trauma but may be only indirectly related to that trauma.

Less common is chronic arthritis with an incidence of 5 to 10 per 100,000 children less than 16 years of age. These diseases are characterized by arthritis persistent for at least 6 weeks in the absence of a defined diagnosis and can be grouped together as chronic idiopathic arthritides of childhood (CIAC). CIAC is much less benign than previously believed, with about 40% of children from all disease subtypes continuing to have active joint inflammation, and 20% of children having severe functional limitations after 10 years or more of follow-up.

EVALUATION AND DECISION

Figure 49.1 depicts an algorithm for the diagnostic approach to the child with joint pain. In evaluating such children, one should inquire about a history of trauma, fever, the specific joint(s) involved, duration, rash, tick bites, sexual risk factors, intravenous drug use, and recent illnesses. Radiographs of the affected joint are particularly useful in the setting of trauma or acute monarthritis without an obvious cause. A complete blood count and erythrocyte sedimentation rate are generally indicated for children with joint pain in the absence of trauma. For the febrile child with monarthritis and a joint effusion, an arthrocentesis will guide the evaluation. Finally, ultrasound is superior to plain radiographs in the detection of a hip effusion.

A key initial point in the history is whether trauma preceded the pain. Because it is easy to be led astray by parents trying to recall what traumatic event could have led to the child's symptoms, one should remember that if the mechanism was not severe enough to immediately prevent the child from continuing an activity, it is unlikely to be the cause of a significantly swollen and painful joint. On the other hand, if there was a definite traumatic event preceding the onset of symptoms, particularly in the absence of fever, one can proceed with that aspect of the evaluation.

TABLE 49.2. Common Causes of Joint Pain

Nongonococcal bacterial (septic)	Postinfectious (reactive)
Gonococcal	Traumatic hemarthrosis
Lyme disease	Serum sickness
Toxic synovitis of the hip	Henoch-Schönlein purpura

TABLE 49.3. Life-Threatening Causes of Joint Pain

Acute rheumatic fever
Kawasaki disease
Malignancy
Leukemia
Neuroblastoma
Bone tumor

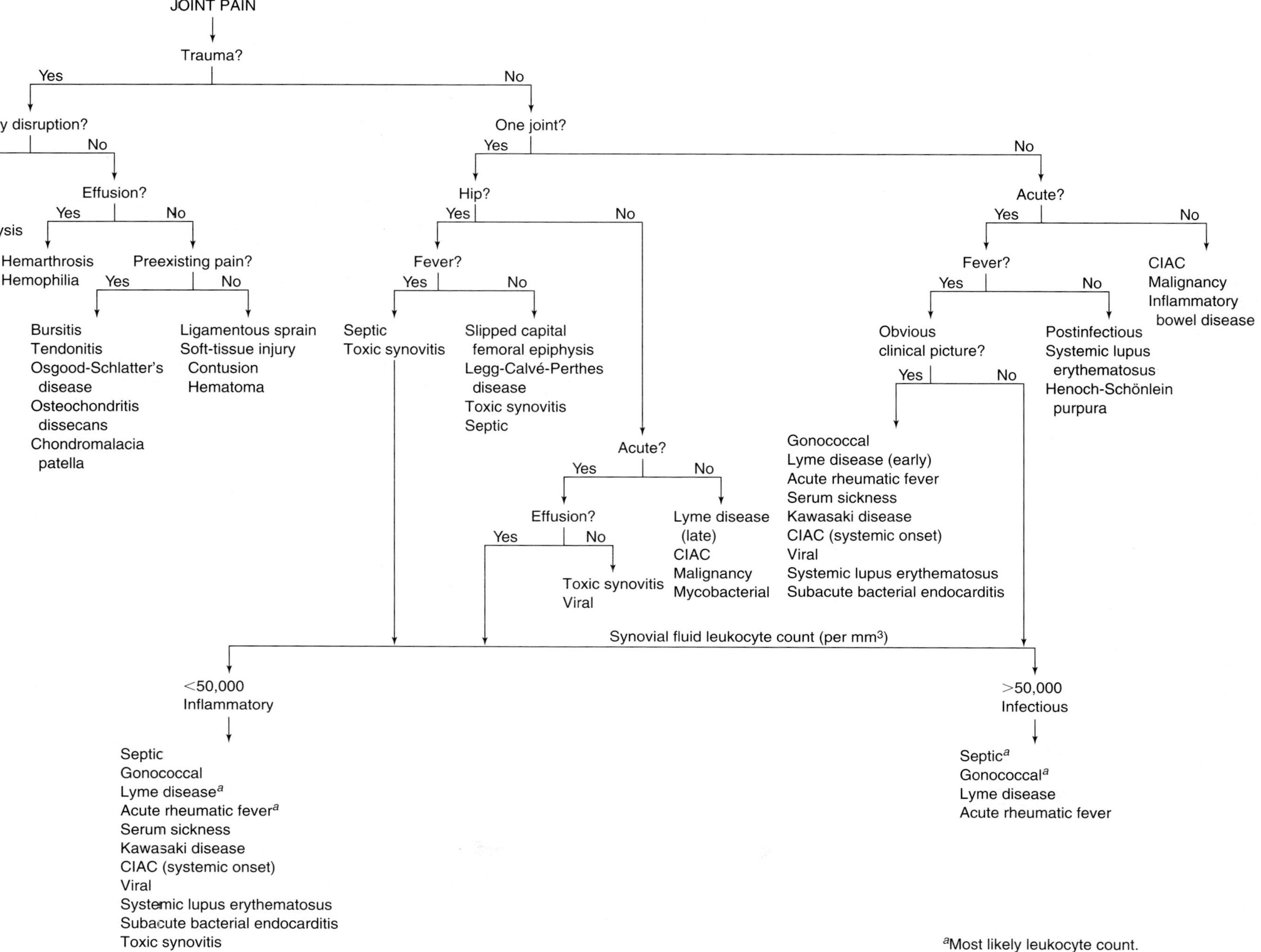

Figure 49.1. A diagnostic approach to joint pain. *CIAC,* chronic idiopathic arthritides of childhood.

A radiograph will detect fractures or a slipped capital femoral epiphysis. Radiographs aid in determining whether associated swelling is caused by a joint effusion or is simply soft-tissue swelling outside of the joint, a distinction that is often difficult to make on physical examination alone. In the setting of acute trauma and in the absence of fever, an effusion is indicative of a hemarthrosis and is rarely a diagnostic or therapeutic indication for performing an arthrocentesis because the patient will typically experience only temporary relief followed by a rapid reaccumulation of blood.

In the absence of an effusion, inquiries about the duration of symptoms should be made. Children with conditions such as bursitis, tendonitis, and Osgood-Schlatter disease typically have chronic, low-grade pain and may inadvertently come to medical attention after minor trauma. New-onset periarticular swelling and pain immediately after acute trauma suggest ligamentous or other soft-tissue injury.

In the absence of trauma, monarthritis of the hip is uniquely problematic. In particular, bacterial infections of this and other joints are the most serious because of the rapidity with which destruction of cartilage can occur. The most important determinant of the outcome of a septic arthritis is the length of delay between the onset of infection and the institution of therapy. Unlike most other causes of fever and arthritis, in more than 90% of affected children, septic arthritis involves only a single joint, usually of the lower extremity; neonates, however, may have polyarthritis. Because just 60% to 70% of children with septic arthritis are febrile at presentation, the absence of fever does not preclude the diagnosis. However, if the child allows full range of motion, the diagnosis is unlikely.

A child with acute onset of monarthritis of the hip or any other large joint, defined by the presence of an effusion and marked by severely restricted range of motion, with or without fever, generally needs an arthrocentesis. The synovial fluid should be analyzed for glucose and protein, cell count and differential, Gram stain, and culture. Most patients with septic joints will have a decreased glucose level and greater than 50,000 white blood cells per cubic millimeter with a neutrophil predominance, but in one study, one-third had counts of less than 25,000/m^3. The erythrocyte sedimentation rate is almost always elevated, with a edian value of 50 mm in one case series.

In contrast to septic arthritis, children with toxic synovitis of the hip typically appear well; often present with a limp; may have only mildly elevated temperatures; allow almost complete range of motion of the affected joint; and the complete blood counts, erythrocyte sedimentation rates, and radiographs are typically normal. Usually, the physician can make a clinical diagnosis of toxic synovitis, but in a small subset, septic arthritis cannot be ruled out before the completion of an arthrocentesis. The disease is self-limited, usually lasting less than 1 week.

A slipped capital femoral epiphysis must not be missed. About half of patients will provide a history of trauma. This condition is most often seen in obese adolescent boys. Most children have chronic pain, although some have an acute limp with hip or knee pain and restricted range of motion. Plain radiographs (frog-leg view of the hip) showing a widened epiphysis and caudal displacement of the femoral head establish the diagnosis.

Legg-Calvé-Perthes disease, a condition of uncertain cause, occurs overwhelmingly in boys, with an onset between 4 and 8 years of age. The pain, which may be localized to the hip or referred to the thigh or knee, is insidious in onset. The aseptic necrosis of the femoral head will be manifest on plain radiographs as a small, osteopenic femoral head with a widened joint space.

TABLE 49.4. Fever and Joint Pain

Usually febrile at presentation	*May or may not be febrile at presentation*
Nongonococcal bacterial (septic)	Leukemia
Gonococcal	Mycobacterial
Acute rheumatic fever	Postinfectious (reactive)
Chronic idiopathic arthritides of childhood (systemic onset)	Lyme disease
Subacute bacterial endocarditis	Systemic lupus erythematosus
Serum sickness	Inflammatory bowel disease
Kawasaki disease	

Historical and physical examination findings help narrow the choices among the many causes of fever and polyarthritis (Table 49.4). The ill-appearing adolescent with migratory arthritis, tenosynovitis involving the extensor tendons of the wrist or ankle, and scattered crops of vesiculopustules on an erythematous base should be strongly suspected for gonococcal arthritis. Joint involvement with Lyme disease has two distinct patterns. In early disseminated disease, the child may develop episodic migratory polyarthritis, affecting mainly large joints. Each episode lasts a few days, helping distinguish it from idiopathic chronic arthritis. Two weeks to 2 years (mean 6 months) after the tick bite, 6% develop an intermittent monarthritis, typically of the knee, ankle, or wrist. The joint is significantly swollen but only mildly painful, and patients are usually afebrile at this stage. Painful migratory joint pain involving five or more joints in a school-age child with recent evidence of a group A streptococcal infection should raise the concern for acute rheumatic fever. Evidence of carditis, erythema marginatum, subcutaneous nodules, and positive serology for antistreptococcal antibodies support the diagnosis. The presence of diffuse urticaria and angioedema accompanying arthralgia or arthritis, especially 3 to 10 days after initiation of an antibiotic, helps distinguish serum sickness from other causes of polyarthritis and fever. Kawasaki disease is characterized by high and persistent fever, conjunctival injection without exudate, mouth and lip swelling and cracking, swelling and erythema of the hands and feet, a nonspecific rash, and lymphadenopathy. Ten days or so after the disease onset, there may be desquamation of the fingers and toes, myocardial dysfunction, and thrombocytosis; about 30% of patients will also develop arthritis or arthralgia. Daily temperature spikes exceeding 40°C (104°F), especially if accompanied by a transient pink rash, suggest one of the CIAC (formerly called Still disease). A common viral-related arthritis is that caused by hepatitis B infection. The arthritis precedes the symptoms of hepatitis and resolves when the jaundice appears. During the 1- to 3-week prodromal phase, polyarthritis may be accompanied by moderate fever and sometimes by an urticarial or maculopapular rash. Parvovirus B19 causes a similar clinical syndrome in young women with a sudden onset of symmetric, self-limited polyarthritis, particularly in the hands. With subacute bacterial endocarditis, musculoskeletal symptoms are variable, ranging from asymptomatic joint effusions to frank arthritis of up to three joints. Preexisting congenital heart disease, a prolonged fever, a new murmur, and splinter hemorrhages may all be clues to the diagnosis of this rare entity in children.

A joint aspiration is rarely necessary to establish a diagnosis for a child with polyarthritis and fever or to rule out a septic process in this setting. If an arthrocentesis is obtained, typically the synovial fluid will be sterile and the leukocyte count will characterize the process as inflammatory (Fig. 49.1).

Postinfectious arthritis is one of the more common causes of acute polyarthritis without fever. One to two weeks after a bout of enteritis or urogenital infection (Reiter syndrome), a child may develop an asymmetric postinfectious (reactive) polyarthritis, predominantly involving large joints of the lower extremities. The severity of the antecedent illness has little correlation with the arthritis, and the intensity of synovitis and fever is mild or absent at this stage.

As with many of the diseases discussed to this point, systemic lupus erythematosus (SLE) has a variable clinical presentation with regard to musculoskeletal involvement. In fact, no two patients have an identical pattern of immune complex formation or clinical disease expression. A symmetric polyarthritis involving peripheral joints of the hands or feet may be seen. However, small effusions of the knee are also common with active disease and the arthritis may be intermittent or migratory as well. Patients with this type of arthritis are usually afebrile, yet high fever may be a prominent finding. Although arthritis is 1 of the 11 diagnostic criteria for SLE established by the American College of Rheumatology, it is uncommon for SLE to present with isolated arthritis. Arthritis of the small joints, a positive test for antinuclear antibodies (ANA), and abnormalities of the skin, kidneys, or central nervous system should raise the clinician's suspicion for SLE.

Henoch-Schönlein purpura (HSP) is rarely a diagnostic challenge thanks to the presence of petechiae and purpura in the characteristic below-the-waist distribution. Classically, children will also have polyarthritis, colicky abdominal pain, and nephritis. As with the rash, periarticular swelling usually involves joints below the waist.

The CIAC are marked by their duration, typically 6 months or longer. That they appear at several points in the diagnostic algorithm reflects their diversity. Some children will have systemic distribution of symptoms, whereas others will have monoarticular or oligoarticular disease, and fever or rash may or may not be present. Tests for rheumatoid factor and ANA in children are unhelpful. When performed as a screen, rheumatoid factor tests are rarely positive and, when positive, are as likely to be in children with other diseases as in children with chronic arthritis.

In the absence of fever, chronic pain of one or more joints may also indicate malignancy. Specifically, leukemia or neuroblastoma can each present with true joint swelling, as can bony tumors. Pallor, weight loss, and other constitutional complaints, as well as anemia or cytopenias, would support this diagnosis.

A large joint oligoarthritis occurs as an extraintestinal complication of inflammatory bowel disease in about one-third of children, usually during times of active disease. Clues to the diagnosis include abdominal pain, hematochezia, anemia, and weight loss.

CHAPTER 50
Pain—Scrotal

Catherine E. Perron, M.D.

Acute scrotal swelling or pain in a child should be considered a potential surgical emergency. The patient with such a complaint should be evaluated promptly. Many diagnoses in cases of scrotal pain are most reliably made clinically, differentiating by age, historical features relating to the evolution of pain and associated symptoms, and physical examination findings.

TABLE 50.1. Causes of Acute Scrotal Swelling

Painful scrotal swelling	Painless scrotal swelling
Torsion of testis	Hydrocele
Torsion of appendage of testis	Hernia
Trauma—hematocele, hematoma, epididymitis, testicular rupture	Varicocele
Epididymitis	Spermatocele
Orchitis	Idiopathic scrotal edema
Hernia—incarcerated	Henoch—Schönlein purpura
Tumor—acute hemorrhage	Kawasaki disease
	Testis tumor
	Antenatal torsion of the testis

DIFFERENTIAL DIAGNOSIS (TABLES 50.1 AND 50.2)

Causes of Painful Scrotal Swelling

TORSION OF THE TESTIS

Testicular torsion is the most significant condition causing acute scrotal pain; it represents a true surgical emergency. It is more common in the newborn period and during the early stages of puberty. Sudden onset of severe scrotal pain and tenderness, often with radiation to the abdomen, and associated nausea and vomiting is typical. These episodes may have onset in the early morning. At other times, they may be associated with sports activity or mild testicular trauma that may be perceived by the patient as the cause of the pain.

With torsion of the testis, typically the testis is acutely swollen and diffusely tender and usually lies higher ("horizontal or transverse lie") in the scrotum than its contralateral mate. Because the pain may be referred to the abdomen, it is essential that the genitalia be examined carefully in every child who complains of abdominal pain. There may be overlying erythema of the skin of the scrotum. The cremasteric reflex is usually absent with testicular torsion but may be present in early or incomplete torsion. Urinalysis is usually negative.

Although the diagnosis continues to be established most reliably by a skilled examiner familiar with acute scrotal lesions in children, diagnostic imaging studies may be valuable. Nuclear testicular scanning or Doppler sonography reveals decreased or absent arterial blood flow within the affected testicle compared with its mate. It must be stressed that if the history and physical examination strongly suggest testicular torsion or if any appreciable time would be lost in arranging for these studies, the preferred course is to proceed with surgical exploration or an attempt at manual detorsion if surgical intervention is not readily available.

The testicular nuclear perfusion scan with technetium-99 pertechnetate is helpful but has limitations. The presence of a

TABLE 50.2. Common Causes of Acute Scrotal Swelling

Infancy	Adolescence
Hydrocele	Epididymitis
Hernia	Torsion of the appendix testes
Childhood	Torsion of the testes
Hernia	Trauma
Torsion of the appendix testes	
Torsion of the testes	
Trauma	

hydrocele, abscess, hematoma, or scrotal hernia may result in decreased counts on that side of the scrotum and may be confused with torsion of the testis. False-negative scans can occur from spontaneous detorsion or in cases of late torsion in which a severe degree of overlying scrotal edema may be associated with sufficient, increased vascularity to obscure the underlying ischemic testis. Doppler flow ultrasound can assess anatomy and blood flow. Limitations associated with Doppler sonography also must be recognized, particularly related to small, lower flow prepubertal testes and the operator-dependent nature of this test. False-negative ultrasounds may occur for reasons similar to those discussed for nuclear scan. Another pitfall encountered with use of both sonography or nuclear scan is incomplete or intermittent torsion in which the study may indicate normal, increased, or decreased flow, depending on timing.

The therapy for testicular torsion is surgical exploration, detorsion, and fixation of both the torsive and contralateral testicles. If a child is seen within a few hours of the onset of his torsion, before severe scrotal swelling has ensued, it may be possible to accomplish detorsion of the spermatic cord manually and thus restore blood supply to the testis. The Doppler ultrasound stethoscope provides a noninvasive evaluation of testicular blood flow and is a useful adjunct in manual detorsion of the testis. Initial examination reveals decreased arterial flow to the affected testis compared with the contralateral one. Intravenous fentanyl (1 to 3 μg per kilogram of body weight) or morphine (0.1 mg per kilogram of body weight) is administered just before attempting detorsion. Because torsion typically occurs in a medial direction, detorsion should be carried out by rotating the testis outward toward the thigh. Relief of pain and reposition of the testis in a lower position in the scrotum suggests a successful outcome, which can be confirmed with the Doppler stethoscope by noting a return of normal arterial pulsations to the testis.

TORSION OF TESTICULAR APPENDAGE

Several vestigial embryologic remnants are commonly attached to the testis or epididymis that may twist around their base, producing venous engorgement, enlargement, and subsequent infarction. Appendage torsion is most common in boys aged 7 to 12 years but can occur at any age. Scrotal pain is the usual presenting feature, although the pain is typically less severe and more indolent in onset than the pain associated with testicular torsion. Although there may be associated nausea, vomiting, and diaphoresis, these symptoms are less common than with torsion of the testis.

If the child is seen early after the onset of pain, scrotal tenderness and swelling may be localized to the area of the twisted appendage, typically on the superior lateral aspect of the testis. It may be possible to hold the testis gently and have the patient point to the specific point of pain. If this site is indicated to be the upper pole of the testis with the remainder of the testis being nontender, the diagnosis of torsion of a testicular appendage is likely. Although the classic "blue dot" sign of an infarcted appendage may be visible, often it cannot be seen because of overlying edema. In some cases evaluated later in the clinical course, the degree of scrotal tenderness and edema increases to the point at which differentiation from torsion of the testis becomes difficult. Nuclear scanning or Doppler sonography demonstrates normal or increased flow to the affected testicle and epididymis compared with the opposite side, representing the inflammation that occurs with torsion of the appendage.

If the examiner is confident in the diagnosis of torsion of an appendix testis, surgical exploration is not needed. The child should be sent home with analgesics and antiinflammatory agents, support to the scrotum, and instructions to rest quietly. The pain usually resolves in 2 to 12 days, but in most cases, the pain should improve somewhat within a few days. The patient should return to the physician in 48 hours, having had nothing to eat or drink on the morning of the return visit. In most cases, the child's pain will have lessened, and nothing further is indicated.

TRAUMA OR HEMATOCELE

In children, most trauma to the scrotum results from a direct blow to the perineum or a straddle injury that forcefully compresses the testicle against the pubic bone. Penetrating injuries are less common, and the small size and greater mobility of the prepubertal testis make testicular injuries rare in this group.

Scrotal trauma includes a spectrum of injuries that ranges from minimal scrotal swelling to rupture of the testis with a tense, blood-filled scrotum. Often scrotal ultrasound examination is useful in differentiating the various injuries. A hematocele, or blood within the tunica vaginalis, may represent severe testicular injury. An obvious ecchymosis of the scrotal wall in the setting of trauma suggests a hematocele. Sonography can identify the fluid collection within the tunica because blood is more echogenic than hydrocele fluid. Scrotal exploration is indicated if testicular rupture is present or in cases of large hematoceles, which heal more readily after surgical drainage. Scrotal trauma also can result in an intratesticular hematoma or laceration of the tunica albuginea. Ultrasound can assist in determining the location of blood. Any question or indication of testicular laceration requires surgical exploration and drainage of the hematoma with repair of the laceration. If the tunica albuginea can be determined to be intact, no surgical intervention is necessary.

Traumatic epididymitis is local inflammation resulting from blunt trauma to the scrotum, which usually occurs within a few days. Typically, short-lived acute pain associated with trauma is followed by a pain-free period, after which pain returns. On examination, scrotal erythema, edema, and tenderness of the epididymis may be found. In this noninfectious variety of epididymitis, the urinalysis is negative. Sonography is helpful to rule out any more severe injury and will demonstrate hyperemia associated with the inflammation.

If a scrotal laceration is present, it is essential that the testis and spermatic cord be evaluated for possible injury. For simple scrotal lacerations, careful hemostasis and closure of the laceration with chromic catgut are sufficient.

EPIDIDYMITIS AND ORCHITIS

Epididmyitis

Epididymitis is an infection or inflammation of the epididymis, which is most commonly seen in adolescents and adults. It is rarely seen in prepubertal boys, in whom it is often associated with a urinary tract infection caused by structural abnormalities of the urinary tract. At any age when epididymitis is associated with a urinary tract infection and in all prepubertal boys with epididymitis, urinary tract imaging with sonogram and voiding cystourethrogram are necessary to rule out a structural problem.

The onset of swelling and tenderness is typically more gradual than with torsion of the testis or a testicular appendage. Associated symptoms of urinary frequency and dysuria may be present. Early on, the epididymis may be selectively enlarged and tender, readily distinguished from the testis. With time, inflammation spreads to the testis and surrounding scrotal wall, making localization impossible. Although elevation of the scrotum relieves pain in epididymoorchitis (Prehn sign) but causes increased pain in torsion, this finding has not been found to be reliable in children. The cremasteric reflex should be preserved.

Although white cells in the urinary sediment are seen more often in epididymitis than in torsion, they are not consistently present. A culture of the urine should always be obtained, as well as a culture of any penile discharge or the urethra in any sexually active male. Color Doppler sonography typically demonstrates an increase in size and blood flow to the affected testis and epididymis. Nuclear scan shows increased activity in the affected testis.

Orchitis

Orchitis is an inflammation or infection of the testis resulting from the extension of epididymitis, rarely as hematogenous spread of a systemic bacterial infection, or following certain viral infections, including mumps. Although rare before puberty, orchitis occurs in about 18% of postpubertal boys with mumps parotitis. In 70% of cases, it is unilateral. It results in testicular atrophy, but not necessarily sterility, in 50% of affected testes.

Causes of Painless Scrotal Swelling

HYDROCELE

An accumulation of fluid within the tunica vaginalis that surrounds the testis—a *hydrocele*—may be seen with torsion of the testis or an appendage, epididymitis, trauma, or tumor. In these cases, examination of the underlying testis is abnormal. If the testis can be felt to be normal and the hydrocele is not associated with any abnormality of the overlying scrotal soft tissues, it is much more likely to be a simple hydrocele. In the infant, this is the result of fluid being left in place after the processus vaginalis has closed. When the size of the hydrocele has no history of waxing or waning, it may simply be observed. Usually, the fluid will be reabsorbed in the first 12 to 18 months of life.

If the hydrocele has a clear history of changing in size (often with crying or exertion), particularly if it is associated with thickening of the cord structures as they are felt against the pubic tubercle (the silk-glove sign), then the processus vaginalis is patent and the diagnosis is that of a communicating hydrocele. Here the patent processus vaginalis does not generally close spontaneously and may enlarge to permit the development of hernia. Occasionally, a hydrocele of the cord presents as a scrotal swelling just above the testis. Differentiation from an incarcerated hernia may be difficult and occasionally may require surgical exploration.

HERNIA

Although most inguinal hernias present in children with a mass in the groin, occasionally the hernia may extend and present as a scrotal swelling. An incarcerated hernia may produce pain in some patients. The diagnosis and treatment of inguinal hernias are discussed in Chapter 103.

VARICOCELE

A usually painless scrotal swelling caused by a collection of abnormally enlarged spermatic cord veins, called a *varicocele*, most commonly is found on routine examination of asymptomatic boys aged 10 to 15 years. Most varicoceles occur on the left, representing spermatic vein incompetence caused by the left spermatic vein draining into the renal vein at a sharp angle, whereas the right spermatic vein drains into the inferior vena cava. On occasion, a varicocele can present with mild pain or discomfort. The hemiscrotum appears full but does not have overlying skin changes. The testis and epididymis should be palpated to be normal. A mass of varicose veins described as "a bag of worms" can be appreciated above the testicle. Standing and supine examinations often reveal the varicocele, which is more prominent when standing. Doppler ultrasound is diagnostic, demonstrating both normal flow to the testis and the collection of tortuous veins.

SPERMATOCELE

Located above and posterior to the testicle in postpubertal boys, spermatoceles are sperm-containing cysts of the rete testes, ductuli efferentes, or epididymis. Multiple or bilateral spermatoceles may occur. On examination, a small, nontender mass that transilluminates may be appreciated distinct from and posterior to the testicle. These masses must be differentiated from a hydrocele or tumor. Sonography may confirm the location distinct from the testis and help distinguish a spermatocele from tumor.

IDIOPATHIC SCROTAL EDEMA

Idiopathic scrotal edema is a rare entity that represents only 2% to 5% of acute scrotal swellings in otherwise normal children. Typically, a prepubertal child presents with the rapid onset of painless but notable edema of the scrotal wall that may be bilateral and may extend up onto the abdominal wall. The skin of the scrotum may be erythematous. The child is usually afebrile and urinalysis is negative. Through the edematous scrotum, the testes can be felt to be normal in size and nontender. This edema of the scrotal wall is of unknown origin, although it is believed to represent a form of angioneurotic edema. Insect bites, allergic reactions, cellulitis, and contact dermatitis also can contribute to localized scrotal swelling. No specific therapy has been demonstrated to be effective. Children spontaneously begin to improve within 48 hours, regardless of treatment. Occasionally, scrotal edema is seen secondary to diseases that cause generalized edema or ascites, such as nephrosis and cirrhosis.

HENOCH–SCHÖNLEIN PURPURA

Occasionally, a child may be seen with a petechial rash on the scrotum as the initial presentation of this systemic vasculitic syndrome characterized by nonthrombocytopenic purpura, arthralgia, renal disease, abdominal pain, and gastrointestinal bleeding. More typically, the rash begins on the lower extremities or buttocks and later may involve the scrotum. If the associated swelling is not great, the cord structures and testes can be felt to be uninvolved and normal. In other cases with severe swelling, surgical exploration may be necessary to rule out testicular torsion, which rarely has been noted to coexist. When skin lesions are present the diagnosis of Henoch-Schönlein purpura (HSP) must be suspected. Occasionally, the acute scrotum is the dominant presenting symptom. Ultrasound may help rule out testicular torsion in these cases.

KAWASAKI DISEASE

Another vasculitis that can produce scrotal swelling and mild pain is Kawasaki disease, which has characteristic features including fever, adenopathy, rash, conjunctivitis, and irritability. Although discussed in detail elsewhere, it is important to note the association of scrotal swelling with this systemic disease to avoid unnecessary surgical explorations or delay in diagnosis of the underlying vasculitis.

TESTIS TUMOR

Testicular or paratesticular tumors are rare in children. They usually present as painless, unilateral, firm to hard scrotal swellings. Leukemic infiltration of the testis may present bilaterally. There may be an associated hydrocele. In children less than 2 years of age, the tumor usually is a yolk sac carcinoma or teratoma. After puberty, germinal cell tumors, as found in the adult population, are seen. Evaluation of a solid testicular mass involves an initial testicular ultrasound examination usually followed by surgical exploration through a groin incision to permit control of the spermatic vessels and a possible radical inguinal orchiectomy.

ANTENATAL TORSION TESTIS (NEWBORN)

A newborn boy may present with a painless, smooth, testicular enlargement that usually is dark. There should be no or minimal edema of the overlying scrotum. This is extravaginal torsion of the testis and probably occurs during the late period of embryonic development, as the testis descends into the scrotum. At this time, the testicular tunics are not yet attached to the scrotal tissue, and torsion of the entire testis with its tunics can occur.

EVALUATION AND DECISION

The physician should first determine whether the patient has scrotal pain or just swelling, as outlined in Figure 50.1. Testicular torsion, torsion of an appendage, orchitis, epididymitis, and trauma-related injuries to the scrotum or testicles are common causes of painful scrotal swelling. Hemorrhage into a tumor, incarcerated hernias, HSP, and Kawasaki disease may cause either painful or painless scrotal swelling. No one aspect of the history or physical examination may be diagnostic, but collectively the clinical findings often suggest a diagnosis. More recently available adjunctive radiologic studies may be helpful when the clinician is fully aware of the capabilities and limitations of the diagnostic studies.

Initial Approach

As a first step in the evaluation of the child with a complaint of scrotal swelling or pain, the physician should determine whether the child is suffering from a generalized edematous state, such as the nephrotic syndrome. When the problem in localized to the scrotum, patients can be divided into those who have a painless swelling and those who are experiencing pain.

In the immediate neonatal period, antenatal torsion may cause painless scrotal enlargement. Beyond infancy, the most common causes (Table 50.2) are hernias and hydroceles; a hernia is often reducible. The physician also must consider idiopathic scrotal edema, spermatocele, and varicocele. Both Kawasaki disease and HSP may involve the scrotal sac and cause swelling that is either painless or mildly painful. When the swelling is within the scrotum, rather than involving the scrotal sac, possible diagnoses include hydrocele, hernia (reducible if incarcerated and nonreducible), spermatocele, and hydrocele.

Painful swelling may follow a well-documented injury, in which case the likely diagnoses are hematocele, hematoma, testicular rupture, or traumatic epididymitis. The physician should bear in mind that boys with testicular trauma often give a history of having had an incidental minor injury. Nontraumatic scrotal pain raises the suspicion of a testicular torsion, particularly if the testis is tender. Unless the diagnosis of a systemic disorder (HSP, Kawasaki disease) is obvious, the patient is an adolescent with the classic signs of epididymitis, or an incarcerated

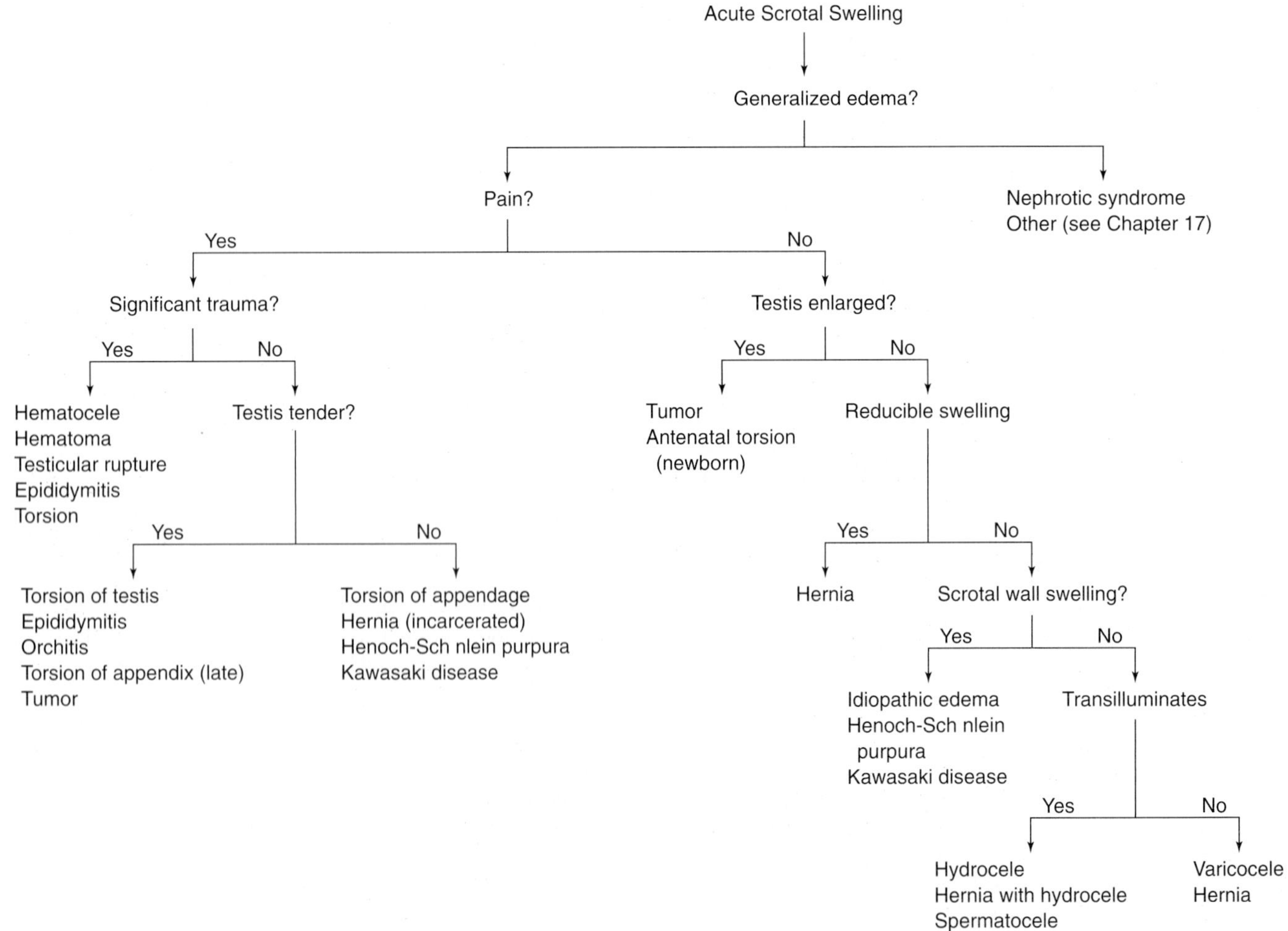

Figure 50.1. Diagnostic approach to acute scrotal swelling.

hernia is reduced, imaging via Doppler ultrasound or nuclear scan usually is indicated.

Physical Examination

Examination of the child with scrotal pain or swelling should be both careful and organized. Initial observations of the patient's gait, resting position, and facial expression are helpful. Writhing or an especially quiet supine posture versus active movement may best indicate the degree of pain. Observation of associated skin changes, presence and location of swelling, and the natural position of the testicle in the scrotum while standing should then be appreciated. The cremasteric reflex elicited by stroking the upper inner thigh should cause the testicle to elevate when intact. Next the lower abdomen, inguinal canal, and cord should be palpated. Finally, the scrotum and its contents should be sequentially palpated. Asking the patient to localize his pain with one finger at this time may be especially helpful. The unaffected hemiscrotum always should be palpated first. Knowledge of the location and specific attempt at palpation of the appendix testis and epididymis are beneficial before palpation of the testis itself. Appreciation of swelling, tenderness, and consistency should be noted for all intrascrotal structures. Transillumination may be helpful in some cases (Fig. 50.1).

CHAPTER 51
Pallor

Alan R. Cohen, M.D.

The development of pallor can be acute and associated with a life-threatening illness, or it can be chronic and subtle, occasionally first noted by someone who sees the child less often than the parents. The degree of pallor depends on the concentration of hemoglobin in the blood and the distribution of blood in the blood vessels of the skin. Any condition that decreases the concentration of hemoglobin or alters the distribution of blood away from the body's surface may present as pallor. Clinically, pallor caused by anemia usually can be appreciated when the hemoglobin concentration is below 8 to 9 g per deciliter, although the complexion of the child and the rapidity of onset can influence this value. Nonhematologic causes of pallor are outlined briefly in Table 51.1.

DIFFERENTIAL DIAGNOSIS

The differential diagnosis of the major hematologic causes of pallor in children is outlined in Table 51.2. The concentration of hemoglobin in the blood can be lowered by three basic mechanisms: decreased erythrocyte or hemoglobin production, increased erythrocyte destruction, and blood loss. The most common causes of pallor and anemia seen in the emergency department are iron deficiency, infections, and blood loss (Table 51.3), but several less common diseases remain important considerations.

TABLE 51.1. Pallor without Anemia

Physiologic ("fair-skinned")	Respiratory distress
Shock: septic, hypovolemic, neurogenic, cardiogenic, anaphylactoid	Skin edema
Hypoglycemia and other metabolic derangements	Pheochromocytoma

Decreased Production of Hemoglobin and Red Cells

NUTRITIONAL ANEMIAS

In children, the most common cause of decreased hemoglobin production is nutritional iron deficiency. This condition usually is seen in the first 2 years of life, at which time the dietary iron content often is insufficient to meet the demands of the rapidly increasing red cell mass. The infant with severe iron deficiency usually is irritable and very pale. The red cells are markedly microcytic and hypochromic in severe iron deficiency anemia. Variation in red cell size and shape usually is present, and elongated, pencil-like cells are particularly common. The percentage of reticulocytes may be elevated moderately, but the absolute reticulocyte count is low. Other nutritional anemias, such as vitamin B_{12} or folic acid deficiency, are uncommon in children in the United States and rarely develop in the absence of a grossly altered diet, extended hyperalimentation, intestinal resection, or chronic diarrhea. Unusual alterations of B_{12} and folic acid absorption and metabolism may cause symptoms similar to those of the nutritional megaloblastic anemias. Megaloblastic anemia is rarely severe enough to be life threatening. The condition is characterized by normochromic, macrocytic red blood cells; hypersegmented neutrophils; and an elevated serum level of lactic dehydrogenase.

HYPOPLASTIC AND APLASTIC ANEMIA

Pallor usually is the first sign of aplastic or hypoplastic anemia. Diamond–Blackfan syndrome is a congenital hypoplastic anemia commonly detected in the first few months of life. The red cells are normocytic or macrocytic. The reticulocyte count is low. The white cell count is low in approximately 10% of affected patients, but thrombocytopenia occurs only rarely. The diagnosis is made by examination of a bone marrow aspirate that shows markedly reduced or absent erythrocyte precursors. The second major congenital hypoplastic anemia is Fanconi anemia, a syndrome characterized by pancytopenia and associated abnormalities, including hyperpigmentation and hypopigmentation, microcephaly, strabismus, small stature, mental retardation, and abnormalities of the thumbs and radii. Unlike Diamond–Blackfan syndrome, all three cell lines of the bone marrow are affected, and the hematologic abnormalities rarely develop before 3 to 4 years of age. The anemia is normochromic and macrocytic.

Acquired aplastic anemia also can present with severe pallor in children. The anemia usually is associated with granulocytopenia and thrombocytopenia.

Transient erythroblastopenia of childhood (TEC) is a condition often associated with a recent viral illness and is characterized by moderate to severe anemia caused by diminished red cell production. The mean corpuscular volume (MCV) usually is normal at the time of diagnosis. The white cell count is normal or moderately decreased; the platelet count is normal. The reticulocyte count is decreased, and the Coombs test is negative. Bone marrow examination shows reduction or absence of erythrocytic precursors initially, followed by erythroid hyperplasia during recovery. Transient erythroblastopenia that occurs in the first 6 months of life may be difficult to distinguish from Diamond–Blackfan anemia. Spontaneous recovery ultimately confirms the diagnosis of TEC.

Hypoplastic anemia can be the presenting symptom of childhood malignancies. The pallor can be severe, and although all

TABLE 51.2. Pallor with Anemia

Decreased erythrocyte or hemoglobin production	Hemoglobinopathies
Nutritional deficiencies	Sickle cell syndromes[a]
Iron deficiency	Unstable hemoglobins
Folic acid and vitamin B_{12} deficiency or associated metabolic abnormalities	Immune hemolytic anemia
Aplastic or hypoplastic anemias	Autoimmune hemolytic anemia[a]
Diamond–Blackfan anemia	Isoimmune hemolytic anemia[a]
Fanconi anemia	Infection
Aplastic anemia[a]	Viral: mononucleosis, influenzas, coxsackie, measles, varicella, cytomegalovirus
Transient erythroblastopenia of childhood	Bacterial: *Escherichia coli, Pneumococcus, Streptococcus,* typhoid fever, *Mycoplasma*
Malignancy: leukemia, lymphoma, neuroblastoma[a]	Drugs: antibiotics
Abnormal heme and hemoglobin synthesis	Inflammatory and collagen vascular disease
Anemia of chronic disease: renal disease, inflammatory bowel disease, collagen vascular disease, thyroid deficiency or thyrotoxicosis, malignancy	Malignancy[a]
Lead poisoning[a]	Microangiopathic anemias
Sideroblastic anemia	Disseminated intravascular coagulation[a]
Thalassemias	Hemolytic uremic syndrome[a]
Increased erythrocyte destruction	Cavernous hemangioma
Erythrocyte membrane defects: hereditary spherocytosis, elliptocytosis, stomatocytosis, pyknocytosis, paroxysmal nocturnal hemoglobinuria	Blood loss
Erythrocyte enzyme defects	Severe trauma[a]
Defects of hexose monophosphate shunt: G6PD deficiency most common	Anatomic lesions
Defects of Embden–Meyerhof pathway: pyruvate kinase deficiency most common	Meckel diverticulum
	Peptic ulcer
	Idiopathic pulmonary hemosiderosis[a]

G6PD, glucose-6-phosphate dehydrogenase.
[a] Conditions that are known to present with acute, life-threatening anemia or are associated with other serious abnormalities.

three cell lines of the bone marrow usually are affected, anemia may be the only notable hematologic abnormality. The diagnosis can be suspected from the presence of other symptoms or findings such as lymphadenopathy, bruising, limb pain, gum bleeding, or an abdominal mass.

Patients with hemolytic anemias such as spherocytosis or sickle cell disease may develop red cell aplasia, usually in association with parvovirus B19 infection. Decreased red cell production in the face of ongoing hemolysis causes an exacerbation of the anemia. The usually elevated reticulocyte count falls to inappropriately low levels, often less than 1%.

Disorders of Heme and Globin Production

Pallor may be the presenting sign of nonnutritional disorders of hemoglobin synthesis, including the sideroblastic anemias and thalassemia syndromes. These disorders are characterized by a microcytic, hypochromic anemia. Sideroblastic anemia may be inherited (sex-linked) or acquired. Iron use within the developing red cell is abnormal, accounting for the presence of diagnostic ringed sideroblasts in the bone marrow. The serum iron and ferritin levels usually are markedly elevated.

In the thalassemias, production of the globin portion of the hemoglobin molecule is defective. Cooley anemia (β-thalassemia major) presents with severe pallor usually between 6 and 12 months of age, as the fetal hemoglobin (HbF) level declines, but the normal rise in adult hemoglobin (HbA) production fails to occur because of reduced or absent β-globin production. Although β-thalassemia is often associated with Mediterranean ancestry, this disease and related disorders (e.g., E-β thalassemia, HbH disease) also are seen commonly in children of Southeast Asian, Indian, Pakistani, and Chinese background. The presence of hepatosplenomegaly and characteristic red cell morphology, including marked variation in red cell shape, makes this diagnosis readily apparent.

Lead poisoning affects heme synthesis, but significant anemia is unusual unless blood lead levels are markedly elevated. Iron deficiency is common in children with increased lead levels and usually accounts for the microcytic anemia found in these patients. If a concomitant hematologic disorder cannot be found in the anemic patient with plumbism, particular care should be given to the possibility of severe lead intoxication.

TABLE 51.3. Relatively Common Causes of Pallor or Anemia

Decreased erythrocyte or hemoglobin production	Increased erythrocyte destruction
Iron deficiency	Sickle cell syndromes
Aplasia	Autoimmune hemolytic anemia
	Viral, bacterial, or parasitic infections
	Blood loss

Systemic Disease

Numerous disorders that are not primarily hematologic may be associated with pallor and anemia. Occasionally, pallor is the only presenting finding of a serious systemic disorder. Chronic inflammatory diseases, such as juvenile rheumatoid arthritis (JRA) and ulcerative colitis, often are accompanied by a normocytic or microcytic anemia related to impaired iron use. Similar clinical and laboratory findings may be associated with chronic infections such as acquired immunodeficiency syndrome (AIDS) and subacute bacterial endocarditis. Other diseases in which anemia may be a prominent component include chronic renal disease, hyperthyroidism, and hypothyroidism.

Increased Red Cell Destruction

The numerous conditions associated with shortened red cell survival can be congenital, as in the case of the hemoglobinopathies and membrane and enzyme defects, or acquired, as in the case of autoimmune hemolytic anemia, drug-associated hemolytic anemias, disseminated intravascular coagulation (DIC), and hemolytic uremic syndrome (HUS). The hemoglobin levels in these disorders can be normal, slightly depressed, or so low as to be life threatening.

An alteration in the patient's ability to compensate for increased red cell destruction may result in a severe life-threatening exacerbation of the underlying anemia. This aplastic crisis, the result of a transient decrease in erythrocyte production in the presence of shortened red cell survival, should be suspected in a patient with a known hemolytic anemia who develops increasing pallor and anemia associated with a reticulocyte count much lower than usual. Unfortunately, when the hemolytic anemia has not been diagnosed previously, the recognition of an aplastic crisis can be difficult because the findings are similar to those of transient erythroblastopenia of childhood or congenital erythrocyte hypoplasia (i.e., anemia with low or absent reticulocytes). Examination of the bone marrow may be helpful in distinguishing these disorders because production of early red cell precursors often resumes shortly after detection of an aplastic crisis.

Membrane Disorders

The degree of pallor associated with anemia caused by erythrocyte membrane abnormalities depends on the hemoglobin level. In rare instances, patients with hereditary spherocytosis, the most common of the membrane disorders, develop significant anemia and pallor in the newborn period. Moderate or severe anemia is less common in the other membrane disorders, such as hereditary elliptocytosis and hereditary stomatocytosis. The anemia of the erythrocyte membrane disorders is accompanied by reticulocytosis. The red cell morphology often permits the diagnosis to be made from the peripheral smear.

Infantile pyknocytosis is a hemolytic anemia seen during the first few months of life and is characterized by distorted and contracted erythrocytes and burr cells. The disorder may be associated with pallor and hyperbilirubinemia. Spontaneous recovery usually occurs by 6 months of age.

Enzyme Disorders

Erythrocyte enzymatic defects, such as pyruvate kinase deficiency and certain variants of glucose-6-phosphate dehydrogenase (G6PD) deficiency, may be associated with pallor from increased red blood cell destruction. In the latter disorder, pallor may be accentuated by acute hemolytic crises after exposure to oxidant stress (e.g., naphthalene-containing mothballs, drugs, acidosis).

Hemoglobinopathies

Pallor may result from the low hemoglobin level found in patients with sickle cell anemia and related hemoglobinopathies. Acute accentuation of pallor can result from an aplastic crisis, a complication of hemolytic disorders that is particularly common in sickle cell anemia. During an aplastic crisis, the normally elevated reticulocyte count may fall to zero, and the hemoglobin level may fall as low as 1 to 2 g per deciliter, resulting in severe pallor and signs of high-output cardiac failure.

The sequestration crisis of sickle cell anemia and related hemoglobin disorders (sickle cell disease, S-β thalassemia, S-β^+ thalassemia) results from acute pooling of red cells and plasma in the spleen. The sudden and severe anemia and the hypovolemia associated with this complication constitute a true hematologic emergency and, if untreated, can rapidly lead to death. The presence of increased pallor and acute enlargement of the spleen in a patient with a sickling disorder should prompt immediate investigation of a possible sequestration crisis. Although this complication rarely occurs in children with homozygous sickle cell disease or S-β thalassemia after the age of 5 years, sequestration crises may occur much later in children with sickling disorders such as SC disease or S-β^+ thalassemia, in which early splenic infarction is less common.

Immune Hemolytic Anemia

Pallor caused by autoimmune hemolytic anemia usually is acute in onset and may be associated with severe anemia. The presence of only moderate anemia (6 to 8 g/dL) at diagnosis should not detract from consideration of this disease as a hematologic emergency because brisk hemolysis may result in a sudden, additional fall in hemoglobin level. Autoimmune hemolytic anemia usually, but not always, is characterized by a positive Coombs test and an increased reticulocyte count. Spherocytes are commonly seen in the peripheral smear. Other causes of immune hemolytic anemia include infections, drugs, inflammatory diseases, and malignancies.

Microangiopathic Anemia

Alterations in the normal flow of blood through the vascular system may cause increased red cell destruction. In DIC, abnormal fibrin deposition within small blood vessels results in mechanical injury to the erythrocytes. Thrombocytopenia and clotting abnormalities, which often herald the onset of DIC, also may contribute to the anemia by causing diffuse bleeding. The main diagnostic findings are red cell fragments in the peripheral blood smear, platelet and clotting abnormalities typical of a consumptive coagulopathy (see Chapter 77), and the clinical features of a disease, such as septic shock, which is associated with DIC.

The increased red cell destruction in HUS and thrombotic thrombocytopenic purpura (TTP) also is caused by intravascular fibrin deposition. Thrombocytopenia and uremia may lower the hemoglobin concentration even further by causing bleeding, impaired red cell production, shortened red cell survival, and increased plasma volume. In some instances, the anemia may be moderately severe when the uremia is only mild and thrombocytopenia is absent, leaving doubt about the correct diagnosis. In more typical cases, however, the diagnosis is readily apparent from the findings of oliguria, central nervous system abnormalities, increased blood urea nitrogen, thrombocytopenia, and abnormalities of red cell morphology, including fragments and helmet cells.

The proliferation of blood vessels within a cavernous hemangioma may trap red cells or initiate a localized consumptive coagulopathy, causing erythrocyte destruction. Anemia is rarely severe unless the thrombocytopenia that is more typical of the disorder causes chronic blood loss.

Blood Loss

Although sudden, massive hemorrhage usually is accompanied by signs of hypovolemic shock, the repeated loss of smaller amounts of blood may be associated with few findings other than pallor. The finding of iron deficiency anemia despite normal dietary iron intake or iron supplementation may be a clue to the presence of chronic blood loss from the gastrointestinal tract or within the lungs.

EVALUATION AND DECISION

If the child with pallor is not acutely ill, a deliberate search for the cause of pallor should be undertaken (Fig. 51.1). A thorough yet relevant history should be obtained, with particular attention to the type of onset of pallor. The slow development of pallor, often noticed only by a family member or friend who sees the child only occasionally, suggests diminished red cell production, as is found in bone marrow aplasia or iron deficiency. The acute onset of pallor is consistent with the brisk hemolysis found in autoimmune hemolytic anemia and often is accompanied by jaundice, dark urine, and cardiovascular changes.

After establishing the type of onset of the anemia, the history can be directed toward more narrow categories of anemia or specific diseases. A detailed dietary history, with particular attention to milk intake, is important in young children with suspected iron deficiency because excessive consumption of cow's milk often results in iron deficiency.

Sources of internal or external blood loss should be carefully sought. Chronic gastrointestinal bleeding may escape detection until iron deficiency anemia develops. Similarly, small pulmonary hemorrhages associated with idiopathic pulmonary hemosiderosis are often mistaken for other pulmonic processes until several recurrences of iron deficiency anemia suggest a hidden site of blood loss.

If increased bruising or bleeding accompanies pallor, multiple blood elements are probably affected. The circulation time of platelets is short compared with that of red cells. Therefore, clinical findings of thrombocytopenia often are present by the time pallor develops in patients with acquired aplastic anemia, Fanconi anemia, and acute leukemia.

The family history helps in the diagnosis of hemoglobinopathies and inherited disorders of red cell membranes and enzymes. Because results of previous hemoglobin testing may have been explained inadequately or recalled inaccurately, a negative family history or newborn screening for hemoglobinopathies should not preclude evaluation of the patient's hemoglobin phenotype if a sickling disorder is suspected. The presence of a microcytic anemia unresponsive to iron in the parents suggests a thalassemic disorder.

A history of splenomegaly, splenectomy, or cholecystectomy in family members may help identify a hemolytic disorder such as hereditary spherocytosis or pyruvate kinase deficiency. Finally, a well-directed review of systems is essential in looking for systemic disorders such as chronic renal disease, hypothyroidism, or JRA. Pallor may be the presenting complaint in these and other disorders.

In the examination of the severely anemic patient, pallor of the skin and mucous membranes usually is readily apparent. When anemia is less severe or when the skin color is dark, pallor may be appreciated only in the nailbeds and palpebral conjunctivae. If anemia or volume loss is mild, tachycardia may be present, but normal blood pressure is preserved. Lymphadenopathy and splenomegaly may suggest a malignancy or an infectious disease such as mononucleosis. When splenomegaly occurs without lymphadenopathy, however, attention is drawn to hemolytic disorders such as hereditary spherocytosis and autoimmune hemolytic anemia or hemoglobinopathies (sickling disorders or thalassemia major). Scleral icterus also may be present in these disorders of shortened red cell survival. The finding of an unusually large and firm spleen in the absence of increasing scleral icterus suggests that red cells are being sequestered (e.g., splenic sequestration crisis of sickle cell disease, hypersplenism).

The skin should be examined for the presence of hemangiomas that might cause microangiopathic anemia. Careful auscultation of the abdomen and head may detect hemangiomas of the viscera. Bony abnormalities associated with red cell disorders include frontal bossing from compensatory expansion of the bone marrow in hemolytic diseases and radial and thumb anomalies found in some patients with Fanconi anemia.

Numerous classifications of anemia have been used to assist the physician in the laboratory investigation of pallor. Historically, the reticulocyte count and the MCV have been helpful measurements in categorizing causes of anemia. The reticulocyte count can be performed rapidly and, as shown in Figure 51.1, distinguishes anemias caused by impaired red cell production (e.g., iron deficiency, hypoplastic anemia) from those caused by shortened red cell survival (e.g., hemoglobinopathies, membrane disorders). The MCV provides a quick, accurate, and readily available method to distinguish the microcytic anemias (i.e., iron deficiency, thalassemia syndromes) from the normocytic anemias (i.e., membrane disorders, enzyme deficiencies, autoimmune hemolytic anemia, most hemoglobinopathies) or macrocytic (i.e., bone marrow or stem cell failure, disorders of B_{12} and folic acid absorption or metabolism) anemias.

The reticulocyte count and MCV should be interpreted with caution. As shown in Figure 51.1, disorders of shortened red cell survival are not always characterized by an increased reticulocyte count. For example, reticulocytopenia may occur in autoimmune hemolytic anemia despite active hemolysis and increased erythropoiesis in the bone marrow. Chronic hemolytic disorders, such as sickle cell anemia or hereditary spherocytosis, may first be detected during an aplastic crisis when the reticulocyte count is low. Unless the underlying disorder is recognized, this finding could mislead the physician. Furthermore, because the reticulocyte count is expressed as a percentage of total red cells, often it must be corrected for the degree of anemia. The easiest way to make this correction is to multiply the reticulocyte count by the reported hemoglobin or hematocrit divided by a normal hemoglobin or hematocrit. For example, a reticulocyte count of 5% in a child with severe iron deficiency anemia and a hematocrit of 6% is not elevated when corrected for the degree of anemia ($5\% \times 6\% / 33\% = 0.9\%$).

As shown in Figure 51.1, the reticulocyte count and MCV help in the initial classification of anemia but leave the physician with broad categories of disease rather than specific diagnoses. In many instances, the history and physical examination, when coupled with these laboratory measurements, permit identification of a particular disorder. Additional laboratory studies and careful examination of the peripheral smear often are required. The application of these procedures to diseases that are commonly encountered or that are associated with unusually severe anemia is discussed next.

Increased Reticulocytes and Low Mean Corpuscular Value

The thalassemia syndromes associated with moderate or severe anemia can be recognized by the distinctive abnormalities of red cell morphology. In Cooley anemia (β-thalassemia major), the

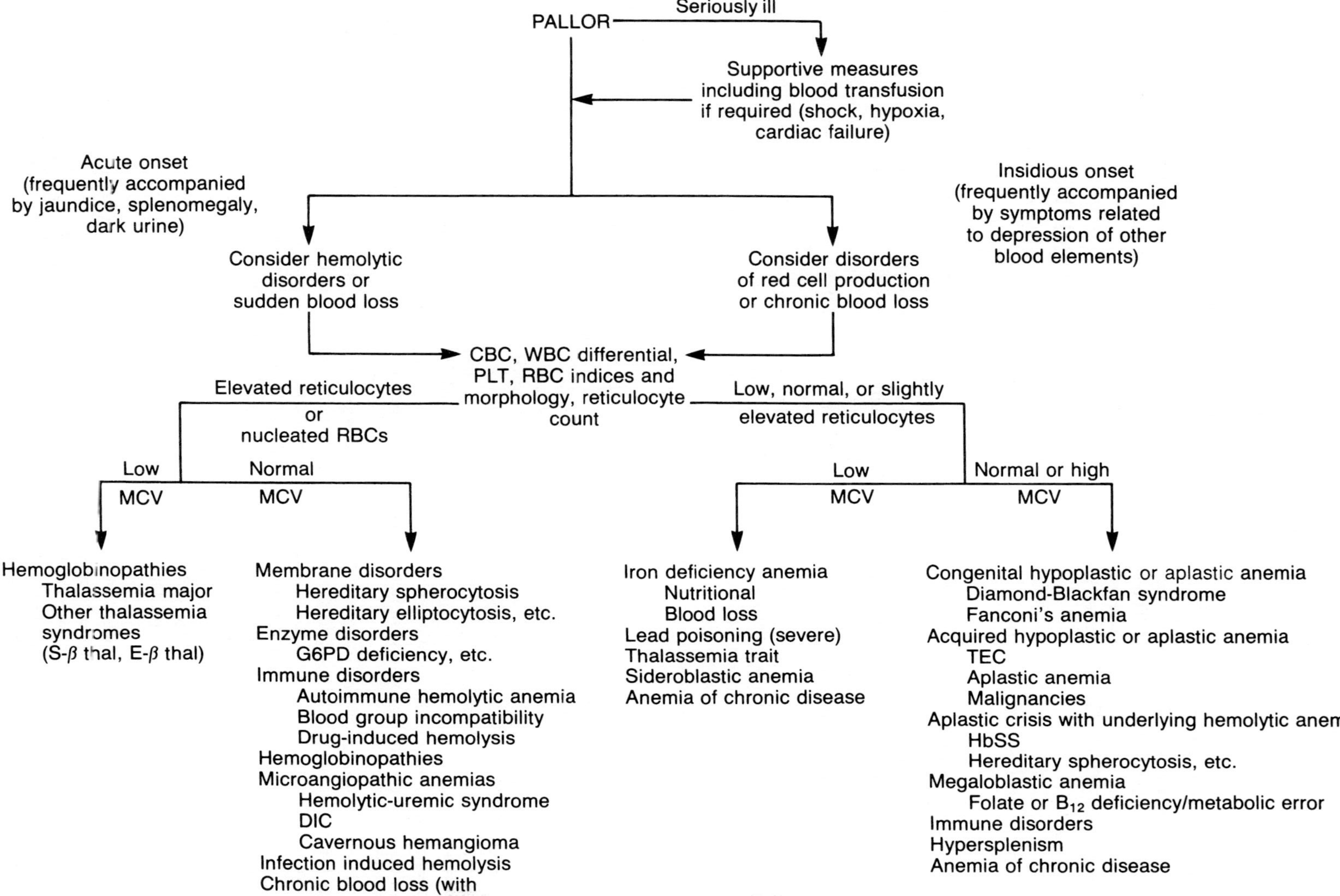

Figure 51.1. The diagnostic approach to pallor. CBC, complete blood count; WBC, white blood cells; PLT, platelets; RBC, red blood cells; MCV, mean corpuscular volume; G6PD, glucose-6-phosphate deficiency; TEC, transient erythroblastopenia of childhood; DIC, disseminated intravascular coagulation.

red cells generally are small but vary markedly in size and shape. Many cells appear to contain little or no hemoglobin; the central pallor extends to the cell membrane. Nucleated red cells, basophilic stippling, and polychromasia reflect active erythropoiesis. The parents of an affected child usually have a low MCV characteristic of thalassemia trait.

Children with HbS-β-thalassemia often have microcytic red cells, although the alterations of red cell morphology are not as dramatic as in Cooley anemia. Sickled forms are often but not always present. Target cells are common. The solubility tests are positive because of the presence of HbS. Hemoglobin electrophoresis reveals HbS and reduced ($< 50\%$) or absent HbA.

Increased Reticulocytes and Normal Mean Corpuscular Value

Most membrane disorders can be readily identified by the characteristic changes in red cell shape that lend their names to the diseases (e.g., spherocytosis, elliptocytosis, stomatocytosis). When the diagnosis of a membrane disorder is uncertain, examination of the parents' peripheral smears may be helpful because, in many cases, the inheritance pattern is autosomal dominant.

Abnormalities of red cell morphology are less striking in erythrocyte enzymatic defects. Blister cells and cells with asymmetric distribution of hemoglobin may be found, however, during episodes of active hemolysis in G6PD deficiency. If transfusion is necessary, a pretransfusion sample should be saved for assay of specific enzymes.

The reticulocyte count usually is markedly elevated in autoimmune hemolytic anemia but may be normal or only slightly elevated during the first days of the disease. In rare instances, reticulocytopenia persists. Spherocytes usually are present on the peripheral smear. Clumping of red cells from agglutination may be seen. This agglutination sometimes causes a falsely elevated MCV because the electronic counter measures the volume of red cell couplets or triplets. The direct Coombs test is positive in 90% of cases. Patients with a negative Coombs test present a challenging diagnostic problem because the initial findings may be similar to those in hereditary spherocytosis.

The recognition of homozygous sickle cell disease usually is accomplished by the finding of sickled red cells on the peripheral smear. Rarely, however, such cells are absent, even during an acute illness. Target cells are commonly found in sickle cell disease but are more prominent in HbSC. Solubility tests are positive. Hemoglobin electrophoresis reveals the presence of the abnormal hemoglobin(s) and the absence of HbA. This confirmatory test takes less than 30 minutes to complete and should be performed when important therapeutic decisions depend on the result.

Red cell fragments are found in diseases characterized by microangiopathic anemia. In HUS or TTP, thrombocytopenia is present, renal or neurologic function is usually impaired, and thrombotic complications may be present. The platelet count also is low in DIC, and clotting studies are abnormal. If intravascular hemolysis is severe, as in anemia associated with certain artificial cardiac valves, hemosiderin may be detected in the urinary sediment.

Low, Normal, or Slightly Elevated Reticulocytes and Low Mean Corpuscular Value

In severe iron deficiency anemia, red cells are markedly microcytic and show substantial variation in size and shape. Elongated red cells (pencil forms) are common. Platelets are often increased.

Anemia is uncommon in lead poisoning but when it is present, resembles the anemia of iron deficiency in its red cell morphology. Basophilic stippling is found in a small percentage of cases. The erythrocyte protoporphyrin is markedly elevated, and the rapid measurement of this compound helps to distinguish severe lead poisoning, which requires hospitalization and intensive chelation, from iron deficiency, which usually can be treated on an outpatient basis.

Low, Normal, or Slightly Elevated Reticulocytes and Normal or Elevated Mean Corpuscular Value

With the exception of mild macrocytosis, red cell morphology usually is normal in childhood disorders of bone marrow or stem cell failure. Thrombocytopenia and neutropenia are present in aplastic anemia and Fanconi anemia. Although the platelet count and white count occasionally may be low in patients with Diamond–Blackfan syndrome, the red cells are most severely affected. Erythropoiesis is most severely affected in TEC and acquired pure red cell aplasia, although neutropenia may accompany the former disorder.

The clinical features at the onset of acute leukemia may closely resemble those of aplastic anemia. Examination of a bone marrow aspirate is sometimes required to distinguish these disorders.

As discussed, children with hemolytic disorders may escape detection until pallor is noted during an aplastic crisis when the reticulocyte count is similar to that found in primary disorders of red cell production. An underlying hemolytic disease such as sickle cell anemia or hereditary spherocytosis usually can be recognized during anaplastic crisis, however, by finding characteristic red cells on the peripheral smear. In the autosomal dominant disorders of the red cell membrane, the presence of abnormal erythrocytes in the peripheral blood of one of the parents may support the diagnosis.

The MCV usually is increased in megaloblastic anemias unless other nutritional disorders are present. Hypersegmentation of the polymorphonuclear leukocytes is characteristic. In severe or long-standing megaloblastic anemia, neutropenia and thrombocytopenia also may be found. In such cases, the findings in the peripheral blood may be similar to those of aplastic anemia or even acute leukemia; examination of the bone marrow and measurement of specific nutrients (B_{12}, folic acid) are necessary to distinguish these disorders.

CHAPTER 52
Polydipsia

Ronald I. Paul, M.D.

Polydipsia, or excessive thirst, is an uncommon complaint in children. Although fluid consumption varies greatly among individuals, pathologic conditions exist when excessive drinking of fluids interferes with daily life or is accompanied by bizarre behavior, such as drinking from a toilet bowl.

TABLE 52.1. Causes of Polydipsia

Diabetes mellitus	Infection
Electrolyte imbalances	Aneurysm
Hypercalcemia	Intraventricular hemorrhage
Hypokalemia	Hereditary
Bartter syndrome	Drugs
Catecholamine excess	Methylxanthines
Pheochromocytoma	Diuretics
Neuroblastoma	Lithium
Ganglioneuroma	Renal causes
Cystinosis	Renal tubular acidosis
Diabetes insipidus (antidiuretic hormone deficient)	Nephrogenic diabetes insipidus
	Sickle cell trait
Craniopharyngioma	Sickle cell diseases
Pituitary adenoma	Interstitial nephritis
Histiocytosis	Obstructive uropathy
Head trauma	Primary polydipsia
Sarcoidosis	Psychogenic polydipsia
Leukemia	Neurogenic polydipsia

DIFFERENTIAL DIAGNOSIS

Diabetes mellitus (DM) is the single most common cause of polydipsia (Table 52.1). Additional prominent symptoms of DM include weight loss and polyuria. Other common causes of polydipsia include sickle cell anemia and diabetes insipidus (Table 52.2). In diabetes insipidus, a wide variety of lesions in the hypothalamus and neurohypophysis will result in a deficiency of antidiuretic hormone. Also, a rare inherited form of nephrogenic diabetes insipidus exists that may be autosomal dominant or X-linked recessive.

Less common metabolic and endocrine causes of polydipsia include electrolyte imbalances, catecholamine excess, and cystinosis. Primary renal causes of hyposthenuria include interstitial nephritis, renal tubular acidosis, medullary cystic disease (*nephrophthisis*), and obstructive uropathy. In nephrogenic diabetes insipidus, the renal tubule is unresponsive to antidiuretic hormone. Patients with nephrogenic diabetes insipidus usually have onset of symptoms in infancy and present with recurrent episodes of dehydration, fever, failure to thrive, and psychomotor retardation. Pharmacologic causes of polyuria and polydipsia include methylxanthines and diuretics. In addition, chronic lithium therapy may result in nephrogenic diabetes insipidus.

Primary polydipsia is diagnosed when the ingestion of water is in excess of that needed to maintain water balance. It can be caused by an inappropriate psychologic thirst drive (psychogenic polydipsia or compulsive water drinking) or by hypothalamic damage that alters thirst but not antidiuretic hormone release (*neurogenic polydipsia*).

Potentially life-threatening conditions may be seen (Table 52.3). Patients with diabetes insipidus or nephrogenic diabetes insipidus may develop severe dehydration if water is withheld for prolonged periods. Conversely, urgent management of hypernatremia is usually unnecessary if patients are able to drink and may be harmful if it is of chronic duration. Diabetic ketoacidosis may be an initial presentation of patients with DM and can result in extreme electrolyte and acid–base imbalances. Patients with primary polydipsia who overload their kidneys' ability to excrete free water may present with hyponatremic seizures. Many of the brain lesions that cause diabetes insipidus can become life threatening. In fact, diabetes insipidus often is seen in dying patients with severe brain injury.

TABLE 52.2. Common Causes of Polydipsia

Diabetes mellitus	Diabetes insipidus (antidiuretic hormone deficient)
Sickle cell anemia	

TABLE 52.3. Life-Threatening Causes of Polydipsia

Diabetes insipidus (antidiuretic hormone deficient)	Diabetes mellitus
Nephrogenic diabetes insipidus	Primary polydipsia

EVALUATION AND DECISION

When evaluating a child with polydipsia, the physician should seek information from the parent that would characterize the quantity of fluid taken each day and whether the child has used any unusual methods to satiate thirst. A history of nocturnal polydipsia and polyuria is helpful because most children with psychogenic polydipsia do not wake in the middle of the night for fluids. Inquiries should be made about known causes of polydipsia such as sickle cell disease, DM, chronic kidney disorders, head trauma, and medications (Fig. 52.1). The physical examination should include a careful evaluation for known systemic and intracranial causes of diabetes insipidus.

If the history and physical examination are not revealing, a urinalysis should be obtained. In almost all cases of polydipsia, the urine specific gravity will be low (< 1.010). A specific gravity greater than 1.020 usually represents an appropriate level of thirst. If the urinalysis is abnormal, DM, sickle cell disease or trait or an intrinsic renal disorder should be suspected. If the urinalysis is normal, electrolytes, calcium, and renal function tests may reveal conditions associated with electrolyte imbalances. Patients with diabetes insipidus or nephrogenic diabetes insipidus may have hypernatremia if they are examined when they are dehydrated. A hemoglobin electrophoresis may be needed to determine whether the patient has sickle cell disease or trait; however, patients with sickle cell disease usually have the diagnosis confirmed before the development of tubular dysfunction and polydipsia. Computed tomography and magnetic resonance imaging scans may be necessary to diagnose intracranial abnormalities.

Patients suspected of having primary polydipsia, diabetes insipidus, and nephrogenic diabetes insipidus require further testing; however, such testing be dangerous. These tests should be done under controlled settings and usually are inappropriate in the emergency department.

Patients with primary polydipsia should respond to a water-deprivation test by increasing their urine gravity and osmolality. Patients with diabetes insipidus and nephrogenic diabetes insipidus should have rapid weight loss while continuing to excrete urine with a low specific gravity. A trial of intranasal desmopressin (DDAVP) should distinguish between diabetes insipidus and nephrogenic diabetes insipidus because patients with antidiuretic hormone-deficient diabetes insipidus will respond to the exogenous hormone.

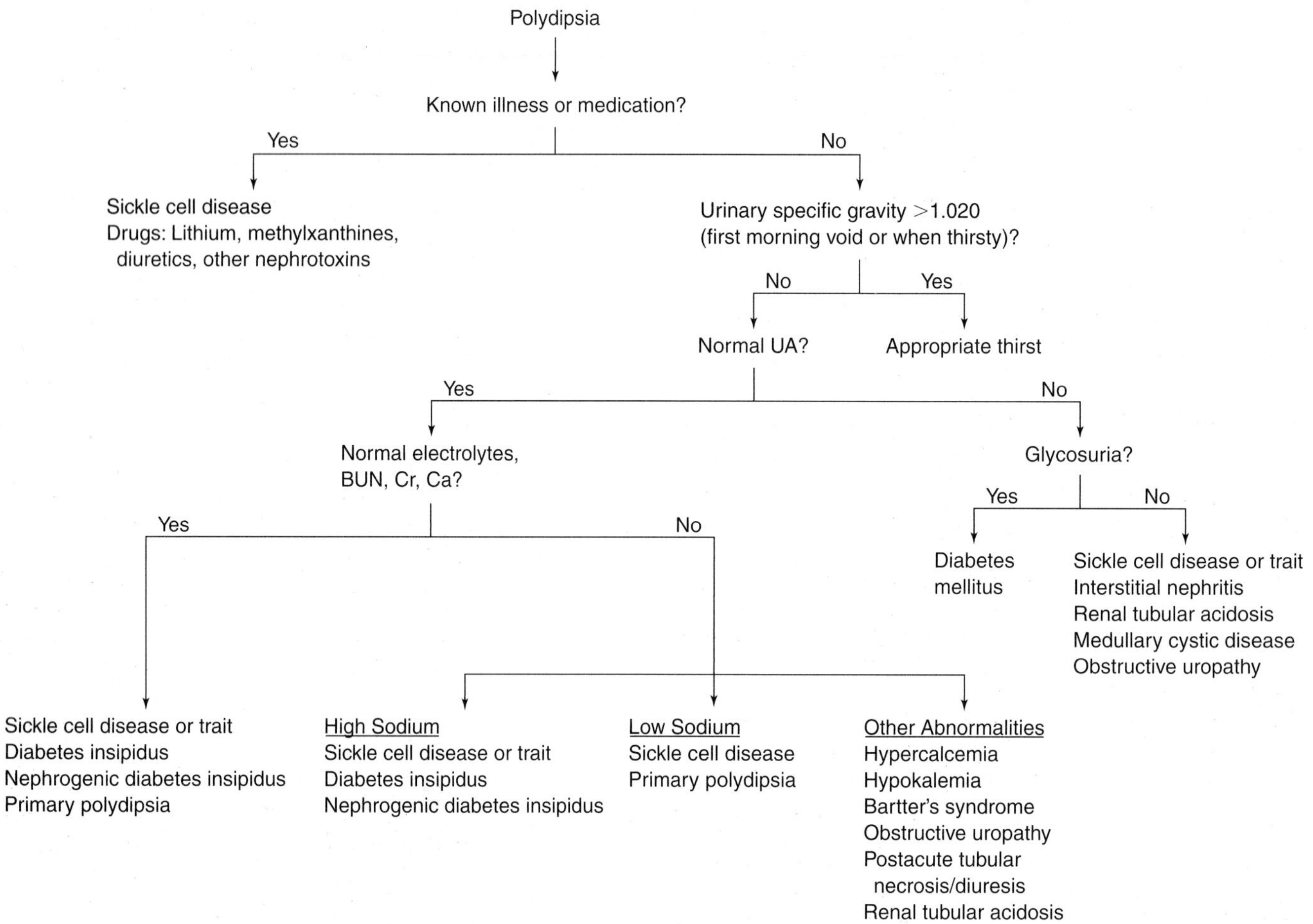

Figure 52.1. Diagnostic approach to a child with polyuria.

CHAPTER 53
Rash—Maculopapular

Karen Gruskin, M.D.

A *papule* is a small, solid, mostly elevated lesion that is usually smaller than 1 cm in diameter. *Macules* are circumscribed flat lesions that differ from surrounding skin because of their color. Both papules and macules may have any size, shape, or color. Commonly, a rash may have papular and macular components, which leads to the term *maculopapular rash.* The causes of maculopapular rashes are diverse (Table 53.1) and range from benign to life threatening (Table 53.2). Common causes include viral exanthems, contact dermatitis, insect bites, and scabies (Table 53.3). The diagnostic approach to these disorders is based on the presence or absence of fever, characteristic clinical appearance, location, and chronicity (Fig. 53.1). Some of these conditions have characteristic clinical appearances (Table 53.4); however, manifestations of these illnesses can be sufficiently variable that some cases will be difficult to diagnose.

DIFFERENTIAL DIAGNOSIS

Presence of Fever

The potentially life-threatening maculopapular rashes (Table 53.2) are all acute illnesses most commonly associated with fever and significant systemic symptoms. Hence, most patients with these illnesses will appear toxic. Erythema multiforme (EM) and rubeola have recognizable clinical appearances, whereas Kawasaki disease, Rocky Mountain spotted fever, and dengue fever require a high level of clinical suspicion. Other, less severe, febrile illnesses associated with maculopapular rashes are listed in Figure 53.1.

Potentially Life-Threatening Illnesses

ERYTHEMA MULTIFORME

Erythema multiforme is believed to result from an immune-mediated acute hypersensitivity reaction to exposure to a sensitizing antigen (see Chapter 88). Common offenders include drugs, especially trimethoprim–sulfasoxazole, cefaclor, and phenytoin; foods, especially nuts and shellfish; and infections by any number of viral, bacterial, protozoal, or fungal organisms. Herpetic and *Mycoplasma pneumoniae* infections rank among the infectious causes.

The rash of EM is characterized by diffuse erythematous macules with central clearing often called a *target* or *iris* lesion. Lesions also may include erythematous papules, macules, urticarial raised lesions, vesicles, and bullae. The distribution is most commonly symmetric and may be noted anywhere on the body, but it has a predilection for the hands and feet, including the palms and soles. Lesions may appear in isolation or as a more confluent rash. Based on severity, patients are classified as having EM minor or EM major, or Stevens–Johnson syndrome. EM major is characterized by extensive skin and mucosal in-

TABLE 53.1. Maculopapular Rash: Etiologic Classification

Infectious	Fungal
Viral	Tinea versicolor
Roseola infactum	Other infections
Rubeola	Rocky Mountain spotted fever
Rubella	Mycoplasma (15% of cases)
Erythema infectiosum (fifth disease)	Etiology uncertain but thought to be viral
Varicella (early manifestations before bullae)	Pityriasis rosea
	Kawasaki disease
Epstein–Barr virus (10%–15% of cases have macular or maculopapular rash)	Papular acrodermatitis
	Noninfectious
Molluscum contagiosum (papules)	Bites and infestations
Dengue	Insect bites
"Nonspecific" viral	Scabies
Enterovirus	Miscellaneous
Echovirus	Drug reaction
Coxsackievirus	Allergic contact dermatitis
Adenovirus	Irritant contact dermatitis
Bacterial	Papular urticaria
Scarlet fever	Erythema multiforme
Syphilis	Guttate psoriasis
Disseminated gonorrhea	Pityriasis lichenoides
	Lichen nitidus

volvement associated with significant systemic symptoms, including fever, chills, and malaise. Skin involvement can progress to sloughing with significant extravascular fluid losses. Conjunctivitis and keratitis are common features of the major form and can lead to permanent corneal scarring. Pulmonary, cardiac, and renal involvement may occur in especially severe cases.

KAWASAKI DISEASE

Kawasaki disease is a well-described illness of unknown cause assumed to be infectious in origin because of its epidemiologic and clinical presentation. The diagnosis is based on an unremitting fever of at least 5 days' duration and four of the five following features: (1) rash; (2) nonexudative bulbar conjunctivitis with limbal sparing; (3) red cracked lips, strawberry tongue, and erythematous oropharynx; (4) erythema, swelling, or induration of peripheral extremities; and (5) a solitary unilateral cervical lymph node with a diameter greater than 1.5 cm.

The most commonly associated rash is a generalized pruritic urticaria-like exanthem with raised erythematous plaques; however, the rash also may present with an erythematous maculopapular, morbilliform, scarlatiniform, or erythema marginatum-like pattern. The exanthem may be fleeting or persist for 2 to 3 days. During the later stages of the acute phase, periungual desquamation and peeling of the palms, soles, or perineal area develops. Laboratory tests often show a persistently elevated erythrocyte sedimentation rate and a markedly elevated platelet count ($> 750{,}000/mm^3$).

MEASLES (RUBEOLA)

In its classic form, measles has a highly characteristic natural history. Prodromal symptoms are cough, fever, coryza, and conjunctivitis. Two to three days after the onset of the prodrome and 12 to 24 hours before onset of the exanthem, pathognomonic Koplik spots occur in the mouth. Most typically, they occur on the buccal mucosa opposite the molars as pinpoint white lesions on a red base. However, Koplik spots may be seen on any of the mucosal surfaces of the oral cavity except the tongue.

The measles exanthem begins on the head as reddish maculopapules and spreads downward during the next 4 to 5 days. Within 1 to 2 days of the onset of a rash on any body part, the discrete maculopapular lesions coalesce to produce the confluent phase of the rash. Hence, within 2 to 3 days of onset, the rash on the face becomes confluent, whereas the rash on the lower extremities still consists of individual maculopapules.

ROCKY MOUNTAIN SPOTTED FEVER

Rocky Mountain spotted fever is caused by *Rickettsia rickettsii* transmitted by the bite of a tick (see Chapter 74). Although initially confined to the Rocky Mountain states (hence its name), confirmed cases have been reported from all parts of the United States with varying ticks as vectors. The rash of Rocky Mountain spotted fever begins on the third or fourth day of a febrile illness as a maculopapular eruption on the extremities, most commonly the wrists and ankles. Over the next 2 days, the rash becomes generalized by spreading centrally to involve the back, chest, and abdomen. Initially, the rash consists of erythematous macules that blanch on pressure; they then become more confluent and purpuric. Notably, the hemor-

TABLE 53.2. Potentially Life-Threatening Illnesses Associated with Maculopapular Rash

Rocky Mountain spotted fever	Dengue fever
Kawasaki disease	Rubeola
Erythema multiforme	

TABLE 53.3. Common Disorders Associated with Maculopapular Rash

Generalized rash	Scarlet fever
Nonspecific viral disease	Pityriasis rosea
Enteroviruses	Localized rash
Adenoviruses	Contact dermatitis
Roseola infantum	Irritant dermatitis
Erythema infectiosum (fifth disease)	Scabies
Hand–foot–mouth disease	

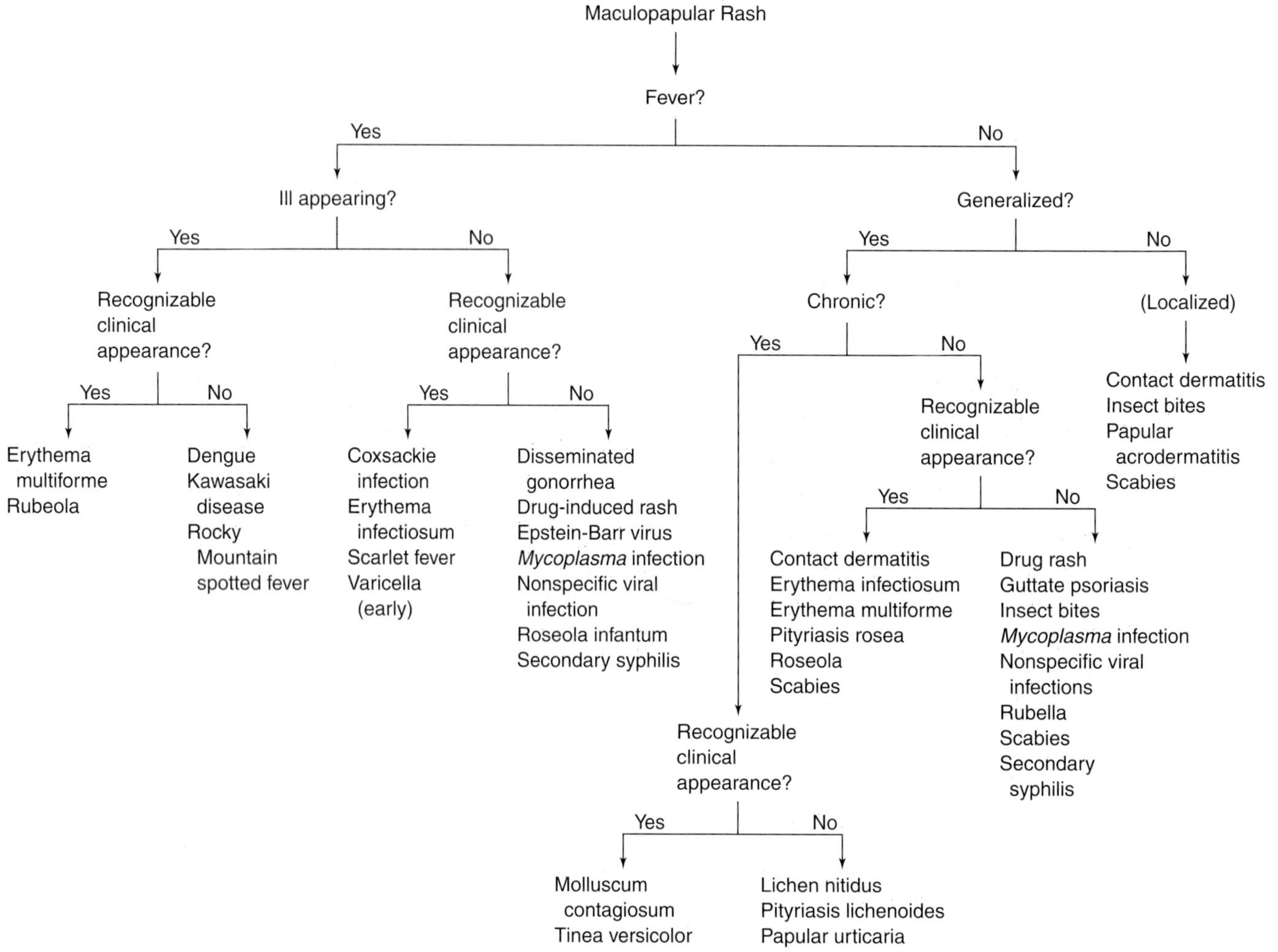

Figure 53.1. Diagnostic approach to maculopapular rash.

rhagic rash remains more peripherally distributed with involvement of the palms of the hands and the soles of the feet. The severity of the rash is proportional to the severity of the disease.

All patients with Rocky Mountain spotted fever have some degree of vasculitis that is the basis for many of the associated systemic symptoms. An overall toxic appearance is common. Systemic symptoms include fever; headache; myalgia; conjunctivitis; periorbital, facial, or peripheral edema; disseminated intravascular coagulation or purpura fulminans; shock; seizures; myocarditis; and heart failure. Diagnosis is most commonly presumptive, based on clinical presentation with a history of potential tick exposure.

TABLE 53.4. Maculopapular Rashes that Often Have Characteristic Clinical Appearances

Rubeola	Tinea versicolor
Erythema infectiosum (fifth disease)	Pityriasis rosea
Hand–foot–mouth disease (coxsackievirus A 16)	Roseola infantum
Molluscum contagiosum	Insect bites
Scarlet fever	Erythema multiforme

DENGUE FEVER

Dengue fever, a biphasic febrile illness caused by several arthropodborne dengue viruses, is seen in tropical and subtropical areas of almost all continents (including areas of Puerto Rico and the Caribbean basin). Initial constitutional symptoms include sudden onset of high fever, severe headache, myalgia, arthralgia, and abdominal pain. During the course of fever that lasts 2 to 7 days, back and leg pain may be severe, hence the disease's nickname of "breakbone" fever. A hemorrhagic vasculitis can develop in some infections that may lead to shock and death.

Two distinct rashes may be seen, which coincides with the disease's biphasic fever pattern. The first rash is a generalized, transient, macular rash that blanches under pressure and is seen within the first 24 to 48 hours of the onset of systemic symptoms. The second rash coincides with or occurs 1 to 2 days after defervescence and is a generalized morbilliform or maculopapular rash, sparing the palms and soles.

Causes of Other Maculopapular Rashes Associated with Fever

Among the other illnesses that are not life threatening but associated with fever are coxsackievirus infections, erythema infectiosum, scarlet fever, and early varicella. Harder to diagnose are rashes associated with Epstein–Barr virus (EBV), *Mycoplasma* infections, roseola infantum, disseminated gonorrhea, secondary syphilis, nonspecific viral eruptions, and drug-induced rash. It is particularly important to consider the diagnoses of disseminated gonorrhea and secondary syphilis in sexually active or potentially abused children.

COXSACKIEVIRUS INFECTIONS

Coxsackievirus infections of groups A and B (multiple types) can all cause maculopapular exanthems. The classic exanthem of coxsackievirus A16 infection, also appropriately called hand–foot–mouth disease, is common and easily recognized. Infections may occur in epidemics, most commonly in the late summer or early fall. Multiple infected members within a household are common. Coxsackievirus A16 infection begins with a prodrome of low-grade fever, anorexia, mouth pain, and malaise, followed within 1 to 2 days by an oral enanthem and then shortly thereafter by a maculopapular exanthem. The oral lesions begin as small red macules, most often located on the palate, uvula, and anterior tonsillar pillar, which evolve into small vesicles that ulcerate and heal over a 1- to 6-day period. The exanthem begins as maculopapular lesions that develop into small crescent or football-shaped vesicles on an erythematous base. These vesicles, which may be pruritic or mildly tender, are usually located on the dorsal and lateral aspects of fingers, hands, and feet but may develop on the buttocks, arms, legs, and face.

The other types of coxsackievirus all cause similar or even indistinguishable exanthems, which may more commonly involve the face, trunk, and proximal extremities. Often, children with these exanthems will be diagnosed with nonspecific viral infections. Other symptoms attributed to coxsackievirus infection include aseptic meningitis and less commonly myopericarditis, encephalitis, or paralysis.

ERYTHEMA INFECTIOSUM (FIFTH DISEASE)

Erythema infectiosum is a benign disease caused by parvovirus B19, the same virus that can cause aplastic crises in patients with sickle cell anemia. For the normal, nongravid host, fifth disease is of no consequence, with the only systemic symptom being fever in 15% to 30% of cases. On the face is a characteristic, intensely erythematous, "slapped cheek" rash. In addition, a symmetric maculopapular, lacelike rash is seen on the arms then trunk, buttocks, and thighs. In its acute phase, the rash usually lasts only for a few days but can wax and wane in intensity with environmental changes (e.g., exposure to heat or sunlight) for weeks and sometimes months.

SCARLET FEVER

Scarlet fever is caused by phage-infected group A streptococcus that makes an erythrogenic toxin. This disease is still seen with regularity but does not appear to be any more serious than group A streptococcal infection without rash. Scarlet fever is most commonly associated with streptococcal pharyngitis but may occur in association with pyoderma or an infected wound.

The diagnosis of scarlet fever can be made in a child with signs and symptoms of pharyngitis and a fine, raised, generalized maculopapular rash. The skin has a coarse or sandpaper feel on palpation. Typically, there is sparing of the circumoral area, leading to circumoral pallor. There usually is a bright erythema of the tongue and hypertrophy of the papillae, leading to the term *strawberry tongue*. Pastia lines, bright red, orange, or even hemorrhagic lines, occasionally are seen in the axillae or antecubital fossa. The rash generally lasts 3 to 5 days, followed by brownish discoloration in association with peeling of the skin. The peeling may range from small flakes to entire casts of the digits. A rapid streptococcal test or throat culture should be sent to confirm infection. Various antibiotic regimens provide effective treatment (see Chapter 74).

VARICELLA (CHICKENPOX)

Although varicella is an easily recognizable vesiculobullous eruption, on occasion, the earliest phase can be confusing. The initial skin manifestations of varicella virus infection are small, red macules. Some of them remain as macules but most progress to the characteristic papules and then umbilicated, tear-shaped vesicles. The earliest lesions appear on the chest and spread centrifugally, but there are many exceptions to the pattern of spread. Occasionally, a child with mild chickenpox may have only a few scattered macules with only one or two progressing to the more typical vesicular lesions of chickenpox. Of children receiving varicella vaccine, 7% to 8% may develop a mild maculopapular or varicelliform rash within 1 month of vaccination (see Chapter 74).

EPSTEIN–BARR VIRUS

Between 5% and 15% of patients with EBV infection, the cause of infectious mononucleosis, will have an erythematous maculopapular eruption. Infection in young children is usually inapparent, nonspecific, or so mild that diagnosis is not sought. The older patient, between the age of 15 to 25 years, more commonly presents for evaluation. In addition, 50% to 100% of patients with infectious mononucleosis receiving concurrent ampicillin will develop a maculopapular rash.

The illness begins insidiously with headache, malaise, and fever, followed by sore throat, membranous tonsillitis, and lymphadenopathy. Splenomegaly is common. The exanthem occurs within 4 to 6 days as a macular or maculopapular morbilliform eruption and is most prominent on the trunk and proximal extremities. An enanthem consisting of discrete petechiae at the junction of the hard and soft palate occurs in approximately 25% of patients. Diagnosis often is presumed clinically but may be supported by a positive heterophile antibody (Monospot) test or confirmed by serology. The heterophile antibody test is less sensitive in children younger than 4 years of age.

MYCOPLASMA INFECTIONS

Infections with *Mycoplasma pneumoniae* may cause maculopapular rashes in up to 15% of cases. The classic clinical presentation is of a child with malaise, low-grade fever, and prominent cough. The cough is initially nonproductive but may become productive, particularly in older children, and may persist for 3 to 4 weeks. Physical examination may show bilateral rales. Roentgenographic examination of the chest, if abnormal, most commonly shows diffuse nonspecific infiltrates.

Diagnosis can be suggested by serum cold hemagglutinins, which are present in more than 50% of patients by the beginning of the second week. If further confirmatory studies are needed, acute and convalescent serum sera should be assayed for specific mycoplasmal antibodies by complement fixation or immunofluorescence.

ROSEOLA INFANTUM

Roseola infantum, also called exanthem subitum or sixth disease, has recently been attributed to herpes simplex virus (HSV)-6. The illness is characterized by the onset of a maculopapular rash following a 3- to 4-day febrile illness. The fever is characteristically high. The rash is widely disseminated, appearing as discrete, small, pinkish macules that rarely coalesce. These macules begin on the trunk and then extend peripherally. The occurrence of the rash within 24 hours of defervescence rather than the morphologic appearance of the rash leads to the correct diagnosis. The rash can appear very similar to that seen in measles, but the child with roseola is well appearing and no longer febrile.

DISSEMINATED GONORRHEA

Disseminated *Neisseria gonorrhoeae* should be considered in sexually active or potentially abused children, especially if associated with a history of vaginal or penile discharge (see Chapter 74). A distinct minority of patients develop disseminated gonorrhea infection through hematogenous spread. Disseminated gonorrhea may cause a range of cutaneous lesions, including small erythematous papules, petechiae, or vesicle–pustules on a hemorrhagic base. These cutaneous lesions usually develop on the trunk but may occur anywhere on the extremities. An etiologic diagnosis can be established by demonstrating the organism on Gram stain of the skin lesion, positive blood culture, or positive culture of oral or genital sites.

SECONDARY SYPHILIS

One needs a high level of suspicion when viewing rashes in sexually active (or potentially abused) children to make the diagnosis of secondary syphilis, caused by the spirochete *Treponema pallidum* (see Chapter 74). Manifestations of secondary syphilis usually occur 6 to 8 weeks after the appearance of the primary lesion, which may have gone unnoticed. The exanthem extends rapidly and is usually pronounced, lasting for only hours or persisting for several months.

The rash is characterized by a generalized cutaneous eruption, usually composed of brownish, dull-red macules or papules that range in size from a few millimeters to 1 cm in diameter. They are generally discrete and symmetrically distributed, particularly over the trunk, where they follow the lines of cleavage in a pattern similar to pityriasis rosea. Papular lesions on the palms and soles as well as the presence of systemic symptoms such as general malaise, fever, headaches, sore throat, rhinorrhea, lacrimation, and generalized lymphadenopathy help differentiate secondary syphilis.

Acquired syphilis is sexually contracted from direct contact with ulcerative lesions of the skin or mucous membranes of an infected individual. Diagnosis may be presumed after a positive nontreponemal test, such as the Venereal Disease Research Laboratory (VDRL) slide test, rapid reagin (RPR) test, or the automated reagin test (ART). Diagnosis should be confirmed by a treponemal test such as the fluorescent treponemal antibody absorption (FTA-ABS) test, the microhemagglutination test for *T. palladium* (MHA-TP), or the *T. palladium* immobilization (TPI) test. Definitive diagnosis also can be made by identifying spirochetes by microscopic dark-field examination or direct fluorescent antibody tests of lesion exudate or tissue.

NONSPECIFIC VIRAL EXANTHEMS

Many times, a specific diagnosis cannot be made even after considering such factors as exposure history, history of preceding illness, description of eruption, time and site of onset, character of initial lesion, progression, distribution patterns, and occurrence of mucosal lesions. This should not be surprising, given the large number of viruses that can be associated with macular or maculopapular eruptions. One usually arrives at the diagnosis of nonspecific viral exanthem in a child in whom other diagnoses have been excluded and who may have signs of associated illness or systemic features such as fever.

DRUG-INDUCED RASH

Multiple drugs can cause maculopapular rashes in susceptible patients. Most commonly, these rashes have an abrupt onset, are generalized, and may be accompanied by systemic signs such as fever, arthralgia, lymphadenopathy, and hepatomegaly. It is often difficult to distinguish drug eruptions from viral exanthems. This is specially true because the emergency physician often is faced with a child who recently was started on one or several medications (often including an antibiotic) who now presents with the emergence of a rash associated with or following a viral-type illness.

The diagnosis of drug eruption depends on a carefully obtained history, including the duration and frequency of all medications taken by the child during the week preceding the onset of the rash. The presence of eosinophilia suggests, but does not confirm, the diagnosis. Often, the final diagnosis is left to the intuition of the physician. In the case of a severe eruption, the potentially offending drug should be discontinued. In milder cases, which more closely resemble nonspecific viral exanthems, a physician may opt to continue therapy as long as the rash does not worsen. The disadvantage of simply discontinuing any potentially offending drug is that the patient is often labeled as "allergic" to the drug for life. In addition, reactions may be caused by preservatives or dyes in a drug preparation and not by the drug itself.

Illnesses Associated with Maculopapular Rashes without Fever

Maculopapular rashes associated with nonfebrile illnesses tend to be benign. Erythema infectiosum, EM, *Mycoplasma* infections, roseola infantum, secondary syphilis, and nonspecific viral exanthems, which in mild cases may not be associated with fever, have been previously discussed. In approaching the acute afebrile disorders associated with maculopapular rash, it is useful to distinguish between those that cause generalized eruptions and those that cause localized ones. Disorders not usually associated with fever but that cause generalized eruptions include rubella, guttate psoriasis, and pityriasis rosea. Disorders that cause mostly local eruptions include papular acrodermatitis (Gianotti–Crosti syndrome), contact dermatitis, insect bites, and scabies. Some of the maculopapular rashes not associated with febrile illnesses are chronic entities, and their duration can help with their diagnosis; examples include lichen nitidus, molluscum contagiosum, papular urticaria, pityriasis lichenoides (Mucha–Habermann disease), and tinea versicolor. Molluscum contagiosum, pityriasis rosea, tinea versicolor, and forms of contact dermatitis also present with clinically recognizable rashes.

GENERALIZED ERUPTIONS ASSOCIATED WITH AFEBRILE ILLNESSES

Guttate Psoriasis

About one-third of cases of psoriasis begin in the first two decades of life among individuals with a genetic predisposition. The guttate form is even more likely to occur in younger age groups. The rash is characterized by multiple small, discrete, round or oval macules or papules (up to 1 cm in diameter) with a loosely adherent scale. The lesions develop predominantly on the trunk, but the face and scalp may be involved. The distal extremities, palms, and soles are usually spared. The lesions of guttate psoriasis are not as hyperkeratotic as other types of chronic psoriatic plaques and may respond better to standard psoriasis therapy.

Pityriasis Rosea

Pityriasis rosea follows a characteristic clinical course. The initial lesion, the herald patch, is an oval-shaped plaque that occurs in about 80% of cases. The center of the lesion is flat, whereas the borders are raised, red, and scaly. The herald patch can occur anywhere on the body but is most commonly seen on the trunk, neck, or proximal extremities. The herald patch is often mistaken for tinea corporis. One to two weeks later, a more generalized, sometimes pruritic, rash erupts. The rash is most dense on the trunk, neck, and proximal limbs. The face and distal extremities are relatively spared but may be involved in younger children. Individual lesions are erythematous papulosquamous ovals that often resemble smaller versions of the herald patch. The orientation of the long axis of the ovals tends to conform to the skinfold lines of the trunk, giving characteristic "Christmas tree" pattern of distribution when looked at on the patient's posterior trunk. Atypical distributions (predominantly peripheral) and forms of the individual lesions (papules, vesicles, pustules, urticarial or purpuric lesions) can occur.

Rubella

In a classic case of rubella, the rash—as with measles—begins on the head and spreads downward. The progression occurs over 2 to 3 days, and typically the rash is entirely gone by the fourth day. The rash always remains macular and never becomes confluent, an important distinguishing characteristic. A rubella rash may show extensive variation in location, progression, and duration, at times disappearing within 12 hours or being localized to one part of an extremity without any progression. Unlike measles, in which systemic toxicity and fever are the rule, fever is uncommon. Associated symptoms and complaints in rubella include joint pain in about 25% of cases and adenopathy (most commonly suboccipital, postauricular, and cervical). Arthralgia that occurs with a viral exanthem is relatively specific for rubella. Diagnosis is based on clinical presentation, and treatment is supportive.

LOCALIZED ERUPTIONS ASSOCIATED WITH AFEBRILE ILLNESSES

Contact dermatitis, insect bites, papular acrodermatitis, and scabies usually have a localized distribution; however, in extensive cases, all may appear as a more generalized eruption.

Contact Dermatitis

Contact dermatitis may be produced by either a local exposure to a primary irritating substance or by an acquired allergic response to a sensitizing substance (see Chapter 88). When the dermatitis results from a nonallergic reaction of the skin, it is termed an *irritant contact dermatitis;* when it results from a delayed hypersensitivity to a contact allergen, it is termed an *allergic contact dermatitis.* Although distinct in etiology, both reactions usually have a localized distribution of the rash, which often assumes the pattern of the irritating or sensitizing agent, and there is generally a sharp demarcation between involved and uninvolved areas of skin. Involved areas are erythematous with variable numbers and combinations of macules, papules, vesicles, or bullae.

Irritant dermatitis arises from contact with primary irritating agents such as detergents, soaps, acids, alkalis, or rough sheets and clothes. This disorder is commonly seen in infancy, when the skin is relatively thin and susceptible to mechanical or chemical irritation. Allergic contact dermatitis, typified by rhus dermatitis (e.g., poison ivy, poison oak) or nickel dermatitis (from jewelry or wristwatches), occurs most commonly in older children.

Insect Bites

Virtually all children experience insect bites. Mosquitoes, fleas, and bedbugs are the most common offenders. Diagnosis depends on the season, the climate, exposure to animals, and distribution and appearance of the lesions. In temperate climates, mosquito bites occur exclusively in the warmer months of the year, whereas flea and bedbug bites occur year round as a result of indoor exposure. Often, a series of bites occurs in groups of bites, which causes a maculopapular appearance. Local reactions can be extensive and take several days to resolve.

Papular Acrodermatitis (Gianotti–Crosti Syndrome)

Papular acrodermatitis is an eruption of unclear cause that has been associated with hepatitis B and other viral infections in young children. Of affected children, 85% are less than 3 years old. The eruption may follow a low-grade fever or mild upper respiratory symptoms. The eruption consists of flesh-colored papules that occur anywhere on the body but often concentrate on the extensor surfaces of the arms, legs, and buttocks. Lesions are particularly prominent over the elbows and knees. The rash usually lasts 2 to 8 weeks and then disappears.

Scabies

Scabies is a contagious infestation of the *Sarcoptes scabiei* female mite that selects a favorable body site, burrows beneath the stratum corneum, and deposits eggs along the way. In older children and adults, the usual sites of infestation are the anterior axillary lines, the areolae, the lower part of the abdomen, buttocks, genitals, wrists, interdigital webs, and ankles. In young children, the lesions are usually more diffuse and may also occur on the palms, soles, scalp, and neck (see Chapter 88). The pathognomonic primary lesion may be visible as a linear, gray–brown, threadlike burrow a few millimeters in length, with a central black dot (the mite). The more usual lesions are erythematous papules that may be excoriated and possibly secondarily infected because of intense pruritus. Diagnosis is usually based on clinical suspicion, although definitive confirmation can be made by identifying the adult mite on microscopic examination of a scraping of suspicious burrows.

CHRONIC ERUPTIONS ASSOCIATED WITH AFEBRILE ILLNESSES

Chronic eruptions are defined as those that are usually present for a minimum of 2 weeks.

Lichen Nitidus

Lichen nitidus is a relatively rare, benign skin disorder that occurs most often in preschool and school-aged children. It is thought to perhaps be a variant of lichen planus. The eruption consists of groups of tiny, shiny, flesh-colored papules. The lesions commonly occur in lines of local trauma (Kobner phenomenon) and are most often seen on the trunk, abdomen, forearm, and genitalia. There is no known effective treatment, and the eruption can last for years.

Molluscum Contagiosum

Molluscum contagiosum is caused by a viral infection and consists of discrete flesh-colored papules, usually 2 to 3 mm in diameter, with umbilicated centers (see Chapter 88). Axillary lines of the trunk, the abdomen, genital region, inner aspect of the thighs, and the face are the most common sites of presentation, although any nonhairy surface may be involved. Usually, a child will have approximately 10 scattered lesions; however, on occasion, some may have many more. The lesions tend to persist anywhere from 2 weeks to 1 years and may be spread by autoinoculation. Spread can occur between individuals involved in contact sports. The lesions are asymptomatic, with the exception of a minority of patients who develop an inflammatory reaction.

Papular Urticaria

Papular urticaria, a benign condition seen most commonly in young children, is manifested by a chronic or recurrent papular eruption caused by a sensitivity reaction to insect's bites. The lesions are usually papules with a central punctum that may rest on a urticarial base. The lesions are most commonly seen in the warm months, when exposure to insects is most intense. Diagnosis is usually made clinically.

Pityriasis Lichenoides (Mucha–Habermann Disease)

Pityriasis lichenoides, or Mucha–Habermann disease, is a relatively rare disorder of unknown cause that can appear in childhood and young adulthood. There are two forms: acute and chronic. The acute disease is characterized by a macular, papular, or papulovesicular rash that often is distributed most heavily on the trunk and upper arms. The lesions occur in successive crops rapidly evolving into vesicular, necrotic, and even purpuric lesions. Lesions may leave pocklike scars. Resolution occurs spontaneously but may take several weeks to months, and recurrences may occur. Parents may describe these recurrences as "he keeps getting the chickenpox."

Tinea Versicolor

Tinea versicolor is a superficial skin disease caused by the fungus *Pityrosporum orbiculare* (see Chapter 88). Although adolescents and young adults are most commonly affected, the disorder can occur at any age. The distribution of scaly macular lesions is patchy and occurs most commonly over the upper trunk and proximal arms. Occasionally, the face and other areas of the body can become involved. In summer, affected areas are relatively hypopigmented compared with unaffected skin because the organism blocks the normal tanning of sun-exposed skin. In winter, the affected areas often are relatively darker than unaffected skin because the fungus causes a mild erythema. This phenomenon of variable coloration of the affected skin gives the disease its name. Microscopic examination of scrapings will demonstrate characteristic hyphae and spores in grapelike clusters ("spaghetti and meatballs" appearance).

EVALUATION AND DECISION (FIG. 53.1)

Acutely Ill-Appearing Patients

Rubeola and EM both have characteristic rashes that often are associated with oral involvement. Patients with rubeola may have a history of an ill contact and several days of cough, coryza, conjunctivitis, and escalating fever. EM may present with a history of the recent introduction of a medication. Kawasaki disease should be considered in children who have been febrile for more than 5 days and who have or have had conjunctivitis, red lips and strawberry tongue, a solitary enlarged cervical lymph node, and a rash. Clues to the possibility of Rocky Mountain spotted fever or dengue fever may be obtained from a travel history or known cases within the geographic location. Patients with Rocky Mountain spotted fever may have a history of a tick bite, and the hemorrhagic rash characteristically remains more peripherally distributed involving the palms and soles. Dengue fever should be considered in patients with a biphasic fever pattern and musculoskeletal pain.

Other Generalized Febrile Eruptions

An acute, generalized febrile maculopapular exanthem usually is the result of a nonspecific viral or streptococcal (scarlet fever) infection. The disorders that are seen in acutely ill-appearing patients, discussed previously, may present as milder versions and should be considered as possible causes in less acutely ill febrile children with generalized eruptions. Other viral and bacterial infections may require a higher index of suspicion and confirmatory studies. Nonspecific viral exanthems most characteristically consist of multiple, closely spaced small papules. The finding of pharyngitis, a strawberry tongue, or intensely erythematous lines in the antecubital fossae points to scarlet fever; however, a throat culture or rapid screening test for streptococcal infection should still be obtained.

Coxsackievirus infections, erythema infectiosum, and early varicella should be able to be diagnosed based on their clinical appearance. It should be remembered that the eruption of varicella initially is maculopapular; however, close inspection usually reveals a few vesicles by the time the child is brought to medical attention.

The final considerations in febrile patients with generalized maculopapular rash are EBV infections (infectious mononucleosis), *Mycoplasma* infections, roseola infantum, disseminated gonorrhea, and secondary syphilis. The exanthem of infectious mononucleosis should be suspected in the child or, more commonly, in the adolescent who has streptococcal negative pharyngitis or history of taking ampicillin or a closely related antibiotic. For children with nonspecific viral symptoms with prominent cough, *Mycoplasma* infection may be the diagnosis. Roseola infantum should be considered in the child who develops maculopapular rash after fever has defervesced. Last, disseminated gonorrhea and secondary syphilis should be considered in sexually active adolescents and appropriate tests sent for confirmation.

Generalized Afebrile Eruptions

Although nonspecific viral illnesses that cause rash are more often than not associated with fever, a few children with viral exanthems will remain afebrile. Often, no specific diagnosis is possible. Again, the appearance of a diffuse rash in an infant or toddler immediately after the defervescence of a high fever indicates the clinical diagnosis of roseola. Similarly, pronounced posterior occipital lymphadenopathy in an unvaccinated child suggests rubella. If a child is taking any medications, drug rash must be considered. Because a drug reaction is difficult to exclude initially, consideration for discontinuing medications is warranted in severe cases. Also common, pityriasis rosea is distinguished by its characteristic predominantly truncal distribution along the skin folds. Rarely does guttate psoriasis present acutely with a diffuse maculopapular eruption.

Localized Eruptions

The most common causes for acute, localized maculopapular eruptions are contact dermatitis and insect bites. Contact dermatitis may be caused by irritation or allergy. History may be helpful in establishing a diagnosis, as in the case of a child who returns from camp with an allergic dermatitis on the arms and legs (rhus dermatitis or poison ivy) or of a teenager who gets an irritant dermatitis of the wrist after wearing a new watch. Irritant reactions are usually exclusively maculopapular, whereas allergic eruptions may become vesicular or eczematous and may have a characteristic linear appearance. The papules of insect bites usually are isolated lesions, as opposed to the confluent rash seen in contact dermatitis. In temperate climates, insect bites occur most commonly in the summer, but the possibility of bedbugs or fleas should not be overlooked during the colder months. Scabies is a relatively common and potentially difficult diagnosis. Linear lesions and involvement of the web spaces are characteristic, but often a diagnostic scraping or presumptive therapy is indicated. Gianotti–Crosti syndrome is a rare disorder that produces primarily an eruption limited to the distal extremities. Any of the causes of localized eruptions may appear more generalized in extensive or severe cases.

Chronic Eruptions

The most commonly seen of the chronic maculopapular eruptions are papular urticaria, molluscum contagiosum, and tinea versicolor. Papular urticaria is most common in warm weather but may occur at any time of the year; the characteristic lesions have an urticarial wheal around a central papule. The papules of molluscum contagiosum have an easily recognizable umbilicated central core. Tinea versicolor consists of hypopigmented and hyperpigmented areas, predominantly on the trunk. This diagnosis can be confirmed by microscopy or culture. Although uncommon, secondary syphilis needs to be considered in any sexually active patient and a serologic test performed as indicated.

CHAPTER 54
Rash—Papular Lesions

Paul J. Honig, M.D.

Often parents will consult physicians because of concern about "bumps" on their child's skin. The following algorithm is used to help practitioners diagnose varying papular lesions (Fig. 54.1 and Table 54.1).

PAPULES WITH A CHARACTERISTIC CLINICAL APPEARANCE

Many conditions can be diagnosed on sight. The experienced eye can easily distinguish milia from molluscum contagiosum (MC) and warts from the uncommon xanthoma. Papules caused by bites are localized to exposed surfaces (face and extremities). Several clues make the process of separating these entities from one another easier (see section on noncharacteristic clinical appearance).

Milia

Milia are 1- to 2-mm firm, white papules. Newborns often have milia on their face, which disappear by the age of 1 month. Milia can be seen in scars after burns and in healed wounds in patients with epidermolysis bullosa. Persistent milia may be a manifestation of the oral–facial–digital syndrome or hereditary trichodysplasia.

Molluscum Contagiosum

For additional information about MC, see Chapter 88.

Warts

For additional information about warts, see Chapter 88.

Xanthomas

Papules, plaques, nodules, and tumors that contain lipid are called *xanthomas*. These lesions can appear on any skin surface and often are associated with disturbances of lipoprotein metabolism. The most interesting, but the rarest, of hyperlipidemias that arise in the pediatric (infancy to adolescence) age group are type I hyperlipidemias. Fifty percent of patients experience episodic abdominal pain that may be acute at times. Malaise, anorexia, fever, and leukocytosis may be present. The cause of the pain is unclear; however, pancreatitis and splenic infarcts have been hypothesized. Eruptive xanthomas occur in more than 50% of the patients. These are 1- to 4-mm yellow papules that appear in crops on the face, extremities, and buttocks. Their sudden appearance causes significant concern. Hepatosplenomegaly also is commonly present, as are lipemia retinalis and creamy plasma. Patients have increased chylomicrons, slightly elevated cholesterol, and significantly elevated triglycerides. Secondary diseases include pancreatitis and diabetes.

The homozygous form of type IIa hyperlipidemia is seen in children. An elevated low-density lipoprotein, significantly elevated cholesterol, and mildly elevated triglycerides characterize this disorder. Tendinous and tuberous xanthomas and xanthelasmas are seen clinically. The plane xanthomas (xanthelasmas) may be misinterpreted as flat warts when seen in skin areas away from the eyelids. Secondary disorders include hypothyroidism and nephrotic syndrome. Patients die of atherosclerotic coronary artery disease in their twenties and thirties.

Insect Bites

For additional information about insect bites, see Chapter 88.

PAPULES WITH A NONCHARACTERISTIC CLINICAL APPEARANCE

When the diagnosis is not obvious, the algorithm presented in Figure 54.1 must be used.

Presence of White or Translucent Core

Milia and MC have white cores. Side lighting and a magnifying glass may be needed to see the core within the central portion of the papule in MC. Therefore, it is essential to sidelight all papules about which one is not sure. The obvious white core in milia fills the entire papule rather than a small central portion of the papule (as in MC). The other differentiating point is that milia are hard and beady white and in MC, more fleshy.

Absence of White or Translucent Core

RAPID GROWTH OF HEMANGIOMA-LIKE LESIONS

Hemangiomas generally present within the first month of life. Two lesions that may mimic hemangiomas generally manifest after this period. These lesions are the pyogenic granuloma and Spitz nevus. They are differentiated by the fact that the Spitz nevus has a red, smooth, dome-shaped surface, as opposed to the crusted granular surface of a pyogenic granuloma. The last differentiating point is the common occurrence of bleeding of pyogenic granulomas following minor trauma. Juvenile xanthogranulomas (JXGs) can be red and appear suddenly. They are firm rather than spongy (like a hemangioma), and when blanched, the underlying color usually is yellow.

Spitz Nevus

Spitz nevi appear suddenly between 2 and 13 years of age. Preferred sites of growth include the cheek, shoulder, and upper extremities. The lesion has a pink to red surface because of numerous dilated blood vessels. Pressure produces blanching of this pink to red color. The lesions can reach a size of 1.5 cm in diameter but are completely benign.

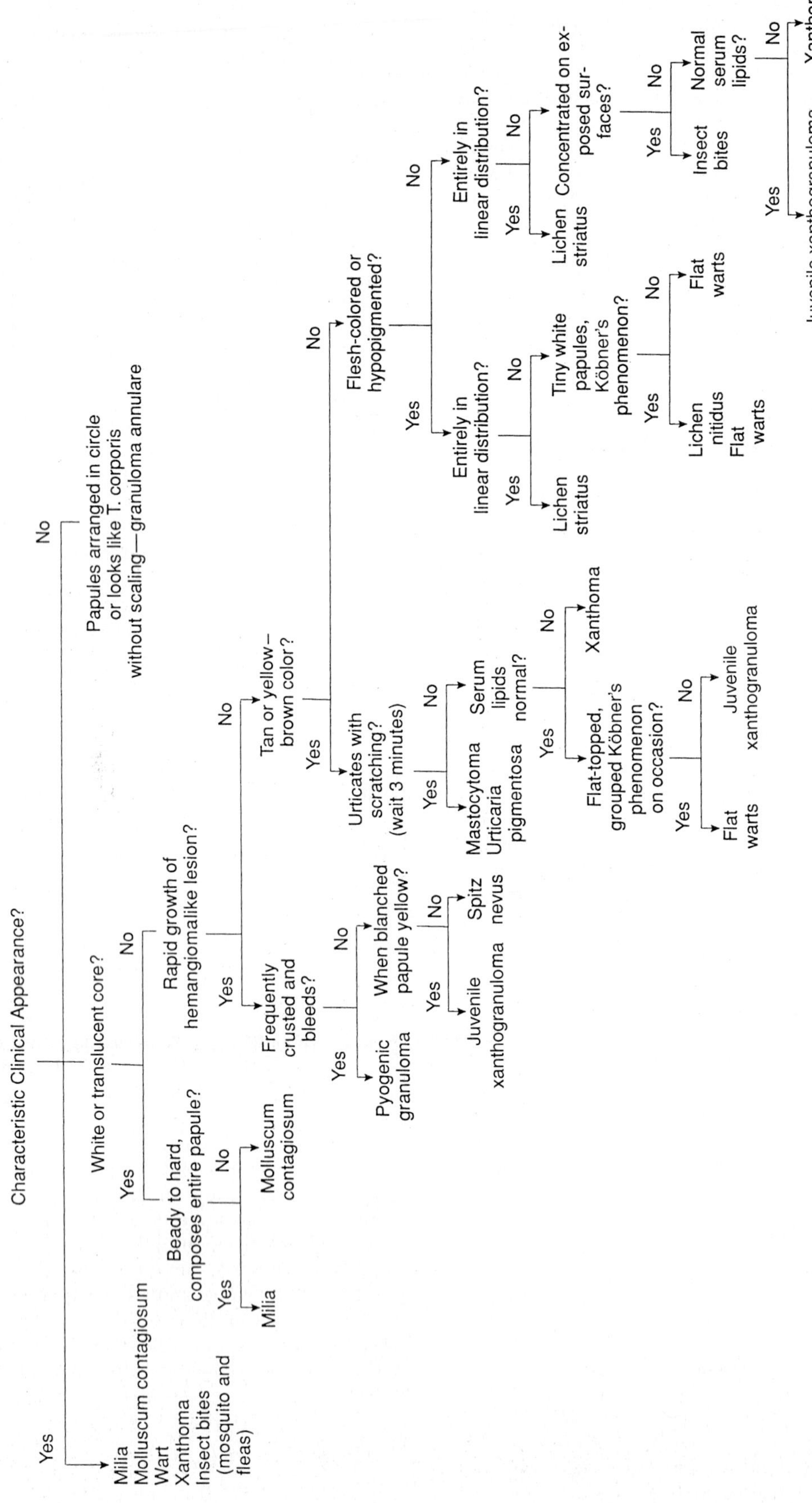

Figure 54.1. Approach to the diagnosis of papular lesions.

TABLE 54.1. Papular Lesions

Granuloma annulare (common)	Molluscum contagiosum (common)
Insect bites (common)	Pyogenic granuloma (common)
Juvenile xanthogranuloma	Spitz nevus
Lichen nitidus	Warts (common)
Mastocytomas, urticaria pigmentosa	Xanthomas
Milia (common)	

Pyogenic Granuloma

For additional information about pyogenic granulomas, see Chapter 88.

Juvenile Xanthogranuloma (JXG)

Juvenile xanthogranuloma can be confused with urticaria pigmentosa or xanthomas. Numerous yellow or reddish-brown papules appear on the face and upper trunk in the first year of life. The number of lesions may increase until the child is 18 months to 2 years of age. Serum lipid levels are normal, and the Darier sign (urtication after scratching—see mastocytoma) is negative.

NO HEMANGIOMA-LIKE LESION

Yellow, Tan, or Brown Papule

The yellow, tan, and brown papules include the lesions seen in urticaria pigmentosa (a single, large lesion is called a *mastocytoma*), flat warts, xanthomas, insect bites, and JXGs. A first step to differentiate the various papules from one another is to scratch them. If urtication (hives) occurs (Darier sign) within a short period (3 to 5 minutes), the lesion must contain mast cells (i.e., a mastocytoma or urticaria pigmentosa). It is important to scratch normal skin to rule out the presence of dermographism. The latter condition will produce a false-positive Darier sign. When no urtication occurs, blood should be drawn to check lipid levels. If lipid levels are normal, the next step is to differentiate two of the entities (i.e., flat warts and JXGs). Flat warts tend to be grouped, are flat-topped, and can be autoinoculated in scratch lines (pseudo-Kobner phenomenon). Lesions characteristic for JXGs are not flat-topped, tend to be singular in number (or when multiple are scattered about), and do not demonstrate the Kobner phenomenon. (This condition is discussed in greater detail later.) The JXG lesions also may look like xanthomas. Unlike xanthomas, however, abnormal lipid levels do not occur with JXGs.

Mastocytoma, Urticaria Pigmentosa

Parents who bring children with mastocytomas or lesions of urticaria pigmentosa to the physician generally describe a single yellow–tan–brown lesion that was present at birth (*mastocytoma*) or multiple pigmented papules that erupt during the first year of life (*urticaria pigmentosa*). One important clue is a history of these lesions becoming red, hivelike, or blistered. The lesions may ooze and form crusts much like impetigo; however, they do not respond to antibacterial preparations.

Physical examination of the lesion provides the next clue. At times, the surface has a peau d'orange appearance. Some papules are very yellow and are easily mistaken for xanthomas. When they are tan to brown, they are thought to be raised moles. The clincher is finding a positive Darier sign (histamine-induced erythema, swelling, and urtication secondary to scratching and subsequent degranulation of mast cells).

Table 54.2 lists medications and physical stimuli that cause mast cell degranulation and histamine or prostaglandin D_2 release. These agents should be avoided.

When massive amounts of mediators are released, generalized flushing, persistent diarrhea, or hypotension may ensue. Children with these symptoms require therapy directed against histamine and prostaglandin D_2. The H_1-receptor antagonists (chlorpheniramine) and H_2-receptor antagonists (cimetidine) may be required. In addition, indomethacin is required to inhibit prostaglandin biosynthesis.

Juvenile Xanthogranulomas

For additional information about JXGs, see the previous section in this chapter.

Warts and Xanthomas

For additional information about warts and xanthomas, see previous sections of this chapter.

LESIONS THAT ARE NOT YELLOW, TAN, OR BROWN: FLESH-COLORED LESIONS

Three entities may present as flesh-colored papules: lichen striatus, lichen nitidus, and flat warts. When the papules are arranged linearly, streaming down an extremity or across the face or neck, lichen striatus should be considered. If the papules are not arranged linearly but are tiny pinpoint, flesh-colored papules, lichen nitidus should be considered, especially if a Kobner phenomenon is present. Flat warts may be flesh-colored.

Lichen Striatus

Lichen striatus is an asymptomatic eruption of unknown cause. The flat-topped papules are arranged linearly and may be confluent. The lesions are flesh-colored to erythematous in white patients and hypopigmented in African Americans. The eruption follows the long axis of an extremity or may involve any other part of the skin surface (especially the face).

Lichen Nitidus

Lichen nitidus is characterized by tiny, pinpoint, flat-topped, flesh-colored papules. The papules often are grouped and are found in scratch lines. Although any skin surface may be involved, the trunk and genitalia are common sites.

Flat Warts

See previous section about flat warts.

NON-FLESH-COLORED LESIONS

Lichen striatus can be composed of hypopigmented or erythematous papules arranged linearly. Red papules not arranged linearly and concentrated on exposed surfaces usually indicate the presence of insect bites. JXGs can be yellow or reddish brown. They can be hypopigmented and brown–orange in

TABLE 54.2. Medications and Physical Stimuli to Be Avoided in Patients with Urticaria Pigmentosa

Medications	Physical stimuli
Alcohol	Rubbing of the skin
Aspirin	Extremes of water temperature
Opiates	
Polymyxin B	
Procaine	
Scopolamine	

African-American children. Xanthomas may be yellow or yellow–red. As discussed previously, the serum lipid levels are normal in patients with JXG and elevated in children with xanthomas.

NONCHARACTERISTIC PAPULES

Papules are arranged in circles and look like tinea corporis without scaling.

Granuloma Annulare

Granuloma annulare is thought to be an idiosyncratic response to trauma. The location of the changes (i.e., the shins, forearms, back of hands, ankles, and dorsum of the feet) seems to confirm this hypothesis. This skin change may begin as a flesh-colored or violaceous papule that clears centrally as the margins advance, or it may appear as a group of papules arranged in a ringlike configuration. The central portion of the lesion is dusky or hyperpigmented. The key point on physical examination is the lack of scaling. This physical finding distinguishes granuloma annulare from tinea corporis and cannot be stressed enough. The border is firm on palpation, unlike tinea corporis. The rings can be 5 cm in diameter or larger.

CHAPTER 55

Rash—Papulosquamous Lesions

Paul J. Honig, M.D.

PAPULOSQUAMOUS ERUPTIONS

Of the skin conditions seen in a pediatric dermatology clinic, 10% are papulosquamous (i.e., have a papular and scaling component). The algorithm contained in this chapter should be used as a guide to differentiate these disorders (Table 55.1 and Fig. 55.1). Each key point that distinguishes one disease from another is discussed here.

PRESENCE OR ABSENCE OF PRURITUS

The initial symptom that should be considered is pruritus. Pruritus is absent in the six conditions listed in Table 55.2.

TABLE 55.1. Papulosquamous Skin Disorders

Acrodermatitis enteropathica[a]	Pityriasis rosea (common)
Drug eruption, papulosquamous (common)[a]	Pityriasis rubra pilaris
Lichen nitidus	Psoriasis (common)
Lichen planus	Reiter syndrome
Nummular eczema (common)	Seborrheic dermatitis
Parapsoriasis	Syphilis, secondary (common)

[a] Potentially life-threatening.

Palmar involvement is prominent in secondary syphilis and papulosquamous drug eruptions but is rare in pityriasis rosea. A positive rapid plasma reagin (RPR) test helps to differentiate syphilis from pityriasis rosea and a drug eruption. Pityriasis rosea begins with a herald patch, followed by a truncal eruption in a "Christmas tree" distribution. Finally, the Kobner phenomenon separates lichen nitidus from other entities.

Conditions that Lack Pruritus

DRUG ERUPTION—PAPULOSQUAMOUS

The diagnosis of a drug eruption is based on the history of current or recent intake of a medication and the disappearance of the eruption after discontinuation of the medication. Drug eruptions may mimic lichen planus, pityriasis rosea, pityriasis rubra pilaris, psoriasis, seborrheic dermatitis, and syphilis (Table 55.3).

LICHEN NITIDUS

Lichen nitidus is a common disorder of children, seen especially in African Americans. There is a 4:1 male-to-female predominance. Lichen nitidus involves the abdomen, genitalia (shaft and glans), and extremities with tiny, pinpoint, sharply demarcated, flat-topped, flesh-colored papules. Often, these lesions are closely grouped and are linear. Linear grouping of lesions is caused by the Kobner phenomenon.

NUMMULAR ECZEMA (XEROSIS)

For more information about nummular eczema, see Chapter 88.

PARAPSORIASIS

Parapsoriasis is an uncommon pediatric skin condition. When it occurs, however, the course is chronic and, on rare occasions, may progress to cutaneous lymphoma. The appearance of this eruption is easily mistaken for nummular eczema, psoriasis, tinea corporis, or a lichenoid change. Small oval scaling, erythematous to yellow–brown macules are concentrated on the trunk. The skin lesions are asymptomatic, and the patient feels healthy.

PITYRIASIS ROSEA

For more information about pityriasis rosea, see Chapter 88.

SECONDARY SYPHILIS

The secondary phase of syphilis is a great mimicker. The eruption may be localized to the trunk, palms, and soles as well as to any other skin surface. Other clues should be sought by history and physical examination (a primary chancre, condyloma lata, or white mucous patches on the tongue, buccal, and labial surfaces). Generalized lymphadenopathy usually is present. It may be difficult to differentiate secondary syphilis and pityriasis rosea; however, Table 88.8 (see Chapter 88) may be helpful in separating the two entities clinically. A positive RPR or fluorescent treponemal antibody (FTA) makes the diagnosis. Remember, a false-negative RPR can occur with antibody excess (the prozone phenomenon).

COLOR OF THE SKIN ERUPTION AND PRURITUS

The eye can discern subtle differences in color. A pruritic papulosquamous eruption that does not look erythematous should suggest four disorders. First, a violaceous (bluish red) or purple appearance generally indicates lichen planus or a lichenoid drug eruption. Tones of yellow or salmon (orange–red), however, suggest the presence of seborrheic dermatitis or an unusual disorder called pityriasis rubra pilaris (PRP). The latter two diseases can

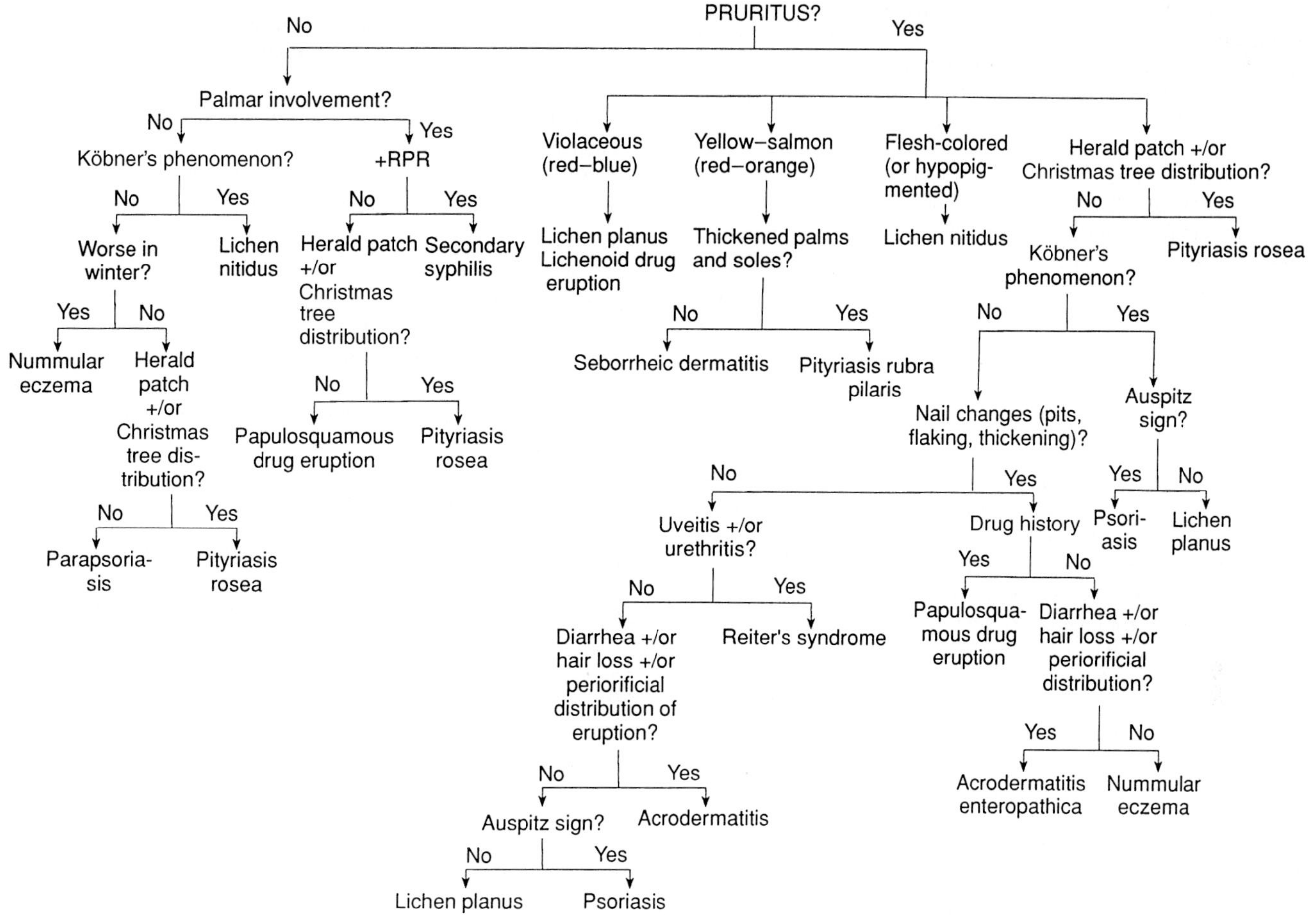

Figure 55.1. Algorithm to distinguish papulosquamous lesions.

be differentiated by looking for yellow thickening of the palms and soles (i.e., in PRP) or by knowing that seborrheic dermatitis occurs before 6 months of age or after puberty. Lichen nitidus is obvious when tiny, discrete, flesh-colored papules (white papules in African Americans) are found, with some arranged linearly (Kobner phenomenon).

Violaceous or Yellow- or Salmon-Colored (Orange–Red) Eruptions or Flesh-Colored (Nonerythematous) Eruptions

LICHEN PLANUS

Lichen planus is seen occasionally in pediatric patients as a chronic, pruritic, reddish blue (violaceous) to purplish eruption. The eruption generally involves the flexors of the wrist, forearms, and legs, especially the dorsum of the foot and ankles. The

TABLE 55.2. Nonpruritic Papulosquamous Skin Disorders

Drug eruption–papulosquamous	Parapsoriasis
Lichen nitidus	Pityriasis rosea
Nummular eczema	Secondary syphilis

TABLE 55.3. Drug Eruptions That May Mimic Various Papulosquamous Lesions

Lichen planus	Pityriasis rosea
β-Blockers	Barbiturates
Isoniazid	β-blockers
Captopril	Captopril
Naproxen	Gold
Carbamazepine	Griseofulvin
d-Penicillamine	Ketotifen
Chloral hydrate	Metronidazole
Phenytoin	Penicillin
Diazoxide	Tripelennamine
Spironolactone	Psoriasis
Furosemide	Antimalarials
Tetracyclines	β-Blockers
Gold	Lithium
Griseofulvin	? Nonsteroidal antiinflammatory drugs
Hydrochlorothiazide	
Pityriasis rubra pilaris	
β-Blockers	
Seborrheic dermatitis	
Contraceptives with progesterone (derived from 19-nortestosterone)	
Testosterone	
Syphilis	
Any drug	

lesions appear as small, violaceous, shiny, flat-topped, polygonal papules. The surface of these papules may have white crosshatching, called *Wickham striae*. Lesions may occur in sites of trauma or injury. The scalp may be involved, often resulting in a scarring alopecia, called *pseudopelade*. It is important to examine the buccal mucous membrane for a reticulated or lacelike pattern of white papules or streaks. This finding is characteristic for lichen planus. The nails are often pitted, dystrophic, or ridged (pterygium nails). The lesions in lichen planus can be vesicular or bullous. Hypertrophic and linear lesions occur but are less common. Persistent, severe, postinflammatory hyperpigmentation is common in African Americans.

SEBORRHEIC DERMATITIS

For more information about seborrheic dermatitis, see Chapter 88.

PITYRIASIS RUBRA PILARIS

Pityriasis rubra pilaris is characterized by follicular papules and yellow–orange skin that surrounds islands of normal skin. Onset of the disease is gradual, beginning in the scalp and spreading to involve the face and ears. Acuminate follicular papules with keratotic plugs occur on the back of the fingers, side of the neck, and extensors of the extremities. The skin is generally salmon-colored and scaling. As the eruption progresses, it surrounds islands of normal skin. Yellow thickening of the palms and soles is characteristic.

Differentiating the Pruritic, Red Papulosquamous Lesions

Pityriasis rosea also should be included in this part of the algorithm. Because the rash of pityriasis rosea may or may not itch, the first differentiating point is to inquire about a history of a herald patch and look for the characteristic Christmas tree distribution. If one or both is present, a diagnosis of pityriasis is made. If not, one must look for the Kobner phenomenon.

A clue to the presence of psoriasis is the finding of abnormal nails (e.g., nail pits, flaking, thickened nails). Reiter syndrome and acrodermatitis enteropathica also may manifest nail abnormalities. These entities can be differentiated from one another by a history or finding of uveitis or urethritis (Reiter syndrome) or diarrhea or hair loss (acrodermatitis enteropathica).

PSORIASIS

Psoriasis is a chronic papulosquamous disease that makes up 4% of all skin disorders encountered in children. There is a predisposition for involvement of the scalp, perineum, and the extensor surfaces of the body, particularly the elbows and knees. Psoriasis occurs in three forms during childhood: guttate, erythrodermic, and pustular. Any or all of these types may develop with silvery scales into the chronic, plaque-type psoriasis. When a scale is removed, pinpoint areas of bleeding occur on the surface (Auspitz sign). Guttate psoriasis is the most common form in childhood. Guttate or drop-like erythematous papules are scattered over the body. The characteristic silvery scale is only minimally expressed, and the lesions may appear quite red. This form often is preceded by a streptococcal infection. Infants often have involvement in the diaper area as well. Erythrodermic psoriasis is less common and more severe. Onset may be abrupt or gradual, with a diffuse erythema and severe desquamation. In the growing child, there may be associated failure to thrive. Pustular psoriasis is rare and the least commonly occurring form of psoriasis seen in children. Various sized sterile and superficial pustules develop on an erythrodermic background. Characteristically small, pitted lesions are seen on the nails in 25% to 50% of patients in all forms of the condition. Eighty percent of children have scalp involvement, especially at the hair margins. A few patients develop arthritis between 9 and 12 years of age; some develop it before the onset of the skin eruption. The distal interphalangeal joints of the hands and feet are involved most often.

TABLE 55.4. Acrodermatitis Enteropathica: Differential Diagnosis

Mucocutaneous candidiasis	Histiocytosis X
Biotin deficiency	Multiple carboxylase deficiency
Essential fatty acid deficiency	Psoriasis
Glucagonoma syndrome	Seborrheic dermatitis

REITER SYNDROME

The skin changes seen in Reiter syndrome look much like those in psoriasis. A symmetric arthritis of major joints, uveitis, and urethritis complete the syndrome. Although most cases occur in young adult men, on occasion the syndrome is seen in adolescents. Only ten cases have been reported in children under 12 years of age. The palms and soles are the major sites of involvement. Yellow, scaly, hyperkeratotic lesions appear on an erythematous base in those locations. The skin lesions may begin as macules, vesicles, or pustules. The palmar plantar changes have been called *keratoderma blennorrhagicum*. The scalp and penis also are characteristically involved with psoriasiform lesions. Erythema and superficial ulcerations may be present in the mouth. Abnormalities of the nails (e.g., dystrophy, onycholysis) are common.

ACRODERMATITIS ENTEROPATHICA

Acrodermatitis enteropathica is characterized by skin rash, diarrhea, and alopecia. The condition is caused by poor absorption of zinc, with plasma zinc levels under 50 g per deciliter. The disease generally begins around 9 months of age (1 week to 20 months). The infant usually presents with a psoriasiform diaper eruption, followed by similar involvement of periorificial (eyes, ears, nose, and mouth) and acral skin. The skin often is eroded and crusted. These changes may be confused with a severe candida infection (Table 55.4) or impetigo. Because of involvement of the digits and periungual tissues, nail dystrophies often are present. Hair is lost from the scalp, brows, and lashes. The children are irritable, photophobic, and apathetic. Growth retardation is common.

CHAPTER 56
Rash—Purpura

Alan R. Cohen, M.D.

Blood in the skin or mucosal membranes is referred to as *purpura*. When the onset of purpura is accompanied by massive hemorrhage or by bleeding in a critical site, such as the central nervous system, the patient is easily recognized as being dangerously ill and appropriate measures are taken rapidly. When purpura is the only presenting complaint, however, the patient should still be considered as having the potential for life-threatening sequelae of disordered hemostasis. The cause of purpura should be established as rapidly as possible because early treatment may lead to a more favorable outcome.

DIFFERENTIAL DIAGNOSIS

A purpuric eruption can result from loss of vascular integrity, thrombocytopenia, disorders of platelet function, or deficiencies of clotting factors. Myriad disorders may cause purpura, but only a few are particularly common (Table 56.1), including trauma, infections, Henoch–Schönlein purpura (HSP), and idiopathic thrombocytopenic purpura (ITP).

Loss of Vascular Integrity

Purpura can be caused by numerous disorders that disrupt vascular integrity (Table 56.2). The most common cause of purpura from vascular injury in children is trauma. Most active children have bruises, particularly on the anterior aspect of the lower extremities. Occasionally, however, a parent will bring a child to a physician with the complaint that the child bruises unusually easily. A thorough history and physical examination often are sufficient to distinguish the patient who requires further evaluation from the patient who requires only reassurance about normal childhood bruising from trauma. The child's level of activity should be correlated with the degree of bruising. Ecchymoses that might be acceptable in a child who enjoys climbing trees would be most surprising in a child who spends most of his or her leisure time reading. In addition, bruising on an area of the body rarely exposed to trauma (e.g., chest, abdomen, back) or bruising disproportionate to the degree of trauma should be evaluated further. Large, raised ecchymoses rarely are seen in the absence of significant trauma that is easily recalled. A history of sudden onset of excessive bruising without an associated change in activity also suggests an underlying disorder. Even when the history indicates that the ecchymoses can be attributed to repeated episodes of minor trauma, the finding of numerous bruises may be a clue to a subtle neurologic disorder that causes unusual clumsiness.

Foremost in the mind of a physician who cares for children must be the consideration that bruising is caused by child abuse. Suspicion should be raised if the child has had unexplained bruising or suspicious injuries in the past; if explanations of the bruises are inconsistent; if bruises are confined to the buttocks, back, or face; if bruises conform to the shape of a belt or cord; or if bruises are in various stages of resolution (see Chapter 111).

Purpura can be the initial manifestation of numerous infectious processes. The purpura may result from a disruption of the vascular integrity by the infecting agent or from the body's reaction to the agent, an infection-induced thrombocytopenia, or disseminated intravascular coagulation (DIC) initiated by the septic process. Capillary damage that results in petechiae or ecchymoses can occur with the viral exanthems and is especially common with rubeola. The child with infectious mononucleosis, bacterial endocarditis, a rickettsial infection, or a streptococcal infection can present with purpura in the absence of coagulation or platelet abnormalities. Rocky Mountain spotted fever should be strongly considered when the patient is from an area in which the disease is endemic or when there is a history of tick exposure, especially in the months of April through October.

TABLE 56.1. Common Causes of Purpura

Disruption of vascular integrity	Platelet deficiency or function disorders
Trauma	Idiopathic thrombocytopenic purpura
Viral infections	Sepsis
Henoch–Schönlein purpura	Drug-associated disorders
Rickettsial infection	Factor deficiencies
	Hemophilia

TABLE 56.2. Causes of Purpura in Children Secondary to Disruption of Vascular Integrity

Trauma: accidental; child abuse[a]
Infection: viral exanthems, infectious mononucleosis, bacterial endocarditis,[a] rickettsial disease,[a] streptococcal infection
Drugs and toxins[a]
Henoch–Schönlein purpura
Vitamin C deficiency
Letterer–Siwe disease
Ehlers–Danlos syndrome
Miscellaneous: acute glomerulonephritis, rheumatic fever, collagen vascular diseases

[a] Conditions that may be life threatening.

The most serious infection that can cause purpura is meningococcemia, and this disorder always must be considered in a child with purpuric lesions. The rapidity with which meningococcemia can progress may warrant the institution of antibiotic therapy in any moderately ill child with purpura until results of cultures are available.

Numerous drugs and toxins can cause purpura as a result of increased capillary fragility or vasculitis. The parents of a child with purpura should be questioned closely regarding the recent use of any medications, including over-the-counter drugs and "home remedies." Drugs that have been implicated include the sulfonamides, iodides, belladonna, bismuth, mercurial compounds, the penicillins, phenacetin, and chloral hydrate. Corticosteroid treatment can cause the appearance of benign purpura, especially striated purpuric lesions just above the buttocks. The appearance of these lesions in a child not taking corticosteroids should cause the physician to search for endogenous corticosteroid production, as in Cushing disease. Vitamin C deficiency also can present with purpura that ranges from scattered petechiae to substantial ecchymoses, particularly on the lower extremities.

Purpura that results from an aseptic vasculitis within the corium may be the presenting symptom of HSP. The purpuric lesions often are accompanied by pink or brownish pink macules or maculopapules that later may develop central areas of hemorrhage. They tend to coalesce and usually are located on the lower extremities, buttocks, and lower back. The platelet count is normal in uncomplicated HSP, as are the prothrombin (PT) and partial thromboplastin (PTT) times. Anaphylactoid purpura that resembles HSP also can accompany acute streptococcal infections, rheumatic fever, acute glomerulonephritis, and collagen vascular disorders.

Rare disorders of childhood that may be associated with purpura from loss of vascular integrity include Letterer–Siwe disease and Ehlers–Danlos syndrome. The former disease is a histiocytic disorder with brown, crusted vesiculopapular skin lesions that often are purpuric. Petechiae also may be present.

Platelet Disorders

THROMBOCYTOPENIA

Increased Platelet Destruction

The most common form of thrombocytopenia in childhood is ITP. This immunologic disorder usually is characterized by the acute onset of petechiae and ecchymoses, although symptoms occasionally occur more gradually. Epistaxis occurs in 10% to

20% of cases. Other bleeding manifestations are much less common. Although ITP occurs in children of all ages, most cases are seen between the ages of 2 and 6 years. The disorder is associated with human immunodeficiency virus, infectious mononucleosis, cytomegalovirus (CMV) infection, rubeola, mumps, and varicella. A similar relationship between ITP and rubeola and rubella immunization has been observed. ITP may be the first manifestation of a systemic immunologic disorder such as systemic lupus erythematosus (SLE). A careful search for this association is particularly important in older children. The association of ITP with autoimmune hemolytic anemia or neutropenia is called Evans syndrome.

Thrombocytopenia from shortened platelet survival may be caused by fibrin deposition and platelet consumption as found in DIC and also in hemolytic uremic syndrome (HUS), which is characterized by a microangiopathic anemia and uremia. In this, pallor, purpura, and signs of renal failure usually follow a prodrome of abdominal pain and diarrhea. Thrombotic thrombocytopenic purpura (TTP) is a disorder that resembles HUS in its hematologic aspects but occurs more commonly in adults than in children.

Infants with Wiskott–Aldrich syndrome, an X-linked recessive immunodeficiency disorder, may develop thrombocytopenic purpura beginning in the newborn period. Shortened platelet survival in this disease comes from an intrinsic platelet abnormality. Numerous drugs have been reported to cause thrombocytopenia by the formation of platelet antibodies with resultant increased platelet destruction. The drugs that cause thrombocytopenia that are most commonly used in children include sulfa compounds (including trimethoprim–sulfamethoxazole), valproic acid, phenytoin, acetazolamide, carbamazepine, and quinidine.

Decreased Platelet Production

Diseases associated with decreased amounts of functional bone marrow also may present with thrombocytopenia and purpura. Most notable in this group are the leukemias, neuroblastoma, histiocytosis, and osteopetrosis. Decreased platelet production also may be the result of abnormalities of development of the hematopoietic stem cell (aplastic anemia, Fanconi anemia, and thrombocytopenia and absent radii), ineffective megakaryocyte development (megaloblastic anemias), or, rarely, the absence of a humoral factor (presumed thrombopoietin deficiency). Although pancytopenia often is present at the time of diagnosis of bone marrow disorders such as leukemia and aplastic anemia, thrombocytopenia may precede notable alterations in other elements in the peripheral blood.

Numerous drugs have been associated with thrombocytopenia because of decreased platelet production. Any drug capable of causing general bone marrow suppression can produce thrombocytopenia (most antibiotics, anticonvulsants, thiazide diuretics, and the like). Drugs that specifically inhibit megakaryocyte production include chlorothiazide, estrogenic hormones, ethanol, and tolbutamide.

PLATELET SEQUESTRATION

Splenomegaly that comes from numerous causes (e.g., portal hypertension, storage diseases) can result in sequestration of platelets and thrombocytopenia. The spleen is markedly enlarged and very firm in these disorders. Purpura that comes from platelet sequestration alone is rare because the platelet count usually does not fall below 40,000mm^3. Bleeding may occur, however, when the platelet sequestration is associated with liver disease and clotting abnormalities. Platelet sequestration and consumption also can occur in large hemangiomas (Kasabach–Merritt syndrome).

Disorders of Platelet Function

A clinical picture similar to that seen with thrombocytopenia can occur with a normal platelet count in the presence of a qualitative or functional platelet abnormality. These disorders can be congenital or acquired and, when they are congenital, can present in infancy with prolonged oozing from venipuncture sites or the umbilical cord, ecchymoses, and petechiae. Glanzmann thrombasthenia is an autosomal recessive disorder in which the platelet count is normal but the bleeding time is prolonged, clot retraction is poor, and platelet aggregation and adhesion are absent. Other inherited abnormalities of platelet metabolism (storage pool disease, aspirin-like defect, Bernard–Soulier syndrome) may be associated with purpura, although bleeding is generally not as severe as it is in Glanzmann thrombasthenia. In addition to shortened platelet survival, platelet dysfunction is found in Wiskott–Aldrich syndrome.

Acquired platelet dysfunction with purpura can occur in the presence of uremia or liver dysfunction and also can be caused by certain medications. Aspirin is the best known of the drugs that cause platelet dysfunction; a single dose of aspirin can alter platelet function for as long as 9 to 10 days. Platelet dysfunction also has been associated with antihistamines, propranolol, phenothiazine, glycerol, guaifenesin, and carbenicillin. These drugs interfere with the release of endogenous adenosine diphosphate and inhibit platelet aggregation and adhesion. Unlike aspirin, however, they cause few, if any, clinical problems.

Factor Deficiencies

Purpura can be the presenting symptom of a congenital or acquired deficiency of coagulation factors. The most commonly encountered congenital deficiencies are von Willebrand disease, hemophilia A (factor VIII deficiency), and hemophilia B (factor IX deficiency, Christmas disease). Although the last two disorders have an X-linked recessive mode of inheritance, the *de novo* appearance of coagulopathy is not uncommon, particularly in children with severe hemophilia A (factor VIII activity $<1\%$). Therefore, a family history of affected males may be helpful in establishing the diagnosis of hemophilia, but the absence of such a history does not eliminate this diagnostic possibility.

Congenital Deficiencies

Often hemophilia is detected in children when they develop purpura either spontaneously or after mild trauma. The diagnosis of hemophilia also should be entertained in newborns who develop excessive bleeding after circumcision and in infants with prolonged bleeding from lacerations of the lip, tongue, or frenulum. Prompt recognition of the disorder at this early age allows careful surveillance, appropriate treatment, and early genetic counseling for parents.

Coagulation tests in children with hemophilia A and B reveal a prolonged PTT and normal PT. The bleeding time is usually normal. Specific factor assays will define the particular abnormality. Special care should be taken in establishing the diagnosis of factor IX deficiency in the young infant because the low factor IX levels found in normal infants in the first few days of life may overlap with the factor IX levels found in mild hemophilia B.

Less common congenital factor deficiencies that may cause purpura in children include fibrinogen and factors II (prothrombin), V, VII, X, XI, and XIII. As in hemophilia, specific factor assays will identify the particular abnormality. Alterations in fibrinogen function (dysfibrinogenemias) also are associated with purpura. Fibrinogen levels determined by clotting assay usually are reduced moderately in these disorders.

Von Willebrand disease is a common bleeding disorder caused by an alteration that adversely affects platelet function as well as clotting. The severity of this autosomal dominant disorder is extremely variable among affected persons. Although some patients may have spontaneous purpura, others remain asymptomatic and the disorder is discovered only after the diagnosis of von Willebrand disease in a close relative leads to laboratory investigation of other family members. Occasionally, von Willebrand disease is uncovered when an acquired alteration of hemostasis is superimposed on the inherited abnormality. For example, bruising occurs very easily after aspirin ingestion in many patients with von Willebrand disease. As in other disorders that affect platelet function, bleeding from mucosal surfaces (epistaxis, menorrhagia) is prominent. The laboratory abnormalities in von Willebrand disease are variable and may fluctuate from week to week in the same patient. In its classic form, the disease is characterized by prolongation of the bleeding time, increased PTT, decreased levels of factor VIII coagulant activity and von Willebrand factor antigen, and diminished aggregation of normal platelets when ristocetin is added to the patient's plasma (von Willebrand or ristocetin cofactor activity). In practice, however, only one or two of the laboratory abnormalities may be found. Indeed, several determinations may be required to detect an abnormality or to confirm the diagnosis of von Willebrand disease.

Acquired Deficiencies

Causes of acquired deficiencies of clotting factors include DIC, liver disease, vitamin K deficiency, circulating anticoagulants, uremia, and cyanotic congenital heart disease. DIC is a potential complication of infection (bacterial, viral, or rickettsial), extensive burns, severe trauma, malignancies (especially acute promyelocytic leukemia), snake and insect bites, shock, and heat stroke. In DIC, the intravascular consumption of clotting factors may cause purpura because of factor depletion and, in severe cases, may lead to widespread, rapidly progressing purpuric lesions (purpura fulminans) associated with thrombosis or emboli. Although other signs of serious illness usually are present in the child with purpura caused by DIC, fever and purpura may be the only significant findings in the early stages of severe bacterial infections such as meningococcemia. Further investigations and appropriate therapy should proceed rapidly in such instances.

Coagulopathies caused by severe hepatocellular disease or vitamin K deficiency can present with some of the same clinical and laboratory findings as DIC. A comparison of the laboratory values in these three disorders is shown in Table 56.3. Hepatocellular disorders that may cause purpura include Reye syndrome, Wilson disease, and toxic or infectious hepatitis. Vitamin K deficiency may be associated with malabsorption and chronic diarrhea. Purpura caused by warfarin (Coumadin) therapy or ingestion can resemble vitamin K deficiency clinically. Hemorrhagic disease of the newborn that comes from decreased vitamin K stores at birth can be prevented by the administration of vitamin K routinely following delivery. This important step in normal newborn care may be overlooked, however, when other problems develop in the delivery room, and a careful review of the records may be necessary to ensure that the young infant with purpura actually received vitamin K.

Circulating anticoagulants in children are associated with viral infections, malignancies, and collagen vascular disorders. They usually are characterized by a prolonged PTT that fails to correct with the addition of normal plasma. Because most acquired inhibitors in children, particularly lupus anticoagulants, are not associated with increased bleeding, the identification of an inhibitor in a patient with purpura should not preclude an investigation of other coagulation abnormalities.

Numerous coagulation abnormalities have been demonstrated in vitro in patients with renal disease. Most commonly, however, bleeding is related to altered platelet function rather than to defects in the fluid phase of coagulation. Abnormalities that resemble those found in DIC have been associated with cyanotic congenital heart disease.

EVALUATION AND DECISION

The evaluation of a child with purpura must combine speed and skill. The diagnostic approach is outlined in Figure 56.1. Purpura can be the initial sign of a life-threatening meningococcal infection, requiring immediate treatment, or the first sign of child abuse, requiring patient, thorough investigation. The initial approach should be dictated by the general appearance of the child and the presenting vital signs.

If the child with purpura appears well or if the more seriously ill child has been given appropriate emergency care, evaluation of the purpura can proceed in an orderly fashion. The recent and past medical history should be reviewed carefully with the parents and child. Acute onset of purpura after a recent viral illness or immunization is consistent with an acquired disorder such as ITP or a circulating anticoagulant. Recurrent purpura since infancy, however, suggests an inherited abnormality of platelets or clotting factors.

The family history should be reviewed for purpura or bleeding disorders. A positive family history in male relatives on the maternal side suggests factor VIII or factor IX deficiency. A history of bleeding or bruising in numerous family members of both sexes suggests a condition with dominant inheritance such as von Willebrand disease. As noted earlier, however, a negative family history does not preclude the diagnosis of von Willebrand disease or hemophilia.

TABLE 56.3. Comparison of Laboratory Values in Disseminated Intravascular Coagulation (DIC), Liver Disease, and Vitamin K Deficiency

	PT	PTT	Fibronogen	FSP	Platelet count	Factor V	Factor VII	Factor VIII
DIC	↑	↑	↓	↑	↓	↓	↓	↓
Vitamin K Deficiency	↑	↑	N	N	N	N	↓	N
Liver disease	↑	↑	N to ↓	N to ↑	N to ↓	↓	↓	N to ↑

PT, prothrombin time; PTT, partial thromboplastin time; FSP, fibrin split products; DIC, disseminated intravascular coagulation ↑, increased or prolonged; ↓, decreased; N, normal.

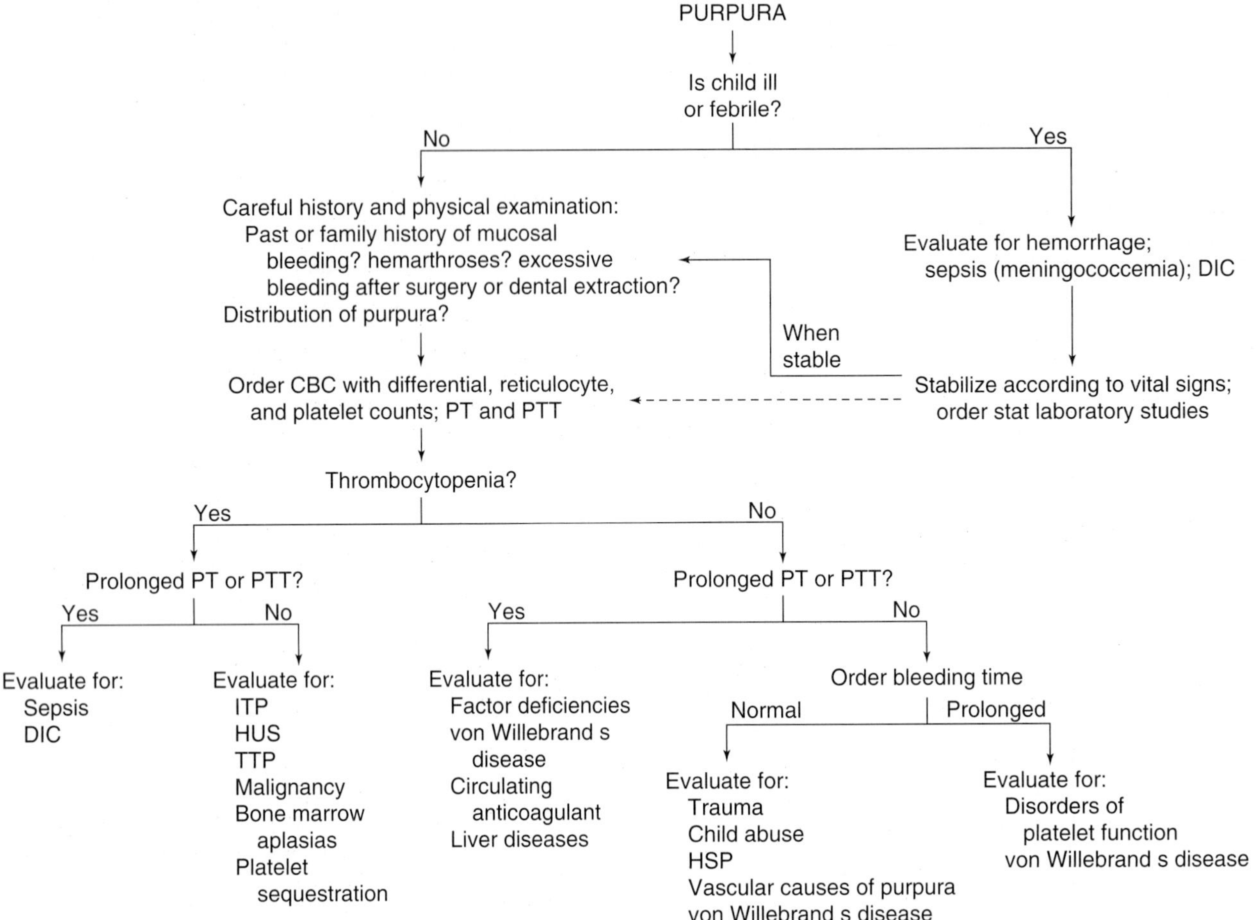

Figure 56.1. The approach to the child with purpura. CBC, complete blood count; PT, prothrombin time; PTT, partial thromboplastin time; DIC, disseminated intravascular coagulation; ITP, idiopathic thrombocytopenic purpura; HUS, hemolytic uremic syndrome; TTP, thrombotic thrombocytopenic purpura; HSP, Henoch-Schönlein purpura.

TABLE 56.4. Tests Commonly Used in the Initial Evaluation of Purpura or Suspected Bleeding Disorders

Platelet count (normal, 150,000–500,000/mm^3)
 Decreased: Increased platelet destruction, drcreased platelet production, platelet sequestration, some platelet function disorders (see Table 56.5)
Prothrombin time (normal range may vary between laboratories)
 Prolonged: Disseminated intravascular coagulation; vitamin K deficiency; warfarin ingestion; deficiencies of factors II, V, VII, X; abnormalities of fibrinogen; liver disease; renal disease; congenital heart disease
 Activated partial thromboplastin time (normal range may vary between laboratories)
 Prolonged: Disseminated intravascular coagulation; von Willebrand's disease; deficiencies of factors II, V, VIII, IX, X, XI, XII; abnormalities of fibrinogen; vitamin K deficiency; heparin therapy or sample contamination; liver disease; congenital heart disease
Fibrinogen (normal >150 mg/100 mL)
 Decreased: Disseminated intravascular coagulation, liver disease, L-asparaginase therapy, dysfibrinogenemia, afibrinogenemia
Fibrin split products (normal <1:20)
 Increased: Disseminated intravascular coagulation, liver disease
Bleeding time (modified Ivy): (normal <8 min, 30 sec)
 Prolonged: Idiopathic thrombocytopenic purpura (early) and other thrombocytopenias, von Willebrand disease, platelet function disorders

The distribution of purpura should be noted. Purpura on the lower extremities and buttocks suggests HSP, and purpuric lesions on the palms and soles often are seen with rickettsial infections. When the purpuric lesion has an unusual shape, such as a folded cord, child abuse should be suspected. Lymphadenopathy may be present in certain malignancies (leukemias) or viral infections (infectious mononucleosis, CMV) that can present with purpura. Hepatomegaly may signal an underlying hepatic disorder that can cause a coagulopathy. Splenomegaly can be seen in infectious mononucleosis, leukemia, hepatic disease, and the storage diseases. Inflammation or synovial thickening of the large joints is consistent with the hemarthroses seen in hemophilia.

Every child who presents with purpura should have a complete blood count with a differential and platelet count, a PT, and a PTT. A decreased hematocrit or hemoglobin concentration may indicate past or present blood loss or bone marrow failure or replacement. The white blood cell count can give information regarding the possibility of sepsis or leukemia. If sepsis is suspected, the smear should be examined for the presence of toxic granulation, vacuolization, or Dohle bodies. Atypical lymphocytes are seen with many viral infections, especially mononucleosis. Causes of abnormal screening coagulation studies (platelet count, PT, PTT, bleeding time) are outlined in Table 56.4 and 56.5.

TABLE 56.5. Causes of Childhood Purpura Secondary to Platelet and Coagulation Abnormalities

Platelet disorders
- Thrombocytopenia
  - Decreased platelet survival
    - Immune-mediated
    - Idiopathic thrombocytopenic purpura[a]
    - Collagen vascular diseases[a]
    - Drug-induced[a]
    - Sepsis[a]
  - Disseminated intravascular coagulation[a]
  - Hemolytic uremic syndrome[a]
  - Thrombotic thrombocytopenic purpura[a]
  - Wiskott–Aldrich syndrome[a]
- Decreased platelet production
  - Malignancies (leukemia, neuroblastoma)[a]
  - Sepsis: viral and bacterial[a]
  - Drugs (bone marrow suppression)[a]
  - Aplastic anemia, Fanconi anemia[a]
  - Megaloblastic anemias
  - Osteopetrosis[a]
  - Histiocytosis[a]
- Platelet sequestration
  - Congestive splenomegaly
  - Large hemangiomas
  - Storage disease (Niemann–Pick disease, Gaucher disease)
- Disorders of platelet function
  - Congenital
  - Glanzmann thrombasthenia[a]
  - Storage pool diseases
  - Bernard–Soulier syndrome
  - Acquired (drug-induced): aspirin, antihistamines, phenothiazines, glycerol, guaifenesin, carbenicillin

Factor deficiencies
- Congenital: Deficiencies or alterations of every coagulation factor have been reported. Von Willebrand disease, factor VIII deficiency (hemophilia A) and factor IX deficiency (hemophilia B) are most common.[a]
- Acquired: Disseminated intravascular coagulation, vitamin K deficiency, warfarin therapy, liver disease, renal disease, congenital heart disease, circulating anticoagulants (associated with malignancies and viral diseases).[a]

[a] Conditions that are known to present with acute, life-threatening bleeding or are associated with other serious abnormalities.

CHAPTER 57
Rash—Urticaria

William J. Lewander, M.D.

Urticarial lesions appear as erythematous papules or wheals from edema in the upper dermis with a surrounding flare of erythema caused by vasodilation. They are pruritic, multiple, and of varying sizes and shapes. Individual lesions are transient, usually lasting 12 to 24 hours or less. They often appear suddenly, resolve almost completely, and may reappear. Urticaria may be accompanied by angioedema and is associated with systemic symptoms from direct visceral involvement or from symptoms secondary to the release of circulating chemical mediators. The respiratory, cardiovascular, and gastrointestinal systems may be involved, resulting in a potential life-threatening reaction. Signs and symptoms may include hoarseness, stridor, shortness of breath, wheezing, and general respiratory distress (from laryngospasm and bronchospasm) as well as hypotension, nausea, vomiting, diarrhea, and abdominal pain.

DIFFERENTIAL DIAGNOSIS

As shown in Table 57.1, urticaria may be classified on the basis of the mechanism responsible for its formation or, if this mechanism is unknown, as idiopathic. The most frequent causes of urticaria are listed in Table 57.2. Although idiopathic urticaria is the most common form, it is a diagnosis reached mainly by exclusion. Any variety of urticaria that involves the airway or cardiovascular system is potentially a life-threatening condition.

EVALUATION AND DECISION

Urticaria is diagnosed by its characteristic appearance and only rarely is confused with erythema multiforme, certain vasculitides (e.g., Henoch-Schönlein purpura), urticaria pigmentosa, or

TABLE 57.1. Classification of Urticaria and Angioedema

Immunologic
- IgE-dependent
- Specific antigen sensitivity
- Physical: dermographism, cold, cholinergic, heat, solar
- Contact
- Complement-mediated
- Serum sickness
- Reaction to blood products
- Hereditary angioedema
- Systemic lupus erythematosus

Nonimmunologic
- Direct mast cell–releasing agents
  - Opiates
  - Radiocontrast media
- Agents that alter arachidonic acid metabolism
  - Aspirin and nonsteroidal antiinflammatory agents
  - Azo dyes and benzoate preservatives
  - Angiotensin-converting enzyme inhibitors

Idiopathic

IgE, immunoglobulin E.
Adapted from Soter NA. Acute and chronic urticaria and angioedema. *J Am Acad Dermatol* 1991;25:146–154, with permission.

TABLE 57.2. Common Causes of Urticaria/Angioedema[a]

Foods	Insect bites
Peanuts	Hymenoptera venom
Eggs	Infections
Chocolate	Hepatitis
Shellfish	Streptococcus
Milk	Infectious mononucleosis
Strawberries	Upper respiratory infection
Food dyes and preservatives	Physical agents
Drugs	Cold
Penicillin	Heat
Opiates	Dermographism
Radiocontrast media	Latex
Aspirin and nonsteroidal antiinflammatories	
Angiotensin-converting enzyme inhibitors	

[a] Essentially all may be life threatening if accompanied by systemic reaction (see text).

infectious exanthems. Following clinical recognition, the patient should be evaluated for the presence of an associated systemic reaction that involves cardiopulmonary compromise (outlined in Fig. 57.1). After stabilization, evaluation for a specific cause should begin with a thorough history and physical examination. The cause often remains unknown; however, Tables 57.1 and 57.2 outline the general classifications and most common identifiable causes of urticaria. In the context of acute onset, the patient must be questioned about specific precipitants, including drugs, foods, and *Hymenoptera* stings. Febrile patients must be examined for clinical findings suggestive of viral and streptococcal infection, mononucleosis, and hepatitis. Latex allergy is uncommon in the general population, but health care workers and children with spina bifida appear to be at risk for latex allergy. These patients may experience urticaria, conjunctivitis, bronchospasm, and anaphylaxis after contact with or inhalation of latex antigens. Patients with chronic urticaria must be questioned about exposure to parasites or hepatitis as well as about a family history of urticaria and must be examined for findings suggestive of collagen vascular disease. Laboratory tests generally are not helpful or necessary in the evaluation of acute urticaria.

Laboratory tests that may be useful in the evaluation of chronic urticaria include complete blood count with differential, erythrocyte sedimentation rate, urinalysis, Monospot, antinuclear factor, and liver function tests. Decreased levels of C_1 esterase inhibitor are found in hereditary angioedema. Stool for ova and parasites should be sent if eosinophilia is present or if symptoms are consistent with this diagnosis. Provocative tests may be tried cautiously if certain physical urticaria is suspected.

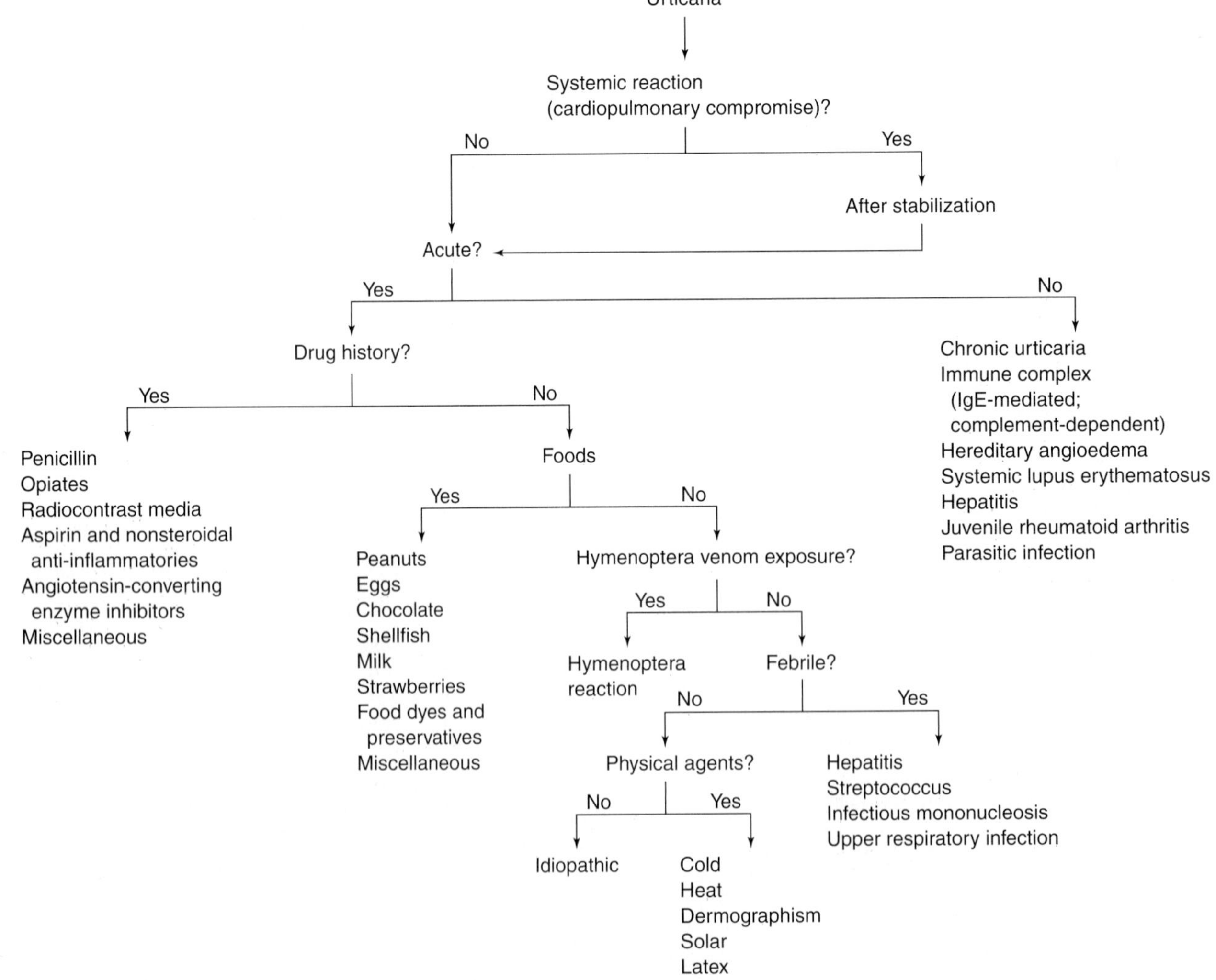

Figure 57.1. Algorithm for the evaluation of urticaria.

CHAPTER 58
Rash—Vesicobullous

Paul J. Honig, M.D.

An approach to vesicobullous eruptions is outlined in Figure 58.1. The key features used in this algorithm to distinguish the various entities are a characteristic clinical appearance, chronicity or presence at birth, associated fever or systemic illness, distribution of lesions, and the child's age. The diagnosis of vesicobullous lesions in children younger than 1 month of age is not discussed in this chapter. Figure 58.1 also outlines the frequency and potential severity of these diseases.

CHARACTERISTIC CLINICAL APPEARANCE

Many times, the appearance of a rash is so characteristic that a diagnosis becomes obvious. Such is the case with the conditions

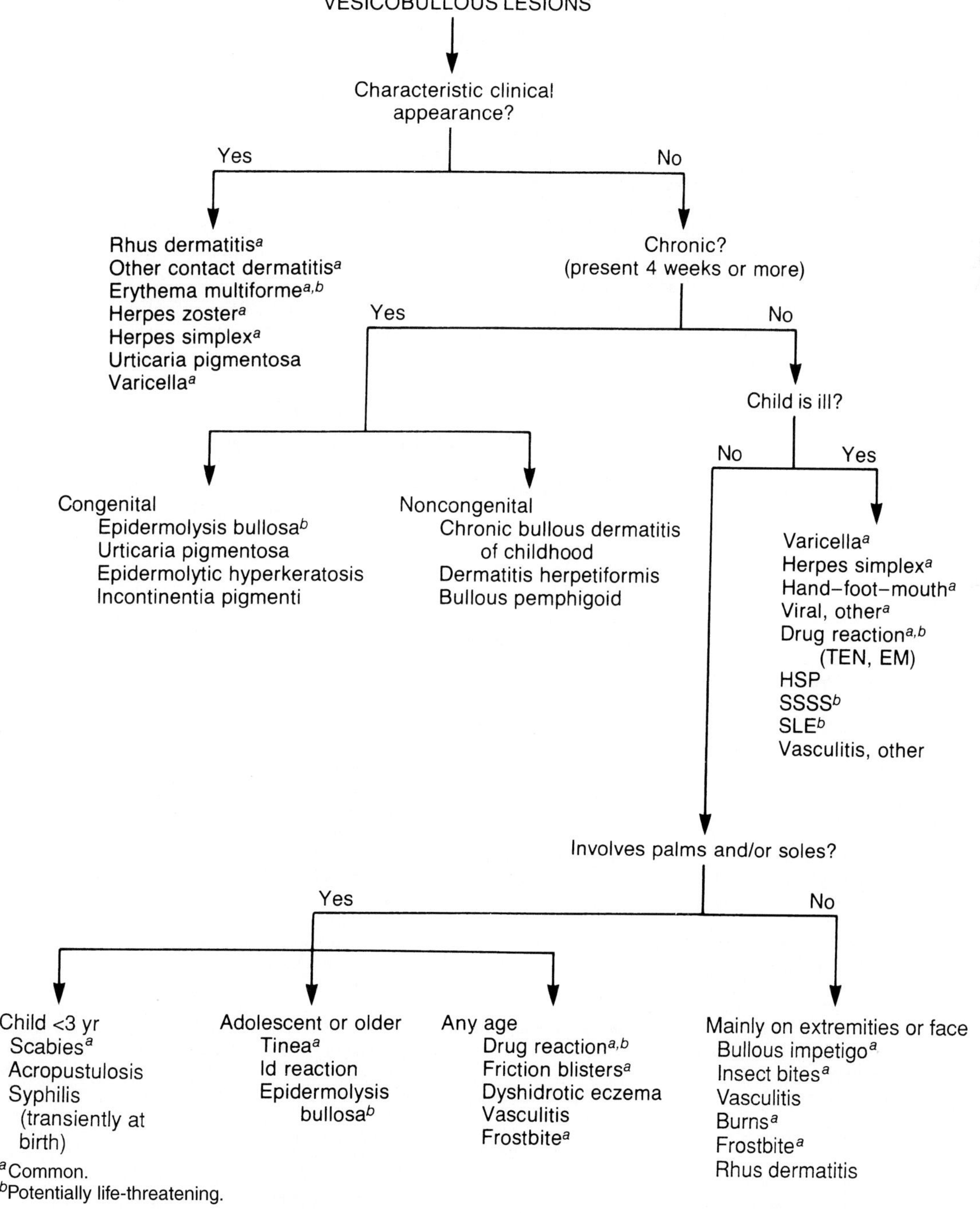

Figure 58.1. The diagnostic approach to the child with vesicobullous lesions. TEN, toxic epidermal necrolysis; EM, erythema multiforme; HSP, Henoch-Schönlein purpura; SSSS, staphylococcal scalded skin syndrome; SLE, systemic lupus erythematosus.

TABLE 58.1. Vesicobullous Rashes with Characteristic Clinical Appearance

Rhus dermatitis	Urticaria pigmentosa
Other contact dermatitides	Herpes simplex
Erythema multiforme	Varicella
Herpes zoster	

TABLE 58.2. Congenital Blistering Disease

Epidermolysis bullosa	Epidermolytic hyperkeratosis
Urticaria pigmentosa	Incontinentia pigmenti

listed in Table 58.1. Linear or geometric areas of vesiculation are the best clues to the presence of allergic contact dermatitis (see Chapter 88). Because children brush against poison ivy leaves, vesicles often are in a line and on exposed surfaces (e.g., the face, extremities). A round group of vesicles on the back of the wrist would point to contact sensitivity to nickel contained in the metal case of a wristwatch. Dermatomal distribution of vesicles or bullae usually indicates the presence of herpes zoster. On rare occasions, in infants, the same appearance may represent herpes simplex infections. Target or iris lesions are pathognomonic of erythema multiforme. The lesion has a dusky center that may blister and has successive bright red bordering rings. At times, a doughnut-shaped blister occurs. Pigmented lesions that blister after stroking or trauma (Darier sign) indicate the release of histamine from a mast cell collection. This collection may be isolated (mastocytoma of the wrist) or generalized (urticaria pigmentosa). Blistering of such lesions generally occurs only until 2 years of age. After this time, only urtication occurs. A delicate "teardrop" vesicle is characteristic of varicella (chickenpox). Lesions usually begin on the upper trunk and neck. A progression through papules, vesicles, and crusts occurs rapidly (6–24 hours). All stages are present in an area at any given time. Mucous membranes are involved. Fever and malaise usually are present but are variable.

DURATION

Chronic Rash (Duration of 4 Weeks or Longer)

If the blistering disease has been present since birth (*congenital*), consider the diagnoses listed in Table 58.2.

Epidermolysis Bullosa Syndromes

Blisters usually occur in areas predisposed to trauma or friction. See Table 58.3 for differentiation of the various types.

Urticaria Pigmentosa

Mast cell disease (mastocytoma or urticaria pigmentosa) may cause blistering in children aged up until 2 years. The pigmented solitary lesion most often occurs on the arm near the wrist. Lesions may be generalized. When a pigmented lesion feels infiltrated, the physician should think about its cause. Gentle mechanical irritation of such lesions causes urtication or blistering (Darier sign).

Epidermolytic Hyperkeratosis (Congenital Bullous Ichthyosiform Erythroderma)

Epidermolytic hyperkeratosis, an autosomal dominant trait, is categorized as an ichthyotic syndrome. Children with this

TABLE 58.3. Epidermolysis Bullosa Syndromes

	Type	Inheritance	Clinical features	Electron microscope
Nonscarring	Epidermolysis bullosa simplex	Autosomal dominant	Bullae present at birth or early infancy; in areas of trauma; improves in adolescence; no mucous membrane involvement; nail involvement (20%)	Cleavage through basal cell layer above the basement membrane
	Recurrent bullous eruption of hands and feet (Weber–Cockayne disease)	Autosomal dominant	May present in first 2 yr of life but usually not before adolescence or early adulthood	Epidermal cleavage may be anywhere from the suprabasal to lower granular cell layer
	Junctional epidermolysis bullosa (Herlitz disease)	Autosomal recessive	Usually at birth; spontaneous bullae and large areas of erosion	Cleavage at junction of dermis and epidermis (above the basement membrane)
Scarring	Dominant dystrophic epidermolysis bullosa (dominant dermolytic bullous dermatosis)	Autosomal dominant	Early infancy and later; little or no involvement of hair and teeth; mucous Membrane lesions and nail dystrophy	Dermal–epidermal separation beneath basement membrane
	Recessive dystrophic epidermolysis bullosa (recessive dermolytic bullous dermatosis)	Autosomal recessive	Present at birth; widespread scarring and deformity; severe involvement of mucous membranes and nails	Separation at dermal–epidermal junction (beneath the basal lamina)

TABLE 58.4. Noncongenital Chronic Blistering Disease

	Bullous disease of childhood	Bullous pemphigoid	Dermatitis herpetiformis
Type of lesions	Large, tense, clear bullae; annular plaques with active vesicular borders	Large, tense bullae	Grouped papulovesicles, bullae or urticarial lesions
Distribution	Scalp, lower trunk, genitals, buttocks, inner thighs	Trunk and flexor surfaces of extremities	Back, buttocks, scalp, extensor surface of extremities, often symmetric
Pruritus	None to severe	Mild	Intense
Mucous membrane involvement	No	Yes	No
Duration	Months to years	Months to years	Months to years
Immunofluorescence	+ or − Linear IgA basement membrane (+ circulating IgA)	+ Linear IgG on basement membrane (+ circulating IgG)	+ Granular IgA at tips of dermal papilla of uninvolved perilesional skin
Treatment	Sulfapyridine or dapsone	Corticosteroids	Sulfapyridine or dapsone

IgA, immunoglobulin A; IgG, immunoglobulin G.

problem have recurrent bullous lesions during infancy and childhood. The skin has a background of erythema, scales, and peels. The flexures are always affected, as are the palms and soles.

Incontinentia Pigmenti

Incontinentia pigmenti, a rare condition, occurs almost exclusively in female patients. Inflammatory bullae erupt in crops in a linear distribution for the first several weeks to months of life. These affected areas then go on to a warty stage. Finally, swirl-like pigmentation occurs but not necessarily in the areas previously involved with warty or blistering lesions. During the vesicobullous stage, a high degree of peripheral eosinophilia occurs.

If the blistering is noncongenital, chronic bullous dermatosis of childhood, dermatitis herpetiformis, and bullous pemphigoid should be considered. These conditions can be differentiated as outlined in Table 58.4.

CHILD WHO IS ILL

When the blistering lesions occur acutely, it must be determined whether the child is febrile or ill. Conditions that cause such systemic findings with associated blisters include those listed in Table 58.5.

TABLE 58.5. Blistering Diseases Associated with Fever or Systemic Illness

Chickenpox	Herpes simplex
Hand–foot–mouth	Staphylococcal scaled-skin syndrome
Viral (nonspecific) + other	Systemic lupus
Drug reaction (TEN, EM)	Atypical measles
Henoch-Schönlein purpura	Smallpox
Nonspecific vasculitis	

TEN, toxic epidermal necrolysis; EM, erythema multiforme.

Varicella (Chickenpox)

For more information about varicella, see the preceding section.

Hand–Foot–Mouth Disease

Caused by coxsackievirus A16, hand–foot–mouth disease is fairly characteristic. Vesicles are present on the palms, on the soles, and in the mouth. Other parts of the body may be involved. Fever, malaise, and abdominal pain may be present.

Viral (Nonspecific) and Other Causes

Vesicles have been described in association with other coxsackievirus types (A4, A5, B1, B4), echovirus, reovirus, and *Mycoplasma pneumoniae* infections. These children usually are ill.

Drug Reactions

The presence of vesicles or bullae may indicate a drug reaction. Involvement of palms, soles, mucous membranes, or the presence of target lesions are other possible clues that this problem exists. Therefore, the intake of prescribed and over-the-counter preparations must be investigated.

Drug-induced toxic epidermal necrolysis may be associated with blisters. Histology that shows separation of dermis from epidermis excludes the staphylococcal-induced problem. Also, the staphylococcal scalded skin syndrome rarely occurs in children older than 6 years of age. A drug reaction should be considered in children older than 6 years old. Children with severe drug reactions may be very toxic. High fevers, malaise, joint problems, and the like can occur.

Henoch-Schönlein Purpura

Children with Henoch-Schönlein purpura (HSP) may have blisters because of the severe involvement of blood vessels (vasculitis) in the typical distribution that occurs in this condition. Associated systemic problems include arthritis, abdominal pain, kidney disease (hematuria or proteinuria), and seizures.

Nonspecific Vasculitis

Children with vasculitic blisters, at times hemorrhagic, may be sick with fever, malaise, and other symptoms. Some go on to well-defined collagen vascular disease, whereas others smolder, with no diagnosis ever being made.

Herpes Simplex

Primary infection with this virus may cause fever and regional lymphadenopathy. The first encounter for young children usually is herpetic gingivostomatitis. Vesicles involve the lips and the rest of the mouth. These children often are uncomfortable and commonly refuse to eat or drink.

Herpes progenitalis may produce fever and local lymphadenopathy as well. Characteristic clusters of vesicles occur on an erythematous base. Often, erosions or ulcerations evolve on the vulva or penis. Diagnosis can be confirmed by a Tzanck smear that shows aggregates of multinucleated giant cells (see Chapter 88) or a rapid slide test (immune-specific immunofluorescent antibody placed on cells scraped from the blister base).

Systemic Lupus Erythematosus

Although not characteristic, bullous lesions can occur in systemic lupus erythematosus (SLE). Multisystem involvement suggests the diagnosis. Laboratory confirmation, which may include a skin biopsy and lupus band test, in conjunction with the complete clinical picture, is necessary for diagnosis.

Palm and Sole Involvement

If the child is not ill, the physician should search for blisters on the palms and soles. The child's age helps differentiate some disorders (Table 58.6).

CHILD YOUNGER THAN 3 YEARS OF AGE

Scabies

Infants and very young children can have vesicobullous lesions on the palms, soles, head, and face. It is important to not be misled by this distribution and appearance. Generally, the mother is infested as well and exhibits the typical appearance of this disorder.

TABLE 58.6. Acute Vesicobullous Diseases Involving Palms and Soles

Child <3 years old	Any age
Scabies	Drug reaction
Acropustulosis of infancy	Friction blisters or burns
Syphilis (transiently at birth)	Dyshidrotic eczema
Adolescent or older	Vasculitis (e.g., Henoch–Schönlein purpura)
Tinea pedis or manus	Frostbite
"Id" reaction	
Epidermolysis bullosa of hands and feet	

Acropustulosis of Infancy

In African-American children, the appearance of pruritic vesicopustules in infants between 2 and 10 months of age on the palms and soles suggests acropustulosis of infancy. Vesicles often involve the lateral aspects of the fingers, palms, and soles. This condition was commonly diagnosed as dyshidrotic eczema in the past. Cyclic eruptions occur every 2 to 3 weeks, lasting 7 to 10 days.

Syphilis

Congenital syphilis may produce transient blisters on the palms and soles immediately after birth. "Snuffles," rhagades, condyloma lata, and violaceous to reddish brown macules should be sought on the palms and soles. Hepatosplenomegaly is often present. Osteochondritis is an early and common sign. Severe tenderness of a limb may cause pseudoparalysis of Parrot. The serologic test for syphilis is always positive in children with clinical manifestations.

ADOLESCENT OR OLDER

Tinea Pedis or Manus

Certain organisms that cause tinea pedis or manus (e.g., *Trichophyton* mentagrophytes) induce a severe inflammatory reaction on the hands and feet. Vesicobullous lesions erupt on the palms, instep, or medial aspect of the foot. A potassium hydroxide (KOH) preparation confirms the presence of hyphae in either location.

"Id" Reaction

If an adolescent's palms have blisters, the physician should look at the feet. Patients with tinea pedis may have allergic reactions to dissemination of antigen.

Epidermolysis Bullosa of the Hands and Feet

For more information, see Epidermolysis Bullosa Syndromes in this chapter (Table 58.3).

ANY AGE

Drug Reaction

For more information about drug reactions, see the section entitled "The Child Who Is Ill" in this chapter.

Friction Blisters or Burns

Blistering on the palms and soles appears after trauma to the skin. The trauma often is related to a new activity (e.g., golfing, rowing, football) or to new, possibly poorly fitted, shoes. Occasionally, accidental burns or burns secondary to child abuse are seen. Abused children may have had cigarette burns or have had their feet dipped in scalding water.

Dyshidrotic Eczema (Pompholyx)

A recurrent rash with episodes of vesicles that involve the palms, soles, and lateral aspects of the fingers is called *dyshidrotic eczema*. On occasion, large bullae occur. The problem generally is bilateral. Often there is a personal or family history of atopy. A KOH preparation or fungal culture of scrapings from the palms or soles generally is negative.

Vasculitis

Vasculitis may involve the palms or soles or both. See the section entitled "The Child Who Is Ill" in this chapter for more information.

Frostbite

Fingers, toes, feet, nose, cheeks, and ears are affected by extreme cold. After exposed areas are damaged by the cold temperature, symptoms occur on rewarming. Erythema, swelling, and burning pain occur at first, followed by vesicles and bullae (at times hemorrhagic) within 24 to 48 hours.

Extremities

If there is no involvement or minimal involvement of the palms and soles and the rash is concentrated on the extremities, insect bites, vasculitis, burns, frostbite, and bullous impetigo should be considered.

Insect Bites

Insects generally bite exposed skin surfaces. Therefore, the heaviest involvement occurs on the head, face, and extremities. Mosquito bites occur in the warm weather months, whereas flea bites occur during the whole year. Historical information includes contact with pets, camping trips, and involvement in outdoor activities. When blisters are present, the more characteristic urticarial papules usually are present in other locations. If not, confusion with bullous impetigo is easily ruled out with a Gram stain (negative for bacteria).

Vasculitis

Concentration of hemorrhagic bullae on the extremities and buttocks indicates HSP. The lower extremities most often are involved because of settling of immune complexes, cryoglobulins, and so forth in that location.

Burns

Exposed areas are commonly involved. Children accidentally rub against hot objects, causing burns and blistering. In cases of child abuse, children are burned intentionally with cigarettes (often mistaken for lesions of impetigo) or other heated objects. At times, children are submerged in scalding water. Usually, both lower extremities are involved.

Bullous Impetigo

In bullous impetigo, *Staphylococcus aureus* usually is present in pure culture. The bullae initially are filled with a clear fluid that rapidly becomes cloudy. The lesions tend to spread locally. Regional lymph nodes usually are not enlarged.

CHAPTER 59
Respiratory Distress

Debra L. Weiner, M.D., Ph.D.

Young children are at particular risk of respiratory distress because of their respiratory anatomy and physiology. Rapid evaluation and aggressive treatment of respiratory distress, as well as anticipation and prevention of impending respiratory distress and failure, are essential to optimize outcome.

DIFFERENTIAL DIAGNOSIS

Establishing a diagnosis for respiratory distress depends in part on localizing the source of the distress to a particular organ system. Respiratory distress may result directly from a disturbance of the upper or lower respiratory system. It also can be caused by the inability of the central or peripheral nervous system to interpret or process respiratory requirements or of the musculoskeletal system to perform the work of breathing. Alternatively, disease or dysfunction of other organ systems may result indirectly in respiratory disturbance by compromising respiratory system function or by stimulating compensatory respiratory mechanisms (Tables 59.1 through 59.3). Treatment of the underlying cause is essential for definitive treatment of the respiratory distress.

Respiratory System

Upper-airway obstruction is common in infants and young children, in part because of their airway anatomy and physiology. Manifestations of upper airway obstruction include nasal flaring, stertor or snoring, gurgling, drooling, dysphagia, aphonia, hoarseness, stridor, retractions, and paradoxical chest and abdominal wall movement. In neonates, the common causes include nasal obstruction, congenital upper-airway anomalies (particularly laryngotracheomalacia), and congenital or postintubation subglottic stenosis. Common causes for acquired upper-airway obstruction in infants and children include adenotonsillar hypertrophy, peritonsillar abscess, croup, foreign body, retropharyngeal abscess, tracheitis, and airway edema from trauma or allergic reaction. Epiglottitis, although less common, is one of the most life-threatening causes of respiratory distress and is a true emergency. The incidence of epiglottitis has declined significantly since routine immunization against *Haemophilus influenzae* B, the pathogen that was responsible for at least 75% of cases. Epiglottitis should be suspected in children who have abrupt onset of fever, dysphagia, drooling, muffled voice, labored respirations, and stridor. Peritonsillar and retropharyngeal abscess may present with symptoms similar to epiglottitis but have more gradual onset. Croup or laryngotracheobronchitis is the most common cause of upper-airway obstruction in children 3 months to 3 years of age. Croup causes subglottic narrowing and is characterized by a barklike cough, inspiratory stridor, and hoarseness that are worse at night. Viral croup, most often caused by parainfluenza, has an insidious onset following several days of upper respiratory infection symptoms with normal temperature or low-grade elevation. Spasmodic or allergic croup has acute onset, usually with wakening during the night, in a child who was well before going to sleep. Children with recurrent or pro-

TABLE 59.1. Causes of Respiratory Distress

Respiratory system
Upper airway obstruction
Nasopharynx (craniofacial anomalies, choanal atresia, adenotonsillar hypertrophy, nasal congestion, foreign body, trauma, mass)
Oropharynx (macroglossia, micrognathia, midface hypoplasia, tonsillitis, peritonsillar abscess, Ludwig angina, trauma)
Larynx (laryngomalacia, hemangioma, papilloma, webs, cysts, laryngoceles, laryngotracheal cleft, subglottic stenosis, croup, epiglottitis, retropharyngeal abscess, tracheitis, anaphylaxis, angioneurotic edema, thermal or chemical burn, foreign body, vocal cord paralysis, trauma)
Trachea (tracheomalacia, stenosis, tracheoesophageal fistula, foreign body)
Bronchi (bronchomalacia, stenosis, bronchogenic cyst, bronchitis, foreign body)
Lower airway obstruction/acinar/interstitial disease
Bronchioles (asthma, bronchiolitis, allergy, angioneurotic edema, bronchiectasis)
Acinic/interstitium
- Disorders of lung maturity (transient tachypnea of newborn, respiratory distress syndrome, bronchopulmonary dysplasia, persistent fetal circulation, Wilson–Mikity)
- Congenital malformation (congenital emphysema, cystic adenomatoid malfunction, sequestration, pulmonary agenesis/aplasia/hypoplasia, pulmonary cyst)
- Aspiration (meconium, foreign body, near drowning, gastroesophageal reflux, vomiting)
- Infection (pneumonia, bacterial, atypical bacteria, viral, chlamydia, pertussis, fungal, pneumocystis)
- Pulmonary collapse, fluid, mass (atelectasis, edema, hemorrhage, embolism, mass)
- Environmental/trauma (high-altitude pulmonary edema, thermal or chemical burn, smoke, carbon monoxide, hydrocarbon, drug-induced pulmonary fibrosis, bronchopulmonary traumatic disruption, pulmonary contusion)

Central nervous system
Structural abnormality (agenesis, hydrocephalus, mass, arteriovascular malformation)
Dysfunction/immaturity (apnea, hyperventilation/hypoventilation)
Infection (meningitis, encephalitis, abscess)
Inherited degenerative disease
Intoxication (alcohol, barbiturates, benzodiazepines, opiates)
Seizure
Trauma (birth asphyxia, hemorrhage)
Spinal cord (congenital anomaly, tetanus, trauma)
Anterior horn (poliomyelitis, transverse myelitis, spinal muscular atrophy)

Peripheral nervous system
Peripheral motor nerve (phrenic nerve injury, Guillain–Barre, multiple sclerosis, tick paralysis, heavy metal, organophosphate, porphyria)
Neuromuscular junction (myasthenia gravis, botulism, snake bite, organophosphate, antibiotic)
Muscle (muscular/myotonic dystrophies, inborn error of metabolism, carnitine deficiency, poly/dermatomyositis, fatigue)

Chest wall/intrathoracic
Air leak (pneumothorax, tension pneumothorax, pneumomediastinum, pneumopericardium)
Space-occupying (esophageal foreign body, pleural effusion, empyema, chylothorax, hemothorax, anomalies great vessels, diaphragmatic hernia, cyst, mass)
Boney and/or muscular deformity or dysfunction (congenital bone/muscle absence, spine deformity, pectus excavatum/carinatum, diaphragmatic hernia, contusion, rib fractures/flail chest, burn)

Cardiovascular
Congenital (structural defect, arrhythmia)
Acquired (myocarditis, myocardial ischemia or infarction, pericardial effusion, pericardial tamponade, aortic dissection or rupture, mass, coronary artery dilation/aneurysm, congestive heart failure)

Gastrointestinal
Distension/pain (necrotizing enterocolitis, mass, obstruction, perforation, laceration, hematoma, contusion, appendicitis, infection, inflammation, ascites)

Metabolic/endocrine
Acidosis (exercise, fever, hypothermia, dehydration, sepsis, shock, IEM, liver disease, renal disease, diabetic ketoacidosis, salicylates)
Hyperammonemia (IEM, liver failure)
Serum chemistry disturbance (hyperkalemia/hypokalemia, hypercalcemia/hypocalcemia, hypophosphatemia, hypermagnesemia/hypomagnesemia)
Respiratory chain disturbance (cyanide)
Endocrine (hyperglycemia/hypoglycemia, hyperthyroidism/hypothyroidism, hyperparathyroidism, adrenal hyperplasia)

Hematologic
Anemia, abnormal hemoglobin (inadequate erythrocyte numbers, decreased production, loss, hemoglobinopathy, carboxyhemoglobin, methemoglobin)
Polycythemia

IEM, ineffective esophageal motility.

TABLE 59.2. Most Common Causes of Respiratory Distress

Neonate	Infant or child
Nasal obstruction	Peritonsillar abscess
Congenital airway anomalies	Croup
Transient tachypnea	Tracheitis
Respiratory distress syndrome	Foreign body
Meconium aspiration	Bronchiolitis
Pneumonia	Asthma
Sepsis	Allergy
Congenital heart disease	Pneumonia
	Fever
	Sepsis
	Gastroenteritis/dehydration

longed croup may have an underlying fixed or functional airway abnormality, most commonly subglottic stenosis or hemangioma. Children with chronic stridor, particularly those younger than 2 years, are also likely to have an underlying congenital anomaly. Foreign-body aspiration, which has a peak age of occurrence 1 to 5 years, may cause obstruction of the upper or lower airway and is a leading cause of accidental death in toddlers. A history of abrupt onset of choking or gagging is suggestive. Drooling, dysphagia, and stridor suggest an upper airway foreign body, whereas unilateral wheeze, particularly first-time wheeze with acute onset, suggests lower airway position. Other common causes of lower airway obstruction involve inflammation and bronchospasm and include asthma, allergy, and bronchiolitis. Wheeze, most often diffuse, is usually a predominant feature of these conditions (see Chapter 71). Asthma may be triggered by infection, exercise, environmental irritants, or stress. Bronchiolitis, most often caused by respiratory syncytial virus, presents with wheeze in children younger than 2 years. Other causes of lower-airway obstruction include filling the airway lumen by excessive secretions (e.g., from inflammation, infection, toxin such as organophosphate) or aspirated fluids and decreasing of lumen diameter as a result of the loss of radial traction of the airway wall as with emphysema and masses.

Alveolar and interstitial disease is characterized by tachypnea, cough, grunting, crackles, rhonchi, wheeze, and decreased or asymmetric breath sounds with or without fever. In neonates, transient tachypnea of the newborn and meconium aspiration are common causes. Pneumonia is one of the most common causes of lower airway disease in neonates, infants, and children. Findings are more likely to be localized in the setting of bacterial pneumonia, whereas patients with viral and atypical pneumonias, such as *Mycoplasma, Chlamydia*, and pertussis, tend to have diffuse peribronchial, interstitial processes. Less commonly, aspiration, hemorrhage, and pulmonary edema cause fluid collection in the acini and interstitium. *Atelectasis*, or airway collapse, resulting from loss of air from the pulmonary parenchyma, often occurs secondary to other processes, including pneumonia, particularly viral; bronchospasm; and inadequate lung expansion, most often resulting from pain, neuromuscular disease, or inactivity. Structural and/or functional abnormalities include bronchopulmonary dysplasia, hyaline membrane disease, or respiratory distress syndrome, bronchiectasis (most commonly seen in cystic fibrosis), congenital or acquired emphysema, and pulmonary fibrosis (usually from radiation and chemotherapy).

TABLE 59.3. Most Common Acute Life-Threatening Causes of Respiratory Distress

Foreign body	Pericardial tamponade
Tension pneumothorax	Epiglottitis

Nervous System

Central nervous system (CNS) disturbances may result in hypoventilation or hyperventilation, loss of protective airway reflexes, or airway obstruction from loss of pharyngeal tone. These conditions include CNS malformation, immaturity, infection, degenerative disease, seizures, mass, trauma, and intoxication. Focal neurologic deficits, visual disturbances, pupillary abnormalities, papilledema, abnormal muscle tone, and altered level of consciousness suggest CNS processes. Spinal cord trauma and anterior horn cell disease cause bulbar and respiratory muscle dysfunction, which results in airway obstruction or hypoventilation. Peripheral neuromuscular (i.e., peripheral nerve, neuromuscular junction, muscle) disorders result in muscle weakness or paralysis. Physical findings that suggest significant chest wall weakness may include hypotonia, hyporeflexia, muscle weakness, weak cry, hoarse voice, cough, gag, shallow or irregular respiratory pattern, and inability to lift the head or extremities.

Chest Wall and Thoracic Cavity

Musculoskeletal deformity or disease involving the support structures of the chest may severely restrict lung expansion, limiting normal ventilatory efforts or attempts at compensatory ventilation for respiratory dysfunction and other systemic disturbances. Intrathoracic conditions that may produce respiratory distress include air leak and space-occupying lesions, including fluid collections and masses. Air leak is most commonly caused by pneumothorax or tension pneumothorax, which may be traumatic or spontaneous. Pneumothorax, in addition to nonspecific signs of respiratory distress, is suggested by chest-wall hyperexpansion, decreased breath sounds, and hyperresonance on the side of the air leak. With tension pneumothorax, jugular venous distension (JVD) and deviation of the trachea and mediastinum away from the air leak also can occur. The most commonly occurring space-occupying lesion is pleural effusion, which may be caused by infection, inflammation, ischemia, trauma, malignancy, major organ failure, drug hypersensitivity, or venous or lymphatic obstruction. Pleural effusion is suggested on physical examination by decreased breath sounds and a pleural rub. Mass lesions include congenital or traumatic diaphragmatic hernia, esophageal anomalies, benign or neoplastic masses, and vascular malformations.

Cardiovascular

Congenital and acquired heart disease may result in respiratory distress from decreased cardiac output, reduced oxygen saturation, or congestive heart failure (CHF). Compromised cardiac output, most commonly caused by congenital structural heart defects, cardiac arrhythmias, myocarditis, pericardial effusion, pericardial tamponade, or hypotension, may result in insufficient tissue oxygen delivery to meet metabolic demands. Pericardial tamponade causes decreased cardiac output as a result of compromised cardiac filling and can be recognized on physical examination by Beck triad of arterial hypotension, JVD, and distant heart sounds. It can be caused by infection, inflammation, trauma, or surgery. Acute tamponade may be immediately life threatening and must be relieved expeditiously by pericardiocentesis. Cardiac anomalies with right-to-left shunting of deoxygenated blood result in reduced oxygen saturation of blood entering the systemic circulation, hence causing hypoxia with cyanosis. Cardiac defects causing left-to-right shunting result in pulmonary overcirculation, pulmonary venous congestion, and pulmonary edema that directly compromises pulmonary function. In children, congenital heart defects are the most common cause of CHF. Other cardiac causes of CHF include valvular heart disease, myocardial dysfunction, arrhythmias, ischemia, and infarction. Metabolic disturbances, sepsis, fluid overload, and severe anemia also can result in CHF. Pulmonary manifestations of CHF include tachypnea, increased work of breathing, dyspnea on exertion, orthopnea, cough, wheeze, and bibasilar rales. Other manifestations include poor feeding, failure to thrive, fatigue, tiring with feeds, diaphoresis, edema, tachycardia, weak thready pulses, JVD, displaced point of maximum impulse, cardiac murmur, gallop, rub, cardiomegaly, and hepatosplenomegaly. Vascular causes of respiratory distress include pulmonary embolism, pulmonary hypertension, and pulmonary arteriovenous fistula.

Gastrointestinal

Abdominal obstruction, perforation of hollow viscous, laceration of solid organs, hematoma, contusion, appendicitis, infection, inflammation, ascites, or mass may result in impaired diaphragmatic excursion secondary to abdominal distension or pain. Prolonged shallow respiration may result in pulmonary hypoventilation. Gastroesophageal reflux or vomiting, particularly in children unable to protect their airway, may result in pulmonary aspiration.

Metabolic and Endocrine Disturbances

Metabolic disturbances often manifest as compensatory alterations in respiratory status. Metabolic acidosis results in rapid, deep breathing. Hyperammonemia directly stimulates the respiratory center to produce tachypnea, which results in primary respiratory alkalosis with secondary metabolic acidosis. Metabolic disruption of oxygen metabolism is another cause for respiratory distress. Endocrine disturbances that cause alterations in metabolic rate or chemical imbalances also may result in respiratory distress.

Hematologic

Inadequate concentrations of hemoglobin or hemoglobin with decreased oxygen-carrying capacity result in deficient oxygen delivery to tissues. Polycythemia results in sludging of blood and therefore compromised oxygen delivery.

EVALUATION AND DECISION

Triage and Stabilization

Every child with significant respiratory distress must be considered to be at potential risk of respiratory collapse. Airway patency, breathing, and circulation should be rapidly assessed and, if compromised, should be established and optimized immediately.

History

Information obtained by history should include a description of respiratory and other symptoms, onset and duration of symptoms, possible precipitating factors, exacerbating factors, therapeutic interventions, history of previous similar symptoms, underlying medical conditions, medications, allergies, and immunizations.

Physical Examination

The physical examination should assess the degree of respiratory distress and should identify the site and likely cause of respiratory distress (Fig. 59.1). General appearance, level of consciousness, vital signs, respiratory rate, respiratory effort, and adequacy of oxygenation and ventilation give immediate information regarding the severity of respiratory distress and possible sites. Table 59.4 provides specific clues to localization by physical examination.

Approach

In approaching children with respiratory distress (Figs. 59.1 and 59.2), the physician first should assess the adequacy of oxygenation and ventilation and then provide appropriate resuscitation. Patients in extremis (Fig. 59.1) are most likely to have sustained an injury, resulting in conditions such as a tension pneumothorax, flail chest, or cardiac tamponade, or have an obstructed airway, either as a result of aspiration of a foreign body or infection.

For patients with mild to moderate respiratory distress, as well as for those in extremis for whom the most likely diagnoses do not provide an explanation, the physician should proceed with a history, a physical examination, and a determination of oxygen saturation and deliver supplemental oxygen as indicated. Respiratory distress of any degree calls for an immediate assessment of the airway. Stridor, altered phonation, or dysphagia suggests partial obstruction, most likely from infection, anaphylaxis, or foreign body. Assessment of the airway is followed by auscultation of the lungs for rales and wheezes. Children with abnormal auscultatory findings and fever are likely to have pneumonia or bronchiolitis, whereas asthma, bronchiolitis, and foreign-body aspiration are common in afebrile patients.

Patients can be further categorized on the basis of tachypnea (Fig. 59.2). Children with rapid respirations and fever are likely to have pneumonia, even in the absence of rales; empyema, pulmonary embolism, and encephalitis are also important considerations. Tachypnea without fever points to trauma, cardiac disease, metabolic disturbances, toxic ingestions, and miscellaneous disorders.

Febrile children without tachypnea may have apnea or bradypnea as late manifestations of CNS infection. In afebrile patients, considerations include the myriad causes of CNS depression, spinal cord injury, neuromuscular disease, and neonatal apnea. Diagnostic tests should be used selectively to rule out diagnoses suggested by history and physical examination (Table 59.5). Nearly all patients with respiratory distress should have oxygenation tested by pulse oximetry. Arterial blood gas, which is more useful for lower than upper respiratory processes, and chest radiograph are the tests most likely to be helpful in the diagnosis of respiratory failure and determination of its cause.

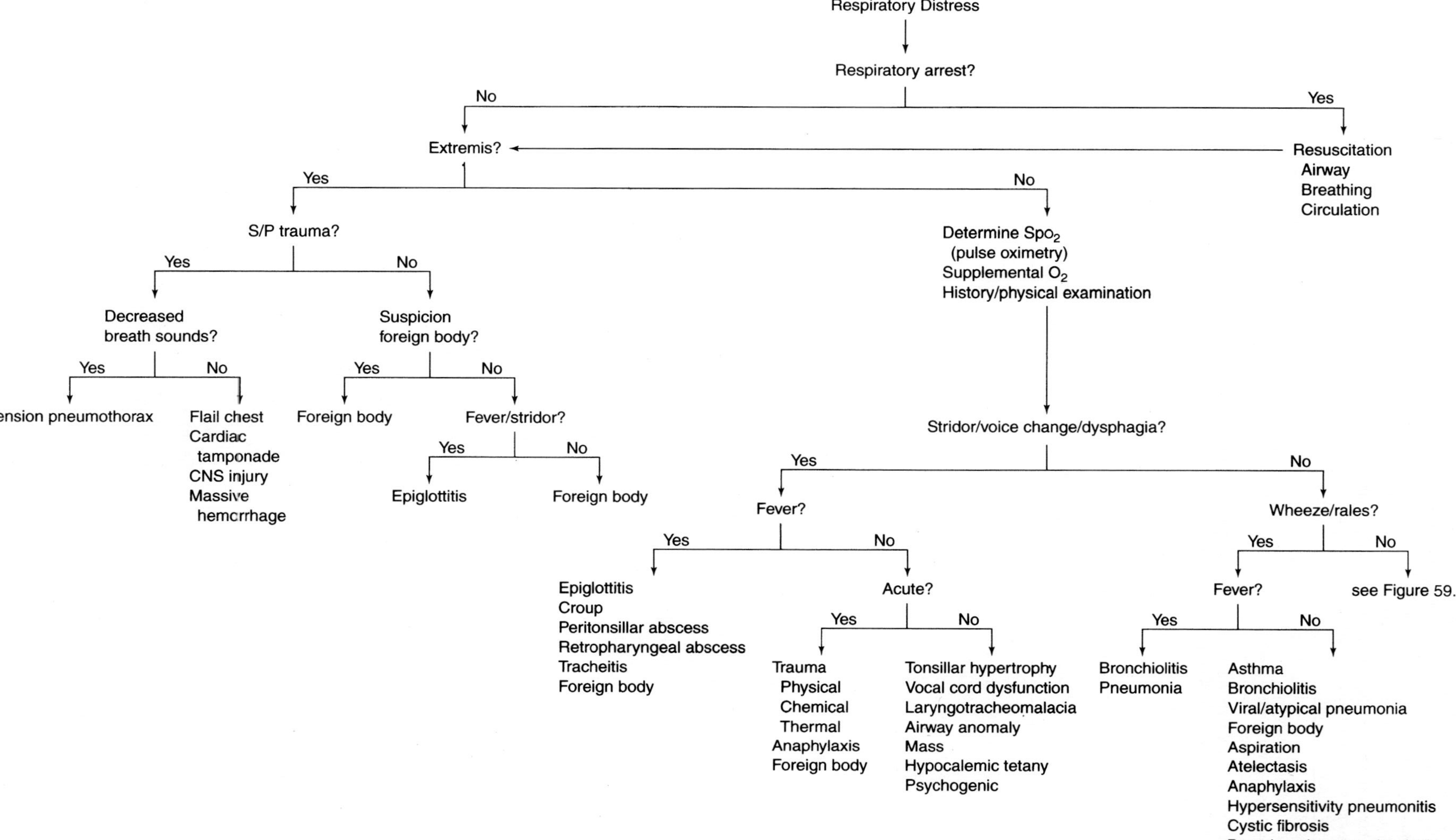

Figure 59.1. Approach to the child with respiratory distress. CNS, central nervous system; Spo_2, percent oxygen saturation; O_2, oxygen.

TABLE 59.4. Localization of Respiratory Distress by Physical Examination Findings

Flaring: reflexive opening of nares during inspiration with upper airway obstruction
Retractions: inward collapse of chest wall as a result of high negative intrathoracic pressure from increased respiratory effort; supraclavicular, suprasternal, subcostal retractions upper airway obstruction, intercostal retractions lower airway obstruction or disease
Stertor: snoring with nasal congestion, adenotonsillar hypertrophy, neuromuscular weakness
Gurgle: inspiratory and expiratory bubbling sounds caused by secretions oropharynx, trachea, large bronchi
Aphonia: vocal cord obstruction, dysfunction
Hoarseness: laryngeal obstruction, dysfunction
Barky cough: subglottic, tracheal obstruction
Stridor: abnormal turbulence over airway obstruction; (1) inspiratory: quiet, high pitched from glottic, subglottic region; (2) expiratory: loud, harsh from carina or below; (3) biphasic: loud, harsh from trachea
Grunt: expiration against a closed glottis to maintain expiratory lung volume with lower airway, gastrointestinal process
Wheeze: continuous, musical; (1) obstructed bronchi, bronchioles—polyphonic (variable, pitched, regional differences) expiratory as in asthma; (2) obstructed central airway—monophonic (low-pitched, same in all lung fields) expiratory ± inspiratory as with tracheal foreign body, tracheomalacia
Crackles (rales): discontinuous, usually high-pitched, inspiratory; moist, from thin secretions in (1) bronchi, bronchioles (medium rales) or (2) alveoli (fine rales)
Rhonchi (coarse rales): discontinuous, usually low-pitched, inspiratory; moist or dry; from exudate, edema, inflammation larger bronchi
Pleural friction rub: loud, low-pitched inspiratory ± expiratory, due to pleural inflammation
Bronchophony, egophony, whispered pectoriloquy: alterations in voice sounds as a result of lobar pneumonia, pleural effusion

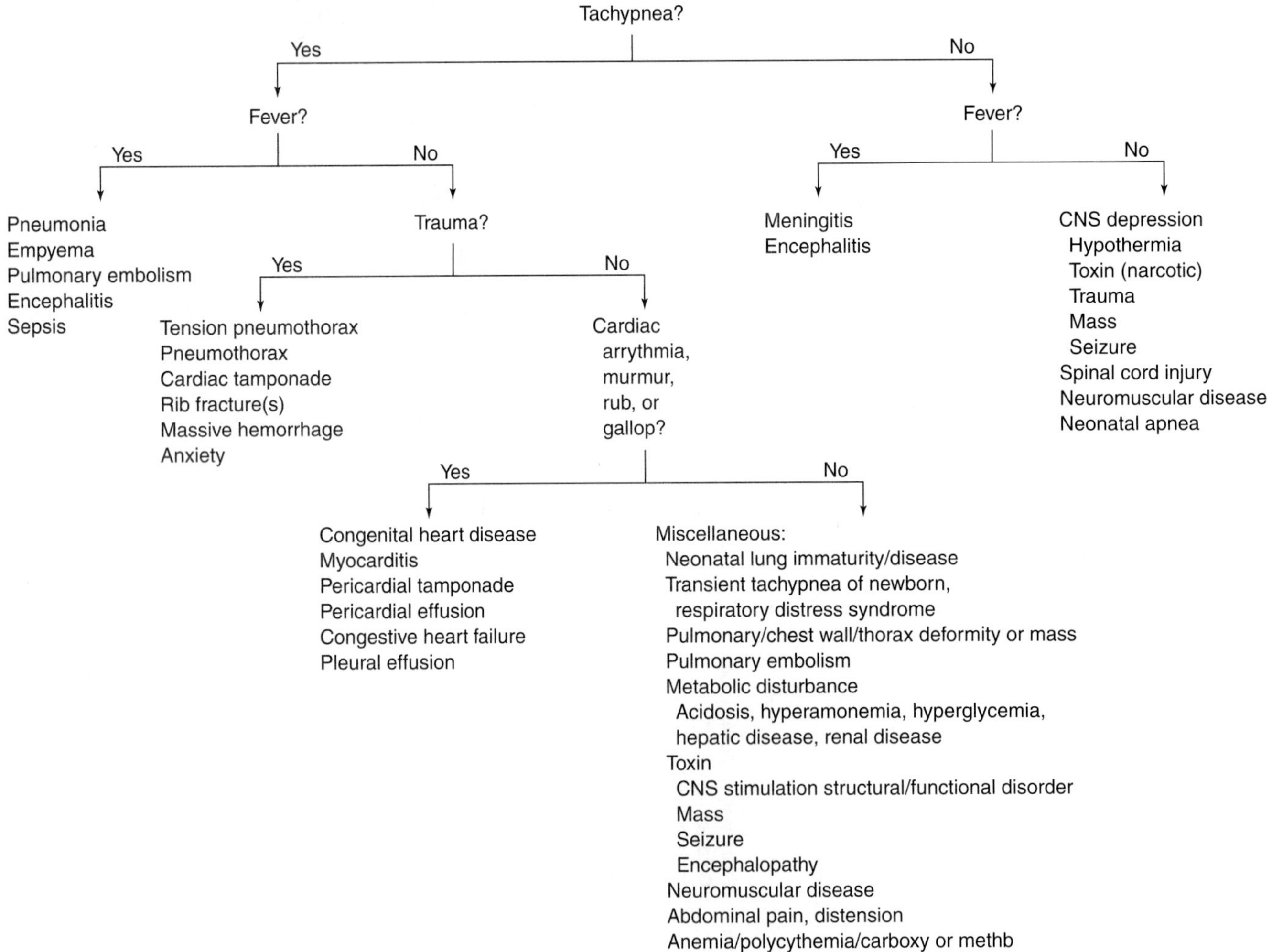

Figure 59.2. Approach to the child with respiratory distress (continued). CNS, central nervous system.

TABLE 59.5. Diagnostic Studies for Evaluation of Respiratory Distress

Test	Indications	Comments
Pulse oximetry	Respiratory distress	Measures oxygen saturation Relative contraindication if agitation will worsen distress Not reliable if severe anemia No information about ventilation
Capnography	Respiratory distress Monitor endotracheal tube placement	Measures end-tidal CO_2 Information about ventilation
ABG	Respiratory failure, acidosis carboxyhemoglobin or methemoglobin	Most useful for lower airway process Relative contraindication if agitation will worsen distress ABG changes occur late and may not be seen until arrest (A-a) O_2 gradient increase suggests ventilation-perfusion mismatch
CBC, blood cx, + CSF analysis, cx, mono spot/EBV titer	Infection, allergy	Relative contraindication if agitation or positioning for lumbar puncture will worsen distress
Electrolytes, BUN, CR, glucose, $CaPO_4$, Mg, LFTs, ammonia, TFTs	Metabolic/endocrine disease, metabolic disturbance	Calculate anion gap May be normal
PT/PTT	Bleeding disorder, pulmonary embolism	
Toxicologic screen blood, urine	Ingestion/intoxication	Central nervous system depressants, neuromuscular blockade, electron transport chain poisons
Nasal, ocular, rectal swab: IFA, cx	Bronchiolitis, chlamydia, pertussis, viral pneumonia	Neonates, infants Adolescents
Sputum: stains, cx	Bacterial, TB, pneumocystis, fungal	
TB skin test	TB	
Radiograph		
Lateral neck	Tracheitis, abscess, foreign body	Not necessary for diagnosis of croup Relative contraindication unstable airway
Chest radiograph (AP/lateral)	Lower respiratory disease, foreign body, barotrauma, effusion, mass, chest wall trauma/deformity, cardiac process	Consider portable if unstable
Forced expiratory or bilateral decubitus	Foreign body	Air trapping behind object
Unilateral decubitus	Distinguish effusion from infiltrate	Effusion layers
AP supine/prone, upright/cross-table lateral	Abdominal mass, obstruction, perforation	
Fluoroscopy	Upper airway obstruction; structural or functional anatomic, foreign body, paralysis vocal cords, diaphragm	
Laryngoscopy/bronchoscopy	Upper or lower airway obstruction; structural or functional, foreign body	Esophagoscopy for esophageal processes
CT scan		
Head	Central mass, hydrocephalus	
Chest	Congenital anomaly, mass—tumor, abscess, diaphragmatic hernia	
Abdomen	Obstruction, mass, appendicitis	
Electrocardiogram	Cardiac anomaly, failure, pericarditis	
Thoracentesis, pericardiocentesis cytology, biochemical, cx	Infection, inflammation, oncologic process chest, heart, lymphatics	Also therapeutic; consider ultrasound guidance
Ventilation–perfusion scan	Pulmonary embolism	
Barium swallow	Tracheoesophageal fistula, vascular ring, reflux	
Pulmonary function tests	Central or peripheral nervous system depression of chest wall function, respiratory system disease	Measures lung volume, flow, compliance
Electromyography	Central respiratory drive depressed, neuromuscular disease	Measures muscle activity generated by neural outflow from respiratory centers
Angiography	Vascular anomaly	

ABG, arterial blood gas; CBC, complete blood count; cx, culture; CSF, cerebrospinal fluid; EBV, Epstein–Barr virus; BUN, blood urea nitrogen; CR, creatinine; Ca^{+}, calcium; Mg, magnesium; LFTs, liver function tests; TFTs, thyroid function tests; PT, prothrombin time; PTT, partial thromboplastin time; IFA, immunofluorescence assay; TB, tuberculosis; AP, anteroposterior; CT, computed tomography.

CHAPTER 60
The Septic-Appearing Infant

Steven M. Selbst, M.D.

A young infant may be brought to the emergency department (ED) because he or she "just doesn't look right" to the parents. To the physician in the ED, such an infant may appear quite ill with pallor, cyanosis, or ashen color. Generally, an ill-appearing infant, such as the one already described, will be considered immediately to have sepsis and will be managed reflexly. Although this approach may be correct in most cases, the physician should remember that several other conditions may cause an infant to appear septic. The purpose of this chapter is to establish a differential diagnosis for infants in the first 2 months of life who appear quite ill. An approach to the evaluation and management of such an infant is discussed.

DIFFERENTIAL DIAGNOSIS

Numerous disorders (Table 60.1) may cause an infant to appear septic. The most common of these disorders (Table 60.2) include certain bacterial infections and viral syndromes. The remaining disorders, although uncommon, demand diagnostic consideration because they are potentially life threatening and yet treatable.

Sepsis

Sepsis (Chapter 74) should always be considered when the emergency physician is confronted with an ill-appearing infant. The signs and symptoms of sepsis may be subtle. The history may vary, and some infants may seem to be ill for several days, whereas others deteriorate rapidly. Likewise, any one or a combination of symptoms, such as lethargy, irritability, diarrhea, vomiting, anorexia, or fever, may be a manifestation of sepsis. Fever generally is an unreliable finding in the septic infant; most septic infants younger than 2 months of age will be hypothermic instead. On physical examination, a septic infant may be pale, ashen, or even cyanotic. The skin is often cool and may be mottled because of poor perfusion. The infant may seem lethargic, obtunded, or irritable. There is often marked tachycardia, with the heart rate approaching 200 beats per minute, and tachypnea may be noted (respiratory rate above 50 breaths per minute).

The laboratory often is helpful in suggesting a diagnosis of sepsis; however, definitive cultures require time for processing. A complete blood count (CBC) may reveal a leukocytosis or left shift. In addition, a coagulation profile may show evidence of disseminated intravascular coagulation (DIC), and blood chemistries may reveal hypoglycemia or metabolic acidosis. If localized infection is suspected, aspiration and Gram stain of urine, joint fluid, spinal fluid, or pus from the middle ear may reveal the offending organism. Similarly, a chest radiograph may show a lobar infiltrate if pneumonia is present.

TABLE 60.2. Most Common Disorders That Mimic Sepsis

Urinary tract infection	Congestive heart failure
Viremia	Gastroenteritis with dehydration

Other Infections

Overwhelming viral infections may mimic sepsis in the young infant. In one study of *enteroviral infections* in the neonate, it was noted that 25% of infants younger than 1 month of age developed a sepsis-like illness. This infection is indistinguishable from bacterial sepsis except that bacterial cultures will be negative, whereas viral isolates from stool and cerebrospinal fluid (CSF) may confirm the offending enterovirus.

Epidemics of *respiratory syncytial virus* (RSV) occur in the wintertime, and infants younger than 2 months old may present with apnea or respiratory distress with cyanosis. Those born prematurely or with previous respiratory or cardiac disorders are especially susceptible to apnea. These infants often appear septic, but knowledge of illness in the community and a pre-

TABLE 60.1. Differential Diagnosis of the Septic-Appearing Infant

Infectious diseases	Inborn errors of metabolism
Bacterial sepsis	Hypoglycemia
Meningitis	Drugs/toxins—aspirin, carbon monoxide
Urinary tract infection	Renal disorders
Viral infections—Enterovirus, respiratory syncytial virus, herpes simplex	Posterior urethral valves
Pertussis	Hematologic disorders
Congenital syphilis	Severe anemia
Cardiac disease	Methemoglobinemia
Congenital heart disease	Gastrointestinal disorders
Supraventricular tachycardia	Gastroenteritis with dehydration
Myocardial infarction	Pyloric stenosis
Pericarditis	Intussusception
Myocarditis	Necrotizing enterocolitis
Kawasaki disease	Appendicitis, volvulus
Endocrine disorders	Neurologic disease
Congenital adrenal hyperplasia	Infant botulism
Metabolic disorders	Shunt obstruction, infection
Hyponatremia, hypernatremia	Child abuse—intracranial hemorrhage
Cystic fibrosis	

dominance of wheezing on chest examination may lead to the suspicion of RSV bronchiolitis. Still, some infants develop wheezing later in the course, and thus, the initial diagnosis is difficult. Chest radiographs may show diffuse patchy infiltrates and, possibly, lobar atelectasis.

Another viral infection to consider is *herpes simplex,* which usually causes systemic symptoms and encephalitis at 7 to 21 days of life. Neonates present with fever, coma, apnea, fulminant hepatitis, pneumonitis, coagulopathy, and seizures, which are often difficult to control. History of maternal genital herpes should lead to suspicion of systemic herpes infection in the neonate. In most cases, however, the mother is completely asymptomatic. Ocular findings such as conjunctivitis or keratitis may be noted as well as focal neurologic findings. If vesicular lesions are present on the skin, this infection should be strongly considered; however, they are present in only one-third to one-half of patients. When this infection is suspected, a Tzanck smear or direct fluorescent antibody staining of a scraped vesicle may provide rapid diagnosis. An electroencephalogram (EEG) or computed tomography scan also may be helpful. The diagnosis is confirmed by culture of a skin vesicle, mouth, nasopharynx, eyes, urine, blood, CSF, stool, or rectum.

Pertussis is another infection to consider when evaluating a very ill infant. Apnea, seizures, and death have been reported in this age group. Parents may report respiratory distress, cough, poor feeding, and vomiting (often posttussive). History of exposure to pertussis may be lacking because the infant usually acquires the disease from older children or adults who have only symptoms of a common upper respiratory infection. Physical examination will distinguish the infection from sepsis if the infant has a paroxysmal cough. The characteristic inspiratory "whoop" after a coughing paroxysm is uncommon in young infants. Auscultation of the chest is usually normal; tachypnea and cyanosis may be present. Initial laboratory studies may not identify the condition. The CBC in young infants may fail to show a marked lymphocytosis as expected in older patients with pertussis. Likewise, the chest radiograph may not show the typical "shaggy right heart border"; atelectasis or pneumonia may be present.

Infants with *congenital syphilis* may present in the first 4 weeks of life with extreme irritability, pallor, jaundice, hepatosplenomegaly, and edema. They may have pneumonia and often have painful limbs. Snuffles and skin lesions are common. Although these infants may appear to be ill on arrival in the ED, their histories reveal that they also have been chronically ill.

Cardiac Diseases

An infant with underlying *congenital heart disease* (CHD), such as ventriculoseptal defect, valvular insufficiency, valvular stenosis, hypoplastic left heart syndrome (HLHS), or coarctation of the aorta, may present with congestive heart failure and clinical findings similar to those of an infant with sepsis. There may be tachycardia and tachypnea as well as pallor, duskiness, or mottling of the skin. Cyanosis is not always present. There may also be sweating or decreased pulses and hypotension caused by poor perfusion; however, a careful history and physical examination may help the physician differentiate CHD with heart failure from sepsis. For instance, a chronic history of poor growth and poor feeding may suggest heart disease. Also, the presence of a cardiac murmur may suggest a structural lesion. Moreover, a gallop rhythm, hepatomegaly, neck vein distension, and peripheral edema may lead one to consider primary cardiac pathology. In a young infant, a difference between upper- and lower-extremity blood pressures suggests coarctation of the aorta. If cardiac output is inadequate, however, pulse differences may not be detected. Normal femoral pulses do not exclude a coarctation because the widely patent ductus arteriosis provides flow to the descending aorta.

Laboratory evaluation is essential in establishing cardiac disease as the cause of an infant's moribund condition. A chest radiograph often shows cardiac enlargement and may show pulmonary vascular engorgement or interstitial pulmonary edema rather than lobar infiltrates (as in pneumonia). The electrocardiogram (ECG) may be helpful in revealing certain congenital heart lesions. For instance, in HLHS, the ECG invariably shows right-axis deviation, with right atrial and ventricular enlargement. The ECG often is a nonspecific indicator of cardiac decompensation however, and an echocardiogram is more helpful. Rarely, an infant with anomalous or obstructed coronary arteries will develop myocardial infarction and will appear to be septic initially. Such young infants may have dyspnea, cyanosis, vomiting, pallor, and other signs of heart failure; however, these infants usually have cardiomegaly on chest radiograph. This will prompt the physician to perform an ECG, which usually shows T-wave inversion and deep Q waves in leads I and aVL. Echocardiogram and cardiac catheterization with contrast are needed to confirm the diagnosis.

In addition to CHD, certain *arrhythmias* may cause an infant to appear ill. For instance, a young infant with *supraventricular tachycardia* (SVT) often presents with findings similar to those of a septic infant. Often SVT will go unrecognized in young infants at home for 2 days or longer because initially they have only poor feeding, fussiness, and some rapid breathing. As this condition goes untreated, however, the infants will develop congestive heart failure and may present with all the signs of sepsis, including shock. Because fever can be a precipitating cause of the arrhythmia, the condition obviously is confused with sepsis. A careful physical examination will make the diagnosis of SVT obvious, however. Particularly, the cardiac examination will reveal such extreme tachycardia in the infant that the heart rate cannot even be counted. It is usual for the heart rate to exceed 250 to 300 beats per minute in such infants. With this information, laboratory aids can confirm the diagnosis. An ECG will show regular atrial and ventricular beats with 1:1 conduction, whereas P waves appear different from sinus P waves and may be difficult to see at all. They are often buried in the T waves. Moreover, a chest radiograph may show cardiomegaly and pulmonary congestion.

Additional cardiac pathologies to consider include *myocarditis* and *pericarditis*. Pericarditis may be caused by bacterial organisms such as *Staphylococcus aureus;* myocarditis usually results from viral infections such as coxsackievirus B. In infants, these often are fulminant infections, and the infant with such a condition will appear critically ill, with fever and grunting respirations often present. A complete physical examination may help the physician distinguish these conditions from sepsis in that signs of heart failure may be seen and unexplained tachycardia is often present. Also, pericarditis may produce neck vein distension and distant heart sounds if a significant pericardial effusion exists. In addition, a friction rub may be present. Laboratory tests may be helpful in that a chest radiograph will show cardiomegaly and a suggestion of effusion if pericarditis is present. The ECG will show generalized T-wave inversion and low-voltage QRS complexes, especially if pericardial fluid is present. Also, ST-T wave abnormalities may be seen. The echocardiogram will confirm the presence or absence of a pericardial effusion and poor ventricular function in the case of viral myocarditis. The CBC will not distinguish these infections from sepsis because leukocytosis is common and a left shift may be present.

Kawasaki disease with associated coronary artery aneurysms is very rare in young infants and is associated with a poor prognosis. A baby with Kawasaki disease may present with cyanosis and shock. Usually, history reveals prolonged and unexplained fever, rash, and mucous membrane inflammation. The physical examination may distinguish this illness from sepsis if there is a diffuse, raised, erythematous rash or cracked red lips, swollen hands and feet, conjunctivitis, and cervical lymphadenopathy. These classic features, found in older infants and children, may be absent in young infants, however. Routine laboratory studies may not differentiate this condition from sepsis either. A CBC may reveal leukocytosis or thrombocytosis. CSF usually shows a pleocytosis, with a lymphocytic predominance. Sterile pyuria is sometimes noted. In some cases, findings consistent with myocardial ischemia or an arrhythmia may be noted on ECG. Normal findings or nonspecific abnormalities are more common. Coronary artery aneurysms may be discovered with an echocardiogram, making the diagnosis highly likely.

Endocrine Disorders

Certain endocrine disorders can mimic sepsis. For instance, infants with *congenital adrenal hyperplasia* (CAH) may present in the first few days or weeks of life with a history of vomiting, lethargy, or irritability. On arrival, signs of marked dehydration may be present, with tachycardia and possibly hypothermia. The recent history may be revealing in that such infants may have been poor feeders since birth and the symptoms may be progressive over a few days. The physical examination can be extremely helpful in establishing the diagnosis in females if ambiguous genitalia are noted. The laboratory evaluation also is helpful in that the presence of marked hyponatremia with severe hyperkalemia should make CAH a likely diagnosis. Other nonspecific laboratory findings in this disorder include hypoglycemia, acidosis, and peaked T waves or arrhythmias on ECG. Specifically, the finding of elevated 17-hydroxyprogesterone and renin with decreased aldosterone and cortisol in the serum confirms the diagnosis of CAH.

Metabolic Disorders

Various metabolic disorders can look like sepsis and should be considered in the differential diagnosis. Prolonged diarrhea or vomiting can produce *dehydration, electrolyte disturbances,* and *acid–base abnormalities* such that an infant will appear quite ill. For instance, young infants with diarrhea may develop marked hyponatremia caused by iatrogenic water intoxication. Such infants may appear extremely lethargic, with slow respirations, hypothermia, and possibly, seizures.

A special cause of hyponatremic dehydration to consider is *cystic fibrosis* (see Chapter 85). The history in these cases may not be helpful initially, except that the infant usually gets very ill in hot weather. The mother may report poor intake, poor growth, and increased lethargy. Only with specific questioning might the mother report that the infant's skin tastes "salty" or that the infant had meconium plug syndrome (transient form of distal colonic obstruction secondary to inspissated meconium) as a newborn or prolonged neonatal jaundice. In some cases, pulmonary symptoms such as cough, tachypnea, or pneumonia may have been treated earlier in life. On examination, the dehydrated infant looks much like any other septic infant; however, laboratory tests that show profound hypoelectrolytemia, especially when not accounted for by gastrointestinal losses, should suggest cystic fibrosis. A sweat test will help confirm the diagnosis.

Likewise, dehydrated infants with *hypernatremia* may be lethargic or irritable, with muscle weakness, seizures, or coma. Infants with persistent vomiting may have hypochloremic alkalosis with hypokalemia, and they may appear weak or have cardiac dysfunction (see Chapter 76). In addition, rare inborn errors of metabolism such as *inherited urea cycle disorders* may produce vomiting in young infants, who then present with lethargy, seizures, or coma resulting from metabolic acidosis, hyperammonemia, or hypoglycemia (see Chapter 87). *Hypoglycemia* also can be secondary to sepsis, certain drugs, or alcohol intoxication. It is thus essential to evaluate the electrolytes, blood sugar, and possibly plasma ammonia levels in young infants with significant symptoms of gastroenteritis, lethargy, or irritability.

Another metabolic problem to consider is that of *toxins* (see Chapter 78). Obviously, young infants are incapable of accidental ingestions, but well-meaning parents may rarely cause salicylism in their attempts to treat fever with aspirin (despite current Reye syndrome warnings). Affected infants then present with vomiting, hyperpnea, hyperpyrexia, or convulsions and coma. In such cases, the history of medication given is crucial because the physical examination will not distinguish this ill infant from one with sepsis. The laboratory evaluation may lead to the suspicion of some metabolic problem because abnormalities of sodium, blood sugar, or acid–base balance often are found. Moreover, hypokalemia can be seen in salicylism as well as in abnormal liver function or renal function studies. An elevated salicylate level in the serum confirms the diagnosis of aspirin poisoning, but in chronic poisoning, the aspirin level may be relatively low despite a fatal course.

Carbon monoxide poisoning may present as an unknown intoxication when families are unaware of a defective heating system in the home. The young infant may have a history of sluggishness, poor feeding, and vomiting. A more careful history generally reveals that other family members are also ill with headache, syncope, or flulike symptoms. Their symptoms may improve after leaving the home environment. The classic "cherry red" skin color may be lacking, and physical examination may reveal only lethargy. Elevation of the carboxyhemoglobin level is diagnostic.

Renal Disorders

A young infant also may appear extremely ill because of renal failure or dysplasia. Such renal failure could be caused by *posterior urethral valves* that cause bladder outlet obstruction, especially in male infants. About one-third of those cases are diagnosed in the first week of life, but more than half will go undetected for the first few months of life. The parents may give a history of vomiting or poor appetite, or they may say that the baby has not grown well or that the infant's abdomen appears swollen. On physical examination, hypertension or an abdominal mass (*hydronephrosis*) may be detected, as well as urinary ascites. Laboratory tests will elucidate the diagnosis further.

Hematologic Disorders

Any infant with severe *anemia* caused by aplastic disease, hemolytic process, or blood loss can look quite ill (see Chapter 77). In addition to anemia, disorders of hemoglobin such as *methemoglobinemia* can cause an infant to appear toxic. Although the chronic forms are uncommon inherited disorders of hemoglobin structure or enzyme deficiency, transient methemoglobinemia in infants occasionally is caused by environmental toxicity from oxidizing agents, such as nitrates found in some specimens of well water. This intoxication presents in very young infants with cyanosis, poor feeding, failure to thrive, vomiting, diarrhea, and then lethargy. In other patients, the oxidant stress is less obvious. Methemoglobinemia has been described in infants with gastroenteritis and acidosis. Often the associated diarrhea is severe, and it has been thought that the infectious agent that causes the diarrhea or the secondary metabolic acidosis may produce an oxidant stress that leads to methemoglobin formation. On examination, such infants have been described as toxic and lethargic, with hypothermia, tachycardia, tachypnea, and hypotension. They often appear mottled, cyanotic, or ashen. One key to the diagnosis of methemoglobinemia is that oxygen administration does not affect the cyanosis, and yet no cardiac problem exists. Also, laboratory tests show a profound acidosis (pH 6.9–7.2), and yet the PA_{O2} is normal despite the cyanosis. Leukocytosis and thrombocytosis are present. The blood itself may appear chocolate brown (most easily noted when a drop of blood on filter paper is waved in t he air and compared with a normal control), and methemoglobin levels will be elevated up to 65% (normal, 0%–2%). Hemoglobin electrophoresis will be normal, except in rare cases of hemoglobin M, as is the glucose-6-phosphate dehydrogenase assay in most cases. Prerenal azotemia may be noted. With appropriate treatment, the methemoglobin level returns to normal; however, death can occur from methemoglobinemia in infants.

Gastrointestinal Disorders

Gastroenteritis, even without electrolyte disturbances, can lead to profound dehydration. In a very young infant with little reserve, this can quickly lead to lethargy and even shock. Bacterial infections such as salmonella and shigella may cause sepsis in a young infant, but viral agents may mimic this. A history of bloody diarrhea may suggest this diagnosis.

Also, *pyloric stenosis* in the young infant causes severe vomiting. This is most often seen in male infants 4 to 6 weeks old. An infant with pyloric stenosis may present with significant dehydration and may be lethargic. Usually, no fever is present. A careful history reveals that vomiting is the predominant feature of the illness, and there may be a positive family history for pyloric stenosis. The physical examination may reveal an abdominal mass, or "olive" in 5% to 10% of cases, which would strengthen the diagnosis of pyloric stenosis. Electrolytes typically show hypochloremia and hypokalemia, and alkalosis is prominent. Plain films of the abdomen, a barium study, or an ultrasound of the upper gastrointestinal tract may be needed to confirm the diagnosis.

Another gastrointestinal disorder to consider is *intussusception.* Although this rarely occurs in infants younger than 5 months old, it has been noted in some infants 2 to 3 months old. These infants may present with vomiting, fever, or signs of abdominal pain (e.g., legs drawn up, irritability). The infant may appear to have spasms of pain during which he or she is fretful. These spasms may be followed by apathy and listlessness. Diarrhea may be seen, and if the typical currant jelly stool is noted, the diagnosis of intussusception should be strongly suspected. On physical examination, an abdominal mass may be palpated or bloody stool found on rectal examination.

Several other unusual but important gastrointestinal disorders must be considered in infants. *Necrotizing enterocolitis* (NEC) occurs in premature infants in the first few weeks of life and can also occur in term infants, usually within the first 10 days of life. A history of an anoxic episode at birth or other neonatal stresses may suggest NEC. These infants are quite ill, with lethargy, irritability, anorexia, distended abdomen, and bloody stools. Radiographs of the abdomen may be helpful and usually show pneumatosis cystoides intestinalis caused by gas in the intestinal wall. Neonatal *appendicitis* is a rare event, but several cases have been reported to closely mimic sepsis. The most common presenting signs include irritability, vomiting, and abdominal distension on examination. There may also be hypothermia, ashen color, and shock as the condition progresses, as well as edema of the abdominal wall, localized to the right flank, and possibly, erythema of the skin in that area. The white blood cell count may be elevated, with a left shift, and there may be a metabolic acidosis, as well as DIC. Abdominal radiographs may show a paucity of gas in the right lower quadrant, evidence of free peritoneal fluid, or a right abdominal wall thickened by edema. Other unusual gastrointestinal emergencies to consider include *volvulus,* perforation caused by *trauma* from enemas or thermometers, and *Hirschsprung enterocolitis.*

Neurologic Diseases

One neurologic process that produces a sepsis-like picture is *infant botulism.* An infant with botulism is often lethargic at presentation, with a weak cry and, possibly, signs of dehydration. These infants usually are afebrile. A thorough history may help distinguish botulism from sepsis. If constipation has preceded the acute illness, botulism should be seriously considered. The disease also is associated with the ingestion of honey, breastfeeding, a recent change in feeding practices, and a rural environment. The parents may note a more gradual progression with this illness. On physical examination, infants with botulism are notably hypotonic and hyporeflexic and may have increased secretions caused by bulbar muscle weakness. Also, the presence of a facial droop, ophthalmoplegia, and decreased gag reflex are consistent with botulism, whereas they remain unusual findings with a septic infant.

A young infant with a ventriculoperitoneal shunt in place because of hydrocephalus can develop serious complications that cause the infant to appear extremely ill. *Shunt infection* could present with fever and irritability in a young infant. Abdominal pain or tenderness may be found on examination, as well as erythema or pus around the shunt itself. The definitive diagnosis is made by shunt aspiration under sterile conditions, but other causes of fever, such as meningitis, should be ruled out first. Shunt obstruction may result in increased intracranial pressure that causes a young infant to present with a history of lethargy or poor feeding. On examination, the infant may have bradycardia, apnea, coma, opisthotonic posturing, bulging fontanelle, or cranial nerve VI palsy. The shunt may be found to pump poorly. Laboratory tests such as radiographic evaluation of the shunt may be helpful if it shows a disconnection. Otherwise, a CT scan will demonstrate ventricle size and indicate the adequacy of shunt function.

Child Abuse

Intracranial hemorrhage that results from child abuse (see Chapter 111) must be considered in the very ill infant. It must be emphasized that the absence of bruises on an infant does not rule out child abuse. Vigorous shaking of an infant, followed by throwing the infant against a soft surface such as a mattress or sofa, can produce subdural or subarachnoid hemorrhages. The history may or may not be helpful in establishing a diagnosis. The parents may note that the child seemed to be in respiratory distress at home; only a few usually admit to shaking the infant.

On examination, the infant may appear gravely ill with apnea, bradycardia, hypothermia, bradypnea, and possibly, seizures. Careful physical examination may suggest abuse rather than sepsis. For instance, bruises may be present elsewhere on the body. More often, no external evidence of trauma is present, but respiratory distress without stridor or lower airway sounds may be apparent, leading to the consideration of a central nervous system cause. The head circumference is often at the 90th percentile, and the fontanelle may be full or bulging. Retinal hemorrhages often are found, strongly suggesting trauma or intracranial hemorrhage rather than meningitis.

Some neurologic signs may be confused with meningitis, such as nuchal rigidity, irritability or coma, seizures, or posturing. The laboratory is helpful in confirming suspicions of intracranial bleeding. Although the CBC often shows a leukocytosis and thus is confusing, the spinal fluid from a shaken baby usually is bloody. A computed axial tomography (CAT) scan or magnetic resonance imaging (MRI) usually demonstrates a small posterior, interhemispheric subdural hematoma. Such shaken babies have a high incidence of serious morbidity and mortality.

EVALUATION AND DECISION

Any infant who is critically ill in the first few months of life should be presumed initially to have sepsis. Because such illness is a life-threatening situation that may respond to early treatment, it is imperative to stabilize the child rapidly (Fig. 60.1). After airway, breathing, and circulation have been restored, vascular access should be obtained. Unless another diagnosis is immediately obvious, it is best to give intravenous antibiotics while pursuing alternative diagnoses. If time permits, cultures should be sent to the laboratory before giving antibiotics. Use of prostaglandins should be considered if cardiogenic shock is suspected.

A complete history should be obtained. It is important to learn of any previous medical problems such as known heart disease or failure to thrive. The time of onset of symptoms, exposure to infection, medications given at home, and specific symptoms noted by the parents must be determined. Next, careful physical examination must be performed because specific findings may

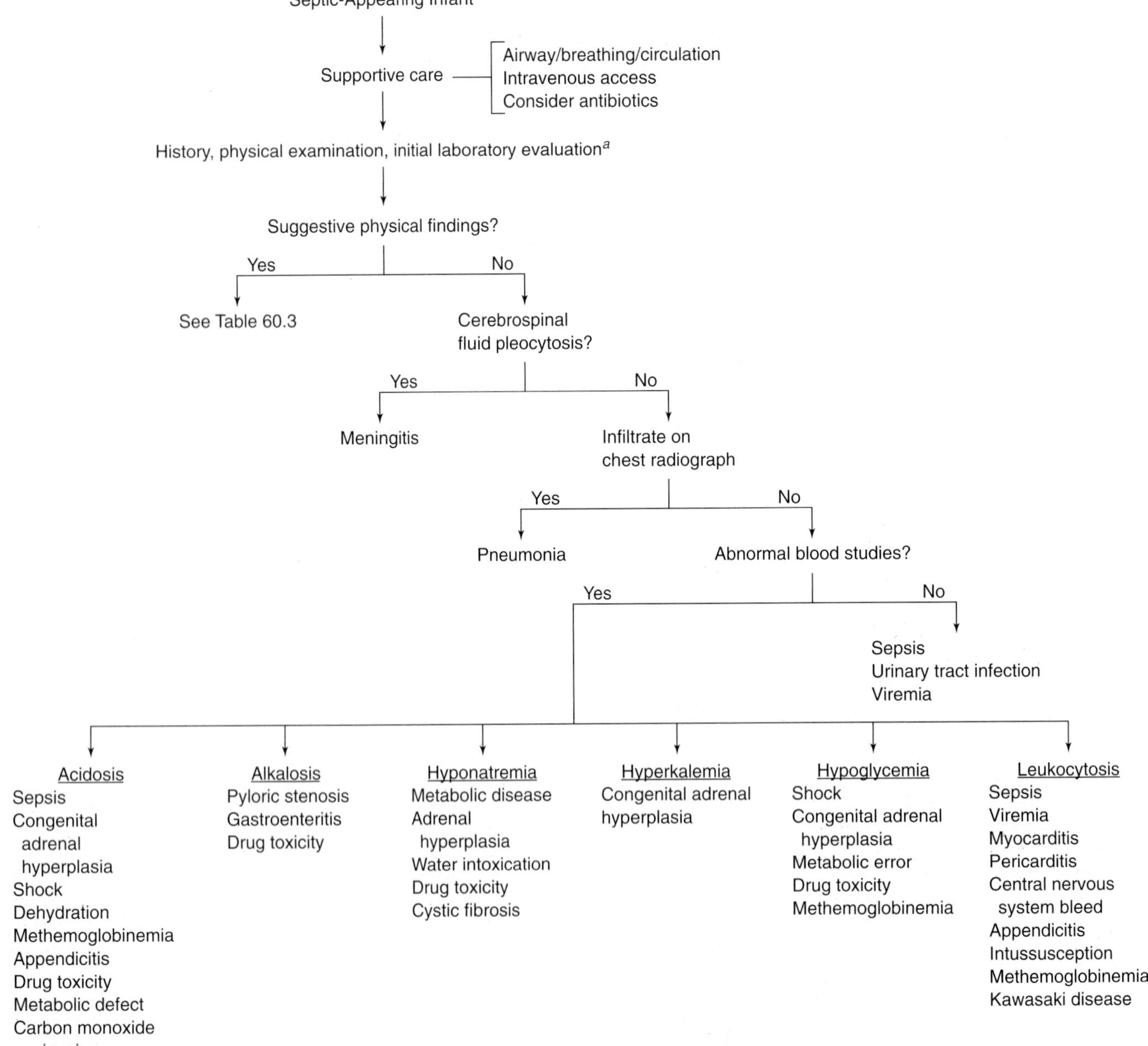

Figure 60.1. Initial approach to the septic-appearing child.

lead to a diagnosis other than sepsis (Table 60.3). After the physical examination, a complete laboratory evaluation should be performed. All sick infants should have a blood culture and urine culture obtained by a urethral catheter or suprapubic bladder tap. A lumbar puncture also should be performed unless the physical findings point strongly to a diagnosis other than sepsis or the infant is too ill to tolerate the procedure. A chest radiograph is also essential to look for pulmonary infection and to evaluate the heart size. A CBC should be obtained; leukocytosis will add support to a suspicion of sepsis but also may be found in various other disorders, including viral infections, myocarditis, pericarditis, intracranial bleeds, NEC, appendicitis, intussusception, and methemoglobinemia. Because metabolic problems (disturbances in acid–base balance, electrolytes, blood sugar) can result from sepsis or be the primary problem that mimics sepsis, all sick infants should have chemistries to evaluate serum sodium, potassium, chloride, glucose, and bicarbonate. If hyponatremia is found, water intoxication, aspirin toxicity, cystic fibrosis, and CAH should be considered. If there is also a marked hyperkalemia, CAH is most likely. If there is hypochloremic alkalosis or alkalosis alone, then pyloric stenosis, aspirin toxicity, or gastroenteritis should be considered. If there is hypoglycemia, it should be considered secondary to poor glucose reserves in an ill infant or related to drug (aspirin) toxicity, inborn errors of metabolism, CAH, or methemoglobinemia. If the serum bicarbonate is low, this should be confirmed with an arterial blood gas. Then, if acidosis is present, poor perfusion caused by shock should be considered, as well as dehydration, drug toxicity, methemoglobinemia, appendicitis, CAH, and inborn errors of metabolism, as primary problems. Finally, if laboratory tests are not revealing for a specific disorder or the patient does not improve quickly as an inpatient receiving antibiotics, stool and CSF isolates for viruses should be considered.

If the physical examination suggests a specific problem, it may be necessary to obtain additional laboratory tests (Table 60.3). For instance, if the examination reveals pallor, cyanosis, or cardiac abnormality (muffled heart sounds, murmur, unexplained tachycardia, or arrhythmia) the physician should consider various cardiac disorders and possibly methemoglobinemia. An ECG, arterial blood to measure Pa_{O2}, and possibly an echocardiogram should be obtained. If there are unusual neurologic findings, such as a bulging fontanelle, a lumbar puncture should be performed to rule out meningitis as well as blood studies mentioned previously. The presence of seizures should prompt a CT scan, EEG, and culture and treatment for herpes simplex virus. Also, if marked hypotonia is present, an electromyogram may help diagnose botulism. Retinal hemorrhages may suggest an intracranial bleed, and thus a CAT scan, MRI, and lumbar puncture would be valuable studies. Likewise, if abdominal distension, rigidity, mass, or bloody stools are present, a gastrointestinal emergency is indicated. In such cases, abdominal radiographs, ultrasound, or barium studies would be important diagnostic aids, but a workup for sepsis may still be indicated.

Furthermore, if the physical examination reveals bruises or purpura, further evaluation for child abuse, coagulopathy, and sepsis should be considered. In addition, long bone radiographs, coagulation profile (including platelet count), and Gram stain of the purpura may then be desirable. If vesicular lesions are seen on the skin, a Tzanck smear and culture for herpes should be obtained. If ambiguous genitalia are noted, blood should be drawn for 17-hydroxyprogesterone, renin, aldosterone, and cortisol to rule out CAH (see Chapter 86). Last, if wheezing is detected on chest examination, a nasopharyngeal swab should be sent for rapid slide detection of RSV or for culture of RSV.

TABLE 60.3. Approach to the Septic-Appearing Infant with Characteristic Physical Findings

Physical findings	Diagnoses to consider	Specific tests
Cardiovascular abnormalities	Congenital heart disease, supraventricular tachycardia, myocarditis, myocardial infarction, methemoglobinemia, Kawasaki disease	ECG Echocardiogram PaO_2, MetHgb level ECG, echo
Neurologic abnormalities	Meningitis, infant botulism, child abuse Shunt malfunction	LP, CAT scan, MRI, EMG
Skin abnormalities	Child abuse, coagulopathy herpes simplex	Gram stain lesion, coagulation profile, CAT scan, Long bone films, Tzanck smear, culture
Genitalia abnormalities	Congenital adrenal hyperplasia	Blood for 17-hydroxyprogesterone, renin, aldosterone, cortisol
Pulmonary abnormalities	Pertussis Pneumonia, bronchiolitis, metabolic acidosis	PCR, chest radiograph, RSV tests, ABG
Renal abnormalities (abdominal mass)	Posterior urethral valves	Abdominal, renal ultrasound, VCUG, BUN, creatinine

ECG, electrocardiogram; LP, lumbar puncture; CAT, computed axial tomography; MRI, magnetic resonance imaging; EMG, electromyogram; PCR, polymerase chain reaction; RSV, respiratory syncytial virus; ABG, arterial blood gas; VCUG, voiding cystourethrogram; BUN, blood urea nitrogen.

CHAPTER 61
Seizures

Vincent W. Chiang, M.D.

A *seizure* is defined as a transient, involuntary alteration of consciousness, behavior, motor activity, sensation, or autonomic function caused by an excessive rate and hypersynchrony of discharges from a group of cerebral neurons. A *convulsion* is a seizure with prominent alterations of motor activity. *Epilepsy*, or seizure disorder, is a condition of susceptibility to recurrent seizures. *Status epilepticus* is the condition of prolonged seizure activity (more than 20 to 30 minutes) or persistent, repetitive seizure activity without recovery of consciousness between episodes.

DIFFERENTIAL DIAGNOSIS

It is important to remember that a seizure does not constitute a diagnosis but is merely a symptom of an underlying pathologic process that requires a thorough investigation (Table 61.1). Although the diagnosis of a seizure is often made in the emergency department (ED) on the basis of the clinical history, other childhood paroxysmal events are often mistaken for seizure activity (Table 61.2). Each episode or "spell" should be evaluated by examining the preceding events, the episode itself, and the nature and duration of the postictal impairment. If any of these features seem atypical, an alternative diagnosis should be considered.

TABLE 61.1. Etiology of Seizures

Infectious	Metabolic
Brain abscess	Hepatic failure
Encephalitis	Hypercarbia
Febrile[a] (nonspecific)	Hyperosmolarity
Meningitis	Hypocalcemia
Parasites (central nervous system)	Hypoglycemia
	Hypomagnesemia
Syphilis	Hyponatremia
Idiopathic	Hypoxia
Withdrawals	Inborn errors of metabolism
Alcohol	Pyridoxine deficiency
Anticonvulsants	Uremia
Hypnotics	Vascular
Toxicologic	Cerebrovascular accident
Anticonvulsant	Hypertensive encephalopathy
Camphor	Oncologic
Carbon monoxide	Primary brain tumor
Cocaine	Metastatic disease
Heavy metals (lead)	Endocrine
Hypoglycemic agents	Addison disease
Isoniazid	Hyperthyroidism
Lithium	Hypothyroidism
Methylxanthines	Obstetric
Pesticides (organophosphates)	Eclampsia
Phencyclidine	Traumatic
Sympathomimetics	Cerebral contusion
Tricyclic antidepressants	Diffuse axonal injury
Topical anesthetics	Intracranial hemorrhage
Degenerative cerebral disease	Congenital anomalies
Hypoxic ischemic injury	

TABLE 61.2. Differential Diagnosis of Paroxysmal Events

Seizure disorders	Movement disorders
Pseudoseizures	Paroxysmal choreoathetosis
Head trauma	Tic disorders
Loss of consciousness	Shudder attacks
Posttraumatic seizures	Benign myoclonus
Syncope	Psychiatric disorders
Hypovolemia	Day dreaming
Hypoxia	Attention-deficit hyperactivity disorder
Reduced cardiac output	Panic attacks
Sleep disorders	Gastrointestinal disorder
Nightmares	Sandifer syndrome (GE reflux)
Night terrors	Abdominal migraines
Narcolepsy	Cyclic vomiting
Sleep-apnea hypersomnia	Breath-holding spells
Somnambulism	Pallid, cyanotic
Atypical migraines	

GE, gastroesophageal.

INITIAL STABILIZATION

The first priority in the seizing patient is to address the ABCs (airway, breathing, circulation) (see Chapter 1). An adequate airway is necessary to allow effective ventilation and oxygenation. The patient's circulatory status also must be closely monitored, as seizure may cause a massive sympathetic discharge that results in hypertension and tachycardia. Continuous cardiac monitoring and intravenous access should be obtained. Blood samples, including rapid blood glucose testing, should be acquired at this time in an attempt to establish a diagnosis.

Once the respiratory and circulatory functions have been assessed and maintained, efforts should be directed at making a diagnosis and stopping any ongoing seizure activity. As long as adequate ventilation and oxygenation are maintained, long-term sequelae are unlikely to result from a transient seizure. Consensus management suggests the initiation of anticonvulsant treatment for anyone who has been seizing for more than 10 minutes. This likely represents all patients who are brought to the ED actively seizing.

EVALUATION AND DECISION (FIG. 61.1)

Once it has been determined that a seizure may have taken place, the initial diagnostic evaluation starts with the history and physical. Laboratory, radiologic, and other neurodiagnostic testing (e.g., electroencephalogram, or EEG) are other tools that can be part of the seizure evaluation. Patients with obvious trauma who are seizing should be treated per Advanced Trauma Life Support (ATLS) guidelines (see Chapter 90), with close attention to possible intracranial injury (see Chapter 92).

Often, patients with a known seizure disorder will present to the ED seizing. Patients known or suspected to be taking anticonvulsants should have drug levels evaluated. A subtherapeutic anticonvulsant level is among the most common reasons for patients to present with seizures. Many different laboratory tests can reveal a cause for a seizure and as a result suggest a potential treatment. A rapid glucose reagent strip should be performed with the initial blood sample. Hypoglycemia is a common problem that can often precipitate seizure activity. If hypoglycemia is documented or a rapid assessment is not available, treatment with 0.25 to 1 g per kilogram of body weight of dextrose is indicated.

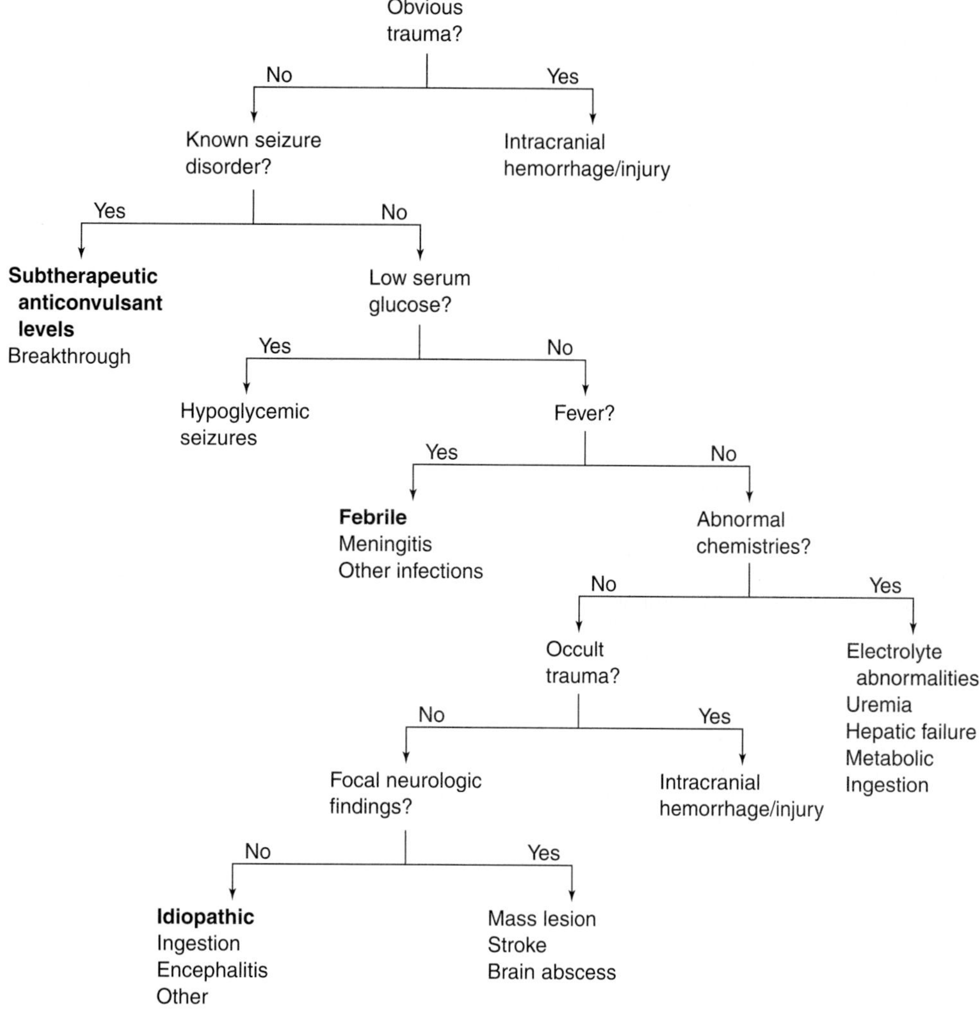

Figure 61.1. Diagnostic approach to seizures. The most common causes are in bold type.

A *febrile seizure* is defined as a seizure caused by a fever, but this is a diagnosis of exclusion. Other infectious etiologies that can be the direct cause of a seizure (e.g., meningitis) must first be ruled out (see Chapters 21 and 74). Furthermore, infections not involving the central nervous system (CNS) still may be the cause of the seizure through the elaboration of fever. The presence of fever or an elevated white blood cell (WBC) count should direct one to look for a potential infectious cause. Blood cultures should be drawn with the initial samples in patients at risk for bacteremia in an effort to identify a specific pathogen. Urinalysis and chest radiographs also can be used to confirm a source of infection.

A lumbar puncture (LP) with analysis of the cerebrospinal fluid (CSF) is the only way to make the diagnosis of meningitis and should be performed when meningitis is being considered. An elevated CSF protein and CSF WBC count and a low CSF glucose are all suggestive of CNS infection. CSF cultures, Gram stain, latex studies, and polymerase chain reaction (PCR) may identify a specific agent. Ideally, CSF cultures should be obtained before antibiotic therapy is initiated. However, in the critically ill or unstable patient, antibiotics should not be withheld until an LP is performed. Furthermore, in cases in which a potential metabolic disease is being considered, CSF lactate, pyruvate, or amino acid determinations can be used to diagnose a specific disorder. In these cases, it is often helpful to collect an extra tube of CSF to be frozen and used for later analysis. In any patient with suspected elevated intracranial pressure (ICP), an LP should not be performed until head imaging can be done.

Electrolyte abnormalities also may cause seizures, with hyponatremia, hypocalcemia, and hypomagnesemia the most common. In general, the routine screening for electrolyte abnormalities in a seizure patient is a low-yield procedure. Unfortunately, seizures caused by electrolyte derangements are often refractory to anticonvulsant therapy, and patients will continue to seize until the underlying abnormality is corrected. Serum electrolytes should be measured in all seizure patients with significant vomiting or diarrhea; with underlying renal, hepatic, neoplastic, or endocrinologic disease; who are taking medications that may lead to electrolyte disturbances; or who have seizures that are refractory to typical anticonvulsant management. One characteristic scenario involves hyponatremic seizures in infants, typically less than 6 months of age, after prolonged feedings of dilute formula ("infantile water intoxication"). Other patients may be evaluated on a case-by-case basis. Intravenous calcium, magnesium, and hypertonic (3%) sodium should be used to treat the appropriate abnormal condition. In the case of hyponatremia, once the seizure activity has been stopped, the rate of sodium correction must be titrated to avoid possible central pontine myelinolysis.

Other chemistries can be helpful in identifying specific organ dysfunction as a cause of the seizure activity or as an assessment of systemic injury. An elevated blood urea nitrogen or creatinine suggests uremia as a potential cause. Elevated liver function tests (transaminases or coagulation times) can be a reflection of hepatic failure. Metabolic acidosis or hyperammonemia can suggest an underlying metabolic disorder. In patients with prolonged seizures, an arterial or venous blood gas can help in assessing adequacy of ventilation, and a creatine kinase can identify possible rhabdomyolysis.

Toxicologic screening also can be helpful in the seizing patient because certain ingestions are managed with specific antidotes or treatments. Typically, the clinical scenario is the young child with a possible accidental ingestion or the adolescent after a suicide attempt. In general, the toxicologic screen should be directed at agents known to cause seizures (Table 61.1) or those suggested by a clinical toxidrome.

Radiologic imaging of the seizure patient generally consists of a computed tomographic (CT) scan in the acute-care setting. The following situations should be considered emergent: (1) a patient who has signs or symptoms of elevated ICP, (2) a patient who has a focal seizure or a persistent focal neurologic deficit, (3) a patient who has seizures in the setting of head trauma, (4) a patient who has persistent seizure activity, and (5) a patient who appears ill. Until cervical spine injury is ruled out, it is important to remember to maintain C-spine immobilization in patients for whom head trauma is a concern. Patients with transient generalized seizures in whom a cause of the seizure activity is identified probably do not require any further head imaging studies. Patients with transient generalized seizures in whom no cause is identified and who appear clinically well can have their head imaging performed on a nonemergent basis.

A magnetic resonance imaging (MRI) study has several advantages over a CT scan. MRI is better at identifying underlying white matter abnormalities, disorders of brain architecture, lesions in the neurocutaneous syndromes, lesions in the posterior fossa and the brainstem, and small lesions. In general, it is used in patients on a nonemergent basis.

Electroencephalography is an important diagnostic tool in the evaluation of seizure types, response to treatment, and prognosis, but it is rarely indicated in the acute-care setting.

Establish ABCs

Identify/correct electrolyte abnormalities
Head trauma/increased ICP management (see Chapter 92)
Identify toxin/provide specific treatment
Identify subtherapeutic anticonvulsant level
Identify/treat infectious cause
Antipyretics

Lorazepam 0.05—0.1 mg/kg

May repeat × 1—2

Consider diazepam PR 0.5 mg/kg of IV preparation (if no IV access)

Fosphenytoin 10—20 mg PE/kg

May give phenytoin 10—20 mg/kg IV at a rate of ≤1 mg/kg/min

Phenobarbital 10—20 mg/kg

Significant respiratory depression may result with benzodiazepine and barbiturate use; be prepared to secure the airway

Consider:
Pyridoxine
General anesthesia*
Barbiturate coma*

Consider pyridoxine in an infant (<1 yr) with refractory seizures or suspected isoniazid toxicity

*EEG monitoring and ICU setting required

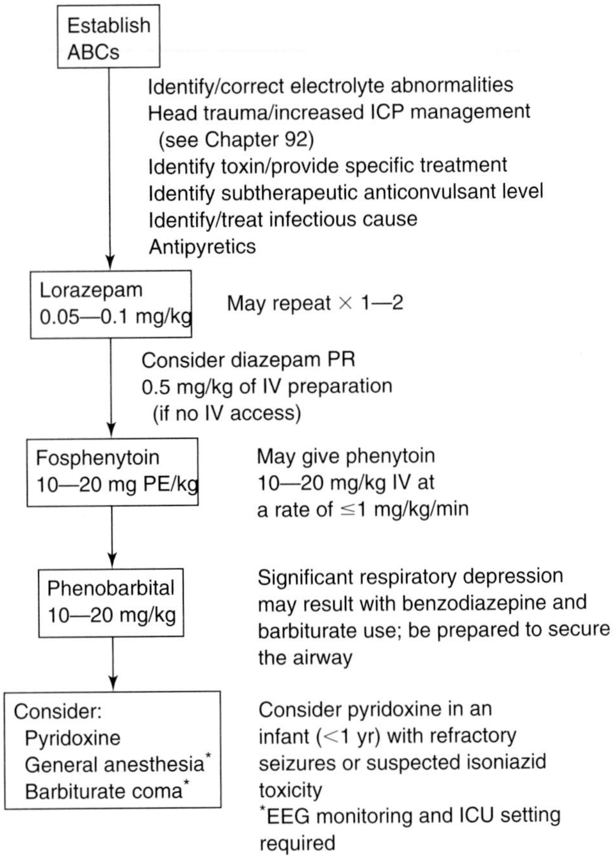

Figure 61.2. Management of status epilepticus. *ICP,* intracranial pressure; PR, per rectum; i.v., intravenous; *PE,* phenytoin equivalent; ICU, intensive care unit.

EMERGENCY TREATMENT

Prolonged seizure activity is a true medical emergency. Thus, following stabilization of the ABCs, further treatment is directed at stopping the seizure activity. Although certain causes of seizures may require a specific treatment, anticonvulsant therapy is initiated simultaneously during the evaluation of the seizing patient (Fig. 61.2). The approach to this subject is detailed in Chapter 73, but some emergency treatment guidelines are reviewed here.

The benzodiazepines are the initial drug of choice for the treatment of seizures. Lorazepam (Ativan) has a rapid onset of action (< 5 minutes) and can be given in the intravenous or intramuscular form. The dose is 0.05 to 0.1 mg per kilogram of body weight with a maximal dose of 4 mg and can be given over 1 to 2 minutes. Diazepam is similar to lorazepam, but it has an advantage in that it can be given rectally, which is useful when a patient does not have intravenous access at a dose of 0.5 mg per kilogram of body weight.

Phenytoin (Dilantin) is a second-line agent for the treatment of seizures. The dose is 10 to 20 mg per kilogram of body weight as an initial load. It must be administered slowly (no faster than 1 mg per kilogram of body weight per minute) because of concerns of cardiac conduction disturbances, which further lengthens its onset of action. It cannot be given in dextrose-containing solutions.

As a result of the limitations in administration of phenytoin, fosphenytoin (Cerebyx) was created. It is a prodrug whose active metabolite is phenytoin. The drug is dosed as phenytoin equivalents (PE) and the loading dose is 10 to 20 mg of PE per kilogram of body weight. The advantages are that it can be given much more rapidly (up to 150 mg of PE per minute) and that it may be given in either normal saline or a 5% dextrose-containing solution or intramuscularly.

Phenobarbital (Luminal) is another second-line agent in the treatment of seizures. The loading dose is 10 to 20 mg per kilogram of body weight. Its advantage over phenytoin is that it can be given much more rapidly (100 mg per minute). With the creation of fosphenytoin, phenobarbital should now be considered a third-line agent.

Pyridoxine deficiency is an uncommon cause of seizures in newborns. One should consider its use in patients less than 1 year of age whose seizure activity is refractory to the other therapies (100 mg). It is also used in the treatment of isoniazid overdose (usual initial dose 70 mg per kilogram of body weight).

If all the described therapies fail, patients may require general anesthesia to abort the seizures. A variety of agents can be used, such as inhalational anesthetics (e.g., halothane, isoflurane) or large doses of short-acting barbiturates (e.g., pentobarbital). The patient needs both to be intubated (if not already done) and to have continuous EEG monitoring in an intensive care unit. The level of anesthesia should be sufficient to maintain either a flat-line or burst-suppression pattern on the EEG. The anesthesia can be then withdrawn slowly to see if any electrical seizure activity persists.

The treatment of a patient who presents during a febrile seizure is identical to that for other seizure types. The primary goal is the establishment of a clear airway; secondary efforts are then directed at termination of the seizure. Because most febrile seizures are brief in duration, however, the typical patient who presents for evaluation of a febrile seizure is no longer seizing on arrival to the ED. In those instances, if the history is consistent with a simple febrile seizure, the patient has no stigmata of a CNS infection, and the patient's neurologic examination is completely "normal" (the patient may be postictal or slightly hyperreflexive), further evaluation for the cause of the seizure is unnecessary. The evaluation should focus on the possible cause of the fever. It is important to note that typical signs of meningitis may be absent in patients less than 12 to 18 months of age. Furthermore, seizure may be the first presentation of meningitis. Thus, one should strongly consider an LP in all patients less than 12 months who present with a simple febrile seizure, and one should maintain a low threshold to perform one in patients 12 to 18 months of age. LP is recommended in patients with complex febrile seizures or a concerning physical or neurologic evaluation.

CHAPTER 62
Sore Throat

Gary R. Fleisher, M.D.

Sore throat refers to any painful sensation localized to the pharynx or the surrounding areas. Because children, particularly those of preschool age, cannot define their symptoms as precisely as adults, the physician who evaluates a child with a sore throat must first define the exact nature of the complaint. Occasionally, young patients with dysphagia (see Chapter 45) that results from disease in the area of the esophagus or with difficulty swallowing because of a neuromuscular disorder will verbalize these feelings as a sore throat. Careful questioning usually suffices to distinguish between these complaints. Most children with sore throats have self-limiting or easily treated pharyngeal infections, but a few have serious disorders, such as retropharyngeal or lateral pharyngeal abscesses.

TABLE 62.1. Differential Diagnosis of Sore Throat in the Immunocompetent Host

Infectious pharyngitis	Other causes
Respiratory viruses	Herpetic stomatitis
Group A streptococci	Irritative pharyngitis
Epstein–Barr virus (infectious mononucleosis)	Foreign body
Human immunodeficiency virus	Peritonsillar abscess
Neisseria gonorrhoeae	Retropharyngeal and lateral pharyngeal abscesses
Anaerobic bacteria	Epiglottitis
Group C and G streptococci (?)	Kawasaki disease
Arcanobacterium haemolyticum (?)	Chemical exposure
Mycoplasma pneumoniae (?)	Psychogenic pain
Chlamydia pneumoniae (?)	Referred pain
Francisella tularensis	
Corynebacterium diphtheriae (diphtheria)	

TABLE 62.2. Common Causes of Sore Throat

Infectious pharyngitis
Respiratory viruses
Group A streptococci
Epstein-Barr virus
Irritative pharyngitis

DIFFERENTIAL DIAGNOSIS

Infectious Pharyngitis

Infection is the most common cause of sore throat and usually is caused by respiratory viruses, including adenoviruses, coxsackievirus A, or parainfluenza virus (Tables 62.1 through 62.3). Several of the respiratory viruses produce easily identifiable syndromes, including hand–foot–mouth disease (coxsackievirus) and pharyngoconjunctival fever (adenovirus). These viral infections are closely followed in frequency by bacterial infections caused by group A streptococcus (*Streptococcus pyogenes*). In the winter months, during streptococcal outbreaks, as many as 30% to 50% of episodes of pharyngitis may be caused by *S. pyogenes*. The only other common infectious agent in pharyngitis is the Epstein–Barr virus, which causes infectious mononucleosis. Although infectious mononucleosis is not often seen in children under 5 years of age, it cannot be considered rare even during these early years of life. More commonly, however, it affects the adolescent. An additional consideration in adolescents with an infectious mononucleosis–like syndrome is human immunodeficiency virus.

Other organisms produce pharyngitis only rarely; these include *Neisseria gonorrhoeae*, *Corynebacterium diphtheriae*, *Francisella tularensis*, and anaerobic bacteria. *N. gonorrhoeae* may cause inflammation and exudate but more often remains quiescent, being diagnosed only by culture. Diphtheria is a life-threatening but seldom encountered cause of infectious pharyngitis, characterized by a thick membrane and marked cervical adenopathy. Oropharyngeal tularemia is rare and should be entertained only in endemic areas among children who have an exudative pharyngitis that cannot be categorized by standard diagnostic testing or persists despite antibiotic therapy. Although unusual, mixed anaerobic infections should be considered in the ill-appearing adolescent with a severe pharyngitis because these organisms occasionally lead to sepsis (Lemierre disease). Other bacteria—group C and G streptococci, *Arcanobacterium hemolyticum*, *Mycoplasma pneumoniae*, and *Chlamydia pneumoniae*—have been implicated as agents of pharyngitis in adults, but in childhood, their roles remain unproved and their frequency is unknown.

Irritative Pharyngitis and Foreign Body

Drying of the pharynx may irritate the mucosa, leading to a complaint of sore throat. This condition occurs most commonly

TABLE 62.3. Life-Threatening Causes of Sore Throat

Retropharyngeal and lateral pharyngeal abscesses
Epiglottitis
Tonsillar hypertrophy (severe) with infectious mononucleosis
Diphtheria
Peritonsillar abscess

during the winter months, particularly after a night's sleep in a house with forced hot-air heating. Occasionally, a foreign object such as a fishbone may become embedded in the pharynx.

Herpetic Stomatitis

Stomatitis caused by herpes simplex usually is confined to the anterior buccal mucosa but may extend to the anterior tonsillar pillars. Particularly in these more extensive cases, the child may complain of a sore throat.

Peritonsillar Abscess

A peritonsillar abscess may complicate a previously diagnosed infectious pharyngitis or may be the initial source of a child's discomfort. This disease is most common in older children and adolescents. The diagnosis is evident from visual inspection, augmented occasionally by careful palpation. These abscesses produce a bulge in the posterior aspect of the soft palate, deviate the uvula to the contralateral side of the pharynx, and have a fluctuant quality on palpation.

Retropharyngeal and Lateral Pharyngeal Abscesses

Retropharyngeal abscess is an uncommon cause of sore throat, usually occurring in children less than 4 years of age. Although most children with this disorder appear toxic and have respiratory distress, a few complain of sore throat and dysphagia without other manifestations early in the course. A soft-tissue radiographic examination of the lateral neck demonstrates the lesion readily, whereas direct visualization often is impossible. If the diagnosis remains uncertain despite adequate radiographs, a computed tomography (CT) scan should be obtained. Lateral pharyngeal abscesses manifest in a fashion similar to retropharyngeal infections but occur less often. To confirm the diagnosis, a CT scan is appropriate.

Epiglottitis

The incidence of epiglottitis, a well-appreciated cause of life-threatening upper-airway infection, has declined significantly since the introduction of vaccination against *Haemophilus influenzae* type b. This disease manifests with a toxic appearance, high fever, stridor, and drooling. In every reported series of cases, sore throat appears on the list of symptoms. Although rarely this may be the primary complaint in a child, other more striking findings almost always predominate. Epiglottitis should be excluded easily as a diagnosis in the patient with a sore throat who is without stridor and appears relatively well.

Kawasaki Disease

Kawasaki disease is characterized by high fever along with at least four of the five following findings: (1) conjunctivitis, (2) mucositis, (3) peripheral erythema or edema, (4) truncal rash, and (5) cervical adenopathy. The mucositis most commonly involves the lips, but occasionally pharyngitis may be a prominent feature.

Miscellaneous

Certain ingestions, such as paraquat and various alkalis, may produce a chemical injury to the mucosa of the pharynx. Usually, these findings occur in the setting of a known ingestion and are accompanied by lesions of the oral mucosa. In addition, several systemic inflammatory conditions (Behçet syndrome and Stevens–Johnson syndrome) may involve the pharynx. Occasionally, pain from inflammation of extrapharyngeal structures is described as arising in the pharynx. Examples include dental abscesses, cervical adenitis, and occasionally otitis media. Some children who complain of a sore throat have no organic explanation for their complaint after a thorough history and physical examination and a throat culture. In these cases, the physician should consider the possibility of anxiety, at times associated with frequent or difficult (globus hystericus) swallowing.

Pharyngitis in the Immunosuppressed Host

Immunosuppressed hosts may develop pharyngitis from any of the previously discussed causes. In addition, these patients exhibit a particular susceptibility to infections with fungal organisms, such as *Candida albicans.*

EVALUATION AND DECISION

The tendency of most clinicians is to assume that one of the common organisms is the cause of pharyngitis in the child with a sore throat. Before settling on infectious pharyngitis, however, the emergency physician should first consider several more serious disorders (Fig. 62.1). Conditions that have immediate life-threatening potential include epiglottitis, retropharyngeal and lateral pharyngeal abscesses, peritonsillar abscess, severe tonsil-

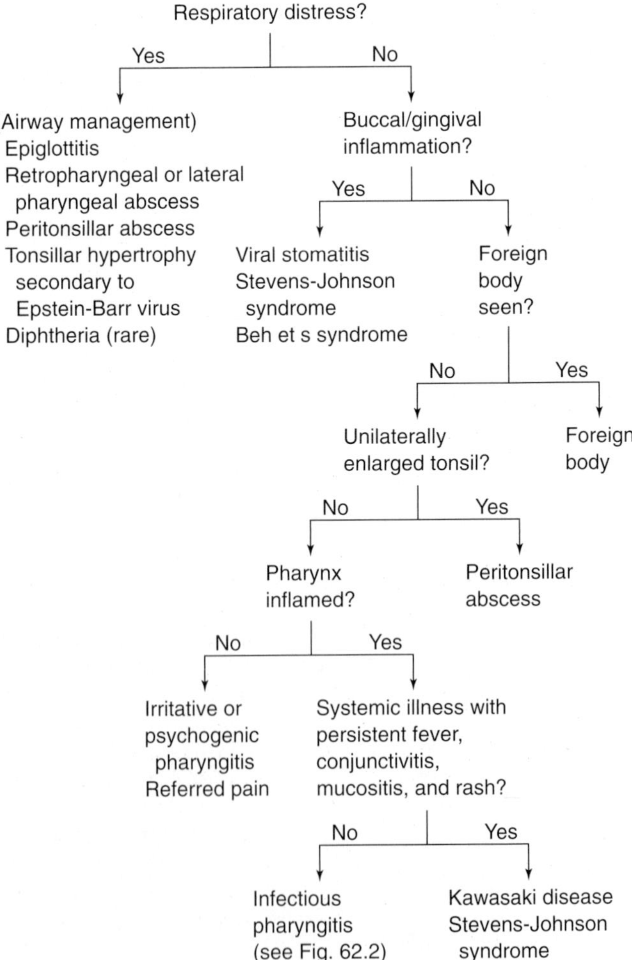

Figure 62.1. Diagnostic approach to the child with sore throat.

lar hypertrophy (usually as an exaggerated manifestation of infectious mononucleosis), and diphtheria. Generally, stridor and signs of respiratory distress accompany the complaint of sore throat in epiglottitis and retropharyngeal abscess. Drooling and voice changes are common in children with these two conditions, as well as in patients with peritonsillar abscess and severe infectious tonsillar hypertrophy. In cases of epiglottitis or retropharyngeal abscess that are not clinically obvious, a lateral neck radiograph, obtained under appropriate supervision, is confirmatory. Peritonsillar abscess and tonsillar hypertrophy can be diagnosed by visual examination of the pharynx. Diphtheria is rarely a consideration except in unimmunized children, particularly those from underdeveloped nations.

The next phase of the evaluation of the child with a complaint of sore throat hinges on a careful physical examination, particularly of the pharynx (Fig. 62.1). The appearance of vesicles on the buccal mucosa anterior to the tonsillar pillars points to a herpetic stomatitis or noninfectious syndromes, such as Behçet or Stevens–Johnson syndrome (erythema multiforme). Uncommonly, a small, pointed foreign body, most commonly a fishbone, becomes lodged in the mucosal folds of the tonsils or pharynx; usually, the history suggests the diagnosis, but an unanticipated sighting may occur in the younger child. Significant asymmetry of the tonsils indicates a peritonsillar cellulitis or, if extensive, an abscess. Clinically, the diagnosis of an abscess is reserved for the tonsil that protrudes beyond the midline, causing the uvula to deviate to the uninvolved side. Kawasaki disease produces a systemic syndrome with a prolonged fever and other characteristic findings that are usually more prominent than the pharyngeal involvement.

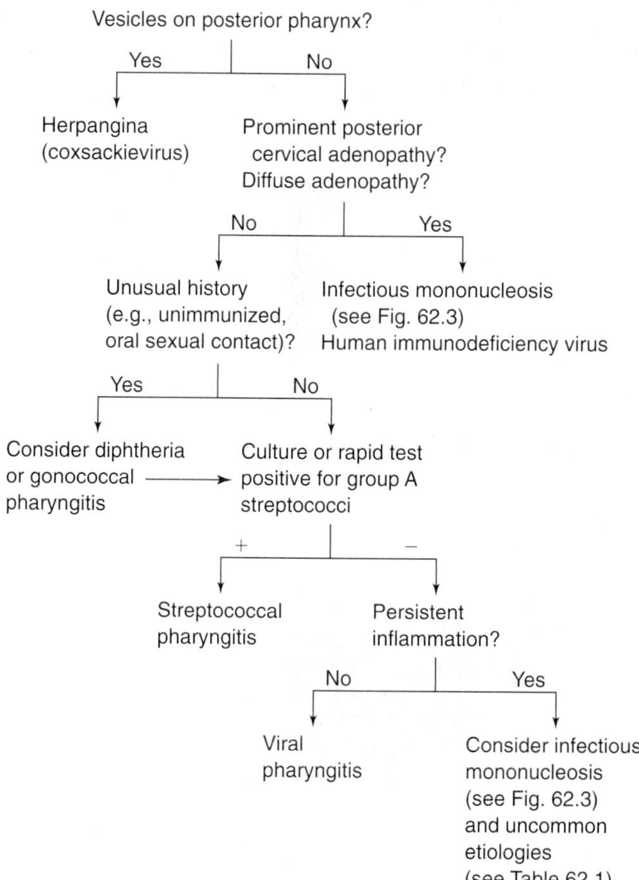

Figure 62.2. Diagnostic approach to infectious pharyngitis in the immunocompetent child.

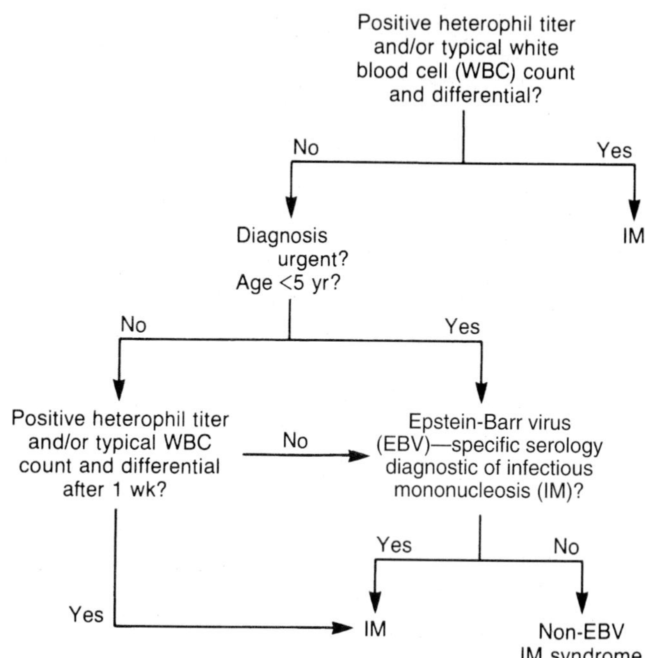

Figure 62.3. Diagnostic approach when findings are clinically suggestive for mononucleosis.

The remaining organic diagnoses, once those already discussed have been eliminated by history, physical examination, and occasionally, imaging, include referred pain, irritative pharyngitis, and infectious pharyngitis. Sources of referred pain (otitis media, dental abscess, and cervical adenitis) usually are identified during the examination. Irritative pharyngitis, seen most commonly during the winter among older children who live in homes with forced hot-air heating, produces minimal or no pharyngeal inflammation. It often is transient, appearing on arising and resolving by midday.

Infectious pharyngitis (Fig. 62.2) evokes a spectrum of inflammatory responses that range from minimal injection of the mucosa to beefy erythema with exudation and edema formation. The three relatively common causes are streptococci, respiratory viruses, and infectious mononucleosis (Fig. 62.2). In a few cases, a viral pharyngitis that results from coxsackievirus infection will be self-evident on the basis of vesicular formation in the posterior pharynx or involvement of the extremities (hand–foot–mouth syndrome). Such patients require only symptomatic therapy. A small number of additional patients will have signs of infectious mononucleosis: large, mildly tender posterior cervical lymph nodes; diffuse lymphadenopathy; or hepatosplenomegaly. In these children, the physician should obtain a white blood cell count with differential and a slide test for heterophil antibody (Fig. 62.3) in an effort to confirm the clinical diagnosis, thereby guiding therapy and discussion of prognosis. Some children, especially those less than 5 years of age, will not have the characteristic lymphocytosis or heterophil antibody response and will require repeated testing or specific serologic assays for antibodies to Epstein–Barr virus. In the rare child with an unusual history, the physician must pursue diagnoses such as gonococcal pharyngitis (sexual abuse, oral sex) or diphtheria (immigration from an underdeveloped nation, lack of immunization).

Ultimately, most children will have a mildly to moderately inflamed pharynx but no specific etiologic diagnosis based solely on the history and physical examination. Although certain symptoms and signs favor streptococcal infection, none is conclusive. Thus, obtaining a rapid test (latex agglutination or optical immunoassay) for group A streptococcus, followed by a culture, if negative, is prudent. Rapid tests are most helpful when positive because specificity of the tests is high; however, a negative test does not exclude streptococcal infection reliably, although some authorities would be satisfied with a negative optical immunoassay alone. With the recent reported rise in the incidence of rheumatic fever, the accurate diagnosis of streptococcal pharyngitis assumes increasing importance.

CHAPTER 63
Stridor

Holly Perry, M.D.

This chapter presents the causes of stridor and provides the emergency practitioner with guidelines for initial evaluation and management.

DIFFERENTIAL DIAGNOSIS

Stridor may occur in a wide variety of disease processes affecting the large airways from the nares to the bronchi, but most often it arises with disorders of the larynx and trachea (Table 63.1). For the purposes of differential diagnosis, it is helpful to categorize the common causes of stridor as acute or chronic in onset and to divide acute onset into febrile and afebrile causes (Table 63.2). In addition, life-threatening causes of stridor must be considered during the earliest phases of evaluation (Table 63.3).

Stridor with Acute Onset in the Febrile Child

Laryngotracheitis (croup) is by far the most common cause of stridor in the febrile child. It is important to consider other diagnoses, however, such as retropharyngeal abscess, epiglottitis, and tracheitis (see Chapter 74).

Laryngotracheitis affects children most often between 6 to 36 months of age but is seen throughout childhood. The illness begins with upper respiratory tract symptoms and fever, usually ranging from 38 to 39°C (100.4 to 102.2°F). Within 12 to 48 hours, a barking, "seal-like" cough and inspiratory stridor are noted. Supraclavicular and subcostal retractions may be present. Symptoms are aggravated by crying and ameliorated by cool mist or nebulized epinephrine. Most children appear only mildly or moderately ill.

Tracheitis closely resembles croup except that affected patients generally appear toxic, tend to be older (4–6 years of age), and do not respond as well to cool mist or nebulized epinephrine. Dysphagia is common, and drooling may be present. The verbal child may complain of anterior neck pain or a painful cough. Less severe cases can more closely resemble croup.

Epiglottitis may be divided into disease caused by *Haemophilus influenzae* or that caused by other pathogens. Patients with *H. influenzae* epiglottitis appear toxic and are febrile. Respiratory distress and a tripod stance are characteristic; drooling is usually present. Epiglottitis caused by pathogens other than *H. influenzae* differs in many important ways from disease caused by *H. influenzae*. It is much more common in adults, has a slower onset, and is more likely to be associated with difficulty swallowing or sore throat. Finally, the risk of airway compromise is also less than with epiglottitis caused by *H. influenzae*.

TABLE 63.1. Causes of Stridor by Anatomic Location

- Nose and pharynx
  - Congenital anomalies
    - Lingual thyroid
    - Choanal atresia
    - Craniofacial anomalies (Apert, Down syndrome; Pierre Robin sequence)
    - Cysts (dermoid, thyroglossal)
    - Macroglossia (Beckwith syndrome)
    - Encephalocele
  - Inflammatory
    - Abscess (parapharyngeal, retropharyngeal, peritonsillar)
    - Allergic polyps
    - Adenotonsillar enlargement (acute infection, infectious mononucleosis)
  - Neoplasm (benign, malignant)
    - Adenotonsillar hyperplasia
    - Foreign body
    - Neurologic syndromes with poor tongue/pharyngeal muscle tone
- Larynx
  - Congenital anomalies
    - Laryngomalacia
    - Web, cyst, laryngocele
    - Cartilage dystrophy
    - Subglottic stenosis
    - Cleft larynx
  - Inflammatory
    - Croup
    - Epiglottitis
    - Tracheitis
    - Angioneurotic edema
    - Miscellaneous: tuberculosis, fungal infection, diphtheria, sarcoidosis
    - Vocal cord paralysis (multiple causes)
  - Neoplasm
    - Subglottic hemangioma
    - Laryngeal papilloma
    - Cystic hygroma (neck)
    - Malignant (e.g., rhabdomyosarcoma)
  - Laryngospasm (hypocalcemic tetany)
- Trachea and bronchi
  - Congenital
    - Vascular anomalies
    - Webs, cysts
    - Tracheal stenosis
    - Tracheoesophageal fistula
  - Neoplasm
    - Tracheal
    - Compression by adjacent structure (thyroid, thymus, esophagus)
  - Foreign body (tracheal or esophageal)

TABLE 63.2. Common Causes of Stridor

Acute, febrile	Chronic
Croup	Laryngomalacia
Tracheitis	Vascular anomalies
Epiglottitis	Adenotonsillar hyperplasia
Retropharyngeal abscess	
Acute, afebrile	
Foreign body	
Caustic or thermal injury to airway	
Spasmodic croup	
Angioneurotic edema	

TABLE 63.3. Life-Threatening Causes of Stridor

Usually febrile	Usually afebrile
Epiglottitis	Foreign body
Retropharyngeal abscess	Angioneurotic edema
Tracheitis	Neck trauma
	Neoplasm (compressing trachea)
	Thermal or caustic injury

The clinical picture of a retropharyngeal abscess is similar to epiglottitis except symptoms appear more gradually. In addition to drooling and stridor, meningismus caused by muscular irritation by the abscess may be present. Physical examination may rarely reveal midline swelling of the pharynx.

Stridor with Acute Onset in the Afebrile Child

A foreign body in either the trachea or esophagus may produce stridor. There may be a history of choking on food or a small object. Physical examination varies, depending on location of the foreign body.

Ingestion of either caustic or hot substances may result in injury to the airway or hypopharynx. Symptoms of airway compromise may be delayed for as long as 6 hours. Drug abuse is yet another potential source of injury: Thermal epiglottitis has been reported after inhalation of crack smoke, a screen from a crack pipe, and a marijuana cigarette.

Other causes include spasmodic croup, angioneurotic edema, and trauma (see Chapter 98).

Chronic Stridor

The age at onset narrows the differential diagnosis. Stridor noted shortly after birth is most likely caused by a structural defect. This type of stridor tends to worsen slowly and is severe only when the infant is stressed, such as during crying. Laryngomalacia is the most common cause of congenital stridor. Stridor associated with laryngomalacia is positional and is ameliorated by placing the infant in the prone position. Other congenital causes of stridor include laryngeal webs, laryngeal diverticula, vocal cord paralysis, subglottic stenosis, tracheomalacia, and vascular anomalies such as a double aortic arch or a vascular sling. Stridor in infants also has been reported to be associated with gastroesophageal reflux.

Stridor in older children may be caused by papillomas or neoplastic processes. Patients with papillomas generally present between 2 to 4 years of age with complaints of hoarseness and stridor. Neoplastic processes causing tracheal compression also can lead to stridor in the older child.

Psychogenic, also called *functional*, stridor is an uncommon cause of stridor in the older child. Cases have been reported in adolescents, with the youngest age being 10 years old. Adolescent girls are diagnosed three times more often with this condition than are boys. More than 50% of patients meet diagnostic criteria for a psychiatric disorder. Characteristically, stridor improves when the patient is unaware that he or she is being observed, and it may clear with cough. The diagnosis can be confirmed only by direct laryngoscopy in the symptomatic patient when the vocal cords are noted to be adducted during inspiration.

EVALUATION AND DECISION

The first priority is to ensure that the airway is adequate by assessing the level of consciousness, color, perfusion, air entry, breath sounds, and work of breathing, including respiratory rate, nasal flaring, and retractions. The child then may be evaluated systematically. In the child with acute onset of stridor, history should focus on associated symptoms such as fever, duration of illness, drooling, rhinorrhea, and history of choking (Fig. 63.1). Immunization status should be verified, particularly *H. in-*

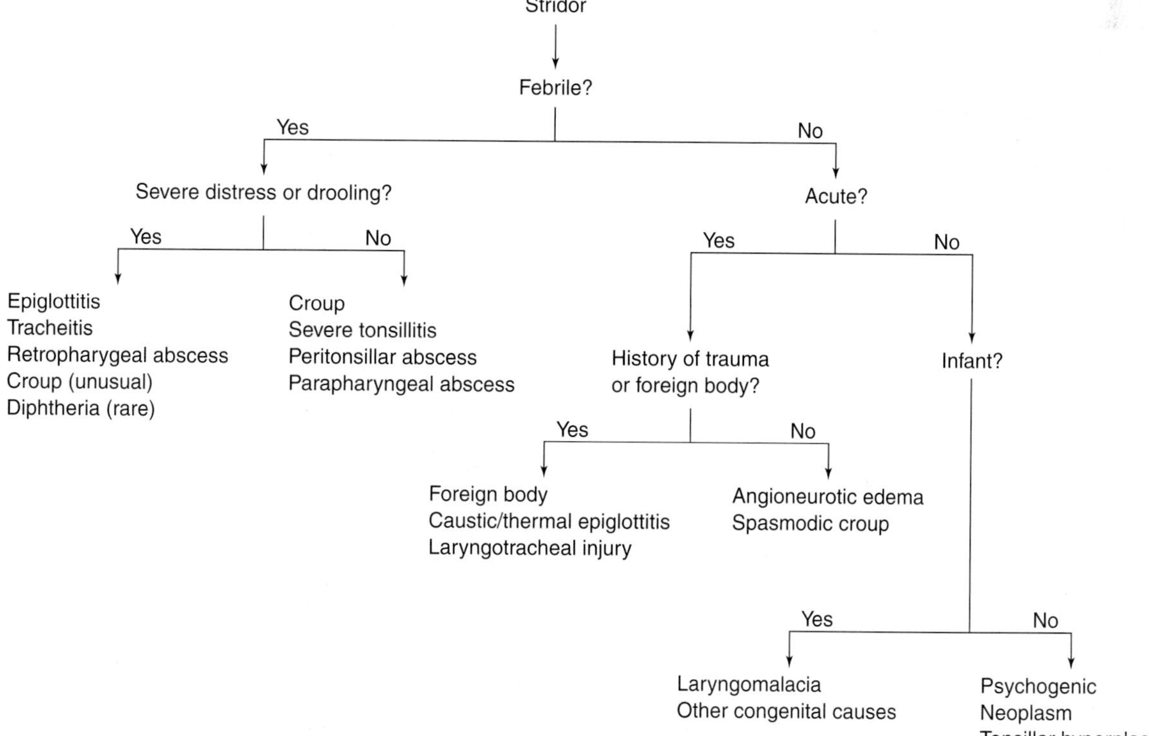

Figure 63.1. Diagnostic approach to stridor.

fluenzae vaccination. In the case of a child with chronic stridor, important historical points include onset and progression of stridor as well as ameliorating and aggravating factors.

Febrile Child

In the febrile child with stridor, the onset is generally acute and the most likely, as well as of the greatest concern, diagnostic possibilities are croup, epiglottitis, and bacterial tracheitis. Radiographs of the neck may be helpful in evaluation and should be considered if the practitioner suspects a diagnosis other than croup. If epiglottitis is strongly suspected, a lateral neck radiograph should be obtained in the emergency department, or the child should be taken to the operating room to have direct visualization of the epiglottis under controlled conditions. Abnormal findings on a lateral neck radiograph include increased prevertebral width (retropharyngeal abscess), swollen epiglottis or aryepiglottic folds (epiglottitis), and irregular tracheal borders or stranding across the trachea (tracheitis). Radiographic findings consistent with croup are a narrowed subglottic area on anteroposterior view (the "steeple sign") and ballooning of the hypopharynx, best appreciated on the lateral view. Airway films must be interpreted with care because they are subject to artifact.

Afebrile Child

In the afebrile child with acute onset of stridor, the duration of stridor, the likelihood of foreign-body aspiration, and the child's age are all key elements to consider. Emergent otolaryngologic or surgical consultation should be obtained in a child with evidence of airway obstruction if either aspirated foreign body or trauma are likely causes of stridor. Angioneurotic edema, an autosomal dominant trait, is characterized by rapid onset of swelling without discoloration, urticaria, or pain. Symptoms may occur in affected patients as young as 2 years of age but usually are not severe until adolescence; they may be precipitated by trauma, emotional stress, or menses. A C_1 esterase inhibitor level should be considered if angioneurotic edema is suspected.

A child with chronic stridor generally does not require an extensive evaluation in the emergency department unless significant respiratory distress is present. The infant with chronic stridor who is otherwise well should be referred back to the private pediatrician or to an otolaryngologist. Once a neoplastic cause is deemed unlikely, the older child with chronic stridor should be referred to otolaryngology for evaluation, including direct visualization of the vocal cords.

CHAPTER 64
Syncope

Carlos A. Delgado, M.D.

From the Greek *synkoptein*, meaning "to cut short," syncope is defined as the temporary loss of consciousness and postural tone, resulting from an abrupt, transient, and diffuse reversible disturbance of cerebral function. Often, the terms *fainting* or *blackout* spells are used. Pathophysiologically, syncope can be explained as a sudden reduction in delivery of substrates such as O_2 or glucose to the brain. Most transient altered consciousness events in children include seizures, syncopes, or hysteric episodes ("fits, faints, or fakes") and the approach to diagnosis of the former is to exclude the latter two.

DIFFERENTIAL DIAGNOSIS

Pathophysiologically, all causes of transient and abrupt onset of alterations of consciousness can be best categorized in three broad groups: (1) true syncope reflecting any mechanism that causes a transient decrease in substrate delivery to the brain (eg, O_2, glucose, blood); (2) all seizures; and (3) hysterical pseudo-loss of consciousness. Most children and adolescents who faint have orthostatic syncope, vasovagal episodes, or breath-holding spells (Table 64.1). The goal in evaluating syncopal episodes must be to accurately identify the common benign events from the occasional warning signs of serious pathology. The causes of true syncope may be classified into three etiologic categories: *autonomic* (vasovagal), *cardiovascular*, and *metabolic*. Table 64.2 lists the major causes of syncope and conditions that mimic it.

Vasovagal Syncope

Vasovagal syncope is also called neurocardiogenic syncope, vasodepressor syncope, or fainting spell. It accounts for more than 50% of cases of childhood syncope. Most episodes occur while the patient is standing or during a rapid change from a supine or sitting position to standing. Syncope represents a cascade of signs and symptoms that begin with a brief prodrome or presyncopal phase. This progresses to a brief and sudden stage of unconsciousness that typically lasts 1 to 2 minutes and ends with arousal to a previous level of consciousness within a short period.

A syncopal episode may be triggered by a wide array of emotional events such as pain, fear, and anxiety, which increase circulatory catecholamines in response to a real or perceived threat. The prodromal symptoms may include light-headedness, dizziness, nausea, shortness of breath, diaphoresis, pallor, and visual changes. Physical conditions such as anemia, dehydration, exertion, hunger, pregnancy, and/or concurrent illness can predispose to a syncopal event. Other factors include confinement to enclosed or poorly ventilated spaces and environmental heat. The patient may remain nauseated, pale, and diaphoretic for several hours after the syncopal episode.

Several other related forms of autonomic syncope are orthostatic hypotensive syncope and situational syncope related to micturition, defecation, cough, and swallow. Orthostatic hypotensive syncope is associated with an excessive and prolonged fall in blood pressure on assuming the erect posture from a recumbent position. An unusual and uncommon condition, micturition syncope, follows rapid bladder decompression, in which reduced cardiac return is associated with both postural effects and splanchnic vascular stasis. Underlying medical conditions such as anemia or pregnancy may exacerbate the tendency toward any of these vasovagal events.

Another common, usually benign, pediatric variant of vasovagal syncope is that of breath-holding spells, which occur in

TABLE 64.1. Common Causes of Syncope

Vasovagal	Hyperventilation
Orthostatic	Breath-holding

TABLE 64.2. Classification of Syncopal Episodes

Syncope
- Autonomic
  - Vasovagal syndrome
  - Excessive vagal tone—athletes
  - Volume depletion (orthostatic)—hemorrhage or anemia, dehydration, diuretic abuse
  - Reflex
    - Breath-holding spells
    - Situational—cough, micturition
  - Pregnancy
- Cardiovascular
  - Structural heart disease
    - Outflow obstruction
      - Hypertrophic cardiomyopathy
      - Valvular aortic stenosis
      - Primary pulmonary hypertension
      - Eisenmenger syndrome
      - Atrial myxoma
    - Dilated cardiomyopathy
    - Pericarditis with tamponade
  - Tachyarrhythmias
    - Long Q-T syndromes
      - Congenital
      - Acquired, including drug/toxin induced (antiarrhythmics, arsenic, tricyclic antidepressants, phenothiazines, antihistaminics, cisapride)
    - Supraventricular tachycardia alcohol, cocaine, and other sympathomimetics
    - Ventricular tachycardia
  - Bradyarrhythmias
    - Atrioventricular block
    - Sinus node disease
  - Vascular
    - Vertebrobasilar insufficiency
- Metabolic
  - Transient hypoglycemia, hypoxia, hyperammonemia, carbon monoxide poisoning

Conditions that mimic syncope
- Psychologic
  - Hysteric faints
  - Malingering
  - Hyperventilation
  - Panic disorder
  - Munchausen syndrome by proxy
- Neurologic
- Seizures
- Migraines

two forms. *Pallid* breath-holding spells result from vagally mediated cardiac inhibition. *Cyanotic* breath-holding spells involve interplay between hyperventilation, Valsalva maneuver, expiratory apnea, and intrinsic pulmonary mechanisms. In pallid breath-holding spells, an inconsequential injury induced by a sudden emotional stimulus such as pain, fright, or anger provokes one or two short cries, followed by pallor and sudden loss of consciousness. In cyanotic spells, the initial result is followed by vigorous crying and breath-holding in expiration, then loss of consciousness. These events typically occur in children between 6 and 18 months of age.

Cardiac Syncope

Syncope caused by significant cardiac or vascular pathology occurs far less often than autonomic syncope. It does not follow the stimuli typical of vasovagal syncope. Hypercyanotic spells, usually associated with tetralogy of Fallot, can occur with any heart defect associated with intracardiac right-to-left shunting. An increase in obstruction to pulmonary blood flow or a fall in systemic vascular resistance can precipitate such a spell. The most common arrhythmia causing syncope with an apparently normal heart structurally is supraventricular tachycardia (SVT), especially in the context of Wolff-Parkinson-White (WPW) syndrome. Arrhythmias occur more often in structurally abnormal hearts. Many drugs and toxins may induce arrhythmias (Table 64.3).

The diagnosis of prolonged Q-T syndrome is made by documenting the prolongation of the corrected Q-T (Q-Tc greater than 0.45 seconds) interval by Bazett's formula (see Chapter 77). Prolonged Q-T syndrome can be congenital or acquired. Syncope occurs because of paroxysmal episodes of rapid ventricular tachycardia (VT). Long Q-T syndromes often present as syncope on exercise or exertion and can also masquerade as a seizure. In acquired forms, the Q-Tc will be prolonged as a result of electrolyte abnormalities (hypokalemia, hypocalcemia), increased intracranial pressure (ICP), or medication use or overdose. A thorough history should include types of medications available at home, possible environmental exposures, and drug use such as psychotropic medications, including tricyclic antidepressants (TCAs) and phenothiazines. Nonsedating antihistamines such as terfenadine (Seldane) and astemizole (Hismanal) or the promotility agent cisapride may be used alone or in combination with other medications such as erythromycin and ketoconazole, which can inhibit the metabolism of these drugs and thus prolong the Q-T interval.

Episodic, complete heart block accompanied by syncope may occur in children and adolescents with baseline abnormalities of cardiac conduction. Children who have undergone surgical repair of ventricular defects, such as in tetralogy of Fallot, are also at risk.

Hypertrophic cardiomyopathy (IHSS), which is associated with recurrent syncope, is a disease that presents with a thickened left ventricular myocardium, resulting in subaortic stenosis that causes obstruction to ventricular outflow. Patients with severe aortic valvular stenosis present with the classic triad of syncopal episodes, anginal chest pain, and dyspnea on exertion.

Noncardiac Syncope and Disorders That Mimic Syncope

Metabolic causes of syncope include hypoglycemia, which often is associated with pallor, dizziness, and diaphoresis and is unrelated to position. Seizures may occur and unconsciousness may be prolonged and will often require the administration of glucose for recovery. Hypoglycemia may be a component of

TABLE 64.3. Differentiating Syncope from Other "Spells"

	Syncope, vasovagal	Metabolic (e.g., hypoxia, hypoglycemia)	Seizure	Breath-holding
Period of unconsciousness	Usually seconds	Variable	Minutes or longer	Seconds
Prodrome	Fright, pain, "feels faint"	Confusion, altered mental status, ↑HR, diaphoresis	Occasional aura	Pain, fright → vigorous cry → apnea → LOC
Incontinence	Absent	Absent	May be present	Absent
Confusion on awakening	Absent or mild	Mild	Marked	Absent
Tonic-clonic movements	Occasionally present, if LOC is prolonged	May occur	Commonly present	Rare, may see 1–2 beats
EEG	Normal	Normal	Often abnormal	Normal

HR, heart rate; LOC, loss of consciousness; EEG, electroencephalogram.

other childhood disorders that include diabetes mellitus, ketotic hypoglycemia, and hepatic enzyme deficiencies. Other metabolic causes of syncope include hypoxia by itself or in association with mild to moderate carbon monoxide poisoning, which is notorious for producing syncope. Recovery occurs when the child is removed from the offending environment. Hyperammonemia may rarely cause syncope by direct cytotoxic central nervous system effect.

Hyperventilation is associated with high anxiety and emotional events, during which the patient will complain of shortness of breath, tachypnea, chest pain, paresthesias, and lightheadedness. It is believed to result from cerebral vasoconstriction in response to self-induced hypocapnia.

Loss of consciousness often occurs with generalized seizures, which may be difficult to distinguish from vasovagal syncope if the event was not witnessed. Seizures are likely to be preceded by an aura and followed by a prolonged postictal state. Neonatal seizures and complex partial seizures may be subtle and particularly difficult to differentiate from syncope (Table 64.3) (see Chapter 61).

Syncopal migraine is rare. It is usually preceded by an aura and followed by severe occipital headache. Basilar artery migraine accounts for 24% of childhood migraines, most often in adolescent girls. It should be considered in patients with severe paroxysmal headaches.

Syncopelike events caused by hysteria are common in the adolescent patient. Characteristic features of the clinical event are helpful in differentiating hysteria from organic causes of true syncope. Hysterical "syncope" may be associated with hyperventilation, usually occurs in the presence of an audience, and lacks true loss of consciousness. No overt or objective prodromal symptoms such as hypotension or bradycardia are recognized. It may occur when the patient is in the supine position, which is virtually unreported with vasovagal syncope. There may be a peculiar fluttering of the eyes behind half-closed eyelids. The patient describes the event in a calm and indifferent manner and vividly recalls the event, suggesting a lack of complete loss of consciousness.

Drug or toxin exposure may be accidental or intentional and, in addition to precipitating arrhythmias as previously noted, may occasionally cause an acute, transient loss of consciousness or gradual altered mental status changes leading to syncope rather than the typical prolonged alterations in consciousness. Such an effect may be more characteristic of carbon monoxide poisoning or abused volatile inhalants (see Chapter 78). Antihypertensives, β-blockers, diuretics, antiarrhythmics, and drugs that decrease cardiac output such as barbiturates, TCAs, and phenothiazines may cause syncope. Substances of abuse such as alcohol, sedative-hypnotics, and opiates can cause alterations in consciousness that mimic syncope but are usually more prolonged.

EVALUATION AND DECISION

A thorough history and physical examination will often suggest the diagnosis. In most cases, an electrocardiogram (ECG) is useful to rule out symptomatic arrhythmias. This approach, emphasizing primarily clinical features of the syncopal episode, supplemented by ECG evaluation is outlined in Fig. 64.1.

The goal in evaluating a syncopal child or adolescent is to identify conditions that are associated with a risk of serious injury or are life threatening. Those potentially life-threatening conditions for which hospitalization is indicated are outlined in Table 64.4.

A thorough history is the most important part of the evaluation. Parents and relatives often contribute important information to the cause of the syncopal event. A typical vasovagal spell is preceded by a prodromal sign or symptom. Most occur while standing. Stressful situations, emotional upset, and mild physical trauma can trigger such an event.

Syncope occurring during intense physical activity may identify those patients with potentially fatal conditions. These patients' symptoms may also suggest vagal tone and/or volume depletion caused by dehydration and heat stress. A detailed evaluation should be considered for patients who have syncope during exercise or have a family history of sudden death, myocardial disease, or arrhythmias. A history of palpitations before syncope should alert the physician to the possibility of tachyarrhythmias. Palpitations are also reported in hyperventilation episodes. History is sought regarding medication use, recent food intake, and intercurrent illnesses to consider additional causes of nonvasovagal syncope. A medical history or family history of cardiac or neurodevelopmental disorders is important to elicit in regard to possible cardiac or neurologic causes of syncope. If there are no suggestive historical features of either vasovagal or the more worrisome causes of syncope, it might be prudent to cautiously consider some psychological assessment questions, particularly in well-appearing adolescents.

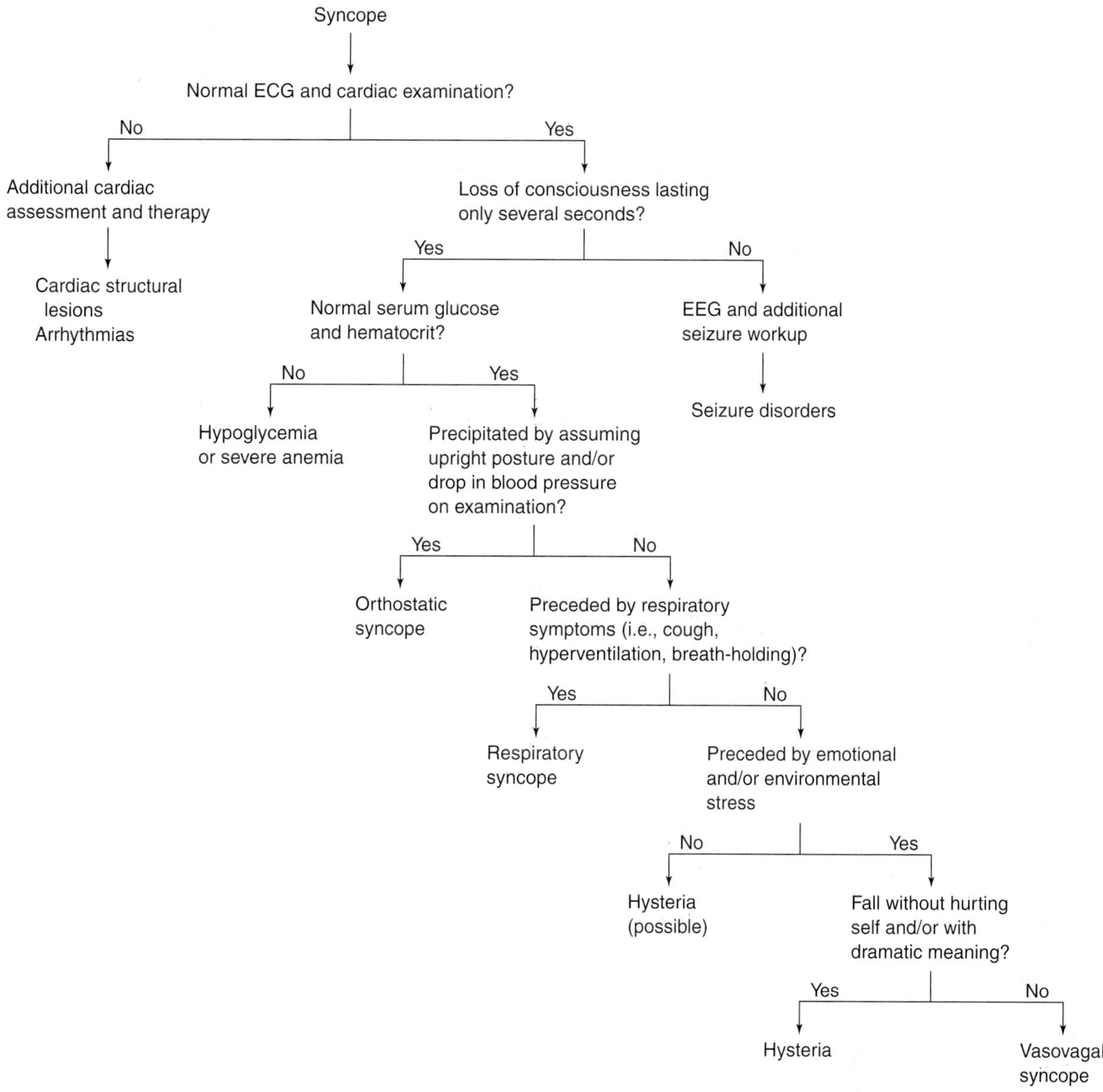

Figure 64.1. The diagnostic approach to syncope. *ECG*, electrocardiogram; *EEG*, electroencephalogram.

On physical examination the heart rate and blood pressure should be measured while the patient is supine and standing. In orthostatic hypotension caused by autonomic dysfunction, dehydration, or blood loss, the patient will have an abnormal decrease in systolic blood pressure (greater than 20 mm Hg) or an abnormal increase in heart rate. Palpation of an abnormal apical impulse or peripheral pulses may suggest a structural heart disease. On auscultation, a loud systolic ejection murmur in the midsternum and upper sternum is present in severe aortic stenosis or IHSS, or the diastolic murmur of a rare left atrial myxoma may be heard. A fourth heart sound may be present in hypertrophic cardiomyopathy. The general physical examination should include a careful neurologic examination, auscultation for cervical and carotid bruits, an assessment of hydration status, and consideration of the presence of any toxidromes.

TABLE 64.4. Life-Threatening Causes of Syncope Requiring Hospitalization

Presence of cardiovascular disease or abnormal cardiovascular examination—congestive heart failure, arrhythmias	Apnea or bradycardic spells requiring vigorous stimulation
Abnormal ECG—prolonged Q-T interval, tachyarrhythmias, atrioventricular or severe bundle branch blocks	Abnormal neurologic findings—focal signs, status epilepticus, signs of meningeal irritation
Chest pain with syncope	Acute toxic ingestions
Cyanotic spells	Orthostatic hypotension resistant to fluid therapy

ECG, electrocardiogram.

Routine Laboratory Testing

The emergency physician must assess the cardiac status of all children who present with a history of a syncopal episode. While in the emergency department, the patient should be placed on a continuous cardiac monitor for evaluation of heart rate, rhythm, and conduction intervals unless an obvious noncardiac cause is revealed by the clinical examination. An ECG should be strongly considered with all initial evaluations for syncope. Particular attention should be paid to the Q-T interval and T-wave morphology for evidence of long Q-T syndrome (see Chapter 72).

Serum laboratory tests, if indicated, may include a complete blood count, serum glucose, and carboxyhemoglobin determinations. Toxicology screens should be performed in patients suspected of ingestion or illicit drug use. In teenage girls, pregnancy should be ruled out.

Several nonemergent studies or devices may contribute to the diagnostic evaluation in selected patients. The use of the *head-upright tilt table* test in pediatric patients is controversial for the diagnosis of vasovagal syncope. It has emerged as a laboratory method for provoking episodes of neurally mediated (vasodepressor) syncope in susceptible individuals. An *echocardiogram* may be a helpful diagnostic test for recognition of hypertrophic cardiomyopathy or obstructive disease. *Holter monitoring* is expensive and rarely diagnostic in children and thus is often not included in an initial workup. *Event recorders,* however, are similar in size and appearance and have replaced Holter monitors in many medical centers for the evaluation of children with syncope. A digitally recorded rhythm strip can be transmitted via a telephone line to a receiving and recording device. Lastly, *electroencephalogram (EEG)* is indicated if a seizure disorder is suspected.

CHAPTER 65

Tachycardia/ Palpitations

James F. Wiley II, M.D.

Palpitations represent a disagreeable perception of the heart beat by the patient. Descriptions commonly given include "pounding," "fluttering," "jumping in the chest," or a sensation of the heart "stopping." A high degree of variation in the sensitivity of patients to changes in the heart rate (HR) or rhythm exists. Severe symptoms may be expressed by a patient who actually experiences trivial cardiac events. However, the absence of palpitations by history does not rule out the possibility of a life-threatening arrhythmia. The challenge to the emergency physician is to determine which complaint can be managed in the emergency department (ED) and which merits further consideration by a cardiologist.

DIFFERENTIAL DIAGNOSIS

Many conditions may produce palpitations (Table 65.1). Most patients with palpitations do not have significant cardiac pathology (Table 65.2), with the exception of patients with supraventricular tachycardia (SVT) and mitral valve prolapse. Many life-threatening conditions can come to medical attention because of abnormal cardiac sensation (Table 65.3). Wolff-Parkinson-White (WPW) syndrome and the prolonged Q-T syndrome are two potentially lethal diseases that may be diagnosed on a resting electrocardiogram (ECG). A patient with palpitations during exercise should also raise the concern of possible hypertrophic cardiomyopathy, SVT, ventricular tachycardia, or myocardial ischemia. Diagnosis of noncardiac causes of life-threatening palpitations, including hypoxemia, hypoglycemia, hyperkalemia, and hypocalcemia, can be made by characteristic ECG changes, serum electrolyte determinations, rapid bedside glucose, and oxygen saturation measurements.

TABLE 65.1. Differential Diagnosis of Palpitations

Hyperdynamic cardiac activity
- Exercise
- Anxiety/hyperventilation syndrome
- Emotional/sexual arousal
- Fever
- Anemia
- Drug-induced (see Table 65.4)
- Hypoglycemia
- Hyperthyroidism
- Pheochromocytoma

Sinus bradycardia
- Sleep
- Drug-induced (see Table 65.4)
- Hypothyroidism
- Advanced physical training (e.g., marathon runners)

True cardiac arrhythmias
- Tachyarrhythmias
  - Supraventricular tachycardia
  - Drug-induced (see Table 65.4)
  - Wolff-Parkinson-White syndrome
  - Congenital heart disease (Ebstein anomaly)
  - Postoperative cardiac repair (especially, Fontan, Mustard, and Senning procedures)
- Ventricular tachycardia
  - Drug-induced (see Table 65.4)
  - Prolonged Q-T syndrome
  - Myocarditis
  - Acute rheumatic fever
  - Mitral valve prolapse
  - Hypertrophic cardiomyopathy
  - Myocardial ischemia/hypoxemia
  - Hyperkalemia
  - Hypocalcemia
  - Postoperative cardiac repair (especially tetralogy of Fallot repair)
- Irregular rhythm or bradyarrhythmia
  - Sinus arrhythmia/respiratory variation
  - Premature atrial contractions
  - Premature ventricular contractions
  - Complete heart block
  - Sick sinus syndrome
  - Postoperative cardiac repair (especially, ventriculoseptal defect, atrioventricular canal repairs)

Hyperdynamic Cardiac Activity

Increased HR and contractility are physiologic responses to catecholamine release, like that which may occur with exercise, emotional arousal, hypoglycemia, and pheochromocytoma. Similarly, increased cardiac work accompanies conditions that increase the basal metabolic rate such as fever, anemia, and hyperthyroidism. Sympathomimetic and anticholinergic drugs are

TABLE 65.2. Common Causes of Palpitations

Exercise	Supraventricular tachycardia
Anxiety/hyperventilation syndrome	Mitral valve prolapse
Emotional arousal	Premature atrial or ventricular contractions
Drug-induced	

TABLE 65.3. Life-Threatening Causes of Palpitations

Cardiac	*Noncardiac*
Wolff-Parkinson-White syndrome	Hypoxemia
Prolonged Q-T syndrome	Hypoglycemia
Hypertrophic cardiomyopathy	Hyperkalemia
Congenital heart disease/ postoperative cardiac repair	Hypocalcemia
Myocarditis/acute rheumatic fever	Pheochromocytoma
Mitral valve prolapse	Drug-induced
Sick sinus syndrome	
Complete heart block	
Myocardial ischemia	

among a group of commonly available substances that directly modulate the autonomic nervous system, causing tachycardia, hyperdynamic cardiac activity, and palpitations (Table 65.4).

Sinus Bradycardia

Low basal metabolic rate associated with hypothyroidism may present with a slow HR and sinus rhythm. Similarly, in the absence of significant sympathetic nervous system input, the HR may slow. This state may be responsible for the sinus bradycardia associated with sleep or with ingestion of drugs such as clonidine, sedative-hypnotics, or narcotics. Advanced physical training results in a highly efficient heart with high ventricular ejection fraction and sinus bradycardia.

True Cardiac Arrhythmias

SVT represents the most common tachyarrhythmia of childhood (see Chapter 72). Possible underlying causes include drug exposure, congenital heart disease, and WPW syndrome. Sympathomimetics in cough and cold preparations are the most common drugs to incite SVT in children. Up to 75% of patients with WPW syndrome have a shortened P-R interval or delta wave on resting ECG (see Chapter 72). However, approximately 50% of children with SVT have no physical findings and no ECG abnormalities between episodes.

Infection, including viral myocarditis and less often acute rheumatic fever, constitutes one of the most common causes of ventricular tachycardia in children with normal cardiac anatomy. Similarly, ingestion of drugs with quinidinelike effects, such as tricyclic antidepressants, phenothiazines, and antiarrhythmic agents, is a preventable cause of torsades de pointes (polymorphic ventricular tachycardia) and unstable ventricular tachycardia in the otherwise normal child (Table 65.4). Syncope or palpitations associated with exercise may be caused by ventricular tachyarrhythmias that occur in conjunction with hypertrophic cardiomyopathy or myocardial ischemia (usually secondary to congenital anomalies of the coronary arteries). Patients with the prolonged Q-T syndrome have a genetically determined predisposition to fatal ventricular arrhythmias that can be detected by calculation of the corrected Q-T interval on a resting 12-lead ECG (see Chapter 72). Patients who have undergone ventriculotomy for tetralogy of Fallot comprise another group who are at high risk for ventricular arrhythmias as a result of the postoperative development of scarring in the right ventricular outflow tract. Finally, electrolyte disturbances, particularly hyperkalemia, hypocalcemia, and hypomagnesemia, may be causative in a child with palpitations and ventricular tachycardia (see Chapter 76).

Premature atrial contractions produce the most common arrhythmia of childhood, with 50% of normal children experiencing at least one premature atrial contraction per day. Premature ventricular contractions (PVCs) also account for many reports of irregular heartbeat. Although this arrhythmia can herald serious underlying pathology, patients with an unremarkable history, normal physical examination, and unifocal PVCs that disappear with exercise do not require further evaluation. Patients with significant sinus or atrioventricular (AV) node dysfunction as a cause of an irregular or slow heartbeat often have a history of syncope or seizure, slow HR (25 to 50 beats per minute) on examination, a pulmonic flow murmur, or signs of congestive heart failure (CHF). Patients who have undergone intraatrial repairs (d-transposition of the great arteries and atrial septal defect) are at highest risk for these potentially life-threatening arrhythmias.

TABLE 65.4. Drugs That Cause Palpitations/Arrhythmias

Sinus or supraventricular tachycardia	Nonsedating antihistamines (astemizole, terfenadine)
Ephedrine, pseudoephedrine	Organophosphate pesticides
Amphetamines	Chlorinated hydrocarbons
Cocaine	Digoxin
Albuterol, metaproterenol	Caffeine, theophylline
Antihistamines	Amphetamines
Phenothiazines	Cocaine
Antidepressants	Arsenic
Tobacco	*Bradycardia*
Caffeine, theophylline	β-Adrenergic blockers
Ventricular tachycardia or torsades de pointes	Calcium channel blockers
Tricyclic antidepressants	Digoxin
Phenothiazines	Clonidine
Antiarrhythmic agents (e.g., quinidine, procainamide, mexilitene, flecanide, encanide)	Sedative/hypnotic agents
Chloral hydrate	Narcotics
	Organophosphate pesticides

EVALUATION AND DECISION

The ill-appearing child with palpitations requires rapid assessment for the presence of hypoxemia, shock, hypoglycemia, or an existing life-threatening arrhythmia. Further evaluation should include measurement of hemoglobin, serum glucose (Dextrostick), serum electrolytes, calcium, and pulse oximetry or arterial blood gas. The presence of heart disease should be assessed by a 12-lead ECG and rhythm strip, followed by continuous monitoring, frequent vital signs, and chest radiographs (Fig. 65.1).

The asymptomatic child with palpitations by history also may have an intermittent or continuing arrhythmia. Continuous cardiac monitoring and a resting 12-lead ECG performed while the patient is in the ED increases the likelihood that this abnormality will be detected. Some patients in this category may benefit from Holter or event monitoring, particularly if there is a history of palpitations. Any patient with a history of syncope, congenital heart disease, or particularly, postoperative or exercise-induced palpitations is at greater risk for having a true cardiac arrhythmia as the cause of his or her symptoms. Similarly, the presence of a short P-R interval with the typical delta wave morphology of WPW syndrome or a prolonged corrected Q-T interval (see Chapter 72) indicates the need for further evaluation and consultation by a pediatric cardiologist.

The presence of fever or an upper respiratory infection should prompt the emergency physician to look for signs and

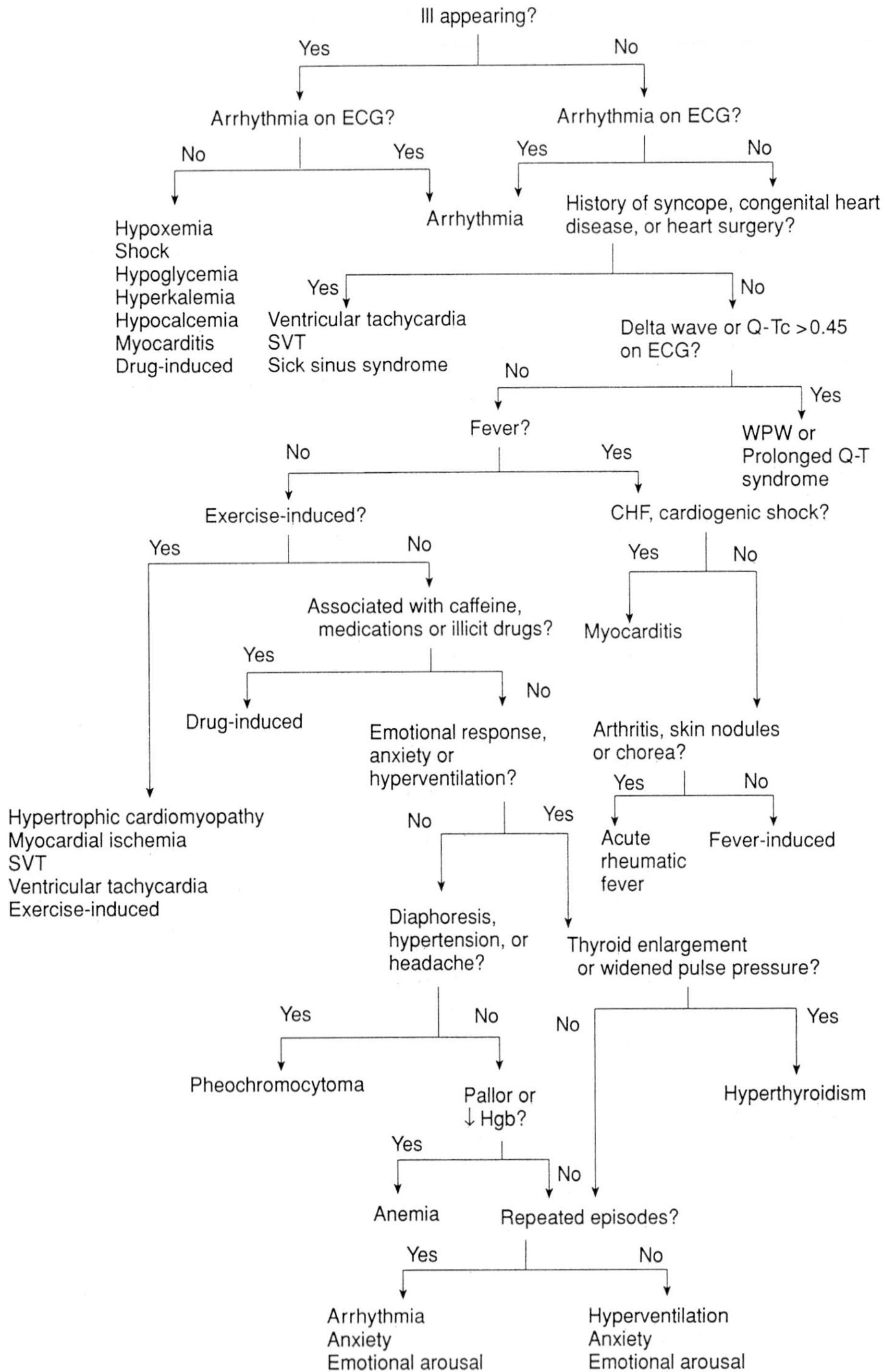

Figure 65.1. A diagnostic approach to palpitations. *ECG,* electrocardiogram; *SVT,* supraventricular tachycardia; *WPW,* Wolff-Parkinson-White syndrome; *CHF,* congestive heart failure; *Hgb,* hemoglobin.

symptoms of myocarditis or acute rheumatic fever. Clinical features of myocarditis are fever, tachycardia out of proportion to activity or degree of fever, pallor, cyanosis, respiratory distress secondary to pulmonary edema, muffled heart sounds with gallop, and hepatomegaly caused by passive congestion of the liver. The ECG findings are nonspecific and include low voltage QRS complexes (less than 5 mm total amplitude in limb leads), "pseudoinfarction" pattern with deep Q waves and poor R wave progression in the precordial leads, AV conduction disturbances that range from P-R prolongation to complete AV dissociation, and tachyarrhythmias such as ventricular tachycardia and SVT.

Acute rheumatic fever follows pharyngeal streptococcal infection and is an inflammatory disease that targets the heart, vessels, joints, skin, and central nervous system (CNS). Diagnosis and management of acute rheumatic fever are discussed in Chapter 72.

A detailed history of recent medications or precipitating events may reveal the cause of palpitations in some patients. Ingestion of caffeinated beverages (including soft drinks), cough and cold preparations, and illicit drugs, as well as a smoking history should be ascertained. The patient's emotional state before the onset of palpitations should be discussed to determine the likelihood of anxiety or emotional arousal as the cause of symptoms. The presence of diaphoresis, hypertension, and headache should encourage the consideration of pheochromocytoma, whereas widened pulse pressure and thyroid enlargement suggest hyperthyroidism (see Chapter 86). Anemia may be the cause of symptoms in a patient with pallor (see Chapter 51).

CHAPTER 66
Urinary Frequency in Childhood

Robert G. Bolte, M.D.

Urinary frequency (pollakiuria) is defined as an increase in the number of voids per day. It is a symptom distinct from polyuria (excretion of excessive amounts of urine). Although the two symptoms can be related, most children with frequency have a normal daily urine output, although the individual voids are frequent and small. Frequency also is distinct from enuresis, which is defined as inappropriate urination at an age when bladder control should be achieved. Urinary frequency is a symptom of several commonly encountered, clinical pediatric problems such as urinary tract infection (UTI), urethritis, vulvovaginitis, diabetes mellitus (DM), drug side effect (with caffeine, theophylline, and diuretics), or psychogenic stress. Moreover, urinary frequency may suggest underlying disease processes with life-threatening potential, such as diabetic ketoacidosis, diabetes insipidus, or congenital adrenal hyperplasia, that require emergent diagnosis and management.

DIFFERENTIAL DIAGNOSIS

A differential diagnosis of urinary frequency is outlined in Table 66.1. Frequency often is associated with UTIs, so this diagnosis always must receive significant consideration in the differential.

The term *urethral syndrome* refers to an entity that can be seen in adolescent girls, characterized by acute onset of frequency and dysuria with "insignificant" bacterial counts (less than 10^5 per mL). Pyuria is generally, but not absolutely, present. Vaginitis is a common cause of the urethral syndrome. *Chlamydia trachomatis* is also a relatively common etiology. The urethral syndrome also can be associated occasionally with *Neisseria gonorrhoeae.* Evidence supports the causal relationship of low-level bacteriuria and symptomatic disease. Therefore, in the context of the urethral syndrome, after all other causes have been excluded, "significant" bacteriuria may be considered as greater than or equal to 10^2 Enterobacteriaceae per mL.

Irritative vulvovaginitis (eg, secondary to poor hygiene or bubble baths) is a relatively common cause of frequency, usually associated with dysuria but not with pyuria. Frequency may be secondary to urethral trauma secondary to straddle injuries, catheterization, masturbation, or sexual abuse. Pinworms *(Enterobius vermicularis)* occasionally may cause frequency in young girls. Children with pinworm infestation may or may not present with perineal itching. Pyuria and dysuria usually are absent.

Frequency may be a presenting symptom of a pelvic appendicitis or appendiceal abscess. Potential for significant morbidity is obvious. Associated abdominal pain, by history and examination, should be present. Rectal examination may be abnormal (differential tenderness, mass). Pyuria, microscopic hematuria, and proteinuria (but generally not bacteriuria) may also be present.

Frequency may be secondary to a partial distal urethral obstruction. The urinary stream in the male infant or child with posterior urethral valves usually is nonforceful and nonsus-

TABLE 66.1. Differential Diagnosis of Urinary Frequency

Bladder/urethra	Intrinsic renal parenchymal disease[b]
Urinary tract infection (bacterial)[a]	Sickle cell anemia or trait[a]
Cystitis (viral)	Hypercalciuria[a]
Cystitis (chemical)	Urinary calculi
Methicillin	Congenital adrenal hyperplasia (salt-losing form)[b]
Cyclophosphamide (Cytoxan)	Hypercalcemia
Urethritis	Chronic hypokalemia
Vulvovaginitis/balanitis (infectious, irritative/abusive, or foreign body)[a]	Diabetes insipidus (nephrogenic)[b]
Meatal ulcerations/local trauma[a]	Diabetes insipidus (central)[b]
Urethral (frequency-dysuria) syndrome[a]	Head injury
Pinworms (*Enterobius vermicularis*)	Brain tumors (e.g., craniopharyngioma, optic nerve glioma)
Urethral foreign body	Septooptic dysplasia
Appendicitis (pelvic/abscess)[b]	Drugs[a]
Posterior urethral valves[b]	Caffeine (colas, coffee)
Neurogenic bladder (spinal cord lesion/injury)[b]	Theophylline
Constipation[a]	Ethanol
Pregnancy[a]	Lithium
Uninhibited (unstable) bladder[a]	Diuretics
Mental retardation/behavioral disorders	Vitamin D
Ectopic ureter	*Psychogenic/stress*
Renal	Extraordinary urinary frequency syndrome[a]
Osmotic diuresis	Water intoxication[b]
Diabetes mellitus[a,b]	Psychogenic water drinking
Excess solute intake (inappropriately concentrated formula)[b]	Munchausen syndrome by proxy
Intravenous contrast	

[a] Relatively common causes of frequency.
[b] Emergent/life-threatening causes of frequency.

tained. Straining to urinate also may be noted. A lower abdominal mass (enlarged bladder) may be palpable.

A neurogenic bladder associated with a spinal cord lesion (eg, tethered cord) may present with urinary frequency. There may be associated lumbosacral abnormalities (hairy patches, cutaneous dimples or tracts, lipoma, or bony irregularities). Decreased anal tone and lower extremity weakness or reflex abnormalities may be noted. An enlarged bladder may be palpable.

It is well recognized that children with urinary tract dysfunction often have associated constipation. Large fecal accumulations may restrict maximal bladder capacity or directly produce symptoms of frequency by stimulating uninhibited bladder contractions. Resolution of the fecal accumulation decreases frequency symptoms.

Pregnancy should always be considered as a cause of frequent urination in the adolescent girl. A lower abdominal mass may be palpable. Adolescent sexual histories are notoriously unreliable.

Uninhibited bladder contractions ("unstable bladder" syndrome) occur involuntarily in children who have failed to gain complete voluntary control over the voiding reflex. Girls may exhibit the so-called curtsey sign, so named because the child squats and attempts to prevent leakage by compressing the perineum with the heel of one foot. This maneuver will usually avoid major incontinence, but generally, small amounts of urine leakage occur. If performed, a screening ultrasound examination would reveal normal (minimal) residual urine volumes. With maturity, spontaneous resolution of uninhibited contractions occurs in most cases. In children with significant mental retardation or behavioral disorders, the infantile pattern of spontaneous bladder contraction may persist. Unstable bladder syndrome may also develop in otherwise normal children who have undergone normal toilet training.

Anatomic anomalies of the urogenital tract may result in chronic leakage of urine. Ectopic ureter is an example of such an anatomic defect.

Uncontrolled DM is a potentially life-threatening condition that can present with frequent urination. Polyuria results from a glucose-induced osmotic diuresis. At initial presentation, polydipsia, polyphagia, Kussmaul respirations, and weight loss also may be present.

In chronic renal failure and in certain diseases of the renal parenchyma (eg, renal tubular acidosis, Fanconi syndrome, and Bartter syndrome), the renal tubules lose their ability to concentrate urine. This leads to polyuria and frequency, with large volumes of relatively dilute urine. A concentration defect also may occur with sickle cell disease or trait and may be evident as early as 6 months of age.

Hypercalciuria has been reported as a significant noninfectious cause of the "frequency-dysuria syndrome" in the pediatric patient, although this association has recently been challenged. Onset of symptoms may present throughout the pediatric age range, generally 2 to 14 years of age. Occasionally, hypercalciuria can present in early infancy, in which irritability is a hallmark symptom. Symptoms often spontaneously resolve within 2 months. There may be a positive family history of calcium urolithiasis. When symptomatic, frequency is almost always associated with dysuria. Hematuria (generally microscopic) and crystalluria are often seen. However, the urinalysis may be normal. If the diagnosis is suspected and symptoms persist, studies of urinary calcium excretion and urologic consultation should be considered.

The salt-losing form of congenital adrenal hyperplasia is a life-threatening, although relatively rare, cause of frequency. Excessive urinary excretion of sodium leads to severe water loss and marked dehydration with associated hyperkalemia and hyponatremia. At the initial presentation in early infancy, however, urinary frequency as a symptom generally is not appreciated. Infant girls may exhibit virilization of the external genitalia. Infant boys may demonstrate increased pigmentation of the external genitalia and/or a relatively enlarged phallus.

Diabetes insipidus (DI) is an uncommon, although life-threatening, cause of frequency. It is clinically characterized by polyuria (with resultant frequency) and polydipsia. Some causes of central DI (eg, septooptic dysplasia) present in the neonatal period. However, most causes of central DI are acquired (eg, head injury, brain tumors) and, therefore, can present at any age. The most common type of nephrogenic DI in childhood is the X-linked recessive type, which presents in boys during early infancy. If fluids are not accessible or if the thirst sensation is impaired, hypernatremic dehydration develops.

Drugs are a relatively common cause of frequency in childhood. Methylxanthines (theophylline, caffeine) and ethanol inhibit production of antidiuretic hormone. Lithium, chronic hypokalemia, hypercalcemia, and Vitamin D are also associated with urinary frequency, interfering with renal responsiveness to antidiuretic hormone. Diuretic agents may cause urinary frequency. These agents represent only a few of the many drugs that can cause urinary frequency as a side effect. Therefore, a detailed pharmacology history should be obtained in the child with urinary frequency.

Frequency may occur secondary to the polyuria of water intoxication. Absence of nocturia and enuresis in the presence of polyuria suggests an excessive fluid intake. The serum sodium and osmolality generally are decreased. Psychogenic water drinking is an extremely unusual diagnosis in young children but may present in adolescents. Water intoxication secondary to Munchausen syndrome by proxy would be an unusual presentation of child abuse.

The "extraordinary urinary frequency syndrome" is a relatively recently described entity but probably represents a common cause of urinary frequency in pediatric primary care settings. Average age of onset is about 6 years (with a range of about 2 to 11 years). Daytime frequency occurs as often as every 5 minutes. Dysuria is not present. Nocturia is present in about half the cases but usually occurs only about 1 to 2 times per night. Polydipsia and polyuria are absent. The physical examination is normal. The urinalysis and other laboratory studies also are normal. If the diagnosis of "extraordinary urinary frequency syndrome" is likely, reassurance and follow-up are indicated. Initial radiologic evaluation and pharmacologic therapy are generally unnecessary. Left untreated, frequent voiding resolves spontaneously, usually in about 2 months. The cause is unclear but often has a psychogenic component, with an apparent "trigger" (eg, school problems, parental death, sibling illness) identifiable in about 40% of cases.

As an isolated symptom, frequency would be an atypical presentation of pediatric sexual abuse. However, urinary frequency may be seen in association with pertinent history or physical findings (eg, vulvovaginal venereal infection or genital trauma), which would be suggestive of sexual abuse.

EVALUATION AND DECISION

The primary role of the emergency physician in evaluating the child with urinary frequency is to exclude significant underlying pathology that may result in morbidity and to identify treatable conditions. The initial history should focus on symptoms related to infection of the urinary tract. Are associated symptoms of dysuria, fever, or flank pain also present? Is there a history of prior UTIs? Questions specifically related to DM also should be included (polyuria, polydipsia, polyphagia, weight loss, family history). The presence or absence of nocturia and enuresis are also important historical points. The urine volume per voiding should be determined (large versus small). Generally, the presence of polyuria (copious volumes of dilute urine) is obvious from the history. The onset and duration of the symptoms and the quality of the urinary stream should be documented.

In addition, other historical features may be pertinent. For example, are there symptoms to suggest central DI (polydipsia, nocturia, intracranial pathology)? Is there a history of poor growth, suggesting renal disease? Is there a family history of sickle cell disease or trait? Is the child taking any medications or drugs (including caffeinated beverages) associated with frequency? Is there a history of chronic constipation, vulvovaginal infection/trauma, or pruritus ani? Are there symptoms of abdominal pain, suggesting the possibility of acute appendicitis or appendiceal abscess? In the young boy, what is the quality of the urinary stream? In an adolescent girl, when was her last menstrual period? Is there a family history of urolithiasis or renal disease?

A complete physical examination should be performed, including an accurate blood pressure measurement. The abdomen should be palpated carefully for the presence of abdominal masses and/or tenderness. Percussion of the flanks should be performed. The lumbosacral area should be examined closely for anomalies (hairy patches, dimples, tracts). Special attention should be focused on the function of sacral nerves II–IV (anal wink and sphincter tone). Unless the diagnosis is readily apparent, a rectal examination should be performed noting tone, tenderness, masses, and the quality and quantity of stool in the rectal vault. The external genitalia should always be thoroughly examined, meticulously searching for signs of infection, trauma, or anatomic abnormalities. Signs of virilization (in the girl) or hyperpigmentation (in the boy) should be evaluated. A thorough neurologic examination with careful attention to the retinal fundi and visual fields is warranted.

The laboratory evaluation is fairly straightforward. A urinalysis (including specific gravity) and urine culture should be performed in all cases. Caution should be exercised in interpreting pyuria and/or bacteriuria from "bag" or "midstream" urine specimens in the infant or toddler. A confirmatory catheterized specimen should be considered in these cases. Glycosuria obviously suggests the diagnosis of DM.

If the diagnosis is not apparent at this point, serum chemistries (including electrolytes, glucose, blood urea nitrogen, creatinine, and calcium) should be obtained. A sickle cell preparation also should be considered in the African-American child, and a pregnancy test should be done in the adolescent girl. This workup generally is sufficient for those children who do not have both daytime and nighttime symptoms, or anatomic and/or neurologic abnormalities.

In the child with progressive or worrisome symptoms or signs (eg, nocturia, persistent dysuria, poor urinary stream, straining to urinate, growth failure, hypertension, fixed low urinary specific gravity, anatomic or neurologic abnormalities), urologic and/or nephrologic consultation is recommended. Additional studies may include a screening ultrasonogram of the urinary tract and abdomen, a voiding cystourethrogram, urinary calcium studies, and possible urodynamic investigation. If the presence of polyuria is in doubt, a 24-hour urine collection may be necessary to establish the diagnosis.

A simplified schematic approach to the evaluation of the child with urinary frequency is outlined in Fig. 66.1.

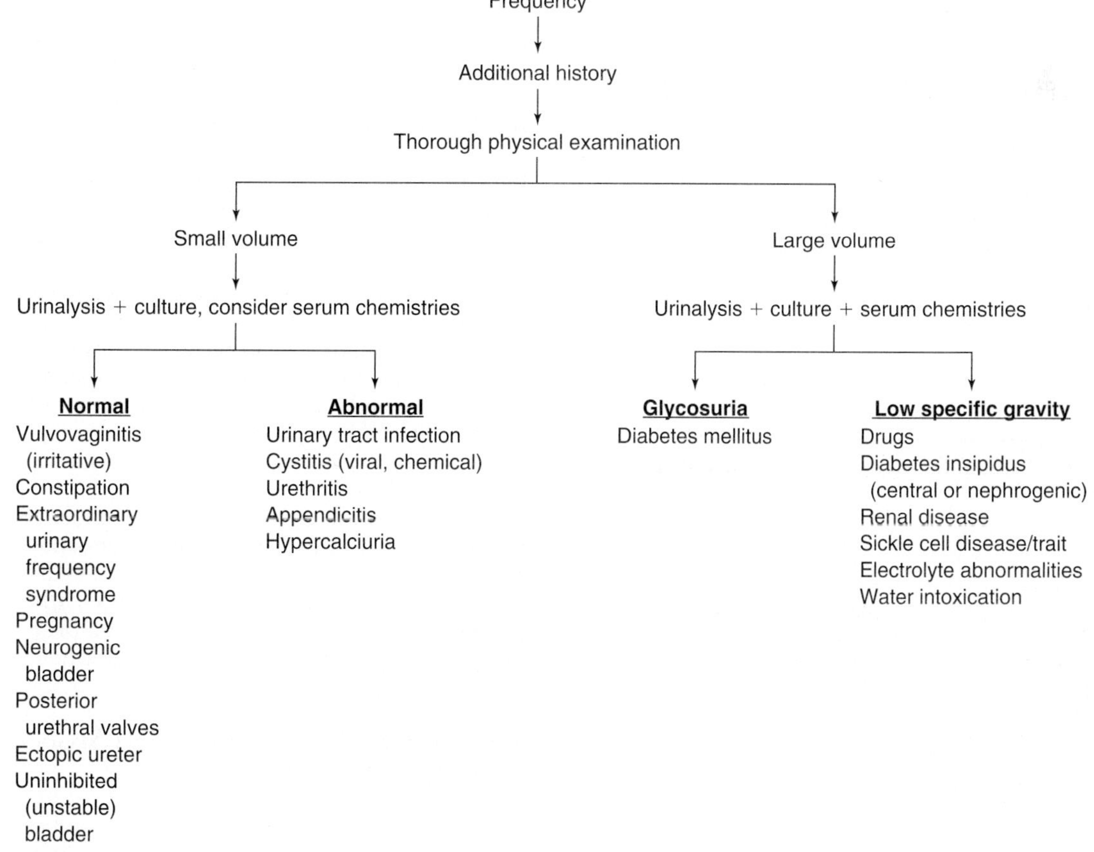

Figure 66.1. Evaluation of urinary frequency.

CHAPTER 67
Vaginal Bleeding

Jan E. Paradise, M.D.

Vaginal bleeding can be either a normal event or a sign of disease and, when pathologic, can indicate variously a local genital tract disorder, endocrinologic or hematologic disease, or a complication of pregnancy. During childhood, vaginal bleeding is abnormal after the first week or so of life and before menarche. After menarche, abnormal vaginal bleeding must be differentiated from menstruation, and in turn, menstrual bleeding must be categorized as either normal or excessive.

Menstrual patterns during the first 2 years after menarche vary widely, but it is possible to set outside limits. Ninety-five percent of young adolescents' menstrual periods are between 2 and 8 days in length. A duration of 10 days or more is abnormal. An occasional interval of less than 21 days from the first day of one menstrual period to the first day of the next is normal for teenagers, but several short cycles in a row are abnormal. Whether the quantity of a patient's menstrual bleeding is normal can be difficult to determine historically. However, it is uncommon for adolescents to soak more than 6 to 8 perineal pads or tampons a day. Normal menstrual bleeding *never* produces an acute fall in hemoglobin or hematocrit.

Because the relative prevalence of disorders that produce vaginal bleeding correlates more strongly with patients' hormonal status than with their chronologic age, the diagnostic approach outlined in this chapter is presented in two sections divided according to patients' menarchal status (Table 67.1).

VAGINAL BLEEDING DURING CHILDHOOD

Evaluation and Decision

During the patient's general physical examination, the emergency physician should be particularly alert for signs of hormonal stimulation—breast development, pubic hair growth, a dull pink vaginal mucosa, or physiologic leukorrhea. For the initial examination of the genitalia, an infant or child should be placed in a frog-leg position either on the parent's lap or on the examining table; a vaginal speculum should not be used. If the vulva is normal, the child should next be placed in the knee–chest position for examination of her vagina.

TABLE 67.1. Differential Diagnosis of Vaginal Bleeding

At any time	After menarche
Trauma	Hormonal contraception
Tumor	Endometritis
Before normal menarche	Dysfunctional uterine bleeding
Hormonal	Bleeding diathesis
Neonatal bleeding	Ectopic pregnancy
Exogenous estrogen	Spontaneous abortion
Precocious puberty	Placenta previa
Nonhormonal	Abruptio placentae
Urethral prolapse	
Genital warts	
Lichen sclerosus	
Infectious vaginitis	
Foreign body	

VULVAR BLEEDING

The vulva consists of several structures: the labia majora, the labia minora, the clitoris, and the vaginal introitus. A premenarchal girl with the complaint of vaginal bleeding whose vulva looks abnormal may have a vaginal disorder, a vulvar disorder, or both (Fig. 67.1A).

Trauma to the vulva often produces lacerations or ecchymoses or both. Any vulvar injury should alert the emergency physician to the possibility of concurrent, potentially serious vaginal or rectal injuries. Vulvar lacerations do not usually bleed excessively, but hematomas can extend widely through the tissue planes, forming large, painful masses that occasionally produce enough pressure to cause necrosis of the overlying vulvar skin. Because even minor periurethral injuries can produce urethral spasm that leads to acute urinary retention, the injured child's ability to void should be checked routinely. The possibility of sexual assault must be considered in the management of every child with a genital injury.

Urethral prolapse (see Chapter 83) is probably the most common cause of apparent vaginal bleeding during childhood. Some patients with urethral prolapse complain of dysuria or urinary frequency, but most have bleeding as their only symptom. A prolapse is diagnosed by its characteristic doughnut shape. The ring of protruding urethral mucosa above the introitus is swollen and dark red with a central dimple that indicates the meatus. When the child is supine, the prolapse is often large enough to cover the vaginal introitus and appears to protrude from the vagina. Bleeding comes from the ischemic mucosa. If the diagnosis is in doubt, one may safely catheterize the bladder through the prolapse to obtain urine.

Genital warts, like a urethral prolapse, can be recognized by inspection and can produce bleeding when they are located on the mucosal surface of the introitus or just inside the hymenal ring. Because the presence of such warts in a child indicates that sexual contact may have occurred, cases should be reported to the state child protective services agency (see Chapter 111).

Vulvar inflammation can be seen in some patients with vaginal bleeding resulting from bacterial or fungal vulvovaginitis. Infections caused by *Shigella* species, group A hemolytic streptococci, *Neisseria gonorrhoeae*, and *Candida albicans* produce vaginal bleeding or bloody discharge in varying proportions of cases. A few children with rectal *Enterobius vermicularis* (pinworm) infestations scratch so vigorously that they excoriate the perineal area and cause bleeding. Pinworm ova can often be discovered by low-power microscopic examination of perianal material that is collected with clear cellophane tape and then attached to a glass slide.

Although bleeding per se is not common, ecchymoses and telangiectasias are frequent clinical manifestations of lichen sclerosus, an uncommon, chronic, idiopathic skin disorder that most often affects the vulva. In this condition, white, flat-topped papules gradually coalesce to form atrophic plaques that involve the vulvar and perianal skin in a symmetric hourglass pattern.

VAGINAL BLEEDING WITHOUT SIGNS OF HORMONAL STIMULATION

Trauma, infection, and foreign bodies are the most common causes of vaginal bleeding during childhood (Fig. 67.1B).

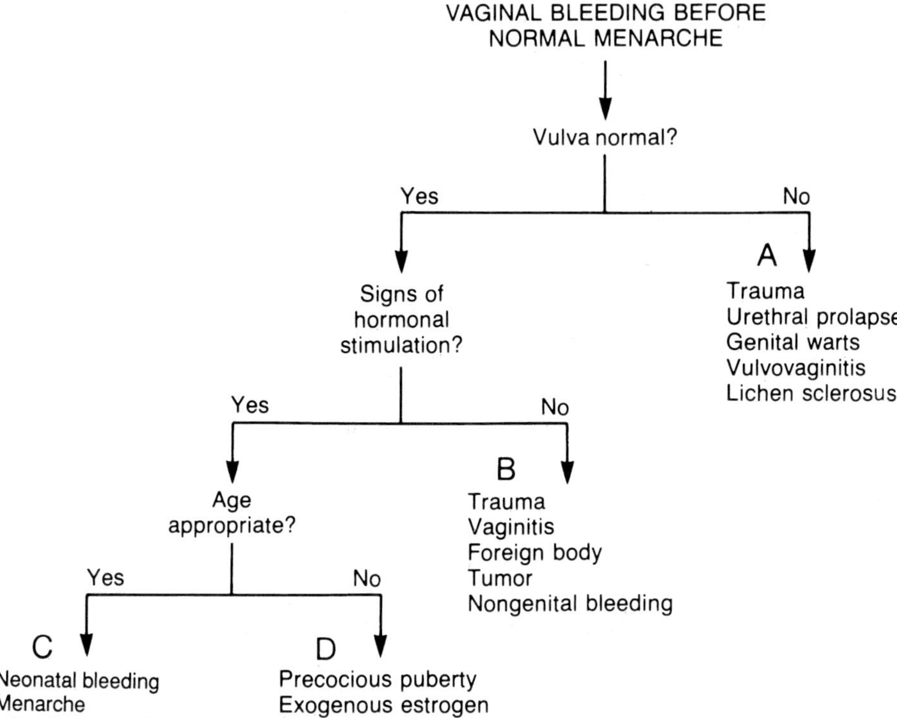

Figure 67.1. Diagnostic approach to vaginal bleeding before normal menarche.

Vaginal bleeding after trauma indicates a potential emergency. A penetrating narrow object can damage the rectum, bladder, or abdominal viscera without producing much external evidence of injury. Because vaginal lacerations do not always produce a great deal of bleeding or pain, the emergency physician cannot rely on the severity of the patient's symptoms to indicate the extent of the injury. When a child sustains a genital injury, the physician must consider the possibility that it was inflicted during a sexual assault.

If the clinician knows or suspects that trauma has occurred, the girl's abdomen should be evaluated carefully. Lower quadrant tenderness may provide a clue to intraabdominal injury. The vulva is inspected for bruises, and a rectal examination is performed to identify any lacerations. A general principle of management is that patients with penetrating genital injuries, even apparently minor ones, should undergo careful vaginal examination.

About half of all patients with *Shigella* vaginitis have bleeding that may be more noticeable than the associated discharge. Most patients do not have concurrent diarrhea. Vaginal infections with group A streptococci, *N. gonorrhoeae,* and *C. albicans* also cause bleeding in some cases. A vaginal culture will provide the diagnosis and guide the selection of an appropriate antibiotic. The manifestations and treatment of vaginal infections in children are discussed in more detail in Chapter 83.

Although a chronic, foul-smelling discharge is generally considered the hallmark of a vaginal foreign body, many girls have intermittent scanty vaginal bleeding alone or with an unimpressive discharge. If a foreign body is strongly suspected but the patient's vagina cannot be visualized when she is placed in the knee–chest position, the patient should receive either gentle vaginal lavage (using saline solution, a 50-mL syringe with the plunger discarded, a red rubber catheter, and gravity) or an examination under conscious sedation or anesthesia. Because the most common foreign body—toilet paper—is not radiopaque, pelvic roentgenography is not likely to be helpful and should be avoided.

Genital tumors are a rare cause of vaginal bleeding. Vaginal bleeding may be the first symptom of this cancer or of another rare malignancy, rhabdomyosarcoma (sarcoma botryoides). Urethral prolapse is sometimes mistaken for a malignant tumor and should be considered in the differential diagnosis.

Occasionally, a patient with a history of bleeding has no abnormalities and no bleeding at the time of the examination. This history should not be dismissed lightly because most parents are good observers, but the patient's urine and stool should also be checked for blood. Vaginal foreign body and inapparent genital trauma are also in the differential diagnosis.

VAGINAL BLEEDING WITH SIGNS OF HORMONAL STIMULATION

During the first 2 to 3 weeks of life, and late in puberty, hormonal fluctuations produce physiologic vaginal bleeding of uterine origin (Fig. 67.1C). Some infants have an endometrial slough that results in a few days of light vaginal bleeding. The bleeding will stop spontaneously and requires no treatment except reassurance for the parents. Occasionally, an adolescent girl is brought to the emergency department (ED) by her family to confirm their belief that she is having her first menstrual period. In this case, if the adolescent's age and degree of pubertal development are appropriate for menarche (Table 67.2), no further evaluation is necessary.

If a girl less than 8 years of age has bleeding that is cyclic or is associated with breast development (thelarche), pubic hair growth (adrenarche), or accelerated linear growth, the various causes of precocious puberty must be given careful consideration in the differential diagnosis (Fig. 67.1D). Such a patient and her parents should be questioned about possible environmental

TABLE 67.2. Chronology of Pubertal Development in Normal Girls

Tanner stage	Breast	Pubic hair	Average age (yr)[a] breast/ pubic hair	Cumulative of percentage girls reaching menarche by each Tanner stage
1	None	None		
2	Breast buds; areolar enlargement	Long, downy, along labia	11.2/11.7	0
3	More growth; no separation of contours	Curly, coarse, along labia	12.2/12.4	25
4	Areola projects beyond breast contour	Covers mons pubis	13.1/13.0	90
5	Mature breast	Adult pattern, extends to thighs	15.3/14.4	100

[a] One standard deviation at each stage is approximately 1 year. Thus, it is uncommon for girls to begin breast growth before 9 years or after 13 years of age.

exposure to feminizing hormones (eg, chronic use of creams or medications containing estrogen). The possibility that a girl early in puberty simply has a nonendocrinologic disorder (foreign body, trauma) must also be considered. If the patient does appear to have precocious puberty, she should be checked in particular for café-au-lait spots (McCune-Albright syndrome) and an abdominal mass (endocrinologically active ovarian tumor or cyst) and referred from the ED to a pediatrician or pediatric endocrinologist for subsequent evaluation and follow-up.

VAGINAL BLEEDING AFTER MENARCHE

Evaluation and Decision

In the discussion to follow, only postmenarchal adolescents with abnormal vaginal bleeding are considered. Accordingly, the first discrimination the emergency physician must make is between those patients whose menstrual bleeding is heavier or more prolonged or more frequent than they would like but is nevertheless normal, and those patients whose bleeding falls outside the limits presented earlier.

Because anovulatory bleeding is almost without exception painless, but approximately 90% of patients with ectopic pregnancy complain of abdominal pain at some time before the diagnosis is established, the physician must inquire carefully about the presence or absence of recent lower abdominal or pelvic pain. Other pertinent historical details include the presence or absence of fainting, fever, easy bruising, sexually transmitted diseases, and trauma.

During the physical examination, the patient's pulse and blood pressure are noted carefully and checked for orthostatic change. If the patient has been injured or is sexually active, a complete pelvic examination is performed. A speculum examination is not necessary for virginal adolescent patients who have not been injured, but a bimanual examination should be carried out routinely because teenagers are not always candid about their sexual activity. If it is more comfortable, bimanual rectoabdominal palpation with the patient in the lithotomy position can be substituted, or the examiner can place one finger intravaginally instead of two. It is advisable to obtain a rapid qualitative urine pregnancy test early in the evaluation of most postmenarchal adolescents presenting to the ED because of vaginal bleeding (Fig. 67.2).

BLEEDING IN LATE PREGNANCY

If the patient is 20 weeks' pregnant or more by history or abdominal examination, potential causes of bleeding that must be identified promptly are a bloody show during labor, premature separation of the placenta (abruptio placentae), and placenta previa (Fig. 67.2).

Because pelvic examination of a patient with placenta previa can provoke uncontrollable hemorrhage, the emergency care of a patient with vaginal bleeding after the twentieth week of pregnancy starts with the management of potential hypovolemic shock (see Chapter 3) rather than with an examination to determine the anatomic site of bleeding. Initial laboratory evaluation should include determinations of the hematocrit, the platelet count, the prothrombin time, and the partial thromboplastin time to screen for disseminated intravascular coagulation, which may be present in moderate and severe abruption. If the patient continues to bleed while in the ED, volume replacement is initiated while blood is typed and cross-matched for use when available. Obviously, an obstetrician should be consulted at the earliest opportunity regarding further ED management of the pregnant patient with second- or third-trimester bleeding.

BLEEDING WITH SHOCK

If the patient with vaginal bleeding is in the first or second trimester of pregnancy and has shock or early signs of cardiovascular instability (pallor, perspiration, vomiting), ruptured ectopic pregnancy must be ruled out. In this case, the treatment of shock and diagnostic measures should be undertaken simultaneously. Pelvic examination is performed, and obstetric consultation should be obtained rapidly. Emergency laparoscopy or laparotomy may be necessary for critically ill patients. If the patient is relatively stable, transabdominal or transvaginal ultrasonography may help to clarify the diagnosis.

EARLY PREGNANCY

The patient with uterine bleeding before 20 weeks' gestation has a pregnancy that is either intrauterine but complicated or ectopic. Vaginal bleeding occurs in 60% to 80% of patients who

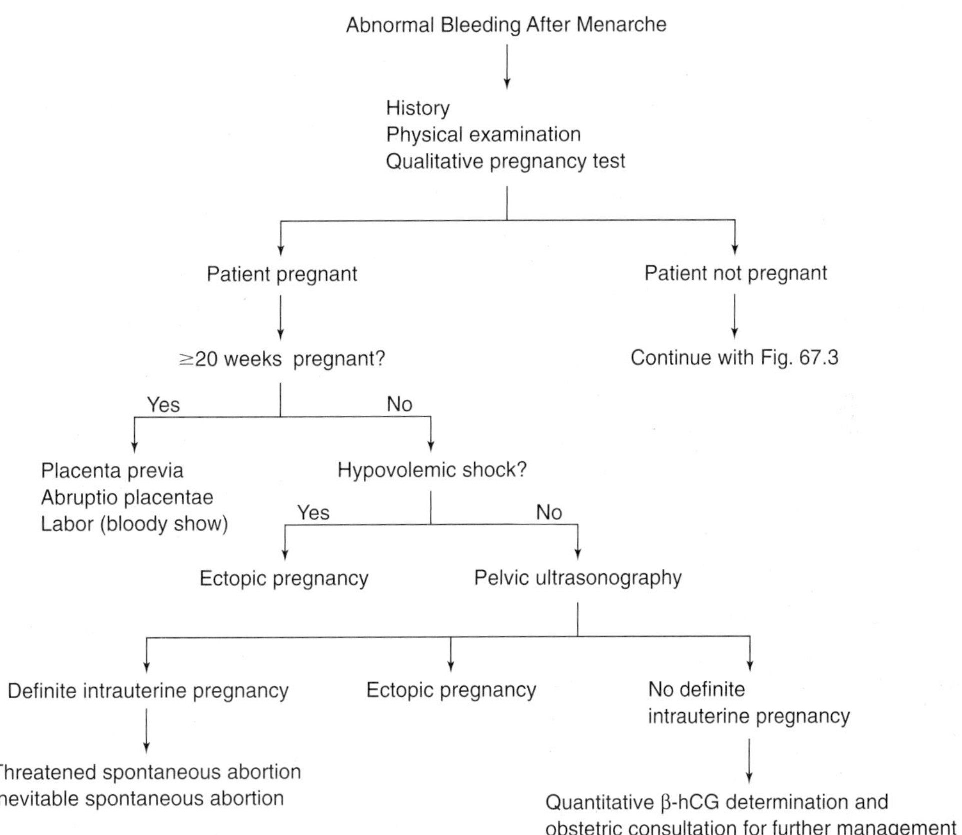

Figure 67.2. Diagnostic approach to abnormal uterine bleeding after menarche: pregnant patients.

have ectopic pregnancies. The bleeding is usually light. The timing of the bleeding sometimes leads the patient to consider it a normal menstrual flow, but about 75% of patients report having missed between one and three menstrual periods. Approximately 90% of patients with ectopic pregnancies experience localized or diffuse abdominal pain that may be present only briefly or for longer than a week before the diagnosis is made. The classic triad of amenorrhea, abdominal pain, and abnormal bleeding occurs in only about 70% of patients with ectopic pregnancy. On examination, the uterus is normal in size or only minimally enlarged because it does not contain the embryo.

Transvaginal or transabdominal ultrasonography is used to guide the management of an adolescent patient with vaginal bleeding and a positive qualitative pregnancy test. If sonography shows that the pregnancy is intrauterine and the fetus is viable, threatened abortion is diagnosed. The bleeding is usually light; some patients have uterine cramps. A spontaneous abortion is considered inevitable or incomplete if the fetal heartbeat is not detectable or if tissue fragments have already been expelled from the uterus. The bleeding is usually heavier, and the patient reports painful uterine contractions. Quantitative β-human chorionic gonadotropin (β-hCG) levels can remain well above 0 for as long as 4 to 6 weeks after spontaneous and induced abortions.

Septic abortion is diagnosed if signs of infection—usually fever, disproportionately severe pelvic pain, and leukocytosis—are present during a spontaneous or induced abortion. After an induced abortion, persistent or heavy bleeding may indicate retained products of conception. In a missed spontaneous abortion, the embryo is not expelled from the uterus within 4 weeks of its death. Dark bleeding is often seen. The patient's symptoms of pregnancy may have regressed, the uterus is smaller than it should be according to her menstrual history, and disseminated intravascular coagulation may occur.

Sonographic signs suggestive of ectopic pregnancy include a solid or complex adnexal mass, a pelvic mass, particulate fluid in the fallopian tube, an endometrial pseudogestational sac, and cul-de-sac fluid. If sonography fails to demonstrate either a definite intrauterine pregnancy or a clearly ectopic pregnancy, a quantitative β-hCG level should be obtained. On ultrasonographic examination, an intrauterine gestational sac should be visible with an abdominal probe when the β-hCG level is above 6000 mIU per mL and with a transvaginal probe when the β-hCG is above 2000 mIU per mL. A fetal heartbeat is detectable by approximately the fifth week of gestation (3 weeks after conception) on transvaginal ultrasonographic examination and by the sixth or seventh week of gestation on transabdominal ultrasonography. Among patients with vaginal bleeding, no definite intrauterine gestational sac on transvaginal sonography, and a β-hCG level of 2000 mIU per mL or higher, about 40% will miscarry, about 55% have ectopic pregnancies, and only about 5% have normal intrauterine pregnancies.

Pregnant patients with vaginal bleeding and indeterminate results on transvaginal ultrasonography should be followed carefully, either by admission to hospital or by close outpatient follow-up with serial quantitations of β-hCG. Obstetric consultation should be obtained in developing an appropriate management plan. In a normal pregnancy, between days 5 and 42 after conception and above an initial level of 100 mIU per mL, the β-hCG level doubles approximately every 2 days. A decline in β-hCG on serial measurement or an increase of less than 66% in 48 hours will suggest a nonviable fetus, but cannot differentiate intrauterine from extrauterine pregnancy.

VAGINAL OR CERVICAL BLEEDING

On pelvic examination, only a few patients will prove to have vaginal or cervical bleeding. The evaluation and management of victims of sexual assault are discussed in detail in Chapters 83 and 111. Hymenal tears produced by coitus rarely require any treatment beyond reassurance for the patient. Bleeding genital warts should not be treated with topical podophylin because toxic amounts of the resin can be absorbed systemically (see Chapter 83). Malignant tumors are a rare cause of vaginal bleeding during adolescence.

Patients are unlikely to be aware of cervical friability or bleeding caused by infection. On examination, however, punctate cervical hemorrhages (a strawberry cervix) can be seen in about 3% of women with trichomonal vaginitis. Cervical bleeding after swabbing and mucopurulent discharge are common manifestations of cervicitis caused by *Chlamydia trachomatis*. Cervical lesions of herpes simplex may also cause a small amount of bleeding.

UNDIAGNOSED UTERINE BLEEDING

Most adolescents with the complaint of vaginal bleeding are not pregnant, and their bleeding is uterine in origin. Each of these patients should receive a complete blood count to screen for anemia and thrombocytopenia. Thrombocytopenia of any cause is the most common coagulation defect responsible for excessive menstrual bleeding. The history and physical examination may now lead the emergency physician to consider as more or less likely each of the several diagnoses discussed below (Fig. 67.3).

ADNEXAL MASS

An adnexal mass in a teenager with abnormal uterine bleeding and a negative pregnancy test may be an ovarian cyst, an abscess, or rarely, a neoplasm. Ancillary investigations should be used to clarify the size, location, and nature of the mass (ultrasonography) and to estimate the likelihood of pelvic infection (leukocyte count, sedimentation rate, cervical tests for gonorrhea and chlamydial infection).

PELVIC TENDERNESS

Pelvic inflammatory disease and ovarian cysts are the likely diagnostic possibilities in a patient with abnormal uterine bleeding and pelvic pain or tenderness. Abnormal bleeding occurs in nearly one-third of patients with pelvic inflammatory disease, probably as a result of endometritis. Pelvic inflammatory disease is discussed in greater detail in Chapter 83. Rarely, an adolescent has spotty midcycle bleeding for 24 hours or less in association with the transient decline in estrogen level that occurs at the time of ovulation. The unilateral pain of mittelschmerz may accompany this brief bleeding episode.

PAINLESS UTERINE BLEEDING

Most patients with painless abnormal bleeding have dysfunctional uterine bleeding (DUB), a consequence of anovulation. Anovulation is an especially likely diagnosis in patients who experience alternating oligomenorrhea and menometrorrhagia. The most common underlying causes of the anovulation itself are functional immaturity of the hypothalamic–pituitary axis, obesity, and polycystic ovary syndrome (see Chapter 40). The management of DUB is detailed in Chapter 83. Hypothyroidism should be considered as a possible underlying cause of dysfunctional uterine bleeding if the patient has other symptoms or signs of thyroid dysfunction.

Hormonal contraception is an important, common cause of dysfunctional uterine bleeding. Of women who use birth control pills containing 35 g or less of estrogen, 5% to 10% will have breakthrough intermenstrual spotting or bleeding, especially during the first 3 months of contraceptive pill use. Breakthrough bleeding is also a common side effect of progestin-only contraceptive pills, injectable medroxyprogesterone, and long-acting progestin implants. Many patients using birth control pills experience estrogen withdrawal bleeding if they forget to take one or several pills.

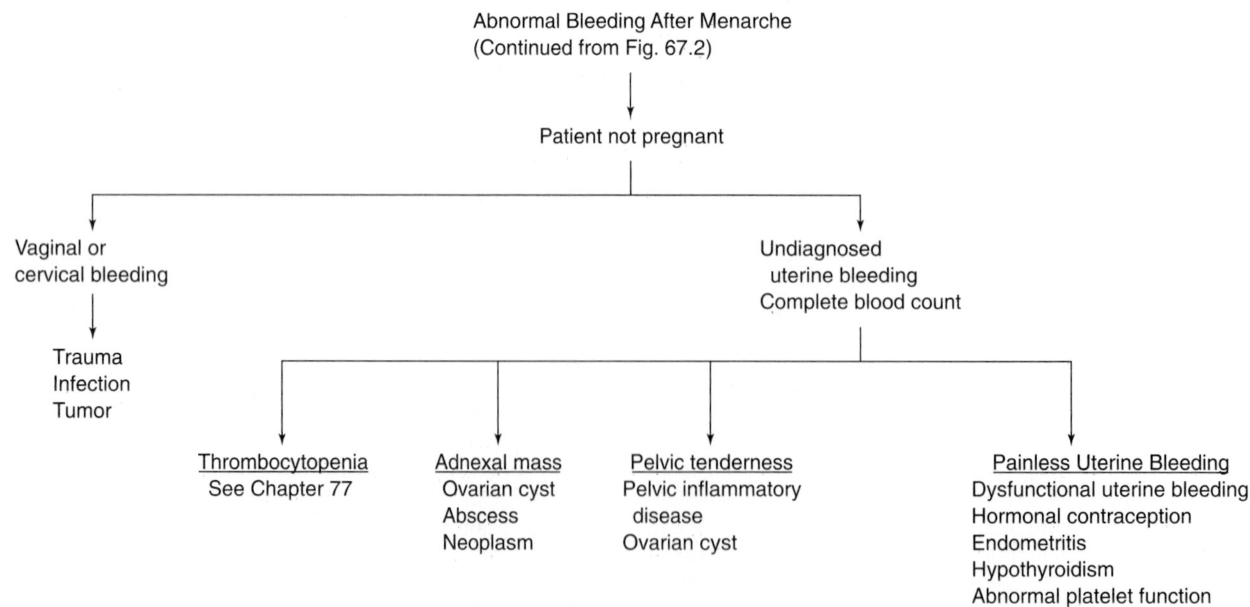

Figure 67.3. A diagnostic approach to abnormal uterine bleeding after menarche: nonpregnant patients.

Less common causes of painless abnormal bleeding include gonococcal and chlamydial endometritis, pharmacologic anticoagulation, and disorders of platelet function (eg, Glanzmann thrombasthenia, von Willebrand disease). Every sexually active patient should be screened for gonorrhea and chlamydial infection. Also to be kept in mind is the possibility, albeit unlikely, of a false-negative urine pregnancy test (as a result of testing too soon after conception, dilute urine, or low hCG production by a blighted or ectopic ovum).

CHAPTER 68
Vaginal Discharge

Jan E. Paradise, M.D.

Normal infants over 1 month of age and prepubertal girls do not have liquid vaginal secretions. Consequently, any vaginal discharge in a female child is abnormal. However, vaginal discharge in neonates and girls who are pubertal may be either normal or abnormal because during these times, estrogen, either maternal or endogenous, stimulates growth of the vaginal epithelium and secretion of mucus by the paracervical glands.

EVALUATION AND DECISION

The patient's age and hormonal status should be considered first in the differential diagnosis of vaginal discharge (Fig. 68.1). For a more detailed discussion of the specific vaginal infections mentioned in this section, the reader is referred to Chapter 83.

Infancy and Childhood

Physiologic leukorrhea is a normal vaginal discharge common among female infants during the first 2 to 3 weeks of life. It is clear or white, slippery when fresh, and sticky when dried. Some neonates have associated withdrawal bleeding when maternal estrogenic stimulation of the uterine endometrium wanes. Trichomonal vaginitis should be suspected if an infant's discharge persists beyond the neonatal period. Occasionally, a baby whose mother has trichomonal vaginitis acquires this infection during delivery. Infected infants may be irritable and have a whitish or yellowish thin discharge. Uncommonly, infants have purulent discharge associated with a congenital malformation of the genitourinary tract (eg, ectopic ureter). A malformation should be suspected if an infant's discharge is accompanied by signs of systemic infection (fever, vomiting, or poor appetite) or if a child with chronic discharge also has had recurrent urinary tract infections (UTIs).

Among older infants and children, a visible vaginal discharge is most likely to indicate a bacterial infection. Cultures for *Neisseria gonorrhoeae* and for other pathogens must therefore be obtained. Gonococcal infection typically produces a whitish to greenish purulent discharge. Bloody discharge occurs in half the cases of *Shigella* vaginitis and is common in vaginitis caused by group A β-hemolytic streptococci. Trichomonal vaginitis occurs virtually exclusively in infants less than 6 months of age and in postpubertal children. Chlamydial infections are nearly always asymptomatic but can produce dysuria, genital discomfort, or a scant mucoid vaginal discharge. Diagnostic tests for *Chlamydia trachomatis* vaginal infection should be reserved for children with histories of sexual abuse and for those whose bacterial cultures already have proved negative because the prevalence of infection is low in unselected populations and because false-positive antigen-detection tests are relatively common. As in adults, diabetes mellitus, broad-spectrum antibiotics, and immunodeficiency are risk factors for the development of candidal vaginitis in children.

An intermittently bloody, foul-smelling vaginal discharge is the classic complaint of the patient with a vaginal foreign body.

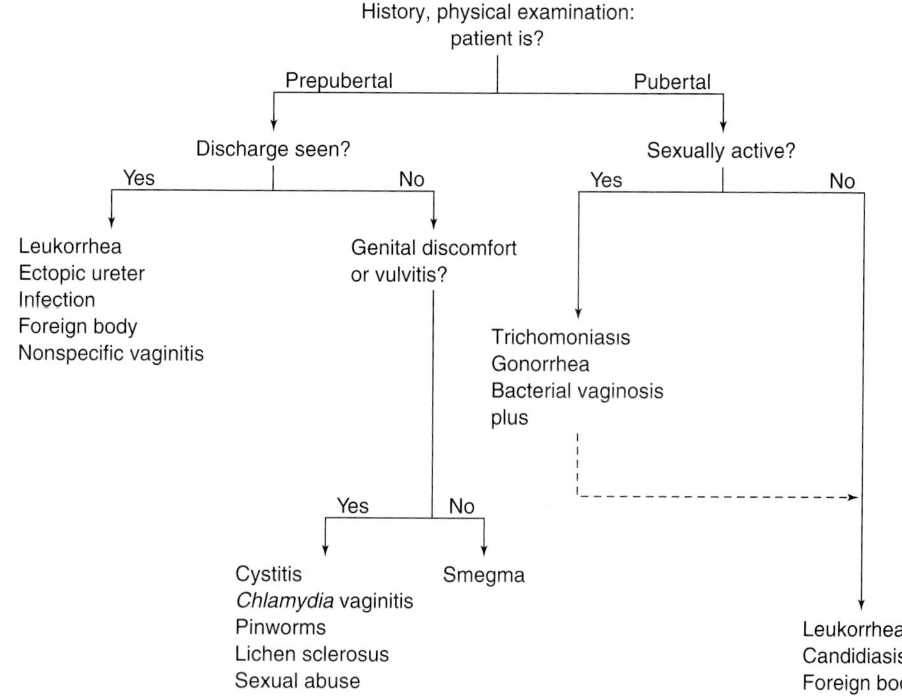

Figure 68.1. A diagnostic approach for vaginal discharge.

Small wads of toilet paper, the most common foreign bodies, are usually easy to see just inside the vaginal vault on knee–chest examination. Rigid foreign bodies—pencil erasers, pins, beads, nuts—are more likely to be palpable during rectal examination but are uncommon.

If examination of the patient discloses vulvar inflammation, excoriation, or hypopigmentation but little or no vaginal discharge, lichen sclerosus and other dermatologic disorders should be considered in the differential diagnosis. Lichen sclerosus is a chronic, idiopathic dermatitis characterized by atrophy, telangiectasia, and hypopigmentation of the perineal skin, often in a figure-of-eight pattern. Perineal excoriation or inflammation secondary to pinworm infestation, varicella, or any generalized dermatitis also can be misinterpreted as primary vulvovaginal disease.

Some girls with complaints of vaginal discharge or discomfort will have no abnormality on genital examination. In these cases, diagnostic possibilities include poor perineal hygiene, smegma, masturbatory behavior, sexual abuse, *Chlamydia* vaginitis, and UTI. Children with vaginal discharge that cannot be ascribed to any of the conditions just discussed generally are considered to have nonspecific vaginitis.

Adolescence

Physiologic leukorrhea (mucous discharge) is normal in postpubertal girls. Postpubertal girls with genital itching are most likely to have candidal vaginitis, even in the absence of any predisposing factor. The associated cheesy discharge may be so scanty that it goes unmentioned by the patient and unnoticed by the clinician. Among postmenarchal patients, birth control pills, broad-spectrum antibiotics, diabetes mellitus, and pregnancy are associated with an increased likelihood of symptomatic vulvovaginal candidiasis. Physical irritants, either mechanical or chemical, should be considered in the differential diagnosis for patients with nonspecific examinations and only polymorphonucleocytes or no abnormality on microscopic examination of the vaginal discharge. Although it is much more common among sexually active adolescents, bacterial vaginosis (see below) occurs occasionally in teenagers who have never had sexual intercourse. A forgotten tampon, the most common intravaginal foreign body, is a rare cause of vaginitis in adolescents.

In girls who have had sexual intercourse, bacterial vaginosis (known previously as nonspecific vaginitis, *Gardnerella* vaginitis, *Haemophilus vaginalis* vaginitis, and *Corynebacterium* vaginitis), trichomoniasis, and gonorrhea are the most likely causes of an abnormal vaginal discharge. Bacterial vaginosis is a clinical syndrome characterized by increased, malodorous vaginal discharge with a pH above 4.5, clue cells but few neutrophils seen on microscopy, and the release of an aminelike odor when potassium hydroxide is added to the discharge. Trichomonal vaginitis is characterized by an increased volume of vaginal discharge associated in some cases with mild pruritus. The discharge is frothy in about 25% of cases. Gonococcal cervicitis or endometritis can produce a noticeable vaginal discharge, but most infected adolescent girls have no lower genital tract symptoms. A pathologic discharge in a girl with gonococcal cervicitis is most likely to be caused by concomitant trichomoniasis or bacterial vaginosis.

Three maneuvers—measurement of the pH of vaginal discharge and microscopic examination of the discharge suspended in 0.5 mL or less of saline solution and in 10% potassium hydroxide—are needed to provide a diagnosis for adolescent patients with vaginitis. To avoid contamination by cervical discharge, specimens should be obtained by swabbing the lateral vaginal wall.

Bacterial vaginosis may be diagnosed when three of four conditions are present (Amsel criteria): (1) a homogeneous, whitish discharge; (2) vaginal pH above 4.5; (3) a fishy odor liberated when potassium hydroxide is added to the discharge; and (4) clue cells. Clue cells are squamous epithelial cells with indistinct borders obscured by granular bacteria, best seen at 400 magnification. On Gram stain, long Gram-positive rods (lactobacilli) are scarce, and short Gram-negative and Gram-variable coccobacilli (*Gardnerella, Prevotella, Mobiluncus* species) are abundant. Trichomoniasis is easily diagnosed if motile flagellates are seen on microscopic examination. However, because microscopy is negative in 20% to 50% of infected women, a rapid DNA probe test or a culture for *Trichomonas* can be helpful for diagnosing patients with suggestive symptoms or signs but negative wet preps. Fungal hyphae are not visible microscopically in over half of patients with symptomatic candidiasis. It is therefore reasonable to recommend empirical antifungal treatment for patients with vulvovaginal pruritus or burning and a vaginal pH less than 5 if a mechanical or physical irritant cannot be identified and if no alternative diagnosis is identified on microscopy.

CHAPTER 69
Vomiting

Molly W. Stevens, M.D. and
Fred M. Henretig, M.D.

Vomiting is defined as the forceful, coordinated act of expelling gastric contents through the mouth. Vomiting may be caused by a number of problems in diverse organ systems. A related complaint, also often heard in the emergency department (ED), is that of young infants who "spit up." Such nonforceful regurgitation of gastric or esophageal contents is most often physiologic and of little consequence, although it occasionally represents a significant disturbance in esophageal function. It is convenient to attempt to organize the many diverse causes of regurgitation and vomiting into age-related categories (Table 69.1).

EVALUATION AND DECISION

General Approach

The approach advocated here focuses on three key clinical features: child's *age*, evidence of *obstruction*, and signs or symptoms of *extraabdominal organ system disease.* Other important points to consider include *appearance* of the vomitus, *overall degree of illness*, and *associated gastrointestinal (GI) symptoms.*

HISTORY AND PHYSICAL EXAMINATION

Evidence of obstruction, including symptoms of abdominal pain, obstipation, nausea, and increasing abdominal girth, are sought in addition to vomiting. Other associated GI symptoms may include diarrhea, anorexia, flatulence, and frequent eructation with reflux. The suspicion of significant extraabdominal organ system disease is raised by neurologic symptoms such as se-

TABLE 69.1. Vomiting and Regurgitation: Principal Causes by Usual Age of Onset and Etiology

- *Newborn (Birth to 2 wk)*
  - Normal variations
  - Gastroesophageal reflux (± hiatal hernia)
  - Esophageal stenosis, atresia
  - Infantile achalasia
  - Obstructive intestinal anomalies
    - Intestinal stenosis, atresia
    - Malrotation of bowel (± midgut volvulus)
    - Meconium ileus (cystic fibrosis)
    - Meconium plug
    - Hirschsprung disease
    - Imperforate anus
    - Enteric duplications
  - Other gastrointestinal causes
    - Necrotizing enterocolitis
    - Cow's milk allergy
    - Lactobezoar
    - Gastrointestinal perforation with secondary peritonitis
    - Gastroenteritis
    - Celiac disease
    - Peritonitis
    - Paralytic ileus
  - Neurologic
    - Subdural hematoma
    - Hydrocephalus
    - Cerebral edema
    - Kernicterus
  - Renal
    - Obstructive uropathy
    - Renal insufficiency
  - Infectious
    - Meningitis
    - Sepsis
  - Metabolic
    - Inborn errors of urea cycle; amino acid, organic acid, and carbohydrate metabolism (phenylketonuria, galactosemia)
    - Congenital adrenal hyperplasia
- *Older infant* (2 wk to 12 mo)
  - Normal variations
  - Gastroesophageal reflux
  - Acquired esophageal disorders (corrosive esophagitis ± stricture, foreign bodies, retroesophageal abscess)
  - Rumination
  - Gastrointestinal obstruction
    - Bezoars, foreign bodies
    - Pyloric stenosis
    - Malrotation (with or without volvulus)
    - Enteric duplications
    - Meckel's diverticulum (complications of)
    - Intussusception
    - Ascariasis
    - Incarcerated hernia
    - Hirschsprung disease
  - Other gastrointestinal causes
    - Gastroenteritis
    - Celiac disease
    - Peritonitis
    - Paralytic ileus
  - Neurologic
    - Brain tumors
    - Other intracranial mass lesions
    - Cerebral edema
    - Hydrocephalus
  - Renal
    - Obstructive uropathy
    - Renal insufficiency
  - Infectious
    - Meningitis
    - Sepsis
    - Urinary tract infection
    - Otitis media
    - Pertussis
    - Hepatitis
  - Metabolic
    - Metabolic acidosis (inborn errors of amino acid and organic acid metabolism, renal tubular acidosis)
    - Galactosemia
    - Fructose intolerance
    - Adrenal insufficiency
  - Drug overdose
    - Aspirin
    - Theophylline
    - Digoxin
  - Respiratory (posttussive)
    - Reactive airways disease (RAD)
    - Respiratory infection
    - Foreign body (FB)
- *Older child (over 12 mo)*
  - Gastrointestinal obstruction
    - Acquired esophageal strictures
    - Foreign bodies, bezoars
    - Peptic ulcer disease
    - Posttraumatic intramural hematoma
    - Malrotation (with or without volvulus)
    - Meckel's diverticulum (complications of)
    - Meconium ileus equivalent (cystic fibrosis)
    - Ascariasis incarcerated hernia
    - Adhesions (postsurgical, peritonitis)
    - Intussusception
    - Hirschsprung disease
    - Superior mesenteric artery syndrome
  - Other gastrointestinal causes
    - Gastroenteritis, gastritis, duodenitis
    - Gastroesophageal reflux
    - Appendicitis
    - Peptic ulcer disease
    - Pancreatitis
    - Peritonitis
    - Paralytic ileus
    - Crohn disease
  - Neurologic
    - Brain tumors
    - Other intracranial mass lesions
    - Cerebral edema
    - Migraine
    - Motion sickness
    - Postconcussion syndrome
    - Seizures
  - Renal
    - Obstructive uropathy
    - Renal insufficiency/renal tubular acidosis
  - Infectious
    - Meningitis
    - Urinary tract infection
    - Hepatitis
    - Upper respiratory infection (postnasal mucous drip)
  - Metabolic
    - Diabetic ketoacidosis
    - Reye syndrome
    - Adrenal insufficiency
    - Inborn error of metabolism (urea cycle or FA oxidation defect; acute, intermittent porphyria)
  - Toxins and drugs
    - Aspirin
    - Ipecac
    - Theophylline
    - Digoxin
    - Iron
    - Lead (chronic)
  - Respiratory (posttussive)
    - Asthma exacerbation
    - Infectious respiratory disease
    - FB
  - Other
    - Pregnancy
    - Psychogenic
    - Cyclic vomiting

vere headache, stiff neck, blurred vision or diplopia, clumsiness, personality or school performance change, or persistent lethargy or irritability; by genitourinary symptoms such as flank pain, dysuria, urgency and frequency, or amenorrhea; by common infectious complaints such as fever, sore throat, or rash; or by respiratory complaints such as cough, increased work of breathing, or chest pain (Tables 69.2 and 69.3).

The appearance of the vomitus often is helpful in establishing the site of pathology. Undigested food or milk should suggest reflux from the esophagus or stomach caused by lesions such as esophageal atresia (in the neonate), gastroesophageal (GE) reflux, or pyloric stenosis. Bilious vomitus suggests obstruction distal to the ampulla of Vater, although it occasionally is seen with prolonged vomiting of any cause when the pylorus is relaxed. Fecal material in the vomitus is seen with obstruction of the lower bowel. Hematemesis usually reflects bleeding in the upper GI tract, as discussed in Chapter 23.

The physical examination should pay particular attention to the abdomen. Are there signs of obstruction such as ill-defined tenderness, distension, high-pitched bowel sounds (or absent sounds in ileus), or visible peristalsis? A complete physical examination must include a search for signs of neurologic, infectious, toxic/metabolic, and genitourinary causes, as well as an evaluation of hydration status (see Chapter 14).

APPROACH TO CHILDREN BY AGE GROUPS

The various approaches to treating children by age group are depicted in Fig. 69.1 and discussed in the following sections.

TABLE 69.2. Life-Threatening Causes of Vomiting

Newborn (birth to 2 wk)
- Anatomic anomalies—esophageal stenosis/atresia; intestinal obstructions (Table 69.1), especially malrotation and volvulus; Hirschsprung disease
- Other gastrointestinal (GI) causes
  - Necrotizing enterocolitis
  - Peritonitis
- Neurologic—kernicterus, mass lesions, hydrocephalus
- Renal—obstructive anomalies, uremia
- Infectious—sepsis, meningitis
- Metabolism—inborn errors, especially congenital adrenal hyperplasia

Older infant (2 wk to 12 mo)
- Gastroesophageal reflux, severe
- Esophageal disorders
- Rumination
- Intestinal obstruction (Table 69.1), especially pyloric stenosis, intussusception, incarcerated hernia, malrotation with volvulus
- Other GI causes, especially gastroenteritis (with dehydration)
- Neurologic—mass lesions, hydrocephalus
- Renal—obstruction, uremia
- Infectious—sepsis, meningitis, pertussis
- Metabolic—inborn errors
- Drugs—aspirin, theophylline, digoxin

Older child (over 12 mo)
- GI obstruction, especially intussusception (Table 69.1)
- Other GI causes, especially appendicitis, peptic ulcer disease
- Neurologic—mass lesions
- Renal—uremia
- Infectious—meningitis, sepsis
- Metabolic—diabetic ketoacidosis, Reye syndrome, adrenal insufficiency, inborn errors of metabolism
- Toxins, drugs—aspirin, ipecac, theophylline, digoxin, iron, lead

Neonates

Newborn babies with the onset of vomiting in the first days of life always should be suspect for one of the common *congenital GI anomalies* that cause obstruction, such as esophageal or intestinal atresia or web, malrotation, meconium ileus, or Hirschsprung disease. If the vomiting is bilious, bright yellow, or green, an urgent surgical consultation is required. All patients in whom the possibility of GI obstruction is entertained must have flat and upright abdominal films. Except for the later presentations of malrotation, most neonates with a congenital basis for their bowel obstruction will present during their initial nursery stay. Neonates or infants with malrotation and volvulus may present with abdominal pain (crying, drawing up their knees, poor feeding), with evidence of obstruction (bilious emesis), or an acute abdomen (abdominal distension or rigidity). The diagnosis of malrotation is confirmed by the abnormal radiographic location of the duodenal–jejunal junction (upper GI series) and/or the cecum (contrast enema).

Other serious causes of neonatal vomiting that may present to the ED include *infection*, such as meningitis, sepsis, pyelonephritis, or necrotizing enterocolitis, *increased intracranial pressure* (ICP) related to cerebral edema, subdural hematoma, or hydrocephalus; *metabolic acidosis* or *hyperammonemia* caused by the rare inborn errors of amino acid and organic acid metabolism; and *renal insufficiency* or *obstruction*. Such infants usually appear ill, with associated lethargy and irritability; sometimes fever, a full fontanel, a diminished urinary stream, an abdominal mass, or respiratory signs will suggest the correct cause. Obviously, any ill neonate with vomiting, even in the absence of obstruction, also requires hospitalization and prompt evaluation for sepsis and neurologic, renal, and metabolic disease.

Commonly, however, a young infant in the first 2 to 4 weeks of life who appears entirely well is brought to the ED with the complaint of persistent vomiting. Usually, a close description of the "vomiting" (or even better, a trial feeding in the ED) reveals the problem to be *physiologic regurgitation* or *reflux*; so-called "spitting up." This is a common (nearly 20% of infants reflux) and insignificant problem, probably representing some normal variation in the developmental maturation of the lower

TABLE 69.3. Common Causes of Vomiting

Newborn (birth to 2 wk)
- Normal variations ("spitting up")
- Gastroesophageal reflux
- Gastrointestinal (GI) obstruction—congenital anomalies
- Necrotizing enterocolitis (premature birth)
- Infectious—meningitis, sepsis

Older infant (2 wk to 12 mo)
- Normal variations
- Gastroesophageal reflux
- Gastrointestinal (GI) obstruction—especially pyloric stenosis, intussusception, incarcerated hernia
- Gastroenteritis
- Infectious—sepsis, meningitis, urinary tract infection, otitis media
- Posttussive—reactive airways disease, respiratory infection, foreign body
- Drug overdose—aspirin, theophylline

Older child (over 12 mo)
- GI obstruction—incarcerated hernia, intussusception
- Other GI causes—gastroenteritis, gastroesophageal reflux, appendicitis
- Infectious—meningitis, urinary tract infection
- Posttussive—asthma, infection, foreign body
- Metabolic—diabetic ketoacidosis
- Toxins/drugs—aspirin, theophylline, iron, lead
- Pregnancy

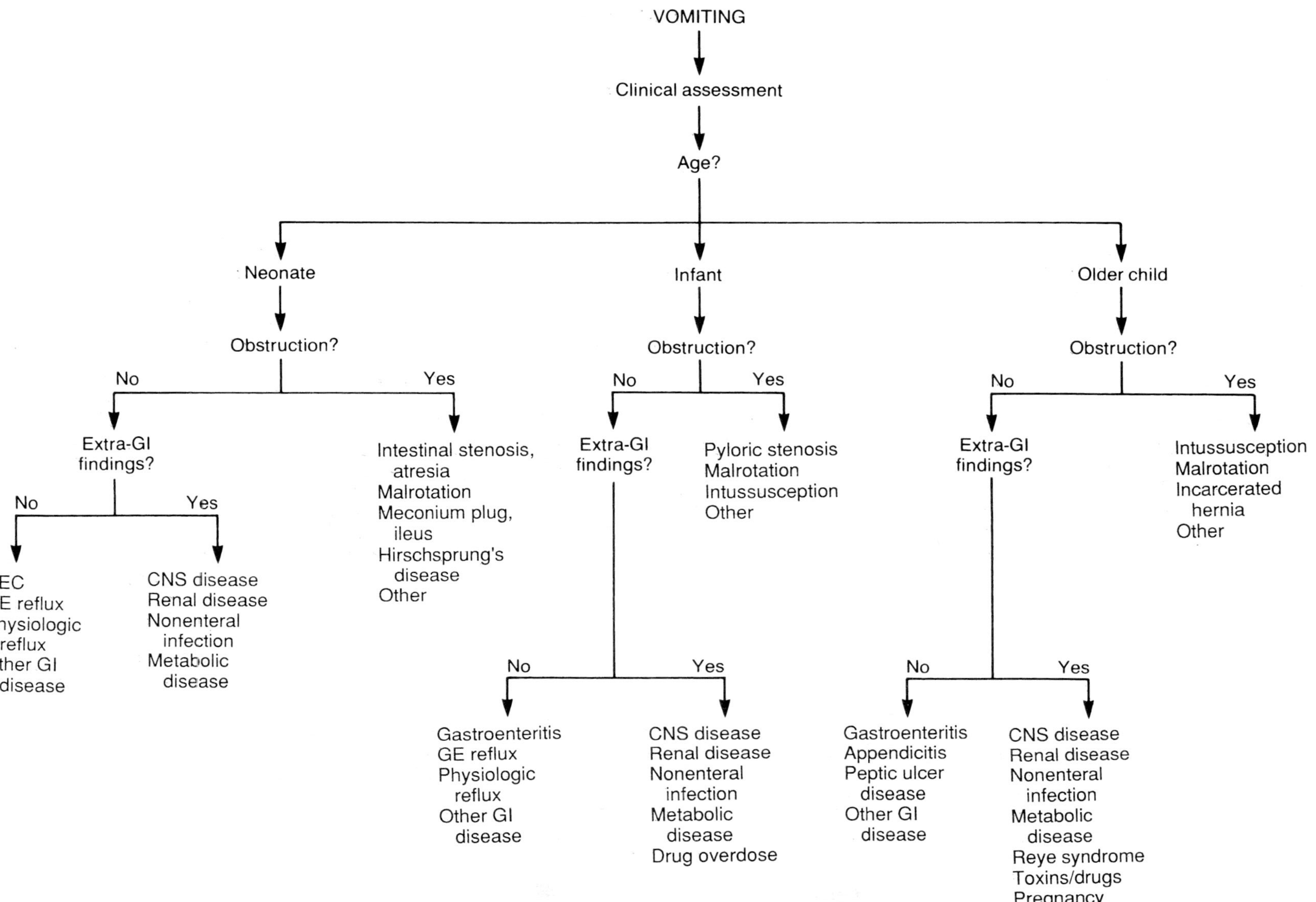

Figure 69.1. Differential diagnosis of vomiting. *GI,* gastrointestinal; *NEC,* necrotizing enterocolitis; *GE,* gastroesophageal; *CNS,* central nervous system (also see Table 69.1).

esophageal sphincter (LES). These infants do not exhibit forceful abdominal contractions but rather reflux milk effortlessly into their mouths, which dribbles out, usually when prone, and often with a burp.

Other infants who regurgitate easily may not be managed so simply. Their course may have more significant symptoms of pain, arching, and high volume and frequency of regurgitation, or it may be complicated by distal esophagitis or gastritis, failure to thrive, esophageal–peptic strictures, pulmonary disease, or rarely, apnea or near-sudden infant death syndrome (SIDS) event. Such infants are diagnosed as having *gastroesophageal reflux disease* (GERD), a more severe or pathologic degree of LES dysfunction that is much less common (1:500). Several imaging and physiologic studies may be used to confirm the diagnosis and to correlate a patient's signs and symptoms with episodes of reflux. A 24-hour intraesophageal pH probe is the most sensitive diagnostic test for GE reflux. Based on the patient's history, evaluation of delayed gastric emptying can be done by GE scintiscan, or by an upper GI series to rule out an anatomic cause for the delay. Endoscopy is used to assess suspected complications (esophagitis or stricture); esophageal manometry is primarily a research tool in this disease. In uncomplicated GE reflux, reassurance, postural management, and dietary measures are usually adequate. For more severe symptoms or with complications, additional medical management includes the use of prokinetic agents (metoclopramide) and acid blockade (ranitidine or cimetidine).

Older Infant

Infants who present with vomiting after the first few weeks of life may still have intestinal obstruction, but the underlying causes are somewhat different than in the neonate. The important lesions responsible for mechanical obstructions in this age group include congenital hypertrophic pyloric stenosis (HPS), malrotation, intussusception, incarcerated hernia, enteric duplications, and complications of Meckel's diverticulum. Occasionally, other anomalies that might be expected to present in the neonate, such as Hirschsprung disease, will appear only after several weeks or months of life. In all cases, these conditions have physical findings suggestive of intestinal obstruction and often are specific for the level of obstruction. Having a high index of suspicion for both common and uncommon forms of intestinal obstruction is important to making a timely diagnosis.

The typical infant with *pyloric stenosis* (see Chapter 103) presents at 4 to 6 weeks of age (95% present by 3 months; rarely after 20 weeks) with a chief compliant of projectile vomiting during or shortly after a feeding. The vomiting in pyloric stenosis is typically crescendo in nature, with increasing frequency and severity over days to weeks. By contrast, vomiting caused by GE reflux tends to be relatively consistent over time; in malrotation, vomiting is sudden in onset and can be episodic. The vomitus is nonbilious, reflecting obstruction at the pylorus, and usually is voluminous, nearly the entire content of the feeding. The infant may become constipated if vomiting has been of sufficient duration. On examination, an olive-sized mass may be palpated (most easily after vomiting has occurred) in the right upper quadrant to the right of the midline and just above the umbilicus. Peristaltic waves may be visualized, moving from left upper to right upper quadrants, again indicating obstruction at the pylorus. Unless the infant is significantly dehydrated, the child usually is vigorous and active, although irritable because of hunger. These infants often develop hypochloremic, hypokalemic metabolic alkalosis, which should be corrected before surgery (see Chapter 76).

The diagnosis of pyloric stenosis is clinical, based on the classic history of projectile, nonbilious emesis, and examination with hyperperistalsis and palpation of a pyloric mass or "olive." Imaging studies (ultrasound [US] or upper GI series) are not necessary if the history and examination are conclusive. In recent years, however, earlier presentations have resulted in a greater number of infants evaluated before the development of the diagnostic clinical hallmarks, and consequently an increased reliance on imaging studies to confirm the diagnosis. US has become the diagnostic modality of choice with characteristic findings in HPS of a thickened pyloric wall (greater than 3 mm) with a lengthened canal (greater than 15 mm).

Between 2 months and about 5 to 6 years of age, the most common cause of obstruction is *intussusception* (see Chapter 103). Most children develop this disorder between 3 months and 2 years of age; the average age was 16 months in a recent large series. Early symptoms usually include paroxysms of colicky abdominal pain and vomiting, suggesting a GI illness. Initially, the infant may appear relatively well between attacks, but some children will fall asleep or seem prostrate at these times. Initially, there may be a normal stool, then occult-positive, but usually within 6 to 12 hours, dark maroon blood is passed per rectum; this blood often is mixed with mucus, earning the label of "currant jelly" stool. However, some infants with intussusception may present primarily with lethargy and decreased responsiveness, without striking GI symptoms (so-called neurologic or painless intussusception). Examination of the abdomen usually reveals a somewhat tender, sausage-shaped mass on the right side. The mass may be more easily appreciated by bimanual rectal and abdominal examination, and a test for occult blood may be positive in the absence of gross blood.

Recommendations for the diagnosis and treatment of suspected intussusception include supine and right-side up decubitus radiographs (decubitus to look for free air or mass at the hepatic flexure region; supine for signs of obstruction such as abnormal air–fluid levels, paucity of gas, or mass effect). US sometimes is used instead of radiographs if experienced personnel are available. Reduction is attempted by contrast (air or liquid) enema if perforation (free air on radiograph or peritonitis) or shock is not evident. Recent success rates for reduction in pediatric centers using air or liquid contrast enemas have improved to the range of 80% to 90%, with some centers reporting their increased success with repeated attempts after short intervals (45 to 60 minutes). Open reduction with laparotomy is reserved for patients with perforation or shock at initial diagnosis or when enema reduction is unsuccessful.

Other important causes of obstruction in the older infant include incarcerated inguinal hernia, volvulus, Hirschsprung disease, or complications related to Meckel's diverticulum. The presence of an incarcerated hernia will be apparent on examination. Volvulus of the bowel is virtually always associated with bilious vomiting. A good clue to diagnosis of Hirschsprung disease is asking, "Has your child ever had a normal (unstimulated) bowel movement?" (see Chapters 10 and 103). The obstructive complications of Meckel's diverticulum include intussusception and volvulus and have similar presentations of these types of obstruction related to other causes.

The principal nonobstructive causes of vomiting in the older infant include GI, neurologic, renal, infectious, and metabolic disorders. Nonobstructive GI disturbances are probably the most common cause for vomiting in this age group. *Viral gastroenteritis*, although usually appearing predominantly as diarrhea associated with vomiting, often begins with a prodromal phase of vomiting alone (see Chapter 74). Physical findings usually are limited to ill-defined and inconsistent abdominal pain and signs of a variable degree of dehydration. Vomiting in older infants also is caused at times by persistent GE reflux, as well as by abdominal disorders uncommon in infancy, such as peptic ulcer disease or appendicitis. Occasionally, vomiting is seen in paralytic ileus related to infection (pneumonia, peritonitis) or electrolyte disorders.

Neurologic causes of vomiting in infancy also include *mass lesions* such as tumor, abscess, and intracranial hematoma (see Chapter 73), as well as *meningitis* and *encephalitis*. There may be evidence of increased ICP: increasing head circumference, bulging fontanel, and split sutures (papilledema is rarely noted during infancy). However, some brainstem tumors cause protracted vomiting by direct effect on the vomiting center without an accompanying increased ICP. Again, it is to be emphasized that meningism rarely is seen with meningitis in infancy and that signs of increased ICP occur late (see Chapter 74). Early findings include fever, vomiting, lethargy, and irritability, especially the paradoxic irritability of increased crying with parental fondling.

Infections outside the GI and neurologic systems may cause vomiting in infants and, occasionally, in older children. The more important such infections are *otitis media* (OM), *urinary tract infection* (UTI), *respiratory infections*, and *viral hepatitis*. Positive physical findings on otoscopic examination are seen in OM, along with mild irritability, and often, fever (see Chapter 74). UTIs may be surprisingly devoid of localizing signs and symptoms in preschool-age children (see Chapter 107); nonspecific GI complaints, including vomiting and abdominal pain, fever, irritability, and anorexia, may be the only presenting symptoms. Urinalysis and culture provide the specific diagnosis. Vomiting also is a common event after the paroxysms of coughing seen in infants with pertussis (see Chapter 74). It is a common symptom in the prodromal phase of infectious hepatitis, usually preceding the onset of jaundice (see Chapter 82). Abnormal liver function tests substantiate this latter diagnosis.

Renal and *metabolic disorders* also cause vomiting in the older infant. Renal failure, renal tubular acidosis, or rarely, diabetic ketoacidosis may be seen in this age group. Hypoadrenalism, hepatic failure, Reye syndrome, and inborn errors of metabolism such as galactosemia and fructose intolerance also may present in infancy and may have vomiting as a prominent symptom in an ill-appearing infant.

Occasionally, parental overzealous use of over-the-counter or prescribed drugs in infants will lead to *intoxication*. Drugs that often produce vomiting in excessive doses include aspirin, theophylline, and digoxin; all of these intoxications are easily verified by associated signs and symptoms and specific drug levels. The problem of accidental ingestion is discussed later in this chapter.

An additional rare cause of regurgitation or vomiting in infants, with onset usually at 6 to 12 months of age, is *rumination*. This severe psychiatric disorder of infancy, related to abnormal maternal–infant relationship, may progress to severe failure to thrive and death. These infants seem to self-induce the reflux, often by gagging themselves, and often appear to partially rechew and reswallow their vomitus.

Older Child

Many of the causes of intestinal obstruction and other important GI diseases described in neonates and older infants, such as volvulus associated with malrotation, Hirschsprung disease, a meconium ileus "equivalent" in the child with cystic fibrosis, and an incarcerated hernia, occasionally may first appear in the older child. Older children with malrotation and/or volvulus will often have a previous episodic history of vomiting or intermittent colicky abdominal pain. In addition, older children often are subjected to blunt abdominal trauma; persistent vomiting after such injury may reflect obstruction related to a duodenal intramural hematoma or ileus secondary to pancreatitis. Gastroenteritis, as in infants, continues to be the most common cause of vomiting in the older child seen in the ED. Two entities that usually occur in older children, appendicitis and peptic ulcers, are discussed here, although they occur rarely in infancy as well.

Appendicitis (see Chapter 103) in a preadolescent child classically begins with periumbilical, crampy abdominal pain and anorexia, often followed by vomiting. Then the pain shifts to the right lower quadrant and fever may develop. Younger children may deviate from this pattern by exhibiting less specific symptoms early in their illness and a more rapid progression to perforation and generalized peritonitis. As peritoneal irritation becomes well established, the child attempts to minimize any motion to the abdomen. Physical examination usually reveals localized involuntary right lower quadrant guarding and tenderness that, when mild, may be easier to elicit by asking the child to cough or to hop on one foot. In addition, there may be rebound and referred rebound tenderness along with a tender fullness high on the right during rectal examination. Atypical positions of the appendix (eg, retrocecal, retroileal, pelvic) will be reflected in atypical areas of maximal tenderness, as well as in confusing symptoms such as diarrhea or dysuria (caused by appendiceal inflammation adjacent to colon or ureter/bladder). Pertinent laboratory findings often include leukocytosis with a left shift in the differential count, but a normal white blood cell (WBC) count in an afebrile patient does not rule out appendicitis. The urinalysis usually is normal. Occasionally, in an atypical patient, abdominal radiographs may be helpful in showing a right lower quadrant fecalith, localized obstruction, a mass effect with a paucity of gas in the right lower quadrant, or lumbar spine scoliosis. Appendicitis is a clinical diagnosis, but when the differential diagnosis is difficult or in early or equivocal cases, imaging studies are helpful. US can be particularly helpful in distinguishing tuboovarian pathology or renal pathology from appendicitis. Computed tomography (CT) scan is widely becoming the imaging study of choice in adults; recent studies show excellent sensitivity of right lower quadrant CT with rectal contrast.

Vomiting as a symptom of *peptic ulcer disease* in children usually is seen in association with abdominal pain (see Chapter 82). In young children, the pain often is nonspecific and not easily related to meals. In adolescents, the pattern becomes more classically related to food or antacids. There may be hematemesis and/or melena. The abdominal examination may be normal or reveal mild to moderate epigastric tenderness. Other inflammatory lesions of the upper GI tract (gastritis, duodenitis, and Crohn disease) can also cause persistent vomiting.

Genitourinary causes of vomiting in the older child include UTI and obstructive urologic disease. An important additional concern in adolescent girls is early *pregnancy* (see Chapter 40). It is common for such patients to offer the chief complaint of persistent vomiting (not necessarily only in the morning) for several weeks, and often sexual activity and/or amenorrhea is initially denied. Physical findings at this stage of pregnancy may be subtle. Thus, prolonged vomiting in a postmenarchal girl should be pursued with the appropriate urine or serum gonadotropin assays (see Chapter 40).

The important extra-GI infectious diseases of the older child that cause vomiting have been discussed for the most part under the neonate and infant headings of this chapter. Serious infections localize symptoms more readily in this older age group. Meningitis usually is accompanied by meningism after the age of 2 years. Lower urinary infections tend to present with dysuria, frequency, and urgency as children approach school age, and pyelonephritis with fever and lower back pain or tenderness. The toddler or school-age child also may vomit with pharyngeal irritation (pharyngitis, postnasal mucous drip) or have posttussive emesis with persistent or severe cough caused by asthma, respiratory infection, or respiratory foreign body.

Neurologic disease that causes vomiting in the older child again represents (primarily) lesions that cause increased ICP or direct irritation of the medullary vomiting center; they usually lead to papilledema and/or abnormal neurologic findings on examination. One important exception is childhood *migraine* (see Chapter 73). Preadolescent children do not usually present with the classic migraine picture with aura, hemicranial headache, and scotomas. More often, they complain of rare but severe, poorly localized headaches accompanied by nausea and vomiting and followed by sleep. The physical examination between attacks usually is normal. Another common but minor form of vomiting on a neurologic basis (caused by labyrinthine stimulation) would be the propensity to motion sickness.

Metabolic aberrations, including hepatic, renal, and adrenal failure, all may cause vomiting in the older child (as well as during infancy). *Ketoacidosis* presenting for the first time in an as yet undiagnosed diabetic occurs more commonly in older children, especially at school entrance age and later as adolescence begins (see Chapter 86). Vomiting may be the chief complaint of such children, although careful questioning usually uncovers a preceding 3- to 4-week history of polyuria, polyphagia, polydipsia, and at times, weight loss.

The other important, but increasingly uncommon, cause of vomiting is *Reye syndrome* (see Chapter 82). Although it may occur at any age, it tends to be seen more commonly in toddlers and school-age children. Typically, these children have had a preceding viral illness within the past 2 weeks (especially varicella and influenza in the United States) from which they have just recovered, or they are recovering at the time of presentation. Generally, about 24 hours of severe, recurrent vomiting is followed immediately by progression through the varying stages of encephalopathy. Abnormal laboratory data in Reye syndrome include elevated serum transaminase and ammonia, prolonged prothrombin time, and often, hypoglycemia; bilirubin usually is normal, making other forms of severe liver disease unlikely. Recent research has emphasized that the differential in cases meeting the criteria for Reye syndrome include Reye-like syndromes: inherited metabolic disorders and viral and toxic diseases.

In children 1 to 4 years of age, *accidental ingestion* is a common problem. Acute poisonings that cause vomiting as a prominent symptom include aspirin, theophylline, digoxin, and iron sulfate (see Chapter 78). Chronic *lead poisoning* also occurs in this pica-prone age group. Early symptoms of lead intoxication are vomiting, colicky abdominal pain, anorexia, constipation, and irritability. Tragically, many such youngsters have been diagnosed as having nonspecific gastroenteritis syndromes initially, only to return days to weeks later with frank encephalopathy and, ultimately, severe neurologic sequelae. The history of pica and lead paint exposure should be sought in every toddler with persistent vomiting. The diagnosis of plumbism can be confirmed with elevated blood levels of lead and erythrocyte protoporphyrins (see Chapter 78).

Finally, the school-age child or adolescent may vomit on a *psychologic* basis. Acutely, brief episodes of vomiting may occur with any emotionally disturbing event. Children with school phobia or other significant psychiatric problems may vomit persistently. Adolescents are at risk for self-induced vomiting in the context of the anorexia nervosa and bulimia syndromes (see Chapter 112).

CHAPTER 70
Weakness/Flaccid Paralysis

Joanne M. Decker, M.D.

A large number of diagnostic considerations exist for the previously well child who presents to the emergency department (ED) complaining of recent onset of weakness or diminished muscle strength (Table 70.1). This chapter limits the discussion to the assessment of the child with acute or subacute onset of weakness and associated flaccid paresis or paralysis on neurologic examination. Although flaccid paralysis or profound weakness in children is an unusual finding in general, relatively common causes are listed in Table 70.2, and serious life- or limb-threatening causes are listed in Table 70.3.

DIFFERENTIAL DIAGNOSIS

The differential diagnosis of acute weakness can be categorized by the different parts of the nervous system that are affected. Upper motor neuron disease involves either the cerebral cortex or the spinal cord. The cerebral cortex can be damaged by a cerebrovascular accident (CVA), leading to sudden weakness, usually unilateral. Children with sickle cell disease have increased risk for cerebral infarction during a vasoocclusive crisis. Cerebrovascular disease associated with the rare metabolic disorder homocystinuria may result in CVA. Hypercoagulable states such as found in pregnancy, malignancy, or severe dehydration can lead to venous thrombosis. Embolic causes are to be considered in patients with congenital heart disease, mitral

TABLE 70.1. Differential Diagnosis of Weakness

Upper motor neuron disease	Lower motor neuron, neuromuscular function, and muscle disease
Cerebral cortex	*Anterior horn cell*
Cerebrovascular accident	Poliomyelitis
Hemorrhage	Hopkins syndrome
Embolic	Werdnig-Hoffman disease
Spinal cord	*Peripheral nerve disease*
Trauma, hemorrhage	Guillain-Barré syndrome
Infection	Heavy metal poisoning
Epidural abscess	Fish toxins
Transverse myelitis	Porphyria
Malignancy	*Neuromuscular junction*
Disc herniation	Organophosphates
Tethered cord	Tick paralysis
	Botulism
	Myasthenia gravis
	Muscle disease
	Inflammatory myopathy
	Periodic paralysis
	Rhabdomyolysis
	Muscular dystrophies

TABLE 70.2. Common Causes of Weakness
Infant botulism
Guillain-Barré syndrome
Viral myositis

valve prolapse, or a history of rheumatic fever. An intracranial hemorrhage may occur after a relatively minor trauma in a child with hemophilia or spontaneously from a previously undiagnosed tumor or arteriovenous malformation (AVM). Finally, cocaine and amphetamine use have been associated with cerebral infarction in previously healthy patients.

Many processes can damage or compress the spinal cord, leading to weakness or paralysis. Trauma, with or without associated vertebral fracture or dislocation, can lead to spinal cord contusion or transection. The trauma often is severe (ie, motor vehicle accident, football injury); however, it may be mild, particularly in children with Down syndrome or juvenile rheumatoid arthritis (JRA) in whom there may be an associated cervical vertebral instability. Neck or back trauma can also cause an epidural hematoma, which compresses the spinal cord as it expands. This is of particular concern in patients with hemophilia or other underlying coagulopathy. Infectious causes of spinal cord compression include epidural abscess and transverse myelitis. In transverse myelitis (see Chapter 73), areas of inflammation and infarction in the spinal cord result in a clinical picture of flaccid paralysis in both legs, along with rectal and bladder incontinence. Other causes of spinal cord compression include hemorrhage from trauma or an AVM, malignancy in the form of a spinal or paraspinal tumor or metastasis, disc herniation, or a tethered cord.

Lower motor neuron disease has more varied origins. The anterior horn cells form the proximal part of the lower motor neuron unit. Anterior horn cell disease involves exclusively the motor neurons, so sensory function is normal. Reflexes are generally lost early in the disease, and muscle atrophy and fasciculations are often noted on physical examination. Cranial nerve nuclei are often affected as well. Poliomyelitis is an example of classic anterior horn cell disease. It generally presents as an asymmetric paralysis, with associated signs of fever and meningeal irritation. Bulbar involvement is often present as well. It is seen in nonimmunized populations or, rarely, as a result of the (live-attenuated) oral polio vaccine. A lumbar puncture reveals cerebrospinal fluid (CSF) protein elevation and pleocytosis.

Mimicking poliomyelitis is the recently reported Hopkins syndrome, also called acute postasthmatic amyotrophy. It presents as the sudden onset of weakness of one limb, preceded by pain, and sometimes associated with meningism. It generally occurs 1 to 2 weeks after an acute asthmatic attack, when the asthma is well under control. The patients are afebrile at presentation, and the preceding asthma attacks have ranged from mild to severe. Because a specific infectious etiology has yet to be demonstrated, it is currently thought to have an immunologic basis.

TABLE 70.3. Life-Threatening Causes of Weakness	
Cerebrovascular accident	Guillain-Barré syndrome
Spinal cord compression	Infant botulism
Organophosphate or heavy metal poisoning	Rhabdomyolysis
Tick paralysis	

Werdnig-Hoffman disease (Type I spinal muscular atrophy) is a disease of the anterior horn cells that presents with gradual weakness of the proximal muscles. There are three types, with onset of symptoms ranging from birth to 2 years of age. Lower cranial nerve involvement occurs early, leading to feeding difficulties and changes in the quality of the cry. The disease is gradually progressive, with deterioration of muscle strength and eventual respiratory insufficiency.

If peripheral axons are the site of the disease process, motor and sensory functions are both impaired with distal changes usually noted first. In children, one of the more common causes of acute peripheral neuropathy is Guillain-Barré syndrome (GBS) (see Chapter 73). It generally presents as ascending symmetric weakness over days to weeks, usually beginning in the legs and progressing proximally. More than half of the patients will have had an upper respiratory or gastrointestinal infection in the 4 weeks before the onset of the weakness. A large majority of children report pain in the first week of the illness, with subsequent weakness developing in the painful muscles. Children, if old enough, may also describe paresthesias or numbness, often in a stocking-glove distribution. Lumbar puncture may show increased protein concentration in the CSF with no pleocytosis. In fact, the cell count is generally less than 10 lymphocytes per mm^3 and always less than 50 lymphocytes per mm^3. Factors that make the diagnosis of GBS less likely include fever at the time of presentation, age less than 1 year, sharp sensory level, or persistence of bowel or bladder symptoms. Other more likely causes in infants with weakness include the anterior horn cell diseases and infantile botulism, discussed below.

Heavy metal poisoning from lead, arsenic, or thallium can also cause peripheral nerve damage. Lead poisoning is associated with anemia, abdominal pain, constipation, and often encephalopathy in children (see Chapter 78). Thallium ingestion may cause ptosis, alopecia, and vomiting in addition to weakness.

Fish toxins can also cause peripheral neuropathy (see Chapter 78). Ciguatera is an illness caused by a toxin from fish that are found generally in the South Pacific, but occasionally near the lower Atlantic states. Nausea and vomiting begin 4 to 36 hours after ingestion of the fish, followed by paresthesias and weakness, and typically reversal of hot/cold sensation. Ingestion of shellfish contaminated during a "red tide" has been associated with paralysis as well. Initial nausea and vomiting are followed rapidly by paresthesias, cranial nerve involvement, and weakness.

Finally, acute intermittent porphyria is a rare autosomal-dominant cause of peripheral neuropathy and paralysis. It is often associated with abdominal pain. Peripheral motor weakness is present and often is more evident in proximal muscles. Central nervous system involvement may be manifested by altered sensorium and hallucinations, and there may be sensory involvement as well. Acute attacks can be precipitated by drugs such as barbiturates, sulfonamides, griseofulvin, estrogens, and alcohol. Detection of increased porphyrin precursors in the urine, as well as familial history, help make the diagnosis.

Diseases involving the neuromuscular junction (NMJ) can be recognized by their association with cranial nerve findings and autonomic processes. Importantly, sensation is *not* affected. Organophosphate exposure is a classic example of NMJ dysfunction. In addition to muscle fasciculations, muscle cramps, and weakness, patients exposed to organophosphates may have symptoms of altered mental status and cholinergic stimulation (see Chapter 78). Tick paralysis is caused by another toxin that is presumed to affect the NMJ, produced by the dog tick *Dermacentor variabilis* and the Rocky Mountain wood tick

Dermacentor andersoni. Because exposure to the tick often precedes the paralysis by 5 to 10 days, travel history is important. The paralysis is typically ascending, and progresses rapidly over 12 to 36 hours to the bulbar area. Although 50% of patients may complain of paresthesias, the sensory examination is usually normal. A third agent that involves the NMJ is the toxin of *Clostridium botulinum*. If contaminated food is the source of the toxin, within 24 to 48 hours of exposure, patients will experience nausea and vomiting, followed by diplopia, photophobia, and then dysphagia and dysarthria from sequential involvement of cranial nerves. Skeletal muscle paralysis follows without any sensory involvement. In wound botulism, a wound is contaminated with soil containing the spores of the clostridium. It presents in a similar manner except that no gastrointestinal symptoms are associated. Peak incidence is between 2 and 3 months. It commonly presents with a history of constipation, lethargy, and feeding difficulties. On physical examination, hypotonia, general muscle weakness, pooling of oral secretions, and a decreased gag reflex are present, and dilated pupils respond poorly to light. Sensory examination is normal. Deep tendon reflexes may be normal or diminished early, and are generally diminished or absent late in the disease. Finally, myasthenia gravis is a disease process involving the transmission of acetylcholine across the synaptic membrane to its receptors. It is recognized by easy fatigability of muscles and worsening weakness over the course of a day. Sensory examination and deep tendon reflexes are normal. Ptosis is often the most easily recognized symptom.

When the muscle itself is the target of the disease, proximal weakness is often noted first, and sensory function is normal. An example of muscle diseases is the group of inflammatory myopathies in which the muscles are often tender. In dermatomyositis or polymyositis, skin and joint manifestations and proximal weakness are usually present. The characteristic rash in dermatomyositis is an erythema of the upper eyelid area, spreading to a malar distribution. Erythema over the extensor surfaces of joints is often present as well. Deep tendon reflexes diminish as weakness progresses and muscles atrophy. In viral myositis, a febrile respiratory illness is associated with significant muscle tenderness and weakness. Deep tendon reflexes are generally present, and sensory examination is normal. Serum creatine kinase is elevated in all of the inflammatory myopathies. Another muscle disease involves periodic attacks of paralysis associated with either decreased or increased serum potassium. The hypokalemic form may be associated with an autosomal-dominant familial disorder, hyperthyroidism, hyperaldosteronism, chronic renal disease, ingestion of large amounts of licorice, or chronic vomiting or diarrhea. The familial form often presents in adolescence with sudden paralysis that may involve all the extremities, usually after a large carbohydrate meal or during rest after strenuous exercise. Sensory examination is normal. Autosomal-dominant familial hyperkalemic paralysis usually is less severe. Improvement of paralysis should ensue after intravenous correction of the potassium imbalance.

Rhabdomyolysis from excessive physical exertion, prolonged seizures, stimulant-drug overdose, or genetic disorders may result in acute weakness. Muscles are generally tender, myoglobin is evident in the urine, and serum creatine phosphokinase (CPK) and AST are elevated.

Finally, the muscular dystrophies, although usually thought of as more slowly progressive, can present to an emergency physician as a recently noticed weakness by the patient or their family. The forms that present in childhood involve the proximal muscles and are primarily X-linked and thus are seen in boys 3 to 15 years of age. Deep tendon reflexes are present early, but disappear later. Sensory examination is normal, and serum creatine kinase is elevated.

EVALUATION AND DECISION

The approach to the child with weakness or flaccid paralysis is depicted in Fig. 70.1.

The first important historical question is whether the patient had neck or back trauma preceding the weakness. If so, the patient should be immobilized, and spinal radiographs should be taken immediately. Cord transections often result in initially flaccid paralysis and sensory loss below the level of the lesion, along with bladder and rectal incontinence. Deep tendon reflexes may be absent early but will become increased over time. If a patient has these symptoms after trauma, radiographs can confirm a fracture or dislocation. However, a patient with persistent symptoms should remain immobilized until further imaging studies are done because negative radiographs do not completely obviate spinal injury (see Chapter 93).

Once it has been confirmed that the patient has had no trauma, a complete history should be taken. A history of acute weakness associated with abdominal pain or vomiting suggests a possible toxin exposure such as botulism or fish poisoning. Gastrointestinal symptoms may also be associated with heavy metal ingestion, either intentional or accidental. Finally, porphyria should be considered as a possible cause of weakness and abdominal pain.

A history of constipation for several days before the onset of weakness in a child less than 1 year of age highly suggests infantile botulism. Parents often also report several days of lethargy and feeding difficulties as well. Ingestion of honey or proximity to an endemic area would further support the diagnosis.

Before proceeding with the physical examination, the physician should be sure that the patient has not had an organophosphate exposure. Generally, this is given in the history or easily recognized by the strong garliclike smell on the patient and the readily apparent cholinergic symptoms. Health care personnel caring for such a patient should be careful to protect themselves from exposure.

Upon beginning a thorough physical examination, the patient's respiratory and cardiovascular status should be assessed. Although rare, some diseases cause rapidly progressive weakness and may quickly involve the respiratory muscles or gag reflex.

One of the main goals of the physical examination in a patient with acute weakness is to locate the site of the disease process. Acute hemiplegia, with or without facial involvement or mental status changes, should direct the physician to an intracranial process such as a cerebral infarction or hemorrhage. Any child suspected of having a CVA should be stabilized and have a computed tomography (CT) scan of the head done promptly. Rarely, seizures or complicated migraines can be associated with hemiplegia, but usually the possibility of an intracranial event must be eliminated first.

When evaluating a patient with a complaint of weakness, a thorough motor examination will help define and locate the disease process. Deep tendon reflexes should be classified as normal, increased, diminished, or absent. A careful sensory examination should be done, both to light touch and to pain, as well as vibratory and position sense. It should be determined whether a spinal level of sensory loss is detectable. The patient's back should be examined for swelling, erythema, loss of normal lordosis, point tenderness, rigidity, or splinting. Cranial nerves should be carefully assessed, looking specifically for ophthal-

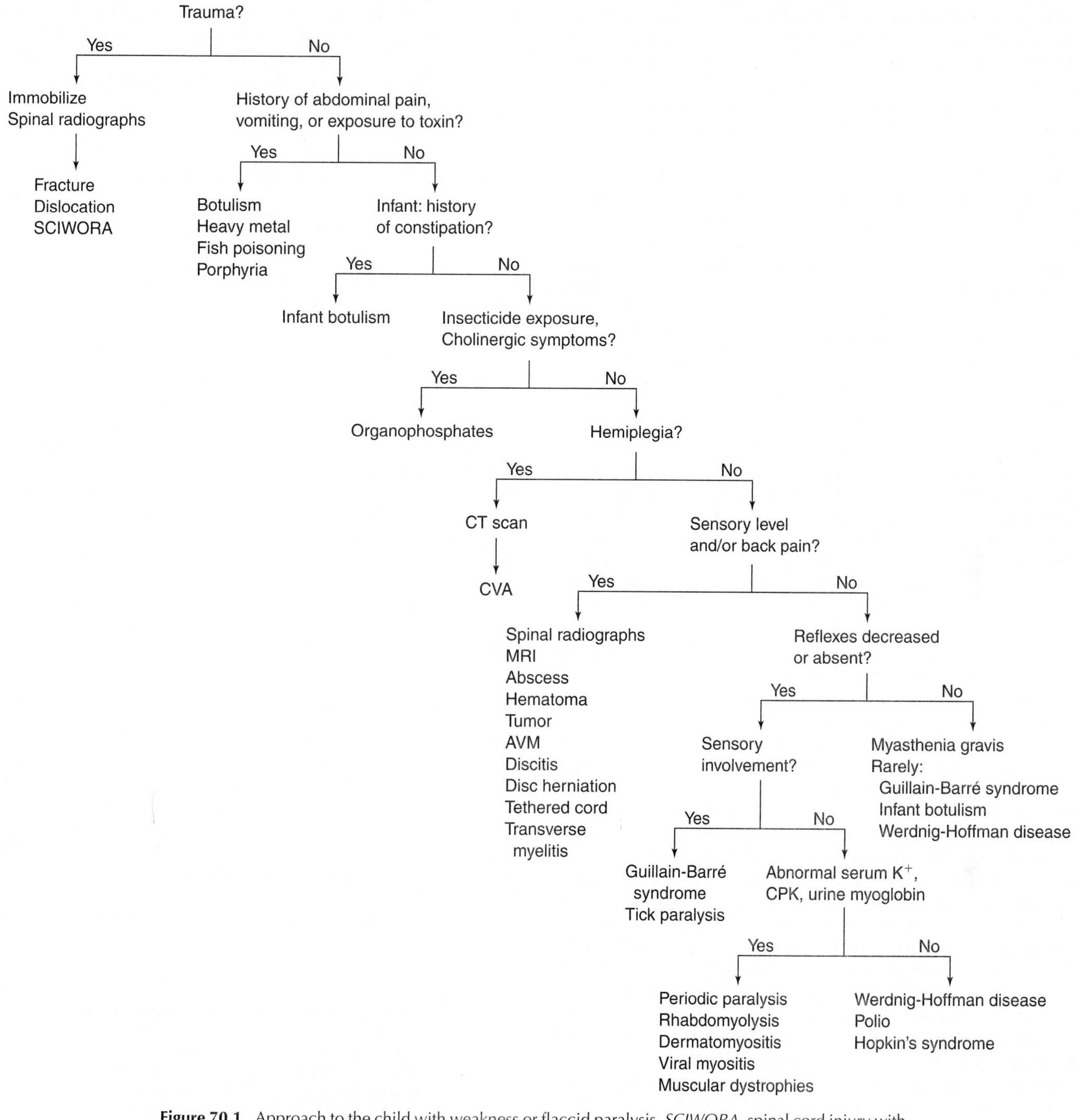

Figure 70.1. Approach to the child with weakness or flaccid paralysis. *SCIWORA,* spinal cord injury without obvious radiographic abnormality; *CT,* computed tomography; *CVA,* cerebrovascular accident; *MRI,* magnetic resonance imaging; *AVM,* arteriovenous malformation; *CPK,* creatine phosphokinase.

moplegia, facial weakness, or bulbar weakness as evidenced by dysphagia, dysarthria, or decreased gag.

Initially, the physician should determine whether the patient has signs and symptoms consistent with an acute or subacute spinal cord compression. Although spinal cord compression may have many etiologies that present similarly, some factors may be helpful in making a diagnosis. Acute onset of symptoms with associated fever and back pain suggests an epidural abscess or transverse myelitis. A patient with an epidural abscess may have point tenderness over the affected area in addition to the paralysis and bowel and bladder dysfunction. In transverse myelitis, prominent sensory loss occurs for pain and temperature, usually with a definable spinal sensory level corresponding to the level of back pain. Acute onset of symptoms without fever may indicate a spontaneous hemorrhage from an AVM. A more subacute presentation may suggest a spinal or paraspinal tumor. Disc herniation is less common in children but may be associated with trauma or symptoms of sciatica. Evidence of spinal dysraphism, such as a hair tuft, dermal sinus, or lipoma, may be a clue to a tethered cord, which also usually presents with a more gradual onset of weakness. Initial evaluation of any patient with signs and symptoms suggesting spinal cord compression should include spinal radiographs, usually followed by magnetic resonance imaging (see Chapter 110).

Assessment of deep tendon reflexes is the next important step in differentiating causes of weakness. Diseases of the NMJ, such as myasthenia gravis, should have normal reflexes. Myasthenia may also be recognized by the involvement of cranial nerves producing dysphagia, facial weakness, and ophthalmoplegia. Rarely, early in their course, other disease processes may present with weakness and normal deep tendon reflexes. However, they can be differentiated from myasthenia gravis by other factors.

Decreased or absent reflexes, when not caused by early spinal cord compression, are a sign of disease in the anterior horn cell, peripheral nerve, or muscle. The physician can use the sensory examination to further distinguish these. If there is abnormal sensation on examination or subjective reporting of paresthesias, the disease is in the peripheral nerves. The most common cause for an acute or subacute onset of ascending flaccid paralysis, with diminished or absent deep tendon reflexes and associated sensory symptoms, is GBS (see Chapter 73). On physical examination, there may be demonstrable sensory loss, as well as loss of position and vibratory sense. Motor weakness, most often asymmetric and distal, is clinically apparent, although 10% to 20% of patients may have descending paralysis or proximal-greater-than-distal weakness. The combination of lower extremity weakness and sensory changes often causes the child to have an abnormal gait, which is often the presenting symptom. Deep tendon reflexes are diminished or absent in the weak muscles, although they may be preserved in less-affected muscles early in the course of the illness. Associated cranial nerve involvement is seen in 30% to 40% of patients, usually manifested by facial weakness or ocular paresis. Pupillary response is not affected, and rarely are the lower cranial nerves involved. Occasionally, children have autonomic symptoms, including arrhythmias and blood pressure lability. These can become severe and, in some cases, life threatening.

Tick paralysis can present similarly to GBS. Any patient with acute onset of ascending paralysis associated with dysesthesias or cranial nerve palsies should be carefully examined for ticks, particularly in the scalp and hairline. Removal of the tick results in dramatic and complete improvement.

In a patient with decreased or absent deep tendon reflexes but normal sensory examination, the disease process is either in the anterior horn cells or in the muscles. Examples of anterior horn cell disease include spinal muscular atrophy (Werdnig-Hoffman disease), enteroviral infection such as polio, and Hopkins syndrome. In Werdnig-Hoffman disease, the infants have no associated pupillary or ocular motility dysfunction but are noted to have tongue fasciculations and a decreased gag reflex. Proximal muscles are weak, and deep tendon reflexes are diminished or absent. Sensory examination is normal.

Polio and Hopkins syndrome both present with a unilateral, asymmetric paralysis. Polio is associated with fever, irritability, and often meningeal signs. There may be an antecedent history of exposure in a person who is not immunized or on oral vaccine administration in a young infant. Hopkins syndrome is associated with a preceding asthma exacerbation, but the patient usually has no other symptoms at the time of presentation of the weakness.

Although infant botulism is a disease process of the NMJ and reflexes should be preserved, it may be confused with anterior horn disease because reflexes may in general be difficult to elicit or appreciate in a young infant. It will otherwise present similarly, with progressive weakness and normal sensory examination. Infant botulism may be distinguished by a history of constipation and the presence of dilated pupils that are poorly reactive to light.

Disease processes involving the muscle present with weakness, decreased reflexes, and a normal sensory examination. These include hypokalemia, hyperkalemia, rhabdomyolysis, inflammatory myopathies, and muscular dystrophies. These can be distinguished from anterior horn cell diseases by history, physical examination, and laboratory evidence of abnormal serum potassium, elevated CPK, or urine myoglobin.

CHAPTER 71
Wheezing

Bruce Rosenthal, M.D.

Wheezes are continuous whistling or musical adventitial sounds that are the hallmark of lower airway obstruction. Table 71.1 provides a simplified pathophysiologic classification of conditions that cause wheezing in children. Table 71.2 outlines the relative prevalence of those conditions associated with wheezing in children with which the emergency physician should be most familiar, and Table 71.3 lists the life-threatening causes of wheezing.

DIFFERENTIAL DIAGNOSIS

Most Common Conditions

Bronchiolitis is an acute viral infection of the lower respiratory tract caused predominantly by respiratory syncytial virus (RSV). Occurring in epidemics between late fall and early spring, this condition primarily affects infants 2 to 6 months of age but may occur in children as old as 2 to 3 years of age. Rhinorrhea and a low-grade fever typically accompany a prominent staccatolike cough and a variable degree of respiratory distress.

Asthma is a chronic inflammatory disorder of the airways,

TABLE 71.1. Causes of Wheezing in Childhood

Extrinsic airway compression	Inflammation
Congenital structural anomalies	Asthma
Cystic malformations of the lung	Bronchiolitis
Vascular ring	Smoke inhalation
Cardiovascular enlargement	Toxocariasis
Mediastinal tumors	Pulmonary hemosiderosis
Teratoma, neuroblastoma, thymoma, ganglioneuroma, pheochromocytoma	Pulmonary aspiration
Enlarged mediastinal lymph nodes	Gastroesophageal reflux
Tuberculosis, sarcoidosis, leukemia, lymphoma	Swallowing disorders
Intrinsic airway narrowing	Tracheoesophageal fistula
Structural anomalies	*Intraluminal airway obstruction*
Tracheobronchomalacia/stenosis	Foreign body aspiration
Bronchopulmonary dysplasia	*Miscellaneous causes*
α_1-Antitrypsin deficiency	Congestive heart failure
Bronchospasm	Immune deficiency
Anaphylaxis	Cystic fibrosis
Organophosphate poisoning	Immotile cilia syndrome

TABLE 71.2. Clinical Classification of Wheezing: Age at Diagnosis and Disease Prevalence

Disease prevalence	<1 yr	>1 yr
Common	Bronchiolitis Asthma	Asthma

Less common	Pulmonary aspiration
	  Gastroesophageal reflux
	  Swallowing disorder
	Foreign body
	Bronchopulmonary dysplasia
	Cystic fibrosis
		Foreign body aspiration
		Anaphylaxis

Uncommon	Congenital heart disease
	Defective host defenses
	  Immune deficiency
	  Immotile cilia syndrome
	Congenital structural anomalies
	  Tracheobronchomalacia
	  Vascular ring
	  Lobar emphysema
	  Cystic abnormalities
	  Tracheoesophageal fistula
		Defective host defenses
		Mediastinal tumors or enlarged lymph nodes
		Parasitic infection
		Pulmonary hemosiderosis
		α_1-Antitrypsin deficiency

characterized clinically by *recurrent* episodes of coughing and/or wheezing. Acute exacerbations of asthma are usually triggered by respiratory infections, allergens, and irritants such as cigarette smoke. Patients with asthma have a higher incidence of associated atopic disease, which includes allergic rhinitis and conjunctivitis and atopic dermatitis.

Less Common Conditions

Pulmonary aspiration is a less common cause of wheezing that occurs in several fairly characteristic clinical circumstances. Recurrent aspiration of oropharyngeal foodstuffs or gastric contents is usually seen in patients with severe developmental delay and a variety of neuromuscular diseases. Repeated aspiration is also seen in children with structural anomalies of the laryngeal complex or an H-type tracheoesophageal fistula. Patients with chronic recurrent aspiration may develop wheezing and respiratory distress in the absence of a well-defined episode of choking or severe coughing because many such patients have depressed cough reflexes or experience "microaspiration." Fever often accompanies pulmonary aspiration, reflecting associated chemical inflammation or infection of the tracheobronchial tree.

In otherwise healthy children, the abrupt onset of respiratory distress, associated with an episode of coughing, choking, or gagging, suggests the pulmonary inhalation of a foreign object (see Chapter 22). Foreign body aspiration is typically seen in toddlers, although older infants may aspirate solid food particles or small objects placed within their reach. The aspiration of a small object or food substance may be unwitnessed and go unrecognized for weeks or months until persistent lower respiratory symptoms trigger a search for an underlying cause. In these circumstances, persistent cough, wheezing, and sometimes recurrent fever is associated with an area of consolidation and/or collapse on radiograph; these symptoms fail to resolve despite seemingly appropriate medical therapy for presumed asthma and/or pneumonia.

TABLE 71.3. Life-Threatening Causes of Wheezing

Asthma (severe)	Mediastinal tumor
Bronchiolitis (severe)	Congestive heart failure
Foreign body	

Wheezing attributable to anaphylaxis is also of sudden onset and usually is accompanied by one or more other clinical findings that include urticaria, angioedema, stridor, and hypotension. When wheezing is the only finding, anaphylaxis may be suspected when the onset of respiratory difficulty is associated closely with Hymenoptera envenomation or food ingestion.

Infants and young children with a history of prematurity, oxygen therapy, and ventilatory support for a variety of conditions occurring in the newborn period may have wheezing caused by bronchopulmonary dysplasia (BPD). This condition is the childhood equivalent of chronic obstructive lung disease and represents a pathophysiologic continuum that includes varying degrees of structural damage and airway inflammation.

Uncommon Conditions

Cardiovascular abnormalities are one of many uncommon causes of wheezing in children. Small airway edema in the setting of congestive heart failure or airway impingement by enlarged cardiovascular structures are the usual pathophysiologic mechanisms. Most such cardiac conditions are associated with other abnormal physical findings, including cyanosis, murmurs, abnormal pulses, poor perfusion, or signs consistent with congestive heart failure. A congenital vascular ring may cause wheezing secondary to extrinsic airway compression. Abnormal cardiac physical findings are generally absent in patients with a vascular ring, although concomitant esophageal compression may result in dysphagia. A right-sided aortic arch is associated with this anomaly.

Children with various defects in host defense mechanisms often present with recurrent wheezing and bacterial pulmonary infections. In addition to respiratory tract involvement, patients with cystic fibrosis (see Chapter 85) will often exhibit steatorrhea and growth failure because of pancreatic insufficiency and malabsorption. Children with cell-mediated or humoral immune deficiency syndromes can have opportunistic infections or repeated extrapulmonary infections, including meningitis, otitis media, otitis externa, furunculosis, and mucocutaneous candidiasis. Similarly, patients with the immotile cilia syndrome develop repeated sinusitis and otitis media, often in association with situs inversus viscerum and bronchiectasis (Kartagener syndrome).

Other uncommon causes of wheezing include extrinsic tracheobronchial compression by an enlarged lymph node or tumor. Mediastinal or hilar lymph node enlargement most often is the result of leukemia, lymphoma, sarcoidosis, or a mycobacterial or fungal infection. Mediastinal tumors most likely to produce pulmonary symptomatology include neuroblastoma, pheochromocytoma, ganglioneuroma, thymoma, and teratoma.

Congenital structural anomalies of the respiratory tract, including bronchogenic cysts, intrinsic stenosis, and webs, are among the rarest causes of wheezing in children. Respiratory symptoms typically begin in the neonatal period or early infancy. The predominant clinical features will be determined by the site of abnormality within the tracheobronchial tree. Stridor and a croupy cough are typical of laryngotracheal constriction, whereas wheezing and recurrent pneumonia are more characteristic of bronchial narrowing. Respiratory findings generally worsen with intercurrent respiratory infection and may accentuate with crying and activity.

EVALUATION AND DECISION

General Considerations

Table 71.4 presents a capsule summary of the clinical features associated with the more prevalent causes of wheezing in childhood. Thorough history taking is the key to arriving at an accurate diagnosis in a child with wheezing. In particular, consideration of the age at onset, course and pattern of illness, and associated clinical features provides a useful framework for approaching a differential diagnosis (Figs. 71.1 and 71.2).

The onset of wheezing in the neonatal period is associated with congenital structural airway anomalies, although a history of prematurity and mechanical ventilation is more suggestive of BPD. The *first episode* of wheezing in an otherwise healthy infant in association with cold symptoms indicates bronchiolitis. *Recurrent episodes* of wheezing precipitated by colds and a variety of other triggers is the hallmark of asthma. On the other hand, *recurrent wheezing beginning in infancy*, or *"difficult to control asthma,"* at any age should lead to a consideration of cystic fibrosis, gastroesophageal reflux, recurrent pulmonary aspiration or a retained airway foreign body, or immune deficiency. *Persistent wheezing* at any age suggests mechanical airway obstruction from a variety of causes, including congenital airway narrowing, pulmonary foreign body, and compression by a mediastinal tumor. The *sudden onset* of wheezing is characteristic of pulmonary aspiration or anaphylaxis.

As indicated previously, the diagnosis of a chronic wheezing disorder, such as asthma, relies on the identification of recurrent episodes of obstructive lower airway disease. Unfortunately, limitations of parental recall combined with the misdiagnosis of previous bronchospastic episodes as infectious illnesses sometimes make it a challenge to reconstruct an accurate history. In particular, subtle manifestations of asthma are often misinterpreted as episodes of bronchitis, pneumonia, or bronchiolitis. Cough as a salient feature in patients with obstructive lower airway disease cannot be overemphasized. In fact, in many patients with asthma, recurrent cough may be the predominant presenting clinical feature and wheezing may be absent despite careful lung auscultation ("cough variant asthma").

TABLE 71.4. Clinical Features and Associated Diagnoses

Clinical features	Associated diagnoses
First episode Winter months Upper respiratory infection (URI) symptoms <12 mo of age	Bronchiolitis
Recurrent episodes URI or environmental trigger Personal history of eczema or hay fever Family history of asthma	Asthma
Developmental delay Cerebral palsy Neuromuscular disease Swallowing dysfunction	Aspiration syndrome
Sudden onset Healthy child >6 mo of age Choking and coughing	Foreign body aspiration
Sudden onset Urticaria and/or stridor Environmental exposure	Anaphylaxis
Prematurity Mechanical ventilation Prolonged oxygen therapy	Bronchopulmonary dysplasia
Recurrent wheezing in infancy Failure to thrive Steatorrhea	Cystic fibrosis
Heart murmur Cardiomegaly Hepatomegaly Failure to thrive	Cardiac disease

Modified from Martinati LC, Boner AL. Clinical diagnosis of wheezing in early childhood. *Allergy* 1995;50:701–710, with permission.

Physical Examination

Wheezing must be distinguished from other causes of "noisy breathing" in children, including the stridor of upper airway obstruction (see Chapter 63), the stertor of nasal congestion, and audible rhonchi. Wheezes tend to be polyphonic in pitch and distributed somewhat unevenly in intensity and location, despite the fact that most disorders causing lower airway obstruction affect both lungs simultaneously. Conversely, wheezes consistently limited to a single lung field suggest a localized obstructive process, such as a foreign body or an extrinsic mass lesion. Key "extrapulmonary" physical findings associated with the more prevalent causes of wheezing in childhood are included in Table 71.4.

Diagnostic Tests

Only a limited number of diagnostic modalities are needed to support the initial evaluation of the wheezing child. Many other necessary investigations can be performed as part of a subsequent inpatient or outpatient workup. The chest radiograph is the most important test obtained in the emergency department. Even so, its value is limited in helping establish a definitive diagnosis in a wheezing child. Rather, the chest radiograph assists in identifying disease complications such as pneumonia, atelectasis, pneumothorax, or pneumomediastinum. Among the few conditions that can be conclusively identified on the basis of plain film findings are heart disease, mediastinal masses, and some foreign bodies of the airway and esophagus.

Varying degrees of hyperaeration, bronchiolar thickening, and subsegmental atelectasis are the most common radiograph findings in patients with bronchiolitis or asthma. Pulmonary infiltrates may reflect the primary viral disease process in bronchiolitis or the complication of airway obstruction in asthma.

Abrupt onset?
No
Yes
Fever/URI symptoms?
Pulmonary aspiration
No
Yes
Neurologic disability, recurrent vomiting?
Prior wheezing episodes?
Yes
No
Asthma
Bronchiolitis
No
Yes
Mechanical ventilation at birth?
Pulmonary aspiration
No
Yes
Recurrent pneumonia, failure to thrive?
Bronchopulmonary dysplasia
No
Yes
Heart murmur, hepatomegaly?
Cystic fibrosis
Immune deficiency
No
Yes
Stridor?
Congenital heart disease
No
Yes
Bronchiolitis
Concurrent croup
Congenital structural anomaly

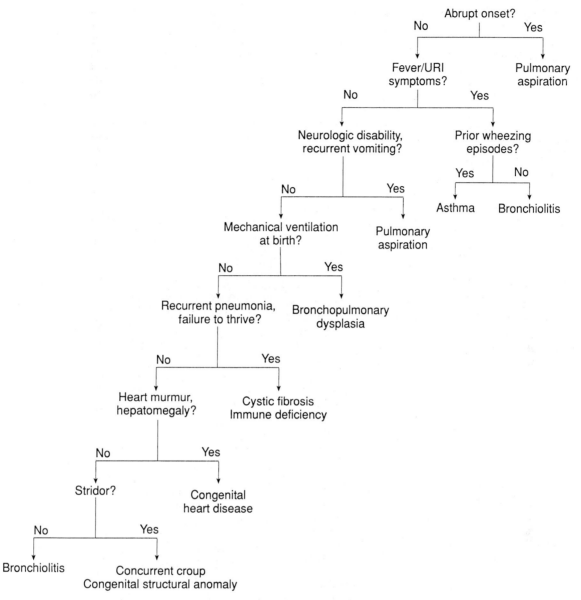

Figure 71.1. Approach to wheezing in children under 1 year of age. *URI,* upper respiratory infection.

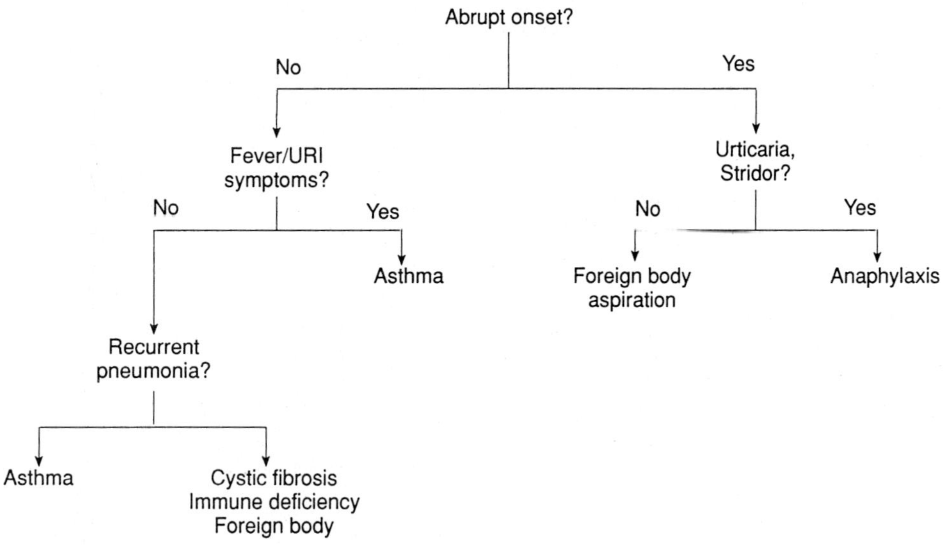

Figure 71.2. Approach to wheezing in children 1 year old or older. *URI,* upper respiratory infection.

When either disorder is suspected, a chest radiograph usually can be avoided if the patient is afebrile and little to no respiratory distress is present.

Patients suspected of having aspirated oropharyngeal or gastric contents should have plain radiographs taken of the chest. Nonspecific findings consistent with lower airway obstruction generally precede the appearance of infiltrates. The location of the latter depends on the position of the patient at the time of the aspiration event. Patients thought to have recurring episodes of pulmonary aspiration subsequently should have further testing to identify swallowing dysfunction, gastroesophageal reflux, or actual tracheobronchial soiling. Such tests might include a barium esophagram, esophageal pH monitoring, esophageal endoscopy and biopsy, or radionuclide scintigraphy ("milk" scan). Fiberoptic bronchoscopy may be required to diagnose patients with a tracheoesophageal fistula.

An immediate and aggressive workup is always justified in patients suspected of having an airway foreign body (see Chapter 22) on the basis of acute and sudden symptomatology. In this setting, chest radiographs are usually normal, although occasionally they can demonstrate a radiopaque object, the faint outlines of a radiolucent foreign body, segmental atelectasis, or a focal area of hyperinflation. Patients with a persistent lower airway foreign body are more likely to show focal collapse and consolidation that is evident on standard chest roentgenograms. Bilateral decubitus views, inspiratory and expiratory radiographs, or airway fluoroscopy may be used to provide additional diagnostic information. Bronchoscopy is the procedure of choice both from a diagnostic and therapeutic perspective when a foreign body is strongly suspected.

Newborn screening should identify most children with cystic fibrosis. Nevertheless, infants with recurrent wheezing and those with failure to thrive associated with chronic diarrhea should be referred for sweat chloride testing.

A patient suspected of having congenital or acquired heart disease should have an electrocardiogram (ECG) and a chest radiograph performed in the emergency department. Definitive diagnosis generally requires echocardiography or cardiac catheterization. A barium swallow is usually sufficient to diagnose the presence of a vascular ring, although angiography is necessary for exact anatomic definition.

Approach

INFANT LESS THAN 1 YEAR OLD

An algorithm for elucidating the cause of wheezing in the child less than 1 year old is presented in Fig. 71.1. The abrupt onset of wheezing, often immediately preceded by an episode of choking, gagging, or vomiting, is highly suggestive of pulmonary aspiration; foreign body aspiration should be considered in the previously healthy older infant, whereas gastroesophageal reflux with aspiration of gastric contents is a more likely cause in early infancy. However, most young infants who present with a first episode of wheezing have bronchiolitis. In this illness, fever and upper respiratory symptoms usually accompany wheezing and respiratory distress during the winter months. A similar complex of physical findings in an older infant with a history of bronchiolitis or wheezing and clear improvement after bronchodilator administration is characteristic of asthma.

The remaining disorders often are found in infants who have overt evidence of chronic or severe underlying illness and who typically present with recurrent or persistent episodes of wheezing and respiratory distress. Neurologic disability predisposes a child to gastroesophageal reflux or a swallowing disorder and recurrent pulmonary aspiration. A report of prematurity and/or respiratory difficulty at birth may be a clue to BPD. Recurrent pneumonia, failure to thrive, and steatorrhea are characteristic of infants with cystic fibrosis, whereas pneumonia in association with repeated extrapulmonary infection is suggestive of an immune deficiency. A heart murmur and other clinical findings consistent with congestive heart failure are indicative of congenital heart disease and pulmonary edema. Wheezing accompanied by stridor commonly indicates the coexistence of viral croup but may reflect intrinsic congenital airway narrowing, such as tracheobronchomalacia or extrinsic compression by a mediastinal structure. In the absence of any of the clinical clues listed, the first episode of wheezing in an otherwise healthy child, especially when it occurs during the winter months, is likely to represent bronchiolitis.

CHILD 1 YEAR OLD OR OLDER

Figure 71.2 outlines an algorithmic approach to the more common causes of wheezing in the child who is 1 year old or older. The sudden onset of respiratory distress and wheezing associated with an episode of choking and coughing is likely to indicate foreign body aspiration, particularly in a toddler who has been eating or playing with a small object. An abrupt onset of wheezing also may accompany stridor, urticaria, and hypotension in the older child with an anaphylactic reaction. However, most first or recurrent episodes of wheezing represent asthma. Typically, such episodes are precipitated by a concurrent upper respiratory infection, and the patient may show responsiveness to bronchodilator administration.

Wheezing and recurrent pneumonia in multiple pulmonary segments are characteristic of patients with defects in host defense mechanisms, such as cystic fibrosis, an immune deficiency syndrome, or the immotile cilia syndrome. Children in this age group who present with these disorders usually have a history of lower respiratory illness that began in infancy, as well as other signs and symptoms suggestive of chronic disease. Repeated pneumonia in the same pulmonary segment in an otherwise healthy child that begins in late infancy or in early childhood is likely to represent a previously unrecognized bronchial foreign body. In the absence of any of the clinical clues previously listed, the first episode of wheezing in an otherwise healthy child is likely to represent asthma.

SECTION

III

Medical Emergencies

CHAPTER 72

Cardiac Emergencies

Michael H. Gewitz, M.D. and
Victoria L. Vetter, M.D.

CONGESTIVE HEART FAILURE

Background

Heart failure is best described as a syndrome in which the heart cannot maintain a level of tissue perfusion adequate to meet metabolic needs. During childhood, these needs also include growth and development. Although the primary cause of congestive heart failure (CHF) in infants and children is congenital heart disease, a number of conditions can be associated with the presentation of CHF in the presence of normal underlying cardiac structures.

CLINICAL MANIFESTATIONS

The clinical manifestations of CHF are directly related to the compensatory mechanisms:

1. Cardiac enlargement usually is the result of ventricular dilation. Although it often may be possible to detect cardiac enlargement by displacement of the cardiac impulse, the chest radiograph remains the most readily available method for assessing ventricular dilation. The other preeminent finding related to mechanical compensatory responses is ventricular hypertrophy, which is easily distinguishable on the electrocardiogram (ECG).
2. A rate of more than 160 beats per minute (bpm) in an infant or 100 bpm in the older child may be a signal for increased adrenergic tone and catecholamine release that is part of the neurohumoral response to diminished cardiac output.
3. The protodiastolic gallop, or third heart sound (S_3), is a sign of decreased ventricular compliance and increased resistance to filling. Less often, the fourth heart sound, or atrial gallop (S_4), can be heard in children. It should be noted that these auscultatory events can be normal findings in children, and thus, the entire clinical picture must be evaluated before defining their significance in any particular situation.
4. Respiratory responses, notably tachypnea, usually are present as part of the total picture of CHF. Often, rales, rhonchi, and wheezing may be heard and should not be confused as signs of pulmonary parenchymal disease rather than heart failure. In contrast, it is not unusual, particularly in infants, for rales to be absent despite the presence of tachypnea or wheezing because considerable alveolar fluid accumulation is necessary for the development of rales. Thus, the presence of rales usually implies severe failure in an infant, whereas pulmonary interstitial fluid collection, which occurs at an earlier stage, may be represented by tachypnea and wheezing alone. In older children, dyspnea with activity and orthopnea also may be present. A chronic cough also can be a sign of pulmonary congestion associated with CHF and not primary lung disease. Associated with these findings are chest retractions that reflect the large negative intrathoracic pressures needed to ventilate stiff, fluid-filled lungs.
5. Growth failure and undernutrition may be important clinical correlates of chronic CHF. Feeding difficulties, which may be associated with the respiratory patterns previously noted, aggravate caloric balance even further.
6. Cool, moist extremities and a generalized pallor also may be present as a result of peripheral vasoconstriction secondary to catecholamine release and the need to maintain blood pressure (BP) in the face of reduced CO.
7. Central and peripheral fluid accumulation with elevated systemic venous pressure also accompanies CHF, reflecting impaired cardiac emptying, as well as impaired sodium and protein balance. Hepatomegaly, jugular venous distension, and peripheral edema represent the clinical manifestations of this aspect of the problem. Peripheral edema, it should be noted, is an unusual finding in young infants.

The child with overt CHF who is seen in the emergency department (ED) may present with nearly all the aforementioned signs and symptoms. If the child is severely ill, pallor will be evident, tachypnea prominent, and intercostal retractions visible. The liver is enlarged and palpable well below the right costal margin; a spleen tip also may be palpable. The pulses are weak and thready, and the skin may be moist and cool to the touch. Auscultation of the chest reveals rales, rhonchi, and sometimes, wheezes. Tachycardia is present, and auscultation of the heart sounds often elicits a gallop rhythm. Murmurs may be strikingly absent unless preexisting heart disease is present. A child with this spectrum of findings deserves immediate attention. Acute heart failure in a child usually implies an unstable situation with possible rapid deterioration.

Laboratory Findings

Usually, a clinical diagnosis of CHF can be made without extensive radiographs or laboratory tests. However, certain objective changes may corroborate the clinical findings:

1. As noted, a chest radiograph shows an increased cardiothoracic ratio, as well as pulmonary congestion. Kerley B lines or platelike atelectasis at the lung bases, which reflect dilated pulmonary lymphatics, may be present. Pleural effusions are common.
2. The ECG is a nonspecific indicator of cardiac decompensation. The precordial voltages decrease in certain conditions associated with CHF, such as myocarditis, but may be normal

or increased in other situations despite overt CHF. The ECG is helpful also for establishing the cause of the CHF, such as cardiac arrhythmia or myocardial ischemia.

3. Echocardiography or radionuclide studies can be helpful in evaluating the child with CHF. The differentiation of an enlarged cardiac silhouette secondary to impaired cardiac performance with ventricular chamber enlargement rather than pericardial fluid accumulation can best be made by ultrasound examination. In addition, functional indices can be obtained as an objective measure of cardiac performance and response to therapy.
4. Blood gas abnormalities may be present. Prolonged tissue hypoperfusion can result in metabolic acidosis of a significant degree, and the pulmonary abnormalities already noted may result in hypoxia.
5. Other abnormalities that may be present include electrolyte changes (hyponatremia and hypochloremia) and a reduction in hematocrit, based on dilutional factors. The erythrocyte sedimentation rate (ESR) usually is lowered in active CHF. In addition, in infants with CHF, serum glucose and calcium should be monitored because deficiencies in either may be responsible in large measure for the impaired cardiac function. In situations of suspected perfusion abnormalities or inflammatory myocardial diseases, cardiac enzymes—creatine phosphokinase (CPK) in particular—may be elevated.

MANAGEMENT

For the patient who requires emergency treatment of CHF, initial medical therapy includes several therapeutic measures as outlined in Table 72.1. First, supplemental oxygen should be given through a humidified system. Second, elevation of head and shoulders is helpful in the face of pulmonary edema, with maintenance of the lower extremities in a dependent position to increase peripheral pooling and thus diminish pulmonary blood volume. Third, morphine sulfate (0.05 to 0.1 mg per kg subcutaneously) can be helpful in the face of agitation and air hunger associated with pulmonary edema. Fourth, positive-pressure respiration by endotracheal intubation is sometimes indicated for severe situations, particularly if arterial blood gas analysis shows respiratory decompensation (Pa_{CO_2} 50 mm Hg). In infants, the use of controlled mechanical ventilation to improve respiratory status greatly enhances survival. Fifth, bicarbonate therapy sometimes is indicated to correct metabolic acidosis that arises from diminished tissue perfusion. It should be remembered that administration of sodium bicarbonate during respiratory decompensation is hazardous because further Pa_{CO_2} elevation can occur. Thus, only for severe acidosis (pH less than 7.2) should bicarbonate be considered and, even then, only if respiratory function is satisfactory (see Chapter 84). Last, an intravenous (i.v.) infusion should be started to aid in the administration of drugs and the strict monitoring and administration of fluids.

Blood products in the form of packed cells should be administered if the child is severely anemic. Antibiotics should be reserved for unequivocal evidence of infection or for situations in which circumstantial evidence is strongly suggestive and appropriate cultures have been drawn. The use of corticosteroids may be indicated at times, particularly for heart failure precipitated by rheumatic heart disease. Treatment of arrhythmias that result in CHF is discussed later in this chapter under "Cardiac Arrhythmias."

Although newer inotropic agents have become available, the mainstay of the medical management of CHF is still digitalis, or other well-tested inotropic agents, to improve contractility and diuretics to manipulate ventricular preload and intrapulmonary fluid. Recently, pharmacologic adjustments of afterload have become an important part of CHF treatment.

Digitalis

The drugs of choice for improving the inotropic condition of the heart, unless the CO is severely compromised and the child is acutely ill, are the digitalis glycosides (Table 72.2).

Parenteral digoxin preparations contain 100 μg per mL, and oral preparations contain 50 μg per mL. In the emergency setting, parenteral administration often is the preferred route. If given i.v., the calculated oral dose is reduced by 25%, and the child should be monitored for sudden changes in heart rate (HR) or rhythm. The total digitalizing dose is given over 24 hours (one-half initially, then one-fourth in 8 to 12 hours, and one-fourth in another 8 to 12 hours). The daily maintenance dosage is one-fourth of the total digitalizing dose divided into twice daily doses.

TABLE 72.1. Emergency Management of Congestive Heart Failure

Define cause, if possible, through history and physical examination.	Perform arterial blood gas determination.
Elevate head and chest.	Achieve rhythm control.
Ensure adequacy of ventilation.	Treat pulmonary edema (e.g., diuretics, morphine sulfate).
Administer oxygen.	Provide inotropic support (digitalis or catecholamines).
Initiate cardiorespiratory monitoring, including frequent blood pressure measurement.	Consider afterload reduction.
Achieve venous access and obtain laboratory studies (e.g., complete blood count, electrolytes).	

TABLE 72.2. Digitalization with Digoxin

I. Usual doses (i.m. or oral)		
	Weight (g)	Dose (TDD)[a]
Premature infants	500–1000	20 μg/kg or 0.02 mg/kg
	1,000–1,500	20–30 μg/kg or 0.02–0.03 mg/kg
	1,500–2,000	30 μg/kg or 0.03 mg/kg
	2,000–2,500	30–40 μg/kg or 0.03–0.04 mg/kg
Term to 12 yr		40–60 μg/kg or 0.04–0.06 mg/kg (no dose greater than 1.5 mg TDD)
II. Alterations in usual doses		
Lower if renal function is impaired		
Lower in presence of poor myocardial function (cardiomyopathy, myocarditis)		
Lower in presence of metabolic imbalance (electrolyte abnormalities, hypoxia, acidosis)		
i.v. dose is 75% of oral or i.m. dose		

i.m., intramuscular; TDD, total digitalizing doses; i.v., intravenous.
[a] Digitalizing regimen usually given as initial dose = one-half of TDD; second dose = one-fourth of TDD, at 8–12 h; third dose = final one-fourth TDD at 8–12 h after second dose. Maintenance is then started as one-eighth TDD every 12 h. (Note: Parenteral preparation contains 100 μg/mL and oral, 50 μg/mL.)

TABLE 72.3. Treatment of Heart Block

Drug	Route	Dose
Epinephrine	i.v.	0.01–0.05 mg/kg (0.1 mL/kg of 1:10,000 solution or 0.01 mL/kg of 1:1,000 solution)
Isoproterenol	Infusion	0.1–2.0 μ/kg/min
	Infusion	0.1–2.0 μ/kg/min

Other Inotropic Agents

In situations of severely compromised CO, isoproterenol or dopamine, both α-receptor agonists, has been used successfully in infants and children. Dobutamine, an analog of dopamine, also has been found to be useful in such circumstances, particularly when impaired myocardial perfusion is part of the underlying problem. Isoproterenol (Isuprel) has vigorous inotropic effects, as well as significant chronotropic effects. The starting dose is 0.1 μg/kg per minute by continuous infusion (Table 72.3). Initial doses of dopamine in pediatric patients range from 2 to 5 μg/kg per minute given by continual infusion. For severe systemic hypotension, 5 to 10 μg per kg per minute may be used as the starting dose. Dobutamine is administered in similar fashion to dopamine with initial doses that range from 2.5 to 5.0 μg per kg per minute.

Diuretics

The so-called loop diuretics are used most commonly for the acute treatment of CHF. Furosemide (Lasix) is the most popular. An initial dose of 1 mg per kg i.v. usually results in adequate urine flow within 1 to 2 hours of administration.

With the proper use of digitalis and diuretic therapy, improvement can be achieved in most children with CHF. Failure to improve an exacerbation of CHF in children already taking these medications requires scrutiny for any of the following: 1) persistent arrhythmia; 2) untreated or unrecognized infection; 3) anemia, especially in the infant with CHF; 4) inadequate or excessive digitalis dose, particularly in the patient with inflammatory myocardial disease; or 5) electrolyte disturbance, such as hypokalemia, which may be worsened with diuretics. If these entities can be ruled out, more intensive treatment is indicated to improve CO.

Other Noncatecholamine Agents

In the patient with CHF in whom standard digoxin and/or catecholamine therapy does not provide improved peripheral perfusion status, use of amrinone (i.v.) should be considered. Infusion rates range from 5 to 10 μg per kg per minute with a bolus dose to start therapy of 0.50 to 2.0 mg per kg given initially over 2 to 5 minutes.

Vasodilators

The management of CHF also includes manipulation of loading conditions, following on the physiologic principles defined earlier in this chapter. Both afterload and preload interventions can be useful. Some of these agents have mixed effects (Table 72.4). In the vasodilator group, the nitrates, particularly nitroprusside, have been most actively used in the acute-care setting. Other drugs used include α-receptor blockers and angiotensin-converting enzyme (ACE) inhibitors, although these are more commonly used in the long-term care setting via the oral route. Calcium channel blockers appear to be most useful for diastolic dysfunction conditions.

NEWBORN WITH OBSTRUCTED SYSTEMIC OR PULMONARY BLOOD FLOW

CLINICAL MANIFESTATIONS

Any newborn with sudden onset of either collapsed systemic circulation or intense cyanosis should be considered at risk for the presence of a ductal-dependent state. Typical conditions that are "ductal dependent" are listed in Table 72.5. In these babies, closure of the ductus unmasks the underlying circulatory insuf-

TABLE 72.4. Afterload Reducing Agents Used in Congestive Heart Failure

Agent	Class	Action	Dosage
Nitroprusside	Nitrate	Mixed dilator	1–10 μg/kg/min i.v. (maximum: 12–15 μg/kg/min)
Nitroglycerin	Nitrate	Venodilator	2–10 μg/kg/min
Hydralazine[a]	Smooth muscle inhibitor	Arteriolar dilator	0.1–0.5 mg/kg/dose q6hr or 0.2–3 mg/kg single bolus i.v.
Prazosin	α Blockade	Mixed dilator	0.01–0.05 mg/kg/dose by mouth q8–12h
Captopril	ACE inhibitor	Mixed	0.1–2.0 mg/kg/dose by mouth q6h
Enalapril	ACE inhibitor	Mixed	8 or 12 h (maximum: 6 mg/kg/d)[b]
Diltiazam	Ca^{2+} channel blocker	Arteriolar dilator	0.2–0.5 mg/kg/dose by mouth or sublingual q8h
Nifedipine	Ca^{2+} channel blocker arteriolar		0.25–1 mg/kg

ACE, angiotensin-converting enzyme; Mixed, both arterial and venous vasoactivity.
[a] Precise mechanism not identified; may inhibit calcium activity.
[b] i.v., Enalapril is available for an every 8-h regimen (enalaprilat), 0.01–0.05 mg/kg/dose.

TABLE 72.5. Ductal-Dependent Cardiac Lesions

Ductal-dependent pulmonary blood flow	Ductal-dependent systemic blood flow
Pulmonary atresia with intact ventricular septum	Coarctation of the aorta
Tricuspid atresia	Aorta arch interruption
Critical pulmonary stenosis	Hypoplastic left heart syndrome (aortic atresia)

Adapted from Gewitz MH. Cardiac disease. In Polin R, Yoder M, Burg F, eds. *Workbook in practical neonatology*, 2nd ed. Philadelphia: WB Saunders, 1993: Ch. 12, with permission.

ficiency resulting in the clinical picture of either severe hypoxemia or shock or both.

MANAGEMENT

Based on the previous principles, prostaglandin E_1 (PGE_1) has become the standard medical intervention used in this urgent situation. Dosage is by infusion at 0.05 to 0.10 μg per kg per minute, after an initial bolus of 0.10 μg per kg. Side effects include bradycardia, apnea, hypotension, and seizures. Rash and hyperthermia also can develop.

CARDIAC ARRHYTHMIAS

General Considerations

CLINICAL MANIFESTATIONS

Many children are not aware of or are unable to express awareness of an abnormal cardiac rhythm. Thus, the physician must suspect the diagnosis from the secondary manifestations. Arrhythmias may surface in the following ways:

1. Symptoms of CHF (see "Congestive Heart Failure" earlier in this chapter).
2. Symptoms related to decreased cerebral blood flow (syncope, dizziness, irritability, and inappropriate behavior).
3. Symptoms related to decreased coronary blood flow (anginal chest pain).
4. Perception of the rhythm disturbance by the child (palpitations, skipped beats).

MANAGEMENT

Cardiac arrhythmias become emergencies when they produce hemodynamic alterations that result in a decreased CO or have the potential to do so. To treat cardiac arrhythmias effectively, one must be able to identify specific arrhythmias, recognize signs and symptoms of cardiac decompensation, and understand which arrhythmias are likely to produce rapid cardiac decompensation. Most infants and children who have symptomatic arrhythmias will require cardiac consultation and admission to the hospital for treatment and observation and continuous ECG monitoring (telemetry or bedside with arrhythmia analysis is preferred). Table 72.6 represents an overview of the emergent management of arrhythmias. Table 72.7 illustrates ranges of rates accepted as normal.

Slow Heart Rates

COMPLETE HEART BLOCK

Complete (third-degree) atrioventricular (AV) heart block is the most common cause of significant bradycardia in infants and children. Complete heart block, which may be congenital or acquired, results from a complete failure of conduction from atria to ventricles. The atrial rate is usually faster than the ventricular rate, which usually is 40 to 80 bpm.

CONGENITAL HEART BLOCK

Congenital heart block may be idiopathic, associated with specific types of congenital heart defects such as l-corrected transposition of the great arteries or left atrial isomerism/polysplenia syndromes (heterotaxy), or associated with collagen disease in the mother associated with the presence of anti-Ro (SS-A) and anti-La (SS-B). The infant with complete heart block who has severe CHF or who is in shock may require intubation for adequate ventilation, oxygenation, and treatment of acidosis. If no improvement is obtained with these measures, infusion of isoproterenol or epinephrine may increase the HR slightly, allowing time for the placement of a temporary pacemaker (Table 72.3).

A hydropic infant may require emergency phlebotomy, as well as a potent diuretic such as furosemide (1 mg per kg i.v.). Distressed infants with congenital heart block generally have HRs below 50 bpm. If an infant is distressed with a rate greater than 50 bpm, one should suspect significant congenital heart disease (CHD) or some other associated problem such as infection or sepsis in addition to the heart block. The infant in extremis from a slow HR may require immediate temporary pacing in the ED. Temporary transvenous pacing is reserved for infants with signs of CHF, most commonly seen with HRs under 50 bpm or with slightly higher rates in association with a structural congenital heart defect. However, an infant with an HR of 45 bpm should not be paced solely on the basis of HR but should be observed for signs of CHF such as tachypnea, poor feeding, or hepatomegaly.

The older child with congenital complete heart block may also present with symptoms associated with CHF. More commonly, dizziness, presyncope, syncope, exercise limitation, or fatigue are the presenting complaints in the older child. At times, the appearance of a ventricular arrhythmia is the presenting sign of difficulty in these patients.

ACQUIRED NONSURGICAL HEART BLOCK

Acquired nonsurgical heart block may be idiopathic or associated with congenital heart defects, infectious diseases such as myocarditis (viral or Lyme) or endocarditis, inflammatory processes (lupus, rheumatic fever), Kawasaki disease, muscle diseases, cardiac tumors, or cardiac sclerosis. The emergency treatment for congenital or acquired nonsurgical heart block is similar.

Pharmacologic therapy plays a role if adequate ventilation, oxygenation, and treatment of acidosis does not produce a normalization of the CO as reflected by the BP and peripheral perfusion. The initial drug to be used should be isoproterenol (Table 72.3) because it is most effective in increasing the HR. Epinephrine may be tried in place of, or in addition to, isoproterenol if bradycardia persists. Temporary transvenous pacing may be required during the acute phase of an infectious process, even when permanent pacing is not needed, as in myocarditis. The presence of CHF is an additional indication for pacing.

POSTSURGICAL COMPLETE HEART BLOCK

All patients with postsurgical permanent complete heart block should have implantation of permanent pacemakers. Emergency treatment of symptomatic postsurgical complete heart block includes pharmacologic support and temporary pacemaker placement until a permanent pacemaker can be placed.

SINUS BRADYCARDIA

Sinus bradycardia is an HR below the normal range for age (Table 72.7). An ECG is necessary to rule out second-degree or complete heart block; P waves with a normal P-R interval must

TABLE 72.6. Emergent Management of Arrhythmias in Children

Arrhythmia	Initial treatment (i.v.)	Secondary treatment (i.v.)
Slow heart rate		
Complete heart block		
Congenital	Isoproterenol (I) infusion: 0.1–2.0 μg/kg/min Epinephrine (E): 0.1–0.5 mg/kg of 1:10,000 dilution Infusion: 0.1–2.0 μg/kg/min	Pacemaker
Acquired, nonsurgical	(I), (E)	Pacemaker
Postsurgical	(I), (E), pacemaker	None
Sick sinus syndrome	(I), (E) Atropine (At): 0.02–0.04 mg/kg (maximum: 1–2 mg)	Pacemaker
Fast heart rate		
Supraventricular tachycardia		
Critical	Adenosine (Ad): 100–400 μg/kg Cardioversion: 1–2 watt-sec/kg	Repeat cardioversion Digoxin 30 μg/kg TDD, amiodarone (Am) 5 mg/kg over 1 h, procainamide (Proc) 5 mg/kg over 5–10 min or 10–15 mg/kg over 30–45 min
Noncritical	Adenosine	Digoxin (see Table 72.2), (Am), (Proc), Esmolol (Es) 500 μg/kg/min over 1 min followed by 50 μg/kg/min over 4 min; repeat in 5 min with 500 μg/kg/min over 1 min, 100 μg/kg/min over 4 min, Propranolol (Prop) 0.05–0.1 mg/kg over 5 min
Wolff-Parkinson-White syndrome	Adenosine	(Am), (Es), (Prop), (Proc)
Junctional tachycardia	Digoxin	(Am), (Proc)
Ventricular tachycardia		
Critical	Cardioversion: 2–5 watt-sec/kg	Lidocaine 1 mg/kg and cardioversion 2–5 watt-sec/kg
Noncritical	Lidocaine: 1 mg/kg	(Am), (Proc)
Ventricular fibrillation	Defibrillation: 2 watt-sec/kg	Lidocaine 1 mg/kg and deibrillation 4–10 watt-sec/kg
Irregular heart rate		
Premature ventricular contractions	Lidocaine: 1 mg/kg	(Am), (Proc)
Second-degree heart block	(I), (E)	Pacemaker

TDD, total digitalizing doses.
Notes: 1. Many arrhythmias require treatment only when symptomatic.
2. Treatment of underlying disorders (electrolyte imbalance, and so on) and supportive therapy (airway management, and so on) are always a first priority.
3. Refer to the text for a more complete discussion.

precede each QRS complex in sinus bradycardia. It often occurs in the athletic child or in the adolescent as a normal variant, especially during sleep. Other causes of sinus bradycardia include hypothyroidism, increased intracranial pressure, and drugs such as propranolol or digoxin. Therapy of the underlying disorder is indicated, but in symptomatic patients atropine may be useful as a temporizing measure (Table 72.8). Isoproterenol or epinephrine also may be given in this emergency setting (Table 72.3).

TABLE 72.7. Normal Heart Rate Ranges

Age	Heart rate (beats per min)
Newborn	80–180
1 wk–3 mo	80–180
3 mo–2 yr	80–160
2 yr–10 yr	65–130
10 yr–adult	55–90

SICK SINUS SYNDROME

Table 72.8 outlines the evaluation of the child with a suspected sick sinus syndrome. The asymptomatic patient with a slow HR can be referred for consultation with a cardiologist. The child with CHF or inadequate perfusion from bradycardia or tachycardia requires therapy directed at the specific arrhythmia and admission to the hospital. Isoproterenol or epinephrine infusions (Table 72.3) may increase the HR temporarily in a child with bradycardia but, in this situation, also may precipitate tachyarrhythmias; thus, these drugs should be administered

TABLE 72.8. Evaluation of Sick Sinus Syndrome

Test	Expected normal response
Atropine (0.02–0.04 mg/kg)	HR >90 bpm >25%–50% increase in HR
Isoproterenol (1–3 μg/min)	>25% increase in HR
Exercise	95% of expected normal rate
Electrophysiology study	Normal CSNRT (<550 msec) Normal SACT (45–105 msec)
24-h ambulatory monitor	Normal low rate for age Pauses <3 sec

bpm, beats per min; CSNRT, corrected sinus node recovery time; HR, heart rate; SACT, sinoatrial conduction time.

cautiously under continuous monitoring. Symptomatic slow rhythms may require temporary or permanent cardiac pacing.

PACEMAKERS

When a pacemaker malfunction is suspected, the specific problem should be identified if possible. A chest radiograph should be obtained to look for wire fractures or lead displacement. Most pacemaker programs now have computerized programmable analysis systems to help identify the problem. An ECG lead that shows the largest possible pacemaker stimulus artifact should be chosen with multiple leads providing more information. A pacemaker stimulus that falls outside the cardiac refractory period and fails to result in a ventricular depolarization indicates a failure of capture. In the currently available pacemakers, the output of the pacemaker may be reprogrammed externally, often resulting in normal capture. As the battery generator is depleted, the rate on most pacemakers decreases to a predetermined end-of-battery life indicator, which reveals impending battery failure. An abnormally long pause or an earlier-than-expected paced complex indicates a sensing failure, either inappropriate sensing of another electrical signal (eg, T wave sensing instead of QRS) or failure to sense the QRS. Sensing errors can be identified and external reprogramming accomplished. Any patient with evidence of pacemaker malfunction should be admitted to the hospital if the problem cannot be resolved in the ED.

Fast Heart Rates

SUPRAVENTRICULAR TACHYCARDIA

Clinical Manifestations

The clinical findings in the patient with supraventricular tachycardia (SVT) depend on the duration of the arrhythmia and the presence or absence of an underlying heart defect or myocardial dysfunction. In the patient with no congenital heart defect or myocardial dysfunction, CHF usually appears only after 24 hours of a rapid rate. The infant with SVT may present with only a fast rate or have varying degrees of CHF (poor feeding, irritability, respiratory distress) or shock. The infant may be acidotic and appear to be septic. The child older than 5 or 6 years of age will usually complain of some symptom such as chest pain or a rapid heartbeat. The child may also present with signs of CHF but is unlikely to be quite as ill when first seen as the infant or young child, unless a congenital heart defect or primary myocardial disease is present.

Management

The main principle of treatment in any cardiac arrhythmia is that the type of therapy is determined by the urgency of the situation. Thus, a different mode of treatment is chosen for the pa-

TABLE 72.9. Treatment of Supraventricular Tachycardia

Clinical status	Treatment
Asymptomatic	Ice, vagal maneuvers i.v. adenosine Pharmacologic agents 1. i.v. digoxin 2. Oral propranolol 3. Oral procainamide
Mild CHF	Ice, vagal maneuvers i.v. adenosine Pharmacologic agents 1. i.v. digoxin 2. Oral procainamide 3. Oral propranolol
Moderate CHF	Ice, vagal maneuvers i.v. adenosine Pharmacologic agents—if i.v. access 1. i.v. digoxin 2. i.v. amiodarone 3. i.v. procainamide Pacing (esophageal or intracardiac)—if no i.v. access or for infants Cardioversion, synchronized
Severe CHF	Cardioversion, synchronized i.v. adenosine Pacing, esophageal or intracardiac Pharmacologic agents 1. i.v. digoxin 2. i.v. amiodarone 3. i.v. procainamide

CHF, congestive heart failure.

tient with tachycardia in shock than for the asymptomatic patient who has only a fast HR (Table 72.9).

When the SVT is caused by reentry using the AV node (AV nodal reentry), or AV reentry using a bypass tract, any intervention that interrupts the critical relationship of conduction and refractoriness in the AV node can interrupt the tachycardia. The patient's response to the drugs or maneuvers is not always predictable. The methods used most often are those that slow AV nodal conduction. In adult patients, carotid sinus pressure or the Valsalva maneuver often can terminate the tachycardia by increasing vagal tone, slowing conduction, and prolonging refractoriness within the AV node. Although these maneuvers often are ineffective in children, the occasional successful attempt justifies their initial use. Ice water or ice bags applied to the face have been used to recruit the diving reflex and stop the SVT. This technique should be reserved for children who are monitored, with particular caution used in applying these techniques in young infants because significant sinus slowing may occur.

Any patient with SVT who presents with shock, acidosis, or severe hemodynamic compromise should be treated immediately. If adenosine (Table 72.10) is not effective, synchronized direct current (DC) cardioversion at a dosage of 1 to 2 watt-second per kg should be used and doubled until effective or until a dosage of 10 watt-second per kg is reached. If ventricular fibrillation should occur, repeat cardioversion generally converts the patient to normal sinus rhythm. The patient should be given a sedative or short-acting anesthetic, and preparations should be made for airway support and ventilation if needed. The underlying acidosis should be treated and adequate ventilation and oxygenation provided because cardioversion may not be successful in the presence of hypoxia or acid-base imbalance. The presence of digoxin in the patient should not prevent the use of cardioversion when needed. Evidence of digoxin toxicity such as ventricular arrhythmia may be treated with lidocaine. Once the patient's rhythm has been converted, the chosen chronic treatment should be initiated immediately.

Children who have only mild to moderate failure may be treated medically, as described earlier, with adenosine if vagal maneuvers fail because most of these patients will convert rapidly after pharmacologic treatment. Agents, other than digitalis, useful for the treatment of SVT are reviewed in Table 72.10. The preferred medical treatment of AV nodal reentrant SVT in children is digoxin, which works by prolonging AV nodal conduction and refractoriness in both the fast (β) and slow (α) path-

TABLE 72.10. Antiarrhythmic Agents

Drug	Intravenous	Oral	Desired level
I. For Supraventricular Tachycardia			
Adenosine	100–400 μg/kg Increase by 50 μg/kg every 2 min to 400 μg/kg or 12 mg maximal dose		
Procainamide	5–15 mg/kg in 30 min—load Infusion 20–80 μg/kg/min	20–100 mg/kg/day in 6 doses	PA 4–8 μg/mL NAPA 4–10 μg/mL
Propranolol	0.05–0.1 mg/kg/dose q6h	0.5–1 mg/kg/dose q/6h	20–150 ng/mL
Esmolol	500 μg/kg/min over 1 min followed by 50 μg/kg/min over 4 min; repeat in 5 min with 500 μg/kg/min over 1 min; 100 μg/kg/min over 4 min	50–200 μg/kg/min	
Phenylephrine	0.005–0.01 mg/kg/dose		NA
Verapamil Not ≤1 yr	0.075–0.15 ng/kg/dose	5–15 mg/kg in 3 doses	NA
Digoxin	See Table 72.2	See Table 72.2	0.5–2.0 ng/mL
II. For Ventricular Tachycardia			
Propranolol	As above	As above	As above
Procainamide	As above	As above	As above
Lidocaine	1–2 mg/kg/dose Infusion: 10–50 μg/kg/min		1–5 μg/mL
Phenytoin	2–4 mg/kg over 5 min not to exceed 1 mg/kg/min	Day 1: 20 mg/kg Day 2: 10 mg/kg Day 3: 10 mg/kg Maintenance 4–10 g/kg/day	10–20 μg/mL
Mexiletine	3–5 mg/kg/dose q8h		0.5 2.0 μg/mL
Bretylium	5 mg/kg/dose q15min Infusion: 5–10 mg/kg over 10 min q6h 1 mg/kg bolus q10min up to 10 doses		NA
Amiodarone		10 mg/kg/day divided b.i.d. (loading; after 7–10 days 0.5 mg/kg once daily)	1.5–2.5 μg/mL
Magnesium	0.25 mEq/kg over 1 min followed by 1 mEq/kg over 5 h to achieve Mg^{++} level of 3–4		

NA, not available for routine clinical use; NAPA, *N*-acetyl procainamide; PA, procainamide.

ways. The usual digitalizing dose appropriate for age is used (Table 72.2). The route (i.v. or i.m.) depends on the status of the patient. Digoxin administered i.v. should be used in the presence of CHF when perfusion is decreased. The interval of time that precedes the second and third doses of the total digitalizing dose should be determined by the patient's status. These additional doses may be required after only 2 to 4 hours. If the tachycardia persists after three doses, one to two additional doses may be given.

Propranolol, which prolongs AV nodal conduction and refractoriness in both α and β pathways, should be used with caution in the ill child because it may depress cardiac function even more. In instances in which cardiac function is preserved, a slow i.v. dose may be given. The dose is 0.1 mg per kg i.v. A shorter-acting β-blocker, esmolol, may be preferred. The doses are shown in Table 72.10.

Procainamide may be used to terminate AV reentrant SVT by blocking retrograde conduction in the fast (β) pathway (Table 72.10). SVT can be converted in the catheterization laboratory by rapid atrial pacing. A less invasive method of esophageal overdrive pacing to terminate SVT in infants and children can be used. A small bipolar electrode catheter is passed by the nasogastric route and positioned in the esophagus behind the left atrium. As with intracardiac methods, esophageal rapid atrial pacing at a rate faster than the SVT can capture the atrium and interrupt a reentrant circuit, terminating the SVT.

The treatment of SVT in Wolff-Parkinson-White (WPW) syndrome or in a concealed bypass tract is similar to the treatment of AV nodal reentrant SVT because the AV node participates in one limb of the reentrant circuit. Propranolol is an exceptionally effective drug because it slows AV nodal conduction and prolongs refractoriness while having no significant effects on the accessory pathway. Digoxin, with similar effects on the AV node, must be used cautiously in patients with WPW syndrome because it can shorten the refractory period of the bypass tract and enhance conduction in the accessory pathway. In a patient with an associated atrial tachyarrhythmia such as atrial flutter or atrial fibrillation, digoxin may predispose to a rapid ventricular response or ventricular fibrillation secondary to rapid conduction of the atrial impulse down the bypass tract. A high percentage of adults with WPW syndrome and SVT also have atrial fibrillation, but the incidence of this association is lower in children. Class IA or IC agents such as procainamide or flecainide are often effective in this type of SVT because they act on the accessory pathway to slow conduction and prolong refractoriness and thus interrupt the retrograde limb of the reentrant circuit.

Verapamil generally should be avoided in patients less than 3 years old. When used, a dose of 0.075 to 0.15 mg per kg is effective. It is important to give the drug slowly, over at least 2 minutes, while monitoring the child's ECG and BP closely. Calcium i.v. (10% CaCl at a dose of 10 mg per kg) and isoproterenol should be available immediately and should be drawn up in the appropriate dose before verapamil is given. Verapamil should not be used in patients who have received i.v. β-blockers and should be used with extreme caution in patients who use any other antiarrhythmic agent.

As soon as the patient converts from SVT, an ECG in sinus rhythm should be obtained. This allows diagnosis of the presence of the WPW syndrome or other abnormalities that might direct chronic therapy to be identified. In general, digoxin is not advised in the presence of WPW syndrome unless one knows that the accessory pathway refractory period is relatively long and is unaffected by the digoxin; this drug might shorten the accessory pathway refractory period and promote rapid ventricular conduction of supraventricular impulses to the ventricle.

ATRIAL FLUTTER AND ATRIAL FIBRILLATION

Atrial flutter and fibrillation occur uncommonly in children. Atrial flutter consists of rapid, regular atrial excitation at rates of 280 to 480 bpm. The ventricular response depends on AV nodal conduction that may allow 1:1, 2:1, 3:1, or 4:1 conduction. The typical ECG reveals saw-toothed flutter waves best seen in leads 2 and V_1. Atrial flutter is most commonly seen in children with CHD, especially postoperatively after Mustard repair for d-transposition of the great arteries or the Fontan repair, but it also can occur idiopathically or congenitally.

Children with atrial fibrillation or flutter raise the same therapeutic problems as those with SVT. If cardiac compromise does not necessitate immediate cardioversion, the initial treatment is digoxin. Adenosine increases the AV block and therefore may help diagnostically, but it usually will not correct the atrial flutter or fibrillation to sinus rhythm. In the child who is stable and has a normal BP and adequate perfusion, the physician should allow 24 hours for a response to digoxin before adding a second drug such as procainamide. Failure to achieve a normal rhythm after an additional 24 to 48 hours calls for cardioversion. Therapeutic drug levels for these agents, which should be obtained in a steady state of drug administration, are listed in Table 72.10.

AUTOMATIC ATRIAL OR JUNCTIONAL TACHYCARDIAS

Automatic atrial or junctional tachycardias may be difficult to control and often are associated with inflammatory states such as myocarditis. Digoxin (at relatively low dosages initially to avoid ventricular arrhythmias in a sensitive myocardium), i.v. procainamide, and i.v. amiodarone have been effective (Table 72.10). Once the abnormal rhythm has converted, chronic therapy must be initiated; otherwise the arrhythmia is likely to recur. Chronic drugs for these arrhythmias include digoxin, β-blockers, procainamide, flecainide, amiodarone, and sotalol.

VENTRICULAR TACHYCARDIA

Ventricular tachycardia (VT) is defined as three or more consecutive premature ventricular contractions (PVCs). The HR usually is 150 to 200 bpm but may be slower or more rapid. These contractions may be hemodynamically inefficient and result in syncope and death. The cause may be electrolyte imbalance, metabolic disturbances, cardiac tumors, drugs, cardiac catheterization or surgery, CHD, cardiomyopathies, acquired heart disease, right ventricular dysplasia, prolonged Q-T syndrome, or idiopathic. VT is being seen more commonly in children who can be divided into three groups: 1) patients with identifiable noncardiac causes (electrolyte imbalance, toxins, drug overdoses, or drug toxicity); 2) patients with no known underlying heart disease and no extracardiac disturbances (may have small Purkinje cell tumors or foci in the right ventricular outflow tract or left ventricle septum); and 3) patients with either congenital or acquired heart disease.

In children with identifiable extracardiac abnormalities (group 1), the underlying disturbance is treated. Children with no known cardiac or extracardiac causes for VT (group 2) require treatment if they have a sustained, rapid arrhythmia. As with SVT patients, the urgency of treatment depends on the clinical status. In cases of shock, impending cardiac decompensation, or cardiac failure, synchronized DC cardioversion at 2 to 5 watt-second per kg up to 10 watt-second per kg should be used. Lidocaine i.v. at 1 to 2 mg per kg also may be effective (Table 72.10); a continuous infusion of lidocaine at 10 to 50 μg per kg per minute may be required. Other effective drugs include amiodarone (i.v.) at 5 mg per kg over the first hour, followed by a 5 to 10 μg per kg per minute i.v. infusion or procainamide (i.v.)

at 10 to 15 mg per kg given over 30 to 45 minutes, followed by a 20 to 80 μg per kg per minute i.v. infusion. Those with Purkinje cell tumors or ectopic foci may be amenable to catheter radiofrequency ablation or surgical ablation in selected cases.

Rapid ventricular pacing may be used for overdrive suppression for conversion to normal rhythm if pharmacologic therapy fails or is contraindicated. Chronic treatment with nadolol, propranolol, mexiletine, amiodarone, procainamide, sotalol, or propafenone has been effective for long-term control of this arrhythmia.

Patients with CHD (group 3) and VT raise a different issue. Often, these patients have some degree of hemodynamic compromise associated with ventricular dysfunction and do not tolerate the VT at all. The emergent and chronic treatment is similar to that outlined previously but may be required even more urgently. All patients with CHD and sustained VT over 150 bpm require therapy because sudden death occurs in up to 30% of patients with CHD who have VT. Some patients in this group with slower VT or nonsustained VT may require treatment, especially if hemodynamic abnormalities exist.

The congenital long Q-T syndrome is a special case. Sudden death occurs in 73% of patients who are not treated. The sudden death is secondary to ventricular tachyarrhythmias (torsades de pointes) of the type that often degenerates to ventricular fibrillation. Any patient who presents with VT, especially of the polymorphic or torsades de pointes type, should have corrected Q-T intervals determined in sinus rhythm.

Emergent treatment of these patients includes lidocaine and synchronized DC cardioversion when needed. If the VT is polymorphic, nonsynchronized cardioversion or defibrillation is indicated. In addition, temporary atrial or ventricular pacing at a rate 10% to 20% faster than the underlying sinus rate may be needed to control the arrhythmia, especially in patients with underlying bradycardia, a common association. Intravenous propranolol, phenytoin, and magnesium have been used successfully in these patients. The class I agents that prolong the Q-T interval in normal patients should be avoided in patients with these long Q-T intervals. In fact, a number of drugs that may produce this form of VT are shown in Table 72.11. This type of drug effect is believed to be related to QTc prolongation with, on some occasions, associated ventricular arrhythmias and bradycardia. Temporary pacing and removal of the offending agent are effective therapies. In acquired long Q-T with ventricular arrhythmias, especially if bradycardia is a prominent factor, an isoproterenol infusion may be therapeutic.

TABLE 72.11. Pharmacologic Agents That Prolong Q-T Intervals

Antiarrhythmic agents	*Psychotropic drugs*
Quinidine	Tricyclic antidepressant
Procainamide	amitriptyline
Flecainide	Phenothiazines
Encainide	Haloperidol
Disopyramide	Risperidone
Amiodarone	Pimozide
Sotalol	Lithium carbonate
Antihistamines	Sertraline hydrochloride
Terfenadine	Nefazodone hydrochloride
Astemizole	Fluvoxamine maleate
Diphenhydramine	*Other*
Antibiotics/antifungal agents	Cisapride
Erythromycin	Probucol
Trimethoprim	*Anthracyclines*
Sulfamethoxazole	*Organophosphates*
Pentamidine	Epinephrine
Ketoconazole	Diuretics
Fluconazole	Potassium loss
Itraconazole	
Clarithromycin	
Azithromycin	

VENTRICULAR FIBRILLATION

Ventricular fibrillation consists of chaotic irregular ventricular contractions with cessation of circulation. Electrical defibrillation with correction of precipitating factors (acidosis, electrolyte imbalance, hypoxia) may result in conversion to normal sinus rhythm. The treatment of cardiac arrest is discussed in Chapter 1.

Irregular Heart Rates

PREMATURE DEPOLARIZATIONS

Clinical Manifestations

PVCs are seen as premature, wide, bizarre-shaped QRS complexes. Generally, the T wave is opposite in direction to the main deflection of the QRS. A compensatory pause usually follows the premature beat, and P waves may reveal AV dissociation or retrograde conduction or may be absent. Children who present with PVCs are often asymptomatic and unaware of their arrhythmia, especially if they are younger than 5 years of age. If the PVC is appreciated, the child may complain of a "skipped" or "hard" beat, a fluttering or pounding in the chest, difficulty breathing, or chest pain. If the PVCs are frequent and/or associated with heart disease (congenital or acquired), the child may note dizziness or a rapid heartbeat. Frequent PVCs in the presence of compromised cardiac function may worsen the CO and produce signs and symptoms of CHF.

Management

The only PVCs that require treatment are those that cause or are likely to cause hemodynamic compromise. This generally is seen in the context of frequent PVCs in a patient with abnormal cardiac function as evidenced by cardiomegaly on chest radiograph, abnormal cardiac function or dilated chamber sizes on echocardiography, or abnormal exercise responses on exercise stress testing. Symptoms of dizziness, chest pain, or presyncope may accompany PVCs in patients with abnormal cardiac function. Such patients may be found to have myocarditis, cardiomyopathy or a congenital heart defect (preoperative or postoperative), and abnormal underlying cardiac function. The treatment may include lidocaine, mexiletine, procainamide, propranolol, or amiodarone (Table 72.10) as outlined previously under "Ventricular Tachycardia." Although digoxin is not generally considered for patients with PVCs or VT, patients with poor myocardial function, as evidenced by the clinical findings of CHF and echocardiographic evidence of abnormal myocardial function, may benefit from digitalization.

Isolated multiform or coupled PVCs or nonsustained VT (rate 150 bpm or less) in an asymptomatic patient with a normal heart may not require treatment, but this decision must be individualized after consultation with a cardiologist. Rarely is emergency treatment of this type of patient required, and investigations that use 24-hour continuous ECG monitors, exercise stress testing, echocardiography, and/or the electrophysiologic catheterization studies may be used to determine the appropriate management. It sometimes is helpful to observe the patient's response to activity. If the PVCs abate completely with sinus tachycardia (140 to 150 bpm), they are likely to be benign in terms of clinical significance and need for therapy, although this is not universally true.

Isolated PVCs in an asymptomatic patient in the presence of a structurally and functionally normal heart do not require treatment. Continuous 24-hour ambulatory monitoring should be performed to rule out the presence of undetected VT or complex ventricular arrhythmias. Restriction of caffeine and other stimulants should be recommended in all patients with ventricular arrhythmias.

Premature atrial contractions (PACs) or PVCs generally do not require treatment. Patients with frequent PACs or PVCs should be evaluated appropriately to rule out myocarditis. Continuous 24-hour ambulatory monitoring should be performed to rule out the occurrence of SVT. Elimination of caffeine or other stimulants such as theophylline, pseudoephedrine, and other sympathomimetic amines may decrease the frequency of PACs. Unless the PACs are demonstrated to initiate episodes of SVT, no treatment is indicated. Variations of normal rhythms commonly seen in children and that do not require treatment include sinus arrhythmia and wandering atrial pacemakers as long as rates remain in the normal ranges.

First-Degree and Second-Degree Heart Block

First-degree heart block reflects slowed conduction from the sinus node to the ventricle and is manifested by a prolonged P-R interval. It is seen with digoxin and other antiarrhythmic drugs; certain types of CHD (primum and secund atrial septal defects); and inflammatory diseases such as rheumatic, viral, or Lyme myocarditis. Second-degree heart block results in the failure of some impulses to traverse the AV node. The Wenckebach phenomenon, a form of second-degree heart block, is a result of progressive slowing of AV conduction and is seen as progressively prolonged P-R interval and eventual dropped beat. Other forms of second-degree heart block include high grade 2:1, 3:1, and 4:1 block. Children with first-degree and second-degree heart block rarely are symptomatic unless the associated HR is low enough to decrease the CO. In such instances, signs and symptoms of CHF may be present. Both first-degree and second-degree heart block may be associated with digitalis toxicity, requiring the digitalis dose be adjusted downward or temporarily held if second-degree AV block is present. Otherwise, first-degree heart block does not need therapy. Second-degree heart block is treated only if it produces an HR sufficiently slow enough to interfere with cardiac output. In this instance, the management is the same as that outlined previously under "Complete Heart Block."

ARRHYTHMIAS ASSOCIATED WITH ELECTROLYTE ABNORMALITIES

Any patient with significant arrhythmias should be evaluated for an electrolyte disturbance. The ECG changes may be characteristic and lead to suspicion of a specific electrolyte abnormality. Normal ECG intervals (P-R, QRS, QTc) are listed in Table 72.12.

Hyperkalemia

Peaked T waves are seen at a serum concentration of 5 to 6 mEq per L, and the QRS widens with a concentration exceeding 6 mEq per L. The Q-T interval increases with the increasing QRS duration. As P wave amplitude decreases, P wave duration increases, and the P-R interval increases above 7 mEq per L. Above 8 to 9 mEq per L, P waves disappear, the ventricular rate becomes irregular, and severe bradycardia with sinus arrest, block, or idioventricular rhythms occur, often with a sinusoidal wave pattern. Ventricular fibrillation or asystole occurs at serum concentrations greater than 12 to 14 mEq per L. Low serum calcium enhances the myocardial toxicity of hyperkalemia. Likewise, acidosis potentiates hyperkalemia by producing potassium ion efflux from cells.

Hypokalemia

Serum potassium concentrations of less than 2.7 mEq per L generally produce typical ECG changes in ventricular repolarization. These changes include a U-wave amplitude greater than 1 mm, seen best in leads V_2 and V_3, and ST-segment depression greater than 0.5 mm. The Q-T interval lengthens and the T wave flattens with progressive hypokalemia. The P-R interval may be prolonged, and intraventricular conduction may be delayed with widening of the QRS complex. With significant hypokalemia, P-wave and QRS amplitude may increase. Other arrhythmias that have been associated with hypokalemia include ectopic atrial and ventricular complexes, ectopic atrial tachycardia with block, AV dissociation, second-degree AV block, ventricular bigeminy, VT, and ventricular fibrillation. Patients taking digoxin who become hypokalemic are especially susceptible to arrhythmias because of the synergistic effects of digoxin and hypokalemia on automaticity and conduction.

Hypocalcemia

Hypocalcemia produces characteristic ECG changes that consist of Q-T interval prolongation secondary to ST-segment prolongation and occasionally, reversal of the T wave. The ECG changes correlate with ionized calcium because the degree of Q-T prolongation generally is proportional to the degree of hypocalcemia. Abnormal rhythms, although uncommon, have

TABLE 72.12. P-R Interval and QRS Duration Related to Rate and Age (and Upper Limits of Normal)

Rate	0–6 mo	1–6 mo	6 mo–1 yr	1–3 yr	3–8 yr	8–12 yr	12–16 yr	Adult
PR								
<60					0.16 (0.18)	0.16 (0.19)	0.17 (0.21)	
60–80					0.15 (0.17)	0.15 (0.17)	0.15 (0.18)	0.16 (0.21)
80–100	0.10 (0.12)				0.14 (0.16)	0.15 (0.16)	0.15 (0.17)	0.15 (0.20)
100–120	0.10 (0.12)			(0.15)	0.13 (0.16)	0.14 (0.15)	0.15 (0.16)	0.15 (0.19)
120–140	0.10 (0.11)	0.11 (0.14)	0.11 (0.14)	0.12 (0.14)	0.13 (0.15)	0.14 (0.15)		0.15 (0.18)
140–160	0.09 (0.11)	0.10 (0.13)	0.11 (0.13)	0.11 (0.14)	0.12 (0.14)			(0.17)
160–180	0.10 (0.11)	0.10 (0.12)	0.10 (0.12)	0.10 (0.12)				
>180	0.09	0.09 (0.11)	0.10 (0.11)					
QRS								
Seconds	0.05 (0.065)	0.05 (0.07)	0.05 (0.06)	0.06 (0.07)	0.07 (0.08)	0.07 (0.09)	0.07 (0.10)	0.08 (0.10)
QTc								
$= QT/\sqrt{R - R}$		Average normal = under 0.450 msec						

been reported and include SVT, 2:1 AV block, complete heart block, and torsades de pointes VT.

Hypercalcemia

Hypercalcemia, with levels above 12 mg per dL, produces a shortened Q-T interval, a shortened ST segment, and normal or prominent U waves. Severe hypercalcemia causes P-R interval prolongation, QRS prolongation, and occasionally, second-degree and third-degree heart block. Elevated serum calcium decreases the effect of hyperkalemia and potentiates digoxin toxicity. Thus, calcium should be administered cautiously to patients taking digoxin and the HR should be monitored.

Hypomagnesemia

Low magnesium levels often are associated with hypokalemia and hypocalcemia. The ECG abnormalities seen may be those associated with any or all of these aberrations and include prolongation of the corrected Q-T interval. Ectopic beats and T-wave changes are commonly noted. Torsades de pointes VT and ventricular fibrillation have been reported.

Hypermagnesemia

Hypermagnesemia of 3 to 5 mEq per L or higher may be associated with a delay in AV and intraventricular conduction.

Treatment of these electrolyte abnormalities is discussed in Chapter 76.

PERICARDIAL DISEASE

CLINICAL MANIFESTATIONS

Table 72.13 reviews some of the principal causes of pericarditis in childhood. A history of onset of respiratory difficulties after resolution of an upper respiratory illness may indicate pericardial disease in some instances. Chest pain, usually a benign symptom in childhood, is common with pericardial inflammation. This pain varies, depending on position. Occasionally, abdominal pain may be the presenting symptom.

The child with significant pericardial effusion may show clinical signs similar to several of those noted in the earlier section in this chapter on "Congestive Heart Failure." Tachypnea secondary to raised pulmonary venous pressures and decreased pulmonary compliance usually is present. This may be associated with intercostal retractions. Reduced CO may result in peripheral vasoconstriction, manifested by cool extremities, pallor, or decreased systemic BP. Elevated systemic venous pressures cause neck vein distension, hepatomegaly, and on occasion in a more chronic picture, protein loss through either the gastrointestinal tract or the urine. Tachycardia is a universal finding and is representative of an effective compensatory mechanism, but only up to a point.

The cardiac auscultatory findings directly relate to the degree of pericardial fluid accumulation. A friction rub—the scratching, harsh sound commonly heard throughout the cardiac cycle—often is not audible in the presence of significant amounts of intrapericardial fluid and may become apparent only after pericardiocentesis. The heart sounds usually are distant, or muffled, and the apical impulse is weak. In general, the presence of a quiet precordium in the face of these previously noted respiratory and circulatory changes should alert the examiner to the possibility of pericardial disease with effusion. The sine qua non of cardiac tamponade is pulsus paradoxus. The finding of a paradoxic pulse greater than 20 mm Hg is unequivocal evidence of circulatory compromise. In addition, most investigators assume that as little as 10 mm Hg is suggestive of hemodynamic impairment.

LABORATORY FINDINGS

The ECG shows diminished precordial voltage in most instances of significant intrapericardial fluid accumulation. With pericarditis, an associated current of injury pattern that reflects myocardial involvement, seen as elevations in the ST segments, also may be present. Diffuse T-wave inversions also are common. The heart size is increased on chest radiograph with pericardial effusion but can be entirely normal if there is no significant amount of intrapericardial fluid. The lung fields may be clear, but one should look for associated bronchopneumonia or pleural effusions that may be helpful for diagnostic considerations. In some situations, as with constrictive pericarditis, the heart size may be relatively small. If the patient has had previous chest radiographs, a sudden increase in heart size always should arouse the suspicion of pericardial effusion. Echocardiography has become the diagnostic procedure of choice for determining the presence and amount of intrapericardial fluid.

MANAGEMENT

For pericarditis without evidence of pericardial effusion, emergency invasive treatment usually is not indicated. Symptomatic therapy for pain should be prescribed, and bed rest in the hospital is advisable. The patient should be followed closely for the

TABLE 72.13. Causes of Diseases of the Pericardium

Infectious	Noninfectious, inflammatory	Traumatic	Oncologic	Chronic
Bacterial	Acute rheumatic	Postpericardiotomy syndrome	Leukemia	Constrictive pericarditis
Viral	Systemic lupus erythematosus	Chest wall injury	Lymphoma	Subacute effusive pericarditis
Fungal	Uremia	Foreign bodies with cardiac contact	Pericardial cyst	Blood dyscrasias
Parasitic	Radiation		Cardiac rhabdosarcoma	
Tuberculous	Juvenile rheumatoid arthritis Drugs (e.g., Minoxidil)			

TABLE 72.14. Purulent Pericarditis: Immediate Management

1. Ensure adequacy of ventilation and cardiac output
2. Administer oxygen
3. Initiate cardiorespiratory monitoring
4. Obtain laboratory studies (simultaneously with step 5)
   Complete blood count, platelet count, electrolytes, blood urea nitrogen, creatinine, glucose, arterial blood gas, blood culture, chest radiograph, electrocardiography, echocardiography
5. Achieve venous access
6. Pericardiocentesis
   Send specimen for laboratory studies: cultures, viral titers, antinuclear antibody, Gram stain, cytology, cell count and differential, chemical profile
7. Administer antibiotics[a]
   Oxacillin (150 mg/kg/d) or nafcillin or methicillin and Chloramphenicol (100 mg/kg/d)
   Aminoglycoside (immunocompromised patient)

[a] Select antimicrobials to cover *Staphylococcus aureus* and *Haemophilus influenzae* at least until specific infection is isolated.

development of complications such as myocarditis, pericardial effusion, and cardiac tamponade. Diagnostic evaluation to identify the cause should be initiated.

For pericardial effusion, a more definitive approach is needed. Diagnostic pericardiocentesis often is required in the de novo presentation, particularly without evidence of other forms of systemic disease; it always is required with the suspicion of a purulent pericardial process. Antibiotic therapy alone is not adequate for treatment of purulent pericarditis. Usually, in the presence of purulent pericarditis, an open drainage procedure is indicated. It is contingent on the emergency physician to ensure cardiovascular stability in the presence of pericardial effusion because tamponade can develop rapidly once maximum pericardial distensibility has been reached (Table 72.14).

The management of cardiac tamponade requires intense medical vigilance. Although it may be possible in relatively mild or highly selected situations to manage the effusion conservatively, it generally is necessary to remove the fluid. This can be a lifesaving technique and, when done successfully, shows clearly the fruitful outcome of appropriate, decisive evaluation and treatment procedures.

TABLE 72.15. Procedures and Endocarditis Prophylaxis

Recommended Endocarditis Prophylaxis

- Respiratory tract
  - Tonsillectomy and/or adenoidectomy
  - Surgical procedures that involve respiratory mucosa
  - Bronchoscopy with a rigid bronchoscope
- Gastrointestinal tract[a]
  - Sclerotherapy for esophageal varices
  - Esophageal stricture dilation
  - Endoscopic retrograde cholangiography with biliary obstruction
  - Biliary tract surgery
  - Surgical procedures that involve intestinal mucosa
- Genitourinary tract
  - Prostatic surgery
  - Cystoscopy
  - Urethral dilation

Not Recommended Endocarditis Prophylaxis

- Respiratory tract
  - Endotracheal intubation
  - Bronchoscopy with a flexible bronchoscope, with or without biopsy[b]
  - Tympanostomy tube insertion
- Gastrointestinal tract
  - Transesophageal echocardiography[b]
  - Endoscopy with or without gastrointestinal biopsy[b]
- Genitourinary tract
  - Vaginal hysterectomy[b]
  - Vaginal delivery[b]
  - Cesarean section
  - In uninfected tissue:
    - Urethral catheterization
    - Uterine dilation and curettage
    - Therapeutic abortion
    - Sterilization procedures
    - Insertion or removal of intrauterine devices
- Other
  - Cardiac catheterization, including balloon angioplasty
  - Implanted cardiac pacemakers, implanted defibrillators, and coronary stents
  - Incision or biopsy or surgically scrubbed skin
  - Circumcision

[a] Prophylaxis is recommended for high-risk patients; it is optional for medium-risk patients.
[b] Prophylaxis is optional for high-risk patients.
Adapted with permission from Dajani A, et al. Prevention of bacterial endocarditis: recommendations by the American Heart Association. *JAMA* 1997;277:1794–1801.

INFECTIVE ENDOCARDITIS

ETIOLOGIC FACTORS

Although the most common setting for this problem is the child with preexisting CHD, variability exists in terms of the types of associated lesions, and it is of concern that a substantial proportion of cases develop in children with no history of cardiac abnormality. Recently, the Committee on Rheumatic Fever, Endocarditis, and Kawasaki Disease of the American Heart Association undertook a major review of the guidelines for endocarditis prevention (Tables 72.15 and 72.16).

CLINICAL MANIFESTATIONS

Often, early signs and symptoms can be subtle and persist for considerable time before the diagnosis is made. As a rule, persistence of fever in any child with CHD should prompt the clinician to consider the possibility of endocarditis. In the clinical context of CHD, certain conditions should prompt a careful evaluation for the presence of endocarditis. These include 1) unexplained fever or a protracted febrile course in a presumed "viral" syndrome, 2) pneumonia, 3) the development of a new neurologic deficit, 4) the onset of hematuria, and 5) signs of systemic or cutaneous embolization.

The classic findings of fever, a change in the cardiac examination, splenomegaly, and evidence of emboli usually are present in severe cases but may require serial examinations. Emboli may be discovered by careful funduscopic examination, by observing for conjunctival lesions, or by meticulous scrutiny of the nailbeds, palms of the hands, soles of the feet, and other skin surfaces. Microscopic hematuria should be recognized as an important sign of endocarditis in the appropriate clinical context. Scrapings of cutaneous emboli may be helpful for rapid identification of infecting organisms.

MANAGEMENT

Treatment of infective endocarditis should be started as early as possible after appropriate evaluation is completed. To facilitate the diagnosis, the physician, particularly one who evaluates a child with heart disease with unexplained fever, must obtain

TABLE 72.16. Cardiac Conditions Associated with Endocarditis

Recommended Endocarditis Prophylaxis
High-risk category
- Prosthetic cardiac valves, including bioprosthetic and homograft valves
- Previous bacterial endocarditis
- Complex cyanotic congenital heart disease (e.g., single ventricle states, transposition of the great arteries, tetralogy of Fallot)
- Surgically constructed systemic-pulmonary shunts or conduits

Moderate-risk category
- Most other congenital cardiac malformations (other than above and below)
- Acquired valvar dysfunction (e.g., rheumatic heart disease)
- Hypertrophic cardiomyopathy
- Mitral valve prolapse with valvar regurgitation and/or thickened leaflets

Not Recommended Endocarditis Prophylaxis
Negligible-risk category (no greater than the general population)
Isolated secundum atrial septal defect
Surgical repair of atrial septal defect, ventricular septal defect, or patent ductus arteriosus (without residuae beyond 6 mo)
- Previous coronary artery bypass graft surgery
- Mitral valve prolapse without valvar regurgitation
- Physiologic, functional, or innocent heart murmurs
- Previous Kawasaki disease without valvar dysfunction
- Previous rheumatic fever without valvar dysfunction
- Cardiac pacemakers (intravascular and epicardial) and implanted defibrillators

Adapted with permission from Dajani A, et al. Prevention of bacterial endocarditis: recommendations by the American Heart Association. *JAMA* 1997;277:1734.

blood for appropriate cultures at an early stage. If the situation requires the initiation of therapy without definition of the microbial agent, many experts recommend the combination of an aminoglycoside such as gentamicin (5 to 7.5 mg per kg per day) and a penicillinase-resistant penicillin such as oxacillin (150 mg per kg per day). Others advocate the use of ampicillin (200 mg per kg per day) and gentamicin for the initial therapy in this particular situation. Cephalosporins such as cefuroxime may also play a role in this context.

Prevention guidelines have been recently modified by the American Heart Association (Table 72.17). As a rule, such measures are practical only in the face of a well-defined, predisposing event. The usual child with heart disease who presents with a routine febrile illness does not require prophylactic antibiotics.

HYPOXEMIC ATTACKS

CLINICAL FINDINGS

Children with cyanotic CHD in which pulmonary blood flow is reduced, such as tetralogy of Fallot, may experience periodic episodes of intense hypoxemia. Diagnosis of a hypoxemic spell usually is self-evident. Aside from the obvious cyanosis and the history of heart disease, there also may be a preceding history of squatting with exertion or of other positional vagaries that parents may recall. During a spell, the child may be irritable and crying or may be lethargic and even unconscious. Hyperpnea is a feature of the syndrome and should be distinguished from tachypnea or other abnormal respiratory patterns that may signal other medical problems associated with cyanosis. During a

TABLE 72.17. Endocarditis Prophylaxis Regimens

Situation	Agent	Regimen
For Dental, Oral, Respiratory Tract, or Esophageal Procedures		
Standard general prophylaxis	Amoxicillin	*Adults:* 2.0 g; *Children:* 50 mg/g p.o. 1 h preprocedure (maximum: 2.0 g)
Unable to take oral medications	Ampicillin	*Adults:* 2.0 g i.m. or i.v.; *Children:* 50 mg/kg i.v. or i.m. within 30 min of procedure
Allergic to penicillins	Clindamycin	*Adults:* 600 mg; *Children:* 20 mg/g p.o. 1 h preprocedure
	Cephalexin or cefadroxil	*Adults:* 2.0 g; *Children:* 50 mg/kg p.o. 1 h preprocedure
	Azithromycin or clarithromycin	*Adults:* 500 mg; *Children:* 15 mg/kg p.o. 1 h preprocedure
Allergic to penicillin and unable to take oral medication	Clindamycin	*Adults:* 600 mg; *Children:* 20 mg/kg i.v. within 30 min of procedure
	Cefazolin	*Adults:* 1.0 g; *Children:* 25 mg/kg i.v. or i.m. within 30 min of procedure
For Genitourinary/Gastrointestinal (Nonesophageal) Procedures		
High-risk patients	Ampicillin plus gentamicin	Ampicillin 50 mg/kg i.m. or i.v. (max 2.0 g) *plus* gentamicin 1.5 mg/kg within 30 min of procedure; 6 h later, ampicillin 25 mg/kg i.v. or i.m. *or* amoxicillin 25 mg/kg p.o.
High-risk allergic to ampicillin and amoxicillin	Vancomycin plus gentamicin	Vancomycin 20 mg/kg i.v. over 1–2 h *plus* gentamicin 1–5 mg/kg complete treatment within 3- min of procedure
Moderate-risk patients allergic to ampicillin/amoxicillin	Vancomycin	Vancomycin 20 mg/kg i.v. over 1–2 h—complete treatment within 30 min of procedure

Total children's doses should never exceed adult doses.
Second dose of vancomycin or gentamicin not recommended.
Adapted with permission from Dajani A, et al. Prevention of bacterial endocarditis: recommendations by the American Heart Association. *JAMA* 1997;277:1794–1801.

TABLE 72.18. Acute Management of Hypoxemic Spells

Knee–chest position	i.v. fluids
Oxygen administration	Vasoconstrictors
Evaluate and treat cardiac arrhythmia	Phenylephrine 0.10 mg/kg bolus, i.m. *or* s.c.; 2–10 μg/kg/min infusion i.v.
Morphine sulfate (subcutaneous) (0.1–2 mg/kg)	Methoxamine 0.10 mg/kg IV
Propranolol i.v. (0.2 mg/kg over 5 min)	Bicarbonate (2–3 mEq/kg, i.v.; ensure adequate ventilation)

spell, there may be a notable absence or lessening of a previously heard heart murmur because pulmonary blood flow through the stenotic right ventricular outflow tract is reduced considerably. Laboratory investigations, such as arterial blood gas analysis, ordinarily should be avoided in the initial evaluation. If the attack is prolonged and associated with deepening sensorium changes, assessment of acid-base balance and ventilatory status may be indicated. Monitoring with peripheral oxygen saturation meters (transcutaneous) may be helpful to chart responses to therapy.

MANAGEMENT

The child with hypoxemic spells requires immediate attention. Appropriate positioning, oxygen, and administration of morphine are the standard initial therapeutic measures, and these usually result in prompt abatement of the attack (Table 72.18). Traditionally, subcutaneous morphine has been used in the treatment of cyanotic spells (0.1 to 0.2 mg per kg), although the precise mechanism of action is unknown. Oxygen should be administered because Pa_{O_2} levels may be low and some benefit in terms of oxygen saturation may be obtained from even relatively small increments in dissolved oxygen. The child should be placed in a knee–chest position and calmed, if possible. If the attack persists, additional therapeutic steps are needed. Sodium bicarbonate may be indicated; the dose depends on arterial pH. Propranolol also has been recognized as efficacious in this situation, and an i.v. dose of 0.2 mg per kg over 4 to 5 minutes may yield relatively prompt improvement.

Intravenous fluids should be administered during the severe spell in maintenance doses at least because pulmonary blood flow and right ventricular output depend on volume. Vasopressors have been advocated as alternates or adjuncts in treating hypoxemic spells. Phenylephrine can be given as a dilute i.v. solution of 10 mg per 100 mL and infused at 2 to 10 μg per kg per minute. HR should be monitored and frequent BP assessment carried out if this type of agent is used. Methoxamine (10 mg per 100 mL) or metaraminol (50 mg per 100 mL) also may be used. By increasing systemic vascular resistance, these drugs reduce intracardiac right-to-left shunting favorably and thus improve systemic oxygenation. Digitalis, epinephrine, or norepinephrine, however, should not be used in this setting. If any underlying condition exists, such as a cardiac rhythm disturbance, prompt correction according to the principles noted under "Cardiac Arrhythmias" may alleviate this situation quickly.

ACUTE RHEUMATIC FEVER

CLINICAL MANIFESTATIONS

The diagnosis of rheumatic fever requires a high index of suspicion. The time-honored Jones criteria (Table 72.19), if unequivocally present, usually establish the diagnosis, but the situation may not be always so clear-cut. Polyarthritis is the most commonly found major criterion. Tenderness, motion restriction, heat, redness, and swelling are the typical signs. In contrast to other forms of collagen disease, joint involvement in rheumatic fever usually is migratory and multiple and tends to localize to the larger joints of the extremities.

Chorea is another major criterion defined by Jones. It is a relatively rare finding limited to children older than 3 years of age and most often occurs some time after the initial streptococcal infection, making accurate diagnosis difficult. Chorea is typified by involuntary purposeless movement of the extremities and facial grimacing. Notable emotional lability is also a part of the picture.

The "minor criteria" defined by Jones are nonspecific indices of inflammatory disease and, often, are sources of overdiagnosis of acute rheumatic fever. The fever associated with acute rheumatic fever is notable for its lack of associated chills or rigor. It typically is low grade, and fevers of greater than 40°C (104°F) or a history of a febrile seizure should point to other illnesses. The wildly fluctuating fever of juvenile rheumatoid arthritis ("quotidian" pattern) usually is not a part of the rheumatic fever picture. Elevation of the ESR or C-reactive protein should be present in acute rheumatic fever, but severe CHF may lower the ESR. A prolonged P-R interval is common in acute rheumatic fever but also is an extremely nonspecific finding. It does not necessarily correlate with the presence of organic murmurs and can be found in other inflammatory cardiac diseases or as a result of certain drugs. Overemphasis of the significance of P-R prolongation is a common cause of improper diagnosis.

It must be emphasized that the modified Jones criteria include evidence of recent streptococcal infection in the history. The widespread use of the multiple antibody test (Streptozyme) has made serologic confirmation of recent streptococcal infection much easier. The antistreptolysin O test (ASO) is still a commonly used single serologic test and is well standardized. Levels above 250 Todd units in older children and above 333 Todd units in younger children are present in active rheumatic fever. As many as 20% of otherwise normal children can have elevated ASO titers, and depending on the time course of the illness, other antibody determinations may be required.

A chest radiograph to assess heart size can be helpful for gauging the severity of carditis, as well as for objectively verifying its presence. An ECG should be taken to ensure that a rapid pulse rate is the result of sinus tachycardia and to enable measurement of P-R interval. If pericardial disease or intracardiac myxoma needs to be ruled out, an echocardiogram can provide highly sensitive information.

TABLE 72.19. Rheumatic Fever Manifestations

Major	Elevated acute phase reactants
Carditis	Erythrocyte sedimentation rate
Arthritis	C-reactive protein
Subcutaneous nodules	Prolonged P-R interval
Erythema marginatum	Supporting evidence of antecedent group A streptococcal infections
Chorea	Positive throat culture of rapid streptococcal antibody titer
Minor	Elevated or rising streptococcal antibody titer
Clinical findings	
Arthralgia	
Fever	
Laboratory findings	

Adapted from Jones TD. The diagnosis of rheumatic fever. *JAMA*, 1944;126:481, as modified in Guidelines for the diagnosis of rheumatic fever. *JAMA* 1992; 268:2069.

MANAGEMENT

Acute rheumatic fever requires admission to the hospital and long-term management. Principles of management include 1) treatment of the active streptococcal infection, 2) rest, 3) antiinflammatory agents, and 4) treatment of chorea. All patients with acute rheumatic fever should receive a course of penicillin to eradicate any streptococci. Intramuscular benzathine penicillin in appropriate dosage for age and weight (see Chapter 74) is preferable. Bed rest may be helpful for as long as evidence of active inflammation is present. It should be initiated at diagnosis and is best implemented during the initial period in a hospital setting. Antiinflammatory drugs (salicylates or steroids) may be indicated, but the tendency to begin such therapy before confirmation of the diagnosis, as outlined already, should be resisted. If arthritis without carditis is present, aspirin usually is sufficient. Treatment of carditis may include steroids in selected cases, but that decision should be undertaken only after the child is hospitalized and a cardiologist has been consulted. Treatment of chorea is also a long-term management issue, with agents such as diazepam or haloperidol currently favored (see Chapter 112). Recent evidence suggests a role for steroids in the treatment of chorea and for the presence of carditis.

Occasionally, the child with acute rheumatic fever may present with significant cardiac compromise that involves CHF associated with a large degree of valvar regurgitation or pericardial effusion that results in cardiac tamponade. Initially, the heart failure or tamponade should be managed as outlined in the previous sections, and then consideration should be given to the rheumatic process.

CHAPTER 73
Neurologic Emergencies

Marc H. Gorelick, M.D., M.S.C.E.

SEIZURES (SEE ALSO CHAPTER 61)

Clinical Manifestations

When the physician is faced with a child with an acute paroxysmal event, the first step is to distinguish seizures from other nonepileptic phenomena. If the event is indeed a seizure, it may be classified according to type. Finally, a specific causative factor should be sought. When a child is actively seizing, the first priority is to provide necessary resuscitation measures and control the seizures (see Chapter 61 and the following text).

NONEPILEPTIC PAROXYSMAL EVENTS

Paroxysmal events other than seizures that involve changes in consciousness or motor activity are common during childhood and may mimic epilepsy (Table 73.1). Breath-holding spells occur in children 6 months to 4 years of age. Breath-holding spells take two forms: cyanotic and pallid.

TABLE 73.1. Nonepileptic Events That May Mimic Seizures

Breath-holding spells	Acute dystonia
Syncope	Gastroesophageal reflux
Migraine	Night terrors
Jitteriness	Sleep paralysis
Benign myoclonus	Narcolepsy
Shuddering attacks	Pseudoseizures
Tics	

Syncope is a brief, sudden loss of consciousness and muscle tone. There are numerous causes of syncope, many of which can be detected on the basis of historical information, physical examination, and simple laboratory tests (see Chapter 64). A syncopal episode can usually be distinguished from a seizure based on the description. The child is typically upright before the event and often senses a feeling of light-headedness or nausea. The child then becomes pale and slumps to the ground. The loss of consciousness is brief, and recovery is rapid. On awakening, the child is noted to have signs of increased vagal tone, such as pallor, clammy skin, dilated pupils, and relative bradycardia.

Single episodes of staring, involuntary movements, or eye deviation have been found to occur commonly in the first months of life, although they rarely lead to the parent seeking medical attention. In some children, however, these episodes occur frequently. Children with benign shuddering attacks have episodes of staring and rapid tremors involving primarily the arms and head, sometimes associated with tonic posturing. The episode lasts only a few seconds, and afterward the child resumes normal activity. Acute dystonia, usually seen as a side effect of certain medications, can mimic a tonic seizure. The child having a dystonic reaction, however, does not lose consciousness and has no postictal drowsiness.

Several paroxysmal events are associated with sleep. Night terrors usually begin in the preschool years. The sleeping child wakes suddenly, is confused and disoriented, and appears frightened, often screaming and showing signs of increased autonomic activity (tachycardia, tachypnea, sweating, dilated pupils). Benign myoclonus is characterized by self-limited episodes of sudden jerking of the extremities, usually upon falling asleep. There is no alteration of consciousness. In sleep paralysis, there is a transient inability to move during the transition between sleeping and waking, also with no change in level of consciousness.

Pseudoseizures are occasionally seen, often in patients with an underlying seizure disorder or with a relative with epilepsy. Some features indicative of pseudoseizures are suggestibility, lack of coordination of movements, moaning or talking during the "seizure," lack of continence, autonomic changes, postictal drowsiness, and poor response to treatment with anticonvulsant agents.

TYPES OF SEIZURES

Clinically, seizures may be divided into partial and generalized seizures (Table 73.2). Generalized tonic-clonic seizures (previously called grand mal seizures) are the type most often seen in acute pediatric care. The onset of generalized tonic-clonic seizures usually is abrupt, although 20% to 30% of children may experience a sensory or motor aura. If sitting or standing, the child falls to the ground. The face becomes pale, the pupils dilate, the eyes deviate upward or to one side, and the muscles contract. As the increased tone of the thoracic and abdominal muscles forces air through the glottis, a grunt or cry may be heard. Incontinence of urine or stool is common. After this brief tonic phase (10 to 30 seconds), clonic movements occur. The child is unresponsive during the seizure and remains so, postictally, for a variable period. After the seizure, there may be weak-

TABLE 73.2. Seizure Types

Generalized	Partial (focal)
Absence (petit mal)	Simple (no impaired consciousness)
Typical	Motor
Atypical	Sensory
Tonic-clonic (grand mal)	Autonomic
Clonic	Psychic
Tonic	Complex (impaired consciousness)
Myoclonic	Partial seizures becoming partially
Akinetic/atonic (drop attacks)	generalized

ness or paralysis of one or more areas of the body (Todd paralysis). In atonic, or akinetic, seizures (drop attacks), there is abrupt loss of muscle tone and consciousness. Myoclonic seizures are characterized by a sudden dropping of the head and flexion of the arms ("jackknifing"); however, extensor posturing also may occur. The episodes occur quickly and frequently, as often as several hundred times daily.

Absence (petit mal) seizures are generalized seizures marked by sudden and brief loss of awareness, usually lasting 5 to 30 seconds. With typical absence seizures, there is no loss of posture or tone and no postictal confusion. There may be a minor motor component such as eyelid blinking.

The child with simple partial (focal) seizures has unimpaired consciousness. Motor signs are most common in children, although sensory, autonomic, and psychic manifestations are possible. The motor activity usually involves the hands or face and spreads in a fixed pattern determined by the anatomic origin of the nerve fibers that innervate the various muscle groups. Focal seizures may become secondarily generalized, in which case there will be alteration of consciousness. Complex partial seizures, also called psychomotor or temporal lobe seizures, exhibit a diverse set of clinical features, including alterations of perception, thought, and sensation. In children, they are usually marked by repetitive and complex movements with impaired consciousness and postictal drowsiness.

ESTABLISHING AN UNDERLYING CAUSE

The first steps in the evaluation of seizures are a thorough history and a physical examination, the results of which are helpful in determining the direction of the search for a specific cause. A complete neurologic assessment to evaluate for signs of increased intracranial pressure (ICP), focal deficits, or signs of meningeal irritation is also essential.

An important distinction is whether the seizure is associated with fever. Simple febrile seizures are those that are single, brief (less than 15 minutes), and generalized. Approximately 20% of febrile seizures are complex, meaning they are focal, prolonged (more than 15 minutes), or occur multiple times during the same illness. In children older than 12 months of age with a typical simple febrile seizure and no evidence of meningeal signs, no further evaluation of the seizure is generally required. Lumbar puncture (LP) is mandatory if meningitis is suspected on the basis of physical findings. An LP should be strongly considered in children younger than 12 months of age, in whom signs of meningitis may be subtle, or when the febrile seizure is complex. In addition, LP should be considered for children with prolonged fever before the seizure, particularly those who have sought medical care in the previous 48 hours and who have been found to be at higher risk.

For the child who presents with a first-time, nonfebrile seizure, laboratory or radiologic evaluation to search for a specific treatable cause of the seizure may be indicated. There is little utility in extensive, routine workups; rather, ancillary test selection should be guided by the results of the history and physical examination. Because hypoglycemia may be clinically difficult to detect, a rapid glucose test should be performed on all children. In young infants, children with prolonged seizures, and those with a suggestive history or physical examination, determination of serum sodium and calcium is also indicated. Other laboratory tests that may be indicated, depending on the clinical picture, include serum magnesium, hepatic transaminases, ammonia, and serum or urine toxicology tests. LP is rarely emergently necessary in the afebrile child without meningeal signs, although it should be considered in neonates even without fever.

In children with a known seizure disorder, subtherapeutic anticonvulsant levels are the most common reason for recurrent seizures. Although many drugs have a therapeutic range (Table 73.3), individual patients may require levels outside that range for adequate seizure control; conversely, dose-dependent toxic effects may be observed in some children even at typically therapeutic levels.

Computed tomography (CT) and magnetic resonance imaging (MRI) allow detailed visualization of the gross anatomy of intracranial structures by a noninvasive technique. Presently, CT is more available on an emergent basis in most institutions. It also is a shorter procedure, and patient monitoring is usually easier. CT (or MRI, if available) is indicated in the emergency evaluation of prolonged or focal seizures, when focal deficits are present, when there is a history of trauma, when the child has a ventriculoperitoneal shunt, or when there are associated signs of increased ICP.

Management

STOPPING THE SEIZURE

It is unusual for the child with a brief seizure to arrive in the emergency department (ED) actively convulsing because, by definition, such seizures last less than 15 minutes. Therefore, the actively convulsing child usually is already in a prolonged or serial seizure state, and pharmacologic intervention to terminate the seizure is required (Fig. 73.1).

Intravenous (i.v.) access is established, and blood is drawn for diagnostic studies. If hypoglycemia is documented by rapid glucose assay or if rapid determination is unavailable, i.v. glucose is given in a dose of 2 to 4 mL per kg of 25% dextrose in water. In neonates or in children with suspected isoniazid toxicity, pyridoxine 100 mg i.v. may be administered.

In most situations, benzodiazepines are the first drug of choice for acute seizures because of their rapidity of action. Lorazepam (Ativan) is the preferred agent. Given in a dose of 0.05 to 0.1 mg per kg i.v. (maximum 4 mg per dose), it has an onset of action of 2 to 5 minutes, and the duration of anticonvulsant effect is 12 to 24 hours. The dose may be repeated after 5 to 10 minutes. An alternative is diazepam (Valium), 0.2 to 0.4 mg per kg i.v. (maximum 10 mg per dose), which has a similarly rapid onset of action but a much shorter duration of anticonvulsant activity, usually less than 30 minutes. Thus, if diazepam is used, another agent for longer-term control, such as phenytoin, is needed to prevent seizure recurrence. If i.v. or intraosseous access cannot be established, diazepam may be administered rectally in a dose of 0.5 to 1.0 mg per kg, instilling the i.v. formulation with a syringe. Intramuscular (i.m.) midazolam (Versed) has also been shown to be effective in a dose of 0.2 mg per kg (maximum 7 mg). Midazolam may also be given i.v.

If the seizures have not been controlled within 15 minutes with benzodiazepines, phenytoin (Dilantin) or fosphenytoin should be given. Phenytoin is administered i.v., at a loading

TABLE 73.3. Commonly Used Anticonvulsant Agents

Drug	Seizure type	Daily dose (mg/kg)	Oral dosage forms	Serum half-life (h)	Therapeutic blood levels (μg/mL)
Carbamazepine (Tegretol)	Generalized motor, partial, complex partial	10–30	Tablets: 100, 200 mg Suspension: 100 mg/5 mL	8–24	4–12
Phenytoin (Dilantin)	Generalized motor, partial, complex partial	3–10	Capsule: 100 mg Chewable tap: 50 mg Suspension: 125 mg/5 mL	10–36	10–20
Phenobarbital	Generalized motor, partial, complex partial	3–6	Tablets: 15, 30, 60, 100 mg Elixir: 20 mg/5 mL	24–96	15–40
Primidone (Mysoline)	Generalized motor, partial, complex partial	10–25	Tablets: 50, 250 mg Suspension: 50 mg/5 mL	12	5–12 (also measure phenobarbital level)
Valproate (Depakote)	Absence, myoclonic, partial complex, generalized motor	20–40	Tablets: 125, 250 mg Sprinkles: 125 mg Syrup: 250 mg/5 mL	6–18	50–100
Ethosuximide (Zarontin)	Absence	20–40	Capsule: 250 mg Syrup: 250 mg/5 mL	20–60	40–100
Lamotrigine (Lamictal)	Partial, atonic, myoclonic, mixed types	10–15	Tablets: 25, 100, 150 mg	24	Not known
Clonazepam (Klonopin)	Atonic, myoclonic, generalized motor	0.05–0.2	Tablets: 0.5, 1, 2 mg	18–50	0.02–0.08 (20–80 ng/mL)

dose of 15 to 20 mg per kg. In patients known to be taking phenytoin chronically, a smaller dose of 5 to 10 mg per kg should be used initially unless the serum level is known to be very low. Each 1 mg per kg of phenytoin administered raises the serum level by approximately 1 mg per mL. Fosphenytoin may also be given i.m., unlike phenytoin. The dose of the two drugs is identical; fosphenytoin doses are expressed as phenytoin equivalents.

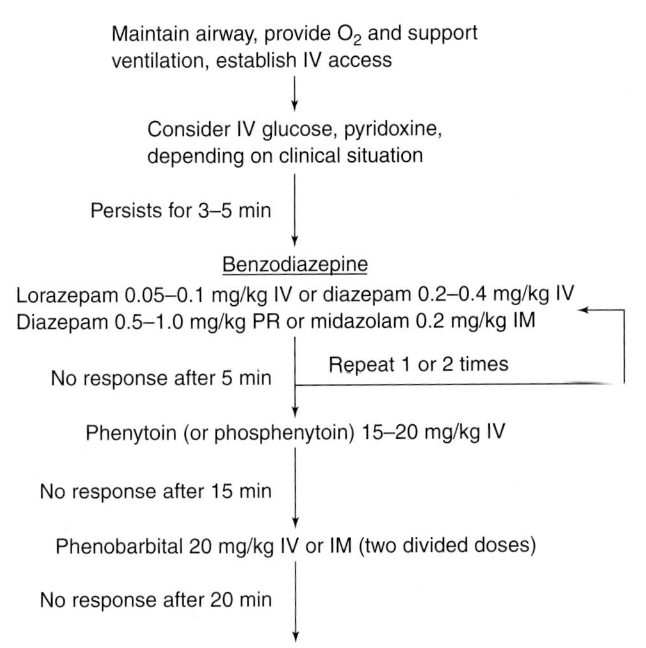

Figure 73.1. Treatment of status epilepticus. *O_2*, oxygen; *IV*, intravenous; *PR*, per rectum; *IM*, intramuscular.

Phenobarbital is the next agent to be added if phenytoin is not effective or contraindicated (eg, allergy, known therapeutic level). The loading dose of phenobarbital is 20 mg per kg, usually given in two divided doses. The drug is given i.v. over 5 to 10 minutes, or i.m. in the absence of i.v. access. Onset of action is usually within 15 to 20 minutes and lasts more than 24 hours.

Patients with status epilepticus that lasts more than 60 minutes present a special problem. Further management should be done in conjunction with a neurologist and with electroencephalogram (EEG) monitoring when possible. Continuous infusion of benzodiazepines may be used. Paraldehyde is often effective but is difficult to handle because of its foul odor, reactivity with rubber and plastic (necessitating the use of glass syringes), and lack of water solubility. A dose of 0.3 mg per kg diluted 1:1 in oil may be given rectally. Other agents potentially useful in the management of refractory status epilepticus include pentobarbital and general anesthetics such as isoflurane, etomidate, and propofol.

Rarely, a child may enter the ED in absence status. In this case, the child may be sitting in a confused or dreamy state. Such attacks may last for hours or even days. The drug of choice in the treatment of absence status is lorazepam or diazepam at the dosages already outlined.

At times, a child may enter the ED with continual focal seizure activity (with or without clouding of consciousness), a condition known as epilepsia partialis continua. In these cases, phenytoin or fosphenytoin in a dose of 18 to 20 mg per kg can be infused slowly. All patients should be admitted to the hospital for further observation and evaluation. Other pharmacologic attempts to control these focal seizures should be performed in the hospital.

INITIATING ANTICONVULSANT MEDICATION

Nonfebrile Seizures

Treatment is seldom started after a single, uncomplicated nonfebrile seizure because most such patients will not experience a seizure recurrence. On the other hand, a patient who has had two or more such seizures should generally receive anticonvulsant therapy. A number of drugs are effective in preventing seizures (Table 73.3). Some are better for certain types of seizures, and all have different profiles of adverse effects. The following principles should guide selection of an anticonvulsant medication:

1. Choose a drug that is effective for the particular type of seizure. When more than one agent is available, choose the least toxic one. Initial therapy should be with a single agent.
2. Start at the low end of the dosage range.
3. Arrange for a serum level of the drug to be measured, when appropriate. This is done after a steady state is anticipated, usually five times the half-life of the drug.
4. If a child is already taking an anticonvulsant medication and has an adequate level, consider adding another agent.

Carbamazepine (Tegretol). Carbamazepine is effective against generalized tonic-clonic seizures as well as simple and complex partial seizures. The effective serum concentrations of carbamazepine range between 4 and 12 μg per mL, but with this drug, there is a variable correlation among clinical efficacy, toxicity, and the serum concentration. Recommended maintenance dosages range between 10 and 30 mg per kg per day, divided into three daily doses. Carbamazepine may cause hepatic and hematologic toxicity but causes little, if any, cognitive dysfunction in most patients.

Phenobarbital. Phenobarbital is another broad-spectrum anticonvulsant useful for generalized tonic-clonic and partial (simple and complex) seizures.. The effective serum concentration ranges between 15 and 40 μg per mL. This serum level usually can be maintained with a dosage of 3 to 6 mg per kg per day in children and 1 to 2 mg per kg per day in adolescents, administered in divided doses twice daily. A loading dosage of approximately twice the maintenance dosage (6 to 10 mg per kg per day in children and 2 to 4 mg per kg per day in adolescents) for 2 to 3 days brings the serum concentration to the therapeutic range within 48 to 72 hours.

Phenytoin (Dilantin). Phenytoin is another agent effective in the treatment of several seizure types, including generalized motor seizures and both simple and partial complex seizures. The effective serum concentration of phenytoin is between 10 and 20 μg per mL. The usual maintenance dosage is 7 to 10 mg per kg per day in children weighing less than 20 kg, 5 to 7 mg per kg per day in children weighing between 20 and 40 kg, and 5 mg per kg per day in children weighing more than 40 kg, given in one or two daily doses. Loading dosages of four times the daily dosage (maximum 20 mg per kg per day) on the first day and two times the daily dosage for the next 2 days will bring serum levels into the therapeutic range within 24 hours; side effects rarely occur with this loading dosage.

Valproate (Depakote). Valproate is highly effective in the treatment of generalized epilepsy, especially absence and myoclonic seizures, as well as simple and complex partial seizures. Doses of 20 to 40 mg per kg usually result in therapeutic levels of 50 to 100 μg per mL. Children younger than 2 years are at particular risk of idiosyncratic fatal hepatotoxicity.

Clonazepam (Klonopin). Clonazepam is used to control myoclonic and atonic seizures. The usual dosage is 0.05 to 0.2 mg per kg per day, given in two to four divided doses. The therapeutic range is 0.02 to 0.08 μg per mL (10 to 80 ng per mL). Patients taking clonazepam may experience drowsiness, ataxia, and drooling.

Ethosuximide (Zarontin). Ethosuximide is indicated for the management of absence seizures. It is given at a dosage of 20 to 40 mg per kg per day divided into twice daily doses, with a usual therapeutic level of 40 to 100 μg per mL. Side effects include headache, nausea, and vomiting; erythema multiforme and a lupuslike syndrome have also been reported.

Lamotrigine (Lamictal). Lamotrigine is a new agent available for treatment of partial seizures, atonic and myoclonic seizures, and intractable mixed seizures (Lennox-Gastaut syndrome). The usual dosage is 10 to 15 mg per kg per day, which is reduced to 5 mg per kg per day when given in conjunction with valproate. Drowsiness, vomiting, and drug rash (including Stevens-Johnson syndrome) are reported side effects.

Other Agents. Several agents are newly available in the United States. These include vigabatrin (Sabril), gabapentin (Neurontin), and felbamate (Felbatol). Because of the risk of severe hepatotoxicity, felbamate is restricted to use in children with intractable seizures refractory to other treatment.

Disposition. Hospital admission is generally required for children who have had a prolonged seizure requiring acute treatment with anticonvulsant medication. Other children, even those with a first-time seizure, can generally be followed as outpatients if they appear well after the seizure, follow-up can be ensured, and the parents are comfortable with home management. Seizure first aid should be explained to the family before discharge. After a simple febrile seizure, hospitalization is seldom necessary, and children may be followed by their primary physician.

DISORDERS THAT PRESENT WITH ENCEPHALOPATHY (SEE CHAPTER 9)

Encephalopathy is an imprecise term that implies diffuse brain dysfunction with or without alterations in the level of consciousness. The emergency physician often must decide whether the child's degree of irritability, uncooperativeness, and lethargy is proportionate to the degree of systemic illness; whether it is caused by fear; or whether it represents cortical dysfunction. Encephalopathy may be a sign of numerous systemic disorders, or it may result from certain primary disorders of the central nervous system (CNS), discussed next.

Encephalitis

CLINICAL MANIFESTATIONS

Encephalitis is an inflammation of the brain parenchyma. When there is an associated leptomeningeal involvement (as often occurs), the term *meningoencephalitis* may be applied, whereas *encephalomyelitis* implies involvement of the spinal cord as well. Viral encephalitides are caused by a wide variety of viruses that lead to clinically similar illnesses (Table 73.4). The clinical picture of viral encephalitis ranges from a mild febrile illness associated with headache to a severe, fulminant presentation with coma, seizures, and death. The onset of encephalitis may be abrupt or insidious. Typical features consist of fever, headache, vomiting, and signs of meningeal irritation. Altered consciousness, ataxia, and seizures are also seen. Focal neurologic deficits occur in certain types of encephalitis, particularly herpes simplex virus (HSV). Flaccid paralysis may be seen in cases of encephalomyelitis, and rarely, respiratory or cardiac dysfunction results from brainstem involvement. Rash or mucous mem-

TABLE 73.4. Agents of Viral Encephalitis

Arboviruses	Varicella-zoster
Eastern equine encephalitis	Epstein-Barr
Western equine encephalitis	Cytomegalovirus
St. Louis encephalitis	Mumps
Japanese encephalitis	Measles
California (LaCrosse) encephalitis	Enteroviruses
	Rabies
Herpesviruses	
Herpes simplex	

brane lesions are often seen with the exanthematous viruses such as measles and varicella; however, cutaneous findings are uncommon with HSV encephalitis.

Laboratory assessment often is nonspecific. The peripheral blood count usually shows a mild polymorphonuclear or mononuclear leukocytosis. With viral encephalitides, cerebral spinal fluid (CSF) pleocytosis is variable and, if present, usually is fewer than 500 cells per mm^3. These cells may be predominantly polymorphonuclear early in the course of the illness; however, a mononuclear predominance is common later. Red blood cells are present in the CSF in approximately 50% of children with herpes encephalitis. Spinal fluid protein and glucose usually are normal with viral encephalitis, but the protein may be greatly elevated in postinfectious encephalomyelitis.

Virus isolation from the CSF may be difficult but should be attempted, as should viral isolation from other body sites, including the nasopharynx, skin lesions, urine, and feces. Serologic evidence for viral infection based on acute and convalescent immunoglobulin G (IgG) titers, although useful later, gives little help in making an immediate diagnosis. Infection with arboviruses may be established more rapidly by detecting virus-specific immunoglobulin M (IgM) in CSF or serum.

Diagnosis of herpes simplex poses a special problem because early diagnosis is important in instituting effective therapy. When available, polymerase chain reaction (PCR) testing of CSF yields rapid evidence of viral nucleic acid and is highly sensitive and specific. Imaging studies, although less sensitive, may also be useful. Either CT or MRI may demonstrate focal parenchymal involvement or edema of the temporal lobes. MRI is more sensitive than CT, although both may be normal in the early stages of disease. Similarly, EEG may demonstrate focal slowing or epileptiform discharges localized to the temporal lobes, but absence of such findings does not rule out herpes encephalitis.

MANAGEMENT

Presently, the treatment of nonherpes viral encephalitis is primarily supportive. Children with very mild manifestations may be followed at home, but those with more significant illness should be hospitalized for observation and monitoring of neurologic status, treatment of increased ICP if present, and fluid restriction and monitoring of urine output and serum sodium because of the risk for inappropriate antidiuretic hormone (ADH) secretion.

Herpes simplex encephalitis causes death or neurologic sequelae in more than 70% of patients. Treatment with acyclovir (30 to 60 mg per kg per day divided three times daily for 14 to 21 days) has resulted in a decrease in mortality and some improvement in morbidity. It must be used early in the disease to achieve maximum benefit. Thus, acyclovir should be considered in all patients suspected of having herpes encephalitis on the basis of clinical or epidemiologic grounds (eg, history of exposure, oral vesicles, focal neurologic or radiographic findings). Because clinical features and laboratory tests are not perfectly sensitive, initial presumptive treatment may be indicated even in the absence of corroborating evidence.

Hemorrhagic Shock and Encephalopathy Syndrome

Hemorrhagic shock and encephalopathy syndrome (HSES), first described in 1983, is a syndrome of catastrophic illness that affects infants less than 1 year of age. It is characterized by the sudden onset of coma, seizures, and shock in a previously healthy infant. The clinical features are similar to those seen in severe bacterial sepsis, although cultures are by definition negative in children with HSES. The syndrome also resembles heat stroke, leading to speculation that an abnormality of thermal regulation may be responsible. Besides the encephalopathy, seizures, and shock, other consistent features of HSES include high fever at the onset, disseminated intravascular coagulation and hemorrhage, and metabolic acidosis. Affected children have a number of characteristic laboratory abnormalities consistent with multiple organ system dysfunction, including elevation of blood urea nitrogen (BUN), creatinine, hepatic transaminases, and creatine phosphokinase (CPK), anemia, thrombocytopenia, and coagulopathy. The laboratory abnormalities peak in the first 48 hours. Brain CT reveals only cerebral edema in the first few days, followed by development of encephalomalacia in severely ill individuals. Treatment of infants with HSES consists of intensive supportive care.

DISORDERS THAT PRESENT WITH HEADACHE

Migraine

BACKGROUND

CLINICAL MANIFESTATIONS

Prolonged (up to 24 to 48 hours), moderate to severe headache is characteristic of migraine. The headaches may be pulsating and unilateral but assume this pattern less often in children than in adults. Migraine is commonly associated with nausea, vomiting, abdominal pain, and photophobia or phonophobia. Auras occur in less than half of children who experience migraines. During the headaches, analgesics are relatively ineffective, and children seek a quiet, dimly lit area to rest or sleep. Occasionally, the attacks awaken the children from sleep. The physical examination usually shows no focal neurologic deficits, although hemiplegia and ophthalmoplegia may occur in complicated migraine. Unless these episodes have occurred previously, their presence warrants further neurologic evaluation, usually in the form of CT or MRI scanning.

A family history of migraine is helpful in diagnosis, and a disproportionate number of children who experience migraines have episodes of motion sickness, dizziness, vertigo, or frank paroxysmal events. Common trigger factors for migraine in children include emotional stress, lighting changes, and minor head trauma. Particularly in adolescents, it is useful to screen for depression or other psychosocial stressors that may warrant separate treatment. Foods, such as lunch meats, which contain nitrates, and cheeses, which contain tyramine, are less common but important triggers.

The diagnosis of migraine is based almost exclusively on the history and is supported by the absence of abnormalities on examination. There are no diagnostic laboratory tests or imaging studies. Given an accurate history, differentiation from tension headaches, sinusitis, and headaches secondary to intracranial lesions usually is possible; studies such as EEG, CT, and MRI are rarely indicated. Of children who experience migraines, 20% to 90% have been reported to have nonspecific EEG abnormalities, but the EEG usually is not helpful in diagnosis.

MANAGEMENT

A number of agents are available for the treatment of acute migraine (Table 73.5). For many children, mild oral analgesics such as acetaminophen or ibuprofen combined with bed rest may provide sufficient relief and should be considered the first-line agents of choice. Ketorolac (Toradol), a nonsteroidal antiinflammatory agent for parenteral use, may be used when nausea or vomiting limits oral intake. A short course of a narcotic analgesic such as codeine may occasionally be needed if nonnarcotic agents have failed, especially if the headache prevents sleep.

When nausea and vomiting are severe, antiemetic medications such as metoclopramide (Reglan), prochlorperazine (Compazine), and promethazine (Phenergan) are useful. In addition to their antiemetic effect, these agents often provide some relief of the headache and may permit the use of other oral medications. All of these agents have the potential to produce dystonic reactions.

Ergot preparations act primarily as cerebral vasoconstrictors and are specifically indicated for aborting acute migraine attacks. Ergotamine tartrate is administered orally or sublingually, but it must be used early in the headache to be effective, preferably at the outset of the prodrome. Because most young children cannot identify an aura, the use of these preparations is limited before adolescence. Common side effects of ergot preparations include nausea, vomiting, cramps, and distal paresthesias, all of which may intensify the symptoms of migraine. Chronic ergotism and dependence may occur with repeated use. Dihydroergotamine (DHE) is an injectable ergot derivative with fewer side effects. Ergotamine preparations with additional drugs such as phenobarbital and caffeine are available; however, there is little evidence to show that they are more efficacious than ergots alone.

For acute migraine, DHE can be given to older children and adolescents in an initial dose of 0.5 mg i.m. or i.v. (no milligram-per-kilogram dose has been established). The initial dose of DHE may be repeated in 1 hour if necessary. One study in adults reported that 3 mg administered intranasally is also effective. Antiemetics may be useful to control the nausea and vomiting that often occur after DHE administration.

Sumatriptan succinate (Imitrex) is a serotonergic agent available for either oral or subcutaneous administration. Its effectiveness in relieving symptoms of acute migraine has been demonstrated in adults, but similar evidence is lacking in children. The dose for children 12 years and older is 6 mg subcutaneously or 100 mg orally. Sumatriptan is generally well tolerated; side effects include irritation at the injection site, flushing, tachycardia, disorientation, and chest tightness that lasts for several minutes after parenteral administration. Sumatriptan should not be used concomitantly with ergotamines. A reasonable approach is to use sumatriptan after a trial of analgesics in an older child, although older children or adolescents with recurrent migraine and a history of successful treatment with sumatriptan in the past may benefit from earlier use of this agent.

If migraines are frequent and severe, prophylactic treatment is possible. Many drugs have been used, but because they require close, serial examination and have no effect on the acute attack, they should not be started in the ED. Among the medications used for chronic suppressive therapy are propranolol, tricyclic antidepressants, cyproheptadine (Periactin), valproic acid, and calcium channel blockers.

TABLE 73.5. Agents for Acute Treatment of Migraine

Drug	Usual dose
Analgesics	
Acetaminophen	10–15 mg/kg/dose p.o. or p.r. q4h
Ibuprofen	5–10 mg/kg/dose p.o. q6h
Ketorolac (Toradol)	30 mg initial dose, then 15–30 mg/dose (0.5 mg/kg) i.v. or i.m., or 10 mg/dose p.o., q4–6h
Codeine	0.5–1 mg/kg/dose p.o. q4–6h
Antiemetics	
Metoclopramide (Reglan)	0.5–2 mg/kg/dose p.o. or i.v. q4–6h
Prochlorperazine (Compazine)	0.1 mg/kg/dose p.o. or i.m. q6h
Promethazine (Phenergan)	0.25–1.0 mg/kg/dose p.o., p.r., i.v., or i.m. q4–6h
Specific antimigraine agents	
Dihydroergotamine	0.5–1.0 mg/dose i.v. or i.m.; may repeat after 1 h
Sumatriptan (Imitrex)	6 mg s.c. or 100 mg p.o.

Idiopathic Intracranial Hypertension (Pseudotumor Cerebri)

CLINICAL MANIFESTATIONS

Headache, of variable severity and duration, is the most common presenting symptom of idiopathic intracranial hypertension (IIH), or pseudotumor cerebri. It is typically worse in the morning. Nausea, vomiting, dizziness, and double or blurred vision also occur. If the process is long-standing, decreased visual acuity or visual field deficits can result. Infants often have nonspecific symptoms of lethargy or irritability. Papilledema is seen in virtually all cases. Other neurologic symptoms and signs are often absent; however, cranial nerve palsies, particularly affecting the sixth cranial nerve, may be seen.

Diagnosis should be considered when a child with a prolonged history of headache is found to have evidence of papilledema without other neurologic findings. Pseudotumor cerebri is a diagnosis of exclusion, and mass lesions and infectious processes must be ruled out. Because posterior fossa tumors and obstructive or nonobstructive hydrocephalus may mimic pseudotumor early in the course of disease, CT or MRI should be obtained in all children with this constellation of findings. In cases of IIH, the ventricles will appear normal or small. If no mass lesion is present, an LP should be performed with a manometer to measure opening pressure. The patient must be recumbent with legs extended to ensure an accurate reading of the opening pressure. Children with pseudotumor have elevated opening pressure (greater than 200 mm H_2O), but normal CSF cell count, protein, and glucose. In children with intermittent symptoms, the opening pressure may be normal when the headache is waning, even though papilledema may persist for several weeks.

MANAGEMENT

Removal of sufficient CSF to normalize ICP usually leads to relief of symptoms. Treatment may then be started with acetazolamide (Diamox) to decrease CSF production (60 mg per kg per day divided four times daily). Although recommended by some authorities, corticosteroids have not been proven to be effective in the management of this condition. However, in cases of IIH following withdrawal of steroid therapy, a course of prednisone or dexamethasone may be beneficial. Patients with mild symptoms and good response to LP may be discharged to home with close follow-up arranged. Children with severe or persistent symptoms or those with visual changes may require hospital admission. Intracranial hypertension may be recurrent or chronic, and long-term monitoring, particularly of visual function, is important.

DISORDERS OF MOTOR FUNCTION (SEE CHAPTER 70)

Every level of the neural axis is involved in the performance of motor tasks. Anatomic localization usually is possible after evaluation of the distribution and character of the deficit (Table 73.6). Paresis refers to partial or complete weakness of a part of the body.

Various clinical designations are used to describe some patterns of weakness: paraplegia (or paraparesis), affecting the lower half of the body; quadriplegia, affecting all limbs; and hemiplegia, referring to weakness of one side of the body. Paraplegia most often results from spinal cord involvement, whereas hemiparesis is most often a sign of cortical disease. Some of the common conditions affecting various levels of the neuromotor system that may present with acute motor dysfunction are discussed next.

Stroke/Cerebrovascular Accident

CLINICAL MANIFESTATIONS

The presentation of stroke in children is highly variable, influenced by the portion of the cerebral vasculature affected as well as the child's age. Hemiparesis is most often observed, with facial weakness typically ipsilateral to weakness in the rest of the body. Involvement of the anterior cerebral artery leads primarily to lower extremity weakness, whereas compromise of the middle cerebral artery circulation produces hemiplegia with upper limb predominance, hemianopsia, and possibly dysphasia. Less commonly, the posterior circulation is affected, which results in vertigo, ataxia, and nystagmus, as well as hemiparesis and hemianopsia. Older children often have concomitant headache, whereas children less than 4 years of age are more likely to have associated seizures. The child with a stroke may also have a diminished level of consciousness.

Investigations in a child with acute hemiparesis should be directed at confirming the diagnosis of stroke and attempting to identify an underlying cause if none is known. Imaging studies are useful. Cranial CT without contrast is the study of choice for identifying acute hemorrhage. However, CT may be normal in the first 12 to 24 hours after an ischemic stroke; MRI, in contrast, may show changes as early as 6 hours after infarction. A usual approach is to obtain a noncontrast CT, followed by MRI if no hemorrhage is seen.

TABLE 73.7. Studies to Consider in the Evaluation of the Child with Acute Stroke

Brain imaging	Erythrocyte sedimentation rate
Computed tomography (noncontrast)	Hemoglobin electrophoresis
Magnetic resonance imaging	Protein C and S quantification
Angiography (standard or magnetic resonance)	Antithrombin III level
Cardiac	*Chemistry*
Electrocardiogram	Blood urea nitrogen
Echocardiogram	Cholesterol and triglycerides
Hematologic	Hepatic transaminases
Complete blood count	Serum amino acids
Prothrombin and partial thromboplastin times	Urine organic acids
Fibrinogen	Toxicology screen
	Lactate
	Lumbar Puncture

In a child without a known predisposing condition, ancillary tests may be revealing of the cause of the stroke. Studies worth considering in such patients, depending on the clinical picture, are listed in Table 73.7. In one large series of 129 children with ischemic stroke, no cause was found in 35%.

MANAGEMENT

Initial treatment after an acute stroke is focused on stabilization and supportive care, including control of any seizures. Several aspects require special attention. Although evident hypotension should be treated with volume expansion, administration of free water should be restricted because of the potential for edema formation. Hypertension, if present, must be treated cautiously, and the blood pressure lowered gradually. Both hypoglycemia and hyperglycemia can exacerbate ischemic stroke, so careful monitoring of serum glucose is important. Fever, which can occur in children with stroke, may also contribute to ischemic damage and should be controlled with antipyretics.

TABLE 73.6. Localizing Level of Neuromotor Dysfunction

	Tone	Distribution	Reflexes	Babinski	Other
Upper motor neuron	Increased (may be decreased acutely)	Pattern (e.g., hemiparesis, paraparesis)	Increased (may be decreased acutely)	Extensor	Cognitive dysfunction possible
Anterior horn cell	Decreased	Distal > proximal Variable, asymmetric	Decreased to absent	Flexor	Fasciculations; no sensory involvement
Peripheral nerve	Decreased	Nerve distribution	Decreased to absent	Flexor	Sensory involvement
Neuromuscular junction	Normal	Fluctuating	Usually normal	Flexor	
Muscle	Decreased	Proximal > distal	Decreased	Flexor	Tenderness, signs of inflammation possible

Further therapy is determined by the type of stroke. With hemorrhagic stroke, neurosurgical intervention may be required to evacuate a hematoma or excise a bleeding arteriovenous malformation (AVM). Catheter-directed embolization may also be possible in cases of AVM. Children with sickle cell disease and stroke should have acute transfusion to decrease the level of hemoglobin S to less than 30%. Thrombolytic and anticoagulant therapies have been shown to be effective in adults with ischemic stroke but remain untested in children. Similarly, novel therapies such as calcium channel blockers and free radical scavengers have not been studied in pediatric patients; their use remains experimental.

Overall, prognosis for children with stroke is better than that in adults. However, regardless of treatment, long-term morbidity of stroke in children is high, with more than 75% of affected children experiencing sequelae such as hemiparesis, seizures, and learning difficulties.

Spinal Cord Dysfunction

BACKGROUND

Dysfunction of the spinal cord may result from any of a variety of disorders, either intrinsic or extrinsic to the spinal cord, with a great deal of overlap in their clinical presentation. Transverse myelitis is an intramedullary disorder, involving both halves of the cord over a variable length, with involvement of motor and sensory tracts. It occurs in children and adults, although it is rare in the first year of life. Transverse myelitis is believed to be a localized form of acute disseminated encephalomyelitis, discussed previously. Like the latter disorder, transverse myelitis may occur after a number of infections; among those commonly reported are Epstein-Barr virus, cytomegalovirus, measles, mumps, *Campylobacter jejuni,* and *Mycoplasma pneumoniae.* Transverse myelitis may also result from systemic autoimmune disorders such as lupus erythematosus or scleroderma. In some older children and adolescents, transverse myelitis is a first manifestation of multiple sclerosis.

Acute spinal cord compression in children usually is caused by trauma, infection, or cancer. Spinal trauma may lead to contusion or concussion of the cord with hemorrhage, edema, and local mass effect, or to development of a spinal epidural hematoma. Parenchymal injury usually presents acutely, but an epidural hematoma may develop over several days after the antecedent trauma. Epidural abscess is the most common infectious cause of spinal cord compression. It is usually caused by hematogenous spread of bacteria, with *Staphylococcus aureus* being the most common pathogen. Neoplastic causes include both primary intraspinal tumors (ependymoma and astrocytoma) and extrinsic lesions such as neuroblastoma or lymphoma.

CLINICAL MANIFESTATIONS

Spinal cord dysfunction from any cause is characterized by paraplegia below the level of involvement, hyporeflexia, and sensory symptoms such as bandlike pain at the level of compression, and sensory loss or paresthesias below the area of damage. If the lower spinal cord is involved (the conus), there usually is early loss of bowel and bladder control. Compression of the cauda equina usually results in asymmetric symptoms, radicular pain, and focal lower extremity motor and sensory abnormalities.

Transverse myelitis may affect any level of the spinal cord, but thoracic involvement is most common. Initial symptoms include lower extremity paresthesia, local back pain, unilateral or bilateral lower extremity weakness, and urinary retention. A preceding respiratory or gastrointestinal illness is usually reported, and at the time of diagnosis, fever and meningism are sometimes seen in children. Characteristically, the insidious onset of paresthesia or weakness of the lower extremities progresses over days or, rarely, weeks, and then is replaced by the abrupt occurrence of static paraplegia or quadriplegia and, in the cooperative child, a detectable sensory level. In other children, the course of progression may be less than 12 hours. The sensory loss generally involves all modalities, although a spinothalamic deficit (pain) may occur without posterior column dysfunction (vibration). The weakness usually is symmetric but may be asymmetric. After a variable interval, initial flaccidity may be replaced by spasticity. Sphincter disturbance of the bowel and bladder occurs in most patients, bladder distension being the most common initial sign of damage.

Traumatic and infectious spinal lesions are usually accompanied by relatively acute onset of local back pain, which is exacerbated by direct percussion of the area. Pain may precede other symptoms for days. With tumors, however, there may be weakness in the absence of pain. Patients with epidural abscess often have systemic signs of infections such as fever, headache, vomiting, and perhaps neck stiffness. Bony tenderness in such a patient may indicate vertebral osteomyelitis or discitis, which can also present with weakness, although usually less severe than is seen with actual spinal cord involvement.

Prompt diagnosis of spinal cord lesions requires a high level of expectation. Detailed neurologic examination is essential, with particular attention to quality of deep tendon reflexes, any asymmetry of reflexes or strength, evaluation for a sensory level, and assessment of anal tone and cremasteric reflexes (in males). Note also any point percussion tenderness.

Diagnosis is confirmed by emergency neuroimaging, with precautions to immobilize the patient as much as possible. Plain spine films are useful initially in trauma. MRI of the spine is the procedure of choice to detect compressive mass lesions, but if not immediately available, plain or CT myelography is an alternative. In transverse myelitis, the cord may be widened at the level of involvement. This is easier to detect with MRI, which in some cases may also reveal evidence of focal intramedullary demyelination.

LP alone should not be performed if a diagnosis of spinal cord compression is entertained. If no mass lesion is noted and transverse myelitis is a diagnostic possibility, LP may be useful, showing a normal or slightly elevated opening pressure and a mild pleocytosis in the CSF in nearly 50% of patients at the time of presentation. The CSF protein is often elevated and may demonstrate oligoclonal bands or increased myelin basic protein, but the glucose usually is normal.

MANAGEMENT

Treatment of children with spinal injury from trauma begins with splinting and immobilization of the spine. If trauma is likely, high-dose methylprednisolone, if given within 8 hours of injury at an i.v. dose of 30 mg per kg followed by infusion at 5.4 mg per kg per hour for 23 hours, improves the quality of neurologic outcome. Neurosurgical consultation should be obtained as soon as possible; however, early surgical attempts to decompress the swollen spine (laminectomy or midline myelotomy) have proven ineffective and, possibly, detrimental.

In cases of possible epidural abscess or tumor-related mass, i.v. dexamethasone at a loading dose of 2 mg per kg (up to a maximum of 100 mg) should be given, followed by 1 to 2 mg per kg per day i.v. in four divided doses over the next 24 hours. In patients with a presumed infectious cause and those with cancer of unknown origin, surgical decompression is indicated on an emergent basis to alleviate pressure and pinpoint diagnosis. Further treatment depends on the organism or exact tumor type found.

Treatment of transverse myelitis is supportive, and some degree of recovery occurs in approximately 80% of cases. All children with this syndrome should be hospitalized. Although systemic corticosteroids are often recommended for treatment of transverse myelitis, there is little evidence of their efficacy.

Treatment with intraspinal steroids or emergency laminectomy has also not been shown to improve outcome. High-dose dexamethasone as described previously may be begun until cord compression by a mass lesion is ruled out.

Acute Polyneuritis (Guillain-Barré)

CLINICAL MANIFESTATIONS

Weakness, commonly with an insidious inset, is the usual presenting complaint. Paresthesias or other sensory abnormalities such as pain or numbness are prominent in up to 50% of cases, particularly in older children. The paresthesias and paralysis usually are symmetric and ascending, although variations may occur. Early in the course of illness, distal weakness is more prominent than proximal weakness. Deep tendon reflexes are depressed or absent at the time of diagnosis. Affected children often have an ataxic gait.

Cranial nerve abnormalities occur during the illness in 30% to 40% of cases and may be the predominant finding, especially in the Miller-Fisher variant of this syndrome, which is characterized by oculomotor palsies, ataxia, and areflexia without motor weakness of the extremities. The most common cranial nerve deficit is seventh (facial) nerve palsy, followed in decreasing frequency by impairment of cranial nerves IX, X, and XI and oculomotor abnormalities. Autonomic dysfunction occurs commonly and results in blood pressure lability, postural hypotension, and cardiac abnormalities; it is a disproportionate cause of morbidity and mortality. Urinary retention, if it occurs, is usually seen late in the illness. As the paralysis ascends, muscles of breathing may become involved, leading to respiratory embarrassment.

The primary aid in diagnosis is LP, which demonstrates an elevated protein, normal glucose, and fewer than ten white blood cells per mm^3—the so-called albuminocytologic disassociation. The protein elevation occurs in almost all cases but may be delayed for weeks, usually peaking in the second or third week of illness. Electrophysiologic evidence for Guillain-Barré syndrome is the presence of nerve conduction velocity delay, which usually is not demonstrable until the second or third week of illness. Emergency electromyography (EMG) and nerve conduction velocity testing are not indicated.

MANAGEMENT

Because of the potential for progression to life-threatening respiratory compromise, the child with Guillain-Barré syndrome should be hospitalized and observed closely. Impending respiratory distress must be anticipated, and routine respiratory monitoring should be aided by specific measures of respiratory function, particularly measurement of negative inspiratory force. Because autonomic dysfunction is common, blood pressure must be monitored closely and abnormalities treated vigorously.

Acute polyneuritis is generally self-limiting, with more than 90% of children in most series having complete or near complete recovery. In mild cases, in which children retain the ability to ambulate, only supportive care is required. However, immunomodulatory therapy may be of benefit in more severely affected children. Plasmapheresis and i.v. immunoglobulin have both been used. Although well-controlled, blinded studies of these treatments in children are lacking, the available data suggest both are effective in reducing the duration and severity of illness in those most severely affected, especially when begun early in the course of the disease. Corticosteroids have not been shown to be beneficial in acute Guillain-Barré syndrome.

Myasthenia Gravis

CLINICAL MANIFESTATIONS

The juvenile form of myasthenia clinically mimics the adult disease. The mean age of onset is 8 years, with a female predominance of approximately 4:1. The onset of symptoms may be insidious or acute. Most cases affect the cranial nerves, and any cranial nerve can be involved in combination or isolation. Bilateral ptosis is the most common cranial nerve deficit, followed in incidence by oculomotor impairment. Generalized truncal and limb weakness is present at onset in up to half of cases and eventually develops in most children with myasthenia. The diagnosis should be suspected if there is a history of worsening weakness during continual activity or if fatigability of muscle strength is demonstrable. Illnesses confused with myasthenia include the muscular dystrophies, congenital myopathies, inflammatory myopathies, acute and chronic polyneuropathies, and in the infant, botulism.

The Tensilon test is the backbone of the diagnosis of myasthenia. In this procedure, the anticholinesterase drug edrophonium (Tensilon), which has a 30-second onset and approximately a 5-minute duration of action, is given slowly by i.v. at a dosage of 0.2 mg per kg, up to a maximum dose of 10 mg. Atropine should be immediately available to treat potential severe cholinergic reactions (eg, bradycardia). Initially, one-tenth of the total dose is given, and if no hypersensitivity or severe reactions are noted, the remainder of the dose is administered. Because edrophonium is short-lived, interpretation of the response requires close monitoring of a muscle or muscle group in which improvement can be seen clearly, such as the eyelid elevators. In small children, this often is impossible and longer-acting anticholinesterases such as neostigmine (0.125 mg in an infant and 0.04 mg per kg in an older child) can be used. EMG provides electrophysiologic evidence for myasthenia gravis, with a decremental response to repetitive nerve stimulation, but may be negative when the disease is confined to the cranial nerves.

MANAGEMENT

Although myasthenia gravis is potentially life threatening, specific management usually can be delayed until after diagnosis is made. If there is evidence of respiratory compromise, ventilatory support is mandatory. Treatment is begun with the use of cholinesterase inhibitors to prolong the availability of acetylcholine at the neuromuscular junction. Presently, the anticholinesterase of choice is pyridostigmine (Mestinon) at a starting dosage of 1 mg per kg by mouth every 4 hours, adjusted according to the clinical response. Other agents, such as corticosteroids or antimetabolites, may be beneficial in selected cases. If there is any concern about respiratory compromise or if severe weakness is present, the child should be hospitalized immediately.

Myasthenia has a fluctuating, unpredictable course that can be exacerbated by intercurrent illness and by certain drugs, particularly the aminoglycoside antibiotics. In a known myasthenic, rapid worsening and respiratory compromise (myasthenic crises) may be difficult to differentiate from deterioration secondary to overdose of anticholinesterases (cholinergic crises) because the muscarinic side effects of the anticholinesterases, such as nausea, vomiting, cramps, and muscle fasciculations, may be absent. At times, differentiation can be made by giving 1 to 2 mg of i.v. edrophonium after ensuring respiratory sufficiency. This should result in rapid improvement in the patient with a myasthenic crisis. This procedure may be falsely positive, however, and if the diagnosis is unclear, the patient should be withdrawn from all anticholinesterases and, if necessary, maintained on mechanical respiration for 48 to 72 hours. Cholinergic crises require the immediate withdrawal of all anticholinesterases. Myasthenic crises respond variably to additional anticholinesterases, and plasmapheresis or steroid therapy may be particularly useful in this situation. Both myasthenic and cholinergic crises mandate admission to the hospital.

Botulism

CLINICAL MANIFESTATIONS

The initial symptom of botulism usually is constipation, followed insidiously by lethargy and feeding difficulties. Physical findings at the time of presentation are hypoactive deep tendon reflexes, decreased suck and gag, poorly reactive pupils, bilateral ptosis, oculomotor palsies, and facial weakness. Differential diagnosis includes all the potential causes of lethargy and poor feeding in infancy, and infants are often misdiagnosed initially. Laboratory studies, including the leukocyte count and LP, are normal. The diagnosis is confirmed by identification of *Clostridium botulinum* toxin (usually type A or B) in the feces or isolation of the organism in stool culture, which is less sensitive. EMG may supply immediate information. Characteristic EMG findings are brief, small-amplitude action potentials; posttetanic facilitation; and normal nerve conduction velocity.

MANAGEMENT

Management of infant botulism is strictly supportive. Affected infants require hospitalization to observe for respiratory compromise. In one large series of 57 patients, 77% required endotracheal intubation because of loss of protective airway reflexes, and 68% received mechanical ventilation for some period. Nasogastric or nasojejunal feedings are usually needed as well. The use of cathartics or other laxatives to reduce the amount of *C. botulinum* present in the intestine has not proved beneficial. Botulinum antitoxin has resulted in anaphylactic reaction in infants and is not recommended. Antibiotics such as penicillin, although widely used, have not been shown to eradicate the organism from the bowel or result in clinical improvement.

Periodic Paralysis

BACKGROUND AND PATHOPHYSIOLOGY

Familial periodic paralysis is a rare illness, inherited in an autosomal-dominant fashion that results in episodes of severe weakness associated with an abnormality of circulating potassium during attacks. Two major forms of illness—hyperkalemic and hypokalemic—are recognized. (A third type, normokalemic, has been described but most likely represents a rare variant of the hyperkalemic variety.) Other disorders that can produce weakness and electrolyte abnormalities, such as use of corticosteroids or diuretics, thyrotoxicosis, hyperaldosteronism, and renal insufficiency, may mimic the periodic paralyses. The serum potassium abnormalities in familial periodic paralysis are thought to be epiphenomena of yet undelineated muscle membrane abnormalities.

CLINICAL MANIFESTATIONS

Many of the clinical features are common to the various forms of periodic paralysis. Characteristically, a previously well patient develops a flaccid weakness in his or her trunk and upper thighs, and the weakness gradually involves the remainder of the skeletal muscles. Deep tendon reflexes are diminished. The attacks last from hours to days, and between the attacks, muscular strength usually is normal, although a minority of patients have residual muscular weakness.

Hypokalemic periodic paralysis, the most common type, occurs primarily in young adults. Trigger factors include vigorous exercise, heavy carbohydrate meals, alcohol, and the cold. During an attack, potassium levels are usually 2 to 2.5 mEq per L, and electrophysiologic examination demonstrates muscles that cannot be stimulated. The hyperkalemic form usually begins in the first decade of life, and attacks occur predominantly during the period of rest after vigorous exercise or after fasting. The episodes are more common than in hypokalemic paralysis, but often last less than a few hours. Myotonia usually is associated with the illness. During the attack, plasma potassium is moderately elevated, although it is often in the upper normal range. In both forms of periodic paralysis, electrocardiogram (ECG) changes consistent with the serum potassium abnormality may be noted, and cardiac arrhythmias may rarely arise.

MANAGEMENT

Emergency treatment of hypokalemic periodic paralysis includes oral, or rarely i.v., potassium. Prophylactically, patients should avoid precipitants such as vigorous exercise or large carbohydrate loads. Recurrences may be prevented with spironolactone or acetazolamide.

Attacks of hyperkalemic periodic paralysis are often brief enough that acute treatment is unnecessary. In severe attacks, i.v. calcium gluconate may be helpful. Acetazolamide, thiazide diuretics, and albuterol have been used for prevention of recurrences.

DISORDERS OF BALANCE (SEE CHAPTER 8)

Acute Cerebellar Ataxia

CLINICAL MANIFESTATIONS

The child develops acute truncal unsteadiness with a variable degree of distal motor difficulty, such as tremor and dysmetria. Dysarthria and nystagmus are variably present. Some children have nausea and vomiting, presumably caused by vertigo. Headache is rare.

When acute ataxia follows varicella in a child with no other neurologic findings, the diagnosis may be made on clinical grounds. In atypical cases, CT or MRI may be necessary to rule out a cerebellar mass. LP is not usually necessary in typical cases; if performed, it reveals a mild CSF pleocytosis in approximately half of the cases.

MANAGEMENT

Treatment is supportive. Resolution of symptoms is complete in most children within 2 weeks of onset, but mild residual neurologic deficits have been reported in 10% to 30% of cases. Varicella-associated cases appear to have the most benign prognosis.

Benign Paroxysmal Vertigo

Benign paroxysmal vertigo is an illness that affects children primarily between 1 and 4 years of age, although it can occur any time during the first decade. It manifests with acute episodes of dizziness and imbalance, lasting seconds to minutes. Between episodes, the child is asymptomatic. During the spell, the child characteristically becomes frightened and pale but does not lose consciousness. He or she may have associated nausea, vomiting, or visual disturbance. The physical examination is usually normal except for nystagmus, which may be present. Although the cause of this illness is unknown, it is thought to be a migraine variant. Many children go on to develop more typical migraine headaches later, and there is often a family history of migraine disease. As the name suggests, the course of benign paroxysmal vertigo is self-limiting and benign, and treatment is supportive.

MOVEMENT DISORDERS

Involuntary movements are components of many CNS disorders and tend to be complex. A classification into specific subtypes, based on the character, predominant anatomic localization, rhythmicity, and frequency, is arbitrary but useful in deducing the cause of the disorder (Table 73.8). Movements such as chorea, athetosis, dystonia, ballismus, and certain types of tremors suggest dysfunction of the extrapyramidal nervous system. Involuntary movements also are caused by damage to the cerebellum or its outflow tract, especially static (on maintaining fixed position) and intention tremors. Myoclonus may occur secondary to cerebral cortex, brainstem, or spinal cord disease. Tics, another form of involuntary movement, may be extremely difficult to distinguish from chorea and are best differentiated by their stereotypic character. They probably represent the most common involuntary movement disorder but are not true neurologic emergencies. Many illnesses may present with involuntary movements and are diagnosed by associated neurologic findings.

Acute Dystonia

Dystonia is marked by involuntary, sustained muscle contractions, typically of the neck and trunk, that cause twisting movements and abnormal postures. In generalized dystonia, the head is usually deviated to the side, and there is grimacing of the face. Acute dystonia in children is nearly always the result of exposure to an antidopaminergic agent such as a neuroleptic, antiemetic, or metoclopramide. Chronic dystonias are rare but may be seen as an isolated disorder or as a manifestation of cerebral palsy. Dystonia must be differentiated from torticollis, an abnormal tilt of the head and neck usually resulting from irritation or spasm of the sternocleidomastoid muscle. Another clinically similar condition is Sandifer syndrome, which describes intermittent arching of the back and neck observed in infants with gastroesophageal reflux.

Acute dystonia resulting from exposure to antidopaminergic drugs is treated with diphenhydramine (1 mg per kg per dose i.v., p.o., or i.m.) or benztropine (Cogentin) (1 to 2 mg per dose i.m.). Because the half-life of many of the precipitating agents is fairly long, treatment should be continued for 24 to 48 hours.

DISORDERS OF CRANIAL NERVE FUNCTION

Optic Neuritis

CLINICAL FINDINGS

On examination, decreased visual acuity and decreased color vision are associated with a relative afferent pupillary deficit to light and a central scotoma in the affected eye. The relative afferent pupil defect is demonstrated by the swinging flashlight maneuver, during which the pupil of the affected eye constricts briskly when light is shone into the contralateral eye (the consensual light reflex) and dilates when light is immediately shone into the affected eye. With bilateral disease, the change in pupillary reflexes may not be apparent. Funduscopic examination discloses a hyperemic, swollen optic disc; in the rare cases of retrobulbar optic neuritis, funduscopic examination is normal.

Optic neuritis must be distinguished from papilledema secondary to increased ICP. Papilledema is almost always bilateral and associated with normal vision and normal pupil reactivity until late in the disease. In cases of bilateral optic neuritis, differentiation may be impossible because funduscopic findings are identical in the two illnesses. If any doubt of increased ICP persists, the patient should undergo evaluation by CT or MRI of the brain and, if normal, CSF analysis. In optic neuritis, the opening pressure is normal, but there may be a mild lymphocytic pleocytosis or elevated CSF protein.

MANAGEMENT

The course of the illness is variable, with most patients recovering to normal or near normal vision over 4 to 5 weeks. Treatment with high-dose systemic corticosteroids, such as prednisone 2 mg per kg per day orally for 7 to 10 days has not been shown to improve the ultimate prognosis but may result in a slightly faster resolution of symptoms.

TABLE 73.8. Categorization of Movement Disorders

Movement	Character	Location	Speed	Rhythmicity	Stereotype
Chorea	Jerky	Anywhere, may be universal	Rapid	Irregular	No
Athetosis	Writhing	Primarily distal	Slow	Irregular	At times
Dystonia	Writhing	Primarily proximal	Slow	Irregular	At times
Ballismus	Flailing	Proximal	Rapid	Irregular	No
Tremor	May be resting, static, or intention	Primarily distal	Variable	Regular	Yes
Myoclonus	Jerky	Anywhere	Rapid	Irregular	Variable
Tic	Jerky	Anywhere (especially face, neck, hands)	Rapid	Variable	Yes

Facial Nerve Palsy

CLINICAL MANIFESTATIONS

Facial weakness may be partial or complete. On the affected side, there is flattening of the nasolabial fold at rest, and the child has difficulty closing the eye or raising the corner of the mouth to smile. In many cases, pain localized to the ear precedes the paralysis. With upper motor neuron involvement, there will be some residual capacity to furrow the brow because of crossed innervation, whereas the entire face is involved with peripheral disease. There may be bilateral involvement in Lyme disease, in contrast to Bell palsy, which is always unilateral.

In children with facial nerve palsy caused by Lyme disease, other manifestations, such as erythema migrans, are rarely seen (27% in one series). Thus, even in the absence of other findings, serologic evidence for systemic Lyme infection should be sought in all children with isolated seventh nerve paresis in endemic areas. An LP should be performed if there is other evidence of meningoencephalitis such as headache; however, the need for LP in a child at risk for Lyme disease with isolated facial nerve palsy is controversial. Other associated neurologic abnormality, specifically in the other cranial nerves, necessitates further evaluation, including CT or MRI.

MANAGEMENT

Treatment for facial nerve palsy not associated with Lyme disease is somewhat controversial, but steroids may be beneficial when started early in the course of the disease. Some authors have recommended a course of prednisone (2 mg per kg per day in two divided doses) over 7 to 10 days if the patient is seen within the first 24 to 48 hours of onset of the disease. A recent study suggests that acyclovir may be of benefit. Regardless of treatment, complete recovery is seen in 60% to 80% of children, beginning during the second to third week of illness. Those with partial paralysis generally have a better prognosis. During recovery period, special care should be taken to protect the cornea by the instillation of bland ointments (eg, Lacrilube). The child should be referred for reexamination to ensure a recovery during the expected time period.

Children with clinical or serologic evidence of Lyme-associated facial nerve palsy should be treated with oral antibiotics (amoxicillin, tetracycline, or erythromycin) for 21 to 28 days. The effectiveness of steroids in such patients has not been evaluated. Parenteral antibiotic treatment is recommended for children who also have evidence of meningitis.

CHAPTER 74
Infectious Disease Emergencies

Gary R. Fleisher, M.D.

BACTEREMIA

Background

Bacteremia refers to the presence of bacteria in the bloodstream. When bacteremia occurs in a young child and produces relatively few signs or symptoms, other than fever, the patient is considered to have the syndrome of occult bacteremia. The presence or absence of toxicity differentiates occult bacteremia, which is relatively asymptomatic, from sepsis, which is accompanied by findings of serious systemic illness. *Streptococcus pneumoniae* causes the majority of primary occult bacteremias but is declining in incidence since the introduction of conjugated vaccine. Less commonly encountered pathogens include *Salmonella*, *Neisseria meningitidis*, group A streptococcus, group B streptococcus, *Haemophilus influenzae* (Hib), and, rarely, others.

Clinical Manifestations

By definition, occult bacteremia causes few symptoms and signs other than high fever in most cases. The complaints are usually those of malaise or an upper respiratory infection (URI). Fever, without evidence of a source, may be the only physical finding, or the patient may have a minor focus of infection, such as otitis media (OM). The white blood cell (WBC) count is usually elevated in children with bacteremia, particularly with *S. pneumoniae.*

Management

The introduction of conjugated vaccines against *H. influenzae* and *S. pneumoniae* has markedly reduced the occurrence of bacteremia in children over the age of 6 months. Thus, for a fully immunized child, a complete blood count (CBC) and blood culture merit consideration primarily in the first 6 months of life.

The decision about whether to treat children who are at risk for occult bacteremia hinges in large part on the balance between unnecessary administration of therapy to many children with no organisms in the bloodstream and prevention of serious complications in the few with bacteremia. Because diagnosis based on clinical and laboratory findings at the time of the visit has limited accuracy, physicians must choose between two alternatives, neither of which is completely satisfactory. Presumptive treatment is particularly appropriate for patients under 6 months of age and for patients aged 6 to 24 months who have a temperature of 39°C (102.2°F) or higher and incomplete immunization, and for those who are at higher-than-average risk (eg, more irritable or lethargic than the usual child with a fever; WBC count 15000–20000/mm^3 or more). For these patients, intramuscular ceftriaxone (50 mg/kg) has been demonstrated to be effective.

The management of patients with proven bacteremia hinges on the identity of the pathogen. If penicillin-sensitive *S. pneumoniae* is isolated, the clinical findings at repeat examination determine the subsequent treatment. Children without fever or evidence of a serious infection (eg, meningitis, pneumonia, cellulitis) should receive oral penicillin 50000 U per kilogram of body weight per day or amoxicillin 50 mg per kilogram of body weight per day for 10 days; those with fever (≥38.5°C, or 101.2°F), clinical toxicity, or a serious focal infection merit initial intravenous antibiotic therapy. Children returning after a blood culture has grown other pathogens (*H. influenzae, N. meningitidis,* penicillin-resistant *S. pneumoniae*) are managed most prudently with intravenous antibiotics in the hospital because even those who remain well and afebrile appear to have some potential for persistent bacteremia or the continued evolution of focal infections. A few recent studies suggested, however, that selected afebrile and well-appearing children with a prior blood culture yielding penicillin-resistant *S. pneumoniae, N. meningitidis,* or *H. influenzae* may be managed with outpatient therapy, such as ceftriaxone (50 mg/kg), pending the results of repeat cultures.

TABLE 74.1. Immediate Management of Sepsis

1. Ensure adequate ventilation and cardiac function.
2. Obtain laboratory studies (simultaneously with step 3): CBC, platelet count, PT, PTT, electrolytes, BUN, creatinine, glucose, arterial blood gas, blood culture, fibrin degradation products, AST, ALT.
3. Initiate hemodynamic monitoring and support: peripheral venous access; urinary catheter; central venous and arterial catheters (as indicated); cardiorespiratory monitors; normal saline, starting at 20 mL/kg.
4. Administer drugs and other therapeutic agents:
   Antibiotics: <2 months: ampicillin (50 mg/kg) and gentamicin (2.5 mg/kg)
   >2 months: ceftriaxone (50 mg/kg) or cefotaxime (50 mg/kg) or both ampicillin (50 mg/kg) and chloramphenicol (25 mg/kg)
   Sodium bicarbonate (pH <7.0) 1–2 mEq/kg
   Glucose (serum glucose <50 mg/dL) 0.25–1 g/kg
   Packed red blood cells (Hgb <10 g/dL) 10 mL/kg
   Platelet concentrates (platelet count <50,000/mm^3) 0.2 unit/kg
   Fresh-frozen plasma (elevated PT/PTT) 10 mL/kg

CBC, complete blood count; *PT,* prothrombin time; *PTT,* partial thromboplastin time; *BUN,* blood urea nitrogen.

SEPSIS

Clinical Manifestations

The duration of the history in a child with sepsis varies. Even though some children are febrile for several days during a preceding bacteremia, others develop a sudden dramatic illness. The interval between the initial fever and death may be less than 12 hours in fulminant meningococcemia. The child progresses with continued sepsis from malaise to profound lethargy and, finally, to obtundation. Although fever is the cardinal sign of infection, children younger than 2 to 3 months of age may remain afebrile with sepsis; hypothermia is common in the first month of life.

A marked tachycardia occurs early in the course of the disease, at times exceeding 200 beats per minute (bpm) in the first 3 months of life, 175 bpm between 4 months and 2 years of age, and 150 bpm in the older child. Hypotension and tachypnea are present. The skin is cold and poorly perfused; in addition, petechiae and purpura may appear, particularly with *N. meningitidis.*

The hemoglobin and hematocrit levels are usually normal, falling occasionally from hemolysis, as seen with disseminated intravascular coagulation (DIC). Although leukocytosis usually accompanies sepsis, an overwhelming infection occasionally produces neutropenia. The WBC count is rarely normal, and the differential is almost always shifted to the left; metamyelocytes and band forms often make their way into the peripheral blood. As the infection progresses, the platelet count decreases. It is distinctly unusual to have evidence of cutaneous hemorrhage from sepsis without thrombocytopenia. Similarly, the prothrombin time (PT), partial thromboplastin time (PTT), and fibrin degradation products rise with the ongoing consumption of the clotting factors. In the infant, hypoglycemia may occur.

Management

Although the initial therapy for sepsis is directed at the preservation of vital functions, every effort must be made to obtain the appropriate diagnostic studies (Table 74.1). Blood should be drawn for culture, CBC, platelet count, PT, PTT, electrolytes, blood urea nitrogen (BUN), arterial blood gas (ABG) analysis, serum aspartate aminotransferase (AST, formerly SGOT), and serum alanine aminotransferase (ALT, formerly SGPT) measurements in conjunction with the immediate insertion of an intravenous catheter. As initial therapy, normal saline, with or without 5% dextrose, is given at 20 mL per kilogram of body weight per hour or more rapidly, depending on the response. The unstable patient may require central venous, arterial, and urinary catheters (see Chapter 3).

For children younger than 2 months of age, ampicillin (200 mg per kilogram daily) and gentamicin (7.5 mg per kilogram daily) are administered; cefotaxime (150 mg per kilogram daily) may be used in place of gentamicin for the newborn. Dosages need to be decreased for premature infants in the first month of life and term infants in the first week (Tables 74.2A and 74.2B). Cefotaxime (200 mg per kilogram daily) or ceftriaxone (100 mg per kilogram daily) alone provides effective monotherapy for the child older than 2 months of age. Vancomycin (40 mg per kilogram daily) may be added for patients who are critically ill or at particular risk of infection with penicillin-resistant *S. pneumoniae,* as in the case, for example, of a patient with sickle cell anemia who is taking daily prophylactic penicillin. In the presence of a focus of infection likely to be staphylococcal, oxacillin (150 mg per kilogram dailoy) can be used together with cefo-

TABLE 74.2A. Intravenous Antibiotic Dosing for Newborn Infants Based on Age and Weight (Total Daily Dose [mg/kg/day] and Dosing Interval)

	Weight <2,000 g		Weight >2,000 g		
Antibiotic	**0–7 days**	**8–28 days**	**0–7 days**	**8–28 days**	**>28 days**
Ampicillin	100 mg q12hr	150 mg q8hr	150 mg q8hr	200 mg q6hr	200 mg q6hr
Cefotaxime	100 mg q12hr	150 mg q8hr	100 mg q12hr	150 mg q8hr	150 mg q8hr
Ceftriaxone	50 mg qd	50 mg qd	50 mg qd	75 mg qd	100 mg qd

qd, daily.

TABLE 74.2B. Intravenous Antibiotic Dosing for Newborn Infants Based on Gestational Age (mg/kg/dose)

Antibiotic	≤26 wk	27–34 wk	35–42 wk	>43 wk
Gentamicin	2.5 mg q24hr	2.5 mg q18hr	2.5 mg q12h	2.5 mg q8hr

taxime; alternatively, the combination of clavulanic acid and ampicillin (200 mg per kilogram daily) may be administered. Chloramphenicol (75–100 mg per kilogram daily) or meropenem (60–120 mg per kilogram daily) should be kept in mind for children with allergies to penicillins and cephalosporins. Corticosteroid therapy is not recommended for sepsis.

Blood components are given as indicated by the results of the initial hematologic studies. If the hemoglobin is lower than 10 g per deciliater, packed red cells are administered at 10 mL per kilogram of body weight. Thrombocytopenia (<50000/mm^3) is corrected with platelet concentrates at 0.2 U per kilogram and decreased clotting factors with fresh-frozen plasma 10 mL per kilogram. For the child with hypoglycemia (glucose <50 mg per deciliter), glucose should be given at a dose of 0.25 to 1 g per kilogram in the form of a 25% solution. Heparin plays no role in the initial emergency care of the child with sepsis but may be useful subsequently to treat severe thrombotic episodes. Specific inhibitors of endotoxin and cytokines, such as bacterial polysaccharide-inhibiting protein, are under investigation but have not been demonstrated to be effective as yet.

CENTRAL NERVOUS SYSTEM INFECTIONS

Bacterial Meningitis

CLINICAL MANIFESTATIONS

The signs and symptoms of meningitis vary with the child's age (Table 74.3). Particularly in the first 3 months of life, the clinician must maintain a high index of suspicion for this disease. In addition, it should be kept in mind that partial treatment with antibiotics may obscure the typical findings.

Before 3 months of age, the history is that of irritability, an altered sleep pattern, vomiting, and decreased oral intake. In particular, paradoxical irritability points to the diagnosis of meningitis. Irritability in the infant without inflammation of the meninges is generally alleviated by maternal fondling; however, in the child with meningitis, any handling, even directed toward soothing the infant, may increase irritability because of its effect on the inflamed meninges. Bulging of the fontanel, an almost certain sign of meningitis in the febrile, ill-appearing infant, is a late finding.

As the child passes beyond the age of 3 months, the symptoms gradually becomes more specific for involvement of the central nervous system (CNS). A change in the level of activity is almost always noticeable. It is only in the child older than 2 years of age, however, that meningitis manifests reliably with complaints of headache and neck stiffness.

The physical examination in the young infant rarely provides specific corroboration, even when the history suggests meningitis. Fever is often absent in these children, despite the presence of bacterial infection. Any child younger than 2 to 3 months of age who is brought to the emergency department (ED) with a documented temperature of 38.0° to 38.5°C (100.4° to 101.2°F) or higher should be considered at particular risk for meningitis. The physical signs are sufficiently elusive that many experts caution that one should not rely exclusively on the examination to rule out meningeal infection.

In children 3 months of age and older, increasing, but not absolute, reliance can be placed on the physical findings; fever is almost inevitably noted. Specific evidence of meningeal irritation often is present, including nuchal rigidity and, less often, Kernig and Brudzinski signs. When a lumbar puncture fails to confirm the diagnosis of meningitis despite the presence of meningeal signs, other conditions must be pursued that can mimic the findings on physical examination. Conditions capable of producing meningismus (irritation of the meninges without pleocytosis in the cerebrospinal fluid, or CSF) include severe pharyngitis, retropharyngeal abscess, cervical adenitis, arthritis or osteomyelitis of the cervical spine, upper lobe pneumonia, subarachnoid hemorrhage, pyelonephritis, and tetanus.

The child with meningitis often has a complicated course beginning in the ED or even preceding arrival at the hospital (Table 74.4). Shock, seizures, and hyponatremia strike at any age, whereas apnea and hypoglycemia predominantly affect infants less than 3 months of age. Although sterile subdural effusions and, rarely, empyemas usually occur later in the disease, they merit consideration in the infant with signs of herniation and a bulging fontanel.

MANAGEMENT

Bacterial meningitis is a medical emergency that requires the immediate institution of therapy (Table 74.5). If meningitis is suspected but attempts to obtain CSF are unsuccessful, this failure should not delay the antibiotic administration. The intramuscular route provides a suitable temporary alternative. The child's age determines the spectrum of microorganisms causing meningitis and the selection of antibiotic therapy (Table 74.5). In addition to the antibiotic administration aimed at the eradication of the offending organism, supportive therapy for complications (Tables 74.4 and 74.5) is an essential ingredient in the care of the child with meningitis. Apneic episodes can occur in the infant. Thus, oxygen, intubation, and assisted ventilation all may be required. Bacteremia, which usually accompanies meningitis, may lead to septic shock. This condition demands vigorous fluid resuscitation with normal saline.

Although many clinicians choose to administer dexamethasone to patients beyond the first 2 months of life in whom the diagnosis of bacterial meningitis appears highly likely, contradictory evidence exists in the literature and expert panels have

TABLE 74.3. Signs and Symptoms of Meningitis

Age (mo)	Symptom	Signs: Early	Signs: Late
0–3	Paradoxical irritability Altered sleep pattern Vomiting Lethargy	Lethargy Irritability Fever (±) Hypothermia (<1 mo)	Bulging fontanelle Shock
4–24	Irritability Altered sleep pattern Lethargy	Fever Irritability	Nuchal rigidity Coma Shock
>24	Headache Neck pain Lethargy	Fever Nuchal rigidity Irritability	Coma Shock

TABLE 74.4. Short-term Complications of Meningitis

Early	Late
Apnea	Hyponatremia
Shock	Subdural empyema
Hypoglycemia	Seizures
Hyponatremia	
Seizures	

TABLE 74.5. Immediate Management of Bacterial Meningitis

1. Ensure adequate ventilation and cardiac function.
2. Obtain laboratory studies (simultaneously with step 3):
   Cerebrospinal fluid: cell count, glucose, protein, Gram stain, culture, latex agglutination (as indicated)
   Blood: complete blood count, platelet count, prothrombin time, partial thromboplastin time, electrolytes, blood urea nitrogen, creatinine, glucose, arterial blood gas, blood culture
3. Initiate hemodynamic monitoring and support.
   Achieve venous access; use cardiorespiratory monitors.
4. Administer drugs.
   Treat septic shock, if present.
   Consider dexamethasone (0.15 mg/kg) before or shortly after antibiotic administration.
   Antibiotics: <1 mo: ampicillin (50 kg) and cefotaxime (50 mg/kg)
   >1 mo: vancomycin (15/mg) and either ceftriaxone (50 mg/kg) or cefotaxime (75 mg/kg)[a]
   Glucose (if serum glucose <50 mg/dL) 0.25–1 g/kg
   Treat acidosis and coagulopathy, if present.

[a] Chloramphenicol (25 mg/kg) or meropenem (25 mg/kg) may be used in place of cephalosporins for children allergic to those agents.

withheld a definitive endorsement. If the decision is made in favor of administration, the drug should be given before antibiotic administration when possible. If dexamethasone is not administered before the initiation of antibiotic therapy, it may be given subsequently but appears to lose its theoretic benefit after an interval or more than 4 hours.

Aseptic Meningitis

CLINICAL MANIFESTATIONS

The signs and symptoms of aseptic meningitis resemble those of bacterial infections of the CNS but are not usually as severe. The infant shows only lethargy and irritability, whereas the older child complains of a headache and stiff neck. Vomiting may occur and may be persistent. There is often a history of a concomitant upper respiratory or gastrointestinal viral illness.

Fever usually occurs but often hovers around 38.5°C (101.2°F). The infant may appear toxic, but the older child may remain remarkably well. Nuchal rigidity in a patient who is alert and conversant suggests aseptic, rather than bacterial, meningitis. Shining a flashlight in the eyes often elicits photophobia. The fontanel of the infant generally maintains a normal configuration but, rarely, may bulge. Aside from occasional positive Kernig and Brudzinski signs, the neurologic examination often shows no abnormalities. An altered level of consciousness or focal neurologic deficit points to meningoencephalitis rather than aseptic meningitis (see Chapter 73).

MANAGEMENT

In addition to the routine CSF studies, children with aseptic meningitis usually require CBC, electrolytes, and a BUN. Most patients need no further tests, but in atypical situations, consideration should always be given to nonviral causes that may mandate additional diagnostic steps or specific therapy. If tuberculosis is suspected based on family contacts, a low CSF glucose, or pulmonary findings, a Mantoux test and chest radiograph are useful for confirmation. In endemic areas, particularly in association with erythema migrans, serologic studies for Lyme disease and antibiotic therapy may be indicated. A computed tomography (CT) scan provides essential information about patients with symptoms or signs of a parameningeal infection or CNS tumors and hemorrhages. Immunosuppressed patients develop infections with a wide variety of unusual bacteria, fungi, and parasites that can be identified in many cases with appropriate examination and culture of the CSF (India ink and acid-fast stains, cryptococcal antigen testing, fungal and mycobacterial cultures). When examining infants, the physician must remain alert to the possibility of a herpetic infection and consider obtaining a polymerase chain reaction (PCR) for herpes simplex virus.

Therapy for the common viral infections does not currently extend beyond supportive care, although an investigational agent is available for enteroviruses. Dehydration from prolonged emesis may necessitate intravenous fluid administration. After any deficit has been corrected, the rate should be set to provide 75% to 100% of the daily maintenance requirement to avoid overhydration and possible aggravation of cerebral edema in the child who develops an encephalitic component.

Because the CSF findings in aseptic meningitis occasionally overlap those in bacterial infections, hospital admission is usually warranted until the CSF culture results are available. The experienced clinician, however, may choose to follow the older child as an outpatient if the family is reliable and nonviral causes (eg, tuberculosis, cryptococcosis) have been excluded. Generally, to qualify for discharge with aseptic meningitis, a patient must have all CSF parameters pointing away from bacterial infection: fewer than 500 cells mm^3, fewer than 50% polymorphonuclear leukocytes, protein levels below 100 mg per deciliter, and glucose levels greater than 30 mg per deciliter.

UPPER RESPIRATORY TRACT INFECTIONS

Nasopharyngitis

Nasopharyngitis (URI), or the common cold, is a viral illness of the upper respiratory tract in children. The most commonly isolated organisms are the rhinoviruses and coronaviruses. Prospective family studies have shown that five or six episodes occur yearly during childhood. The illness is characterized by a fever of less than 39°C (102.2°F) and coryza. There may be a mild conjunctivitis and infection of the pharynx. Although the tympanic membranes may show a slightly dull appearance and decreased mobility, the characteristic features of acute purulent OM (erythema, loss of the landmarks, and bulging) are absent. Therapy is limited to a recommendation for rest, adequate hydration, saline nose drops, and antipyretic agents.

Stomatitis

Stomatitis, an infection of the mouth, is caused by herpes simplex and the coxsackieviruses at any age and by *Candida albicans* ("thrush") in the infant (see Chapters 106 and 109) or in the immunosuppressed child. Viral infections cause vesicular lesions initially and ulcerations and plaques subsequently. Some coxsackieviruses may involve the hands and feet as well as the mouth (coxsackievirus hand–foot–mouth syndrome), and herpetic stomatitis may be complicated by spread of infection to the digits, which is called *herpetic whitlow*. For otherwise healthy patients, treatment is limited to systemic antipyretic and analgesic drugs and the local application of topical analgesics, such as 2% viscous lidocaine (Xylocaine) or the combination of Kaopectate and diphenhydramine. Oral acyclovir hastens the resolution of herpetic lesions in immunosuppressed patients.

C. albicans produces white plaques on the mucosa that bleed if scraped. Nystatin 200000 U four times daily leads to a prompt resolution of this condition. Although either oral ketoconazole or fluconazole is effective, neither treatment is indicated routinely for the immunocompetent host.

Pharyngitis

Pharyngitis (see Chapter 62) is an infection of the throat (including the tonsils). In the immunocompetent child, several viruses, perhaps *Mycoplasma pneumoniae* and *Chlamydia trachomatis,* and only a few bacteria cause pharyngitis. Although many bacteria have been reported as possible causes of pharyngitis, only three organisms have well-defined roles: group A streptococcus, *Corynebacterium diphtheriae,* and *N. gonorrhoeae.* For practical purposes, isolated pharyngitis can be considered as streptococcal (bacterial) or nonstreptococcal (viral). Because the symptoms of the two types overlap, the physician can reliably distinguish the more important streptococcal infections only with the aid of the laboratory. Certain clinical features favor a bacterial cause, however. Such infections more often have an abrupt onset with fever and sore throat; cough and coryza are uncommon. Examination of the pharynx shows an erythematous mucosa, often with exudate and petechiae on the posterior palate. In addition, the cervical lymph nodes often become enlarged and tender.

Although unusual, complications may occur with bacterial pharyngitis; both suppurative and nonsuppurative sequelae can result from streptococcal infections. The latter category includes acute rheumatic fever and glomerulonephritis. Viral pharyngitis resolves spontaneously in 2 to 5 days with the exception of Epstein–Barr virus (EBV), as discussed under "Infectious Mononucleosis."

In the ED, a tonsillar swab for antigen detection by latex agglutination or preferably optical immunoassay, if available, should be obtained from children with pharyngeal inflammation and those who complain of sore throat, unless the diagnosis of a generalized viral syndrome can be confidently established on clinical grounds. If the test for antigen is positive, the infection presumably is caused by group A streptococcus and the child is treated with penicillin. Although a single injection of benzathine penicillin (600000 U if < 28 kg and 1.2 million U if ≥ 28 kg) obviates all problems with compliance, oral phenoxymethyl penicillin (250 mg per dose for children and 500 mg per dose for adolescents, given two to three times per day) provides an acceptable alternative, if prescribed for 10 days. Amoxicillin may be used in place of penicillin but offers no advantage. Erythromycin (40 mg per kilogram daily) is used for penicillin-allergic children; azithromycin for 5 days (10 mg per kilogram on the first day and 5 mg per kilogram on subsequent days) represents a more expensive alternative. Shorter courses of therapy, particularly with oral cephalosporins, have been shown to be effective in limited studies but cannot be enthusiastically recommended at present because of the small number of patients treated in various investigations and a lack of data on the prevention of complications. Antipyretic agents, fluids, and adequate rest should be recommended. In children with pharyngitis suggestive of streptococcal disease for which antigen detection is negative or unavailable, a throat culture is indicated. While awaiting the results of cultures, one may choose to treat presumptively children with severe pharyngitis characteristic of streptococcal disease and those unable to reliably return for follow-up. Because antibiotics shorten the course of streptococcal pharyngitis minimally, there is no reason to give these drugs hastily before confirming a bacterial cause. Institution of a liquid diet and acetaminophen provides some symptomatic relief.

Otitis Media

CLINICAL MANIFESTATIONS

In the young child, the initial manifestation is often not otologic but rather is fever, irritability, or diarrhea. Children beyond the age of 3 years generally, but not invariably, complain of pain in the ear. Less common symptoms include vertigo and hearing impairment. Fever, which occurs in 25% to 35% of children with acute otitis media (AOM), serves only to arouse suspicion of infection in the middle ear. The diagnosis rests in the usual clinical settings on the accurate interpretation of the otoscopic findings, a skill gained only by experience with the pneumatic otoscope.

The tympanic membrane in AOM typically bulges out at the examiner as a result of the positive pressure generated by the production of purulent material in the middle ear cavity. Although the drum is sometimes red, it more often appears yellow because of the exudate behind it. A convex contour of the drum secondary to an effusion in the child suspected of having AOM is sufficient to make this diagnosis, regardless of the color of the tympanum. The diffuse injection of the normal tympanum, which is often exaggerated by crying, should not be confused with the intense erythema of infection.

Difficulty arises in differentiating AOM from otitis media with effusion (OME) and in diagnosing "early" AOM, particularly in the child with a preexisting middle ear effusion. The tympanic membrane has decreased mobility in both AOM and OME; however, it is usually retracted in the latter condition. During the course of a single examination, the physician may be unable to differentiate with any certainty; in such cases, it is safest to assume a bacterial cause.

The WBC count, if it has been obtained, usually falls within the normal range or shows a mild leukocytosis. Occasionally, a young child may have a count of 20000 to 30000/mm^3. Tympanocentesis, when performed as part of a research protocol, yields an organism in 60% to 70% of cases. Blood cultures drawn selectively, most often from highly febrile children in the first 2 years of life, show growth of a pathogen in about 3% of cases.

Acute complications have occurred occasionally in AOM subsequent to the advent of effective antibiotics. Local suppuration may involve the mastoids and rarely leads to meningitis or brain abscess. Perforations generally heal spontaneously (see Chapter 106). A child with OM in the first year or two of life may develop dehydration from vomiting and diarrhea associated with the infection.

MANAGEMENT

Uncomplicated OM in the child older than 1 month should be treated with oral antibiotic therapy on an outpatient basis. Amoxicillin (80 mg per kilogram of body weight per day in three divided doses) is the drug of choice in the United States. The most reasonable alternatives include (1) amoxicillin fortified with clavulanic acid in a 7:1 formulation, 45 mg per kilogram daily of amoxicillin in two divided doses; (2) cefuroxime axetil, 30 mg per kilogram daily in two divided doses; and (3) ceftriaxone, 50 mg per kilogram administered intramuscularly as a single dose. Cephalosporins can be used in children with a history of penicillin allergy. Intramuscular ceftriaxone has an advantage in children with persistent vomiting and perhaps in those at high risk of occult bacteremia and also obviates the issue of compliance in high-risk social situations. Whether the course of therapy must be 10 days (except for single-dose ceftriaxone) or can be shortened is controversial. Most authorities believe that antibiotics administered for 5 days are sufficient in children older than 2 years but prefer the longer course in infants. Antihistamines and decongestants have not hastened the resolution of AOM.

If AOM persists during therapy with amoxicillin or recurs within 2 days of its discontinuance, ampicillin-resistant organisms emerge as likely causes of the infection. All the alternatives to amoxicillin represent reasonable agents for a second course, and no compelling data favor any particular regimen. Failure of such a second course of antibiotics to eradicate the infection necessitates a third trial of antibiotic therapy and merits consideration of a tympanocentesis for culture.

The management of OM in the first month of life has provoked controversy because of (1) the occurrence of gram-negative enteric bacilli and *S. aureus* in-middle ear infections in these children and (2) the decreased ability of the neonate to resist infection (Fig. 74.1). If a child younger than 1 month of age presents with fever or irritability and is found to have OM, admission for intravenous antibiotic therapy provides the safest course pending the outcome of cultures of the blood, urine, and CSF. Afebrile infants in the first month of life may be treated as outpatients with the usual oral antibiotics used for older patients and with careful follow-up.

Otitis Externa

Otitis externa (OE), or swimmer's ear, is an infection of the auditory canal and external surface of the tympanic membrane that spares the middle ear. There is usually a history of recent swimming, but occasional cases are seen in children whose only submersion occurs during normal bathing. The first symptom is itching of the ear canal. The child complains subsequently of an earache that may be unilateral or bilateral, and purulent material often drains from the ear. Fever is never present unless cellulitis or another illness is associated. Unlike AOM, pulling on the ear lobe to straighten the canal in preparation for otoscopic examination elicits marked tenderness. A cheesy white or gray–green exudate fills the canal in more than 50% of patients, often obscuring the tympanum.

Treatment consists of removing the inflammatory debris from the ear canal, eliminating pathogenic bacteria, providing symptomatic relief, and controlling predisposing factors. Usually, dry-mopping the canal with a cotton-tipped wire applicator cleanses the canal adequately; occasionally, gentle suction is also necessary. The patient should be given commercially available otic drops and a mild analgesic, such as aspirin or acetaminophen. Acetic acid solutions (Otic-Domeboro or Vosol), the combination antibiotic–corticosteroid preparations (Cortisporin, Lidosporin), four drops instilled four times daily, or ofloxacin otic, five drops instilled twice daily, are effective. In cases with known or suspected perforations, suspensions (but not solutions) are preferred. For the occasional case of a patient with an edematous canal and thick exudate, a wick should be inserted 10 to 12 mm into the canal after cleansing to facilitate entry of the medications. All patients should be instructed to avoid swimming until cured.

Sinusitis

CLINICAL MANIFESTATIONS

The presentation of acute sinusitis varies in some respects with the child's age. Usually, the infection follows a viral URI. Two features that distinguish sinusitis from a viral URI include persistent (> 10 days) or severe (temperature > 39°C [102.2°F] beyond 3 days) symptoms. Cough occurs in 75% of the patients. Unlike adolescents, young children do not often complain of a headache or facial pain. A fever is noted in about half of children with sinusitis. Nasal discharge occurs in almost all these infections and is often the symptom that prompts a visit. The area of the face that overlies the sinus swells in 10% to 20% of the patients with maxillary disease, and periorbital or orbital edema and cellulitis even more commonly accompany ethmoiditis. The child with chronic sinusitis complains only of chronic cough and rhinorrhea. Fever, headache, and facial pain are unusual. Often, abnormal findings are not seen on examination. The sinus radiograph is abnormal in almost every child with sinusitis; there may be an air–fluid level, complete opacification, or mucosal thickening (> 4 mm). A CT scan is more sensitive for diagnosis than a plain radiograph but is not needed in routine cases.

Although sinusitis usually responds to oral antibiotic therapy, serious complications occasionally result from the local spread of the suppuration. These include orbital infection, brain abscess, epidural or subdural empyema, and cavernous sinus thrombosis. Proptosis and paralysis of the extraocular muscles point to the accumulation of purulent material within the orbit. After intracranial extension, the child appears toxic and usually has a detectable neurologic deficit.

MANAGEMENT

Children suspected of having acute sinusitis with severe symptoms or an uncertain clinical picture should have a radiograph evaluation of their sinuses. Among this group of patients clini-

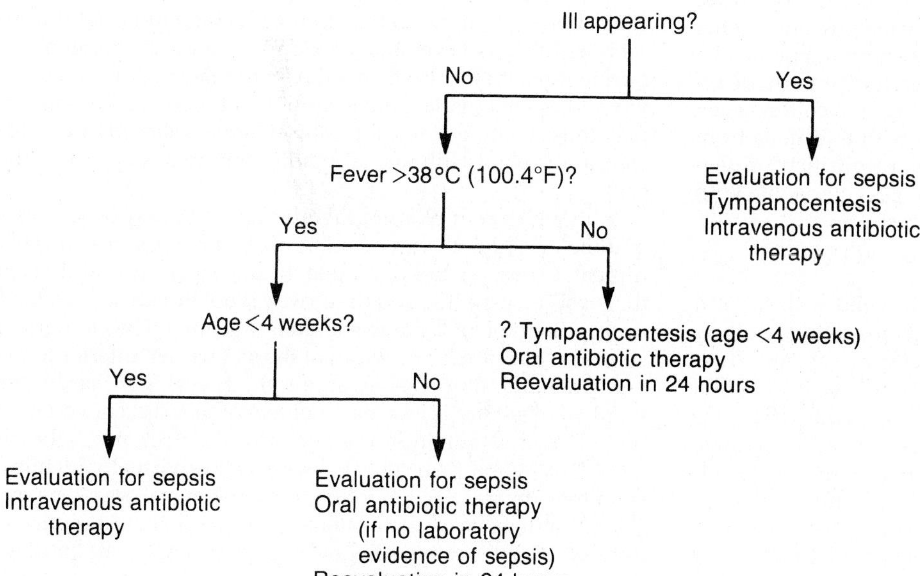

Figure 74.1. Diagnostic approach for the management of acute otitis media in the infant during the first month of life.

cally believed to be at risk for an infection, any abnormality (air–fluid level, opacification, or mucosal thickening) suffices to confirm the diagnosis. Afebrile children with chronic sinusitis diagnosed on the basis of persistent nasal discharge need no laboratory or radiographic evaluation. Possible indications for antral puncture and aspiration of the sinus include (1) associated life-threatening infection, (2) immunocompromise, (3) persistent illness despite therapy, and (4) unusually severe disease. Amoxicillin (40–50 mg per kilogram daily) effectively treats the common pathogens, *S. pneumoniae* and *H. influenzae,* in most cases. Current recommendations call for antibiotic therapy for 10 days, although shorter courses of treatment are under investigation. Alternative drugs for penicillin-allergic children and those with recurrent disease are the same as for OM. Children with acute sinusitis require admission if they appear ill, have facial swelling and tenderness, or develop any complications.

Peritonsillar Abscess

A peritonsillar abscess, or "quinsy," results from the accumulation of purulent material within the tonsillar fossa. Adolescents develop this condition more often than do younger children. The complaints of trismus and difficulty in speaking separate a peritonsillar abscess from the far more common pharyngitis. The voice sounds muffled, and the child drools profusely. Both tonsils may swell, but the enlargement of one is more pronounced. Usually, the abscessed tonsil becomes sufficiently large to push the uvula to the opposite side of the pharynx, and the examiner can palpate a fluctuant mass intraorally. The WBC count is often elevated.

All children with a peritonsillar abscess should have the lesion drained, usually in the ED or after admission to the hospital and receive treatment with antibiotics. Penicillin (100000 U per kilogram daily) or clindamycin (25 mg per kilogram daily in four divided doses) constitute the usual therapy.

Cervical Lymphadenitis

CLINICAL MANIFESTATIONS

The child with cervical lymphadenitis usually is noted to have swelling in the neck. If the child is of a sufficient age, he or she will complain of pain. Fever occurs only occasionally, more often in children younger than 1 year of age. The infected node may vary in size from 2 cm to more than 10 cm. Initially, it has a firm consistency, but it becomes fluctuant in about 25% of cases. The skin overlying the node becomes erythematous, and edema may surround it. The WBC count is usually normal but may be elevated in the younger, febrile child. Aspiration of the node often identifies the organism by both Gram stain and culture, even if fluctuance is not appreciated. Children with infections from *M. tuberculosis* usually react to the standard purified protein derivative (PPD-S) skin test and have changes compatible with tuberculosis seen on radiography of the chest.

MANAGEMENT

Figure 74.2 outlines the management of the child with cervical lymphadenitis. Children with cervical adenitis who are otherwise healthy should receive an antibiotic effective against *S. aureus* and the group A streptococcus. Agents such as dicloxacillin (50 mg/kg per day) and cephalexin (50 mg/kg per day) have activity against both organisms. In more severe infections, oxacillin (150 mg/kg per day in four divided doses) can be administered intravenously. If the node is fluctuant, aspiration provides useful etiologic information and speeds the rate of resolution. All children with lymphadenitis should have a PPD skin test and should be followed until the infection subsides.

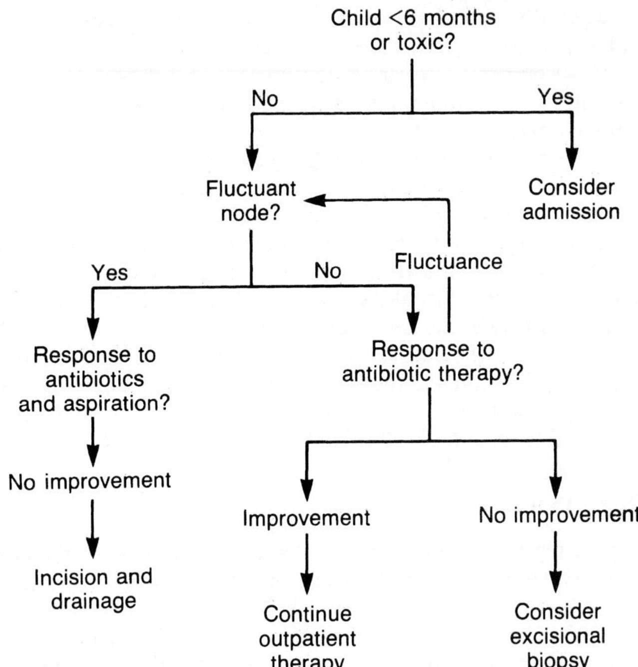

Figure 74.2. Diagnostic approach for the management of the child with presumed bacterial lymphadenitis.

Children less than 3 months of age and those who appear toxic or who have developed a draining sinus are best managed in the hospital. Failure to improve with oral antibiotic therapy or a positive skin test for tuberculosis necessitates subsequent hospitalization.

Retropharyngeal and Lateral Pharyngeal Abscess

A retropharyngeal abscess fills the potential space between the anterior border of the cervical vertebrae and the posterior wall of the esophagus. The usual pathogens are group A streptococcus, anaerobic organisms, and occasionally *S. aureus.* These uncommon infections occur most often in children less than 4 years of age. A lateral pharyngeal abscess occurs in the deep soft tissue space of the neck but not in the midline and is less common than a retropharyngeal infection.

The child with a retropharyngeal abscess presents with a clinical picture similar to that seen with epiglottitis, but the onset is less abrupt. Fever and a toxic appearance are common. As purulent material collects, the fluctuant mass obstructs the larynx and esophagus, leading to stridor and drooling. The abscess may cause meningismus; thus, this diagnosis should be considered in the child with nuchal rigidity but no pleocytosis in the CSF.

Although a retropharyngeal infection can rarely be seen as a midline swelling on examination of the pharynx, it is usually difficult to observe this finding in the uncooperative child. If the diagnosis is suspected and the airway is not threatened, a lateral neck radiograph or CT scan should be obtained. The radiograph shows an increase in the width of the soft tissues anterior to the vertebrae and, on occasion, an air–fluid level. Ordinarily, the width of this space is less than half that of the adjacent vertebral body if the examination is done with the neck properly extended. A lateral pharyngeal abscess causes virtually identical symptoms to an infection in the retropharyngeal area. One important difference is that a lateral pharyngeal abscess, which is not well visualized by radiograph, requires a CT scan for diagnosis.

A retropharyngeal or lateral pharyngeal abscess poses a risk to the patency of the airway. All children with this infection should have careful monitoring in the ED and then be hospitalized in consultation with an otolaryngologist. Unless the airway is in immediate jeopardy, intravenous access should be secured and treatment given with either clindamycin (30 mg per kilogram per day in four divided doses) or a combination of penicillin (100000 U per kilogram of body weight daily) and clindamycin, both in four divided doses. In the event of respiratory compromise, intubation or, less commonly, tracheotomy becomes necessary. Most patients require drainage, either transcutaneously with ultrasound guidance or at surgery, but a few reports indicate that high-dose antibiotics may suffice, particularly when the CT scan shows cellulitis or only a small collection of pus.

Laryngotracheobronchitis (Croup)

CLINICAL MANIFESTATIONS

Croup begins insidiously with the onset of fever and coryza. During the next 1 to 2 days, the infection spreads farther along the airway, producing signs of upper respiratory obstruction. Inspiratory stridor develops at this stage of the illness, and a barking cough is heard. The child may be unable to maintain adequate oral intake. Although the severity of croup varies, most children appear mildly to moderately ill in contrast to the toxic patients with epiglottitis or retropharyngeal abscess. The fever usually ranges from 38° to 39°C (100.4° to 102.2°F). Tachycardia and tachypnea are evident, but the respirations rarely exceed 40 breaths per minute. Suprasternal and subcostal retractions often accompany croup. On auscultation of the chest, the examiner may hear either stridor alone in mild disease or rhonchi and wheezes with more extensive involvement of the respiratory epithelium.

Ancillary studies are indicated only occasionally. The lateral and anteroposterior neck radiographs show subglottic narrowing ("steeple" sign) from soft-tissue edema in severe disease. Most of the radiographic studies of the airway are normal, however, or disclose only ballooning of the hypopharynx. Rather than confirm the diagnosis of croup, radiograph examination more often excludes other illness such as epiglottitis or retropharyngeal abscess.

Both dehydration and upper airway obstruction may complicate croup. Because of the respiratory distress and the toxicity associated with a febrile illness, the ability to maintain normal hydration will decrease in some children. Dehydration then occurs in the face of increased fluid losses through the pulmonary and cutaneous routes. Occasionally, a child with croup develops significant upper airway obstruction. Signs suggestive of impending respiratory failure include (1) hypotonicity, (2) noticeable retractions, (3) decreased or absent inspiratory breath sounds, (4) depressed level of consciousness, (5) tachycardia out of proportion to the fever, and (6) cyanosis. Although an ABG is not needed in the evaluation of children with mild croup, this study plays a role in deciding on the therapy in more severe cases. *Respiratory failure* is defined as a partial pressure of arterial carbon dioxide (P_aCO_2) of 60 mm Hg or higher or a partial pressure of arterial oxygen (P_aO_2) of less than 50 mm Hg in 100% oxygen. Significant respiratory compromise is present in croup when the P_aCO_2 rises over 45 mm Hg and the P_aO_2 falls below 70 mm Hg in room air.

MANAGEMENT

Many children with croup are never taken to seek medical attention. Of those who come to the ED, most can be managed as outpatients. Clear indications for admission are dehydration or significant respiratory compromise. If any of the signs of respiratory failure are noted, hospitalization becomes necessary. Use of a scoring system may be helpful in deciding on disposition (Table 74.6). Neck radiographs and an ABG may be obtained in cases in which the clinical picture is not decisive. In addition, the physician should consider the social milieu of the family. Hospitalization provides the safest course for the child when the parents are unreliable caretakers or transportation to the ED for a reevaluation presents an obstacle to further treatment.

Mist therapy lessens the severity of croup. Racemic epinephrine, or more recently in the United States 1-epinephrine, is indicated for children with moderate to severe croup who will be hospitalized or for whom admission is being considered. The dose is 0.25 mL of racemic epinephrine, mixed with 3 to 5 mL of

TABLE 74.6. Scoring System for Assessing Severity of Croup

A. Croup Score

	0	1	2	3
Stridor	None	Only with agitation	Mild at rest	Severe at rest
Retraction	None	Mild	Moderate	Severe
Air entry	Normal	Mild decrease	Moderate decrease	Marked decrease
Color	Normal	Not applicable	Not applicable	Cyanotic
Level of consciousness	Normal	Restless when disturbed	Restless when undisturbed	Lethargic

B. Croup Severity[a]

Score	Degree	Management
4	Mild	Outpatient—mist therapy
5–6	Mild to moderate	Outpatient if child improves in emergency department after mist, is older than 6 months, and has a reliable family
7–8	Moderate	Admitted—racemic epinephrine
≥9	Severe	Admitted—racemic epinephrine, oxygen, intensive care unit

Modified from Taussig LM, et al. Treatment of laryngotracheobronchitis (croup): use of intermittent positive pressure breathing and racemic epinephrine. *Am J Dis Child* 1975;129:790, with permission.

[a] Any one category with score of three leads to classification as severe disease.

saline, delivered by nebulization. If a response is noted and discharge to home is contemplated, the child should be observed in the ED for at least 2 hours to be certain that the respiratory symptoms do not rebound.

In a study by Leipzig and co-workers, dexamethasone was found to be effective in a controlled study in 1979, and a meta-analysis of the literature in 1989 supported the use of corticosteroids for hospitalized patents. More recently, controlled trials by Klassen, Schuh, and others demonstrated that nebulized budesonide decreases the severity of illness in patients with mild to moderate croup. Budesonide has been shown to be slightly less effective than dexamethasone and to provide a slight additive effect. A single report has suggested that the response to budesonide may be equal to that of racemic epinephrine.

Until more data become available, treatment regimens will remain in flux. A reasonable approach for the present is to tailor therapy to the severity of illness. In rare cases with inadequate gas exchange, management of the airway, at times with endotracheal intubation, takes precedence; tracheal edema may make passage of a tube with the usual diameter impossible, and the physician should be prepared with one a size smaller. Patients in the ED who have upper-airway obstruction that is of concern and a high likelihood of hospitalization will benefit from prompt administration of both racemic epinephrine by nebulization and intramuscular dexamethasone at 0.6 mg per kilogram of body weight. For children with moderately severe croup, when hospitalization is being considered, the response to an initial trial of mist and either intramuscular dexamethasone or nebulized budesonide can be assessed. If the response is adequate, the physician could add either a second steroid (eg, budesonide if dexamethasone was already administered) or racemic epinephrine. Finally, most patients who are mildly ill require only instructions for home care.

Epiglottitis

CLINICAL MANIFESTATIONS

Epiglottitis has an abrupt onset. The duration of illness before presentation is often as short as 6 hours and rarely exceeds 24 hours. Among the 21 children reported by Greenberg and Schisgall, an average of 17 hours elapsed between the first symptom and hospital admission. The parents first note the onset of fever. Shortly thereafter, the child develops stridor and labored respirations. As the disease progresses, the supraglottic edema interferes with the ability to swallow secretions; thus, drooling is a complaint in 60% to 70% of cases. Of the children with epiglottitis, 50% complain of a sore throat. Aphonia, hoarseness, and cough are uncommon. Although both croup and epiglottitis manifest with stridor in a febrile child, the examiner usually can differentiate these two illnesses on the basis of the clinical features (Table 74.7).

TABLE 74.7. Epiglottitis and Croup: A Comparison

	Epiglottitis	Croup
Anatomy	Supraglottic	Subglottic
Etiology	Bacterial: *H. influenzae*	Viral: parainfluenza
Age range (yr)	3–7, adults	0.5–3
Onset (h)	6–24	24–72
Toxicity	Marked	Mild to moderate
Drooling	Frequent	Absent
Cough	Unusual	Frequent
Hoarseness	Unusual	Frequent
White blood cell count	Leukocytosis	Normal

The anxious appearance of most children with epiglottitis strikes the examiner immediately. To maximize air entry, these children assume a sitting position with their jaws thrust forward. Cyanosis may occur in the later stages of the illness. The temperature, almost always elevated, often reaches a level of 40°C (104°F). Tachycardia is a constant feature. Although the patients are universally tachypneic, the respiratory rate rarely exceeds 40 breaths per minute. Stridor can be heard without a stethoscope, but auscultation of the lungs reveals no other adventitious sounds. Marked retractions are seen, predominantly involving the suprasternal and subcostal musculature.

As discussed under "Management," rigorous attempts to visualize the epiglottis are hazardous and should be avoided in the child with suspected epiglottitis; however, the examiner may view the pharynx without the use of a tongue depressor. The mucosa is seen to be erythematous, and pooled secretions are present in about half the children. Occasionally, a swollen, cherry red epiglottis protrudes above the base of the tongue and is visible without instrumentation.

Collection of laboratory specimens is usually delayed until the airway has been secured. The WBC count is elevated in most children with epiglottitis. As in other diseases that result from bacteremia with *H. influenzae,* a leukocytosis in the range of 15000 to 25000/mm^3 and a shift to the left occur in response to the infection.

A lateral neck radiograph is pathognomonic of epiglottitis. There are three characteristic features: (1) a swollen epiglottis, (2) thickened aryepiglottic folds, and (3) obliteration of the vallecula. The normal epiglottis has a thin, curved silhouette that has been likened to a bent finger, convex on one side and concave on the other. As a result of inflammatory edema from infection, it swells and assumes a configuration that is convex on both sides. This has been called the "thumb sign." The airway below the level of the vocal cords appears normal on the lateral neck radiograph of a child with epiglottitis.

The most serious complication of epiglottitis is sudden respiratory obstruction. This may occur unpredictably at any point in the illness, before seeking medical attention, in the ED, or after hospitalization. Although a child with minimal respiratory distress occasionally has a total obstruction, marked retractions and labored breathing should serve as a warning of an impending airway catastrophe. An additional complication of this illness is extraepiglottic spread of the infection. During the course of the bacteremia, seeding may involve the meninges, lungs, pericardium, synovial membranes, and soft tissues. Thus, the initial examination should attempt to elicit signs of infection at these additional sites.

MANAGEMENT

When a child is suspected of having epiglottitis, the thrust of the management plan is to make a definitive diagnosis and institute therapy before the onset of airway obstruction.

The initial steps in management are based on the degree of respiratory distress and the likelihood of epiglottitis, as judged from the clinical features (Fig. 74.3). Some children with epiglottitis have total or nearly total airway obstruction as the initial presentation of their disease. In this situation, treatment precedes any diagnostic evaluation and steps to maintain an adequate exchange of air are taken (see Chapters 1 and 5).

Most children, however, manifest lesser degrees of stridor and respiratory compromise with fever. The clinician must decide whether the constellation of historical and physical features points to croup or epiglottitis. In most children with stridor, the history will favor croup, which is the more common of the two

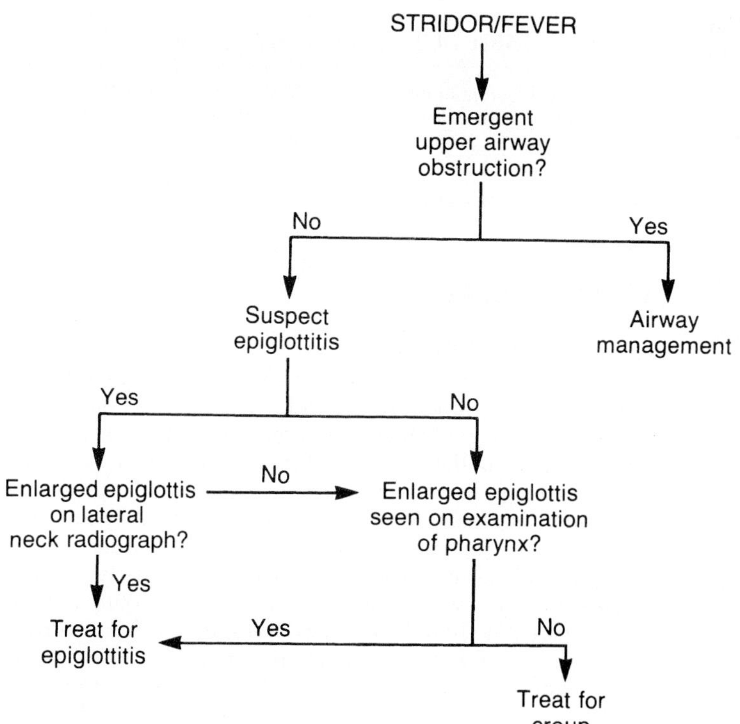

Figure 74.3. Diagnostic approach to the child with suspected epiglottitis.

diseases. The child will not appear toxic or show signs of air hunger. In such situations, a lateral neck radiograph is not indicated. Rather, the pharynx may be visualized directly with a tongue depressor to confirm the absence of a swollen, inflamed epiglottis.

When the findings weigh in favor of epiglottitis, however, further examination should be postponed and immediate preparation should be made for the insertion of an artificial airway; this includes collecting the necessary equipment and summoning additional personnel as needed. Anesthesiologists and otorhinolaryngologists alike, if available, should be involved in the care of children with epiglottitis, in addition to the staff in the ED. Following the appropriate preparations, a physician should accompany the child to the radiology department for a lateral neck radiograph, or a portable radiograph may be obtained. An intravenous infusion using a plastic cannula may be started in the cooperative patient. If the child becomes agitated or the procedure lengthy, however, the radiograph must be obtained quickly, assuming the airway has not been compromised, rather than persisting with attempts to gain intravenous access. The lateral neck radiograph either confirms or disproves the clinical diagnosis. If epiglottitis is verified radiographically, a skilled physician next performs endotracheal intubation, most often in the operating suite. If intubation is not possible, a surgical approach to the airway is necessary (Table 74.8). Ceftriaxone (100 mg per kilogram daily in one or two divided doses) and cefotaxime (200 mg per kilogram daily in four divided doses) serve as single-drug alternatives and are useful particularly for patients allergic to penicillins.

TABLE 74.8. Immediate Management of Epiglottitis

Ensure adequate ventilation	Endotracheal intubation (or tracheostomy)
Gain peripheral venous access, if tolerated by child	Defer laboratory studies until airway is secured

Bacterial Tracheitis

The signs and symptoms of bacterial tracheitis mimic those of acute epiglottitis but have a somewhat slower onset. The temperature is usually greater than 39°C (102.2°F), and the patients have stridor. Toxicity and respiratory distress occur as a rule. On radiograph, there is tracheal narrowing, and a pseudomembrane may be visible within the tracheal lumen; the supraglottic area is normal. Children with bacterial tracheitis often are diagnosed initially as having severe viral croup or epiglottitis. Their management is as outlined for these conditions. The first priority is to secure an adequate airway. If bacterial tracheitis is suspected on the basis of a lateral neck radiograph or the findings at laryngoscopy, antibiotic therapy should be initiated with ceftriaxone (100 mg per kilogram daily in one or two divided doses) or ampicillin–sulbactam (200 mg per kilogram daily of ampicillin in four divided doses).

LOWER RESPIRATORY TRACT INFECTIONS

Bacterial Pneumonia

CLINICAL MANIFESTATIONS

Bacterial pneumonia generally has an abrupt onset with fever, often accompanied by chills. A cough is a common but nonspecific complaint. Occasionally, pleuritic involvement produces pain with respiratory effort. Observation of the child at rest before the examination often provides the key to the diagnosis of pneumonia. Tachypnea out of proportion to the fever is rarely the only sign, particularly in the first year of life. The infant who breathes at a normal rate, however, seldom has a bacterial infection of the lung. A hasty effort at auscultation that disturbs the quiet infant obscures this finding.

Fever is almost universally present, ranging from 38.5° to 41°C (101.2°–105.8°F). Grunting respirations in a young child should arouse a strong suspicion of pneumonia. Localized findings, more often seen in the child older than 1 year, include inspiratory rales, decreased breath sounds (sometimes the only abnormality), and less often dullness to percussion. Gastric dilation may accompany pneumonia; occasionally, the abdominal findings in pulmonary infections mimic appendicitis. With upper lobe pneumonia, the pain may radiate to the neck, causing meningismus; the diagnosis of pneumonia must therefore be considered in the child with nuchal rigidity and normal CSF.

In the ED, a chest radiograph often assists in the management of a child suspected of having bacterial pneumonia. Although occasionally a patient who is dehydrated with pneumonia does not have an infiltrate, the radiographic evaluation confirms or denies the diagnosis of bacterial pneumonia in most cases. This is important in a clinical setting not conducive to continuity of care. In addition, the radiograph may provide information on the disease process. A lobar consolidation is assumed to be of bacterial origin, needing treatment with antibiotics, whereas a minimal, diffuse interstitial infiltrate in a previously healthy toddler suggests a viral infection that can be managed with symptomatic therapy or, in an adolescent, *M. pneumoniae,* calling for treatment with erythromycin or another macrolide. Bilateral involvement, pleural effusion, and pneumatoceles point to more severe disease.

Further laboratory studies are obtained only on specific indications. A WBC count may be helpful in differentiating viral from bacterial disease or in assessing the likelihood of bacteremia in the young child; the count often exceeds 15000/mm^3 and occasionally rises above 30000/mm^3 with bacterial invasion of the pulmonary parenchyma or the bloodstream. Levels of CRP correlate with the bacteremia and lobar infiltrates more closely than the WBC count; however, this test is less readily available than the WBC count.

The most common complication of pneumonia is dehydration, particularly in young children. Electrolytes and a BUN are useful in assessing the degree of fluid loss in a child who appears ill or exhibits dry skin or mucosa. Rarely, extensive pulmonary involvement compromises ventilation, leading to respiratory failure. ABG measurements are indicated for any child with significant respiratory distress or oxygen saturation below 90%. A pleural effusion accumulates in most infections with *S. aureus* and *H. influenzae,* less often with *S. pneumoniae.* Bacteremia may result in additional foci of infection, including meningitis, pericarditis, epiglottitis, and septic arthritis.

MANAGEMENT

Most healthy children with pneumonia respond to outpatient antibiotic therapy. Because most of the infections are caused by *S. pneumoniae,* amoxicillin (50 mg per kilogram of body weight daily given orally in three divided doses) has been the mainstay of therapy. Ceftriaxone (50 mg per kilogram) may be administered intramuscularly at the time of diagnosis, especially if there is any concern about oral intake during the first 24 hours. Alternatively, macrolides, including erythromycin (40 mg per kilogram daily in four divided doses) or azithromycin (10 mg per kilogram as a single dose on the first day and 5 mg per kilogram as a single dose on days 2 to 5) may be used in penicillin-allergic children or when mycoplasmal infection is suspected on the basis of age or radiographic findings. Supportive therapy includes antipyretics and adequate hydration. Antitussives have no place in the treatment of pneumonia. Every child should return within 24 to 48 hours for a second evaluation; patients who do not clinically improve and become afebrile should be evaluated carefully for admission to the hospital. Any child who appears to be toxic (on the basis of the physician's clinical judgment) or is immunocompromised should be hospitalized. Firmer, but not unarguable, indications for admission are listed in Table 74.9.

TABLE 74.9. Indications for Admission

Age <1 yr (lobar infiltrate)	Failure to respond to antibiotic therapy within 24–48 hr
Respiratory compromise	Dehydration
Pleural effusion	
Pneumatocele	

Viral Pneumonia

CLINICAL MANIFESTATIONS

Viral pneumonia generally has its onset over a 2- to 4-day period, being more gradual than with bacterial infection. Cough, coryza, and low-grade fever commonly occur. Particularly with RSV infections in the first 3 months of life, an apneic spell may be the first sign to draw attention to the illness. Fever in viral pneumonia is usually lower than 39°C (102.2°F). As with bacterial infections, tachypnea in the undisturbed child may be the only physical finding. Rales are often audible diffusely throughout the chest, and wheezing also may be present. With more severe disease, the child shows signs of respiratory failure: grunting, cyanosis, and changes in mental status. The WBC count varies widely in viral pneumonia. Although leukocytosis over 15000/mm^3 may occur in some cases, such elevated counts should arouse suspicion of bacterial disease.

The radiographic examination provides useful clues to the type of pathogen that causes pneumonia but never can confirm a viral infection or rule out a bacterial cause. Most typically, the radiograph in a child with viral pneumonia shows bilateral air trapping and peribronchial thickening. A diffuse increase in the interstitial markings is also commonly seen; however, the findings can vary from barely detectable increases in volume to segmental infiltrates. Decubitus films occasionally detect small effusions. Because of the limitations in obtaining reliable cultures for bacteria, it is safest to presume a bacterial cause in the child with clinical evidence of pneumonia and a lobar infiltrate, a pleural effusion, a temperature over 39°C (102.2°F), or signs of clinical toxicity. Particularly in a dehydrated child, the chest radiograph may fail to show a lobar consolidation early in the course of a bacterial pneumonia.

MANAGEMENT

The physician must attempt to make an etiologic diagnosis in pneumonia on the basis of the clinical and radiographic findings without the benefit of definitive laboratory tests. A WBC count should be obtained if there is uncertainty about the likely cause. In such cases, a leukocytosis over 15000/mm^3 would weigh against a viral infection. If a viral pneumonia is strongly suspected, no specific therapy need be given. An example of such a situation would be a well-hydrated 5-year-old child with a gradual onset of cough, a temperature of 38°C (100.4°F), scattered bilateral rales, WBC count of 8000/mm^3 with predominantly lymphocytes, and the finding of hyperaeration on chest radiograph. Treatment in this case could be limited to antipyresis and hydration with a follow-up visit in 24 hours. Because the infant less than 3 months of age may become apneic during the course of viral pneumonia, these young children may benefit from observation in the hospital.

Mycoplasmal Pneumonia

CLINICAL MANIFESTATIONS

Pneumonia caused by *M. pneumoniae* usually begins insidiously with fever and malaise. After 3 to 5 days, the child develops a nonproductive cough, hoarseness, sore throat, and, in one-quarter of cases, chest pain. Fever is almost invariably present and may reach a level of 40°C (104°F). Children seldom develop much respiratory distress, with the exception of those younger than 5 years of age or those who also have sickle cell anemia or an immunodeficiency. Rales are heard in 75% of these infections, often bilaterally. The pharynx may appear inflamed, and some investigators have noted ear infections, particularly bullous myringitis, in association with pneumonia caused by *M. pneumoniae.* In 10% of patients, a maculopapular or, less often, a vesicular rash occurs; rarely, erythema multiforme, urticaria, or petechiae are seen.

The total WBC count is often normal in infections with this pathogen. A cold agglutinin titer of 32 or higher is found in most patients with lobar infiltrates from an *M. pneumoniae* infection but may also occur, although less often, with viral and bacterial illnesses. The organism may be recovered by culture, and specific diagnosis is possible with measurement of antibody titers in acute and convalescent sera; however, these procedures require 1 to 3 weeks and are not readily available. The radiographic findings show considerable variation. Between 10% and 25% of children will have lobar consolidation. Scattered segmental infiltrates, interstitial disease, and combinations of all these patterns may be seen. Pleural effusions occur in 5% of cases.

MANAGEMENT

The diagnosis of mycoplasmal pneumonia is presumptively based on the clinical and radiographic findings and, in some cases, on the cold agglutinin titer. An older child or adolescent with the gradual onset of a mild bilateral pneumonia should be treated for this infection. On the other hand, a lobar infiltrate in a 5-year-old child usually is assumed to be of bacterial origin regardless of the level of the cold agglutinins. The results of cultures and specific serologic assays entail too great a delay to be useful to the clinician in the ED. Erythromycin (40 mg per kilogram daily) provides effective therapy for *M. pneumoniae* infections. The response is more pronounced in the older child with lobar disease than in the younger child with a diffuse infiltrate.

Chlamydial Pneumonia

CLINICAL MANIFESTATIONS

Infancy

Infants with chlamydial pneumonia usually have a staccato cough that may resemble the paroxysms seen in pertussis but is usually less prolonged. In 50% of cases, conjunctivitis precedes the onset of respiratory symptoms. Pneumonia with this organism only rarely produces a fever. Mild retractions, hyperresonance, and diffuse rales are noted on examination of the chest. Hyperaeration of the lungs depresses the liver, allowing the edge to be palpated 1 to 2 mm below the right costal margin.

Although the WBC count is usually in the normal range, the eosinophil count rises slightly (400/mm^3, or 5%–10%) in 75% of these patients. Elevated immunoglobulin levels, although nonspecific, often occur with chlamydial infections, but seldom with viral illnesses. Mild hypoxemia is common. The chest radiograph shows hyperaeration of the lungs and a diffuse increase in the interstitial markings. Lobar consolidations and pleural diffusions are not seen.

Childhood

The spectrum of infection ranges from asymptomatic to severe. Adolescents are more likely to have signs of pneumonia than children, who may have clinical findings that are confined to the upper respiratory tract. Often, a sore throat and hoarseness precede pneumonia, and these usually are accompanied by a brief fever. By the time pneumonia has developed, the fever often resolves. Patients usually have a cough and scattered rales on auscultation. As for the clinical syndrome, the chest radiograph picture resembles that seen with *M. pneumoniae,* consisting of subsegmental lesions rather than lobar consolidation. Leukocytosis is not seen. No specific diagnostic testing is routinely available.

MANAGEMENT

Because of the difficulty in making a definitive etiologic diagnosis and the potential for complications, most young infants with presumed chlamydial pneumonia should be admitted to the hospital. Erythromycin (40 mg/kg daily) may shorten the course and should be given. *C. pneumoniae* infections in older children respond to therapy with macrolide antibiotics, including erythromycin (40 mg/kg per day) or azithromycin (10 mg/kg on day 1 and 5 mg/kg on days 2 through 5).

Bronchiolitis

CLINICAL MANIFESTATIONS

Bronchiolitis begins as a URI with cough and coryza. Over 2 to 5 days, signs of respiratory distress appear. The parents can often hear the child wheezing. Fever occurs in two-thirds of children with bronchiolitis. They often appear ill on overall assessment. The respiratory rate climbs to at least 40 breaths per minute and may reach 80 to 100 breaths per minute. Nasal flaring and retractions of the intercostal and supraclavicular muscles are noted and increase as the disease progresses. In bronchiolitis and other lower respiratory tract infections, the intercostal retractions are more pronounced than the supraclavicular, the opposite of the findings in croup and epiglottitis. Wheezes and a prolonged expiratory phase are heard in all children with bronchiolitis, at times without a stethoscope; rales are usually minimal. As the ventilatory muscles fatigue, the child will have grunting respirations; only in the most severe cases does cyanosis occur. The total WBC count in bronchiolitis is normal. Usually, the chest radiograph shows only hyperaerated lungs, but occasionally areas of atelectasis are present. If respiratory failure supervenes, the P_{aO_2} decreases and carbon dioxide is retained.

The complications of bronchiolitis include dehydration, respiratory failure, and, rarely, bacterial superinfection. Pneumothorax and pneumomediastinum are rarely seen. The increased respiratory effort in bronchiolitis may prevent an infant from maintaining an adequate oral intake. Careful attention should be paid to the details of fluid balance when taking a history. Of infants with bronchiolitis, 10% to 20% develop significant respiratory compromise. Cyanosis (or oxygen saturation <91%), decreased inspiratory breath sounds, and lethargy on examination point to ventilatory failure. Bacterial superinfection is uncommon in the early stages of the illness, occurring occasionally in hospitalized infants; however, lobar consolidation seen on the chest radiograph suggests a potential bacterial pneumonia, although atelectatic patches may be confused with infiltrates.

MANAGEMENT

In the management of children with suspected bronchiolitis in the ED, a chest radiograph should be considered, both to look for findings compatible with this diagnosis and to help exclude other entities such as lobar pneumonia or a foreign body. Pulse oximetry provides an estimate of the degree of hypoxia.

Measurements of WBC count, ABG, and electrolytes are obtained only if the diagnosis is uncertain or the clinical picture suggests that complications have occurred.

Children with bronchiolitis may benefit from nebulized bronchodilators. Although conflicting reports have been published, at least two studies have described an improvement in clinical status and oxygen saturation following albuterol delivered by nebulization. One group of investigators found aerosolized epinephrine to be superior. For the child with moderate to severe distress, treatments can be administered every 20 minutes, starting at 0.1 to 0.3 of a 0.5% solution of albuterol or using 3 mL of 1:1000 epinephrine. Patients who show a favorable response to nebulized therapy are candidates to receive further nebulized treatments. Oral albuterol solution at a dosage of 0.1 mg per kilogram of weight per dose, given every 6 hours, has limited efficacy.

Corticosteroids are not indicated for the treatment of patients with bronchiolitis. In general, it is difficult to differentiate asthma from bronchiolitis during the first 2 years of life; thus, corticosteroids may be given occasionally to some children who may have bronchiolitis or asthma, in accordance with the guidelines for the latter disease.

For the patient who does not respond to nebulized albuterol or has only mild distress, bronchodilators should not be prescribed. Therapy is limited to antipyretics and the encouragement of adequate oral intake, and the infant should be examined again after 24 to 48 hours. Dehydration, secondary bacterial infection, and significant respiratory distress necessitate admission to the hospital. Although not validated in infants with bronchiolitis, a score of 4 or more on the asthma scale (see Chapter 81) suggests significant respiratory compromise. An oxygen saturation level less than 93% or an arterial P_{aO2} less than 70 mm Hg in room air also suggests a need for hospitalization. In addition, children with underlying cardiac or pulmonary disease usually require admission. Ribavirin has proved somewhat useful in ameliorating the course of bronchiolitis when administered by continuous aerosol for 3 to 5 days to severely ill children who are hospitalized. This agent is recommended primarily for patients with underlying cardiac or pulmonary conditions.

Pertussis

CLINICAL MANIFESTATIONS

Although pertussis can be divided into three stages for discussion, a clinically distinct syndrome does not evolve until the disease has progressed to the second stage. Initially, the symptoms mimic a viral URI. This first stage (*catarrhal*) is characterized by a mild cough, conjunctivitis, and coryza and lasts 1 to 2 weeks. An increasingly severe cough heralds onset of the second stage (*paroxysmal*), which continues for 2 to 4 weeks. After a prolonged spasm of coughing, the sudden inflow of air produces the characteristic whoop. Vomiting often occurs after such an episode. When not coughing, the child has a remarkably normal physical examination, except for an occasional subconjunctival hemorrhage. During the third stage (*convalescent*), the intensity of the cough wanes. The WBC count in children usually reaches a level of 20000 to 50000/mm^3 with a marked lymphocytosis, but such changes are not often seen in infants younger than 3 to 6 months.

MANAGEMENT

Except for occasional situations in which fluorescent antibody testing is immediately available, the diagnosis of pertussis rests on clinical grounds. Children with an unmistakable paroxysmal cough followed by a whoop should be assumed to have the disease. When the clinical picture is unclear, a WBC count and chest radiograph may be useful. The radiograph helps eliminate other causes of a severe cough (eg, foreign body, bacterial pneumonia, cystic fibrosis, tuberculosis), and the WBC count provides confirmatory evidence if a leukocytosis with marked lymphocytosis is found. Because of the grave risk of complications, all children younger than 6 months who are diagnosed firmly as having pertussis should be observed in the hospital. Older children who show signs of respiratory compromise, such as cyanosis during paroxysms of coughing, or who develop complications also require admission. Treatment includes erythromycin (40 mg per kilogram daily for 14 days), maintenance of adequate hydration, and a level of respiratory support appropriate to the severity of the disease. Clarithromycin and azithromycin are alternative choices. Household and other close contacts require chemoprophylaxis with erythromycin (40 mg per kilogram daily for 14 days). Children younger than 7 years who are unimmunized or who have received fewer than four doses of pertussis vaccine should have their pertussis immunization initiated or continued as soon as possible after exposure. Children who are fully immunized for age but have received only three doses require a fourth dose. Those who have had four doses need a booster unless the last dose has been within 3 years or they are more than 6 years old. Diphtheria, tetanus, and pertussis vaccine (DTP_a) is preferred.

Tuberculosis

CLINICAL FINDINGS

Most infections by *M. tuberculosis* in children never cause any significant symptoms. Among the many possible clinical presentations, three stand out as particular concerns to the emergency physician: primary pneumonia, miliary tuberculosis, and meningitis. Pneumonia is by far the most common. Of note, these infections may develop despite prior vaccination against tuberculosis with bacille Calmette-Guérin vaccine (BCG).

The onset of primary tuberculosis pneumonia resembles that of bacterial infections of the lungs. It begins with fever and tachypnea; rales and an area of dullness are found on examination of the chest. The WBC count may be elevated with a shift to the left, and the chest radiograph shows a lobar consolidation, often accompanied by hilar adenopathy and less often by pleural effusion or cavitation. Although the primary pneumonia often resolves spontaneously, the child occasionally follows a downhill course caused by local progression. In addition to the epidemiologic risks described, clinical findings that should arouse a suspicion of tuberculous pneumonia in the child otherwise thought to have a bacterial infection of the lung include pleural effusion, cavitation, toxicity, and a failure to respond to antibiotic therapy.

Miliary tuberculosis begins with an abrupt rise in temperature but a paucity of other physical findings; it may mimic sepsis. Subsequently, respiratory symptoms and enlargement of the liver, spleen, and superficial lymph nodes occur. The WBC count is usually in the range of 15000/mm^3. Although the chest radiograph initially shows no lesions, a diffuse mottling of the lung fields appears 1 to 3 weeks after the fever. Miliary tuberculosis is a consideration in a child with a persistent fever and hepatosplenomegaly.

Tuberculous meningitis comes on insidiously with a low-grade fever, apathy, and in 50% of patients, vomiting. After 1 to 2 weeks of nonspecific illness, neurologic signs appear, including drowsiness and nuchal rigidity; if untreated, the child lapses into coma. The CSF shows a mononuclear pleocytosis, an elevated protein concentration, and eventually a low glucose level.

TABLE 74.10. Definition of Positive Criteria for the Standard Mantoux Skin Test (5 Tuberculin Units of PPD) in Children[a]

Induration >5 mm
- Children in close contact with known or suspected cases of active tuberculosis, if adequate and timely treatment cannot be verified
- Children suspected to have tuberculosis based on a consistent chest radiograph or clinical findings
- Children immunosuppressed on the basis of therapy or disease

Induration >10 mm
- Children <4 yr of age
- Children with chronic illness including lymphoma, diabetes mellitus, renal failure, and malnutrition
- Children born in or traveling to regions of the world with a high prevalence of tuberculosis or exposed to adults likely to be infected

Induration >15 mm
- Children ≥4 yr of age without any risk factors

PPD, purified protein derivative.
[a] Applies regardless of previous bacille Calmette-Guérin (BCG) vaccination.
Modified from Committee on Infectious Diseases, 1997 RedBook. Elk Grove Village, IL: American Academy of Pediatrics, 1997, with permission.

MANAGEMENT

A child suspected of having pneumonic, meningeal, or miliary tuberculosis should be admitted to the hospital for evaluation and possible chemotherapy. Among innercity populations, where the risk of tuberculosis is greatest, the routine placement of a tine or Mantoux test in children with lobar pneumonia should be considered. The Mantoux test must be interpreted in accordance with the child's age and the presence of risk factors (Table 74.10). Current treatment for tuberculosis consists of two to four or more drugs (isoniazid, rifampin, pyrazinamide, ethambutol, streptomycin, capreomycin, ciprofloxacin, cycloserine, ethionamide, kanamycin, ofloxacin, para-aminosalicylic acid) for a minimum of 6 months.

Hantavirus

The Hantavirus pulmonary syndrome begins with fever, cough, and myalgias, followed shortly thereafter by tachypnea, tachycardia, dyspnea, and finally, hypotension. A marked leukocytosis is common along with thrombocytopenia and elevated clotting studies. The initial chest radiograph shows an interstitial more often than an alveolar infiltrate, with changes starting or becoming bilateral in the majority of cases. Pleural effusions occur in about one-quarter of the patients. The diagnosis should be considered when a severe pneumonia occurs in combination with systemic deterioration and can be confirmed subsequently by specific viral serology. Treatment is supportive.

GASTROINTESTINAL INFECTIONS

Viral Gastroenteritis

CLINICAL FINDINGS

Children with viral gastroenteritis are usually brought to the ED with a complaint of diarrhea or vomiting or both. The numbers of stools may vary from two or three up to 15 or 20 daily. Most commonly, six to eight bowel movements occur in a 24-hour period; the stools range from semisolid in consistency to watery. Although hematochezia occasionally occurs in viral infections, the presence of blood in the stool should suggest a bacterial gastroenteritis. Vomiting may accompany diarrhea, or it may be the sole manifestation of a viral gastroenteritis. The daily frequency of emesis varies in the same range as for diarrhea. After forceful emesis, streaks of blood may be present in the vomitus. Many children with viral gastroenteritis beyond the age of 2 or 3 years complain of crampy abdominal pain. In more severe illnesses, the parent may relate a history of decreased oral intake and oliguria.

Children with viral gastroenteritis are usually febrile. In the child older than 3 years, however, a temperature over 39°C (102.2°F) may suggest a bacterial enteritis. Tachycardia, hypotension, and lethargy may reflect dehydration in severe episodes. Whereas the respiratory rate is usually normal, tachypnea occurs when acidosis or dehydration is present. The abdomen is soft and is not distended in most cases. Although the child may perceive palpation as uncomfortable, this maneuver does not elicit localized or rebound tenderness. Auscultation reveals hyperactive bowel sounds. The skin turgor is decreased and the mucous membranes are dry only in severe gastroenteritis with dehydration (see Chapters 14, 15, and 76).

No laboratory studies are indicated in the uncomplicated case of gastroenteritis. The CBC, electrolytes, and BUN usually fall within normal range. If oral intake fails to keep pace with the efflux of fluids from the alimentary tract, dehydration occurs. The sodium, usually normal, may drop as low as 110 mEq per liter or rise to 170 mEq per liter, and the bicarbonate is invariably low. With mild dehydration, the serum bicarbonate hovers just below the normal level at 18 to 20 mEq per liter; however, values of 10 to 12 mEq per liter are usually found in the face of prolonged diarrhea. The BUN reflects the state of hydration and the adequacy at the recent intake of protein. It may climb as high as 100 mg per deciliter in children who lose more than 10% of their body weight. In a child who has been maintained on clear liquids, however, the BUN will not accurately indicate the degree of dehydration because urea rises as a breakdown product during protein metabolism. Although the hemoglobin and WBC count are usually normal in the child with viral gastroenteritis, hemoconcentration may occur with dehydration.

MANAGEMENT

Uncomplicated viral gastroenteritis usually remits in 2 to 5 days and does not require treatment in the hospital. All children should be weighed, preferably without clothing, to provide a baseline for follow-up. The vomiting generally responds to a brief cessation of oral intake. After 2 to 4 hours of abstinence, the diet should be resumed gradually. The diarrhea may persist for several days, but hydration can usually be maintained orally after the vomiting has subsided.

Current recommendations for oral therapy emphasize the use of appropriately balanced glucose and electrolyte solutions, as well as the early reintroduction of feedings. Generally, rehydration is initiated, particularly in infants younger than 1 year, with a solution that contains 75 to 90 mEq per liter of sodium in a ratio with glucose of 1:1 (eg, Rehydralyte). Older children often tolerate juices and sodas. Some studies have advocated the use of glucose polymers (eg, Ricelyte) instead of glucose as a means to reduce diarrhea, but significant advantages have yet to be demonstrated for these products. Preparation at home of fluids that contain salt notoriously leads to errors, and this procedure is to be condemned. Similarly, the physician should avoid the use of boiled skim milk, a hypertonic solution that may produce hypernatremia.

Antiemetics are seldom used, but recent studies suggest that ondansetron (0.15 mg per kilogram in a single dose) facilitates discharge from the ED in case where vomiting predominates. Loperamide (0.5 mg per kilogram daily) has been shown to reduce the severity of diarrhea in conjunction with oral rehydration therapy but is indicated only for unusually severe or prolonged cases of gastroenteritis after excluding a cause that would respond to specific therapy.

Dehydration is the only significant complication of viral gastroenteritis. If the physician suspects that a child has developed more than 5% to 10% dehydration, electrolytes and a BUN should be obtained. These tests establish the degree of acidosis and the presence of hyponatremia or hypernatremia. Most children with gastroenteritis tolerate oral rehydration. In underdeveloped countries, even patients with severe dehydration are often managed successfully in most cases by using the oral route. In the ED, treatment for children with moderate to severe dehydration usually is initiated intravenously. As a rule, all patients with dehydration estimated to be greater than 10%, and many cases falling in the range of 5% to 10%, require intravenous fluids.

When intravenous therapy is chosen, a bolus of fluid, such as 10 to 20 mL per kilogram of normal saline, may be administered over 1 hour or more rapidly if needed (see Chapter 3). If rehydration is achieved and the child is capable of subsequent oral intake, treatment may be continued at home (as in the milder cases).

Children who are more than 5% dehydrated or have alterations in the serum sodium (<130 mEq/L or >145 mEq/L) may require hospitalization. Intravenous therapy should be started in the ED, particularly if there is evidence of vascular instability (see Chapters 3, 14, 15, and 76).

Bacterial Gastroenteritis

BACKGROUND

Five pathogens commonly produce gastroenteritis: *Salmonella, Shigella, Yersinia, Campylobacter,* and pathogenic *E. coli.* Together, these organisms cause 10% to 15% of the diarrheal illnesses seen in children coming to the ED. In underdeveloped countries and occasionally in the United States, *Vibrio* species also must be considered. In addition, *A. hydrophila* has been associated occasionally with diarrheal illnesses in children. *C. difficile* causes a toxin-associated colitis, particularly in patients who receive antibiotics.

CLINICAL MANIFESTATIONS

Signs and Symptoms

A careful epidemiologic history often provides a clue to the diagnosis of *Salmonella* infections. Foodborne outbreaks often occur in the summer. After an incubation period of 8 to 48 hours, the child experiences crampy abdominal pain and nausea. The stools are watery and may contain blood, but this is not the rule. Fever is noted in most children. Unless protracted diarrhea has led to clinically apparent dehydration, the physical examination is unremarkable. Abdominal tenderness and distension are usual findings. The leukocyte count is usually 10000 to 15000/mm^3. Methylene blue staining of the stool may show the presence of polymorphonuclear leukocytes, but not in sheets as seen with *Shigella.* A single rectal swab leads to isolation of *Salmonella* from more than 90% of children with this infection.

Shigella organisms may cause an asymptomatic infection, mild gastroenteritis, or bacillary dysentery. Mild illnesses are more common. Children affected in this way complain of frequent watery stools but few constitutional symptoms. Bacillary dysentery begins suddenly with fever and abdominal pain. Diarrhea begins shortly thereafter. The stools, which may average 10 to 12 daily, contain mucus and blood, and tenesmus is common. Children with this form of shigellosis have a fever, often in the range of 39° to 40°C (102.2° to 104°F). Palpation of the abdomen often elicits diffuse tenderness but no evidence of peritoneal irritation.

Occasionally, a *Shigella* infection may produce CNS irritation because of the release of toxin before the onset of diarrhea. Thus, shigellosis must be considered in the differential diagnosis of meningismus in the absence of a pleocytosis in the CSF. A seizure may actually be the first manifestation of the illness.

Certain laboratory abnormalities strongly suggest *Shigella* organisms as the cause of gastroenteritis. The leukocyte count often shows many band forms that exceed the mature neutrophils in number. The total WBC count may show a leukopenia or a leukocytosis but most commonly hovers in the normal range. Because *Shigella* invades the intestinal mucosa, this infection elicits a profound inflammatory response. The exudation of white cells leads to the finding of sheets of neutrophils in the stool after methylene blue staining. A single rectal swab suffices for the isolation of *Shigella* from most children with this illness.

Children with gastroenteritis caused by *Y. enterocolitica* usually have an abrupt onset of diarrhea. The stools are often watery and may contain blood, but vomiting generally remains inconsequential. Patients with this illness often complain of severe abdominal pain, sometimes before the onset of diarrhea. Gastrointestinal infection with *Y. enterocolitica* usually elicits a febrile response. The abdominal examination is usually benign, but palpation produces marked tenderness in the subset of patients with mesenteric adenitis. Arthritis and skin rashes occur in 5% to 10% of patients with this disease.

The mean WBC count in children with yersiniosis is usually normal, although leukocytosis with a shift to the left occurs occasionally. The electrolytes and BUN are normal except in the face of dehydration. Examination of stool stained with methylene blue reveals polymorphonuclear neutrophils. The organism can be recovered from stool culture, but this requires enrichment techniques. Although a single specimen is diagnostic in 70% to 80% of illnesses, a second sample should be obtained in the face of a previous negative culture when the clinical suspicion of disease remains strong.

Campylobacter enteritis is characterized by the abrupt onset of fever and abdominal pain, followed shortly by diarrhea. The temperature often remains normal in children younger than 3 months but ranges up to 40°C (104°F) in the older child. Vomiting occurs uncommonly and resolves rapidly. Two-thirds of children complain of abdominal pain, which may be severe. The number of stools varies from 2 to 20 daily; they are watery and contain blood in at least 50% of cases. Karmali and Fleming found frank blood in the stools of 95% of their patients. The physical examination is generally unremarkable. Although the abdominal pain occasionally simulates appendicitis, palpation of the abdomen elicits minimal tenderness. Signs of dehydration are found only rarely.

The WBC count in *Campylobacter* enteritis usually remains below 12000/mm^3, the highest being 22500/mm^3 in one study; on occasion, there may be a shift to the left. The electrolytes and BUN are usually normal. Maki and colleagues found fecal leukocytes in four of five patients with enteritis caused by *Campylobacter.* The organism is not often isolated from the blood but can be recovered easily from the stool by using appropriate media. When available, phase contrast microscopy can demonstrate the organism in fresh stool specimens.

The clinical picture of diarrhea caused by *E. coli* varies. This organism is suspected most often in the setting of a specific outbreak. In general, features suggestive of a bacterial rather than a viral gastroenteritis include (1) more than 10 stools per day or diarrhea lasting for more than 4 days, (2) blood in the stool, (3) fever of 39.5°C (103°F) or higher, (4) clinical toxicity, and (5) polymorphonuclear leukocytes in the stool. The presence of these findings enhances the likelihood that a bacterial pathogen is involved, although a viral gastroenteritis is not necessarily ruled out.

COMPLICATIONS

The complications of *Salmonella* gastroenteritis include dehydration and spread of infection beyond the confines of the gastrointestinal tract. During bacteremia, focal infections, including meningitis, osteomyelitis, and endocarditis, may develop. Most episodes of bacteremia terminate spontaneously. Dehydration is diagnosed on the basis of the clinical findings: dry mucous membranes, decreased skin turgor, tachycardia, and hypotension. Although the electrolytes are most often normal, both hyponatremia and hypernatremia may occur.

Bacteremia is most common in young children. In a study by Hyams and co-workers, 25% of hospitalized patients with *Salmonella* gastroenteritis had the organism recovered from their blood; however, Torrey and associates noted an incidence of only 6% in an ambulatory population. Although a high fever usually accompanies spread to the circulation, the physical examination is often devoid of any signs of serious illness. In addition, infants in the first 3 months of life often remain afebrile in the face of bacteremia. The WBC count is greater than $15000/mm^3$ in 80% to 90% of patients with bacteremia, and culture of the blood leads to recovery of the organism.

Enteric fever also occurs from the dissemination of certain serotypes of *Salmonella;* if *S. typhi* is isolated, the illness is called *typhoid fever*. The disease is characterized by chills and fever, often rising in a steplike pattern to 40°C (104°F). Diarrhea does not necessarily precede or coexist with the systemic illness. A relative bradycardia in relation to the height of the temperature is a hallmark of enteric fever. Splenomegaly and a macular rash, or rose spots, are detectable in 20% to 30% of patients. Leukopenia characterizes the hematologic picture. Both blood and stool cultures may be negative. The diagnosis may rest on a fourfold rise in the agglutinin titers.

Invasion of the bloodstream may lead to various focal diseases. Meningitis most commonly affects the youngest children. The features are identical to those observed in CNS infections with other purulent organisms. Children with sickle cell hemoglobinopathies have a peculiar predilection for bone and joint involvement. Endocarditis is seen less commonly.

The complications of shigellosis include dehydration, bacteremia, seizures, and colonic perforation. Dehydration often accompanies dysenteric infections and is diagnosed on the basis of the usual clinical findings. Bacteremia and perforation are both rare, occurring in fewer than 1% of gastrointestinal infections.

Most episodes of gastroenteritis with *Yersinia* are self-limiting, resolving before dehydration develops. Appendicitis occasionally results from obstruction of the appendiceal lumen by swollen lymphoid tissue. The incidence is unknown, but 5 of 38 patients in the New York State epidemic underwent removal of appendices that were suppurative. Bacteremia and focal infection follow gastroenteritis almost exclusively in the compromised host, particularly in association with thalassemia.

Campylobacter infections occasionally lead to dehydration but less often than is seen with the other bacterial pathogens in the gastrointestinal tract. Rarely, bacteremic or focal infections occur.

MANAGEMENT

Salmonella gastroenteritis is usually a self-limiting illness. In most cases, the disease is not sufficiently distinct or severe enough to suggest to the clinician the need for a diagnostic evaluation; however, life-threatening complications occur with predictable regularity in infants younger than 6 months and in children with sickle cell hemoglobinopathies.

The treatment of *Salmonella* gastroenteritis should be directed toward the maintenance of adequate hydration. As with viral infections, limitation of the diet to electrolyte solutions ("clear liquids") suffices in most children. Antibiotic therapy neither ameliorates the course of the gastroenteritis nor eradicates the organism from the intestinal tract in the immunocompetent host. In fact, several studies have suggested prolonged carriage after the administration of antibiotics.

The indications for admission of a child with diarrhea suspected or proved to be caused by *Salmonella* species are (1) dehydration, (2) focal infection or bacteremia/sepsis, (3) age less than 3 months or temperature over 39°C (102.2°F) in a child younger than 12 months (unless blood culture is known to be sterile), and (4) sickle cell anemia. If bacteremia is suspected, intravenous therapy with cefotaxime (200 mg per kilogram of body weight daily in four divided doses) or ceftriaxone (100 mg per kilogram daily in two divided doses) should be initiated. Chloramphenicol (75–100 mg per kilogram daily in four divided doses) or, in adolescents, one of the fluoroquinolones (ciprofloxacin, ofloxacin) provides an alternative for cephalosporin-allergic patients. When oral therapy is indicated, trimethoprim–sulfamethoxazole (TMP-SMZ; 8 mg of trimethoprim per kilogram daily in two divided doses) is the drug of choice.

Shigellosis stands alone as the only form of bacterial gastroenteritis for which antibiotics have proved efficacious. Antimicrobial therapy shortens the course of the illness and the duration of excretion of the organisms in the stool. Treatment alleviates the symptoms and signs of the gastroenteritis and limits transmission of the disease. TMP-SMZ (8 mg of trimethoprim and 40 mg of sulfamethoxazole per kilogram daily) is the initial drug of choice while the results of sensitivity tests are pending. Fluoroquinolones and ceftriaxone are alternatives.

Supportive therapy is an important aspect of the management of shigellosis. The initial oral intake should be limited to solutions with physiologic concentrations of glucose and electrolytes. As the diarrhea begins to abate, solid foods can be added. Dietary manipulation leads to resolution of the disease in some children before the organism is isolated. Antibiotic therapy may be omitted in such cases unless there is a particular concern about spread in a closed population. Iaregoric or combinations of diphenoxylate and atropine (Lomotil) are contraindicated.

Most episodes of shigellosis can be handled on an outpatient basis. Indications for admission include (1) age 6 months or younger, (2) dehydration, and (3) bacteremia (rare). Before the definitive diagnosis of shigellosis, particularly with significant bleeding, hospitalization may be required because of a concern about noninfectious entities such as a Meckel diverticulum.

Most children with yersiniosis can be treated as outpatients. Initially, the diet should be limited to electrolyte solutions (clear liquids). Although *Y. enterocolitica* is usually sensitive *in vitro* to tetracycline, chloramphenicol, colistin, gentamicin, and kanamycin, current studies have demonstrated no benefit from antibiotic therapy of uncomplicated gastroenteritis; however, persistent diarrhea may respond to antimicrobial treatment. Suspected or proven sepsis merits intravenous administration of antibiotics such as gentamicin (5–7.5 mg per kilogram daily in three divided doses beyond the neonatal period). The indications for admission include dehydration, severe abdominal pain suggesting appendicitis, and underlying diseases such as thalassemia.

Campylobacter enteritis is a self-limited but prolonged illness; diarrhea persists for more than 1 week in one-third of children.

These organisms exhibit almost universal sensitivity to erythromycin, which can be given orally at a dosage of 40 mg per kilogram of weight daily; ciprofloxacin is an alternative for adolescents. Antimicrobial therapy has not proved to decrease the duration of diarrhea, however.

Antibiotic-associated Colitis

Colitis with *C. difficile* varies widely in severity. Typically, profuse watery or mucoid diarrhea begins after several days of antibiotic therapy. Many older children complain of crampy abdominal pain. On examination, the usual findings include fever and diffuse abdominal tenderness. Often, the WBC count rises above 15000/mm^3. The stool may be guaiac-positive or frankly bloody; leukocytes are found on smears from approximately 50% of patients. An etiologic diagnosis requires the identification of *C. difficile* toxin in the stool; recovery of the organism on culture is suggestive but not sufficient. If *C. difficile* colitis goes unrecognized and untreated, complications, including toxic megacolon, perforation, and peritonitis, may develop.

The treatment for children with colitis caused by *C. difficile* depends on the severity of the disease. Mild cases respond to cessation of antibiotics and supportive therapy with fluids and electrolytes. In particular, children seen with a small amount of diarrhea on oral antibiotics for a minor infection, in whom the suspicion of pseudomembranous colitis is low, do not need an extensive diagnostic investigation or institution of specific antimicrobial therapy. Patients with more severe or persistent antibiotic-associated diarrhea should be evaluated for *C. difficile* with a test for toxin in the stool. Oral metronidazole (30 mg per kilogram daily in four divided doses) or vancomycin (40 mg per kilogram daily in four divided doses) are used most commonly.

Gastritis

Gastritis caused by *H. pylori* manifests in older children and adolescents with persistent epigastric pain, nausea, and vomiting. Often, the stool will test positive for blood. More severe cases are characterized by hematemesis. In younger children and infants unable to verbalize or localize pain reliably, irritability may be the primary manifestation. *H. pylori* can be diagnosed by culture of gastric tissue obtained at biopsy, breath testing, and serology. Only serology has applicability in the setting of the ED. Sensitivity of the serologic assay has been reported to range from 70% to 95%, with greater accuracy being observed in older children.

In most cases, the clinician cannot diagnose *H. pylori* infection in the ED with sufficient certainty to warrant the initiation of treatment with antibiotics. Effective two-drug regimens include clarithromycin–omeprazole, amoxicillin–bismuth, and amoxicillin–omeprazole for 2 to 4 weeks. A 1-week course of omeprazole (20 mg twice daily), clarithromycin (250 mg twice daily), and metronidazole (500 mg twice daily) proved effective in a group of 35 children 10 to 19 years of age.

SKIN, SOFT-TISSUE, AND BONE INFECTIONS

Impetigo

Impetigo is more common in young children, particularly those less than 6 years of age. Typically, a parent will bring a child to the ED complaining of sores on the body. No systemic ailments, such as fever or malaise, are associated. Physical examination shows a healthy child with a normal temperature. The lesions usually ooze serous fluid but may be bullous or crusted as well. Erythromycin (40 mg/kg per day in four divided doses) provides effective oral treatment for the usual pathogens. Other acceptable oral drugs include dicloxacillin (50 mg/kg per day) or cephalexin (50 mg per kilogram daily). Mupirocin applied locally is able to eradicate most cases of impetigo, particularly if the disease is limited in distribution. Combination topical and systemic therapy is unnecessary.

Lymphadenitis

Lymph nodes in any region of the body may become infected. Regardless of the site of involvement, the same considerations apply as discussed under cervical lymphadenitis. *S. aureus* and group A streptococcus are the most common pathogens. The finding of inguinal or axillary adenitis should prompt a meticulous search for a portal of entry for bacteria on the extremities. Locating an impetiginous lesion or other breech in the integument provides reassurance that the lymph node enlargement is caused by infection rather than by neoplasm. History should be requested regarding a cat scratch or bite as a possible etiologic focus. Particularly in the adolescent, inguinal adenitis suggests a need to look for sexually transmitted pathogens. Cat-scratch disease (SCD) is another important consideration. The child with lymphadenitis should be treated with antibiotic therapy and drainage, if fluctuation occurs. Dicloxacillin (50 mg per kilogram daily) and cephalexin (50 mg per kilogram daily) are both effective against the usual pathogens.

Cellulitis

CLINICAL MANIFESTATIONS

The child with cellulitis develops a local inflammatory response at the site of infection with erythema, edema, warmth, pain, and limitation of motion. There may be a history of a prior wound or insect bite. Facial infections are more common during the first 5 years of life. Fever is unusual, except in bacteremic infections or when the lesions are extensive. Only 10% to 20% of children with cellulitis manifest a fever. The lesion itself is erythematous and tender but not fluctuant; red streaks may radiate proximally along the course of the lymphatic drainage. The regional lymph nodes usually enlarge in response to the infection.

With cellulitis caused by *S. aureus* or group A streptococcus, the WBC count is normal in most children. More extensive lesions or bacteremia, seen only occasionally, evoke a leukocytosis. A culture obtained from the central area of the cellulitis will yield a pathogen in 50% of cases, but cultures of the blood usually remain sterile.

Bacteremia accompanies cellulitis caused by *H. influenzae* or *S. pneumoniae*; these organisms are isolated from the blood in 90% of infected patients. The WBC count is greater than 15000/m^3 as a rule, usually with a shift to the left.

The complications of cellulitis, although uncommon, include local and metastatic spread of infection. The organisms may invade deeper tissues, producing septic arthritis or osteomyelitis. During the course of bacteremia with *H. influenzae, S. pneumoniae,* or rarely other organisms, there may be involvement of the meninges, pericardium, epiglottis, or synovial membranes. Multifocal areas of cellulitis should arouse a suspicion of hematogenous dissemination. Occasionally, cellulitis provides a clue to an infection that originates in deeper anatomic structures. As an example, a lesion on the abdominal wall, may be a sign of peritonitis.

MANAGEMENT

Most children with nonfacial cellulitis can receive antibiotic therapy as outpatients, as long as bacteremic disease is unlikely

(Fig. 74.4). Because *S. aureus* and group A streptococcus are most commonly isolated, treatment should be directed at these organisms. Acceptable alternatives include a semisynthetic penicillin, such as dicloxacillin (50 mg per kilogram of body weight daily), cephalexin (50 mg per kilogram daily), or amoxicillin–clavulanic acid (50 mg per kilogram daily of amoxicillin); *S. aureus* is generally resistant to penicillin and ampicillin. A CBC, blood culture, and aspirate culture are not necessary in afebrile patients.

If a child with a nonfacial cellulitis has a high fever [39°C (102.2°F) or higher], the likelihood of a bacteremic infection or lymphangitic spread increases. A WBC count and culture of the blood should be obtained, along with consideration of a culture from the lesion. In cases in which the WBC count is below 15000/mm^3, antibiotic therapy is given as described for afebrile children, and the patient is asked to return the following day. A leukocytosis in association with a temperature of 39°C (102.2°F) or higher points toward intravenous treatment, usually on an inpatient basis, with oxacillin (150 mg per kilogram daily in four divided doses) or cephazolin (100 mg per kilogram daily in three divided doses). For children not immunized against Hib, consider therapy with cefotaxime (200 mg per kilogram daily in four divided doses), ceftriaxone (100 mg per kilogram daily in a single dose), or ampicillin–clavulanic acid (200 mg per kilogram daily of ampicillin in four divided doses). Children allergic to penicillins and cephalosporins can be given clindamycin (40 mg per kilogram daily in four divided doses) alone or with chloramphenicol (75–100 mg per kilogram daily in four divided doses) when *H. influenzae* type b is a concern.

Children with facial cellulitis and fever are particularly likely to be bacteremic, in most cases with *S. pneumoniae* or, less commonly, *H. influenzae* type b, and they are at risk for local complications. Thus, these patients should receive intravenous therapy as listed previously. Those who are afebrile may be managed as outpatients if they do not have risk factors for bacteremic disease: age younger than 3 years, spontaneous cellulitis without a preceding wound, and violaceous discoloration (Fig. 74.4).

Fasciitis

As occurs with cellulitis, the child with fasciitis develops a local inflammatory response at the site of infection, characterized by erythema, edema, warmth, pain, and limitation of motion. Often, the swelling is tense and quite tender.

Fever occurs in almost every case, often exceeding 39°C (102.2°F). In contrast to the usual patient with cellulitis, those with fasciitis almost always appear toxic with a marked tachycardia and, occasionally, hypotension. The family often describes the local lesion as progressing rapidly and generally exhibiting noticeable induration and erythema. Particularly in the presence of varicelliform lesions, the physician should maintain a high index of suspicion for fasciitis, as opposed to cellulitis, in

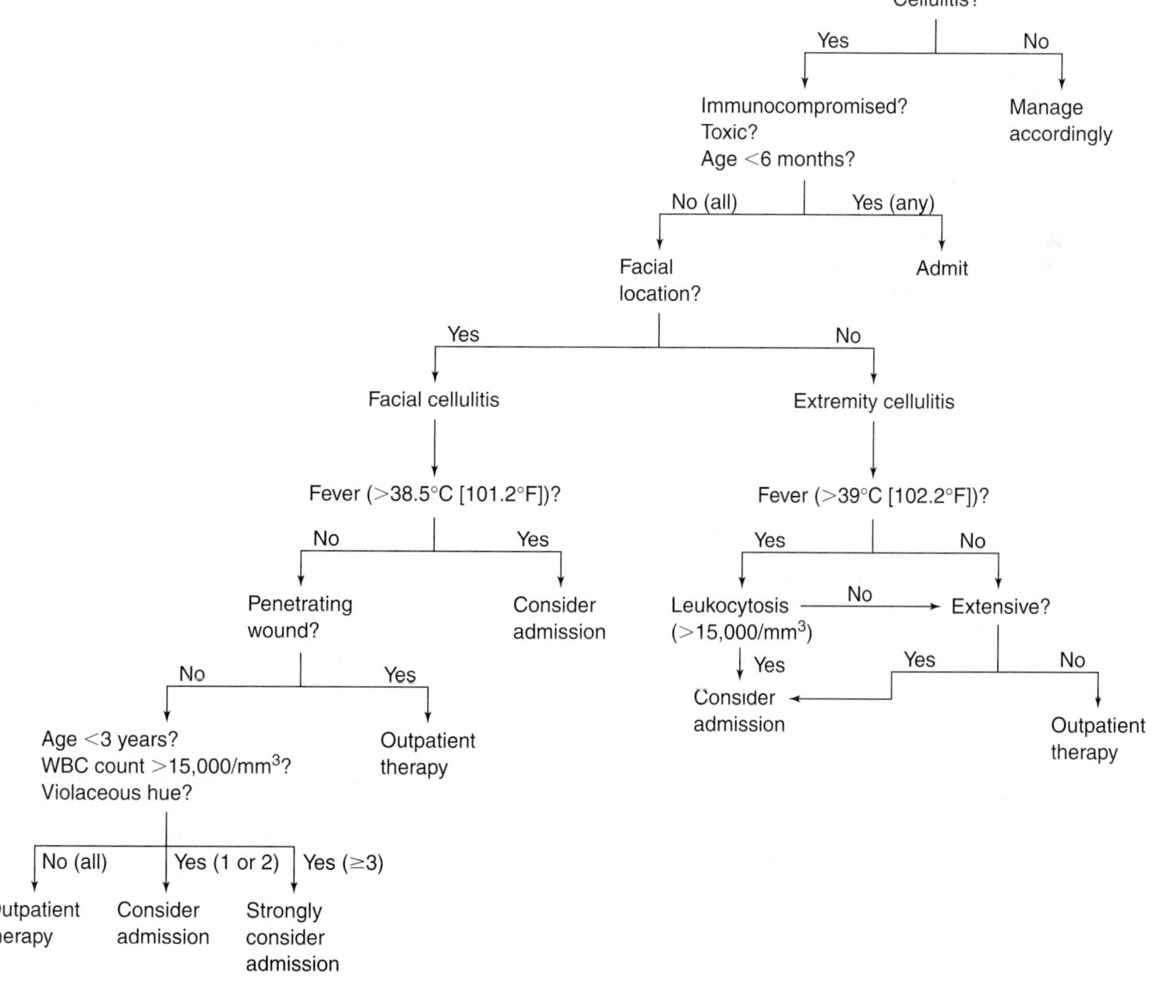

Figure 74.4. Diagnostic approach for the management of the child with soft-tissue swelling and possible cellulitis. WBC, white blood cell.

children with extensive local disease, high fever, and any degree of prostration. The WBC count generally reflects a leukocytosis, and blood cultures yield an organism in most cases.

A confirmed case of necrotizing cellulitis should be considered an emergency. The first priorities include supportive therapy for signs of sepsis and initiation of antibiotics, followed promptly by surgical consultation. Appropriate antimicrobial therapy includes penicillin (500000 U per kilogram daily in four divided doses) and clindamycin (40 mg per kilogram daily in four divided doses administered intravenously). In a large number of cases, the surgical consultant will elect to incise or debride the lesions.

Omphalitis

Omphalitis is characterized first by drainage and later by erythema around the umbilical cord stump. Late in the course of infection, infants manifest the signs of sepsis, including lethargy, irritability, and hypothermia or hyperthermia. Laboratory studies are normal early in the course. Because a small amount of drainage and patchy erythema can occur in the absence of infection, the diagnosis of omphalitis may be difficult. There are no definite clinical criteria for early infections, and laboratory tests are not helpful. The findings suggestive of omphalitis are (1) purulent, foul-smelling drainage from the umbilical cord with any erythema of the anterior abdomen; or (2) any drainage with erythema that completely encircles the umbilicus. Induration and erythema of the anterior abdomen wall are definite indicators of infection.

Infants who appear toxic, have induration and erythema of the abdominal wall, or show signs clearly suggestive of omphalitis (purulence and patchy erythema or light drainage plus circumferential erythema) should be presumed to have a significant infection and require intravenous antibiotic agents. Appropriate therapy is oxacillin (150 mg per kilogram daily in four divided doses) and gentamicin (7.5 mg per kilogram daily in three divided doses for term infants). In some cases, minimal drainage or erythema may be present, but the findings are not sufficient for the diagnosis of omphalitis. The parents of these infants should be instructed to swab the cord after each diaper change and to observe the child for any changes in activity or feeding. Reexamination in 24 hours is advisable if the problem has not resolved.

Neonatal Mastitis

The primary finding in neonatal mastitis is a warm, erythematous, enlarged breast bud. With disease progression, purulent drainage from the nipple may occur, and there is tenderness to palpation. Only 25% of infants are febrile or appear ill. Mastitis in the infant must be distinguished from physiologic hypertrophy, which resolves spontaneously. The normal breast bud that enlarges in response to stimulation by maternal hormones is neither red nor tender; if any drainage is present, the material is milky white, rather than yellow, and does not contain polymorphonuclear leukocytes or bacteria on Gram stain. Culture of the purulent drainage yields the pathogen in most cases, but the blood is usually sterile. Because these infections are well localized, the WBC count is usually in the normal range. Oxacillin (150 mg per kilogram daily in four divided doses) and gentamicin (7.5 mg per kilogram daily in three divided doses) provide appropriate coverage for the expected pathogens. Surgical consultation for possible incision and drainage are advisable in the case of local fluctuance.

Septic Arthritis

CLINICAL FEATURES

Infection within a joint produces pain and limitation of motion. Thus, the site of the arthritis determines the specific complaint. Ninety percent of children have a monoarticular arthritis that involves the lower extremity (hip, knee, and ankle). Thus, limp (see Chapter 36) is the most common initial manifestation. If a joint in the arm is involved, mobility of the upper extremity will be decreased (see Chapter 29). With infections in deeper joints, the pain may radiate to contiguous anatomic structures. Children with a septic hip often complain of an ache at the knee, and sacroiliac arthritis may mimic appendicitis, pelvic neoplasm, or UTI. Although the duration of symptoms in septic arthritis is less than 3 days in more than 50% of children with these conditions, the delay in diagnosis may reach 3 to 4 weeks with sacroiliac arthritis.

The findings are often vague in the first 6 months of life. Pyoarthritis may cause paradoxical irritability and an increase in crying on being fondled, as seen with meningitis. The infant with a septic hip usually lies quietly, holding the leg abducted and externally rotated. Of children with septic arthritis, 60% to 70% have a temperature of 38.5°C (101.2°F) or higher. The absence of fever occurs most commonly in the adolescent with a gonococcal infection or in the neonate. Infants with infections caused by *H. influenzae,* rare since the advent of the conjugated vaccine, almost invariably have a high fever. An erythematous swelling may surround a superficial joint that is infected. Although a temperature difference exists between the affected and unaffected sites, it can be difficult to discern in the febrile child. Inflammation within the joint distends the capsule and produces pain with movement. If a child allows the physician to manipulate an extremity through a full range of motion, septic arthritis is unlikely.

The erythrocyte sedimentation rate and CRP are the most consistently abnormal laboratory study. Molteni observed an elevated ESR in 32 of 37 (86%) children with septic arthritis; the median value was 50 mm. The peripheral WBC count usually varies from less than 5000 to more than 20000/mm^3. Although a leukocytosis with a shift to the left commonly occurs, as many as 20% of children will have a WBC count less than 10000/mm^3. If septic arthritis is diagnosed early, a radiograph of the joint will not show any pathologic changes. The first radiographic alteration to be noted is edema of the adjacent soft tissues, which is not pathognomonic of inflammation in the joint. Later, distension of the capsule becomes visible, and bony destruction may be seen late in the course of the infection.

The thickness of the tissues that surround the hip joint makes the detection of an effusion difficult by physical examination. A radiograph of the hip always should be obtained if infection in this joint is possible. Early in the course, the tendon of the obturator internus is displaced as the muscle passes over the distended hip capsule. Continued accumulation of an inflammatory exudate forces the femoral head laterally and upward, disrupting the arc formed by the femoral head and the pelvis (Shenton's line). The hip may actually dislocate with intraarticular infection in the young infant, but this is an unusual radiographic finding in older children. Ultrasound examination is useful for the detection of a small effusion not apparent on radiograph.

No constellation of laboratory and radiographic results can rule out the diagnosis of septic arthritis; an analysis of the joint fluid is mandatory if the index of suspicion is high. Infection causes an infiltration of polymorphonuclear leukocytes into the joint space. Although intraarticular WBC counts greater than 100000/mm^3 are traditionally associated with infection, a lesser cellular response is often noted. Nelson found a WBC count in the joint fluid below 25000/mm^3 in 9 (34%) of 31 children with proven bacterial arthritis. The joint fluid glucose is reduced to less than 40 mg per deciliter in only 25% to 50% of patients, but the Gram stain of the synovial fluid shows organisms in 75%.

Because inflammatory exudates have bacteriostatic properties, cultures of joint fluid yield an organism in only 60% of cases. A pathogen is recovered from the bloodstream in 40% of children with septic arthritis, more commonly if *H. influenzae* or *S. pneumoniae* is the cause of the disease.

The complications of septic arthritis include both local and distant spread of the infection. Osteomyelitis often accompanies joint infections in the first year of life because of the location of the metaphysis within the joint capsule. During the process of hematogenous dissemination, bacteria may invade sites other than the joint. Simultaneous infections may occur in the meninges, pericardium, or the soft tissues; these are particularly common with *H. influenzae.*

MANAGEMENT

Septic arthritis demands prompt management; in particular, infection in the hip joint should be considered an emergency. The initial treatment is aimed at relieving the pressure within the joint and controlling the infection. At the time of the diagnostic aspiration, as much purulent fluid as possible should be removed. Immediate surgical intervention is needed for hip infections.

If no organisms are apparent on examination of the joint fluid, presumptive antibiotic therapy is begun as follows: (1) infants aged 2 months or younger—oxacillin 150 mg per kilogram daily in four divided doses and gentamicin 7.5 mg per kilogram daily in three divided doses; (2) children aged 2 months to less than three 3 years—cefotaxime 200 mg per kilogram daily in four divided doses, ampicillin–clavulanic acid 200 mg per kilogram daily of ampicillin in four divided doses or, for the penicillin-allergic patient, clindamycin 40 mg per kilogram daily in four divided doses and chloramphenicol 75 to 100 mg per kilogram daily in four divided doses; (3) children aged 3 to 12 years—oxacillin 150 mg per kilogram daily to a maximum of 6 g per day; (4) adolescents—ceftriaxone 100 mg per kilogram daily. Ceftriaxone (100 mg per kilogram once daily) may be used as a single agent for children older than 2 months; as further experience confirms the virtual disappearance of *H. influenzae,* oxacillin (150 mg per kilogram daily in four divided doses) probably will prove sufficient as monotherapy during childhood.

Osteomyelitis

CLINICAL FEATURES

Osteomyelitis causes bone pain as the infection progresses. The site of the osteomyelitis determines the presentation of the disease. In 90% of cases, a single bone is involved. The femur and tibia are the most common bones infected, making limp (see Chapter 36) a common presentation. Osteomyelitis affects the bones of the upper extremity in 25% of cases. These children complain of pain on motion of their upper extremities (see Chapter 29).

The multiplicity of bones that may be involved leads to a wide spectrum of chief complaints. Vertebral osteomyelitis manifests as backache, torticollis, or stiff neck, and involvement of the mandible causes painful mastication. Infection of the pelvis is particularly elusive and may masquerade as appendicitis, neoplasm, or UTI. Infants with osteomyelitis localize the symptoms less well than older children. Initially, irritability may be the only complaint.

Fever exceeds 38.5°C (101.2°F) in 70% to 80% of children with osteomyelitis. The infant with a long bone infection often manifests pseudoparalysis, an unwillingness to move the extremity. Movement may be decreased in the older child, but to a lesser degree. Point tenderness is seen almost always in osteomyelitis; however, it is also found in other conditions such as trauma, may be difficult to discern in the struggling infant, and it does not always occur early in the course of the infection. Percussion of a bone at a point remote from the site of an osteomyelitis may elicit pain in the area of infection.

When purulent material ruptures through the cortex, diffuse local erythema and edema appear. This finding occurs often in infants, but late in the course, and is confined primarily to children in the first 3 years of life (before the cortex thickens sufficiently to contain the inflammatory exudate). Weissburg and colleagues noted swelling of the extremity in 14 of 17 patients than 1 month old who had osteomyelitis.

The ESR or CRP provides a useful screening test for osteomyelitis because bony infection almost always leads to an elevation. Nelson found an ESR less than 15 mm per hour in only 4 of 88 children with osteomyelitis, and the mean value was 70 mm per hour. Although the WBC count may reach a level of 20000/mm^3, it falls within the normal range in two-thirds of cases. Cultures from the blood yield an organism in 50% and from the bone in 70% of children with osteomyelitis.

If osteomyelitis is suspected, radiographs of the affected area always should be obtained, even though they are often normal early in the course. The first change, noted after 3 to 4 days, is deep soft-tissue swelling seen as a subtle shift of the lucent deep-muscle plane away from the bone. Within 3 to 10 days, the muscles swell and obliterate the lucent planes that usually separate them radiographically. Visualization of osseous destruction requires the loss of 40% of the bony matrix in an area at least 1 cm in diameter. This amount of demineralization occurs only after 10 to 12 days of infection. At this stage, lytic lesions and periosteal elevation are apparent on the radiograph.

Radionuclide scanning provides a useful diagnostic tool for the clinician. Uptake of compounds such as technetium is seen at sites of increased metabolic activity, which occurs in an infection before sufficient bony destruction has occurred to be seen on conventional radiographs. If scintigraphy is available, the patient strongly suspected to have osteomyelitis despite a normal radiograph should have this study; however, the absence of increased uptake does not preclude bony infection. Some patients will have decreased uptake because the accumulation of purulent material lessens the flow of blood to the site; occasionally, in children, the scan may be entirely normal early in the course. When scintigraphy is not diagnostic and clinical suspicion persists, magnetic resonance imaging is useful.

MANAGEMENT

All children strongly suspected or known to have osteomyelitis require admission to the hospital for intravenous antibiotic therapy. Those with a low likelihood of bony infection can be reevaluated in 12 to 24 hours and can have a technetium scan at that time if the clinical findings are not definitive. The emergency physician should withhold antibiotics until the orthopedic surgeon has been contacted about culturing the bone at the site of infection. Infants should subsequently receive oxacillin, 150 mg per kilogram daily in four divided doses and gentamicin, 7.5 mg per kilogram daily in three divided doses; older children can be treated with oxacillin alone.

GENITOURINARY INFECTIONS

Urethritis/Cervicitis

CLINICAL MANIFESTATIONS

Urethritis causes dysuria and discharge in the male. Persistent discharge in a young boy or adolescent treated for gonorrhea, in particular, should alert the clinician to infection with *C. trachomatis*. Mucopurulent cervicitis caused by *C. trachomatis* in the adolescent girl is characterized by an erythematous friable cervix and the accumulation of purulent yellow endocervical secretions. Gram stain of the discharge shows more than ten polymorphonuclear leukocytes per microscopic field under 1000 magnification. This organism also causes the "sterile" dysuria–pyuria syndrome; females with this condition complain of dysuria, at times described as originating external to the urethra at the level of the labia, and have pyuria along with a negative urine culture. In prepubertal girls, *C. trachomatis* is a cause of vaginitis, usually with scant or no discharge. An etiologic diagnosis in urethritis–cervicitis relies on the clinical syndrome, Gram stain of any discharge, and specific identification of the organism, either by antigen/detection or culture. In general, culture is preferred for prepubertal children.

MANAGEMENT

If an etiologic diagnosis is not possible based on the clinical findings and the results of Gram stain, treatment should be given for both *N. gonorrhoeae* and *C. trachomatis*. Infections with *C. trachomatis* in adolescents and children older than 8 years are treated with doxycycline (100 mg twice daily) or a single dose of azithromycin (1 g). Children younger than 8 years may be given azithromycin (20 mg per kilogram as a single dose) or erythromycin (40 mg per kilogram daily in four divided doses for 10 days) and should have a "test-of-cure" culture after this course of therapy.

Urinary Tract Infection

CLINICAL MANIFESTATIONS

The manifestations of UTIs vary with age and are particularly nonspecific in infancy. During the neonatal appearance, a septic appearance (see Chapter 60) or fever is often the only finding. UTIs in infants also may cause vomiting, diarrhea, irritability, and reportedly, meningismus. Beyond 2 to 3 years of age, symptoms more often point to the urinary tract. For all practical purposes, strict differentiation between upper and lower tract disease is not feasible for the clinician in most cases, and children who are febrile [38.5°C (101.2°F)] should be assumed to have pyelonephritis. On the other hand, some patients will have typical syndromes that localize disease to the upper or lower tract. Typically, children with cystitis appear relatively well and complain of dysuria and suprapubic pain. On examination, they have a lower-grade fever and tenderness on the suprapubic area. In contrast, patients with pyelonephritis may be toxic and usually have additional symptoms, including vomiting and flank pain. The physician is often able to elicit tenderness to percussion in the costovertebral area, either unilaterally or bilaterally.

The mainstays of diagnosis are the urinalysis and culture of the urine, both of which require the clinician to make an interpretation that is influenced by the method of collection and processing as well as the clinical syndrome exhibited by the patient.

Urine is analyzed directly using both a chemical reagent strip (dipstick) and microscopy, looking most specifically, in regard to infection, for the presence of leukocyte esterase, nitrites, WBCs, and bacteria. Either spun or unspun urine may be studied through the microscope, with or without the aid of a Gram stain. Spinning should be done in accordance with a standardized protocol. When a clean urine specimen is centrifuged at 2000 rpm for 5 minutes and examined under high power (ie, 40), each leukocyte [per high-power field (HPF)] represents 5 to 10 cells/mm^3, with 10 to 50 WBCs/mm^3 (5–10 per HPF) being the upper limit of normal. One organism per HPF seen on Gram stain of a spun specimen correlates with a colony count of 10^5 organisms or more.

In interpreting a urine culture in children, the physician must keep in mind that the guidelines for positivity were developed based on data in adults and that the significance of colony counts applies most explicitly to voided specimens. Given these caveats, it is generally accepted that a colony count of greater than 10^5 on a single sample indicates a probability of infection of 80%, increasing to 90% when repeated once and 95% when done a third time. Colony counts between 10^4 and 10^5 of single organisms are somewhat suggestive of infection and merit another culture. On a catheterized specimen, a result of $\geq 10^4$ organisms points to infection. The criterion for a suprapubic aspirate is greater than 10^3.

In general, a single negative finding on one parameter of the urinalysis does not exclude a UTI. Taken together, however, negative testing for both leukocyte esterase and nitrates by dipstick alone, or even more so in combination with a microscopic examination that shows the absence of pyuria, makes the diagnosis of a UTI (as opposed to asymptomatic bacteriuria) in a male infant older than 6 months of age or a female older than 2 years, highly unlikely. A schema for the use of urinalysis and urine culture is presented in Figure 74.5. As illustrated for older children who are somewhat older but not yet toilet-trained, in the absence of a high likelihood of UTI a priori, the urinalysis may be collected using a bag. If the urinalysis is positive, however, a specimen for culture should preferably be obtained by catheterization or suprapubic aspiration.

Bacteremia accompanies UTIs primarily during the first 6 to 12 months of life. In the young infant, bacteremia may be present in the absence of fever and should be suspected in any children during the first year of life with a temperature 39°C (102.2°F) or higher. Indications for a CBC and blood culture with a suspected UTI include (1) signs of clinical toxicity (extreme tachycardia, low blood pressure, shaking chills); (2) age younger than 3 months; and (3) age 3 months to 1 year and temperature greater than 39°C (102.2?°F). Only children with dehydration require measurement of electrolytes. When a diagnosis of pyelonephritis, as opposed to cystitis, is being entertained, consideration should be given to ascertaining the BUN and creatinine in the serum.

MANAGEMENT

When the diagnosis of UTI has been established as a result of earlier urine culture or is presumed, based on the clinical syndrome and findings on urinalysis, antibiotic therapy is indicated. If available, the results of susceptibility testing should guide the selection of antimicrobial agent. In all other cases, an antibiotic is chosen to cover the most likely pathogens.

Most patients respond to oral antibiotic therapy. Indications for intravenous administration of antibiotics include (1) clinical toxicity; (2) age younger than 3 to 6 months; (3) vomiting, refusal to drink, or other factors making the delivery of oral medications unreliable; (4) adverse anatomic factors, such as an obstruction to urinary flow; and (5) a known positive culture for a pathogen resistant to oral agents.

For ill-appearing patients, intravenous ampicillin (200 mg per kilogram daily in four divided doses) plus gentamicin (7.5 mg per kilogram daily in three divided doses, adjusted for gestation age and weight; see Table 74.2) are given. Options for oral therapy include TMP-SMZ (8 mg per kilogram daily of TMP in two divided doses) or cefixime (8 mg per kilogram daily as a single dose). If the pathogen is susceptible to ampicillin, amoxicillin provides effective oral coverage.

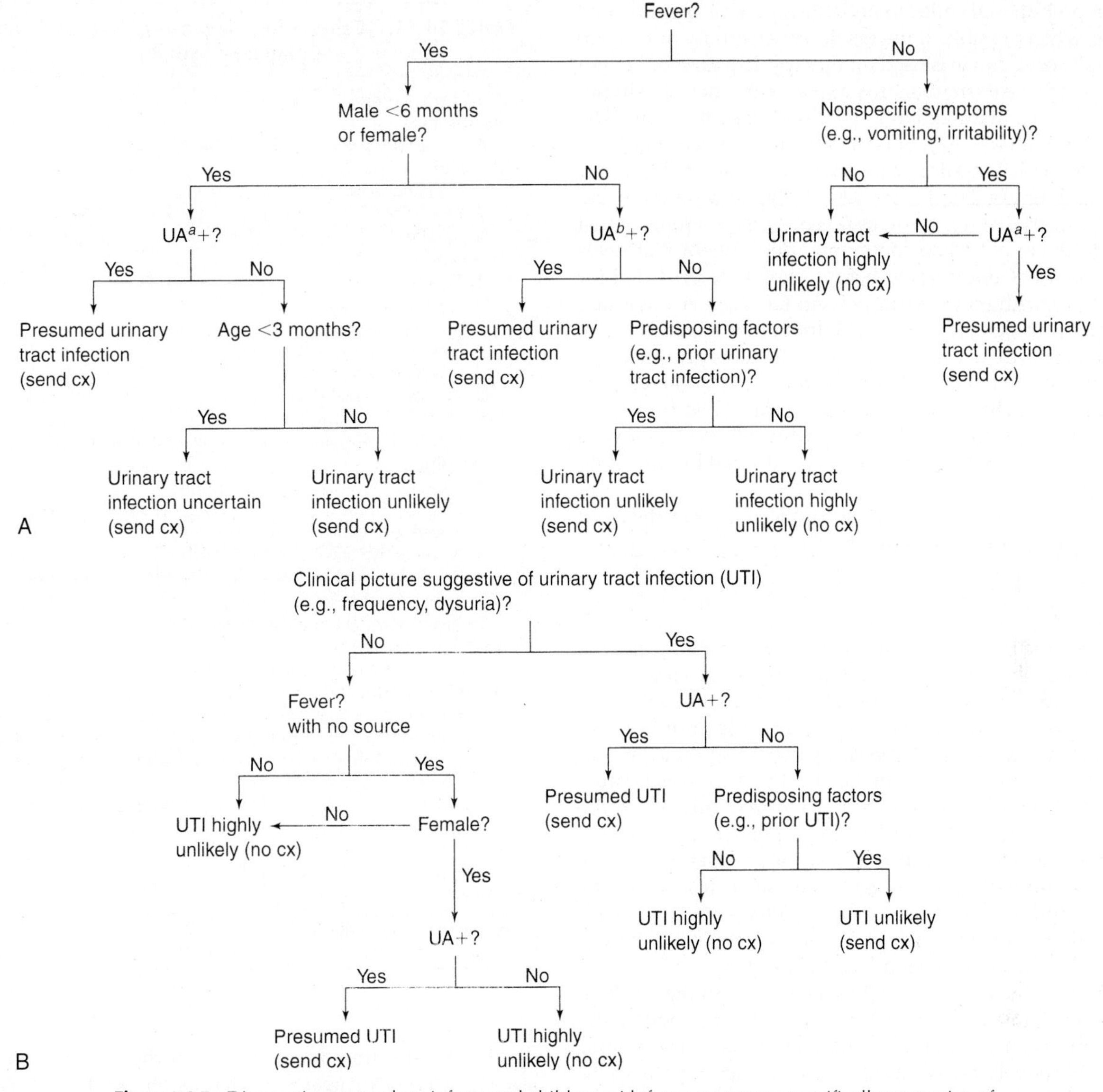

Figure 74.5. Diagnostic approach to infants and children with fever, symptoms specifically suggestive of urinary tract infection (UTI) or nonspecific symptoms and signs compatible with urinary tract infection. Use of urinalysis and culture in the diagnosis of UTI **(A)** in children aged 2 years or younger and **(B)** in those older than 2 years.[a] Urinary analysis (UA) obtained by catheterization or suprapubic aspiration.[b]UA (only) may be obtained using a urine collection bag.

SPECIFIC INFECTIONS

Gonorrhea

CLINICAL MANIFESTATIONS

The most common form of infection with *N. gonorrhoeae* seen among children is infection of the genitals. Prepubertal girls develop a vaginitis, rather than a cervicitis as seen in adult women, because of differences in the vaginal mucosa. Vaginal irritation, dysuria, and a discharge are the most common complaints. Boys have a urethral discharge and occasionally swelling of the penile shaft or urinary retention. Fever, systemic signs and symptoms, and spread to the pelvic organs in females occur rarely.

A Gram stain will show gram-negative intracellular diplococci in most children with gonorrhea. Cultures allow definitive identification of the organism, a crucial issue from the medicolegal standpoint. Pharyngeal and rectal cultures are positive in 5% to 10% of cases in which the organism is not isolated from the genital tract.

Despite the widespread use of prophylactic solutions in the eyes of newborns, gonococcal conjunctivitis continues to appear sporadically. A thick, purulent discharge quickly replaces the initial mild erythema from chemical irritation. Gram stain of the exudate usually shows the organism, and cultures are almost always positive.

Disseminated gonorrhea and pelvic inflammatory disease emerge as problems in the sexually active adult. A complete discussion of these entities is found in Chapter 83.

MANAGEMENT

All children with suspected genital gonorrhea should have cultures of the genitals, pharynx, and rectum, as well as serologic tests for syphilis and human immunodeficiency virus (HIV). Because of the medicolegal considerations, treatment should be delayed in prepubertal children until the diagnosis is confirmed by culture, when possible. If the results of sensitivity testing are not available, ceftriaxone is used for therapy, in a dose of 125 mg intramuscularly. Alternatives for adolescents include single-dose oral therapy with cefixime (400 mg), ciprofloxacin (500 mg), or ofloxacin (400 mg). Spectinomycin is an acceptable alternative for penicillin-allergic patients in a dose of 40 mg per kilogram (maximum 2.0 g) intramuscularly. Because the usual mode of acquisition often involves sexual contact, a report must be made to the appropriate community department that deals with child abuse. Concomitant therapy should be provided for *C. trachomatis,* with either azithromycin (20 mg per kilogram, maximum 1 g) or doxycycline (in children older than 8 years).

In infants less than 1 month of age with conjunctivitis, particularly when purulent, consideration should be given to a Gram stain and culture of the ocular exudate. The finding of gram-negative diplococci on the smear warrants treatment with ceftriaxone (50 mg per kilogram as a single dose) while awaiting culture results.

Therapy for adolescents with uncomplicated gonorrhea and salpingitis is discussed in Chapter 83.

Syphilis

Syphilis is an infection caused by *Treponema pallidum.* Congenital syphilis usually presents with the same clinical picture as other intrauterine infections (rubella and cytomegalovirus). Characteristic features include jaundice and hepatosplenomegaly in an ill-appearing newborn. Some infants, however, have only a few stigmata, and the diagnosis is often overlooked in the nursery. These children may turn up in the first months of life with skin lesions, a persistent nasal discharge, and painful extremities (pseudoparalysis of Parrot). Dark-field examination of cutaneous lesions can identify the spirochetes, and the serologic test for syphilis is positive. In addition, radiographs may show lesions of the long bones. Diagnostic criteria are provided in Table 74.11.

TABLE 74.11. Criteria for Diagnosis of Neonatal and Early Congenital Syphilis

I. Diagnostic Criteria
- A. Absolute
  1. *T. pallidium* seen by dark-field microscopy
- B. Major
  1. Condylomata
  2. Osteochondritis, perichondritis
  3. Snuffles
- C. Minor
  1. Fissures of lips
  2. Cutaneous lesions
  3. Mucous patches
  4. Hepatomegaly, splenomegaly
  5. Lymphadenopathy
  6. Central nervous system signs
  7. Hemolytic anemia
  8. Elevated cell count or protein level in spinal fluid
- D. Serologic
  1. Reactive serologic test for syphilis
  2. Reactive immunoglobulin M (IgM) (FTA-ABS) fluorescent treponemal antibody absorption test
  3. Nonreactive serologic test for syphilis
  4. Reactive serologic test for syphilis STS that does not revert to non-reactive within 4 mo
  5. Rising serologic test for syphilis titer over 3 mo

II. Certainty of diagnosis
- A. Definite: Absolute clinical criterion
- B. Probable: Any of the following: (1) Serologic criterion 4 or 5; (2) one major or two or more minor clinical criteria and serologic criterion 1 or 2; (3) one major and one minor clinical criterion
- C. Possible: Serologic criterion 1 or 2 with only one minor or no clinical criterion
- D. Unlikely: (1) Serologic criterion 3; (2) maternal history of adequate treatment for syphilis during pregnancy

FTA-ABS, fluorescent treponemal antibody absorption test; STS, serologic test for syphilis.
Modified from Mascola L, et al. Congenital syphilis revisited. *Am J Dis Child* 1985;139:575, with permission.

Acquired syphilis appears in the teenager, as in the adult, in the first stage with a chancre and in the second stage with cutaneous or mucosal manifestations. The rash of secondary syphilis may resemble pityriasis rosea, and all sexually active patients diagnosed with this disease, particularly with involvement of the palms or soles, should have a serologic test for syphilis. Other lesions include white patches on the mucous membranes and flat-topped warts (condyloma lata) around moist areas. Such lesions shed spirochetes detectable by dark-field microscopy.

Congenital syphilis rarely is diagnosed in the ED, and the delay involved in confirmation moves the treatment out of the realm of the emergency physician. All such children require admission to the hospital. In acquired disease, benzathine penicillin (2.4 million units) is given intramuscularly in a single dose for early syphilis and in three doses, each separated by 1 week, for syphilis of more than 1 year's duration.

Herpes Genitalis

Herpes simplex can infect the genitals as well as other anatomic sites. Although the most common cause of genital ulceration seen among adolescents and adults at venereal disease clinics, this entity is unusual in prepubertal children. Genital pain is a common complaint with infections caused by herpes simplex and may precede the appearance of the lesions. Characteristically, the virus produces grouped vesicles on an erythematous base; however, erosion of the overlying skin often leaves only painful ulcers at the time of the first visit. Particularly with a primary infection, the inguinal lymph nodes enlarge.

Visual inspection often suffices for the diagnosis in the adolescent. A Tzanck smear (see Chapter 88) positive for giant cells lends further weight to the clinical impression; either immunofluorescent staining of a scraping from the base of a vesicle or a viral culture can verify the diagnosis. In children, a culture always should be obtained because the disease is rarely seen and needs medicolegal confirmation. Serologic tests for syphilis and HIV and bacterial cultures are appropriate to rule out coexisting sexually transmitted infections. Although it is occasionally spread by nonsexual contact, the physician must explore the possibility of sexual abuse when herpes genitalis occurs before puberty. Oral acyclovir therapy is indicated for primary infections; the dosage is 45 to 60 mg per kilogram daily in three divided doses.

SYSTEMIC VIRAL INFECTIONS

Viral Syndrome

The term *nonspecific viral syndrome* is used to refer to a generalized illness presumed clinically to be caused by a virus and characterized by malaise and, usually, fever. Numerous agents, including influenza, enteroviruses, and herpesvirus (roseola), have been implicated. Nonspecific viral syndromes and viral URIs account for most of the febrile visits made by children to the ED.

A viral syndrome begins with malaise and usually with fever

as well. The temperature varies from 37°C (98.6°F) to more than 40°C (104°F); greater elevations occur at times in children less than 2 years old. Particularly with influenza, children who are able to verbalize their discomfort complain of diffuse aching. There may be a cough or occasional bout of emesis. Signs of mild inflammation may be seen in the upper respiratory tract.

The physician arrives at a diagnosis of a nonspecific viral syndrome by excluding other diseases on the basis of the history and physical examination. At times, a WBC count may help the physician determine whether the young child with a high fever is at risk for occult bacteremia. Treatment is limited to antipyresis with acetaminophen (15 mg per kilogram dose) or ibuprofen (10 mg per kilogram per dose) for patients who do not respond to acetaminophen and the maintenance of an adequate oral intake. Antibiotics will not prevent secondary bacterial infections and are not to be prescribed routinely. The parents must be instructed to seek further care if the fever persists for more than 48 hours.

Erythema Infectiosum (Fifth Disease)

Erythema infectiosum, or fifth disease, is an exanthematous illness of childhood caused by parvovirus B19. It occurs most commonly between 2 and 12 years of age. The appearance of a rash marks the onset of the disease; fever or other prodromal symptoms are uncommon. The rash involves the face initially, conferring on the child a "slapped-cheek" appearance. Maculopapular lesions erupt 24 hours later, initially on the upper portion of the extremities, and they then spread both proximally and distally. Fading of the central portion of the lesions gives a lacelike appearance to the rash. Adolescents in particular may develop arthralgia or arthritis, and patients with chronic hemolytic anemias, such as sickle cell disease, are at risk for aplastic crisis. During pregnancy, infection with parvovirus B19 causes fetal hydrops in about 10% of cases. There is no specific therapy in the normal host, but immunocompromised patients may benefit from intravenous gamma globulin.

Infectious Mononucleosis

CLINICAL MANIFESTATIONS

Infectious mononucleosis (IM) begins insidiously with fever and malaise. Three-fourths of children with this illness complain of a sore throat. Although a child may recover from IM in 7 to 10 days, the symptoms usually last for 2 to 4 weeks. Occasionally, the onset resembles that of infectious hepatitis. The child with IM is febrile in 90% of cases at presentation. Enlarged lymph nodes are uniformly palpable; EBV characteristically affects the posterior cervical and submental glands as well as the anterior cervical chain. In 75% of cases, the pharynx is inflamed, often with an exudate. The spleen enlarges in 60% of children, the liver in 25%. Periorbital edema and a diffuse maculopapular rash are seen occasionally.

Although the total WBC count does not often increase much beyond 15000/mm^3, levels up to 30000/mm^3 are seen in 10% to 15% of children. There is an absolute lymphocytosis with many atypical mononuclear cells; however, 16% of children presenting with IM in one series had fewer than 10% atypical lymphocytes. The mainstay for the diagnosis of IM in the adult is the heterophil antibody test, but these antibodies reach levels detectable by routine assays in only 50% of children. Confirmation of a heterophil-negative case of IM requires EBV-specific serologic assays. The AST and ALT levels are elevated in most children.

The most worrisome complications of IM for the emergency physician are splenic rupture and airway obstruction. Even minor trauma can cause a rent in the capsule of the enlarged spleen seen in IM; these children manifest the usual signs of intraperitoneal hemorrhage.

MANAGEMENT

Usually, a WBC count and a heterophil antibody titer suffice for confirmation of the clinical diagnosis. EBV-specific antibodies are indicated only for heterophil-negative cases. Specific therapy is not available. Adequate rest and nutrition should be maintained, and antipyretic agents will increase the child's comfort. The treatment of a child with uncomplicated IM does not require the administration of corticosteroids, but the duration of the illness can be shortened and the patient made more comfortable by judicious use of a short course.

Corticosteroids almost always shrink dramatically the enlarged tonsils of the child with airway obstruction. Prednisone is given at 2 mg per kilogram of body weight for the first day and tapered over 5 days.

Measles

Measles begins with fever, cough, coryza, and conjunctivitis, followed by Koplik spots on the buccal mucosa and a morbilliform rash. The clues gathered from the history and physical examination suffice for the diagnosis of measles by the experienced clinician; however, serologic studies are required. Measles runs a self-limited course. Bed rest and antipyretic therapy help keep the child comfortable. Antitussives, antihistamines, and topical ophthalmic preparations have no role. Prophylaxis against secondary bacterial infections with antibiotics is not warranted. Children with uncomplicated measles or superficial secondary infections such as otitis and cervical adenitis can be treated as outpatients. Hospitalization is required when significantly severe laryngotracheobronchitis is evident, as discussed earlier in this chapter. Lower respiratory tract or CNS involvement necessitates admission to the hospital.

Measles is a preventable disease. Otherwise healthy, susceptible contacts should receive immune serum globulin, 0.25 mL per kilogram of body weight; the dose is increased to 0.5 mL per kilogram for immunocompromised patients. Within 72 hours of infection, vaccine is indicated in addition, unless the patient is younger than 6 months or is immunocompromised.

Roseola

Roseola infantum, or exanthem subitum, is a common, self-limiting, viral infection of infants caused in most cases by human herpesvirus-6; recently, reports indicate that human herpes virus, which occurs less often, produces a similar syndrome in slightly older children. The child, usually under the age of 3 years, presents with a high fever, ranging up to 40.5°C (104.9°F), and a paucity of physical findings. There may be mild irritability but no coryza, pharyngeal infection, or conjunctivitis. After 2 to 4 days of illness, the fever drops precipitously and a rash appears. The lesions are discrete, pink maculopapules, 2 to 3 mm in diameter. They fade with pressure and do not coalesce. The exanthem appears on the trunk initially and spreads outward. Roseola resolves without complications other than an occasional febrile convulsion. The diagnosis of roseola is made on the basis of the clinical course, often in retrospect. If a WBC count is obtained, leukopenia with lymphocytosis will be seen. Treatment is limited to antipyretic agents.

Varicella/Zoster

CLINICAL FINDINGS

Varicella

A mild prodrome that lasts 1 to 3 days often precedes the exanthem of varicella; however, the first sign of illness may be the rash. Most children develop fever, usually less than 39.5°C (103.1°F) and may complain of malaise. The fever usually subsides within 24 hours of the appearance of the skin lesions. Recurrence of significant fever should serve as a warning sign for suspicion of complications. Lesions erupt initially on the upper trunk, neck, or face and spread centripetally. Pruritus is universal.

The abnormal findings on physical examination are limited to the elevated temperature and lesions of the skin and mucous membranes. Initially, the exanthem consists of erythematous papules that evolve into vesicles and then pustules over 6 to 8 hours. The early vesicles have a diameter of 2 to 4 mm and a "dewdrop-like" appearance. Because new lesions erupt in crops for 2 to 4 days, papules, vesicles, and pustules are usually seen together. An exanthem involves the mucosa of the oropharynx and occasionally the vagina. The severity of the cutaneous manifestations varies widely, and there may be from 1 to more than 1000 lesions. There are few laboratory derangements in varicella. The WBC count occasionally shows a leukocytosis, and the AST and ALT may be mildly elevated. In adolescents, the chest radiograph reveals an interstitial infiltrate in 5% to 10% of patients, even though there may be no respiratory symptoms.

Varicella runs a self-limited course in most cases but is occasionally a more serious illness. Complications include encephalitis, pneumonia, hepatitis, bacterial superinfection, and rarely except with aspirin administration, Reye syndrome. Simultaneous streptococcal pharyngitis can occur.

Encephalitis takes two forms: (1) a diffuse cerebritis with coma and seizures and (2) a cerebellitis with ataxia. Both varieties may occur before, during, or after the cutaneous eruption. Because bacterial meningitis also can complicate varicella, an analysis of the CSF should be done even if viral encephalitis is suspected. There will often be a mild pleocytosis (10–300 cells) and a slight elevation of the protein (40–80 mg per deciliter). If the encephalopathy is thought to be related to Reye syndrome, serum ammonia should be measured.

Starting in approximately 1990, a number of investigators reported an increasing incidence of group A streptococcal complications with varicella, including primarily sepsis and necrotizing fasciitis. The diagnosis of streptococcal sepsis should be considered for patients who appear toxic, remain febrile for 5 days or more, or develop a fever after being afebrile for more than 48 hours.

ZOSTER

Zoster appears suddenly in most children without any warning symptoms (pain or pruritus). The lesions are grouped vesicles on an erythematous base in a dermatomal distribution. In 15% to 20% of cases, extradermatomal cutaneous dissemination is seen. Spread to the viscera does not occur in the immunocompetent child, however. If the eruption follows the ophthalmic branch of the trigeminal nerve, the cornea may be involved. The appearance of vesicles on the tip of the nose should evoke a suspicion of ocular involvement that can be best seen after fluorescein staining of the eye.

MANAGEMENT

Visual inspection suffices for the diagnosis of varicella; no laboratory studies are indicated. Acetaminophen is given to control the fever, and antihistaminic drugs provide some relief from the pruritus. Aspirin is contraindicated because of an association with Reye syndrome. Although some investigators have speculated about a relationship between the use of ibuprofen and the development of fasciitis, this remains unproved. Diphenhydramine (5 mg per kilogram daily), hydroxyzine (2 mg per kilogram daily), or other antihistamines may be used to decrease pruritus. The child cannot attend school for 1 week after the eruption of the first lesion.

Immunosuppressed children with varicella require hospitalization to receive intravenous acyclovir, which has been shown to prevent visceral dissemination; recent reports on the use of high-dose oral acyclovir in children with mild immunosuppression await further confirmation before this approach can be routinely recommended. Complications that mandate admission to the hospital for immunocompetent patients include fasciitis, Reye syndrome, pneumonia, and encephalitis, except in the mildest cases. Superficial bacterial infections such as impetigo, cellulitis (if fasciitis is thought to be unlikely), and adenitis can be treated with oral antibiotic therapy such as dicloxacillin 50 mg per kilogram daily, cephalexin 50 mg per kilogram daily, or erythromycin 40 mg per kilogram daily. Children with deeper bacterial infections (ie, septic arthritis) should receive intravenous antibiotics.

For immunocompetent children, oral acyclovir (80 mg per kilogram daily in four divided doses) given within 24 hours of the onset of the rash reduces the duration of fever and the number and duration of skin lesions. Indications for use have not been formalized, but consideration is warranted for patients who are at some risk for a particularly severe course: infants younger than 6 months, adolescents (older than 12 years), children receiving long-term aspirin therapy or being treated with oral or inhaled steroids, patients with chronic cutaneous (eg, atopic dermatitis) or pulmonary (eg, cystic fibrosis) disorders, and those with fever above 40°C (104°F), and those in whom a large number of lesions are noted as early as the first day of the eruption (particularly if case follows a household contact). Oral acyclovir should be considered for the pregnant adolescent, but its use remains controversial in this situation.

Zoster usually requires no specific therapy. Although famciclovir and valacyclovir are recommended for adults, they have not been shown to be efficacious in children. Antipruritic and antipyretic agents provide symptomatic relief. Immunocompromised children should be admitted to the hospital. Intravenous acyclovir therapy benefits immunocompetent children with unusually severe disease and reduces the incidence of dissemination in immunocompromised patients. Ocular involvement merits consultation with an ophthalmologist.

Anyone likely to experience a severe episode of varicella should receive prophylaxis after a significant exposure to a patient contagious for varicella–zoster virus (household or close contact for more than 1 hour in a closed environment). Varicella-zoster immunoglobulin (VZIG), 1 vial (125 U) per 10 kg, is indicated for susceptible normal adults, pregnant women, and immunocompromised children. Newborns whose mothers have had onset of varicella within 5 days before or 2 days after delivery should receive 125 U as soon as possible.

MISCELLANEOUS INFECTIONS

Botulism

CLINICAL MANIFESTATIONS

Botulism from the ingestion of toxin causes vomiting in 50% of cases. The patients complain of weakness and a dry mouth; constipation and urinary retention may occur. Paralysis is noted within 3 days, usually affecting the cranial nerves first and then the extremities. Patients are alert and afebrile. Abnormalities of the neurologic examination include ptosis, extraocular palsies, fixed dilated pupils, symmetric weakness, and hyporeflexia. Both the ileus and urinary retention seen in this disease may lead to abdominal distension.

Infantile botulism occurs in children in the first 6 months of life who are otherwise healthy. The duration of symptoms before hospitalization ranges from 1 to 20 days. Breast-fed, white infants from middle-class families are primarily affected. Constipation is the first symptom of the disease but may not be sufficiently severe to draw attention to any underlying illness. After several days, mild lethargy, weakness, and a decreased appetite are noted. Occasionally, the onset of lethargy and weakness may be so precipitous as to resemble bacterial sepsis or meningitis.

On examination, the infant is quiet, with little discernible movement, and has a weak cry. Fever is not a part of this syndrome. The child sucks on a nipple with difficulty and may be unable to swallow. The absence of a gag reflex, profound hypotonia, and hyporeflexia in infantile botulism helps distinguish this illness from bacterial sepsis.

The WBC count is normal in botulism. Organisms may be recovered by anaerobic culture techniques from the gastrointestinal tract in infantile or wound botulism, but identification of the toxins requires the specialized facilities of the public health department. Children with botulism have an electromyogram that shows a characteristic pattern of brief duration, small amplitude, overly abundant motor unit action potentials.

Respiratory failure is a potential life-threatening complication in botulism of any variety, and ventilatory support is often required. The profound bulbar weakness in infantile botulism often prevents an adequate fluid intake; dehydration occurs frequently.

MANAGEMENT

Because no test is immediately available to diagnose infantile botulism, the initial evaluation of these infants aims at excluding other causes of lethargy and weakness, such as sepsis, poliomyelitis, myasthenia gravis, neuropathy, and drug ingestion. A lumbar puncture is often performed in the ED to rule out meningitis, and electrolytes and a BUN are useful to assess hydration.

These children all require admission to the hospital (Table 74.12). Monitoring of pulse and respiratory rate should start in the ED. An intravenous line should be started for the administration of fluids to correct dehydration and in anticipation of a possible respiratory arrest. Neither antibiotics nor antitoxin can ameliorate the course of infantile botulism. Because they may potentiate the neuromuscular blockade, aminoglycoside antibiotics should be avoided when treating for possible sepsis.

Children with foodborne and wound botulism also require admission to the hospital. Antitoxin is available from the Centers for Disease Control and Prevention (CDC) and should be administered after consultation with the staff at this agency.

Cat-scratch Disease

This infection is caused by *Bartonella henselae*. Approximately 80% of cases occur in patients younger than 20 years. Traditionally, this disorder has been thought of primarily as an infection of regional lymph nodes (typical CSD), but the spectrum of the disease has been expanded to include infections of other organ systems by *B. henselae* (atypical CSD). In addition, this same agent causes severe infections (bacillary angiomatosis and peliosis hepatis) in patients with HIV (see Chapter 75).

More than 90% of children with typical CSD have a history of exposure to cats. The most complete form of the illness begins with the appearance of a pustule at the site contact, 7 to 10 days after exposure. Lymphadenopathy follows within 1 to 6 weeks. The regional nodes enlarge and become mildly to moderately tender on palpation. In one-third of cases, the glands become fluctuant. The epitrochlear, axillary, inguinal, and cervical nodes are commonly affected.

In typical cases with a history of exposure, particularly to a kitten, and characteristic lymph node enlargement, no specific diagnostic studies are needed. In atypical disease or with lymphadenopathy that is not characteristic, serum should be sent to a reference laboratory for an indirect fluorescent antibody test. Various antibiotics have been reported to have some efficacy for CSD, including rifampin, TMP-SMZ, ciprofloxacin, and azithromycin. The only controlled study of patients with typical CSD found that azithromycin (10 mg per kilogram in a single dose on day 1, followed by 5 mg per kilogram once daily on days 2–5) shortened the duration of adenopathy. Nodes that persist and become fluctuant usually resolve after needle aspiration.

TABLE 74.12. Infantile Botulism: Immediate Management

Ensure adequate ventilation	Achieve venous access and maintain hydration
Administer oxygen, as indicated	Obtain laboratory studies
Initiate cardiorespiratory monitoring	

PARASITIC INFESTATIONS OF THE GASTROINTESTINAL TRACT

Table 74.13 summarizes the clinical symptoms and treatment of gastrointestinal parasites in children.

Rabies

The decision of whether to give prophylaxis for rabies is influenced by the species of animal, the condition of the animal, the ability to study the animal, the type of exposure, and the prevalence of rabies in the region (Fig. 74.6). The incidence of rabies in the area should be available from the local health department. If a sleeping or preverbal child has had close exposure to a bat in an area where rabies is endemic in this species, prophylaxis is indicated even in the absence of a visible bite wound because of the occurrence of several pediatric cases in this circumstance. When the physician determines that prophylaxis is necessary, human rabies immune globulin (HRIG) 20 IU per kilogram of body weight and human diploid cell vaccine (HDCV) are used. After cleaning the wound, half the HRIG is given locally and the remainder at a distant site. Vaccine must be given in the deltoid muscle (not the thigh or buttock) in a different extremity then that used for the HRIG.

Rocky Mountain Spotted Fever

CLINICAL MANIFESTATIONS

The incubation period of Rocky Mountain spotted fever (RMSF) ranges from 2 to 10 days but usually lasts 1 week. The initial symptoms of headache and malaise are followed by fever. The rash erupts on the third or fourth day of illness. In more than half the cases reviewed by Vianna and associates, the exanthem appeared first on the wrists and ankles and then spread inward toward the trunk. The initial lesions are maculopapular but become hemorrhagic in the ensuing 24 to 48 hours if the disease remains unchecked.

The findings on examination vary with the duration of the disease. Early in the course of the illness, the child remains alert. Conjunctivitis and a rash may be the only signs. Edema begins in the periorbital regions and involves the extremities as the vasculitis progresses. Mild splenomegaly is found in one-third of cases.

TABLE 74.13. Parasitic Diseases

Parasite	Disease	Clinical manifestations	Treatment (uncomplicated disease)
Ancyclostoma braziliense	Cutaneous larval migrans	Serpiginous rash	Thiabendazole topically or 50 mg/kg/day in 2 divided doses
Ascaris lumbricoides	Ascariasis	Abdominal pain, passage of large (20 cm) worm	Mabendazole 100 mg twice daily for 3 days
Balantidium coli	Balantidiasis	Abdominal pain, vomiting, bloody diarrhea	Metronidazole 35–50 mg/kg/day in 3 divided doses
Cryptosporidium parvum	Cryptosporidiosis	Diarrhea	No proven therapy
Entamoeba histolytica	Amebiasis	Abdominal pain, bloody diarrhea, extraintestinal abscesses	Metronidazole 35–50 mg/kg/day in 3 divided doses
Enterobius vermicularis	Enterobiasis (pinworms)	Perianal pruritus Observation of small (1 cm) worm	Mebendazole 100 mg once; repeat in 2 wk
Giardia lamblia	Giardiasis	Diarrhea, malabsorption, abdominal pain	Furazolidone 8 mg/kg/day in 4 divided doses or metronidazole 15 mg/kg/day in 3 divided doses
Necator amercanus	Hookworm	Initial pedal rash, then diarrhea and eosinophilia, later anemia	Mebendazole 100 mg twice daily for 3 days
Taenia saginatum/solium	Taeniasis (adult)/cystericosis (larvae)	Diarrhea, tapeworm segment in stool, seizures (cystercicosis)	Taeniasis: praziquantel 10 mg/kg once Cystercicosis: praziquantel 50 mg/kg/day in 3 divided doses
Toxocara canis	Visceral larval migrans	Hepatosplenomegaly	Thiabendazole 50 mg/kg/day in 2 divided doses
Trichinella spiralis	Trichinosis	Abdominal pain, vomiting, myalgias, periorbital edema, eosinophilia	Mebendazole 300 mg 3 times daily

Vomiting is common. Although the sensorium is clear initially, obtundation and, finally, coma develop after several days of illness.

The WBC count remains normal or rises slightly with RMSF. Thrombocytopenia occurs in 75% of patients during the first stages of the disease; later, DIC may develop with a prolonged PT and PTT, as well as elevated fibrin split products. Most patients have hyponatremia but no other electrolyte abnormalities. Bradford and Hawkins noted a decrease in the serum sodium among 88% of children. Immunofluorescent staining has been used to identify rickettsiae in the endothelial cells of dermal vessels from skin biopsies but is not routinely available for diagnosis. Even when myocarditis remains clinically silent, the electrocardiogram may show signs of cardiac dysfunction. The earliest changes consist of an elevation of the ST segment; later, the P-R interval may become prolonged and arrhythmias may occur. In some cases, mild increases in the CSF cell count and protein concentration are seen.

MANAGEMENT

A CBC, platelet count, electrolytes, PT, PTT, and serologic titers should be obtained on the child with suspected RMSF. These studies help pin down the diagnosis and influence the management. Because no routinely available test confirms the diagnosis of RMSF early in its course, treatment must be initiated presumptively. The mildly ill child with a fever, maculopapular exanthem, and a history of a tick bite can be treated as an outpatient. Chloramphenicol (50 mg per kilogram of body weight daily) is the drug of choice for patients less than 8 years of age and tetracycline (50 mg per kilogram daily) in older youths.

Admission is indicated when there is (1) clinical evidence of toxicity, (2) encephalitis, (3) thrombocytopenia (platelet count $<150000/mm^3$) or derangements in the clotting studies, and (4) hyponatremia (Na less than 130 mEq per liter). In the ED, an intravenous infusion should be started and sufficient fluids administered to maintain an adequate blood pressure as discussed under "Septic Shock" (see Chapter 3). Chloramphenicol (50 mg per kilogram daily) can be given alone if the illness is clearly felt to be RMSF; in practice, however, broader antibacterial coverage (eg, chloramphenicol plus ampicillin or oxacillin) is often used because bacterial sepsis cannot be excluded.

Tetanus

For prevention, both tetanus toxoid (0.5 mL) and human tetanus immunoglobulin (250 U) may be indicated, depending on the wound and the immunization history (Table 74.14). Tetanus-prone wounds include punctures, crush injuries, and injuries contaminated by animal excreta or those left untreated for more than 24 hours.

Toxic Shock Syndrome

CLINICAL MANIFESTATIONS

Toxic shock syndrome (TSS) begins suddenly with high fever, vomiting, and watery diarrhea. Pharyngitis, headache, and myalgias also may occur, and oliguria rapidly develops. Within 48 hours, the disease progresses to hypotensive shock. The patient has a fever, usually 39° to 41°C (102.2° to 105.8°F), a diffuse, erythematous maculopapular rash, and hyperemia of the mucous membranes. Often, marked disorientation evolves. The WBC count is elevated, with a shift to the left. Thrombocytopenia commonly occurs, being present in more than 75% of children reported by Todd. Most patients develop DIC and have an elevated PT and PTT. Additional abnormalities in the laboratory studies may include an elevated AST, ALT, BUN, creatinine, and creatinine phosphokinase. The serum calcium and phosphate may be decreased.

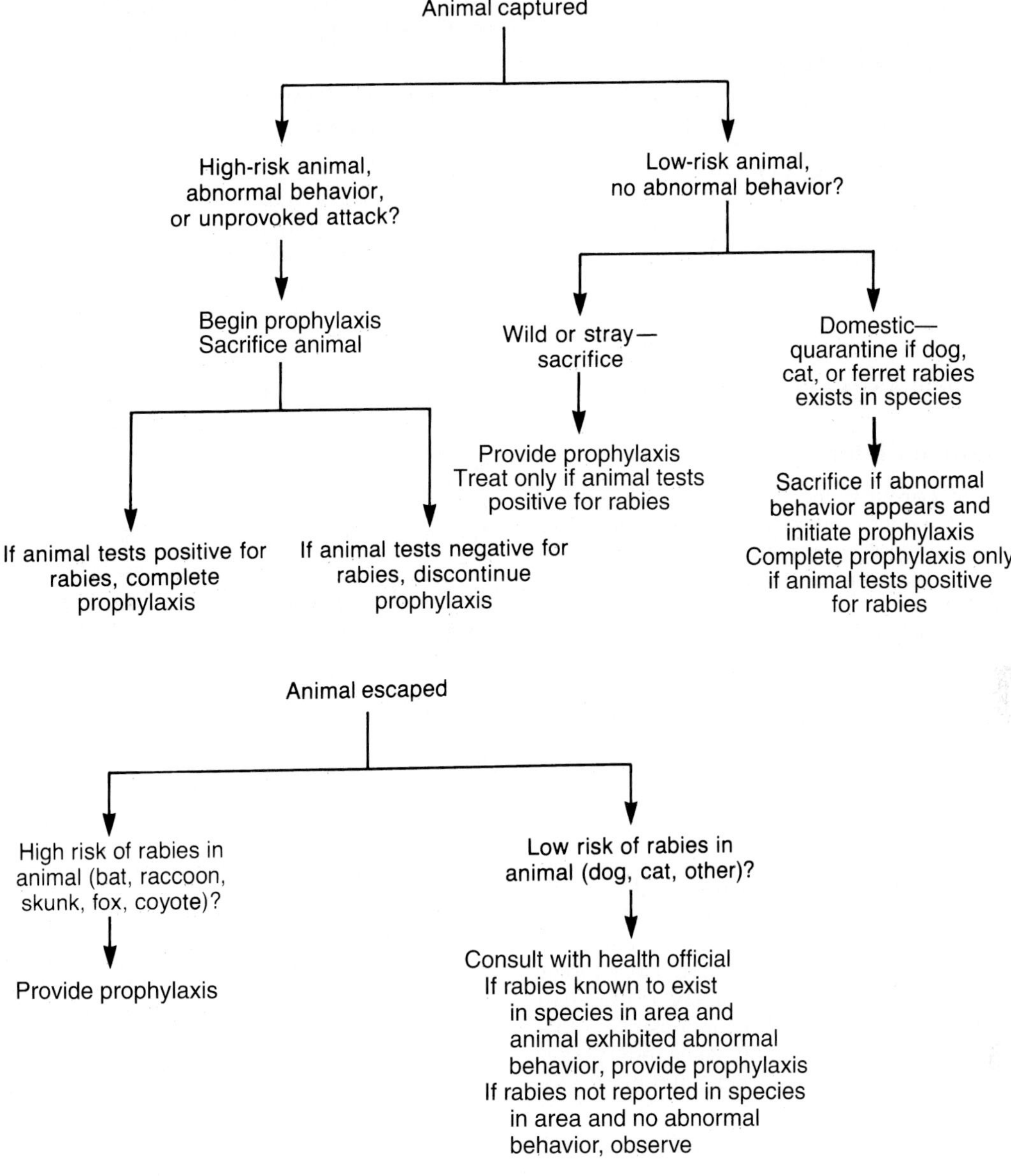

Figure 74.6. Diagnostic approach for the management of the child with a mammalian bite wound.

TABLE 74.14. Guidelines for Tetanus Prophylaxis

No. of primary immunizations	Years since last booster	Type of wound	Recommendation
≤2	Irrelevant	Low risk	T
		Tetanus prone	T + TIG
3	10	Low risk	T
		Tetanus prone	T
3	5–10	Low risk	No treatment
		Tetanus prone	T
3	<5	Low risk	No treatment
		Tetanus prone	No treatment

T, tetanus toxoid; TIG, human tetanus immune globulin.

MANAGEMENT

The initial diagnosis of TSS rests on the constellation of clinical and laboratory findings. The following laboratory tests should be obtained from all children suspected of having this syndrome: CBC, platelet count, PT, PTT, fibrin-split products, electrolytes, BUN, creatinine, AST, ALT, and creatinine phosphokinase. Cultures of the blood, urine, stool, throat, and vagina serve to isolate *S. aureus* and to rule out other infectious causes of shock. A lumbar puncture often is required to exclude bacterial meningitis. The management of TSS is the same as that for shock caused by other organisms (see Chapter 3). The physician should secure venous access with a plastic cannula and administer sufficient fluids to maintain an adequate blood pressure, beginning with 20 mL of normal saline per kilogram of body weight. Monitoring of the intravascular volume and urine output usually requires the placement of central venous and peripheral arterial lines and a urinary catheter.

CHAPTER 75
Human Immunodeficiency Virus Infection

Marvin B. Harper, M.D.

CLINICAL FINDINGS AND MANAGEMENT

Initial Presentation of Children with HIV

Most pediatric patients are infected perinatally and develop symptoms progressively over time. Although lymphadenopathy, hepatosplenomegaly, and failure to thrive are common clinical features, any organ system can be affected (Table 75.1). Many children show signs of abnormal humoral immune function, such as recurrent or persistent bacterial infection. Some children show early defects in cellular immunity exhibited by persistent candidiasis, chronic diarrhea, or opportunistic infections. Still others may remain relatively asymptomatic for long periods (6% completely asymptomatic at 5 years).

The initial presentation may actually represent acute human immunodeficiency virus (HIV) infection. Within days to weeks of initial exposure to HIV, a syndrome of fever, fatigue, and maculopapular truncal rash can mark acute disease. Myalgia, arthralgia, pharyngitis, lymphadenopathy, headache, nausea, vomiting, and diarrhea are common. Many also have leukopenia and thrombocytopenia. The diagnosis of acute HIV infection cannot be made with standard serologic tests [enzyme-linked immunoabsorbent assay (ELISA) or Western blot] because these tests first become positive 3 to 4 weeks after acute infection. Early detection, when indicated, is possible through the use of p24 antigen testing and plasma viral RNA testing.

Fever

Fever in HIV-infected children can represent simple childhood viral infections, but because of the humoral immunodeficiency of these children, they also commonly suffer from acute bacterial infections. In addition, opportunistic infections must be considered. Some parents may be able to provide a recent CD4 count, but laboratory data that reflect the status of the immune system usually are not available to the emergency physician. The physician should search carefully for a focus (Fig. 75.1).

TABLE 75.1. Signs and Symptoms of Human Immunodeficiency Virus Infection in Children

Lymphadenopathy	Recurrent fevers
Hepatomegaly	Splenomegaly
Failure to thrive	Chronic or recurrent diarrhea
Bacteremia	Wasting syndrome
Oral thrush	Developmental delay
Chronic or recurrent parotitis	Acquired microcephaly
Opportunistic infections	Spastic paresis

EVALUATION OF THE FEBRILE, HIV-POSITIVE CHILD WITHOUT A SOURCE

Evaluation of the Well-appearing, Febrile HIV-positive Child

An evaluation similar to that for febrile children at risk for occult bacteremia is reasonable; however, laboratory testing should be obtained even in children older than 24 months. Thus, even if the older child presents with a temperature of 39°C (102.2°F) or higher, a complete blood count (CBC) with differential and blood culture is recommended. If the child is still in diapers, a urine sample should be obtained for analysis and culture. If the child has any respiratory signs or symptoms, including isolated tachypnea, or if the CBC has an elevated leukocyte count with a shift to left regardless of the presence of respiratory signs, pulse oximetry and a chest radiograph should be ordered. These patients may be started on antibiotics such as amoxicillin, amoxicillin–clavulinic acid (Augmentin), or intramuscular ceftriaxone (Rocephin), pending culture results.

Evaluation of the Ill-appearing, Febrile, HIV-positive Child

The HIV-positive child who comes to the emergency department (ED) with fever and appears ill should be treated like other ill-appearing, febrile children because they are likely to be infected with the same types of organisms that infect immunocompetent children. Ceftriaxone (100 mg per kilogram daily divided every 12 hours) is an appropriate choice because it covers the organisms that most commonly cause sepsis in children. Especially in young children, because of the possibility of Pneumocystis carinii pneumonia (PCP) presenting with fever and ill appearance, trimethoprim–sulfamethoxazole (TMP-SMZ) (5 mg per kilogram of body weight per dose every 6 hours) should be added to the antibiotic regimen if there are respiratory symptoms, with or without a positive chest radiograph.

SOFT-TISSUE INFECTIONS

Cervical adenitis and cellulitis are common and may be accompanied by fever. Parotitis is another common soft-tissue infection that occurs in HIV-positive children, who can have chronic enlargement of the parotid glands secondary to lymphocytic infiltration. If the child appears well and the infection is well circumscribed and does not impinge on a critical structure, such as the airway, outpatient antibiotic therapy active against *S. aureus* and *Streptococcus pyogenes* (eg, cephalexin 60–80 mg per kilogram daily in four divided doses) is appropriate as long as it appears that the caretaker can adhere to the regimen and the child can be reevaluated within 24 to 48 hours.

PULMONARY INFECTIONS

Pneumocystis Carinii Pneumonia

The manifestation of PCP can be as either an acute or a subacute illness. The infant typically is febrile, with marked tachypnea, wheezing, rhonchi, and diminished breath sounds. Rales are not usually part of the PCP picture, and cough may be absent. When coughing is present, it is typically dry and nonproductive. Over hours to days, the patient develops hypoxia and increased respiratory distress. The patient typically has a high (>30 mm Hg) alveolar–arterial (A-a) oxygen gradient and low oxygen saturation, and generally there is marked (>500 IU) elevation of the serum lactic dehydrogenase (LDH). Radiographic findings typ-

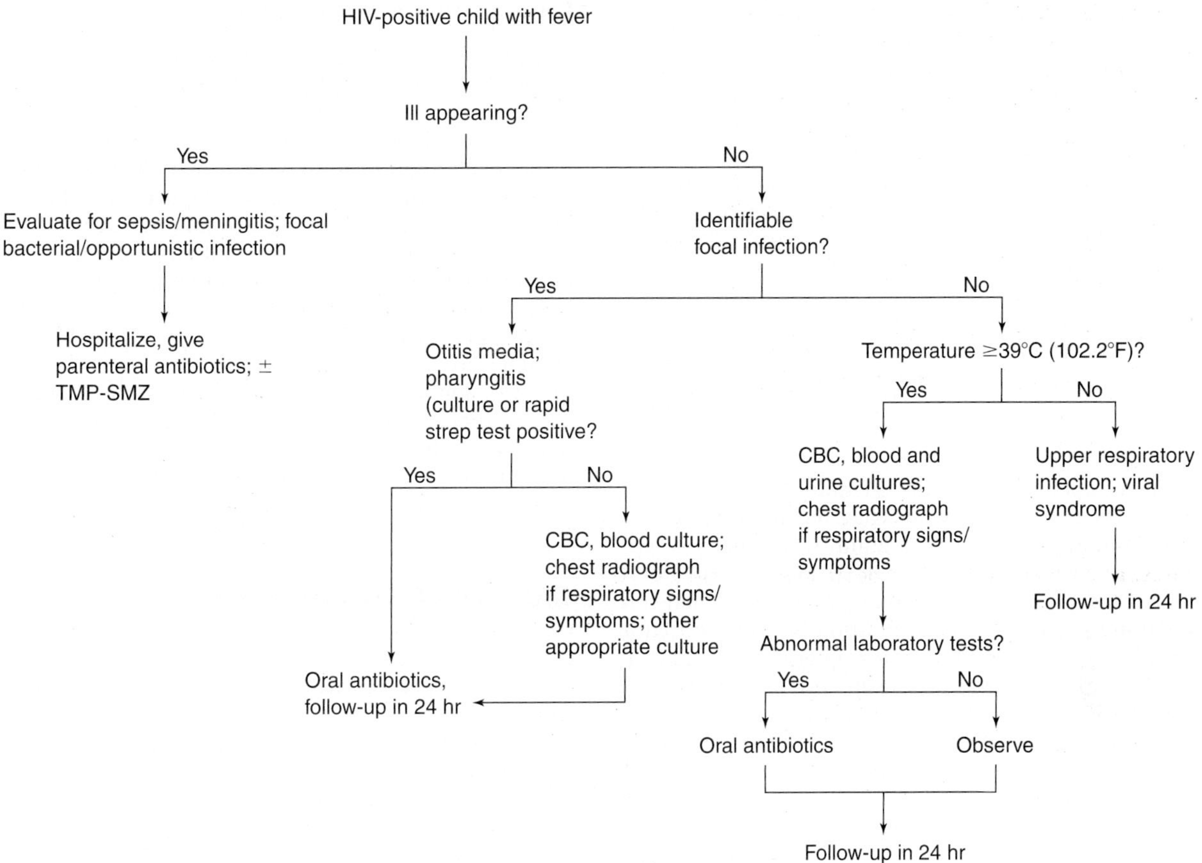

Figure 75.1. Evaluation of the human immunodeficiency virus (HIV)-positive child with fever. TMP-SMZ, trimethoprim–sulfamethoxazole; CBC, complete blood count. (Modified from Dorfman D, Crain E, Bernstein L. Care of febrile children with HIV infection in the emergency department. *Pediatr Emerg Care* 1990;6:308, with permission.)

ically consist of a diffuse interstitial ("ground glass") pattern, but in infants there may be patchy infiltrates or complete opacification of the lung fields. Occasionally, however, there may be clear lung fields with hyperinflation suggestive of bronchiolitis, and in 5% to 10% of patients with PCP, the chest radiograph appears normal. If PCP is suspected on the basis of the history, physical examination, or the results of the laboratory investigation, it is appropriate to start intravenous TMP-SMZ at a dosage of 20 mg of TMP per kilogram divided into four doses. The child should be hospitalized for close observation and further diagnostic evaluation as needed.

Bacterial Pneumonia

The HIV-positive child with bacterial pneumonia is most often infected with the usual organisms: *Streptococcus pneumoniae, Haemophilus influenzae,* group A streptococcus, and *Moraxella catarrhalis.* Hospitalized children or those with indwelling devices may be infected with gram-negative enteric organisms or *S. aureus.* A chest radiograph should be part of the evaluation of the HIV-positive child with fever of unknown origin or with respiratory signs or symptoms. The radiograph can help distinguish bacterial pneumonia from PCP or pulmonary lymphoid hyperplasia (PLH), and in fact, a chest radiograph compatible with bacterial pneumonia in an otherwise well-appearing child suggests that outpatient therapy may be possible if other criteria are met (Table 75.2). The chest radiograph in bacterial pneumonia typically reveals a lobar or segmental infiltrate, and the peripheral white blood cell count is often above $20000/mm^3$. Because it is rare to be confident that a case of pneumonia is not bacterial in origin, children with pulmonary signs and symptoms, especially associated with fever, are commonly given antimicrobial therapy against the common respiratory flora.

Wheezing

Reactive airway disease is the most likely diagnosis in an HIV-positive child with wheezing, with or without fever. If the wheezing is associated with rales, however, the physician needs to consider the possibility of PCP or congestive heart fail-

TABLE 75.2. General Guidelines for Outpatient Therapy of HIV-Positive Children with Pneumonia

Age > 6 mo
Able to tolerate oral fluids and medication
Absence of signs of respiratory distress (e.g., flaring or retractions)
Respiratory rate
<45 respirations/min if age <2 yr
<30 respirations/min if age >2 yr
Oxygen saturation ≥93%
Has not already worsened while receiving oral antibiotic
Close clinical follow-up available and patient able to return
Pneumocystis carinii pneumonia should be considered unlikely

HIV, human immunodeficiency virus.

ure (CHF). CHF is rarely a presenting sign of HIV infection; instead, HIV-positive children with cardiomyopathy can develop CHF when under additional stress caused by an infection or fever. After a rapid but thorough physical examination to evaluate the degree of wheezing and air movement, the presence and location of retractions, and any other focus for fever, it should be noted whether the child responds to bronchodilator therapy. If so, reactive airway disease is the likely diagnosis, and the child can be treated accordingly. Pulse oximetry should be performed before the patient is discharged; although an oxygen saturation less than 95% is not an absolute indication for admission, a saturation of 95% or greater is reassuring. Five days of prednisone therapy (2 mg per kilogram daily divided into two doses, 60 mg daily maximum) can be given if it would be used for an immunocompetent child with the same clinical findings.

If the child has high fever (> 39°C, or 102.2°F), a chest radiograph should be obtained to look for an infiltrate or evidence of PCP or CHF. The febrile child with wheezing and rales or evidence of pneumonia on chest radiograph who otherwise appears well enough for outpatient therapy may be given oral amoxicillin (60–80 mg per kilogram daily) or intramuscular ceftriaxone (50 mg per kilogram) in addition to bronchodilator therapy. Children with clinical or radiographic evidence of PCP or congestive heart failure should be hospitalized. A first dose of intravenous TMP-SMZ should be given to infants suspected of having PCP, and CHF should be treated with afterload reducers and diuretics in addition to bronchodilators (see "Cardiology" section).

Lymphocytic Interstitial Pneumonitis

Lymphocytic interstitial pneumonitis (LIP) is an insidious condition that causes a slowly progressive hypoxia typically in children who are older than 1 year. Table 75.3 contrasts the findings in LIP with those associated with PCP. The approach to the evaluation of the HIV-infected child with respiratory signs and symptoms is outlined in Figure 75.2. Chest radiography commonly reveals an interstitial nodular pattern that can be diagnostic. Fever is an important differentiating point in the management of HIV-positive children thought to have LIP. If the P_aO_2 is less than 65 mm Hg, LIP is treated with 1 to 2 mg of prednisone per kilogram of body weight daily to a maximum of 60 mg for 2 to 4 weeks and subsequently tapered as necessary to maintain the P_aO_2 above 70 mm Hg. If the patient is febrile, tuberculosis or MAI must be ruled out before beginning steroid therapy; these entities can appear similar to PLH both clinically and radiographically, but steroid therapy is contraindicated.

GASTROINTESTINAL TRACT

Chronic or recurrent oral thrush or esophageal candidiasis are common and can be treated with nystatin, clotrimazole, or fluconazole.

Because diarrhea can be such a problem in HIV-infected children, the physician should seek to identify the cause. A stool test for blood, a stool smear for polymorphonuclear leukocytes, and

TABLE 75.3. Findings in HIV-Positive Children with Lymphoid Interstitial Pneumonitis/Pulmonary Lymphoid Hyperplasia vs. *P. carinii* Pneumonia

	LIP/PLH	PCP
Age	>20 mo most common	Infancy most common
Onset	Chronic, progressive	Acute, subacute
Fever	Afebrile	Febrile
Tachypnea	Mild	Marked
Cough	Common	±
Auscultatory findings		
Wheezes	Rare	Common
Rhonchi	Rare	Common
Rales	Intermittent	Rare
Diminished breath sounds	Rare	Common
Lymphadenopathy	Marked	Mild
Parotitis	Common	Rare
Digital clubbing	Common	Rare
Hypoxia	Mild to moderate	Moderate to severe
A-a O_2	Mild to moderate	Marked
LDH elevation (normal <250 IU/L)	Moderate	Marked
Chest radiograph	Diffuse nodular pattern; widening of mediastinum + hilum	Diffuse interstitial pattern (can be clear, hyperinflated in 10%)
Biopsy	Peribronchiolar lymphoid nodular aggregates; ± evidence of Epstein-Barr virus DNA or HIV RNA in lung tissue	Organisms on silver stain in alveoli (biopsy or bronchoalveolar lavage)
Treatment	Steroids for PaO_2 <65	Antibiotics, steroids
Prognosis	Better long-term prognosis	Poor—death common in first 2 yr

HIV, human immunodeficiency virus; LIP, lymphoid interstitial pneumonia; PLH, pulmonary lymphoid hyperplasia; PCP, *Pneumocystis carinii* pneumonia.
From Cunningham S, Crain E, Bernstein L. Evaluating the HIV infected child with pulmonary signs and symptoms. *Pediatr Emerg Care* 1991;7:34, with permission.

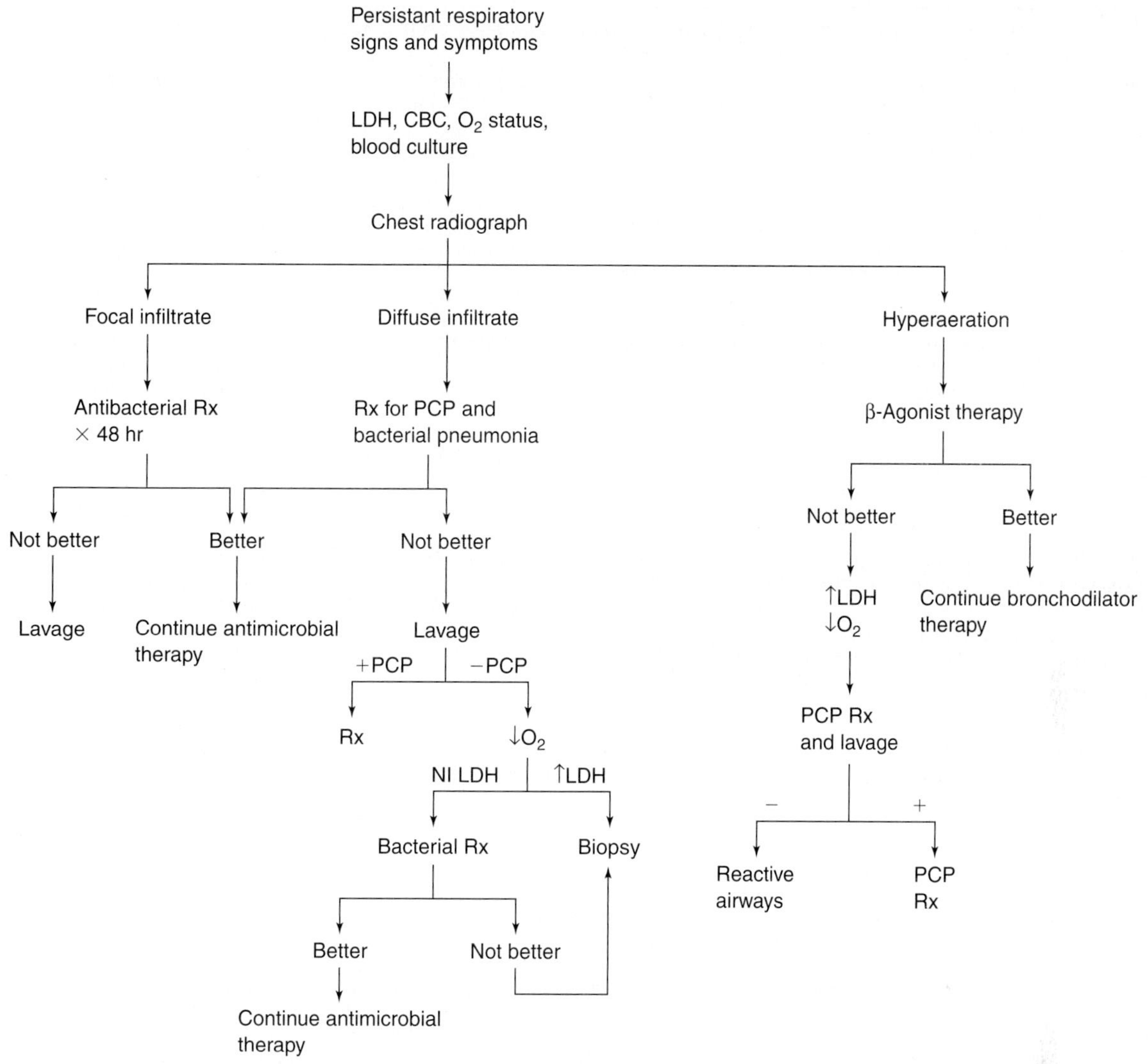

Figure 75.2. Evaluation of persistent respiratory signs and symptoms. LDH, lactate dehydrogenase; CBC, complete blood count; Rx, treatment; PCP, Pneumocystis carinii pneumonia. (Modified from Cunningham SJ, Crain EF, Bernstein LJ. Evaluations of the HIV-infected child with pulmonary signs and symptoms. *Pediatr Emerg Care* 1991; 7:32–37, with permission.)

a stool culture (for *Salmonella, Shigella, Yersinia, Campylobacter, Escherichia coli* species) should be done, with consideration given to sending stool to test for parasites and *Clostridium difficile.* The child who is afebrile, appears to be well hydrated, and has no blood or leukocytes in the stool can be treated symptomatically with dietary management and close follow-up. In febrile children with gastroenteritis, although viral causes are still most common, *Salmonella* is the primary bacterial pathogen of concern and is a major cause of bacteremia in HIV-positive children. If there is blood or more than five leukocytes per high-power field are found on examination of the stool smear, but the child has normal vital signs and looks well, he or she should be treated with TMP-SMZ and reevaluated the next day.

RASH

Measles can be particularly severe in HIV-positive children. The illness may be associated with the characteristic clinical signs and symptoms of generalized rash, coryza, conjunctivitis, cough, and Koplik spots, or it may occur without the typical rash. If the child is taking liquids well and breathing comfortably, he or she may be sent home with careful instructions to return for reevaluation if the child's status worsens. All HIV-positive children who have been exposed to measles should receive gamma globulin (0.5 mL per kilogram with a maximum of 15 mL given intramuscularly), whether or not they have been vaccinated against measles.

Varicella-zoster immunoglobulin should be given to HIV-infected children after exposure to chickenpox (1 vial containing 125 U for each 10 kg of body weight with any opened vial used completely; maximal dose, five vials). Once clinical illness has started, these children should initially be treated with intravenous acyclovir (10 mg per kilogram every 8 hours). Children with local zoster infection may be treated with oral acyclovir (20 mg per kilogram per dose given every 6 hours).

More than 10% of children infected with HIV will have thrombocytopenia associated with high levels of circulating immune complexes and antiplatelet antibodies that may manifest as petechiae or easy bruising. Patients with fewer than 50000 platelets per liter should be considered for hospital admission and treatment. Febrile or toxic-appearing HIV-positive children with petechiae must be considered to have septicemia (see

TABLE 75.4. Anti-Human Immunodeficiency Virus Medications

Drug	Dosage	Dosage forms	Common adverse effects
Nucleoside reverse transcriptase inhibitors			
Abacavir (Ziagen)	8 mg/kg/dose b.i.d. up to 300 mg/dose	20 mg/mL solution, 300 mg tablet	Malaise, nausea, vomiting, headache, uncommon but potentially severe hypersensitivity reaction
Didanosine (ddI, Hivid)	100 mg/m2/dose b.i.d. up to 200 mg b.i.d.; adult: 125 mg if <60 kg; 200 mg b.i.d. for ≥60 kg; taken on an empty stomach	10 mg/mL suspension, 25-, 50-, 100-, 150-mg chewable tablets; powder for oral solution in packets containing 100, 167, or 250 mg;	Pancreatitis, peripheral neuropathy, diarrhea, rarely retinal changes and optic neuritis, increased liver enzymes
Lamivudine (3TC, Epivir)	3 mo to 12 yr: 4 mg/kg/dose b.i.d. (up to 150 mg b.i.d.); adult: 150 mg b.i.d. unless <50 kg then 2 mg/kg/dose b.i.d.	10 mg/mL oral solution; 150-mg tablets	Generally well tolerated, used in combination with other agents may accentuate hematologic effects, rare pancreatitis, neuropathy
Stavudine (d4T, Zerit)	1 mg/kg/dose up to adult dosing of 30 mg/dose b.i.d. if <60 kg and 40 mg/dose b.i.d. if ???60 kg	1 mg/mL oral solution; 15-, 20-, 30-, 40-mg capsules	Peripheral neuropathy, pancreatitis, myalgias, nausea, vomiting, abdominal pain, diarrhea, rash, insomnia
Zidovudine (ZDV, AZT, Retrovir)	0–6 wk of age 2 mg/kg/dose q.i.d.; >6 wk 120–160 mg/m²/dose t.i.d. up to adult dose of 200 mg/dose t.i.d.	10 mg/mL syrup: 100-, 300-mg tablets	Anemia, granulocytopenia, myopathy, increased liver enzymes, macrocytosis, anemia, nausea, vomiting, headache, lactic acidosis
Zalcitibine (ddC, Hivid)	0.01–0.02 mg/kg/dose t.i.d. up to adult dose of 0.75 mg t.i.d.	0.1 mg/mL syrup; 0.376, 0.75-mg tablets	Peripheral neuropathy, pancreatittis, mouth sores, lactic acidosis, dysphagia, abdominal pain, rash, headache
Combivir (a fixed combination of zidovudine)	≥12 yr of age 1 tablet twice daily	150 mg lamivudine, 300 mg zidovudine per tablet	See lamivudine and zidovudine
Nonnucleoside reverse transcriptase inhibitors			
Nevirapine (NVP, Viramune)	Pedi 120 mg/m²/dose b.i.d. up to adult dose of 200 mg/dose b.i.d.	200-mg tablets	Rash, increased liver enzymes (both can be severe)
Delavirdine (DLV, Rescriptor)	Adult dose is 400 mg/dose t.i.d. on an empty stomach	100-mg tablets	Decreased hepatic metabolism or other medications, rash, increased liver enzymes, nausea
Etavirenz (Sustiva)	10–15 mg/kg/dose qD to 600 mg/dose	50-, 100-, 200-mg capsule	Rash, dizziness, headache, impaired concentration
Protease inhibitors			
Indinavir (IDV, Crixivan)	Pedi dose 500 mg/m²/dose t.i.d. up to adult dose of 800 mg/dose t.i.d. on an empty stomach	200-, 400-mg capsules	Crystalluria and nephrolithiasis, nausea, vomiting, headache, indirect hyperbilirubinemia
Nelfinavir (Viracept)	20–30 mg/kg/dose t.i.d. up to adult dose of 750 mg/kg/dose t.i.d. taken with food	Oral powder 50 mg/g 1 scoopful mixed in liquid; 250-mg tablets	Flatulence, diarrhea
Ritonavir (Norvir)	400 mg/m²/dose b.i.d. up to adult dose of 600 mg/dose b.i.d. taken with food	80 mg/mL oral solution; 100-mg capsules	Significant decreases in hepatic metabolism of other medications, nausea, vomiting, diarrhea, paresthesias, taste perversion
Saquinavir (Fortivase, Invirase)	Adult dose is 1,200 mg t.i.d. of the Fortivase formulation taken with food	200-mg capsules	Nausea, diarrhea, abdominal discomfort

TABLE 75.5. Approximate Risk of Human Immunodeficiency Virus Acquisition after a Single Exposure Listed by Source

Exposure	Risk of infection (per 1,000)
Transfusion with positive blood unit	950
Intravenous drug use	7
Percutaneous exposure (needlestick)	3
Receptive anal intercourse	3
Receptive vaginal intercourse	1
Receptive oral sex	Low but reported
Perinatal exposure without zidovudine	250
Perinatal exposure with zidovudine	80
Breast-feeding (not single exposure)	120

Chapter 74), and they should receive parenteral antibiotics pending culture results.

NEUROLOGIC MANIFESTATIONS

These children exhibit developmental delay or developmental regression, acquired microcephaly, and pyramidal tract signs. Although growth and development are often affected by any serious illness in a child, acquired immunodeficiency syndrome (AIDS) encephalopathy may occur in patients with no signs of opportunistic infections and few signs of immunodeficiency. AIDS encephalopathy may manifest itself as a static, progressive, or indolent encephalopathy with periods of plateaus in cognitive and motor development. Physical examination of the patient often reveals microcephaly. Younger children will be hypotonic with persistence of the Moro or tonic neck reflexes after 4 months of age. Older children may have symmetric ankle clonus and extensor plantar responses. As the condition progresses, pyramidal signs of varying severity, including a pure spastic quadriparesis with signs of pseudobulbar palsy, dysphagia, and dysarthria, are seen. Ataxia may be seen in children old enough to walk.

The diagnosis of AIDS encephalopathy involves obtaining a history suggestive of developmental delay or regression in an HIV-infected child. Management is more complicated when these children come to the ED with fever because it may be difficult to evaluate their mental status. In general, a lumbar puncture is necessary to rule out bacterial meningitis, unless the physician can be confident on a clinical basis that the child is behaving at baseline and that the fever is not secondary to central nervous system infection.

MANAGEMENT

Overview of Anti-HIV Medications

Many effective anti-HIV medications are now available (Table 75.4). Because HIV has the capacity rapidly to develop resistance to individual antiviral agents, combination therapy using three to four agents has now become the treatment standard.

Prevention of Acquisition

Current strategies for preventing HIV infection take advantage of the finding that it may take several hours after exposure (or possibly in some cases days) for HIV infection to become established. The risks of acquisition from exposures to HIV are listed in Table 75.5.

A patient with a significant exposure to HIV, such as receptive or penetrative anal or vaginal sex, receptive oral intercourse with ejaculation, or needle sharing involving a partner who is HIV positive or who is in a known risk group, should be considered for postexposure prophylaxis (PEP). Accidental community-acquired needlestick exposures also require attention. When considered appropriate (Fig. 75.3), PEP should be instituted as quickly as possible after exposure. Most researchers would limit PEP to exposures within 72 hours of exposure (preferably <24 hours). Patients receiving PEP should receive first doses of medication in the ED and will need follow-up with clinicians knowledgeable about antiviral therapies and able to provide intensive emotional and behavioral counseling to help cope with the immediate event and to help them avoid situations likely to result in future exposure. The medications, which must be taken for 4 weeks, can have significant side effects.

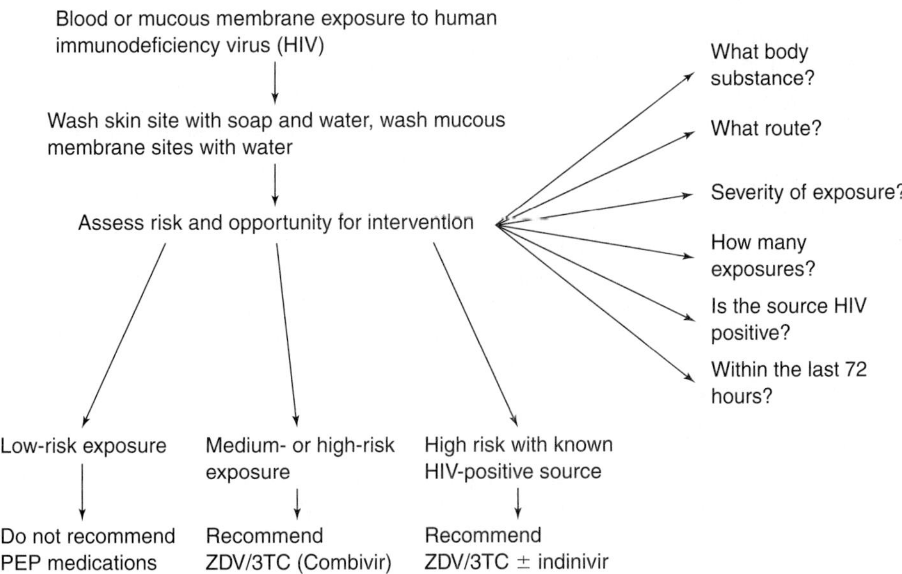

Figure 75.3. Postexposure prophylaxis for possible community-acquired exposures to human immunodeficiency virus. When available, additional information regarding the source individual may alter recommendations. PEP, postexposure prophylaxis.

CHAPTER 76
Renal and Electrolyte Emergencies

Kate Cronan, M.D., and
Michael E. Norman, M.D.

DEHYDRATION

Isotonic Dehydration

Fluid loss occurs commonly in pediatrics, and most children have isotonic dehydration. Appropriate treatment of dehydration requires an understanding of maintenance and deficit fluid and electrolyte calculations.

Weight (kg)/Fluid/24 Hours	
<10 kg	100 mL/kg
11–20 kg	100 mL × 10 + 50 mL for each kg > 10 kg
>20 kg	100 mL × 10 + 50 mL × 10 + 20 mL for each kg > 20 kg

The maintenance requirement for electrolytes relates directly to the caloric expenditure, which also determines the requirement for water. For Na, this is 2 to 3 mEq per 100 mL and for potassium (K), 2 mEq per 100 mL. As an example, a 30-kg child would have a daily maintenance requirement for fluid of 1700 mL (100 mL per kilogram × 10 kg + 50 mL per kilogram × 10 kg + 20 mL per kilogram × 10 kg). The requirement for Na would be 34 to 51 mEq, and for K, 34 mEq.

CLINICAL MANIFESTATIONS

A careful history taken from the parents of a child with isotonic dehydration helps to establish the cause for the fluid loss and to estimate the degree of depletion. The physical examination should begin with a careful weighing of the child—the most accurate clinical indicator of dehydration. The signs of dehydration become increasingly severe as the degree of dehydration progresses (see Table 14.4). With a 5% loss of body weight, the skin and mucous membranes feel dry, but there are no signs of vascular instability. Tachycardia and hypotension appear as the loss of fluid exceeds this mark, and the skin turgor shows deterioration. The development of acidosis leads to tachypnea and contributes to poor peripheral perfusion. If the child has lost more than 10% of body weight in a brief time, signs of shock, including a rapid, thready pulse; marked hypotension; and cold, clammy skin, may appear (see Chapter 3).

MANAGEMENT

In all children with significant dehydration (5%–10%), an intravenous infusion should be started and blood sent to the laboratory for measurement of electrolytes and blood urea nitrogen (BUN). An initial fluid bolus of 20 mL of physiologic saline per kilogram of body weight given rapidly over 30 to 60 minutes is the treatment of choice. With lesser degrees of dehydration, the optimal type and rate of fluid infusion are calculated on the basis of the child's estimated ideal weight and degree of dehydration. Sufficient fluids are administered in the first 24 hours to fulfill the maintenance requirement and correct the total deficit; half the deficit is replaced in the first 8 hours.

EXAMPLE

A 5-month-old infant has a 3-day history of diarrhea and a decreased oral intake. One week previously, she weighed 5.0 kg in the pediatrician's office. Now she weighs 4.5 kg and has a temperature of 37.0°C (98.6°F), a pulse of 120 beats per minute, a respiratory rate of 30 breaths per minute, and blood pressure (BP) of 80/40 mm Hg. The child's skin and mucosa are dry, and the skin shows "tenting" if lifted. The urine specific gravity is 1.028, and the serum electrolytes are as follows: [Na] 135 mEq per liter; [K] 4.0 mEq per liter; [Cl] 90 mEq per liter; and [HCO_3] 9.0 mEq per liter. The BUN is 30 mg per deciliter.

This infant has lost 10% of her body weight. Because acute decreases in weight reflect fluid loss, the fluid deficit is 500 mL. Dehydration occurred over 3 days, indicating that 60% of the loss is from the extracellular fluid (ECF) and 40% from the intracellular (ICF). Thus, the Na and K deficits are calculated as follows:

$$\text{Na deficit} = 135\ \text{mEq}/1000\ \text{mL} \times 0.6 \times 500\ \text{mL} = 40\ \text{mEq}$$

$$\text{K deficit} = 150\ \text{mEq}/1000\ \text{mL} \times 0.4 \times 500\ \text{mL} = 30\ \text{mEq}$$

The maintenance requirements for this infant are 500 mL of fluid (100 mL × kilogram = 5 kg), 15 mEq of Na (3 mEq/100 mL × 500 mL), and 10 mEq of K (2 mEq/100 mL × 500 mL) for each 24-hour period.

Half of the fluid and Na deficits are replaced during the first 8 hours of rehydration. Thus, the infant would receive 250 mL of deficit fluid with 20 mEq of Na. In addition, one-third of the maintenance requirement, or 175 mL of fluid with 5 mEq of Na, would be given during that 8-hour period, for a total of 425 mL of fluid with 25 mEq of Na.

Only half of the K deficit is corrected during each of the first 2 days, and this is done at a constant rate. Because the maintenance K for this infant is 15 mEq and the deficit is 30 mEq, the amount of K administered would be 30 mEq daily (or 10 mEq for each 8-hour period) for the first 48 hours. The solution also would need to contain an appropriate amount of bicarbonate. A maintenance amount of bicarbonate is 2 mEq per kilogram of body weight daily.

Hypotonic Dehydration

The pathophysiology and clinical findings for hypotonic (hyponatremic) dehydration are discussed in the section under "Disorders of Sodium Homeostasis: Hyponatremia." An example follows.

EXAMPLE

The 5-month-old infant described under the previous section on isotonic dehydration might well have presented with more pronounced clinical manifestations of dehydration and the following serum electrolytes:

[Na] 128 mEq/L; [K] 4.0 mEq/L; [Cl] 90 mEq/L; and [HCO] 9.0 mEq/L. The BUN is 30 mg/dL

Deficits of Na and K are calculated in the same fashion as given in the previous example of isotonic dehydration. Maintenance requirements are also the same. What is different about the calculations in this example is the added Na requirement in the deficit fluids to bring the serum Na from 128 to 135 mEq/L. The calculation should be as follows:

1. Additional mEq of Na =
   [135 − 128 mEq/L] × 5.0 × 0.6
   "ideal" − "observed" "healthy" body weight (kg) Na space
2. Additional mEq of Na =
   7.0 mEq/L × 5 kg × 0.6 = 7.0 × 3.0 L (kg)
3. Additional mEq of Na = 21 mEq

This extra Na is added to the previously calculated 40 mEq Na in the deficit fluids, but the rate of repair may be staged in the same fashion as for isotonic dehydration.

Hypertonic Dehydration

The background, pathophysiology, clinical manifestations, and management of hypertonic (hypernatremic) dehydration are discussed under "Hypernatremia."

ELECTROLYTE DISORDERS

Disorders of Sodium Homeostasis: Hyponatremia

CLINICAL MANIFESTATIONS

The multiple causes of hyponatremia are grouped into four categories (Table 76.1). Symptoms and signs of hyponatremia are related to the absolute level and the rate of fall of serum Na from the normal range, but they tend to be somewhat nonspecific (Table 76.2). Signs and symptoms are usually seen at serum Na lower than 120 mEq per liter, but specific symptoms and signs do not correlate with specific levels of serum Na. The clinical examination can help in limiting the possible diagnoses to explain the hyponatremia. It is especially critical to note the presence of edema and hypovolemia. Complications of hyponatremia that require urgent diagnosis and treatment include Cheyne-Stokes respirations and seizures; however, a clouded sensorium and pathologic reflexes are often warning signs of seizures.

TABLE 76.1. Causes of Hyponatremia

Normal total body water and Na (hyperosmolar hyponatremia)
Hyperglycemia[a]
Mannitol, glycerol therapy
Increased total body water and Na (edema-forming states)
Congestive heart failure
Nephrosis
Cirrhosis
Acute renal failure
Decreased total body water and Na (Hypovolemic States)
Gastrointestinal losses (vomiting, diarrhea, fistulas)
Renal losses (diuretics, renal tubular acidosis, primary interstitial disease)
Adrenal (mineralocorticoid deficiencies)
Third-space losses (ascites, burns, pancreatitis, peritonitis)
Increased total body water but normal total body Na
Syndrome of inappropriate antidiuretic hormone secretion
Water intoxication
Miscellaneous (reset osmostat, hypothyroidism, glucocorticoid deficiency)
Pseudohyponatremia
Extreme hyperlipidemia or hyperproteinemia

Na, sodium.
[a] For every 100 mg/dL rise in plasma glucose concentration above normal, there is a corresponding decrease in plasma sodium concentration of approximately 1.6 mEq/L.

TABLE 76.2. Symptoms and Signs of Hyponatremia

Symptoms	Signs
Anorexia	Clouded sensorium
Nausea	Decreased tendon reflexes
Muscle cramps	Pathologic reflexes
Lethargy	Cheyne–Stokes respiration
Apathy	Hypothermia
Disorientation	Pseudobulbar palsy
Agitation	Seizures
Acute respiratory failure	

MANAGEMENT

Armed with a working knowledge of pathophysiology, the clinical history and examination, and the few simple laboratory tests, the emergency physician should be able to diagnose rapidly the specific cause of hyponatremia in most cases. A specific diagnosis is necessary because therapies differ significantly depending on the cause of the hyponatremia. A working schema is outlined in Figure 76.1.

In the patient with hyponatremia in the face of obvious contraction of ECF volume (diarrhea or vomiting), reexpansion with isotonic saline is appropriate. The volume and rate of infusion are dictated by estimates of fluid loss (ie, weight loss) made from the history and physical examination. In shock, 20 mL of isotonic saline per kilogram of body weight can be administered rapidly over 1 hour or more as needed and then repeated as necessary until BP and peripheral circulation return to normal. Underlying diseases, such as renal tubular acidosis (RTA) and adrenal insufficiency, can be treated most effectively by specific replacement therapy. Diuretics, if previously given, should be discontinued promptly.

In water intoxication, restriction of daily free water administration by 25% to 50%, depending on the chronicity and severity of the hyponatremia, is the treatment of choice. In the acutely ill patient with neurologic symptoms and signs, immediate relief may be accomplished temporarily by rapidly elevating the serum Na by 10 mEq per liter up to 125 mEq per liter with intravenous administration of 3% sodium chloride as follows: mL 3% NaCl (0.5 mEq per milliliter) to give = 10 mEq per liter body weight (kg) × 0.6 (ECF space). Alternatively, 10 to 12 mL of 3% NaCl per kilogram of body weight can be infused over 1 hour. In adults, the rapid overcorrection of hyponatremia (eg, an increase in serum Na of more than 2 mEq per liter per hour) may be dangerous, producing the crippling or even fatal osmotic demyelination syndrome. The risk of this is greatest when a rapid overcorrection is made in a case of chronic hyponatremia.

In simple water intoxication, the normal kidney responds with maximal urinary dilution, which, when coupled with restriction of water intake, rapidly restores Na concentration to normal. In the syndrome of inappropriate secretion of antidiuretic syndrome (SIADH), water restriction is the initial treatment of choice but is not always effective. In the edema-forming states and acute renal failure (ARF), hyponatremia is usually mild and water restriction usually suffices. In some patients, di-

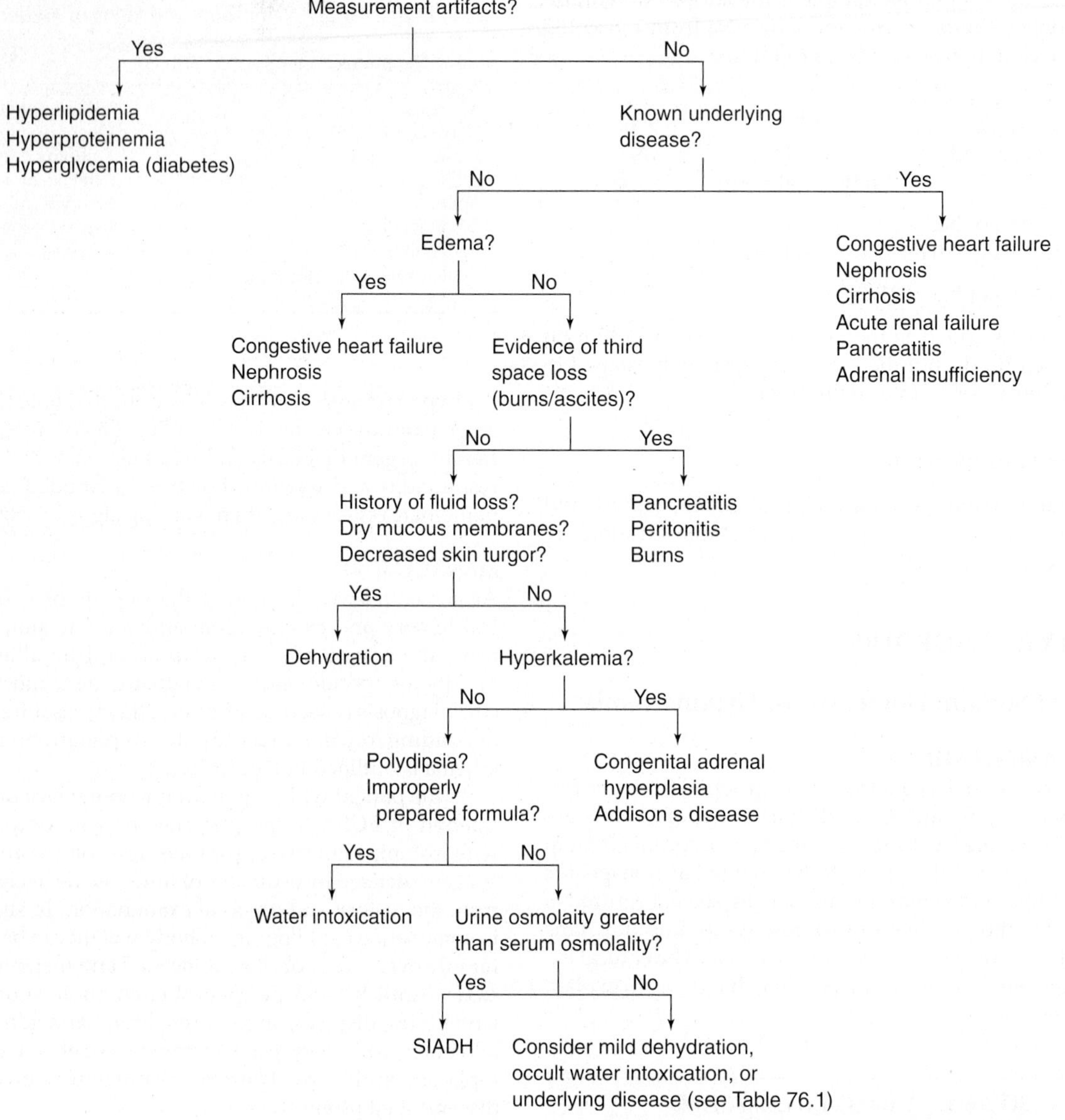

Figure 76.1. Diagnostic approach to hyponatremia. *SIADH,* syndrome of inappropriate secretion of antidiuretic hormone.

uretics may be necessary to treat the underlying disease. In such situations, free water excretion is increased but at the risk of inducing ECF volume contraction through increased Na excretion. Admission to the hospital is recommended for any patient with symptomatic hyponatremia or hyponatremia per se (<130 mEq per liter) when the cause is not obvious.

Disorders of Sodium Homeostasis: Hypernatremia

CLINICAL MANIFESTATIONS

As with hyponatremia, the causes of hypernatremia can be grouped into four major categories (Table 76.3) on the basis of net changes in total body water and Na. Symptoms and signs range from lethargy and irritability to muscle weakness, convulsions, and coma. Because ECF volume is defended early in the course of a dehydrating illness associated with hypernatremia, the classic physical sign of decreased skin turgor is absent until total fluid losses are severe (≈10%–15% of body

TABLE 76.3. Causes of Hypernatremia

Increased total body Na or increased total body Na greater than increased total body water
Na poisoning (accidental; Na bicarbonate therapy)
Hyperaldosteronism (rare in children)
Normal total body Na; "pure" water loss
Insensible losses—respiratory and skin renal (central and nephrogenic diabetes insipidus) inadequate access to water
Decreased total body Na less than decreased total body water
Extrarenal (gastrointestinal)[a] renal (osmotic diuretics; glucose, mannitol, urea) obstructive uropathy
Normal total body Na and water with abnormal central osmotic
Regulation of water balance
Essential hypernatremia

Na, sodium.
[a] In diarrheal states, hypernatremia usually results from a combination of relatively greater water than Na losses coupled with relatively greater Na than water replacement.

weight). The major complications of hypernatremia that require urgent diagnosis are seizures and coma.

MANAGEMENT

As in the hyponatremic states, the emergency physician should be able to reach a specific category of disease or diagnosis armed with a working knowledge of pathophysiology, clinical evaluation of the status of ECF volume, and a few simple serum and urine tests. The algorithm in Figure 76.2 provides a working schema.

For patients who are severely dehydrated and in shock, reexpansion with isotonic saline is the appropriate initial therapy (see "Hyponatremia"). Osmotic diuretics, if previously given, must be stopped. Replacement of water and Na losses with hypotonic electrolyte solutions is appropriate, but in the case of diarrhea, serum Na should be lowered slowly (usually no more than 10 to 15 mEq per liter per 24 hours) to guard against brain edema. In hypertonic dehydration, a free-water deficit of 4 mL per kilogram for every 1 mEq per liter of serum Na greater than 145 mEq per liter should be replaced over 48 to 72 hours.

For example, a 5-month-old infant has a 3-day history of diarrhea. Last week she weighed 5.0 kg but now she weighs 4.5 kg. She has been receiving undiluted skim milk and "salt water" orally. Vital signs are normal. Electrolytes are as follows: [Na] 160 mEq/L; [Cl] 120 mEq/L; [CO_2] 10 mEq/L; and [K] 3.5 mEq/L. This patient has lost 10% of her body weight but is asymptomatic because of relative preservation of the ECF space in hypernatremia. That percentage of the total fluid deficit (ie, 500 mL) that is to be replaced as solute-free water is calculated as follows:

$$\text{Free water (mL)} = [160 - 145\ \text{mEq/L}] \times 4\ \text{mL/kg} \times 5\ \text{kg} = 300\ \text{mL}$$

This is given slowly over 2 days to lower serum Na by approximately 10 mEq per liter. The other 200 mL of the deficit are also given slowly over 2 days as solute-containing fluid. Calculation of the Na deficit (ie, the amount of Na to put in the remaining 200 mL of volume deficit) can be made from any one of a number of general formulas based on certain fundamental assumptions about fluid and electrolyte physiology as discussed elsewhere (see Chapter 14). If one views the solute-containing fluid deficit as coming 40% from the ICF and 60% from the ECF, then deficits of Na and K are as follows:

1. ECF: 60% × 200 mL × 145 mEq/L, [Na] = 17 mEq
2. ICF: 40% × 200 mL × 150 mEq/L, [K] = 12 mEq

For patients with increased insensible water losses, simple free water replacement with glucose solutions is all that is required. Here, monitoring weight and serum Na concentrations are useful guides to the adequacy of therapy. Correction can usually be given over several days.

The emergency treatment of the diabetes insipidus syndromes is free water replacement, monitoring vital signs and clinical signs of dehydration, and serum Na concentration as guides to the rate and volume of replacement. There is no place for the various antidiuretic agents that promote ADH release or mimic its actions in central diabetes insipidus or for thiazide diuretics in nephrogenic diabetes insipidus as initial therapies.

Children who are victims of acute salt poisoning and who are severely symptomatic can safely have serum Na concentrations lowered rapidly, either by a combination of loop diuretics (furosemide 0.5–2 mg per kilogram every 12 hours) and glucose water administration or, rarely, peritoneal dialysis against a Na-free dialysate. The latter procedure should be carried out only in consultation with a nephrologist. Admission is recommended for any patient with symptomatic hypernatremia or severe hypernatremia per se (>160 mEq per liter) when the cause is not obvious.

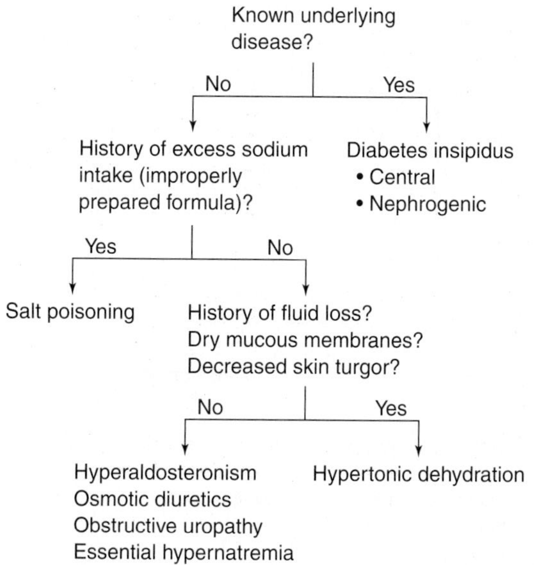

Figure 76.2. Diagnostic approach to hypernatremia.

Disorders of Potassium Homeostasis: Hypokalemia

CLINICAL MANIFESTATIONS

The cause of hypokalemia (Table 76.4) usually can be suspected as belonging to one particular diagnostic category after obtaining a careful history. Potassium depletion can result in

TABLE 76.4. Causes of Hypokalemia

Apparent potassium deficit (transcellular shifts)
Alkalosis
Familial hypokalemic periodic paralysis
Insulin
β_2 catecholamines
Decreased intake
Anorexia nervosa
Unusual diets (rare in pediatrics)
Extrarenal losses
Protracted vomiting (e.g., pyloric stenosis, gastric suction)
Protracted diarrhea
Ureterosigmoidostomy
Laxative abuse (rare in pediatrics)
Increased sweating (cystic fibrosis)
Renal losses
Diuretic abuse (naturetic, osmotic agents)
Renal tubular acidosis
Diabetic ketoacidosis
Excessive mineralocorticoid effect
Primary or secondary hyperaldosteronism
Bartter syndrome
Licorice abuse (rare in pediatrics)
Cushing syndrome (rare in pediatrics)
Excessive administration of "impermeant anions" (carbenicillin)

TABLE 76.5. Pathophysiological (Clinical) Consequences of Hypokalemia

Muscle cell dysfunction (rhabdomyolysis)
Cardiac cell dysfunction (myocardiopathy, arrhythmias)
Neuromuscular dysfunction (weakness/paralysis, ileus, tetany, encephalopathy with underlying liver disease)
Renal (polydipsia, polyuria, concentration defect)

widespread disturbances in cellular physiology and function, although symptoms are usually not seen at serum K concentrations above 3 mEq per liter. The major abnormalities and their clinical consequences are listed in Table 76.5. Impulse formation and propagation and the resultant muscle contraction are impaired in both striated and smooth muscle, leading to ileus, tetany, skeletal muscle weakness, and if severe enough, paralysis and areflexia.

Hypokalemia may cause rhabdomyolysis with myoglobinuria. Alteration of the cardiac action potential by slowing the rate of repolarization leads to conduction abnormalities and arrhythmias (see Chapter 72). Although the signs and symptoms of hypokalemia generally parallel its rate of development and its severity, electrocardiogram (ECG) changes often fail to correlate with serum K. They are helpful if present but not reassuring if absent. In the presence of digitalis, however, hypokalemia is much more likely to produce cardiac arrhythmias. Complications that require urgent diagnosis include acute respiratory failure from muscle paralysis, cardiac arrhythmias, and myoglobinuria, which can lead to ARF.

Generally, in situations of total body K depletion, a 1 mEq per liter fall in serum K concentration reflects a 100- to 200-mEq K deficit. The blood glucose rises in diabetes mellitus and creatinine phosphokinase with rhabdomyolysis. An increased BUN reflects contraction of ECF volume. If the electrolytes reveal a hyperchloremic hypokalemic metabolic acidosis with a normal anion gap and an alkaline urine pH, RTA should be suspected. When there is a hypochloremic metabolic alkalosis, the urine electrolytes are helpful. A urine chloride level less than 10 mEq per liter suggests vomiting, cystic fibrosis, or diuretic abuse as the cause of hypokalemia. A urine chloride greater than 20 mEq per liter points to one of the disorders that lead to mineralocorticoid excess. When the urinary K is less than 10 mEq per liter, several conclusions can be drawn. First, the K deficiency has probably been present for at least 2 weeks. Second, the kidney can be excluded as the route of K depletion. An elevated urinary K concentration, however, suggests either K wasting of short duration or a primary renal loss. In similar fashion, a urinary concentrating defect that persists in the face of a stimulus to concentrate bespeaks chronic K depletion.

MANAGEMENT

To manage hypokalemia in the ED effectively, one must delineate the source of the condition, as shown in Figure 76.3. When hypokalemia results from simple transcellular shifts in response to alkalosis without an accompanying K deficit, correction of the pH is all that is required. It is estimated that for every 0.1-U change in pH, there is an average inverse change in the serum potassium of 0.6 mEq per liter. In periodic paralysis, K supplementation with 2 to 6 mEq per kilogram of body weight per day is recommended, along with careful monitoring of serum K to avoid hyperkalemia as paralysis subsides. In most circumstances, K repletion should be slow (over days) and given by the oral route once urine flow is confirmed. Intravenous loading should be avoided except under special conditions. Despite the fact that ECF K concentration does not reflect accurately total body K deficits, serum K concentration is the only practical way

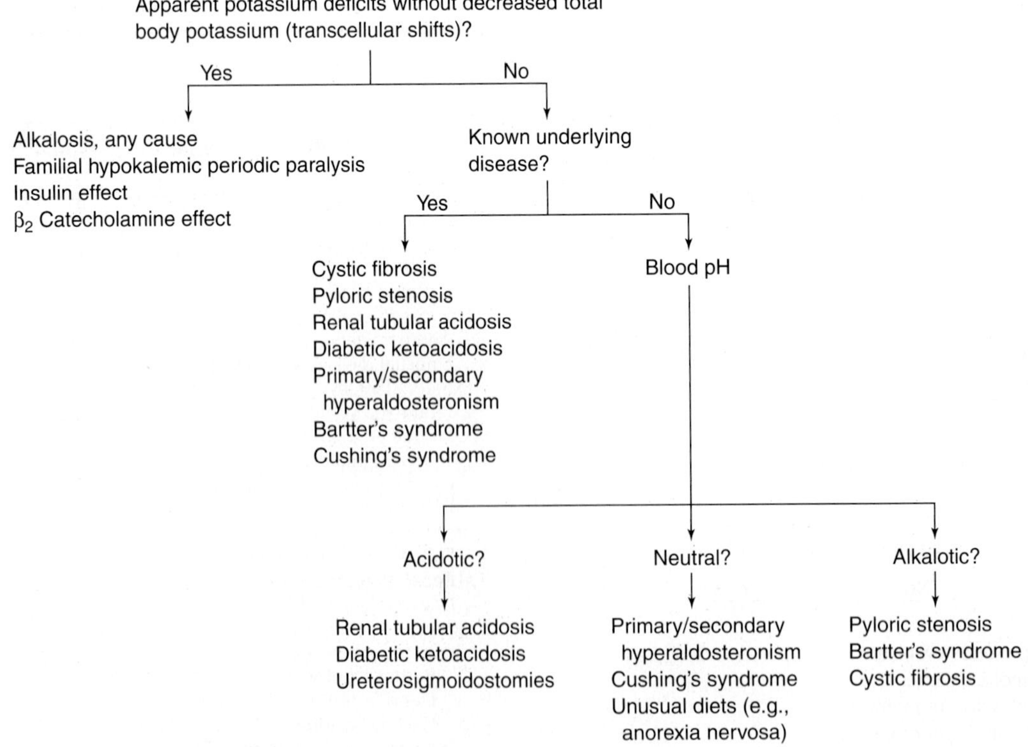

Figure 76.3. Diagnostic approach to hypokalemia.

TABLE 76.6. Twenty-kg Child; Total Body Potassium =40–50 mEq/kg or 800–1,000 mEq

Serum K (mg/L)	Plasma pH	K deficit (%)
2.9	7.6	18
2.5	7.5	15
3.0	7.4	10
3.5	7.3	10

K, potassium.

to assess adequacy of replacement and avoid unwanted complications. An estimate of the K deficit is generally obtained from the degree of hypokalemia and the blood pH, and it can be replaced over 2 to 3 days (assuming no ongoing losses) (Table 76.6). If intravenous replacement must be used, no more than 40 mEq per liter of K should be given by peripheral vein and 80 mEq per liter by central vein. In terms of the quantitative rate of repair, this should be no more than 0.2 to 0.3 mEq K per kilogram per hour. If, however, potentially life-threatening conditions such as cardiac arrhythmias or respiratory paralysis are evident, up to 1 mEq per kilogram per hour can be given by infusion pump with continuous ECG monitoring. Finally, selection of the specific K salt used in repairing deficits is important. Generally, potassium chloride should be used if alkalosis is present, and potassium bicarbonate or its equivalent should be used if there is acidosis. In states of ECF volume depletion from any cause, volume replacement with isotonic saline is as important as K replacement in normalizing serum K and turning off renal K wasting. The child with symptomatic hypokalemia requires admission for therapy and monitoring (and possibly for diagnostic workup), as do most children with a serum K of less than 3.0 mEq per liter.

Disorders of Potassium Homeostasis: Hyperkalemia

CLINICAL MANIFESTATIONS

The categories of hyperkalemia are shown in Table 76.7. The predominant symptoms and signs are neuromuscular. Paresthesias are followed by weakness and even flaccid paralysis. Major toxicity is reflected in the ECG. The earliest change is symmetric peaking of the T wave and then widening of the P-R interval. First-degree heart block, loss of the P wave, ventricular arrhythmias, and cardiac standstill may follow. In general, the ECG changes parallel the degree of hyperkalemia when it has developed acutely. The presence of any ECG changes associated with hyperkalemia mandates urgent diagnosis and therapy.

Although hypokalemia may cause rhabdomyolysis, hyperkalemia is often an early and life-threatening consequence of rhabdomyolysis from other causes. Elevated BUN and creatinine levels point to ARF. The urinary electrolyte pattern of the untreated patient can be helpful if adrenal corticoid deficiency is suspected. In acute adrenal insufficiency, urine Na concentration is inappropriately high and urine K concentration is inappropriately low for their respective serum concentrations.

TABLE 76.7. Causes of Hyperkalemia

Pseudohyperkalemia (hemolysis, extreme leukocytosis, or thrombocytosis)
- Apparent K excess (transcellular shifts)
  - Acidosis

Increased intake
- Endogenous (rhabdomyolysis, massive hemolysis)
- Exogenous (suicide attempt with K salts)

Decreased excretion
- Acute or chronic renal failure (oliguria)
- Adrenal corticoid deficiency (acute adrenal insufficiency, hyporeninemic hypoaldosteronism)
- Use of K-sparing diuretics in renal failure or in conjunction with dietary K supplements
- β-blockers converting enzyme inhibitors

K, potassium.

MANAGEMENT

Determining the origin of hyperkalemia is crucial before managing this life-threatening condition. Figure 76.4 provides an algorithm for ascertaining the cause. Three general techniques are used (Table 76.8) to lower serum K levels to normal: (1) reverse the membrane effects, (2) transfer K into cells, and (3) enhance renal excretion of K. If patients are asymptomatic, serum K is less than 6.5 mEq per liter, and the ECG is normal or reveals only peaked T waves, all that may be required is discontinuation of K intake, removal of K-sparing diuretics if they are being used, and treatment of acidosis. Exceptions occur in acute oliguric renal failure and rhabdomyolysis, in which the serum K level may rise to much higher levels precipitously, and a more aggressive therapeutic approach is indicated.

When ECG changes are more widespread or serum K is greater than 7.0 mEq per liter, several available therapies are designed to move K into cells acutely, including glucose and insulin combination and Na bicarbonate. The latter agent is effective even in the absence of acidosis.

With the onset of cardiac arrhythmias or a serum K level greater than 8.0 mEq per liter, urgent therapy is needed. Under continuous ECG monitoring, intravenous calcium is given first to reverse potentially life-threatening arrhythmias without altering serum K. Calcium accomplishes this by restoring a more normal differential between the threshold and resting transmembrane potentials. This then may be followed by glucose and insulin and Na bicarbonate.

For more long-term control of hyperkalemia, the cation exchange resin Na polystyrene sulfonate (Kayexalate) can be administered. Finally, for patients with oliguric renal failure, peritoneal dialysis removes potassium, although the immediate fall in serum levels may reflect redistribution caused by the alkalinizing effect of dialysis and the glucose load in the dialysate itself. The dosages of drugs used to treat hyperkalemia, the recommended rates of administration, and onset of action are detailed in Table 76.8.

Any child with symptomatic hyperkalemia or a serum K level greater than 6.5 mEq per liter on a nonhemolized sample deserves admission for therapy and additional workup.

Disorders of Acid-Base Homeostasis: Metabolic Acidosis

CLINICAL MANIFESTATIONS

Table 76.9 enumerates the causes of metabolic acidosis, and Figure 76.5 offers an approach to the diagnosis. The clinical manifestations of metabolic acidosis usually reflect the predisposing illness and are not unique in themselves. Nonetheless, in some patients, the presenting complaints appear to result primarily from the acid-base disturbance in that they resolve after bicarbonate therapy. The signs and symptoms include tachypnea with or without hyperventilation, abdominal pain, vomiting, unexplained fever, and lethargy. Tachypnea and hy-

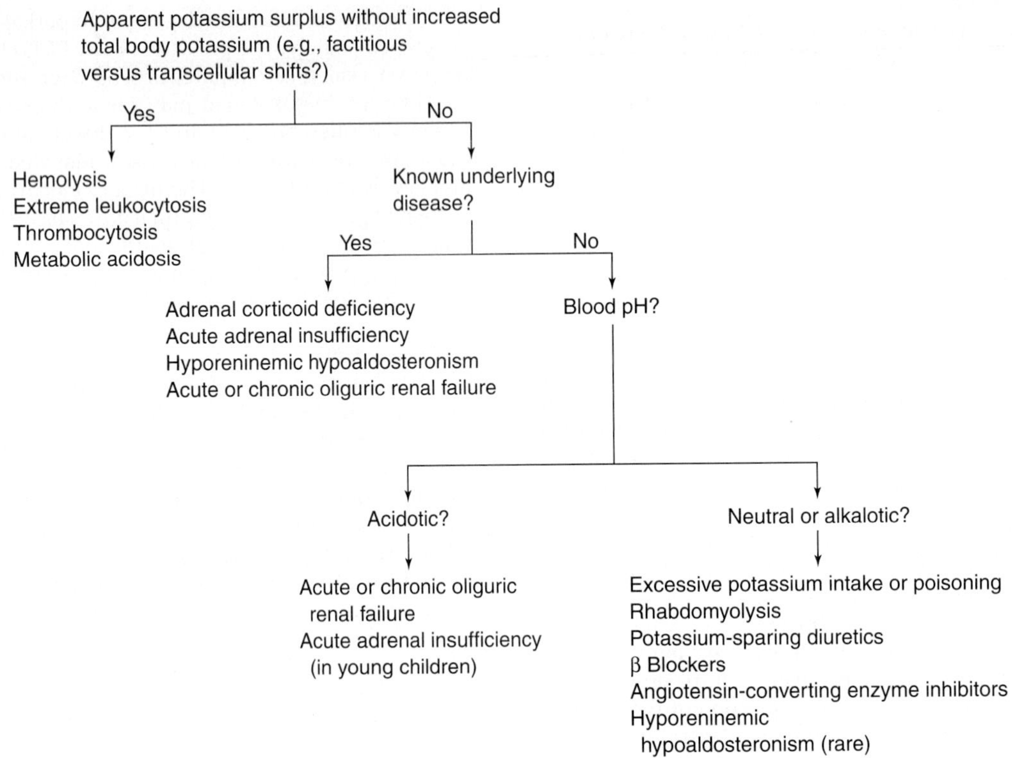

Figure 76.4. Diagnostic approach to hyperkalemia.

perpnea are characteristic of severe lactic acidosis, and coma may ensue if the pH is significantly depressed. There is often an associated but unexplained leukocytosis. A measurement of pH is needed to assess the potential urgency of alkali therapy, and the remainder of the arterial blood gas analysis is needed to assess the adequacy of respiratory compensation. The simultaneous measurement of blood and urine pH provides a clue to the diagnosis of RTA; this diagnosis is also suspected in the patient who has hypokalemia rather than normokalemia or hyperkalemia.

MANAGEMENT

The choice of therapy is alkali, and the preferred agent is almost always $NaHCO_3$. Sodium lactate, given as lactated Ringer's solution, is an acceptable alternative, provided liver function is normal and lactic acidosis is ruled out. Patients require treatment if the serum HCO is less than 15 mEq per liter or the pH is less than 7.20, unless the underlying disorder is simple diarrheal dehydration. In that case, discontinuing oral intake and administering intravenous fluids are usually the only therapies required. The diarrhea usually stops, and the kidney corrects the acidosis.

Of equal importance to the choice of alkali therapy is the amount of bicarbonate to use and the rate of repair. The bicarbonate or buffer deficit requires some estimate of the "bicarbonate space," which in health equals the ECF space of 20% of body weight in liters. Experimental studies in dogs, however, have suggested that the bicarbonate space is increased in severe metabolic acidosis to as much as 50% and, in lactic acidosis, even to 100%. The proposed reason for this is the movement of excess H^+ ions out of the ECF into other body compartments. Calculations of the HCO deficit therefore may be as follows:

Mild/moderate acidosis (pH 7.20–7.37):

HCO deficit in mEq = ("normal" serum [HCO] − "Observed" serum [HCO]) × 20% of total body weight in liters

TABLE 76.8. Emergency Treatment of Hyperkalemia

Technique	Agent	Dose	Rate of administration	Onset/duration of action	Comment
Reversal of membrane effects	10% Calcium gluconate	0.5 mL/kg	2–5 min i.v.	Min/30–60 min	ECG monitor; discontinue if pulse rate < 100
Movement of K into cells	Na bicarbonate, 7.5% (1 mEq ≈ 1 mL);	2–3 mL/kg	30–60 min	30 min/1–4 h	May use in the absence of acidosis;
	Glucose 50% plus insulin (regular)	1 u for every 5–6 g glucose	Same	Same	Monitor blood glucose
Enhanced excretion of K	Kayexalate	1 g/kg	Can be given in 10% glucose (1 g in 4 mL) every 4–6 h	Hours/variable	Can be given p.o. or by rectum

i.v., intravenous; ECG, electrocardiogram; K, potassium; Na, sodium; p.o., orally.

TABLE 76.9. Cause of Metabolic Acidosis

Elevated anion gap acidosis
- Diarrheal dehydration
- Diabetic ketoacidosis
- Renal failure (acute or chronic)
- Inborn errors of metabolism
- Poisons (e.g., salicylates, ethanol, ethylene glycol)
- Lactic acidosis (e.g., hypoxia, sepsis, idiopathic)

Normal anion gap acidosis
- Hypernatremic dehydration (older children)
- Renal tubular acidosis
- Hyperalimentation
- Enteric fistulas (e.g., pancreatic) or enterostomies
- Ureterosigmoidostomy
- Drugs (e.g., Sulfamylon, ammonium chloride, amphotericin, acetazolamide)
- Early renal failure (chronic interstitial nephritis)
- Dilution (rapid volume expansion)

Severe acidosis (pH < 7.20):

HCO deficit in mEq = ("normal" serum [HCO] − "Observed" serum [HCO]) × 50% of total body weight in liters

If the volume of infused solution must be limited, 7.5% $NaHCO_3$ (1 mEq/mL) is used; otherwise, lesser concentrations should be used. Full correction of serum HCO never should be attempted; a reasonable goal is to increase serum HCO in increments of 5 to 10 mEq per liter until a level of 15 to 18 mEq per liter is achieved or a pH of 7.25 or greater. At this point, maintenance HCO therapy can be continued at roughly 2 mEq per kilogram of body weight daily unless the underlying cause of the acidosis has been successfully treated. Overzealous alkali therapy is risky and can lead to a variety of complications, as outlined in Table 76.10. Any child who requires intravenous alkali therapy should be admitted to the hospital.

TABLE 76.10. Complications of Alkali Therapy in Metabolic Acidosis

Hypokalemia
- K^+ losses as part of the disease process (e.g., renal tubular acidosis, diabetic ketoacidosis)
- K^+ shifts into cells

Alkalosis
- Overcorrection
- Persistent hyperventilation
- Endogenous manufacture of HCO_3

Cerebrospinal fluid acidosis
- Delay in equilibrium of HCO_3 across the blood-brain barrier

Sodium overload

Hypocalcemic tetany
- Ca^{2+} binding to protein
- Ca^{2+} incorporation into bone

K^+, potassium; HCO, bicarbonate; Ca^{2+}, calcium.

SPECIFIC RENAL SYNDROMES

Nephrotic Syndrome

CLINICAL MANIFESTATIONS

Nephrotic syndrome is the clinical expression for a variety of primary and secondary glomerular disorders, the hallmarks of which are (1) hypoproteinemia (serum albumin <3.0 g per deciliter); (2) heavy proteinuria, initially or at some point in the illness (more than 40 mg/m^2 per hour in a 24-hour urine); (3) edema; and (4) less consistently, hyperlipidemia (predomi-

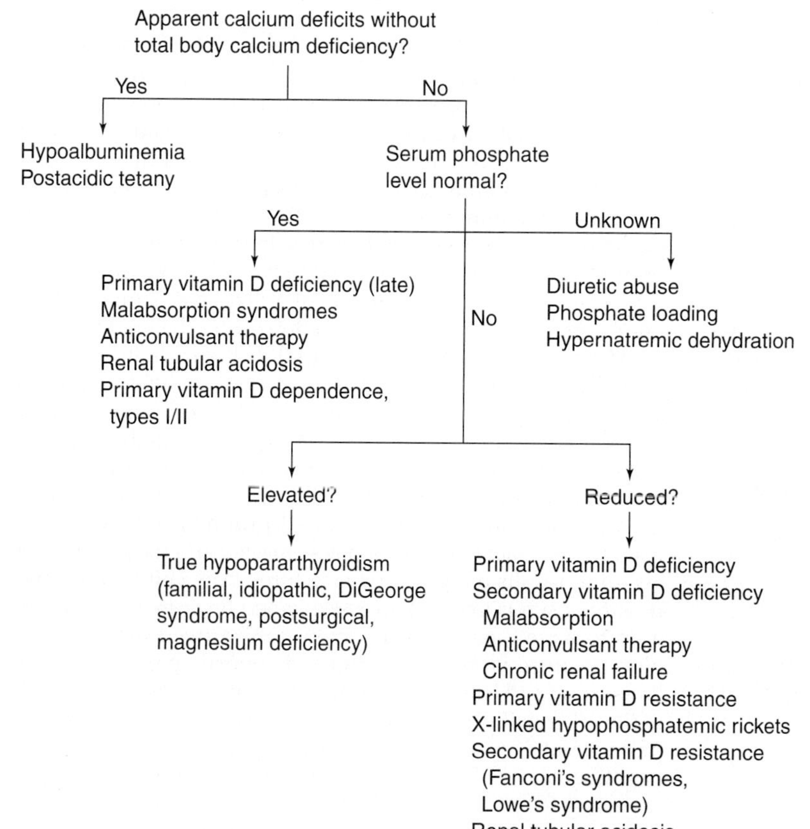

Figure 76.5. Diagnostic approach to metabolic acidosis (reduced serum bicarbonate for age).aAnion gap = serum [Na]mEq/L − [Cl$^-$ + HCO_3]mEq/L. Normal range in children = 16 ± 4 mEq/L.

nantly triglycerides and cholesterol). *Primary nephrotic syndrome* is the term applied to diseases limited to the kidney. These diseases are further classified according to the response to corticosteroid therapy and histology on renal biopsy. *Secondary nephrotic syndrome* is the term applied to multisystem disease in which the kidney is involved. Occasionally, nephrotic syndrome develops as a consequence of exposure to environmental agents, including heavy metals and bee venom.

PRESENTATIONS

The major presenting complaint is edema, which may be localized or diffuse. The degree of edema also depends on and varies inversely with the urine output, which is typically reduced in the full-blown case. In fact, in some patients true oliguria (<300 mL/m_2 per day) may be seen, although it almost never signifies ARF. Rarely, salt and water retention is abrupt and massive, leading to respiratory distress because of a combination of hydrothorax and ascites with elevation of the diaphragm. Ascites also may be associated with various abdominal complaints, such as anorexia, nausea, and vomiting, which are thought to result from edema of the intestinal wall because they disappear with successful treatment of the edema.

COMPLICATIONS

The acute complications of nephrotic syndrome occur in two groups of patients: (1) those who present *de novo* or in relapse but are not taking steroids and (2) those who present in relapse or remission while still receiving pharmacologic doses of steroids (Table 76.11). Bacterial infections are noted with increased frequency in both groups, although they are more common in the steroid-treated children. The types of infections include cellulitis, peritonitis, sepsis, pneumonia, meningitis, and arthritis. The typical signs and symptoms of infection may be masked in the steroid-treated nephrotic child, especially when the dose of steroid is high (eg, 2 mg of prednisone per kilogram daily).

Symptomatic hypovolemia, which can progress to shock despite the presence of edema, results from injudicious fluid restriction, excess diuretic administration, or a combination of both. This complication should rarely happen once the patient is under medical management. The problem is not total body water or salt depletion but intravascular depletion that results from the abnormal distribution of what amounts to excess total body salt and water in the interstitial spaces. The signs and symptoms are those that are common to any child with hypovolemic shock.

In steroid-treated children, acute rises in BP with symptoms of headache, blurred vision, or frank encephalopathy may occur at any point in the clinical course. The diagnosis of hypertensive encephalopathy does not require a specific level of systolic or diastolic BP. Rather, it is the degree of BP change and rate of rise that cause symptoms. Acute mood changes, ranging from euphoria to depression, are associated with the introduction, sudden increase, or decrease of steroid therapy. Symptomatic complaints include irritability with a low frustration level, hyperwakefulness at night, and emotional lability with crying and withdrawal. Abrupt reductions in steroids may lead to benign intracranial hypertension characterized by headaches, vomiting, and occasional papilledema, which are not associated with arterial hypertension.

TABLE 76.11. Acute Complications of Nephrotic Syndrome

Without steroid therapy	Hypercoagulability[a]
Bacterial infection	Respiratory embarrassment
Hypovolemia	Hypertension
Hypercoagulability (thromboembolic phenomena)	Altered behavior
Respiratory embarrassment	Steroid withdrawal (benign intracranial hypertension)
With steroid therapy	
Bacterial infection[a]	
Hypovolemia[a]	

[a] These complications occur more often after steroid therapy.

MANAGEMENT

Acute management of nephrotic syndrome can be divided into two categories: specific and supportive. In the ED, the primary goal is usually to restore and preserve intravascular volume or to treat symptomatic edema.

Despite the presence of peripheral edema, shock is treated in the usual way, with 20 mL of normal saline per kilogram of body weight per hour until circulation is restored (see Chapter 3). If the child is clinically dehydrated and hemoconcentrated (hematocrit >50%) but not in shock, a trial of Na-deficient fluids orally at twice maintenance is preferable to an immediate start of hypotonic intravenous solutions (ie, 5% dextrose in 0.25 N salt solution). Fluids should be given in small amounts (1–4 ounces) at frequent intervals (1 to 4 hours) to avoid vomiting caused by an edematous gut. Although Na restriction is indicated for an edematous nephrotic child, water restriction is rarely indicated and only further decreases a usually low urine output. The ongoing state of intravascular hydration can be assessed by serial hematocrit tests.

If the patient is well hydrated but symptomatic from massive edema, a trial of diuretics is warranted. Symptoms include difficulty in ambulating, abdominal discomfort, skin breakdown, and respiratory distress. Furosemide, 1 to 2 mg per kilogram per day in two divided oral doses, can be used. If there is no response, additional diuretics that act at other sites in the tubule (thus enhancing the diuretic effect) may be added. Commonly used agents are spironolactone and hydrochlorothiazide, both starting at 1 mg per kilogram per day in two doses. Diuretics do not usually work, however, if the serum albumin concentration is less than 1.5 g per deciliter. When it appears urgent to remove some edema fluid, a combination of albumin infusions followed 30 minutes later by intravenous furosemide is often effective. The dose of albumin is 0.5 to 1.0 g per kilogram given as 25% salt-deficient albumin followed by 0.5 to 1.0 mg of furosemide per kilogram. Paracentesis is rarely indicated but may bring prompt relief of severe respiratory distress from massive ascites.

Prednisone is generally begun at a dosage of 2 mg per kilogram daily in two or three divided doses after the workup is initiated and a tuberculin test is placed. If the patient has previously been responsive to prednisone and is on either no drug or a maintenance program, a return to full therapy is indicated, provided frank relapse is obvious. If not, a quantitative 24-hour urine test should be ordered. Concurrent administration of a low-sodium antacid may reduce the risk of gastric irritation.

Antibiotics are not administered prophylactically but are used when a bacterial infection is suspected and the physician is awaiting results of appropriate cultures. Any child with active nephrotic syndrome and an unexplained fever must be considered to have a bacterial infection until proved otherwise. A blood culture is indicated, and a diagnostic paracentesis for Gram stain and culture is appropriate in the presence of obvious ascites. Penicillin has been the appropriate first choice in the past to treat *S. pneumoniae.* In view of reports of increased Gram-negative bacterial infections in nephrotic children, it may be necessary to broaden this initial coverage with ampicillin, one of the newer cephalosporins, or an aminoglycoside.

TABLE 76.12. Hypertension

	Upper limit (mm Hg)	
Age (yr)	Systolic	Diastolic
0–2	110	65
3–6	120	70
7–10	130	75
11–15	140	80

Hypertension

CLINICAL MANIFESTATIONS

Hypertension reflects an elevation of blood pressure above the upper limits of normal (Table 76.12) and arises from numerous causes (Table 76.13) Hypertension usually presents in one of four ways. First, there is the asymptomatic or mildly symptomatic child with mild to moderate elevations in BP (130–150 mm Hg systolic; 80–94 diastolic). Acute symptoms are usually nonspecific and may include headaches, abdominal pain, epistaxis, and irritability. If the hypertension is chronic, failure to thrive, irritability, personality changes, and deteriorating school performance may be prominent complaints.

Malignant hypertension is characterized by marked elevations in systolic or diastolic BP or both (eg, 160 mm Hg or higher systolic for those aged <10 years; ≥170 mm Hg systolic for those aged >10 years; ≥105 mm Hg diastolic for those aged <10 years; ≥110 mm Hg diastolic for those aged >10 years) and often is associated with spasm and tortuousity of the retinal arteries, papilledema, and hemorrhages and exudates on funduscopic examination. This condition is seen much more commonly in adults than in children. *Accelerated hypertension* is defined as an acute rise in systolic or diastolic BP or both superimposed on previously existing hypertension. In both malignant hypertension and accelerated hypertension, the patient may present with dramatic symptoms and signs such as heart murmur, congestive heart failure (CHF), lower motor neuron facial palsy, and hematuria.

TABLE 76.13. Causes of Hypertension

Primary
- Essential hypertension

Secondary
- Renal
  - Acute or chronic glomerulonephritis
    - Postinfectious
    - Henoch-Schönlein purpura
    - Systemic lupus erythematosus
    - Membranoproliferative nephritis
  - Hemolytic uremic syndrome
  - Pyelonephritis (reflux nephropathy)
  - Obstructive uropathy (with or without urinary infection)
  - Segmental hypoplasia (Ask-Upmark kidney)
  - Renal vascular disease (renal artery stenosis, embolus)
  - Hemodialysis or renal transplant patients
- Endocrine
  - Pheochromocytoma
  - Cushing syndrome
  - Treatment with adrenocortical steroids
  - Hyperthyroidism
- Cardiac
  - Coarctation of the aorta
  - Congestive heart failure (multiple causes)
- Neurologic
  - Central nervous system infection, drugs, tumor
- Miscellaneous drugs or poisons

TABLE 76.14. Malignant Hypertensive Encephalopathy

Nausea, vomiting
Headaches
Altered mental status (neuropsychiatric symptoms, confusion, stupor, coma)
Visual disturbances (blurry vision, decreased visual acuity, diplopia)
Seizures, stroke

Hypertensive encephalopathy is often seen in malignant hypertension and consists of a combination of symptoms and signs that often vary from patient to patient (Table 76.14). No single symptom or sign is diagnostic of this syndrome; the diagnosis is confirmed by demonstrating a rapid improvement in the symptoms and signs after the BP is lowered. Although there is no generally agreed-on level of systolic or diastolic BP at which encephalopathy occurs, most investigators believe that the rate of rise in the BP is as important as the actual level itself. In this, as in all forms of severe hypertension (which are almost always secondary), the presenting complaints are usually attributable to the hypertension itself and not to the underlying disease.

Ascertaining the cause for increased BP in the acutely hypertensive child with an abnormal neurologic examination presents a difficult challenge (Table 76.15). In general, when there is primary neurologic disease with secondary hypertension, the hypertension is usually mild and predominantly systolic. To determine whether the hypertension caused the neurologic abnormalities or vice versa, the physician first must observe the neurologic response to lowering the BP. If signs and symptoms clear rapidly, he or she is probably dealing with true hypertensive encephalopathy. In addition, primary neurologic disease can be screened for by a spinal tap (if a mass lesion is not suspected) or computed tomography (CT) scan (if a mass lesion or intracranial bleeding is suspected).

When confronted with newly diagnosed hypertension in the child, the physician should ask three important questions: (1) Is the hypertension primary or secondary? (2) Is there evidence of target organ injury? and (3) Are there associated risk factors that would worsen the prognosis if the hypertension were not treated or were treated unsuccessfully?

MANAGEMENT

Acute Management of Hypertension

The spectrum of hypertension that presents to the pediatric ED ranges from mild and asymptomatic to a true hypertensive emergency (see Chapter 28). A brief but careful history and physical examination aim to classify the severity of the hypertension. When the hypertension is severe, this evaluation should progress only after the ABCs (airway, breathing, and circulation) of resuscitation have been accomplished. After several determinations of BP, a focused physical examination should be performed immediately. Emphasis should be placed on the neurologic examination, searching for any evidence of dysfunction.

TABLE 76.15. Differential Diagnosis of Hypertensive Encephalopathy

Head trauma	Brain tumor
Cerebral hemorrhage or infarction	Uremic encephalopathy
Meningitis, encephalitis	

TABLE 76.16. Drugs Used in Hypertensive Emergencies

Drug	Initial dosage	Administration	Onset of action	Interval to repeat or ↑ dose (min)	Duration of action	Acute side effects
Nitroprusside	0.5 μg/kg/min	i.v. infusion	Instantaneous	30–60	Only during infusion	Headache; abdominal pain; chest pain; NaCl, H_2O retention
Diazoxide	3–5 mg/kg (max. 150 mg/dose)	Rapid i.v. push into vein	Minutes	15–30	4–12 hr	Hyperglycemia; hyperuricemia; NaCl, H_2O retention
Hydralazine	0.1–0.5 mg/kg (max. 20 mg)	i.v. infusion over 15–30 min	30 min	10	4–12 hr	Tachycardia; flushing; headache; vomiting, NaCl, H_2O retention
Labetalol	0.25 mg/kg (max. 3–4 mg/kg)	i.v. infusion while supine	5 min	10	To 24 h	GI upset; scalp tingling; headache; sedation
Nifedipine	0.25–0.5 mg/kg (max. 20 mg)	Bite and swallow or sublingual (may aspirate from capsule, if necessary)	15–30 min	30–60	6 h	Dizziness; facial flushing; nausea
Phentolamine	0.1 mg/kg/dose	i.v.	Instantaneous	30	30–60 min	Tachycardia; abdominal pain

IV, intravenous; NaCl, sodium chloride; GI, gastrointestinal.

It is the presence or absence of acute end-organ dysfunction discovered in the history, physical examination, or laboratory studies and not the height of the BP that distinguishes a hypertensive urgency from a hypertensive emergency. Classifying the hypertensive episode as urgent or emergent governs the approach to treatment.

Hypertensive Emergency

In a hypertensive emergency, an intravenous line should be placed immediately to allow administration of medications and fluid resuscitation if indicated. It is important to note that many patients in hypertensive crisis have volume depletion most likely caused by vomiting, diarrhea, or a diuresis of unclear origin. A cardiac monitor and urinary catheter should be used from the outset. Continuous BP monitoring must be provided, preferably by arterial catheter. Any serious complications must be managed before or as the hypertension is treated (eg, anticonvulsants should be administered to a seizing patient along with hypertensive medications). Numerous medications are available for hypertensive emergencies, and the drug(s) chosen will depend on several factors. The following factors must be considered: the patient's clinical condition, the presumed cause, whether there is a change in CO (propanolol would be contraindicated in the presence of CHF) or TPR, and whether there is end-organ involvement (nifedipine would be contraindicated in the presence of intracerebral bleeding).

In a hypertensive emergency, the goal is to lower the BP promptly but gradually. The mean arterial pressure should be lowered by 25% over several minutes to several hours, depending on the nature of the emergency. For example, a patient who is seizing or herniating must have the BP reduced immediately. This is not so for a patient who presents with headache or vomiting. Once antihypertensive therapy is begun, the patient's condition must be assessed frequently, giving special attention to the BP and neurologic status. Precipitous decreases in BP can lead to avoidable neurologic deficits. Therefore, the preferred drugs are those that allow close monitoring of BP reduction (eg, those given in incremental infusions). Most hypertensive emergencies can be controlled given the availability of new classes of potent antihypertensive agents and the expertise to use them. In general, physicians treat hypertensive emergencies most effectively by becoming expert in the use of a few agents. Each of the most commonly used medications offers distinct advantages and disadvantages. Each clinical situation dictates the precise mode of therapy, but some general guidelines are usually applicable.

The medications described next are recommended for use in the emergency setting (Table 76.16). Sodium nitroprusside is an arteriolar and venous vasodilator that is invariably effective. After antihypertensive therapy has been instituted and the patient's end-organ disease has been stabilized, the patient must be admitted to the intensive care unit for close monitoring and further hypertensive management.

Hypertensive Urgency

A *hypertensive urgency* is defined as severe hypertension without evidence of end-organ involvement. Patients with known hypertension who present in an urgent hypertensive crisis may not

TABLE 76.17. Drugs Used in Hypertensive Urgencies

Drug	Dosage	Administration	Onset	Duration (hr)
Nifedipine	0.25–0.5 mg/kg	Bite and swallow or sublingual	15–30 min	6
Captopril	Age <6 mo 0.05–0.5 mg/kg; age >60 mo 0.3–2.0 mg/kg	p.o.	15–30 min	8–12
Minoxidil	2.5–5.0 mg	p.o.	2 h	12

p.o., orally.

TABLE 76.18. Causes of Acute Renal Failure[a]

Prerenal
- Decreased cardiac output (cardiogenic shock)
- Decreased intravascular volume (hemorrhage, dehydration, "third-spacing")

Renal
- Primary renal parenchymal disease
  - Vascular (acute glomerulonephritis, HUS)
  - Interstitial (pyelonephritis, drug-induced)
- Acute tubular necrosis
  - Ischemic injury
  - Nephrotoxic injury (antibiotics, uric acid)
  - Pigmenturia (myoglobinuria, hemoglobinuria)

Postrenal
- Obstructive uropathy
  - Posterior urethral valves
  - Intraabdominal tumor
  - Nephrolithiasis (rare)
- Renal vein thrombosis (rare outside of the neonatal period)

HUS, hemolytic uremic syndrome;
[a] Major pediatric causes of acute renal failure are listed in parentheses.

require hospitalization if the therapy in the ED is successful and adequate follow-up can be ensured. Often, oral antihypertensive agents will be sufficient (Table 76.17), although on some occasions parenteral therapy will be indicated.

A 4- to 6-hour period of observation should follow administration of the antihypertensive agent in the ED. This should be done to identify any untoward effects of the medication, such as orthostasis. Patients should be discharged on the same medication used in the ED.

When hypertension is discovered by accident and is not the reason for the patient's visit, medical follow-up for repeated BP measurements is indicated before therapy is begun, especially if the elevation is mild (no more than 5–10 mm Hg above the upper limits of normal for systolic and diastolic pressures given in Table 76.12). If the BP is moderately elevated but the patient is asymptomatic, two options exist. Arrangements can be made for an outpatient workup in the future and a thiazide diuretic or a β blocker may be initiated at a low dosage. Alternatively, the patient may be admitted to begin an evaluation and therapy under hospital observation.

Acute Renal Failure

CLINICAL MANIFESTATIONS

Presentation

The presentation of ARF varies and usually relates to the underlying disorder (Table 76.18) Typical symptoms and signs are given in Table 76.19, together with the likely diagnosis. Most children are oliguric or give a history of "decreased urination." If solute retention is severe and has persisted for days to weeks before seeking medical attention, the clinical manifestations of uremia may ensue and obscure, for the moment, the underlying diagnosis (Table 76.20). One consideration that always must be raised in a patient with suspected ARF is whether it has occurred *de novo* or is superimposed on preexisting chronic renal failure. Clinical clues that may lead to the latter diagnosis are failure to thrive, a history of polyuria or polydipsia, continued good urine output despite historical and physical evidence of dehydration, and physical evidence of renal rickets. Relevant laboratory data to support the diagnosis of chronic renal disease are reviewed later in this chapter.

COMPLICATIONS

It is the immediate or, occasionally, the delayed complications of ARF, not ARF itself, that confront the emergency physician with the most important diagnostic and therapeutic challenges. The major complications in terms of frequency and threat to life are disturbances in serum tonicity and water balance; severe hyperkalemia with impending or actual cardiac arrhythmia; CHF with pulmonary edema, usually secondary to hypertension; malignant hypertensive encephalopathy with seizures; urinary tract infection with associated urinary obstruction; and metabolic seizures.

LABORATORY AND RADIOLOGIC STUDIES

Of particular importance in differentiating the three anatomic forms of ARF are the urinalysis and the so-called urinary indices. In the critically ill patient who has not passed urine, a sterile straight catheterization of the bladder is appropriate to obtain a sample. The urinalysis is most helpful in separating glomerulonephritis from the other causes of ARF. In the typical case of acute glomerulonephritis, the dipstick shows large amounts of blood and protein, and red blood cells (RBCs), granular, and cel-

TABLE 76.19. Acute Renal Failure Presenting Symptoms and Signs

Symptoms	Signs	Likely diagnosis
Nausea, vomiting		Gastroenteritis (ATN)
Diarrhea	Dehydration, shock	Gastroenteritis (ATN)
Hemorrhage	Shock	ATN
Fever	Petechiae, bleeding	Sepsis, DIC (ACN)
Melena		HUS
Sudden pallor		HUS
Grand mal seizures		HUS
Fever, chills	Flank tenderness	Pyelonephritis
Fever, skin rash	Erythema multiforme, purpura	AIN
		HSP nephritis
Sore throat	Hypertension	PSGN
Pyodema	Edema	PSGN
Grand mal seizures	Congestive heart failure	PSGN
Trauma	Muscle tenderness	Myoglobinuria
Myalgia	Myoedema	Myoglobinuria
Antibiotics, diuretics		Nephrotoxic acute renal failure
Variable urine output	Suprapubic mass	OU

ATN, acute tubular necrosis; DIC, disseminated intravascular coagulation; ACN, acute cortical necrosis; HUS, hemolytic uremic syndrome; AIN, acute interstitial nephritis ("hypersensitivity nephritis"); HSP, Henoch-Schönlein purpura nephritis; PSGN, poststreptococcal glomerulonephritis; OU, obstructive uropathy.

TABLE 76.20. Acute Renal Failure: Clinical Uremia

Gastrointestinal	Neurologic
Nausea, vomiting, diarrhea	Apathy, fatigue
Hiccoughs, fetid odor	Psychiatric disturbance
Hematemesis, melena	Seizures
Cardiovascular	Asterixis
Pericarditis	Coma
Dermatologic	Peripheral neuropathy
Puritus	
Uremic "frost"	

lular (ie, RBC) casts are in the spun sediment. Patients with prerenal ARF and those with acute tubular necrosis typically have little blood or protein by dipstick and an unremarkable sediment save for hyaline casts. Occasionally, the latter group will have prominent numbers of renal tubular epithelial cells and epithelial cell casts in the sediment, but this is generally unhelpful.

The major differentiation of prerenal ARF from acute tubular necrosis is by urine concentration as measured by specific gravity. Typically, the patient with prerenal ARF has a concentrated urine (specific gravity >1.025), whereas the patient with acute tubular necrosis tends to have an isosthenuric urine (specific gravity 1.005–1.015). Hematuria by dipstick examination without corresponding RBCs in the sediment suggests hemoglobinuria or myoglobinuria as the cause of ARF, especially if pigmented granular casts are also seen. Renal tubular and bladder epithelial cells and epithelial cell casts are commonly seen in nephrotoxic ARF or drug-induced (hypersensitivity) acute interstitial nephritis. Eosinophils on a Wright's stained urine sediment make the latter diagnosis much more likely. Marked pyuria, leukocyte casts, and a positive Gram stain of the urine all support the diagnosis of acute pyelonephritis, with or without coexistent obstruction.

Urinary indices refer to the ratios of the simultaneously measured solutes sodium, creatinine, and urea, and osmolality in "spot" samples of blood and urine. The primary purpose of these indices is to assist in differentiating prerenal ARF from acute tubular necrosis (Table 76.21). Other diagnostic studies are outlined in Table 76.22.

MANAGEMENT

When confronted in the ED with a child who has ARF, the examining physician should always ask the following questions about therapy: (1) Is this prerenal renal failure and can parenchymal ARF be prevented by the appropriate fluid therapy? (2) Are there any life-threatening complications evident at this time that must be treated immediately? (3) Is there urinary tract infection with associated obstruction that must be relieved immediately? and (4) Are there indications for immediate peritoneal dialysis or hemodialysis?

1. If prerenal ARF is suspected from the clinical history, physical examination, and urinary indices, fluid resuscitation should be used. Confirmation of this diagnosis requires a resumption of normal urine flow and a decrease in solute retention after restoration of euvolemia. An approach to fluid resuscitation is outlined in Table 76.23. A single exception to this approach might be the patient who is euvolemic or even hypervolemic but in cardiogenic shock. In the critically ill, unconscious, or uncooperative patient with an uncertain urine output, placement of an indwelling urinary catheter helps monitor urine output accurately. One clinical condition that demands the use of mannitol and furosemide is myoglobinuria or hemoglobinuria. Here the purpose of therapy is to prevent tubular obstruction by pigmented proteins after ECF volume is restored. The order of therapy in Table 76.24 is revised; 1 to 2 mg of intravenous furosemide per kilogram of body weight is given initially followed 5 to 10 minutes later by 0.5 g mannitol per kilogram. After urine flow is established, an infusion of 5% mannitol in one-quarter strength saline can be administered as milliliter-for-milliliter replacement of urine until the pigmenturia has resolved. Finally, as indicated in Table 76.23, failure to respond to a fluid challenge or a fluid plus diuretic challenge has one of three explanations: (1) volume losses have been underestimated, (2) there is coexistent urinary obstruction, or (3) the patient has already developed parenchymal ARF. The major risk of mannitol occurs in a parenchymal ARF because if not excreted, it will recirculate and may cause ECF volume expansion.

2. Regarding life-threatening complications of ARF, the therapy of hypertensive emergencies has been discussed previously. Hyponatremia is common but rarely symptomatic in ARF unless it is the result of ECF volume depletion. In euvolemic or clinically edematous patients, the treatment is fluid restoration and no extra sodium. Hypocalcemia is also common but rarely symptomatic in ARF and should not be treated with supplemental calcium until and unless the serum phosphorus concentration is known. Failure to take this precaution may result in raising the Ca $\times$ P_i product and risk ectopic calcification or further renal damage. Metabolic acidosis does not need correction unless the serum bicarbonate is less than 15 mEq per liter, and only then with slow replacement with 1 mEq per kilogram per

TABLE 76.21. Acute Renal Failure: Urinary Indices[a]

	Acute renal failure	
Indices	**Prerenal**	**Intrinsic[b]**
Older children and adults		
U/P urea nitrogen	>8	<3
U/P creatinine	>40	<20
U/P osmolality	>500 mOsm/kg H_2O; >1.5	<350 mOsm/kg H_2O; <1.5
FENa (%)[c]	<1.0	>1.0
Neonates and infants		
U/P urea nitrogen	Variable	Variable
U/P creatinine	Variable	Variable
U/PO osmolality	>1.0	<1.0
FENa (%)[c]	>2.5	<2.5

[a] *Ux/Px* refers to simultaneously measured urine and plasma concentrations of *x*.
[b] Refers to classical acute tubular necrosis from various causes.
[c] Fractional excretion or filtered sodium = (U/P)Na/(U/P) creatinine × 100.

TABLE 76.22. Acute Renal Failure Laboratory Tests for Diagnosis

Test	Diagnosis
Blood	
Platelet count	HUS, DIC
Blood smear	HUS, DIC
Coagulation profile	HUS, DIC
Blood culture	DIC, acute pyelonephritis
Streptococcal serologies	PSGN
C3 complement	PSGN
Antinuclear antibody	Systemic lupus erythematosus-nephritis
IgE, eosinophil count	AIN
Aminoglycoside level	Nephrotoxicity
Creatine phosphokinase (CPK)	Myoglobinuria
Haptoglobin, "pink" plasma	Hemoglobinuria
Urine	
Culture	Acute pyelonephritis
Protein (24 hr)	Acute nephritis
Uric acid (24 hr or U_{uric}:$U_{creatinine\ ratio}$)	Uric acid nephropathy
Radiology	
Renal ultrasound	Obstructive uropathy
Intravenous pyelogram	Obstructive uropathy, pyelonephritis
Voiding cystourethrogram (VCUG)	Underlying chronic renal disease, obstructive uropathy
Renal flow scan	Acute tubular necrosis (cortical necrosis), renal vascular insult

HUS, hemolytic uremic syndrome; DIC, disseminated intravascular coagulation (bacterial sepsis); PSGN, poststreptococcal glomerulonephritis; AIN, acute interstitial nephritis ("hypersensitivity" nephritis).

day of bicarbonate and frequent monitoring. "Overshoot" alkalosis can easily occur in the face of a rapidly changing glomerular filtration rate (GFR) and urine flow. Also, a sudden shift of the pH toward normal or an alkaline range can convert asymptomatic hypocalcemia into frank tetany. Treatment of hyperkalemia is often the most urgent goal in ARF. Specifics of therapy for varying levels of serum K are outlined in Table 76.24.

3. If the clinical picture, urinalysis, and Gram stain suggest urinary tract infection, then coexistent obstructive uropathy must be ruled out rapidly. It can be suspected immediately because acute pyelonephritis in the unobstructed patient rarely causes ARF. Absence of a history of difficulty voiding or failure to palpate an enlarged bladder does not rule out obstruction, and a renal ultrasound should be obtained.

TABLE 76.23. Acute Renal Failure (ARF): Immediate Therapy of Prerenal ARF

Dehydration with shock
- 20 mL/kg/hr of crystalloid solution[a] until vital signs stable and urine flow reestablished (6–10 mL/kg/h)
- Repeat hourly if necessary for 1–2 doses
- After hour 2 or 3, if no urine flow, catheterize
- If no urine in bladder, give furosemide, 2 mg/kg i.v.[b]
- If no urine flow, treat as parenchymal ARF

Hemorrhage with shock
- 20 mL/kg/hr of plasma, or if unavailable, crystalloid solution as listed in *I.A*
- Transfuse when blood available (whole fresh blood or packed red blood cells plus fresh-frozen plasma)
- After hour 2 or 3, if no urine flow, catheterize
- If no urine in bladder, give furosemide, 2 mg/kg i.v.[b]
- If no urine flow, treat as parenchymal ARF

[a] Normal saline; 5% dextrose in normal saline; 10% dextrose in one-quarter strength sodium chloride plus one-quarter strength sodium bicarbonate (37.5 mEq/L each).
[b] Mannitol can be substituted for furosemide at a dose of 0.5 g/kg (2.5 mL/kg of a 20% solution) infused over 10–20 min. A urine flow of 6–10 mL/kg/hr should be established in the first several hours.

4. The indications for dialysis are outlined in Table 76.25. Generally, peritoneal dialysis is favored over hemodialysis, although the latter may be more efficient at removing certain nephrotoxins and potassium. The reasons for favoring peritoneal dialysis are its ready availability, the relatively simple technique used, and its safety in terms of preserving cardiovascular stability or minimally disturbing cardiovascular instability. It is generally not recommended in patients with generalized vasculitis, heat stroke, or recent abdominal surgery.

Hemolytic Uremic Syndrome

CLINICAL MANIFESTATIONS

Historical features of diarrhea-associated hemolytic uremic syndrome (HUS) include abdominal pain and diarrhea. Fever and vomiting may also be present, but it should be noted that *E. coli*

TABLE 76.24. Acute Renal Failure: Emergency Treatment of Hyperkalemia

1. Serum [K] 5.5–7.0 mEq/L (normal ECG): Kayexelate 1 g/kg po or per rectum[a]
2. Serum [K] >7.5 mEq/L or >7.0 mEq/L with abnormal ECG[b]
   - Step 1. Calcium gluconate 0.5 mL/kg as 10% solution over 2–4 min with ECG monitoring; stop when pulse rate falls 20 beats/min or to <100 beats/min
   - Step 2. Sodium bicarbonate 3.3 mL/kg of 7.5% solution
   - Step 3. Glucose 1 mL/kg as 50% solution; hyperkalemia persists, infuse a 20–30% glucose solution with 0.5 unit regular insulin/kg; keep blood sugar <300 mg/dL
3. Serum [K] persistently >6.5 mEq/L: Dialysis

ECG, electrocardiogram.
[a] Kayexelate exchanges 1 mEq K for 1 mEq Na and lowers serum [K] by approximately 1 mEq/L within 4 hr. It can be administered orally with food or beverage, by nasogastric tube, or per rectum in 10% glucose/water (1 g in 4 mL) or in 20% sorbitol (50–100 mL). It must be retained for at least 30 min.
[b] Serum [K] >7.0 with a normal ECG can be treated as outlined in step 1.

TABLE 76.25. Acute Renal Failure: Indications for Peritoneal Dialysis

Uremic syndrome
Blood urea nitrogen >100 mg/dL
Persistent hyperkalemia (serum [K] >6.5 mEq/L)
Persistent metabolic acidosis (serum $[HCO_3]$ <10 mEq/L)
Persistent congestive heart failure
Oliguric acute renal failure secondary to hemolytic uremic syndrome or rhabdomyolysis with myoglobinuria

O157:H7 infection rarely results in fever. There may also be blood in the stool, and this is seen more often in *E. coli* O157:H7 infections. Within the first week after the development of these symptoms, the patient will experience an abrupt onset of pallor, listlessness, irritability, and oliguria. The onset of HUS is relatively explosive, particularly the change in skin color. Physical examination reveals a sallow complexioned, listless, dehydrated child who may have edema hypertension, petechiae, or hepatosplenomegaly. Neurologic manifestations may be striking in HUS; some degree of encephalopathy is present in most patients. Specific findings include obtundation, hemiparesis, seizures, and brainstem dysfunction. The initial impression may be that of a surgical abdomen, primary colitis, or intussusception when hematochezia is the predominant complaint; in these cases, a barium enema is often the first diagnostic test ordered.

Diagnosis of HUS is based on the clinical profile of hemolytic anemia, thrombocytopenia, and ARF. The anemia is severe in many cases with a hemoglobin of 5 to 9 g per deciliter. The reticulocyte count is mildly elevated, and the platelet count can drop as low as 20000/mm^3. The peripheral smear shows helmet cells, burr cells, and schistocytes, confirming the microangiopathic process. The urinalysis reveals hematuria, sometimes gross, with variable degrees of proteinuria and leukocyturia. Granular and hyaline casts often are seen in the urine sediment. Chemical studies reveal azotemia, metabolic acidosis, hyperbilirubinemia, and an increased lactate dehydrogenase (LDH). Routine stool cultures will not reveal *Escherichia coli* O157:H7. The presence of O157 antigen must be detected with a specialized antiserum directed at the antigen.

MANAGEMENT

The cornerstone of treatment remains early recognition and supportive care. Oliguric ARF is best managed by dialysis when any one or a combination of the following complications occurs: (1) BUN more than 100 mg per deciliter, (2) CHF, (3) encephalopathy, and (4) hyperkalemia, particularly if associated with an arrhythmia. Peritoneal dialysis has been shown to be as effective as hemodialysis. Treatment of the intrarenal coagulation with heparin or streptokinase is discouraged. The microangiopathic process is managed with transfusions of blood and platelets as clinically indicated. There has been no efficacy demonstrated in the use of fresh-frozen plasma (FFP) or plasmapheresis in the diarrhea-associated form of HUS; however, success has been reported after infusion of FFP in patients with the nondiarrheal form of HUS.

Acute Glomerulonephritis

CLINICAL MANIFESTATIONS

Various causes can lead to acute glomerulonephritis. These causes can be divided into conditions that affect the kidney and conditions that are more systemic in nature that may present with renal manifestations. The typical story is that of a 5- or 6-year-old boy who, 1 to 2 weeks after a sore throat, develops the sudden onset of brown, tea-colored, or grossly bloody urine in association with peripheral edema, particularly around the eyes, and a decreased urinary output. There may be associated cough and congestion. On physical examination, hypertension, both systolic and diastolic, is found. Some children are completely asymptomatic and present merely with abnormally colored urine. Rarely, patients may develop acute CHF or acute malignant hypertensive encephalopathy, dramatic complications of a sudden rise in BP caused by an acute reduction in GFR, with consequent retention of salt and water. These patients are particularly challenging for the emergency physician because the complications often mask the underlying disease. The history may or may not be positive for an antecedent infection. Generally, however, there is a latent period of 10 to 14 days after a sore throat and 14 to 20 days after pyoderma in poststreptococcal glomerulonephritis; 75% of children have edema and abnormally colored urine. This edema is usually firm in texture. The incidence of hypertension and oliguria varies from 25% to 33% of patients. ARF and nephrotic syndrome occur, but much less commonly.

The emergency physician always must consider an underlying chronic nephritis with an acute exacerbation when making the diagnosis of acute glomerulonephritis *de novo*. Underlying chronic nephritis may be suspected initially by the absence of a latent period between the antecedent infection and the onset of urinary abnormalities, an anemia disproportionate to the degree of renal glomerular insufficiency, and changes in the optic fundi of chronic hypertension. Poor linear growth is also a clue to the duration of glomerulonephritis and attendant renal insufficiency.

The findings on urinalysis are the most important in categorizing glomerulonephritis. Proteinuria, although a function of urinary concentration, is almost always greater than 2 on the dipstick, indicating that the protein present is not merely a result of the hematuria itself. RBC casts are the hallmark of acute glomerulonephritis from any cause. Leukocyturia also may be seen. In girls, urinary tract infection can present with proteinuria and hematuria, and so a urine culture always should be obtained in the initial workup. Routine electrolytes may reveal hyponatremia secondary to water retention, hyperkalemia secondary to oliguria, and, of course, azotemia with a raised BUN and creatinine. In nephrotic patients, serum albumin is reduced.

MANAGEMENT

The goals of the emergency physician are to recognize the diagnosis and to treat life-threatening emergencies secondary to hypertension. If CHF is noted, the head-up position, supplemental oxygen, and 0.5 to 1.0 mg of Lasix per kilogram of body weight administered intravenously are recommended. Hypertension may be treated with 0.25 to 0.5 mg of sublingual nifedipine per kilogram of body weight, 2.5 to 5.0 mg of intravenous diazoxide per kilogram administered by push, or 0.5 mg of hydralazine per kilogram given intravenously over several minutes. Nitroprusside is rarely required. Encephalopathy usually requires antihypertensive therapy only if the link between severe hypertension and the neurologic abnormalities was noted immediately.

Any child with acute glomerulonephritis who is oliguric or hypertensive should be admitted for close observation. In the mildly affected patient, discharge from the ED is reasonable if the patient is instructed to follow a low-sodium diet. A follow-up appointment with the primary physician is advised within 48 to 72 hours, and instructions are given to the family on following urine output and weight and observing for the signs and symptoms of hypertension.

Henoch–Schönlein Purpura

Antecedent upper respiratory tract infections are noted in one-third to three-quarters of patients with Henoch–Schönlein purpura (HSP), which is characterized by rash, joint swelling, abdominal pain, and renal involvement. The abdominal pain is described as colicky but often severe. The arthritis is migratory, affecting the larger joints. Swelling may not be present around these joints. The rash is symmetric and purpuric and most noticeable over the extensor surfaces of the arms, legs, and buttocks. Other rashes, including erythema multiforme, also may be noted. Renal involvement is variable but typically occurs in the first month of illness. Asymptomatic microhematuria occurs most commonly in 80% of affected patients. Azotemia is usually transient. The older the child and the later the onset of renal involvement, especially if there is nephrotic-range proteinuria or renal insufficiency, the worse the prognosis. Hypertension is uncommon. Routine laboratory studies that include complete blood count (CBC), electrolytes, serum proteins, and C3 complement are usually normal. The diagnosis is primarily based on clinical findings. There is no specific therapy for HSP other than the use of corticosteroids used acutely to treat the severe abdominal pain or arthritis that occurs in selected patients.

Renal Tubular Acidosis

Renal tubular acidosis is a syndrome characterized by a persistent hyperchloremic nonanion gap metabolic acidosis. In this disorder, the renal regulation of the bicarbonate reabsorption or regeneration is deranged. A child with RTA may confront the emergency physician in one of several clinical settings: (1) an acute urinary tract infection, (2) muscle weakness or an adynamic ileus of the bowel secondary to profound hypokalemia, and (3) least common, acute renal colic secondary to the passage of renal calculi.

MANAGEMENT

The immediate treatment of RTA in the ED depends on the severity of signs and symptoms of hypokalemia (see "Hypokalemia"). Therapy of this disorder is best carried out in conjunction with a nephrologist. Administration of alkali is the treatment of choice for most types of RTA. Overzealous intravenous alkali therapy should not be attempted, however, because a rise in blood pH often lowers serum potassium and may exacerbate symptoms of weakness or cardiac arrhythmia.

The most commonly used alkalis are sodium bicarbonate and sodium citrate. For patients with hypokalemic RTA, a portion of the alkali can be given as $KHCO_3^-$ or K^- citrate. Plasma bicarbonate and serum potassium levels should be determined every 2 to 4 days initially. For patients with hyperkalemic RTA (type 4), furosemide occasionally is required to return the potassium to normal. Rarely, exchange resins are indicated.

Urolithiasis

CLINICAL MANIFESTATIONS

Children with urolithiasis rarely present with the excruciating pain of stone passage as seen in adults. Pain occurs in the abdomen or flank in 50% of patients. In infants, such pain may be confused with colic, and occasionally a diaper that is stained or shows crystals will provide a clue. Hematuria, either microscopic or macroscopic, occurs in at least 90% of children with urolithiasis. Other symptoms include urinary frequency, dysuria, and, at times, urinary retention. A history of urinary tract infection is variably present. A family history of urolithiasis can be elicited in 50% of patients. Colic and hematuria episodes are most characteristic of calcium stones. The physical examination may reveal tachycardia and an increase in BP because of pain; fever may be seen in 15% of patients. Costovertebral angle or flank tenderness may be present.

MANAGEMENT

If the history and physical examination are suggestive of urolithiasis, one should proceed to the detection of the calculus (Fig. 76.6). A urinalysis is an essential diagnostic screen for stone disease. In most affected children, there will be microscopic or macroscopic hematuria; pyuria and bacteriuria also may be found. Crystal formation, if present in the urinary sediment, is an additional supportive and often diagnostic finding. Definitive detection of a radiopaque calculus relies on an imaging study. It is estimated that 95% of urinary calculi are radiopaque and can therefore be identified on a plain abdominal radiograph. Ultrasonography and spiral CT are usually definitive.

Once a calculus has been detected in the ED, attention should be focused on the recognition and treatment of the potential acute complications that may accompany urolithiasis. Such complications include pain (at times severe), urinary tract infection, or urinary obstruction. If a urinary calculus is not found

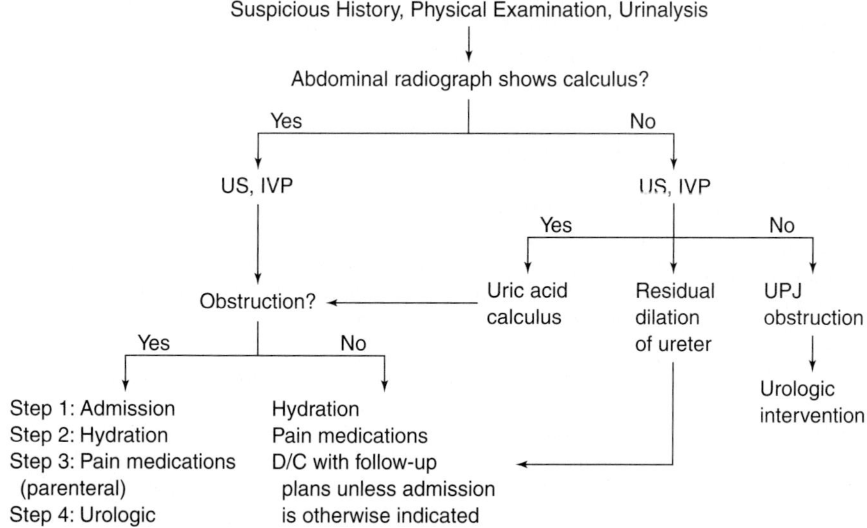

Figure 76.6. Diagnostic approach for evaluation for urinary calculi. *US,* ultrasound; *IVP,* intravenous pyelogram; *D/C,* discharge; *UPJ,* ureteropelvic junction.

with the aforementioned studies, but the history is suspicious of calculus disease, it is likely that the patient has already passed the stone and presently is suffering from the aftermath of stone passage (ie, spasm and dilation of the ureter). In this scenario, one must carefully examine the urine for crystalluria and hematuria as well as search for an increased Ca:Cr ratio.

For severe pain, relief should be provided promptly. Narcotic analgesics such as morphine sulfate or meperidine may be necessary. Nonsteroidal antiinflammatory medicines such as ibuprofen may have an important role in pain management if the patient can tolerate oral medications. Some patients may be unable to drink, and intravenous hydration may be required to ensure an adequate urine flow rate. If there is no evidence of urinary obstruction or renal insufficiency, fluids should be run at twice the maintenance requirement. When an associated urinary tract infection is suspected, appropriate antimicrobials should be initiated after culture. If urinary obstruction is entertained, a sonogram should be performed urgently and a urologic consultation should be obtained. Immediate treatment of an obstruction-inducing calculus includes extracorporeal shock wave lithotripsy, percutaneous nephrostolithotomy, or open stone surgery. All urine should be strained to assist in collecting gravel or stone particles for analysis. If a patient is known to have renal insufficiency, the management of superimposed urolithiasis should be done in conjunction with a pediatric nephrologist. Numerous indications exist for the admission of patients with urolithiasis (Table 76.26). If the patient does not fit into one of these categories, outpatient management is appropriate.

TABLE 76.26. Urolithiasis—Indications for Admission

Urinary obstruction	Solitary kidney
Intractable pain	Renal insufficiency
Dehydration	Inability to tolerate oral fluids

Chronic Renal Failure

CLINICAL FINDINGS

Many patients are not known to have CRF when they present acutely to the ED. Clues in the history are excessive fatigue, anorexia, vomiting, short stature, skeletal pain, polyuria, and polydipsia. On physical examination, signs of anemia, a fetid breath, chronic changes of hypertension, asterixis, and peripheral neuropathy are tell-tale clues. Signs and symptoms of CRF usually begin at a GFR 20% of normal or less and virtually always when the GFR reaches 10% of normal. Rapid falls in GFR may exacerbate the clinical picture.

MANAGEMENT

Disturbances in fluid electrolyte and acid–base balance, calcium and vitamin D metabolism, and cardiovascular and neurologic function predominate in end-stage renal failure (ESRF) and are outlined in Table 76.27. Anemia in ESRF has been managed successfully with a combination of effective dialysis and recombinant erythropoietin injections. CHF may be aided by improving the hemoglobin level and restricting or removing extra salt and water, either with diuretics or dialysis. Uremic pericarditis is less commonly seen in children than in adults and appears to correlate with the level of serum creatinine. The careful monitoring of water intake is required to avoid hyponatremia and hypernatremia because the kidneys' ability to modulate urinary water excretion is greatly reduced. Some patients also may exhibit a Na-wasting state despite the low GFR. Potassium retention is a significant risk in ESRF, particularly for patients who have not yet started dialysis. Uremia may block transcellular K transport in these patients. Accumulation of organic acids and the inability of the damaged kidney to regenerate new bicarbonate buffer explain the metabolic acidosis of ESRF. Modest doses of alkali normally correct this problem unless the patient is "Na-sensitive"; in that case, dialysis is indicated to avoid fluid overload.

TABLE 76.27. Metabolic and Clinical Abnormalities in End-Stage Renal Failure

Anemia
- Decreased erythropoietin production
- Hemolysis
- Blood loss (bleeding tendency)[a]

Cardiovascular
- Congestive heart failure[a]
- Uremic pericarditis[a]

Fluid, electrolyte, acid-base balance
- Reduced free water clearance, obligatory isothermia[a]
- K balance lost when glomerular filtration rate ??? 10 mL/min, hyperkalemia common[a]
- Metabolic acidosis (increased anion gap)[a]
- Vitamin D/Ca metabolism
- Hypocalcemia; hyperphosphatemia[a]
- Secondary hyperparathyroidism
- Osteomalacia (aluminum bone disease)

Immune function
- Increased risk of infection[a]
- Impaired host defense (white blood cell function)

Neurologic Function[a]
- Inability to concentrate, loss of memory
- Headache, drowsiness, coma
- Weakness, tremors, seizures
- Peripheral neuropathy
- Autoimmune dysfunction (sweating, swings in blood pressure)

[a] Improved with dialysis.

The neurologic disturbances noted in ESRF are what usually define the *uremic state*. Clinical manifestations are diverse but often respond dramatically and rapidly to efficient dialysis. Of particular note is the dialysis disequilibrium syndrome, characterized by headache, nausea and vomiting, visual disturbances, disorientation, wide swings in BP, and seizures. This condition is less common in children than in adults, but it occurs when initial dialysis (usually hemodialysis) lowers a significantly elevated BUN ($\geq$150 mg per deciliter) too rapidly, allowing water to move into brain cells and cause cerebral edema. Rapid infusion of mannitol is often effective in reversing these signs and symptoms.

Rhabdomyolysis

CLINICAL MANIFESTATIONS

Rhabdomyolysis may be caused by a number of disorders, including trauma, intoxications, seizures, infections, endocrinopathies, and metabolic defects, may lead to significant injury of skeletal muscle (Table 76.28). The classic triad of complaints in rhabdomyolysis consists of myalgias, weakness, and dark urine. In mild cases, particularly early in the course, myalgias may be the predominant manifestation, with or without mild weakness. The emergency physician should inquire about preceding viral infections, exercise, environmental conditions, injuries, bite wounds, ingestions, and medication use. Important considerations in the medical history include seizures, thyroid disorders, and diabetes.

TABLE 76.28. Causes of Rhabdomyolysis

Trauma	Amphetamines
Extensive muscle injury	Aspirin
Crush injury	Neuroleptic agents
Compartment syndrome	Monoamine oxidase inhibitors
Strenuous exertion	Succinylcholine
Infections	Envenomations
Influenza	Endocrinopathies
Sepsis	Hyperthyroidism
Toxic shock syndrome	Hypothyroidism
Rocky Mountain spotted fever	Diabetic ketoacidosis
	Inherited disorders of muscle enzymes
Tetanus	Miscellaneous
Hyperthermia	Polymyositis
Prolonged seizure	
Toxins/medications	
Ethanol	
Cocaine	

On examination, findings specific to rhabdomyolysis include tenderness of the muscles to palpation, decreased strength, and, less commonly, edema. The vital signs may be revealing of the cause in the case of hyperthermia. In some cases, trauma may be apparent, as in the form of a crush injury; however, patients with muscle injury secondary to vigorous exercise may manifest no local signs or minimal tenderness and edema.

The most reliable test for rhabdomyolysis is elevation of the CPK level to at least five times the upper limit of normal. The release of CPK occurs rapidly after injury to the muscle, peaks at 24 to 36 hours, and persists for several days. Levels as high as 50000 to 100000 U per milliliter are not unusual. The urine from patients with rhabdomyolysis may appear dark and test positive for blood with a reagent strip, but RBCs are not increased on microscopy. Other laboratory abnormalities include hyperphosphatemia, hypocalcemia, acidosis, hyperuricemia, and elevations of BUN and creatinine.

The major potential complication of rhabdomyolysis is ARF, resulting at least in part from myoglobin casts obstructing renal tubules. Renal failure manifests with oliguria or anuria and worsens the biochemical profile of the patient by increasing the plasma levels of hydrogen ions, phosphate, potassium, BUN, and creatinine.

MANAGEMENT

In addition to general supportive care of critically ill patients, when possible, steps should be taken to eliminate the inciting event. As an example, anticonvulsants are administered to interrupt status epilepticus and cooling is indicated for the patient with hyperthermia. Initial measurement of muscle enzymes and electrolytes is appropriate, and vital signs should be monitored. Therapy is directed at restoring vascular volume, when compromised, and facilitating blood flow to the kidneys in an effort to preserve renal function. Management begins with the delivery of a 20 mL per kilogram bolus of normal saline. In more severe cases, diuresis is achieved either with mannitol (1 g per kilogram) or furosemide (1 mg per kilogram). Depending on their severity, acidosis and electrolyte disorders may need specific treatment; occasionally, dialysis is required. Patients with significant rhabdomyolysis, as defined by markedly elevated levels of creatine phosphokinase (CPK) or myoglobinuria, require admission to the hospital.

CHAPTER 77
Hematologic Emergencies

Alan R. Cohen, M.D.

DISORDERS OF RED BLOOD CELLS

Severe anemia is a pediatric emergency that requires rapid evaluation and treatment to prevent hypoxia, congestive heart failure, and death. The classification of causes of anemia according to 1) blood loss, 2) increased red cell destruction, and 3) decreased red cell production is familiar to most physicians and provides an excellent starting point for the evaluation of the anemic child. In Chapter 51, these categories are used for the differential diagnosis of hematologic causes of pallor and for the appropriate selection of initial laboratory studies. In the section that follows, the same classification is applied to the emergency management of specific hematologic disorders.

Increased Red Cell Destruction

MEMBRANE DISORDERS

The anemia in disorders of the red cell membrane (hereditary spherocytosis, hereditary elliptocytosis, stomatocytosis, liver disease) is rarely severe enough to constitute a hematologic emergency. However, the hemoglobin level may fall even further when red cell destruction increases (hemolytic crisis) or red cell production slows (aplastic crisis). Hemolytic crises are usually associated with acute infections and are self-limiting. Most aplastic crises accompany parvovirus infection; anemia may be the only manifestation of the infectious process.

METABOLIC ABNORMALITIES

Like the red cell membrane disorders, erythrocyte metabolic abnormalities usually do not cause severe anemia. However, episodes of acute and sometimes life-threatening hemolysis can occur in many variants of glucose-6-phosphate dehydrogenase (G6PD) deficiency, including the A^- variant found in 10% of African-American boys, after exposure to drugs or chemicals (Table 77.1) or during an infectious illness. Ingestion of naphthalene-containing mothballs is the most common cause of severe hemolysis in children in the United States with G6PD deficiency, and parents should be asked about the presence of mothballs as part of the evaluation of any child with an acute hemolytic anemia. The acute intravascular hemolysis of G6PD deficiency usually occurs within 1 to 3 days of oxidant exposure and is characterized by pallor, malaise, fever, scleral icterus, abdominal and back pain, and dark urine. The anemia is accompanied by an increased reticulocyte count, and diagnostic blister cells are present on the peripheral smear. Treatment should include removal of the offending agent and fluid administration to prevent renal tubular damage. When hemolysis is severe, red cell transfusions may be required. However, if the diagnosis is uncertain, a pretransfusion blood sample should be saved for measurement of specific enzyme levels. Because enzyme levels are higher in younger red cells, the diagnosis of G6PD or other enzyme deficiencies may be obscured at the time of acute hemolysis and a high reticulocyte count.

TABLE 77.1. Drugs and Substances Associated with Acute Hemolysis in Children with Glucose-6-Phosphate Dehydrogenase (G6PD) Deficiency

- Antimalarials (primaquine)
- Sulfonamides (including sulfasalazine and trimethoprim–sulfamethoxazole)
- Nalidixic acid and nitrofurantoin
- Naphthalene (mothballs)
- Fava beans
- Aspirin (does not cause acute hemolysis with G6PD deficiency in African Americans when used in therapeutic doses)

AUTOIMMUNE HEMOLYTIC ANEMIA

Clinical Manifestations

Although this disorder may occasionally be indolent and may go undetected for days or weeks, autoimmune hemolytic anemia (AIHA) is usually associated with the sudden onset of pallor, jaundice, and dark urine. The hemoglobin level may be as low as 1 to 2 g per dL at the time of diagnosis. When the anemia is this severe, the child may appear moribund and desperately ill. Signs of congestive heart failure may be prominent.

The anemia is usually accompanied by reticulocytosis, although the reticulocyte count may be below 5% during the first few days of the illness. Occasionally, patients remain reticulocytopenic for prolonged periods. Spherocytes are often found on the peripheral smear, and red cell fragments may sometimes be present. Free hemoglobin in the urine produces a positive dipstick reaction for blood in the absence of red cells on microscopic urinalysis. When hemolysis is severe enough to exceed the renal clearance of hemoglobin, the plasma will be pink, and careful inspection of the plasma layer of a spun hematocrit may provide an early diagnostic clue. The direct Coombs test using broad-spectrum Coombs serum (immunoglobulin G [IgG], immunoglobulin M [IgM], and complement) is usually positive in childhood AIHA. Acute hemolysis is most commonly associated with IgG antibody and/or complement but may also occur with IgM-mediated disease. Although the antibody may appear to have specificity *in vitro* (usually in the Rh system), the shortened survival of "compatible" blood suggests the presence of wider activity of the identified antibody or the presence of additional undetected antibodies in many cases. However, certain specific antibodies are associated with infectious causes of AIHA, such as *Mycoplasma* (anti-I) or infectious mononucleosis (anti-i).

Management

The management of the child with AIHA should be aggressive because the hemoglobin level may fall precipitously (Table 77.2). Hospitalization for careful observation and treatment is usually necessary. The immediate institution of corticosteroid therapy (prednisone 2 to 4 mg per kg per day or equivalent doses of parenteral preparations) may prevent or reduce the need for red cell transfusions. Alternatively, the patient may be treated with γ-globulin 1 g per kg by intravenous (i.v.) infusion. For life-threatening AIHA, the use of steroids and γ-globulin should be considered. The response to steroids or γ-globulin in AIHA usually occurs within a few hours or days.

Red cell transfusions are hazardous in patients with AIHA and should be reserved for children with severe anemia and signs of hypoxia or cardiac failure. The presence of a nonspecific antibody in the patient's serum makes it difficult to find a unit of donor blood compatible in the major cross-match (donor cells and patient serum). The use of the "least incompatible" unit is a common practice, although data to support this approach are lacking. The best policy is to avoid transfusion when possible. If red cells are required and a compatible donor unit can be found, this unit should be used. Otherwise, ABO- and, if possible, Rh-compatible units should be administered despite the incompatibility *in vitro*. The recognition of the risks of transfusion in children with AIHA should not lead to the withholding of "incompatible" blood when transfusion therapy is required to prevent severe morbidity or death.

In rare instances, the hemoglobin level continues to fall despite steroids, γ-globulin, and red cell transfusion, necessitating alternative therapeutic attempts to sustain life. Plasmapheresis may remove sufficient antibody to reduce the destruction of the patient's erythrocytes and to allow improved survival of transfused red cells. If this measure fails, emergency splenectomy may be required.

NONIMMUNE ACQUIRED HEMOLYTIC ANEMIA

Acute hemolytic anemia in children may be caused by infections, chemicals, or drugs that damage the red cell directly. These disorders resemble AIHA in their clinical presentation and should be considered in the child with acquired hemolytic anemia and a negative Coombs test. Treatment is directed at elimination of the offending agent. Red cell transfusions are usually unnecessary unless anemia is severe (hematocrit less than 15%) or accompanied by signs of cardiovascular compromise.

ERYTHROCYTE FRAGMENTATION SYNDROMES

Red cells undergo fragmentation and lysis when subjected to excessive physical trauma within the cardiovascular system. Hemolytic anemias as a result of red cell fragmentation have been associated with abnormalities of the heart (valve homografts and synthetic prostheses, uncorrected valvular disease), great vessels (coarctation of the aorta), and small vessels (hemolytic uremic syndrome, thrombotic thrombocytopenic purpura, collagen vascular disease, hemangiomas). When hemolysis is a result of small vessel disease, treatment of the underlying disorder (eg, collagen vascular disease) or primarily affected organs (eg, renal failure in hemolytic uremic syndrome) is the first priority. Red cell transfusions should be reserved for the treatment of symptomatic anemia.

TABLE 77.2. Treatment of Severe Autoimmune Hemolytic Anemia

- Maintain normal or increased urine output with intravenous (i.v.) fluids.
- Immediately begin corticosteroid therapy with prednisone 2 mg/kg/day or a parenteral preparation in an equivalent dose.
  - Alternatively, administer γ-globulin 1 g/kg by i.v., alone or in combination with corticosteroid.
- Administer red cell transfusions when severe anemia is accompanied by signs of hypoxia or cardiac failure.
  - Give first 5 mL in 10–15 min and observe for symptoms of acute hemolysis.
  - Check plasma layer of a spun hematocrit for pink color indicative of hemolysis of the transfused red cells.
  - If symptoms or signs of worsening hemolysis are present, try a different unit of red cells.
- If hemoglobin level does not increase after transfusion:
  - Increase steroid dosage to 4 mg/kg/day; *or*
  - Administer i.v. γ-globulin 1 g/kg; *or*
  - Begin plasmapheresis or exchange transfusion; *or*
  - Perform splenectomy.

Decreased Red Cell Production

APLASTIC AND HYPOPLASTIC ANEMIAS

The differential diagnosis of aplastic and hypoplastic anemias is discussed in Chapter 51. Most of these disorders have a protracted course and, after initial stabilization of the patient, require intensive diagnostic evaluation and careful assessment of chronic therapy rather than emergency management. Transfusion should be used with particular caution in the initial management of patients with hypoplastic and aplastic anemias because exposure to human leukocyte antigen (HLA) and other antigens may adversely affect engraftment of transplanted bone marrow in patients who might otherwise have benefited from this procedure. If transfusions are required for severe anemia (hemoglobin less than 3 to 4 g per dL) and signs of cardiac failure or poor oxygenation, the goal of treatment should be relief of symptoms, not restoration of a normal hemoglobin level. When possible, filtered red cells should be used to decrease exposure to donor white cells, which contribute significantly to refractoriness to platelet transfusions. Related family members should not be used as blood donors. If the patient is cytomegalovirus (CMV)- seronegative, the use of filtered blood or blood from CMV-seronegative donors may decrease the likelihood of CMV-related complications if a bone marrow transplant is performed later.

NUTRITIONAL ANEMIAS

Nutritional anemias in children constitute more of a public health problem than a hematologic emergency. However, on occasion, the hemoglobin level may be very low at the time of diagnosis. Severe iron deficiency occurs mainly in 1- to 2-year-old children who drink 1 quart or more of cow's milk daily and have little room for other foods richer in iron. Adolescent girls make up another group at high risk for iron deficiency because a diet normally marginal in iron content becomes totally inadequate in the face of menstrual blood losses. The presenting complaint in severe iron deficiency anemia is usually pallor, lethargy, irritability, or poor exercise tolerance. In megaloblastic anemias such as Vitamin B_{12} deficiency in an infant exclusively breastfed by a vegetarian mother or in folic acid deficiency caused by impaired folate absorption, nonhematologic symptoms such as diarrhea, slowed development, or coma may be more prominent than the symptoms of anemia.

Stabilization and improvement can usually be achieved with replacement of the deficient nutrient. Nucleated red cells or reticulocytes usually appear within 48 hours of replacement therapy in folic acid or Vitamin B_{12} deficiency and within 72 hours of therapy in severe iron deficiency anemia. Because of this rapid response, red cell transfusions are rarely required unless symptoms associated with the anemia pose a serious threat. A response to replacement therapy should not preclude further investigation of the origin of the anemia, especially when the dietary history is inconclusive. For example, iron deficiency anemia may result from repeated small pulmonary hemorrhages or chronic bleeding from an intestinal lesion rather than from inadequate iron intake. Similarly, megaloblastic anemias may be caused by deficient intrinsic factor or abnormalities of folic acid transport rather than from a seriously altered diet.

Iron replacement therapy consists of 3 to 6 mg per kg per day of elemental iron given orally as ferrous sulfate in two or three divided doses. Parenteral iron is painful and dangerous. Moreover, the hematologic response to intramuscular or i.v. iron dextran is no faster than the response to oral iron. Replacement doses of 1 mg of folic acid and 100 g of Vitamin B_{12} daily are undoubtedly excessive, but their common use reflects the safety and the concentrations of the available compounds.

DISORDERS OF HEMOGLOBIN STRUCTURE AND PRODUCTION

Sickle Hemoglobin Disorders

CLINICAL MANIFESTATIONS/MANAGEMENT

Presentation

The diagnosis of sickle cell disease should be considered in African-American children with unexplained pain or swelling (especially of the hands or feet), pneumonia, meningitis, sepsis, neurologic abnormalities, splenomegaly, or anemia. The hemoglobin level and reticulocyte count are inadequate screening tests for the sickle hemoglobinopathies because values in affected patients (especially those with hemoglobin sickle cell disease and S-β-thalassemia) may overlap with normal values. Similarly, the peripheral smear may be devoid of sickled cells. Definitive testing for sickling disorders can be accomplished quickly by hemoglobin electrophoresis, isoelectric focusing, or high-pressure liquid chromatography (HPLC). If these tests are not available, standard solubility tests can be used to identify the presence of sickle hemoglobin. However, solubility tests do not distinguish patients with sickle cell trait, hemoglobin sickle cell disease, or other sickle variants from patients with sickle cell anemia (hemoglobin SS). Therefore, the results of solubility screening tests must be considered in the context of the clinical presentation and other laboratory studies. In addition, whether the screening test is positive or negative, confirmatory testing by hemoglobin electrophoresis or another method is mandatory in all patients with hematologic or nonhematologic emergencies that may be related to sickle cell anemia.

Sepsis

A combination of impaired immunologic functions, including early loss of normal splenic activity, contributes to the significantly increased frequency of sepsis in patients with sickle cell disease and the fulminant nature of this complication. The period of greatest risk is between the ages of 6 months and 3 years.

The treatment of the very ill-appearing child with sickle cell disease and probable sepsis should include the rapid institution of antibiotic therapy and aggressive management of septic shock. Because of the emergence of penicillin-resistant strains of *Streptococcus pneumoniae,* children in whom sepsis is strongly suspected should receive a third generation cephalosporin (cefotaxime or ceftriaxone). In areas with a high incidence of highly resistant *S. pneumoniae,* vancomycin may be added.

In many centers, children with sickle cell disease and fever who do not appear to be seriously ill, but who nonetheless are at increased risk for sepsis, continue to be admitted to the hospital for at least 48 hours. Ampicillin or a third-generation cephalosporin is usually administered i.v. until the cultures are confirmed to be negative. As an alternative to conventional inpatient management, other centers now treat selected children with sickle cell disease and fever as outpatients. This approach is usually restricted to children who do not appear acutely ill and who, on physical examination, do not have findings such as pallor, rales, or increased spleen size that indicate additional problems. Those children who do not appear to be seriously ill and who, on the basis of physical findings and results of laboratory tests, are judged to be at low risk for bacteremia, are treated in the emergency department (ED) with a long-acting cephalosporin such as ceftriaxone (75 mg per kg) and then discharged. A key component of the outpatient management of children with sickle cell disease and fever is a return visit or telephone report within 24 hours after discharge from the ED or short-stay unit.

Other Infections

Children with sickle cell disease are affected more often with infections other than sepsis in comparison with their hematologically normal counterparts. Meningitis, pneumonia, septic arthritis, and osteomyelitis may be responsible for substantial morbidity and mortality unless promptly recognized and appropriately treated. The level of suspicion for meningitis should be particularly high in the young, irritable child with sickle cell disease and unexplained fever. Antibiotic therapy of meningitis is similar to that recommended for hematologically normal children with this disorder (see Chapter 74). Exchange transfusion to lower the percentage of sickle hemoglobin may reduce the risk of intracerebral sickling and infarction in areas of local swelling and possible red cell sludging.

Acute chest syndrome, which includes pneumonia as well as pulmonary infarction, is one of the most common reasons for hospital admission for children with sickle cell anemia. The affected patient is usually tachypneic, even after antipyretic therapy. Rales, rhonchi, and physical findings of lobar consolidation may be present. However, in some children, particularly those who are somewhat dehydrated, physical findings may be far less striking. Rales may be heard only after several hours of rehydration. Because acute chest syndrome may escape detection on physical examination, a chest radiograph should be obtained in children with sickle cell disease and unexplained fever or chest pain. A decrease in oxygen saturation, readily measured in the ED and compared with baseline values, may identify patients with early acute chest syndrome.

Because a responsible organism for acute chest syndrome is nearly never known at the outset, treatment is begun with i.v.-administered ampicillin or a third generation of cephalosporin and modified according to the clinical response. In the very ill child, the identification of the causative organism should be pursued more vigorously with tracheal aspirate, aspiration of pleural fluid when present, or aspiration of lung tissue. Initial therapy of the child with severe acute chest syndrome should also include erythromycin. Oxygen should be administered to children with acute chest syndrome who have evidence of respiratory distress or hypoxia. Red cell transfusions or exchange transfusion should be used very early in the course when the patient is severely anemic (eg, hemoglobin less than 5 g per dL), is hypoxic, or has radiologic or other evidence of severe or rapidly progressive disease.

Septic arthritis and osteomyelitis present particularly difficult diagnostic problems in children with sickle cell disease because the clinical findings so closely resemble those found in infarctions of the bone. Closed or open bone aspiration should precede the institution of antibiotic therapy in the patient with suspected osteomyelitis. Similarly, aspiration of an affected joint should be performed if septic arthritis is strongly suspected. In most instances, swollen, warm, and tender joints are caused by local infarction. The presence of other sites of concurrent infarction and the patient's description of the pain as typical "crisis pain" may be helpful in identifying the cause as vasoocclusion. The total white cell count and differential count of the joint fluid may be similar in both septic arthritis and sterile effusion secondary to infarction. Therefore, the Gram stain and culture are especially important.

Vasoocclusion

Infarction of bone, soft tissue, and viscera may occur as a result of intravascular sickling and vessel occlusion. Children may have only pain or may have symptoms related to the affected organ (eg, hematuria in papillary necrosis, jaundice in hepatic infarct, seizures or weakness in central nervous system ischemia, respiratory distress in pulmonary infarction). Initial management usually centers around control of pain, general supportive measures, and differentiation of vasoocclusion and disorders unrelated to the hematologic abnormality.

The treatment of the child with a painful crisis requires an objective assessment of the severity of the discomfort and an appropriate use of analgesic therapy (Table 77.3). Once nonsickling disorders have been ruled out, hydration should be undertaken with D5 normal saline solution (NSS) or D5 NSS at a rate of 1.5 maintenance fluid requirements (see Chapters 4 and 76). The choice of analgesic is aided by familiarity with the patient's previous crises. Hesitancy to use parenteral narcotics may result in inadequate pain relief, mounting anxiety, and a loss of trust between physician and patient. For moderate or severe vasoocclusive pain, morphine sulfate (0.10 to 0.15 mg per kg) should be administered by i.v., and further therapy should be based on the degree of pain and the duration of pain control. Admission to the hospital is necessary if continuing parenteral analgesic therapy is required, fluid intake is inadequate, or the child has had several visits for the same problem.

Several specific areas of vasoocclusion deserve special attention. Between 6 and 24 months of age, dactylitis is a common manifestation of sickle cell disease. Infarction of the metacarpals and metatarsals results in swelling of the hands and feet. These episodes recur frequently. Pain usually resolves after several days, but swelling may persist for 1 or 2 weeks. Treatment is similar to that described for a painful crisis.

Infarction of abdominal and retroperitoneal organs may produce clinical findings that closely resemble the findings in a variety of nonhematologic diseases. The distinction between occlusion of the mesenteric vessels and appendicitis or other causes of an acute abdomen is, at times, particularly difficult. Hepatic infarction may also create a diagnostic dilemma because the acute onset of jaundice and abdominal pain that characterize this disorder are similar to the symptoms of hepatitis, cholecystitis, and biliary obstruction. The major emergencies related to vasoocclusion within the genitourinary tract are hematuria that results from renal papillary necrosis and priapism. Alkalinization of the urine may reduce bleeding but is difficult to accomplish and usually unnecessary. Administration of antifibrinolytic drugs such as ϵ-aminocaproic acid (EACA) (Amicar) (100 mg per kg every 6 hours) or tranexamic acid (25 mg per kg every 6 to 8 hours) may stop bleeding but carries a risk of ureteral clot formation. Priapism is an unusually painful and frightening form of vasoocclusion. The initial treatment consists of fluid therapy and analgesics (Table 77.4). Once again, red cell transfusions or exchange transfusion may promote resolution, but these forms of therapy should be reserved for patients without a rapid response to other measures.

Infarction of the central nervous system is a catastrophic form of vasoocclusion. The initial presentation varies from the

TABLE 77.3. Management of Vasoocclusive Crisis in Sickle Cell Crisis

Mild or moderate pain
Hydration—1 $^{1}/_{2}$ × maintenance with oral fluids or i.v. dextrose 5% (D5) 5$^{1}/_{4}$ normal saline solution (NSS) or D5$^{1}/_{2}$ NSS
Analgesia—Acetaminophen with or without codeine
Disposition—Admit if pain worsens, oral fluid intake is inadequate, or repeat visits to the emergency department have occurred
Severe pain
Hydration—1 $^{1}/_{2}$ × maintenance with i.v. D5$^{1}/_{4}$ NSS or D5$^{1}/_{2}$ NSS
Analgesia—Morphine sulfate, 0.10–0.15 mg/kg i.v.
Disposition—Admit unless pain is markedly reduced and patient can take oral fluids

TABLE 77.4. Management of Priapism in Sickle Cell Anemia

Hospitalize if erection persists or if pain is severe.
Intravenous hydration with dextrose 5% (D5)$^1/_4$ normal saline solution (NSS) or D5$^1/_2$ NSS at 1$^1/_2$–2 × maintenance for 24–48 h.
Consider aspiration of the corpora.
If swelling does not decrease, transfuse with red cells to raise hemoglobin level to 9–10 g/dL.
If no improvement after simple transfusion, institute exchange transfusion to reduce hemoglobin S to less than 30% of total hemoglobin.
Reserve shunting procedures for patients who have failed other forms of therapy in the first 72 h.

TABLE 77.6. Splenic Sequestration Crisis

Symptoms	*Laboratory findings*
Left upper quadrant pain	Severe anemia
Pallor	Increased reticulocytes
Lethargy	Mild to moderate thrombocytopenia and neutropenia
Signs	*Management*
Hypotension	Immediate volume replacement
Tachycardia	Transfusion with packed red cells or whole blood
Markedly enlarged and firm spleen	

mild and fleeting symptoms of a transient ischemic attack to seizures, hemiparesis, coma, and death. Physical findings usually define, and magnetic resonance imaging usually confirms, the area of cortical infarction. Supportive therapy should be instituted immediately (Table 77.5). A 1.5 or 2 volume exchange transfusion should begin as soon as the blood is ready. This procedure reduces the likelihood of further intravascular sickling and may prevent extension of cortical damage.

Splenic Sequestration Crisis

The sudden enlargement of the spleen with resulting sequestration of a substantial portion of the blood volume is a life-threatening complication of sickle cell disease. Because this crisis requires the presence of vascularized splenic tissue, it usually occurs before 5 years of age in patients with homozygous sickle cell disease but may occur much later in children with milder sickling disorders such as sickle cell trait or S-β^+-thalassemia. The patient undergoing a severe sequestration crisis may first complain of left upper quadrant pain (Table 77.6). Within hours, the patient becomes very pale, lethargic, and disoriented, and appears ill. The physical examination shows evidence of cardiovascular collapse; hypotension and tachycardia are often present. The level of consciousness falls. The hallmark of a severe sequestration crisis is a spleen that is significantly enlarged in comparison with previous examinations and is unusually hard. The hematocrit or hemoglobin level is much lower than during routine visits, and the reticulocyte count is usually increased (Fig. 77.1). Mild neutropenia or thrombocytopenia may be present.

Recognition of this complication should be immediate so that lifesaving therapy begins without delay. The rapid infusion of large amounts of normal saline or albumin is necessary to restore intravascular volume. Although a sufficient number of red cells to relieve tissue hypoxia may be released by the spleen after initial fluid resuscitation, transfusion with packed red cells (2 to 10 mL per kg) is often required in more severe cases. Whole blood transfusion may help relieve the dual problems of intravascular volume depletion and impaired tissue oxygenation. Reversal of shock and a rising hematocrit signal improvement of a sequestration crisis. The spleen gradually becomes less firm and smaller.

TABLE 77.5. Management of Stroke in Sickle Cell Anemia

1. Obtain computed tomography scan or magnetic resonance imaging to identify an area of infarction or to rule out a ruptured cerebral aneurysm or other intracranial bleed.
2. Immediately begin 1$^1/_2$–2 volume exchange transfusion to reduce hemoglobin S below 30% of total hemoglobin.
   a. Use whole blood less than 3–5 days old or use packed red cells less than 3–5 days old reconstituted with fresh-frozen plasma.
3. Reserve pretransfusion blood sample for characterization of red cell antigens in preparation for chronic transfusion program.

Aplastic Crisis

Increased bone marrow erythroid activity (as reflected by the elevated reticulocyte count and presence of nucleated red cells in the peripheral blood) partially compensates for the shortened red cell survival in sickle cell anemia and other hemolytic disorders. If erythropoiesis slows or ceases, this precarious balance is disturbed, and the hemoglobin level may gradually fall (Table 77.7). The event that most commonly causes erythroid aplasia is a parvovirus infection. Progressive pallor is unaccompanied by jaundice or other signs of hemolysis. If a red cell transfusion is required, a small aliquot is usually sufficient to raise the hemoglobin concentration to a level that ensures adequate oxygenation until red cell production recovers.

Hemolytic Crisis

Worsening anemia and increasing reticulocytosis may accompany viral and bacterial infections in children with sickle cell disease (Table 77.7). Scleral icterus is more prominent than usual. The findings are consistent with an increasing degree of active hemolysis. The hemoglobin level rarely falls low enough to require specific therapy. Hematologic values return to the usual level as the infection process resolves.

Thalassemia Major (Cooley Anemia)

CLINICAL MANIFESTATIONS

Children with thalassemia major usually develop a sallow complexion and increasing fatigue between 6 and 24 months of age. Weight gain and linear growth may be retarded. Physical examination shows pallor and enlargement of the liver and spleen. The hemoglobin level may be as low as 3 or 4 g per dL, and the mean corpuscular volume (MCV) is usually low. The red cells are hypochromic and microcytic with striking variation in size and shape; nucleated red cells are present in the peripheral smear. Thalassemia major is readily distinguishable from severe nutritional iron deficiency. In the latter disorder, the dietary history is grossly abnormal, organomegaly is uncommon, changes in red cell morphology are less impressive, and nucleated red cells are rarely seen in the peripheral smear. The diagnosis of thalassemia major should be considered in a child with severe microcytic anemia and an appropriate ethnic background. Although severe anemia is extremely rare in heterozygous thalassemia disorders, thalassemia trait and concomitant iron deficiency may be particularly difficult to distinguish from a homozygous thalassemia disorder.

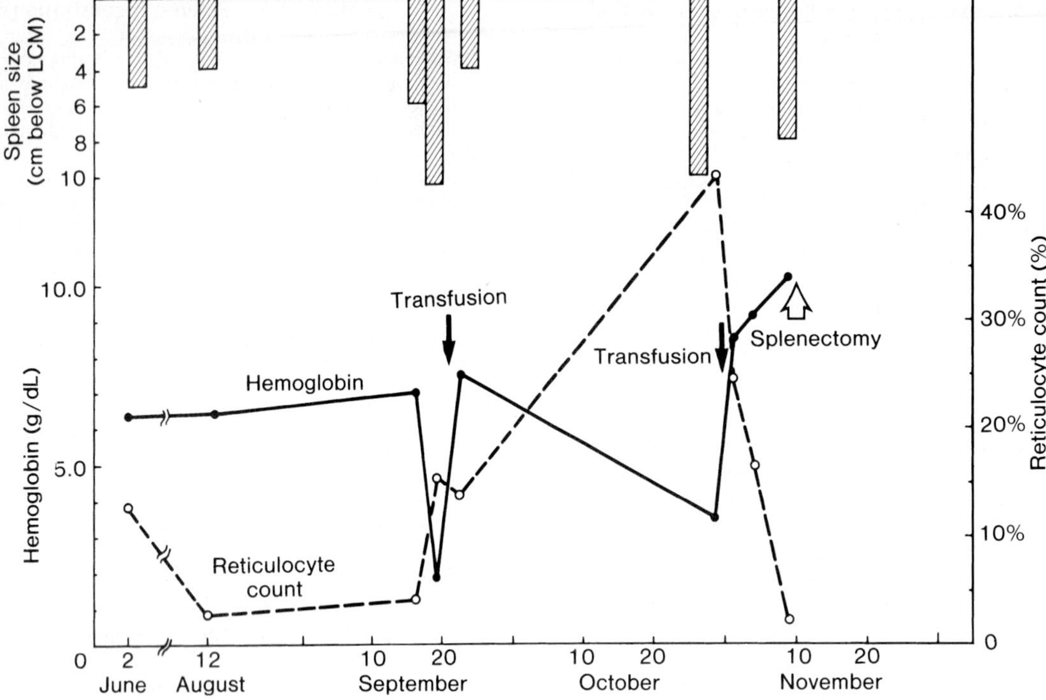

Figure 77.1. Clinical course of a 6-year-old girl with hemoglobin S-β^+-thalassemia and two splenic sequestration crises that were characterized by abdominal pain, increased splenic size, and a rapid fall in hemoglobin concentration.

MANAGEMENT

The moderate anemia usually apparent at presentation allows sufficient time for a careful diagnostic evaluation and outpatient transfusion therapy. However, when anemia is severe and congestive heart failure is present or imminent, the need for red cell transfusion may be urgent. In such instances, pretransfusion blood should be saved for appropriate diagnostic studies (hemoglobin electrophoresis) and initial red cell antigen typing. If transfusion is necessary, small aliquots of red cells (2 to 3 mL per kg) should be given. The administration of a rapid-acting diuretic (furosemide 1 mg per kg per dose) may diminish the risk of fluid overload. Partial exchange transfusion has also been recommended for patients with severe anemia to prevent further increases in intravascular volume and myocardial stress. Because patients with thalassemia major and severe anemia invariably have a lifelong dependence on red cell transfusions, the use of non–cross-matched blood should be scrupulously avoided at the time of presentation to prevent sensitization to foreign red cell antigens.

Methemoglobinemia

CLINICAL MANIFESTATIONS

Symptoms depend on the concentration of methemoglobin (Table 77.8). The diagnosis should be strongly suspected when oxygen administration fails to affect cyanosis. To eliminate an anatomic abnormality as a cause of oxygen-unresponsive cyanosis, an attempt should be made to oxygenate the patient's blood *in vitro*. As a rapid screening test, a drop of blood is placed on filter paper. After the filter paper is waved in the air for 30 to 60 seconds, normal blood appears bright red, whereas blood from a patient with methemoglobinemia remains reddish-brown. Arterial blood oxygen saturation is low when measured directly by blood oximetry rather than calculated, even though Po_2 is normal. Although blood oximetry measures oxyhemoglobin as a percent of total hemoglobin, including methemoglobin that is nonfunctional, pulse oximetry devices measure oxygen saturation of only that hemoglobin that is available for saturation. Thus, a patient with methemoglobinemia and obvi-

TABLE 77.7. Comparison of Findings in Sequestration, Aplastic, and Hemolytic Crises in Sickle Cell Disease

	Sequestration crisis	Aplastic crisis	Hemolytic crisis
Onset	Sudden	Gradual	Sudden
Pallor	Present	Present	Present
Jaundice	Normal	Normal	Increased
Abdominal pain	Present	Absent	Absent
Hemoglobin level	Very low	Low or very low	Low
Reticulocytes	Unchanged or increased	Decreased	Increased
Marrow erythroid activity	Unchanged or increased	Decreased	Increased

TABLE 77.8. Symptoms and Signs According to Severity of Methemoglobinemia

Methemoglobin level	Symptoms
10%–30%	Cyanosis
30%–50%	Dyspnea, tachycardia, dizziness, fatigue, headache
50%–70%	Lethargy, stupor
70%	Death

ous cyanosis may have normal oxygen saturation as measured by pulse oximetry. Spectrophotometric assays can be used for confirmation of methemoglobinemia as well as for determination of the level of methemoglobin.

MANAGEMENT

The treatment of methemoglobinemia depends on the clinical severity (Table 77.9). In all cases, an attempt should be made to identify an oxidant stress and, once identified, to remove the causative substance. If symptoms are mild after oxidant exposure, therapy is unnecessary. If the symptoms are severe, 1 to 2 mg per kg of methylene blue as a 1% solution in saline should be infused over 5 minutes. A second dose can be given if symptoms are still present 1 hour later. Because methylene blue can act as an oxidant at high dosages, the total dosage should not exceed 7 mg per kg. Failure of methylene blue to improve the course of methemoglobinemia may be a result of concomitant G6PD deficiency because the therapeutic effect requires an intact hexose monophosphate shunt. For patients with G6PD deficiency, ascorbic acid (500 mg orally) may be of some value, but if symptoms are severe, exchange transfusion or hyperbaric oxygen may be required. Even if treatment with methylene blue or ascorbic acid in the ED is successful, any child with symptomatic methemoglobinemia should be admitted to the hospital for close observation and further evaluation of the underlying abnormality or causative agent.

DISORDERS OF WHITE BLOOD CELLS

Neutropenia

The most common forms of neutropenia and abnormal neutrophil function are listed in Table 77.10. When the neutrophil count falls below 500 per mm^3, the patient exhibits an increased susceptibility to infection.

TABLE 77.9. Treatment of Methemoglobinemia

Methemoglobin level	Treatment
<30%	Not needed
30%–70%	Methylene blue, 2 mg/kg of a 1% solution, infused intravenously over 5 min[a]
Severely ill and no response to methylene blue	Hyperbaric oxygen or exchange transfusion

[a] If no response to two doses of methylene blue in a noncritically ill patient or a patient with known glucose-6-phosphate dehydrogenase deficiency, use ascorbic acid 500 mg orally.

The management of localized infection or unexplained fever in the child with neutropenia depends in large part on the underlying disorder and on the patient's history of infection. In neutropenic states associated with repeated, severe infections, an aggressive attempt to identify a causative organism should be undertaken. Blood and urine cultures, along with appropriate cultures from identified areas of infection (eg, skin abscess, cellulitis), should be obtained. The cerebrospinal fluid should be examined and cultured when central nervous system infection is suspected. If the child appears ill or toxic, broad-spectrum i.v. antibiotic therapy should be instituted with modification of therapy when culture results are available. Initial treatment should include antibiotics effective against *Staphylococcus aureus* and other Gram-positive organisms as well as Gram-negative bacteria, including *Pseudomonas aeruginosa.* If no source of fever is identified and the child appears well, observation in the hospital without antibiotic therapy may be considered.

Decisions regarding admission to the hospital and treatment are often more difficult in children with more benign neutropenic states. Although infections are usually mild and localized in these patients, severe infections rarely may occur. A white cell count and differential may be valuable because, in some children, the white count will rise to normal or near-normal levels during acute infection. Further laboratory investigation and treatment once again depend on the physical examination of the child and the history of infection. In most instances, antibiotic therapy can be reserved for children with a specific source of bacterial infection. However, careful follow-up is required for untreated children in whom fever is unexplained or attributed to probable viral infection.

A particularly perplexing problem arises when a child is found to be neutropenic during an evaluation of fever. In most instances, both the fever and neutropenia are results of a viral illness. Under these circumstances, serious secondary bacterial infections are unlikely to occur, and admission to the hospital and antibiotic therapy are probably unnecessary. However, because the neutropenia usually cannot be attributed with certainty to a viral illness, other causes of neutropenia should be carefully sought.

DISORDERS OF PLATELETS

Idiopathic Thrombocytopenic Purpura

CLINICAL MANIFESTATIONS

The diagnosis of idiopathic thrombocytopenic purpura (ITP) is made readily in the child with newly acquired petechiae and ecchymoses, thrombocytopenia, normal or increased megakaryocytes in the bone marrow, and the absence of any underlying disease. Epistaxis, gum bleeding, and hematuria occur less commonly than simple bruising and petechiae, but when persistent, these hemorrhagic manifestations can lead to moderate or even severe anemia. In teenage girls with ITP, heavy and prolonged menstrual bleeding can also cause a severe fall in the hemoglobin level. Fortunately, the development of anemia in children with ITP is gradual; acute, massive blood loss is extremely rare. The major life-threatening complication of ITP is intracranial hemorrhage.

MANAGEMENT

Controversy continues to surround the management of the patient with newly diagnosed ITP who has no serious bleeding. Until recently, the three approaches have included withholding therapy, i.v. γ-globulin, and corticosteroids. In many centers, patients are treated with γ-globulin at a dosage of 0.8 to 1.0 g per kg

TABLE 77.10. Causes of Neutropenia and Disorders of Neutrophil Function in Children

Congenital neutropenia
- Kostmann syndrome (infantile agranulocytosis)
- Chronic benign neutropenia
- Neutropenia associated with immunoglobulin disorders
- Reticular dysgenesis
- Neutropenias associated with phenotypic abnormalities (metaphyseal chondrodysplasia, cartilage-hair hypoplasia)
- Cyclic neutropenia

Acquired neutropenias
- Drugs and chemical toxins
- Infection (bacterial, viral, rickettsial, and protozoal)
- Bone marrow infiltration (leukemia, neuroblastoma, lymphoma)
- Nutritional deficiencies (starvation, anorexia nervosa, Vitamin B_{12}, folate, and copper deficiencies)
- Immune neutropenias (collagen vascular diseases, Felty syndrome, neonatal isoimmune neutropenia, autoimmune neutropenia, transfusion reactions)

Disorders of neutrophil function
- Cellular defects of chemotaxis (Job syndrome, "lazy leukocyte" syndrome, congenital icthyosis, chronic renal failure, diabetes, rheumatoid arthritis, bone marrow transplantation, malnutrition, infection)
- Secondary defects of chemotaxis (Chediak-Higashi syndrome, hypogammaglobulinemia, chronic mucocutaneous candidiasis, Wiskott-Aldrich syndrome, chronic granulomatous disease)
- Complement abnormalities and congenital absence of opsonin system
- Disorders of degranulation (Chediak-Higashi syndrome)
- Defective peroxidative killing of bacteria and fungi (chronic granulomatous disease, myeloperoxidase deficiency)
- Acquired disorders of phagocytic dysfunction (severe iron deficiency, malnutrition, malignancies, severe burns)

by i.v. infusion, with a second dose 24 hours later if the platelet count remains below 40000 to 50000 per mm^3. Unfortunately, one of the more common side effects of i.v. γ-globulin is headache, and when this symptom persists despite slowing the rate of infusion, imaging studies of the brain may be necessary to investigate possible intracranial bleeding. An alternative approach to the treatment of the stable patient with ITP is a 4- to 8-week course of prednisone, beginning with 2 mg per kg per day. Some physicians have argued that a bone marrow aspirate to confirm the diagnosis of ITP is unnecessary in the patient with typical findings of the disorder and an absence of neutropenia or anemia.

Currently, the most common option for treatment of acute ITP is the administration of antibody directed against the d-antigen of red cells. The effect of anti-d, usually given at a dosage of 50 μg per kg by i.v. infusion, is slightly delayed compared with γ-globulin, and the peak platelet count may be somewhat lower. However, anti-d has the advantage of being administered over minutes rather than hours, and it rarely causes severe headache. Mild to moderate hemolysis may follow the administration of anti-d with a fall in hemoglobin level of 0.5 to 2.0 g per dL. This therapy is effective only in Rh-positive patients.

For the patient with ITP and active bleeding, local therapeutic measures may be helpful until corticosteroids or infusions of γ-globulin or anti-d raise the platelet count to a hemostatic level or when these drugs become ineffective. Nasal packing and topical phenylephrine are useful for persistent epistaxis. Excessive menstrual bleeding may require hormonal therapy. If bleeding does not stop despite these measures, plasmapheresis should be undertaken and, if necessary, followed by a transfusion of 0.2 unit per kg (maximum 10 to 12 units) of platelets.

Intracranial hemorrhage, the major cause of death in ITP, requires immediate recognition and therapy. The child with mild head trauma and no symptoms or signs of intracranial bleeding should be observed carefully. Whether to treat the asymptomatic child is a common and perplexing problem. Although no firm rules exist, management should be based on the duration of ITP, tendency to bleed as demonstrated by petechiae or ecchymoses, platelet count, and likelihood of careful follow-up (Table 77.11). If the head trauma has occurred within 1 week of diagnosis, the patient is still having spontaneous bleeding, the platelet count is less than 20000 per mm^3, or follow-up is uncertain, one or two i.v. infusions of γ-globulin (0.8 to 1.0 g per kg) or anti-d (50 μg per kg) may be given.

If severe head trauma has occurred or if neurologic abnormalities are present, hydrocortisone (8 to 10 mg per kg) and γ-globulin (0.8 to 1.0 g per kg) should be administered by i.v. and random donor platelets (0.4 unit per kg, maximum 20 units) should be infused immediately thereafter. If necessary, the volume of plasma in the platelet preparation can be reduced by centrifuging the platelets, removing a portion of the plasma, and resuspending the platelets.

TABLE 77.11. Management of Head Trauma in Idiopathic Thrombocytopenic Purpura (ITP)

Mild head trauma without neurologic findings
- Observe carefully
- Administer γ-globulin 0.8–1.0 g/kg by intravenous (i.v.) infusion or anti-D 50 μg/kg if:
  - Platelet count is 20,000/mm^3
  - Signs of easy or spontaneous bleeding (e.g., bruises, petechiae)
  - Patient is within 1 wk of diagnosis of ITP
  - Follow-up is uncertain

Severe head trauma or neurologic abnormalities
- Hydrocortisone 8–10 mg/kg by i.v.
- γ-Globulin 0.8–1.0 g/kg by i.v. infusion
- Platelet transfusion 0.4 U/kg
- If neurologic changes are severe or progressive or if no response to earlier measures:
  - Splenectomy
  - Exchange transfusion or plasmapheresis, followed by platelet transfusion

If the platelet count of a patient with ITP and intracranial bleeding does not increase after steroids, γ-globulin, and platelet transfusions, or if the initial neurologic changes are severe, the patient should undergo splenectomy and, if appropriate, neurosurgical exploration. If the spleen has been removed previously and if steroids, γ-globulin, and platelet transfusions have failed to raise the platelet count, an exchange transfusion or plasmapheresis with subsequent platelet transfusion should be performed. However, this is a desperate situation and full recovery is unlikely.

DISORDERS OF COAGULATION

Inherited Bleeding Disorders

CLINICAL MANIFESTATIONS AND MANAGEMENT

Joint Bleeding

Hemarthroses are a common complication in hemophilia that often occur in the absence of known trauma in severe disease. Initial replacement therapy should be designed to raise the factor level to 30% to 50% (Table 77.12). Some centers treat all joint bleeds with one or two additional doses of factor replacement, whereas others reserve further treatment for patients with persistent pain or increasing swelling. Initial immobilization of the joint is often helpful and can be easily accomplished with a splint.

Bleeding in the hip is a particularly serious problem. As the joint becomes distended, blood flow to the femoral head may be impeded, resulting in aseptic necrosis. A radiograph of the hip shows widening of the joint space, and ultrasonography may demonstrate fluid. Because of the importance of achieving and maintaining hemostasis in this joint, initial correction to 70% to 100% is usually followed by several days of continuing replacement therapy (30% to 50% correction every 12 hours for factor VIII deficiency or every 24 hours for factor IX deficiency). Hospitalization may be required for immobilization, using either strict bed rest or traction.

TABLE 77.12. Specific Factor Deficiencies and Replacement Therapy

Factor deficiency	Replacement therapy
Fibrinogen (I) (also dysfibrinogenemias)	Cryoprecipitate Fresh-frozen plasma
Prothrombin (II)	Fresh-frozen plasma Prothrombin complex concentrate
Factor V	Fresh-frozen plasma
Factor VII	Fresh-frozen plasma Prothrombin complex concentrates Factor VIIa (recombinant) concentrate
Factor VIII	Factor VIII concentrates DDAVP
Factor IX	Prothrombin complex concentrates Factor IX concentrates
Factor X	Fresh-frozen plasma Prothrombin complex concentrates
Factor XI	Fresh-frozen plasma
Factor XIII	Cryoprecipitate Fresh-frozen plasma
von Willebrand disease	DDAVP Certain factor VIII concentrates

DDAVP, 1-deamino-8-D-arginine vasopressin.

Muscle Bleeding

Most muscle bleeding is superficial and easily controlled with a single dose of replacement therapy to achieve 30% to 50% correction. However, emergencies may arise when substantial blood loss occurs or when nerve function is impaired. Extensive hemorrhage is most commonly found in retroperitoneal bleeds (eg, ilealpsoas) or thigh bleeds. Retroperitoneal bleeds are often accompanied by lower abdominal pain. A mass is sometimes palpable deep in the abdomen, and sensation in the distribution of the femoral nerve may be diminished. Loss of the psoas shadow may be seen on an abdominal radiograph, and a hematoma may be demonstrated by ultrasonography. The hemoglobin level should be measured initially and, if bleeding persists, at regular intervals thereafter. Treatment consists of hospitalization, bed rest, initial correction to 70% to 100%, and maintenance of a 30% to 50% factor level until pain has resolved and ambulation has been successfully achieved.

Nerve paralysis and contracture are associated with bleeding into the volar compartment of the forearm or the lower leg. Consequently, hemorrhage in these areas should be treated with an initial correction of 70% to 100% and, if abnormal muscle or nerve function is present or if swelling increases, maintenance of factor levels above 30% to 50% until resolution of symptoms. Orthopedic consultation should be obtained to help assess the pressure in the soft-tissue compartment and to determine the possible role of surgical decompression. Patchy sensory loss is often associated with compression of superficial nerves and may persist for several months before normal sensation reappears.

Subcutaneous Bleeding

Hemorrhage under the skin may cause extensive discoloration but is rarely dangerous and usually requires no therapy unless compression of critical organs occurs. However, pressure on the airway from a subcutaneous bleed of the neck may be life threatening, requiring steps to ensure airway patency, such as placement of an endotracheal tube, in addition to correction of the factor level to 100%. Careful observation of children with bleeding in the muscles of the neck is mandatory because airway obstruction may be sudden.

Oral Bleeding

Mouth bleeds are particularly common in young children with hemophilia. The site of bleeding should be identified. If a weak clot is present, it should be removed and dry topical thrombin placed on the site. Initial correction should be 70% to 100%. Often, one or more additional treatments are necessary to achieve adequate clot formation and to prevent rebleeding when the clot falls off. The antifibrinolytic agents, EACA and tranexamic acid, are useful adjuncts in the treatment of oral bleeding. EACA should be administered orally for 5 days at a dosage of 100 mg per kg every 6 hours, with a maximum of 24 g per day. Tranexamic acid is administered orally at a dosage of 25 mg per kg three or four times daily. Because children may swallow a substantial amount of blood, acute, actual blood loss may be underestimated by the patient or family, and measurement of the hemoglobin level is helpful, particularly if bleeding has persisted for more than 24 hours. As in bleeds of the neck muscles, careful evaluation of airway patency is essential. Complete airway obstruction may result from extensive bleeding in the tongue.

Gastrointestinal Bleeding

Hemorrhage from the gastrointestinal (GI) tract is rarely severe in hemophilia unless an anatomic lesion such as a duodenal ulcer or diverticulum is present. Maintenance of the factor level above 30% to 50% for 2 or 3 days after initial correction to 70% to 100% is usually sufficient. If bleeding persists, appropriate diagnostic studies are necessary. A careful search for infectious causes of GI bleeding is important in human immunodeficiency virus (HIV)-positive hemophiliacs.

Urinary Tract Bleeding

Atraumatic, painless hematuria is the most common manifestation of renal bleeding in children with hemophilia. In the absence of trauma or a demonstrable lesion, several approaches to ensuring hemostasis seem equally effective. Bed rest without replacement therapy is often successful. In some centers, one or more doses of factor replacement (70% to 100%) are used in combination with bed rest for at least 24 hours after gross hematuria has ceased. A brief course of orally administered prednisone has also been effective. When the child with hemophilia develops hematuria or flank tenderness after trauma, a more aggressive approach to diagnosis and treatment is required.

Intracranial Hemorrhage

In practical terms, however, head trauma in children with hemophilia is common, whereas intracranial hemorrhage is comparatively rare. Thus, the physician must be able to recognize as well as treat the child at risk without exposing other patients to unnecessary hospitalization, diagnostic studies, or therapy.

The management of the hemophiliac child with head trauma but no neurologic signs requires careful attention to the severity of the bleeding disorder, type of trauma, history of intracranial bleeding, and likelihood of close follow-up. Children with seemingly insignificant trauma may develop the first obvious signs of intracranial bleeding several days later when concern has diminished. To prevent such occurrences, every child with severe hemophilia and reported head trauma is treated with at least one dose of replacement therapy in some centers. However, this approach carries the risk and expense of frequent therapy. Moreover, in an effort to prevent yet another visit to the ED, the child or parent may fail to report a serious episode of trauma. Consequently, other centers use an approach that is still conservative although slightly less rigid. If the trauma is mild (eg, a light bump on the forehead), the child is observed at home for the usual signs of intracranial hemorrhage or increased intracranial pressure. When the trauma is somewhat more substantial (eg, falling down two or three carpeted stairs), the child with severe hemophilia is evaluated by the physician, given replacement therapy to achieve a level of 70% to 100%, observed for several hours in the office or ED, and, if well, is discharged. The child with mild hemophilia usually does not need replacement therapy under these circumstances, whereas the child with moderate hemophilia needs particularly careful attention to the type of trauma and bleeding history for the physician to decide whether to use replacement therapy. A computed tomography (CT) scan may be useful in identifying intracranial bleeding that requires more intensive and prolonged treatment. However, the imaging study should not be used to decide on administration of an initial dose of replacement factor that should, in fact, always be given before the study is performed to avoid unnecessary delays.

If more severe trauma (eg, hitting the head on the dashboard, falling off a changing table onto a hard floor) has occurred in any hemophiliac child, hospital admission and repeated doses of replacement therapy are essential. The initial dose of replacement should be administered as soon as it is available. A CT scan should be performed after initial correction to search for intracranial bleeding and help determine the duration of treatment.

The management of the patient with hemophilia who has neurologic findings in the presence or absence of head trauma begins with replacement therapy and those measures required for life support and treatment of increased intracranial pressure. Levels of the appropriate factor should be raised to 100%. The indications for surgery are similar to those for children without coagulation disorders, provided an appropriate correction of clotting abnormalities has been achieved.

Acute neurologic changes, such as decreasing level of consciousness or seizures, may result from direct HIV infection of the brain or from associated infections that affect the immunocompromised host (see Chapter 75). In the HIV-positive hemophiliac patient, these changes may mimic the signs and symptoms of intracranial hemorrhage. Similarly, changes in vision that result from retinitis caused by CMV may be similar to visual changes caused by intraocular bleeding. The physician evaluating an HIV-positive hemophiliac patient with new neurologic findings should consider both infectious and hemorrhagic causes, and the absence of demonstrable hemorrhage on imaging studies should prompt careful attention to HIV-related disorders.

Bleeding in von Willebrand Disease

The sites of bleeding in mild von Willebrand disease resemble those found in patients with platelet disorders. Epistaxis, oral bleeding, and menorrhagia are common while joint bleeding is very unusual. Children affected with more severe forms, in which the factor VIII level is very low, may have bleeding problems that resemble those found in both hemophilia and von Willebrand disease.

REPLACEMENT PRODUCTS

Factor Concentrates

Recombinant factor VIII and factor IX products are presently used as a treatment for hemophilia for almost all newly diagnosed children and for most older children as well.

Prothrombin complex concentrates are used primarily for the treatment of patients with factor VIII deficiency and inhibitors (see below) and for the treatment of the relatively rare disorders of factor II, VII, or X deficiency. The use of this product for factor IX deficiency has diminished since the pure factor IX concentrates became available. Activated prothrombin complex concentrates are used exclusively in the management of patients with inhibitors.

Fresh-Frozen Plasma

Fresh-frozen plasma contains all plasma clotting factors and is therefore particularly useful when a child with a previously undiagnosed bleeding disorder presents to the ED with a hemorrhage that requires therapy before the specific factor deficiency can be ascertained. The recent availability of fresh frozen plasma that has been treated with a solvent-detergent solution to inactivate viruses with lipid envelopes (eg, HIV, hepatitis C) has increased the safety of this product. Nonetheless, its use is generally restricted to the treatment of an unknown inherited factor deficiency or a deficiency of a factor such as factor XI for which there is no available factor concentrate.

Cryoprecipitate

When plasma is frozen and then slowly thawed, the precipitate contains enriched factor VIII coagulant activity, von Willebrand protein, fibrinogen, and factor XIII. The availability of recombinant factor VIII and, to a lesser degree, plasma-derived concentrates with an excellent safety record, makes cryoprecipitate, which does not undergo virucidal treatment, an unsuitable choice for the treatment of factor VIII deficiency and a very unlikely choice for the treatment of von Willebrand disease.

Calculation of Dosage

Two formulas are commonly used for determining the number of units of factor VIII or factor IX necessary to achieve a specific level:

Factor VIII

1. Weight of patient (kg) × desired level of correction (%) × 0.5 (for recombinant) or 0.5–1.0 (for plasma-derived concentrate) = number of units
2. One unit of factor VIII per kg raises the measured factor level by 2% for recombinant product ([desired level/2] × weight of patient [kg] = number of units) or by 1–2% for plasma-derived concentrate ([desired level/1–2] × weight of patient [kg] = number of units)

Factor IX

1. Weight of patient (kg) × desired level of correction (%) × 1.2 (recombinant factor IX) or 1.0 (plasma-derived factor IX) = number of units
2. One unit of factor IX per kg raises the measured factor IX level by 0.83% for recombinant factor IX or by 1% for plasma-derived factor IX ([desired level/1.0 × weight of patient [kg] = number of units):([desired level/0.83] × weight of patient [kg] = number of units)

In the treatment of major hemorrhages, the achieved level of factor activity should be measured directly because the recovery *in vivo* varies widely among patients and because inadequate hemostasis may lead to severe morbidity or death. In addition, the dose of plasma-derived factor VIII required in children to achieve a particular factor VIII level may be 50% to 100% greater than in adults. If a minor bleed fails to respond to conventional dosing, the posttreatment factor level should be measured to be certain that the desired level is being achieved.

When children with von Willebrand disease are treated with concentrate or rarely with cryoprecipitate, doses of 15 to 25 units of factor VIII activity per kg and 30 to 50 units of factor VIII activity per kg are commonly used for the treatment of minor and major hemorrhages, respectively.

1-Deamino-8-D-Arginine Vasopressin

After the administration of 1-deamino-8-D-arginine vasopressin (DDAVP), levels of factor VIII coagulant activity, von Willebrand antigen, and ristocetin cofactor activity increase by about threefold in most people. This activity makes DDAVP an excellent alternative to blood products for the treatment of minor bleeding episodes in patients with mild hemophilia and for the treatment of most bleeding episodes in patients with the common form (type I) of von Willebrand disease The dose of DDAVP is 0.3 μg per kg administered by i.v. over 30 minutes. Side effects include facial flushing, headache, and rarely, hypertension, hypotension, and water retention. Hyponatremic seizures have occurred, and the patient should avoid excessive water intake. Subsequent doses may be less effective because the drug acts by releasing factor VIII and von Willebrand protein rather than by increasing their synthesis. In patients with severe factor VIII deficiency, DDAVP is ineffective. This is also true for many patients with severe (type III) von Willebrand disease because the baseline factor VIII level is so low. In the rare type IIB von Willebrand disease, DDAVP may cause or aggravate thrombocytopenia and therefore should be used with caution.

MANAGEMENT OF PATIENTS WITH INHIBITORS

For serious bleeding in patients with factor VIII deficiency and relatively low inhibitor titers (less than 10 Bethesda units), large doses of factor VIII may be sufficient to overwhelm the antibody and raise the factor VIII level to hemostatic levels. Doses as high as 100 to 200 units per kg may be necessary.

If the initial inhibitor titer in a patient with critical bleeding is too high to warrant a trial of factor VIII therapy, or if no response to factor VIII is obtained, alternative approaches should be initiated. Porcine factor VIII can achieve hemostatic levels in patients whose inhibitor does not cross-react with this animal protein.

Another approach to the treatment of serious bleeding in the patient with factor VIII deficiency and inhibitors is the administration of prothrombin complex concentrate or activated prothrombin complex concentrate. However, neither product is uniformly effective, and treatment cannot be monitored by the PTT or factor levels but only by clinical response. A new option for the treatment of bleeding in children with high-titer inhibitors is recombinant factor VIIa. This product is not derived from plasma and therefore should have little or no risk of viral transmission. However, factor VIIa has a very short half-life and must be administered every 2 hours. As with the prothrombin complex concentrates, success of treatment must be judged clinically rather than by changes in laboratory values.

Occasionally the condition of the patient with inhibitors will worsen despite factor therapy. In such instances, plasmapheresis may remove sufficient antibody to allow a response to factor VIII administration. However, because 50% of the IgG inhibitor is tissue-bound and will rapidly return to the plasma, further infusions of factor VIII will be unsuccessful unless preceded by additional plasmaphereses.

Minor bleeds in the patient with factor VIII deficiency and inhibitors can be treated with any of the products described above for use with major bleeds. Factor VIII is the product of choice for patients with low titer inhibitors who can achieve hemostatic factor VIII levels without anamnesis.

Inherited Hypercoagulable Conditions

The three major proteins that serve as brakes on the coagulation pathway are antithrombin III, protein C, and protein S. Homozygous protein S is rarer but may have similarly severe and early clinical manifestations. The most common inherited cause of thrombosis, factor V Leiden, is a single gene mutation that alters the amino acid composition of factor V and makes this coagulation protein resistant to the antithrombotic activity of protein C. Patients who are heterozygous for antithrombin III, protein C, protein S deficiency, or factor V Leiden and who develop a venous thrombosis should be treated with heparin by i.v. infusion. Treatment is usually initiated with a bolus injection of 50 to 100 units per kg body weight followed by a constant infusion of 25 units per kg per hour. The heparin dose should be adjusted to maintain the PTT between 1.5 and 2.0 times normal. Once adequate anticoagulation with heparin has been achieved, warfarin should be given orally.

Newborns with homozygous protein C deficiency and purpura fulminans should receive fresh-frozen plasma 8 to 12 mL per kg body weight every 12 hours. Long-term therapy includes regular infusions of fresh-frozen plasma or oral anticoagulation. Cryoprecipitate plays an analogous role in the acute and chronic therapy of homozygous protein S deficiency.

CHAPTER 78
Toxicologic Emergencies

Kevin C. Osterhoudt, M.D.,
Michael Shannon, M.D., M.P.H.,
and Fred M. Henretig, M.D.

GENERAL APPROACH TO THE POISONED CHILD

The management approach to the poisoned child attempts to prioritize critical assessment and, at times, simultaneous management interventions (Table 78.1). The initial phase (or "primary survey") addresses traditional ABCs of airway securement and cardiorespiratory support, with a slight additional emphasis on emergent toxicologic considerations. The more specific evaluation and detoxification phase (or "secondary survey") is aimed at simultaneously initiating generic treatment while assessing the actual extent of intoxication (in cases of known or presumed exposures) and/or identifying the actual toxins involved (in unknown, but highly suspected intoxications).

Initial Life Support Phase

The general approach to recognition and support of vital airway and cardiorespiratory functions (or "ABCDs") is well known to most readers and is covered in detail in Chapter 1. In the context of the poisoned child, a few points deserve special emphasis. In addition to the usual signs of airway obstruction, the physician must pay special attention to evidence of disturbed airway protective reflexes. Many poisoned patients will vomit or undergo procedures such as gastric lavage or administration of charcoal, which pose an aspiration risk. Elective endotracheal intubation (see Chapter 5) may thus be indicated at a slightly lower threshold in this context than in another child with comparable central nervous system (CNS) depression.

Evaluation and Detoxification Phase

HISTORY

For a known or highly suspected toxin, an attempt is made to estimate the total amount ingested (number of pills missing, ounces left in the bottle, dosage of pills, concentration of alcohol, and so forth). The best estimate of time elapsed since ingestion is also sought.

General historical features that suggest the possibility of poisoning include 1) acute onset; 2) age range of 1 to 5 years; 3) history of pica or known, unintentional ingestion; 4) substantial environmental stress, either acute (eg, arrival of a new baby, serious illness in a parent) or chronic (marital conflict, parental disability); 5) multiple organ system involvement; 6) significant alteration in level of consciousness; and 7) a clinical picture that seems especially puzzling.

TABLE 78.1. General Approach to the Known or Suspected Intoxication

Initial Life Support Phase	Social: Grandparents visiting
Airway: Maintain patency, assess protective reflexes	Holiday parties, and so on
Breathing: Adequate tidal volume?	*Physical examination*
ABG?	Vital signs
Circulation: Secure i.v. access, assess perfusion	Level of consciousness, neuromuscular status
Disability: Level of consciousness (AVPU or GCS)	Eyes—pupils, extraocular movements, fundi
Pupillary size, reactivity	Mouth—corrosive lesions, odors
Drugs: Dextrose (± rapid bedside test)	Cardiovascular—rate, rhythm, perfusion
Oxygen	Respiratory—rate, chest excursion, air entry
Naloxone	GI—motility, corrosive effects
(Other ALS medications)	Skin—color, bullae or burns, diaphoresis, piloerection
Decontamination: Ocular—copious saline lavage	Odors
Skin—copious water, then soap and water	*Laboratory* (individualize)
GI—consider options	CBC, cooximetry
Evaluation and Detoxification Phase	ABG, serum osmolarity
History—Brief, focused	ECG/cardiac monitor
Known toxin: Estimate amount	Chest radiograph, abdominal radiograph
Elapsed time	Electrolytes, BUN/creatinine, glucose, calcium, liver function panel
Early symptoms	Urinalysis
Home treatment	Rapid overdose toxicologic screen
Significant underlying conditions	Quantitative toxicology tests (especially acetaminophen)
Suspected but unknown toxin—consider poisoning if:	*Assessment or severity/diagnosis*
Patient: Acute onset of illness	Clinical findings
Pica-prone age	Laboratory abnormalities (with consideration of anion, osmolar gaps)
History of pica, ingestions	Toxidromes (see Table 78.3)
Current household "stress"	*Specific detoxification*
Multiorgan system dysfunction	Reassess ABCDs
Significantly altered mental status	Institute appropriate GI decontamination (if not already under way)
Puzzling clinical picture	Urgent antidotal therapy
Family: Medications at home	Consider excretion enhancement
Recent illness (under treatment)	Continue supportive care

ABG, arterial blood gas; AVPU, *A*lert, *V*erbal, *P*ain, *U*nresponsive; GCS, Glasgow Coma Scale; ALS, advanced life support; GI, gastrointestinal; CBC, complete blood count; ECG, electrocardiogram; BUN, blood urea nitrogen.

The focused physical examination should begin with a reassessment of vital functions and complete recording of vital signs, including core temperature (Table 78.2) With secure airway and cardiorespiratory function confirmed, the examination should then focus on the central and autonomic nervous systems, eye findings, changes in the skin and/or oral and gastrointestinal (GI) mucous membranes, and odors on the breath or clothing of the patient. These features represent those areas most likely affected in toxic syndromes and, when taken together, often form a constellation of signs and symptoms referred to as toxidromes (Table 78.3).

LABORATORY EVALUATION

The comprehensive drug screen that requires blood and urine samples may be useful for patients who are seriously ill with an occult ingestion or for the occasional intentional overdose adolescent patient whose clinical picture does not fit with the stated history. Often of greater help is the critical interpretation of routine measurements of serum chemistries and osmolarity in patients with altered mental status. The presence of hypoglycemia or aberrations of serum electrolytes may be crucial information about the poisoned patient. In certain circumstances, tests of liver or renal function, urinalysis, creatine phosphokinase levels, and other select tests may be useful. Metabolic acidosis with a high anion gap is found in many clinical syndromes and toxidromes, reflected by the often-cited mnemonic *MUDPILES*, for *m*ethanol and *m*etformin; *u*remia; *d*iabetic and other ketoacidoses; *p*araldehyde; *i*soniazid, *i*ron, and *i*nborn errors of metabolism; *l*actic acidosis (seen with hypoxia, shock, carbon monoxide, cyanide, and many drugs that cause compromised cardiorespiratory status or prolonged seizures); *e*thanol and *e*thylene glycol; and *s*alicylates. Differences between calculated and measured serum osmolarity (Calculated = 2 × [Serum Na] + blood urea nitrogen/2.8 + glucose/18 with normal osmolarity = 290 mOsm/kg) may suggest

TABLE 78.2. Clinical Manifestations of Poisoning

I. Vital Signs
  A. Pulse
    1. Bradycardia
       Digoxin, narcotics, organophosphates, cyanide, plants (lily of the valley, foxglove, oleander), clonidine, β-blockers, calcium channel blockers
    2. Tachycardia
       Alcohol, amphetamines and sympathomimetics, atropinics, tricyclic antidepressants, theophylline, salicylates, phencyclidine, cocaine
  B. Respirations
    1. Slow, depressed
       Alcohol, barbiturates (late), narcotics, clonidine, sedative-hypnotics
    2. Tachypnea
       Amphetamines, barbiturates (early), methanol, salicylates, carbon monoxide
  C. Blood pressure
    1. Hypotension
       Cellular asphyxiants (methemoglobinemia, cyanide, carbon monoxide), phenothiazines, tricyclic antidepressants, barbiturates, iron, theophylline, clonidine, narcotics, β-blockers, calcium channel blockers
    2. Hypertension
       Amphetamines/sympathomimetics (especially phenylpropanolamine in over-the-counter [OTC] cold remedies, diet pills), tricyclic antidepressants, phencyclidine, monoamine oxidase inhibitors (MAOIs), antihistamines, atropinics, clonidine, cocaine
  D. Temperature
    1. Hypothermia
       Ethanol, barbiturates, sedative-hypnotics, narcotics, phenothiazines, antidepressants, clonidine, cabamazepine
    2. Hyperpyrexia
       Atropinics, quinine, salicylates, amphetamines, phenothiazines, tricyclics, MAOIs, theophylline, cocaine

II. Neuromuscular
  A. Coma
     Narcotic depressants, sedative-hypnotics, anticholinergics (antihistamines, antidepressants, phenothiazines, atropinics, OTC sleep preparations), alcohols, anticonvulsants, carbon monoxide, salicylates, organophosphate insecticides, clonidine, gamma hydroxybutyrate
  B. Delirium/psychosis
     Alcohol, phenothiazines, drugs of abuse (phencyclidine, LSD, peyote, mescaline, marijuana, cocaine, heroin, methaqualone), sympathomimetics and anticholinergics (including prescription and OTC cold remedies), steroids, heavy metals
  C. Convulsions
     Alcohol, amphetamines, cocaine, phenothiazines, antidepressants, antihistamines, camphor, boric acid, lead, organophosphates, isoniazid, salicylates, plants (water hemlock), lindane, lidocaine, phencyclidine, carbamazepine
  D. Ataxia
     Alcohol, barbiturates, carbon monoxide, anticonvulsants, heavy metals, organic solvents, sedative-hypnotics, hydrocarbons
  E. Paralysis
     Botulism, heavy metals, plants (poison hemlock), ticks, paralytic shellfish poisoning

III. Eyes
  A. Pupils
    1. Miosis
       Narcotics, organophosphates, plants (mushrooms of the muscarinic types), ethanol, barbiturates, phenothiazines, phencyclidine, clonidine
    2. Mydriasis
       Amphetamines, atropinics, barbiturates (if comatose), botulism, cocaine, methanol, glutethamide, LSD, marijuana, phencyclidine, antihistamines, antidepressants
  B. Nystagmus
     Diphenylhydantoin, sedative-hypnotics, carbamazepine, glutethimide, phencyclidine (both vertical and horizontal), barbiturates, ethanol, MAOIs

IV. Skin
  A. Jaundice
     Carbon tetrachloride, acetaminophen, naphthalene, phenothiazines, plants (mushrooms, fava beans), heavy metals (iron, phosphorus, arsenic)
  B. Cyanosis (unresponsive to oxygen, as a result of methemoglobinemia)
     Aniline dyes, nitrites, benzocaine, phenacetin, nitrobenzene, phenazopyridine
  C. Pinkness to redness
     Atropinics and antihistamines, alcohol, carbon monoxide, cyanide, boric acid

V. Odors
  A. Acetone: acetone, isopropyl alcohol, phenol and salicylates
  B. Alcohol: ethanol (alcoholic beverages)
  C. Bitter almond: cyanide
  D. Garlic: heavy metal (arsenic, phosphorus and thallium), organophosphates
  E. Oil of wintergreen: methylsalicylates
  F. Hydrocarbons: hydrocarbons (e.g., gasoline, turpentine)

Modified with permission from Mofenson HC, Greensher J. The unknown poison. *Pediatrics* 1974;54:336.

TABLE 78.3. Toxidromes

	Sympathomimetics (amphetamines, cocaine)	Anticholinergics (antihistamines, many others)	Organophosphates (insecticides, nerve cases)	Opiates/ clonidine	Barbiturates/ sedative-hypnotics	Salicylates	Theophylline
Mental status/CNS	Agitation, delirium, psychosis, convulsions	Delirium, psychosis, coma, convulsions	Confusion, fasciculations, coma	Euphoria, somnolence, coma	Somnolence, coma	Lethargy, convulsions	Agitation, tremor, convulsions
Heart rate	Increased	Increased	Decreased (or increased)	Decreased			Increased
Blood pressure	Increased	Increased		Decreased	Decreased		Decreased
Temperature	Increased	Increased		Decreased	Decreased	Increased	
Respirations			Increased	Decreased	Decreased	Increased	Increased
Pupils	Large, reactive	Large, sluggish	Small	Pinpoint			
Bowel sounds	Present	Diminished	Hyperactive				
Skin	Diaphoresis	Flushed, dry	Diaphoresis				
Miscellaneous			"SLUDGE"[a]			Vomiting	Vomiting

CNS, Central nervous system.
[a] SLUDGE is a mnemonic representing salivation, lacrimation, urination, defecation, gastric cramping, and emesis.

intoxication with ethanol, isopropanol, or more rarely in pediatric patients, methanol or ethylene glycol.

An immediate determination of quantitative levels is helpful in making management decisions for some drugs, and these are outlined in Table 78.4. Furthermore, many important causes of coma and altered vital signs are not detected on even the most sophisticated "comprehensive" toxicology panels (which are usually biased toward psychoactive medications and illicit drugs). An overview of such agents is presented in Table 78.5. An electrocardiogram (ECG) should be performed in all seriously ill patients in whom poisoning is being considered. Detectable conduction delays may precede life-threatening cardiac rhythm disturbances.

SPECIFIC DETOXIFICATION

Gastrointestinal Decontamination

Simple Dilution. Dilution may be indicated only when the toxin produces local irritation or corrosion. Water or milk is an acceptable diluent.

TABLE 78.4. Frequently Useful Quantitative Toxicology Tests in Pediatric Patients

Drug/toxin	Optimal time after ingestion
Acetaminophen	4 h
Carbamazepine	2–4 h
Carboxyhemoglobin	Immediate
Digoxin	4–6 h
Ethanol	1 h
Ethylene glycol	1 h
Iron	4 h
Lithium	2–4 h[a]
Methanol	1 h
Methemoglobin	Immediate
Phenobarbital	1–2 h
Phenytoin	1–2 h
Salicylates	2–4 h[a]
Theophylline	1–2 h[a]

[a] Repeat levels over 6–12 h may be necessary with sustained-release preparations.
Modified with permission from Weisman, RS, Howland MA, Flomenbaum, NE. The toxicology laboratory. In: Goldfrank LR, Flomenbaum NE, Lewin NA, et al., eds. *Toxicologic emergencies.* Norwalk, CT: Appleton & Lange, 1990.

Gastric Emptying. The utility of gastric emptying diminishes with time and is most effective if done within the first hour. In certain circumstances, such as the delayed gastric emptying accompanying intoxication with anticholinergic drugs, benefit may be noted longer after ingestion. *Emesis* was once a favored means of gastric emptying, but currently induction of emesis is typically limited to first aid in the home setting.

An alternative to ipecac-induced emesis for emptying the stomach is *gastric lavage.* This procedure is usually reserved for patients who have ingested a potentially life-threatening amount of a poison, in cases where the procedure can be performed safely within 60 minutes of ingestion and charcoal alone is not believed to be adequate.

Activated Charcoal. Charcoal administration has become the decontamination strategy of choice for most pediatric poisonings and is most effective when used in the first few hours after ingestion. A number of notable compounds, such as iron and lithium, do not adsorb well to activated charcoal (Table 78.6). The usual dose of activated charcoal is 1 g per kg; adolescents and adults should receive 50 to 100 g.

Whole Bowel Irrigation. An additional technique of GI decontamination that has been developed over the past several years is that of intestinal irrigation with large volumes and flow

TABLE 78.5. Important Drugs and Toxins Not Detected by Most Drug Screens

Coma-causing	Hypotension-causing
Bromide	β-Blockers[a]
Carbon monoxide	Calcium channel blockers[a]
Chloral hydrate	Clonidine[a]
Clonidine	Colchicine
Cyanide	Cyanide
Organophosphates	Digitalis[a]
Tetrahydrozoline (in over-the-counter eye drops)	Iron

[a] Hypotension often is seen with bradycardia.
Modified with permission from Wiley JF II. Difficult diagnoses in toxicology: poisons not detected by the comprehensive drug screen. *Pediatr Clin North Am* 1991;38:728–737.

TABLE 78.6. Activated Charcoal

Substances poorly (or not) adsorbed:
Common electrolytes
Iron
Mineral acids or bases
Alcohols
Cyanide
Most solvents
Most water-insoluble compounds (e.g., hydrocarbons)

rates of a polyethylene glycol-balanced electrolyte solution such as Colyte or GoLYTELY. Whole bowel irrigation (WBI) has been found to be particularly useful in pediatric iron overdoses in which gastric lavage may be limited by tube size and the substance is not bound to charcoal. It has been used for other metal ingestions (eg, lead), for overdoses of sustained-release medications (eg, lithium, theophylline) with increasing levels after initial decontamination, and for ingestions of crack vials or cocaine packets. It might also be useful in particularly massive and/or late-presenting overdoses for which the efficacy of gastric emptying and/or charcoal is expected to be suboptimal. The technique may be used by mouth in cooperative patients or by nasogastric tube; the usual recommended dosing is 500 mL per hour in toddlers and 2 L per hour in adolescents and adults.

GASTROINTESTINAL DECONTAMINATION STRATEGIES

Figure 78.1 summarizes one approach to GI decontamination. When gastric decontamination is warranted, the administration of activated charcoal, without gastric emptying, is most often the appropriate choice. WBI is of theoretic benefit to body packers and stuffers, and patients who have ingested toxic amounts of sustained-release preparations or agents not adsorbed well by activated charcoal.

Antidotal Therapy

Antidotes that should be available for immediate administration include sodium bicarbonate (cyclic antidepressants), sodium nitrite/sodium thiosulfate (cyanide), atropine and pralidoxime

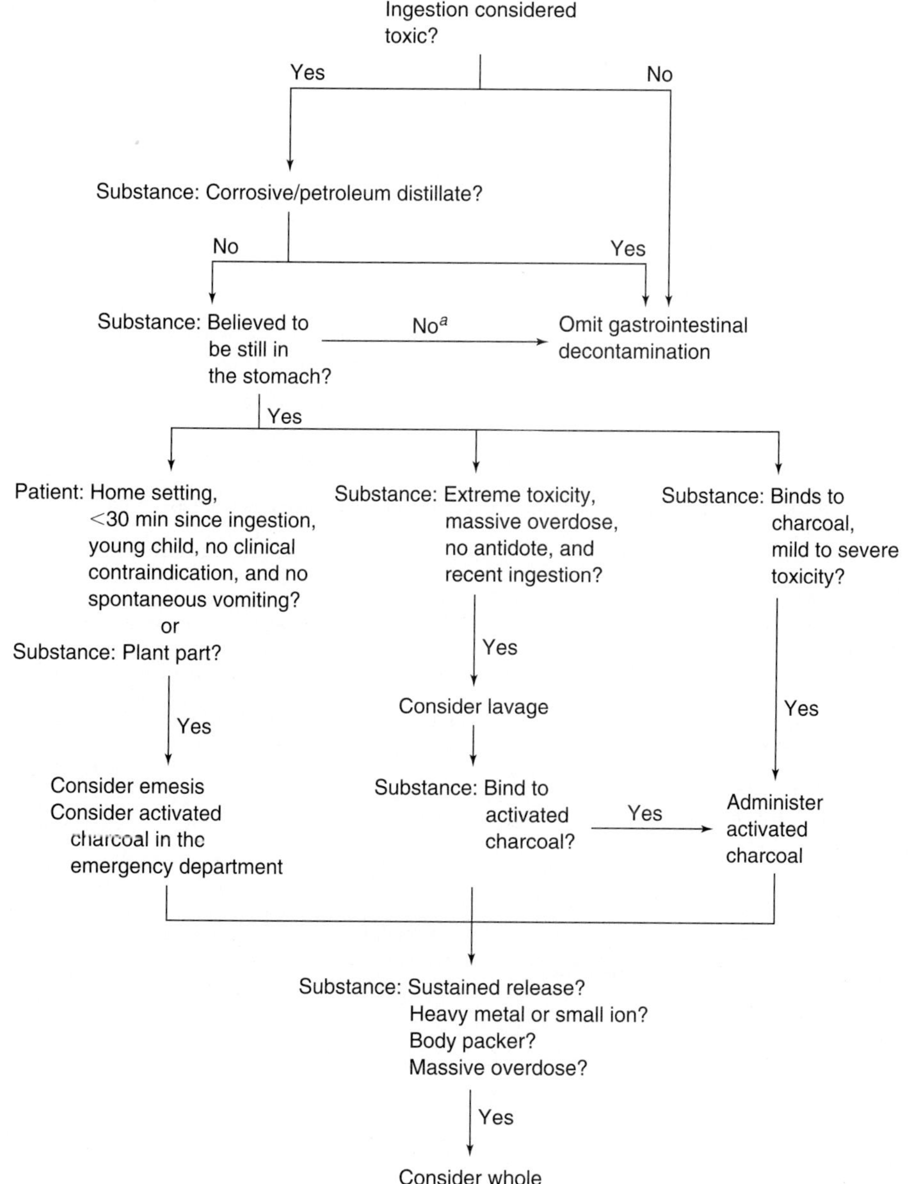

Figure 78.1. Approach to gastrointestinal decontamination. [a]For patients in whom the toxin is no longer believed to be in the stomach, activated charcoal administration and/or whole bowel irrigation might still be valid considerations.

TABLE 78.7. Summary of Antidotes

Poison	Antidote
Acetaminophen	*N*-Acetylcysteine (Mucomyst) initial dose of 140 mg/kg p.o. in water, fruit juice, or soda; then, 70 mg/kg every 4 h for 17 doses (see text regarding i.v. *N*-acetylcysteine)
Anticholinergics	Physostigmine (adult, 2 mg; child, 0.5 mg) i.v.; may repeat in 15 min until desired effect is achieved; subsequent doses every 2–3 p.r.n. (*Caution: May cause seizures, asystole, cholinergic crisis;* see text)
Anticholinesterases	Atropine, 2–5 mg (adults): 0.05–0.1 mg/kg (children) i.m. or i.v.; repeated every 10–15 min until atropinization is evident
Organophosphates	Pralidoxime chloride 1–2 g (adults); 25–50 mg/kg (children) i.v.; repeat dose in 1 h p.r.n., then every 6–8 h for 24–48 h (consider also constant infusion; see text)
Carbamates	Atropine, as above; pralidoxime for severe cases (see text)
Benzodiazepines	Flumazenil, 0.01 mg/kg i.v. (estimated pediatric dose; see text)
Beta-adrenergic blockers	Glucagon, 50 μg/kg i.v.
Calcium channel blockers	Calcium chloride 10%, 10 mL (adult); 0.2 mL/kg (pediatric) i.v. or calcium gluconate 10%, 30 mL (adult); 0.6 mL/kg (pediatric) i.v. Glucagon, 50 μg/kg i.v.
Carbon monoxide	Oxygen 100% inhalation, consider hyperbaric for severe cases
Cyanide	*Adult:* Amyl nitrite inhalation (inhale for 15–30 sec every 60 sec) pending administration of 300 mg sodium nitrite (10 mL of a 3% solution) i.v. slowly (over 2–4 min); follow immediately with 12.5 g sodium thiosulfate (2.5–5 mL/min of 25% solution) i.v. *Children* (Na nitrite should not exceed recommended dose because fatal methemoglobinemia may result):

Hemoglobin	Initial Dose 3% Na Nitrite i.v.	Initial Dose 25% Na Thiosulfate i.v.
8g	0.22 mL(6.6mg)/kg	1.10 mL/kg
10g	0.27 mL(8.7mg)/kg	1.35 mL/kg
12g(normal)	0.33 mL(10mg)/kg	1.65 mL/kg
14g	0.39 mL(11.6mg)/kg	1.95 mL/kg

Poison	Antidote
Digitalis	Fab antibodies (Digibind): dose based on amount ingested and/or digoxin level (see text, package insert)
Ethylene glycol	4-Methylpyrazole: Load 15 mg/kg; maintenance 10 mg/kg q12h 4 doses, then 15 mg/kg q12h thereafter (little experience in children) (see Methanol)
Fluoride	Calcium gluconate 10%, 0.6 mL/kg i.v. slowly until symptoms abate, serum calcium normalizes; repeat p.r.n.
Heavy metals/usual chelators Arsenic/BAL Lead/BAL, EDTA, penicillamine, DMSA Mercury/BAL, DMSA	*BAL* (dimercaprol): 3–5 mg/kg/dose deep i.m. every 4 h for 2 d, every 4–6 h for an additional 2 d, then every 4–12 h for up to 7 additional days *EDTA:* 50–75 mg/kg/24 h deep i.m. or slow i.v. infusion given in 3–6 divided doses for up to 5 d; may be repeated for a second course after a minimum of 2 d; each course should not exceed a total of 500 mg/kg body weight (see text) *Penicillamine:* 100 mg/kg/d (max 1 g) p.o. in divided doses for up to 5 d, for long-term therapy do not exceed 40 mg/kg/d *DMSA (succimer):* 350 mg/m^2 (10 mg/kg) p.o. every 8 h for 5 d, followed by 350 mg/m^2 (10 mg/kg) p.o. every 12 h for 14 d
Iron	Deferoxamine: 5–15 mg/kg/h i.v.; use higher dosage for severe symptoms (see text) and decrease as patient recovers
Isoniazid	Pyridoxine 5%–10%, 1 g per gram of INH ingested (70 mg/kg up to 5 g if dose unknown) i.v. slowly over 30–60 min
Methanol (and ethylene glycol)	Ethanol loading dose: 0.75 g/kg infused over 1 h Maintenance: 0.1–0.2 g/kg/h infusion; adjust as needed with target level 100 mg/dL Folate 1 mg/kg i.v. every 6 h (methanol) Thiamine .5 mg/kg and pyridoxine 2 mg/kg (ethylene glycol)
Methamoglobinemic agents	Methylene blue 1%, 1–2 mg/kg (0.1–0.2 ml/kg) i.v. slowly over 5–10 min if cyanosis is severe or methemoglobin level >40%
Opioids	Naloxone 1–2 mg i.v., i.m., sublingual or by ETT; may repeat up to total 8–10 mg in adolescent/adult (see text)
Phenothiazines (dystonic reaction)	Diphenhydramine, 1–2 mg/kg i.m. or i.v.; or Benztropine, 1–2 mg i.m. or i.v. (adolescents)
Tricyclic antidepressants	Sodium bicarbonate, 1–2 mEq/kg i.v.
Warfarin (and "superwarfarin" rat poisons)	Vitamin K_1 10 mg (adult); 1–5 mg (pediatric) i.v., i.m., subcutaneous, p.o.

Animals	For Envenomation (see Chapter 80)	Antivenin[a]
Snake, Crotalidae (all North American rattlers and moccasins)		Antivenin (Crotalidae) Polyvalent (Wyeth)
Snake, coral		Antivenin (*Micrurus fulvius*), monovalent (Wyeth)
Spider, black widow		Antivenin *Latrodactus mactans* (Merck, Sharp and Dohme)

[a] See package insert for dosage and administrations

(cholinesterase inhibitors), ethanol or 4-methylpyrazole (ethylene glycol and methanol), deferoxamine (iron), dextrose (ethanol, salicylates, oral hypoglycemics), methylene blue (methemoglobinemic agents), oxygen (carbon monoxide), flumazenil (benzodiazepines), and naloxone (opioids). Table 78.7 summarizes a list of commonly used antidotes, suggested doses, and their indications for use.

Enhancing Excretion

DIURESIS

Although it is important to maintain high glomerular filtration rates in the presence of rhabdomyolysis or when chelating with agents such as ethylenediaminetetraacetic acid (EDTA), forced diuresis has limited value in the treatment of acute poisoning. Ionized diuresis takes advantage of the principle that excretion is favored when a drug is in its ionized state. Urinary alkalinization promotes excretion of salicylate (a weak acid) and may also enhance clearance of phenobarbital, chlorpropamide, and chlorophenoxy herbicides. Urine alkalinization can be initiated with sodium bicarbonate at a dose of 1 to 2 mEq per kg by intravenous (i.v.) over a 1- to 2-hour period. The rate of bicarbonate infusion can be adjusted to maintain a urinary pH of 7.5 to 8.5.

DIALYSIS

Dialysis is indicated for selected cases of severe poisoning or when renal failure is present. Indications for dialysis depend on patient-related and drug-related criteria. Patient-related criteria include 1) anticipated prolonged coma with the high likelihood of attendant complications, 2) development of renal failure or impairment of normal excretory pathways, and 3) progressive clinical deterioration despite careful medical supervision. Drug-related criteria are 1) satisfactory membrane permeability, 2) a correlation between plasma drug concentration and drug toxicity of the agent, 3) plasma levels in the potentially fatal range or the presence of a significant quantity of an agent that is normally metabolized to a toxic substance, and 4) significant enhancement of clearance. Hemodialysis is the most effective means of dialysis.

HEMOPERFUSION

Table 78.8 summarizes the generally accepted common drugs and drug concentrations for which hemodialysis and hemoperfusion should be considered, in light of the previous discussion regarding clinical criteria.

TABLE 78.8. Drugs and Their Plasma Concentrations for Which Hemodialysis or Hemoperfusion Should Be Considered

Hemodialysis	Hemperfusion
Lithium, 4.0 mEq/L	Phenobarbital, 100 mg/L
Ethylene glycol, 50 mg/dL	Theophylline, 6–10 mg/dL (60–100 mg/L)
Methanol, 50 mg/dL	Paraquat, 0.1 mg/dL
Salicylates, 100 mg/dL	Glutethimide, 4 mg/dL
	Methaqualone, 4 mg/dL
	Ethchlorvynol, 15 mg/dL
	Meprobamate, 10 mg/dL

Modified with permission from Winchester JF. Active methods for detoxification. In: Haddad LM, Winchester JF (eds). *Clinical management of poisoning and drug overdose.* Philadelphia: WB Saunders, 1983:162–166.

MULTIPLE-DOSE ACTIVATED CHARCOAL (GASTROINTESTINAL DIALYSIS)

Several studies have shown significant increase in clearance for a number of drugs when repeated doses of 0.5 to 1.0 g per kg of activated charcoal are given every 4 to 6 hours. To be safe and effective, this technique requires active peristalsis and an intact gag reflex or a protected airway. Common pediatric poisonings for which repetitive charcoal dosing may be indicated include phenobarbital, carbamazepine, phenytoin, digoxin, salicylates, and theophylline. Cathartics, such as sorbitol, should be administered no more frequently than every third dose.

NONTOXIC INGESTION

Table 78.9 provides a list of nontoxic ingestions.

Acetaminophen (*N*-acetyl-*p*-aminophenol, APAP)

CLINICAL FINDINGS

Initially, the signs and symptoms of APAP ingestion are vague and nonspecific but include nausea and vomiting, anorexia, pal-

TABLE 78.9. Products That Are Nontoxic When Ingested In Small Amounts

Abrasives	Hand lotions and creams
Adhesives	Hydrogen peroxide (medicinal 3%)
Antacids	Incense
Antibiotics	Indelible markers
Baby-product cosmetics	Ink (black, blue)
Ballpoint pen inks	Laxatives
Bath oil	Lipstick
Bathtub floating toys	Lubricating oils
Bleach (less than 5% sodium hypochlorite)	Magic Markers
Body conditioners	Matches
Bubble-bath soaps	Mineral oil
Calamine lotion	Newspaper (black and white pages)
Candles (beeswax or paraffin)	Paint (indoor, latex)
Caps	Pencil (graphite)
Chalk	Perfumes
Cigarettes (less than 3 butts)	Petroleum jelly
Clay (modeling)	Phenolphthalein laxatives (Ex-Lax)
Colognes	Perous-lip marking pens
Contraceptive pills	Putty (less than 2 oz)
Corticosteroids	Rubber cement
Cosmetics	Shampoos (liquid)
Crayons (marked AP, CP)	Shaving creams and lotions
Dehumidifying packets (silica or charcoal)	Soap and soap products
Detergents (phosphate)	Suntan preparations
Deodorants	Sweetening agents (saccharin, cyclamates)
Deodorizers (spray and refrigerator)	Teething rings (water sterility)
Elmer's Glue	Thermometers (mercury)
Etch-A-Sketch	Thyroid tablets
Eye makeup	Toothpaste
Fabric softener	Vitamins (without iron)
Fertilizer (if no insecticides or herbicides added)	Warfarin (rat poison; excludes "superwarfarins")
Glues and pastes	Watercolors
Grease	Zinc oxide (Dasitin)
Hair products (dyes, sprays, tonics, excludes "relaxers")	Zirconium oxide

Adapted from Mofenson HC, Greensher J. *Pediatrics* 1974;54:336.

lor, and diaphoresis. These manifestations usually resolve within 12 to 24 hours, and the patient appears well for 1 to 4 days. The potential severity of an acute intoxication may be predicted by the amount ingested, if accurately known, and the plasma level of APAP. APAP in single doses of less than 150 mg per kg in children is likely to be harmless. However, the only reliable indication of the potential severity of the hepatic damage is the plasma APAP level, taken at least 4 hours after ingestion. A nomogram (Fig. 78.2) is available for using this value in the prediction of likely toxicity.

MANAGEMENT

For most cases of acetaminophen overdose per se, and particularly for those typically seen 2 to 4 hours after ingestion, charcoal alone is probably effective and should not significantly alter the ability to use *N*-acetylcysteine (NAC) several hours later. In cases that present after 4 hours have elapsed, gastric decontamination is usually not warranted.

NAC, given orally, essentially prevents the occurrence of hepatotoxicity when instituted within 8 hours of ingestion. It also lessens the severity of hepatic damage if used within 16 hours. Antiemetic therapy with metoclopramide or ondansetron may also be helpful. An i.v. preparation is also available. The protocol for NAC therapy may be summarized as follows:

1. Consider GI decontamination options as already noted.
2. If patient presents less than 4 hours after ingestion, wait to draw 4-hour level and base therapeutic decision on nomogram (assumes rapid turnaround time so that level will be available by 8 hours after ingestion); if necessary, initiate treatment as described next. For extended-release preparations, McNeil Consumer Products Co., a manufacturer of

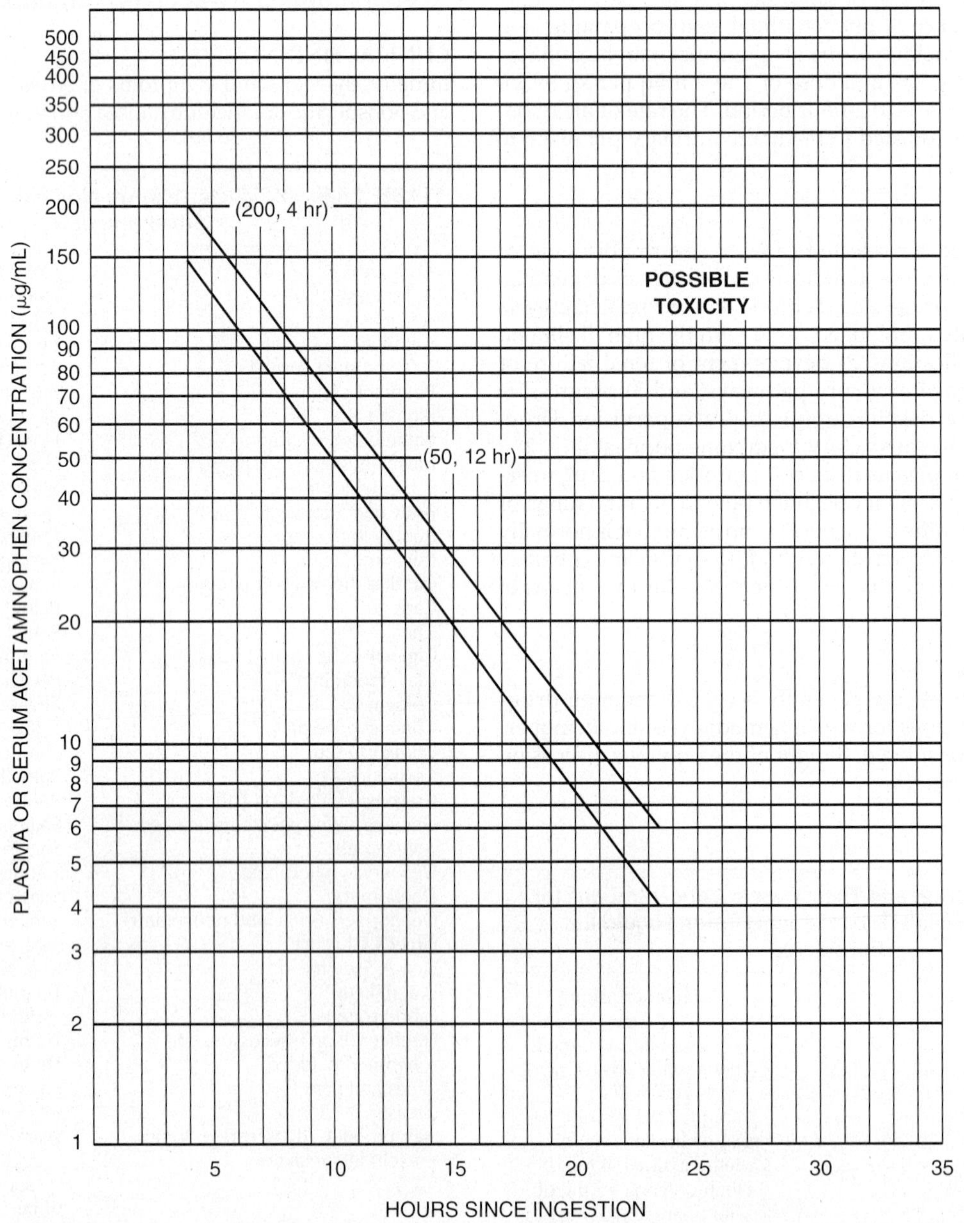

Figure 78.2. Nomogram for estimating severity of acute acetaminophen poisoning. (Modified with permission from Rumack BH, Matthew H. *Pediatrics* 1975;55:871–876. Copyright, American Academy of Pediatrics, 1975.)

acetaminophen, suggests a second APAP level drawn 4 hours after the first; antidotal therapy is to be instituted if either level suggests possible toxicity.

3. If patient presents more than 6 to 8 hours after ingestion, give a loading dose of NAC, 140 mg per kg orally (regardless of time since ingestion, consider increasing dose by 40%, or repeating the loading dose, if charcoal had been given within the preceding 1 to 2 hours). Obtain level and base subsequent course of therapy on nomogram.
4. If level plots out above the lower line on the nomogram, admit the patient to hospital and continue NAC at 70 mg per kg orally every 4 hours for a total of 17 doses. Monitor complete blood count (CBC), renal, and liver function tests.
5. Treatment for patients who present more than 24 hours after ingestion is controversial, as is treatment for patients with subacute, repetitive overdosing over several days. We generally advise treatment for children who receive more than 150 mg per kg per day for 1 to 2 days or more and/or patients with levels above 10 μg per mL who present more than 24 hours after ingestion.

Alcohols and Glycols

ETHANOL

After ingesting ethanol, children may develop nausea, vomiting, stupor, and ataxia. Coma and death from apnea may occur if significant quantities are consumed. In adolescents, blood concentrations of less than 50 mg per dL rarely result in sensory or motor impairment. Values of 100 to 150 mg per dL are consistent with intoxication and cause mild neurologic findings. Lethal blood alcohol concentrations are generally greater than 500 mg per dL. Infants and toddlers who ingest ethanol have a clinical course that is significantly different from that in adolescents and adults; a triad of coma, hypothermia, and hypoglycemia appears once ethanol levels exceed 50 to 100 mg per dL. This triad may be accompanied by metabolic acidosis.

The blood ethanol level may be estimated by calculating the osmolol gap (measured serum osmolality − [2 × Serum Na + blood urea nitrogen/2.8 + Serum glucose/18]). An osmolal gap of 22 to 25 mOsm per kg H_2O exists for every 100 mg per dL of ethanol in the serum. The amount of an ethanol-containing liquid that is of concern when ingested by a child depends on the alcohol concentration. However, a rough rule is that ingestion of 1 g per kg of ethanol is sufficient to raise blood alcohol to 100 mg per dL.

The management of ethanol ingestion in children begins with prompt recognition and evaluation of blood glucose. Airway or ventilatory compromise should be treated with endotracheal intubation. If seizures result from hypoglycemia, they should be promptly treated with 10% to 50% (0.25 to 1.0 g per kg) i.v. glucose and anticonvulsants if necessary. Warming techniques should be instituted to increase core temperature. Because ethanol is rapidly absorbed from the gut and is not adsorbed by activated charcoal, there is rarely a role for GI decontamination if the patient presents more than 1 to 2 hours after ingestion. However, if presentation is earlier, gastric lavage should be performed. Because of the high risk of drug coingestion, activated charcoal should be administered to adolescents. The institution of hemodialysis may be useful in those patients who have impaired liver function or a blood alcohol concentration greater than 450 to 500 mg per dL.

METHANOL

Although methanol has little or no inherent toxicity, its metabolism by alcohol dehydrogenase to form formaldehyde and formic acid creates highly toxic compounds. Formic acid is a potent organic acid that results in severe metabolic acidosis and ocular symptoms. Ingestions approaching 100 mg per kg should be considered dangerous. The clinical effects of a methanol ingestion usually occur after a latent period of 8 to 24 hours. In large ingestions, acute methanol poisoning may cause severe CNS depression, metabolic acidosis, and a number of reversible or irreversible optic changes. In the early stages of intoxication, funduscopic examination may be remarkable for hyperemia.

Management

The treatment of methanol ingestion consists of supportive care, administration of specific therapies, and enhancement of elimination. Laboratory assessment includes serial arterial blood gases, electrolytes, blood urea nitrogen (BUN), creatinine, glucose, toxin screen, serum osmolality, and methanol level. Serum methanol concentration in milligrams per deciliter can be estimated by the formula (osmolal gap × 3). There are three specific treatments for methanol intoxication: sodium bicarbonate, folic acid, and ethanol (or 4-methylpyrazole—see the following). Sodium bicarbonate should be administered aggressively to correct metabolic acidosis. Folate is provided because of its role in formic acid disposition within the tetrahydrofolate cycle. Customary doses are 1 mg per kg i.v. every 6 hours.

Because serum methanol levels of 20 mg per dL or greater are associated with toxicity if untreated, higher levels require treatment to prevent its metabolism and/or interventions to enhance its elimination. Ethanol, which has a higher affinity for alcohol dehydrogenase than methanol, is provided to "block" further production of toxic metabolites. 4-Methylpyrazole, another alcohol dehydrogenase antagonist, shows promise as an antidote for methanol intoxication. Currently, in the United States, it has received indication for use only in adult ethylene glycol poisoning (see the following section, "Ethylene Glycol").

Ethanol should be instituted if the calculated or measured methanol concentration is 20 mg per dL or greater. It is administered with the goal of maintaining serum ethanol concentrations at 100 mg per dL or greater. Ethanol may be given by continuous i.v. infusion (600 mg per kg bolus followed by a 110 mg per kg per hour) or by oral administration. Intravenous ethanol is preferred but has the problems of being often unavailable, hyperosmolar (preventing its administration in small veins), and requiring large fluid volumes. Therefore, the oral route must often be used in children. Given orally, any beverage that contains ethanol may be used. It must be remembered that proof designation of a beverage is twice the alcohol concentration expressed as a percentage (eg, 80 proof equals 40% alcohol). Children must be closely monitored for the complications of ethanol administration, including mental status depression, hypoglycemia, and hypothermia. Patients who have a blood methanol concentration of 50 mg per dL or greater require hemodialysis in addition to ethanol administration. During hemodialysis, the infusion rate of the ethanol must be doubled because hemodialysis will also remove ethanol.

ETHYLENE GLYCOL

The clinical syndrome of ethylene glycol intoxication appears in three different stages. The first stage consists predominantly of CNS manifestations and is accompanied by a profound metabolic acidosis. In this early stage, mild hypertension, tachycardia, and a leukocytosis are often present. Nausea and vomiting commonly occur, and with larger doses, coma and convulsions may appear within a few hours. Another common finding is the presence of hypocalcemia. Hypocalcemia may be severe enough to cause tetany and cardiac conduction disturbances. Urinalysis usually reveals a low specific gravity, proteinuria, microscopic hematuria, and crystalluria. The second distinct state is ushered in by coma and cardiopulmonary failure; it is usually the result of acidosis and hypocalcemia. The third stage usually occurs after 24 to 72 hours. Here, renal failure emerges as the dominant problem. Usually, a picture of acute tubular necrosis develops with either polyuria or anuria. Urine sediment contains blood, protein, and casts. Patients often require dialysis for extended periods and may be left with permanent renal insufficiency.

Consideration of ethylene glycol poisoning should be based either on the history or, in the absence of diabetic ketoacidosis, the presence of any of the following criteria: 1) alcohol-like intoxication without the odor of alcohol; 2) large anion-gap metabolic acidosis; 3) an elevated osmolar gap in the absence of ethanol or methanol ingestion; or 4) a urinalysis that demonstrates oxalate crystals. Another diagnostic tool is to perform a Woods lamp examination of urine. If the ingested substance is radiator antifreeze, the fluorescein dye that it contains will be excreted in urine and fluoresce under Woods lamp. Arterial blood gases should be obtained frequently because of the rapid evolution of metabolic acidosis.

Gastric emptying is the only decontamination measure that is effective after ethylene glycol ingestion and should be performed if the patient arrives within 1 hour of ingestion. Activated charcoal negligibly adsorbs ethylene glycol and is unnecessary. As with methanol intoxication, treatment of ethylene glycol poisoning falls into three areas: supportive care, administration of pharmacologic agents, and enhancement of elimination.

Pharmacologic therapy is subdivided into four areas: administration of sodium bicarbonate, calcium, pyridoxine with thiamine, and ethanol or 4-methylpyrazole. Correction of acidosis should begin immediately with the administration of sodium bicarbonate and appropriate ventilation. Hypocalcemia may present as skeletal muscle disturbances (tetany) or cardiac dysfunction (prolonged Q-T interval). These may be alleviated by the prompt institution of calcium (eg, 10% calcium gluconate, 0.3 to 0.6 mL per kg). Thiamine and pyridoxine are vitamins that act as cofactors in the nontoxic metabolic pathways of ethylene glycol and, theoretically, divert its metabolism toward formation of nontoxic metabolites. Therefore, thiamine (0.25 to 0.5 mg per kg) and pyridoxine (1 to 2 mg per kg) are recommended for the first 24 hours of treatment.

Ethanol administration is one option to inhibit ethylene glycol metabolism by alcohol dehydrogenase (previously discussed under "Methanol"). It should be initiated as soon as possible to interrupt further formation of organic acids. As with methanol, ethanol is indicated for ethylene glycol concentrations of 20 mg per dL or greater. For serum ethylene glycol concentrations of 50 mg per dL or greater, both ethanol and hemodialysis are recommended. Hemodialysis is also indicated if there is renal failure or severe electrolyte disturbances, regardless of the serum ethylene glycol concentration.

4-Methylpyrazole is a competitive inhibitor of alcohol dehydrogenase recently approved for the treatment of ethylene glycol poisoning in adults. Currently, use of ethanol is recommended in children; but if available, 4-methylpyrazole could be considered. 4-Methylpyrazole is an oral or i.v. agent with quick onset of action, and unlike ethanol, its use is not associated with CNS depression. The loading dose is 15 mg per kg i.v. The maintenance dose is 10 mg per kg every 12 hours for four doses, then 15 mg per kg every 12 hours thereafter. During hemodialysis, additional doses may be required.

Antihistamines

Antihistamines may depress or stimulate the CNS. Used therapeutically, CNS depression is most commonly seen as drowsiness or dizziness. With increasing doses, stimulation results in insomnia, nervousness, and restlessness. In antihistamine overdose, the CNS stimulatory effects of the drug predominate. In children, CNS stimulation causes excitement, tremors, hyperactivity, hallucinations, and with higher dosages, tonic-clonic convulsions. Children are also more likely to have signs and symptoms of anticholinergic poisoning: flushed skin, fever, tachycardia, and fixed dilated pupils. The nonsedating antihistamines terfenadine (no longer available in the United States) and astemizole have caused cardiac arrhythmia after overdose and as a result of drug–drug interactions. Cetirizine, loratadine, and fexophenadine have not produced this complication. Death from antihistamine ingestion in children usually is the result of uncontrolled seizures that progress to coma and cardiorespiratory arrest.

Options for GI decontamination include gastric emptying and the use of activated charcoal, as described in general previously. Overdoses with the sustained-release preparations may benefit from WBI. Patients with seizures (see Chapters 61 and 73) require anticonvulsant therapy immediately. Preferably, short-term control may be gained using diazepam, in a dose of 0.1 to 0.2 mg per kg i.v. Severely agitated patients with a clear anticholinergic toxidrome may have improved sensorium after administration of physostigmine. This is usually administered in an initial dose of 0.5 mg i.v. slowly over 3 minutes. The 0.5-mg dose may be repeated every 10 to 15 minutes (maximum 2 mg) to establish the effective total dose. This minimal effective dose may be repeated in several hours if necessary. It should be noted that when administered too rapidly or in too large a dose, physostigmine may precipitate seizures or asystole. Physostigmine would be particularly dangerous to use in the context of any coingestants that might affect intracardiac conduction, such as tricyclic antidepressants. A 12-lead ECG should be examined for conduction delays before physostigmine is given. Cardiac rhythm should be monitored closely during antidote infusion, and atropine should be available to reverse severe cholinergic effects that may also occur with physostigmine use. The potential risks encountered with physostigmine may favor use of a benzodiazepine for treatment of anticholinergic delirium.

Some patients may develop extreme hyperthermia and thus require aggressive measures to reduce core body temperature, including ice water baths and fans.

Aspirin

CLINICAL FINDINGS

The initial clinical signs and symptoms, the estimate of dose ingested, and the measurement of salicylate levels all serve to gauge the severity of a given acute aspirin poisoning. However, in cases of chronic therapeutic salicylism, the clinical picture is the most useful guideline. Because of the nonspecific nature of symptoms with salicylism, the initial differential diagnosis is broad and may include diabetic ketoacidosis, iron intoxication, and ethylene glycol ingestion.

Acute ingestion amounts of 150 to 300 mg per kg are associated with mild symptoms, 300 to 500 mg per kg are associated with moderate toxicity, and more than 500 mg per kg are associated with death. With mild toxicity (serum concentrations 30 to 50 mg per dL), manifestations may be confined to GI upset, tinnitus, and mild tachypnea. With moderate salicylate poisoning (serum level 50 to 100 mg per dL), more visible signs of toxicity—fever, diaphoresis, and agitation—appear. After severe salicylate poisoning (serum concentrations greater than 100 mg per dL), signs and symptoms are primarily neurologic and consist of dysarthria, coma, and seizures. Pulmonary manifestations, particularly pulmonary edema, may appear in severe cases. In victims of chronic salicylism, these same conditions appear at significantly lower serum salicylate concentrations. Death from salicylism results from severe CNS toxicity with complete loss of function in cardiorespiratory centers, leading to respiratory and/or cardiac arrest. A nomogram that strives to correlate clinical toxicity with serum salicylate levels and the time of ingestion exists. This nomogram has many shortcomings that diminish its clinical utility. Severity of salicylate intoxication is best assessed by physical examination, electrolytes, and blood gas analysis.

MANAGEMENT

Specific therapeutic goals in salicylate intoxication include correction of fluid and electrolyte disturbances and the enhancement of salicylate excretion. Fluid therapy should be aimed at restoring hydration and electrolyte balance and at promoting renal salicylate excretion. For patients with symptomatic salicylate intoxication, urine alkalinization should be combined with fluid resuscitation. The initial fluid should contain 5% dextrose with 50 to 100 mEq per L of sodium bicarbonate. In cases of severe acidosis, additional bicarbonate may be necessary. Because hypokalemia impairs the ability of the urine to create an alkaline urine and is exacerbated by administration of sodium bicarbonate, potassium must be added to i.v. fluids. Both urine alkalinization and repetitive oral charcoal should be continued until salicylate concentration falls below 30 to 40 mg per dL and symptoms resolve.

Salicylate elimination can also be enhanced by hemodialysis or hemoperfusion. Hemodialysis should be reserved for seriously ill patients. Specific indications include 1) serum salicylate levels greater than 100 mg per dL after acute ingestion, 2) a serum salicylate level of 60 to 70 mg per dL or greater after chronic salicylism, 3) severe acidosis or other electrolyte disturbance, 4) renal failure, 5) persistent neurologic dysfunction, and/or 6) progressive clinical deterioration despite standard treatment.

Cardiac Drugs

BETA-ADRENERGIC BLOCKERS AND CALCIUM CHANNEL BLOCKERS

Both beta-blockers (BBs) and calcium channel blockers (CCBs) may present with fulminant cardiovascular and neurologic findings after a large overdose. Typical presentations of both agents include marked bradycardia and hypotension; particularly with the CCBs, common additional findings are those of abnormal atrioventricular (AV) node conduction, with AV block or accelerated junctional rhythm. The CNS may also be affected, with coma and/or convulsions that occur in either category of overdoses. Metabolic disturbances include hypoglycemia with BBs and hyperglycemia and metabolic acidosis with CCBs. Bronchospasm may complicate BB toxicity further in patients with underlying reactive airway disease.

Management begins with aggressive gastric decontamination for both types of agents. Bradycardia and hypotension may improve with standard treatment such as atropine, fluid boluses, and pressors; however, many cases prove resistant to these measures. Additional therapy includes calcium infusion for the CCBs, with the recommended adult initial dose being 10 mL of 10% calcium chloride, or 30 mL of 10% calcium gluconate, which may be repeated two or three times as necessary (eg, an initial pediatric dose of approximately 0.2 mL per kg calcium chloride or 0.6 mL per kg of calcium gluconate). Serum calcium should be monitored if several doses are used to avoid severe hypercalcemia. Glucagon has been used with success to improve heart rate and blood pressure in overdoses of both types of agents. The usual adult dosing regimen is 3 to 5 mg by i.v. bolus, which may be repeated to a total dose of 10 mg, followed by infusion at 2 to 5 mg per hour. Such dosing translates to 50 to 150 μg per kg boluses and similar amounts per hour for pediatric patients.

CLONIDINE

Ingestions of small amounts of clonidine can potentially lead to significant toxicity in children. Initial toxic manifestations include altered mental status that may range from lethargy to coma. Victims also may develop significant hypothermia. In severe intoxications, coma, miosis, and respiratory depression may appear. The cardiovascular changes that accompany clonidine intoxications may range from profound hypotension and bradycardia to hypertension. Clonidine-induced hypertension occurs uncommonly and is thought to result from α-adrenergic effects at peripheral vascular receptors that override the central, antihypertensive effect. The clinical picture of clonidine intoxication typically lasts 8 to 24 hours.

Because patients with severe intoxication often have coma and respiratory depression, emergency endotracheal intubation may be necessary. Hypotension should be treated with fluids and vasopressors as needed. Hypertension is generally uncommon, very transient, and would rarely require specific treatment. GI decontamination may be ineffective more than 2 hours after ingestion because clonidine is rapidly absorbed from the GI tract. However, the potential benefits of activated charcoal administration far outweigh any of its risks.

Because naloxone is a benign agent and may potentially improve mental status to the extent that intubation becomes unnecessary, a trial dose of 1 to 2 mg should be administered. Large amounts of naloxone (up to 8 mg) must be provided before it can be concluded that the intoxication is not responsive to this therapy.

DIGOXIN

The therapeutic serum digoxin concentration (SDC) is less than 2 ng per mL. A concentration in the slightly higher range often does not correlate with clinical manifestations and may be of limited value. However, when SDC exceeds 4 ng per mL, some evidence of intoxication usually appears. This toxicity is influenced by many host factors, including patient age, underlying illness, and disturbances in serum potassium, magnesium, and calcium.

With significant intoxication, the symptoms of digoxin poisoning include nausea, vomiting, and visual disturbances. With more severe intoxication, additional symptoms, including lethargy, disorientation, electrolyte disturbances, and cardiac disturbances, appear. The hallmark of severe acute digoxin toxicity is hyperkalemia, the result of profound inhibition of sodium-potassium adenosine triphosphatase activity. The typical pattern of cardiac toxicity with digoxin overdose initially is prolonged AV dissociation that appears as heart block that ranges from first to third degree. These conduction disturbances can lead to the development of ventricular or supraventricular escape rhythms. In patients with chronic digoxin intoxication, these symptoms may be more striking than in those with acute, single digoxin overdoses. In fact, children with acute digoxin intoxication rarely develop life-threatening illness if their peak SDC remains below 10 ng per mL.

Management

The management of the patient with digoxin intoxication begins with evaluation of the vital signs, particularly hemodynamic status. Patients should have an ECG followed by continuous cardiac monitoring. If significant cardiac arrhythmias are already present, they are treated initially according to advanced cardiac life support protocols. GI decontamination should include administration of activated charcoal with a cathartic. Clinical assessment requires an ECG, electrolytes (including magnesium and calcium), urinalysis, and SDC. Electrolyte disturbances should be treated aggressively because they will aggravate any digoxin-induced arrhythmias.

Some digoxin-specific antibody fragments have become specific antidotal therapy for reversing the toxic manifestations. These antibody fragments are indicated in the following circumstances after digoxin poisoning: 1) progressive signs and symptoms of intoxication, 2) life-threatening cardiac arrhythmias, or 3) severe hyperkalemia (defined as a serum potassium of 5.5 mEq per L or greater). The dose of antibody fragments is calculated on the basis of ingested digoxin dose (in the case of acute intoxication) or on the basis of SDC (in the case of chronic intoxication). Each 40-mg vial of digoxin-Fab will bind 0.6 mg of digoxin. The total dose of Fab needed (in vials) may be estimated by dividing a known ingested dose by 0.6, or calculated for the steady state context as body load of digoxin:

$$\text{No. of vials} = \text{SDC (ng/mL)} \times \text{wt (in kg)}/100$$

Household Cleaning Products and Caustics

CLINICAL FINDINGS

Ingestions of acid and alkali corrosives cause immediate severe burning of exposed surfaces, usually with intense dysphagia. Associated glottic edema may cause airway obstruction and asphyxia. Severe acid ingestions most often cause gastric necrosis and may be complicated by gastric perforation and peritonitis. With alkalis, severe damage is more commonly found in the esophagus; deep-tissue injury may quickly lead to esophageal perforation, mediastinitis, and death. As already noted, alkalis also produce severe esophageal strictures in survivors.

MANAGEMENT

The approach to management of cleaning products and caustic ingestions, as outlined in Figs. 78.3 and 78.4, begins with rapid clinical assessment of cardiorespiratory function, neurologic status, and evidence of GI hemorrhage. Life support measures may be needed emergently to secure the airway and to treat shock or metabolic acidosis. Even patients with minimal symptoms and the absence of oral lesions may have significant esophageal injury; thus, all patients with a convincing history of exposure to a caustic substance need esophagoscopy to be evaluated fully for the presence of esophageal burns.

If the eyes are involved (something that should always be considered if a caustic has splashed on the face), copious irrigation should be provided and carried out for at least 15 minutes,

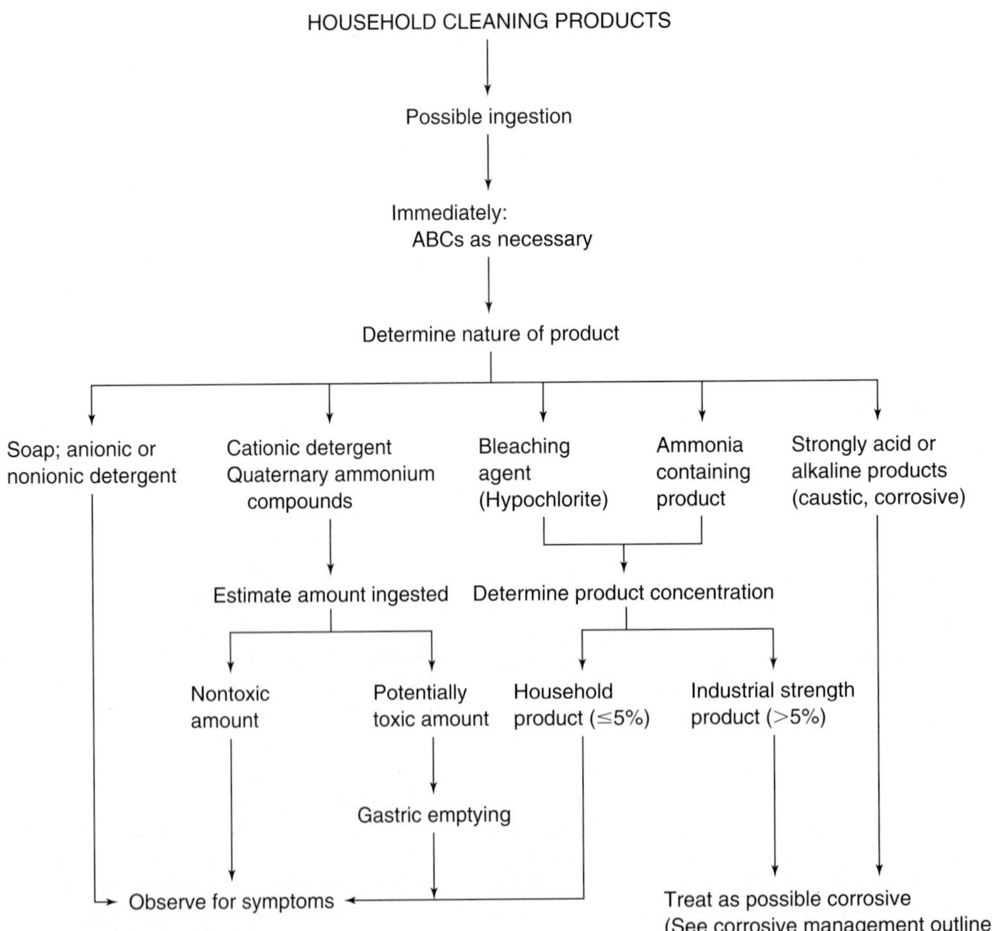

Figure 78.3. Algorithm for management of household cleaning product ingestion. (Modified with permission from Temple AR, Lovejoy FH Jr. *Cleaning products and their accidental ingestion*. New York: Soap and Detergent Association, 1980.)

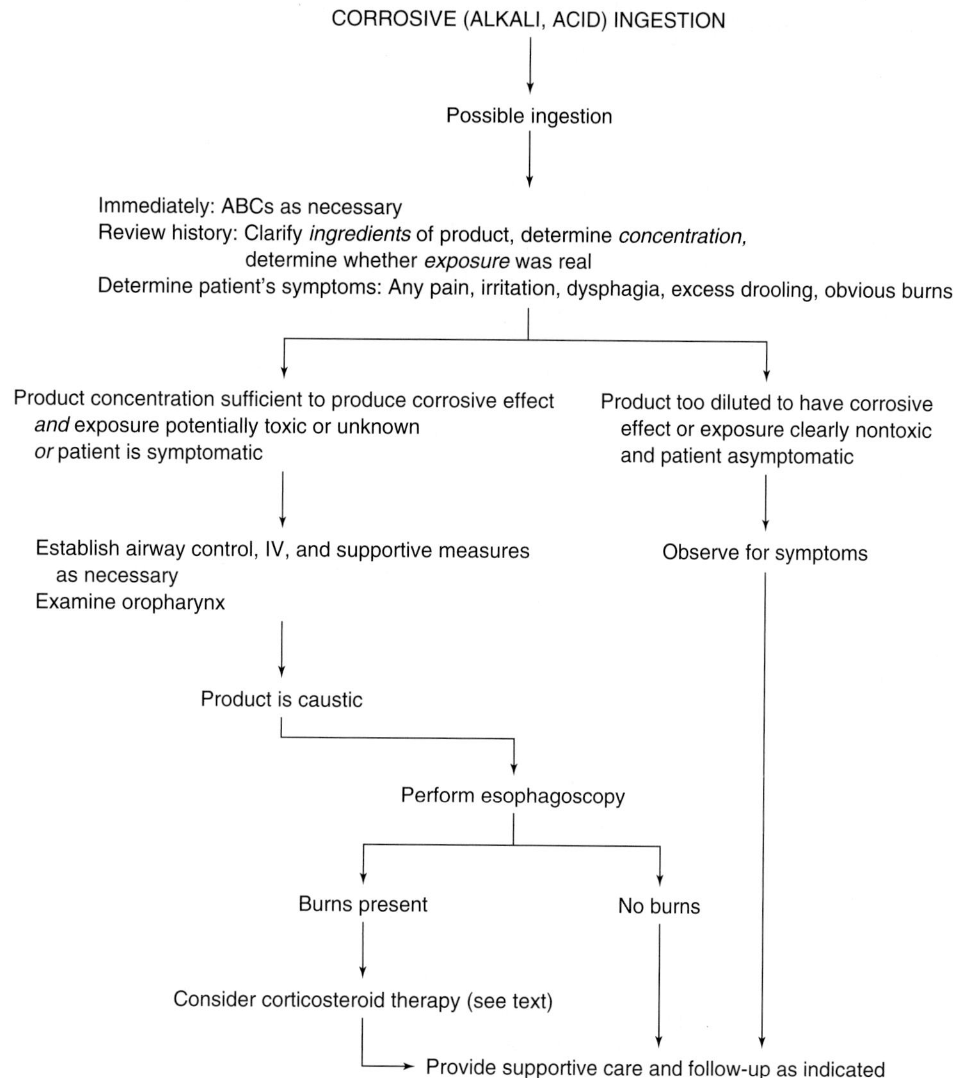
CORROSIVE (ALKALI, ACID) INGESTION
Possible ingestion
Immediately: ABCs as necessary
Review history: Clarify ingredients of product, determine concentration, determine whether exposure was real
Determine patient's symptoms: Any pain, irritation, dysphagia, excess drooling, obvious burns
Product concentration sufficient to produce corrosive effect and exposure potentially toxic or unknown or patient is symptomatic
Product too diluted to have corrosive effect or exposure clearly nontoxic and patient asymptomatic
Establish airway control, IV, and supportive measures as necessary
Examine oropharynx
Observe for symptoms
Product is caustic
Perform esophagoscopy
Burns present
No burns
Consider corticosteroid therapy (see text)
Provide supportive care and follow-up as indicated

Figure 78.4. Algorithm for management of corrosive ingestion. (Modified with permission from Temple AR, Lovejoy FH Jr. *Cleaning products and their accidental ingestion*. New York: Soap and Detergent Association, 1980.)

with longer periods for crystalline caustics. The physician should perform pH testing of fluids in the ocular cul-de-sac after irrigation to confirm that corrosives have been neutralized; the normal pH of tears is 7.

Hydrocarbons

The major toxicity of hydrocarbons varies from class to class. However, the feature that these agents have in common is a low viscosity that permits them to spread freely over large surface areas, such as the lungs, when aspirated. This property (plus their solvent actions) leads to a necrotizing, often fatal chemical pneumonitis when these compounds are aspirated. The high volatility of these substances is responsible for alterations in mental status, including narcosis, inebriation, and frank coma. In addition to these toxicities, the solvents possess additional toxicities, including the risk of bone marrow injury (in the case of benzene). Finally, with the toxic hydrocarbons, additional toxicities may occur as a result of actions such as cardiotoxicity or as a result of the pharmacologic properties of the other agents contained within these compounds. The major toxicity of hydrocarbons is classified in Table 78.10.

TABLE 78.10. Classification of Hydrocarbons
Nontoxic (unless complicated by gross aspiration)
Asphalt, tars
Mineral oil
Liquid petrolatum
Motor oil, axle grease
Baby oils, suntan oils
Systemic toxicity
Halogenated (carbon tetrachloride, trichloroethane)
Aromatic (benzene, toluene, xylene)
Additives (camphor, organophosphates, heavy metals)
Aspiration hazard (without significant systemic toxicity unless ingested in massive quantity)
Turpentine
Gasoline
Kerosene
Mineral seal oil (furniture polish)
Charcoal lighter fluid
Cigarette lighter fluid
Mineral spirits

TABLE 78.11. Guidelines for Chelation Therapy of Lead Poisoning

Condition, BPb (μg/dL)	Regimen	Comment
Encephalopathy	BAL 450 mg/m²/d + CaNa2EDTA 1,500 mg/m²/d[a]	75 mg/m² i.m. every 4 h for 5 d Continuous infusion, or 2–4 divided i.v. doses, for 5 d (start 4 h after BAL)
Symptomatic, BPb > 70	BAL 300–450 mg/m² day + CaNa2EDTA 1,000–1,500 mg/m²/d[a]	50–75 mg/m² every 4 h for 3–5 d Continuous infusion, or 2–4 divided i.v. doses, for 5 d (start 4 h after BAL)
Asymptomatic, BPb 45–69	Succimer 700–1,050 mg/m²/d or CaNa2EDTA, 1,000 mg/m²/d[a]	350 mg/m² t.i.d. for 5 d, then b.i.d. for 14 d Continuous infusion, or 2–4 divided i.v. doses, for 5 d

BPb, blood lead (μg/dL); i.m., intramuscular; i.v., intravenous.
[a] Doses expressed in mg/kg: BAL 450 mg/m² (24 mg/kg); 300 mg/m² (18 mg/kg); CaNa2EDTA 1,000 mg/m² (25–50 mgkg); 1,500 mg/m² (50–75 mg/kg); Succimer 350 mg/m² (10 mg/kg).

The amount of a hydrocarbon that has been ingested by a pediatric patient is often difficult to quantify. However, any degree of aspiration results in signs, including coughing, gagging, or tachypnea. Less than 1 mL of some compounds, when aspirated directly into the trachea, may produce severe pneumonitis and eventual death. When ingested, these compounds are poorly absorbed from the GI tract. In a retrospective study of hydrocarbon ingestions in children, most children (880 of 950) developed no symptoms.

Clinical manifestations of hydrocarbon ingestion depend largely on the specific profile of toxicity of the ingested substances. All these agents cause significant GI irritation that may be associated with nausea and bloody emesis. CNS effects may range from inebriation to coma. Hemolysis with hemoglobinuria has been reported after significant ingestions. Finally, hydrocarbon ingestion may be associated with the development of fever and leukocytosis in up to 15% of patients in the absence of clinically evident pneumonitis.

Because most hydrocarbons cause clinical toxicity only when aspirated, the mainstay of treatment is to leave ingested compounds in the gut (when possible) and to prevent emesis or reflux. Gastric emptying is generally reserved only for those compounds with the potential for systemic toxic effects (Table 78.10). These compounds include the halogenated hydrocarbons (eg, trichloroethane, carbon tetrachloride) and aromatic hydrocarbons (eg, toluene, xylene, benzene). In addition, all petroleum distillates, regardless of their viscosity, should be evacuated from the GI tract if they contain dangerous additives, such as heavy metals or insecticides. Finally, gastric emptying should be considered when a huge amount of hydrocarbon has been ingested, as in a suicide attempt.

Patients who have aspirated may exhibit immediate choking, coughing, and gagging as the product is swallowed and then vomited after ingestion. Aspiration of the product may also occur at the time of the initial swallowing. Emergency department (ED) management of these patients is outlined in Fig. 78.5. If the patient has any cough or respiratory symptoms upon arrival to the ED, a chest radiograph should be obtained immediately. Because there is a gradual evolution of abnormal radiographs, an initially negative chest radiograph should be repeated at 4 to 6 hours after ingestion. All patients with abnormal chest radiographs or persistent respiratory symptoms after 4 to 6 hours of ED observation should be admitted to the hospital for observation. Patients who are asymptomatic after this period of observation may be discharged. Because pneumonitis occasionally appears 12 to 24 hours after exposure, detailed instructions should be provided for warning signs of respiratory dysfunction.

Iron

CLINICAL MANIFESTATIONS

The clinical effects of iron poisoning are classically divided into four phases. Phase I represents the effects of direct mucosal injury and usually lasts 6 hours. Vomiting, diarrhea, and GI blood

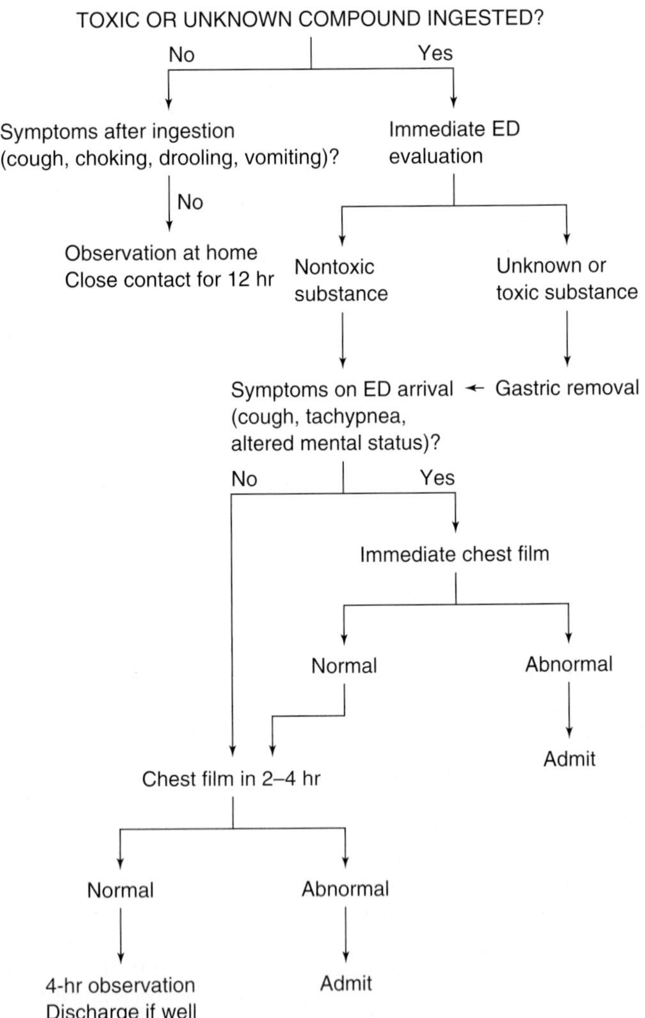

Figure 78.5. Management of petroleum distillate ingestion. (Modified with permission from Shannon M. *Petroleum distillate poisoning*. Harwood-Nuss A, ed. Philadelphia: JB Lippincott, 1991.)

loss are the prominent early signs; when severe, the patient may lapse into early coma and shock caused by volume loss and metabolic acidosis.

Phase II, which lasts from 6 to 24 hours after ingestion, is marked by diminution of the GI symptoms. With appropriate therapy to replace fluid and/or blood losses, the child may seem relatively well and often goes on to full recovery without any subsequent symptoms. However, this remission may be transient and may be followed by phase III, characterized by cyanosis and profound metabolic acidosis. The child may develop coma, seizures, and intractable shock. This phase is believed to represent hepatocellular injury with consequent disturbed energy metabolism; elevated levels of lactic and citric acids are noted in experimental iron poisoning before cardiac or respiratory failure occurs. Jaundice and elevated transaminases are noted in this phase. A phase IV has been described in survivors of severe iron poisoning, marked by pyloric stenosis that results from scarring and consequent obstruction.

Laboratory abnormalities often associated with severe iron intoxication include metabolic acidosis, leukocytosis, hyperglycemia, hyperbilirubinemia and increased liver enzymes, and a prolonged prothrombin time. If fluid loss is significant, there will be hemoconcentration and elevated BUN. Abdominal films may show radiopaque material in the stomach, but the absence of this finding does not indicate a trivial ingestion.

MANAGEMENT

Serum iron levels have been shown to correlate with the likelihood of developing symptoms (usually a reflection of the serum iron that exceeds the iron-binding capacity and results in free-circulating iron). Usually, iron levels below 350 μg per dL, when drawn 3 to 5 hours after ingestion, predict an asymptomatic course. Patients with levels in the 350 to 500 μ per dL range often show mild phase I symptoms but rarely develop serious complications. Levels higher than 500 μ per dL suggest significant risk for phase III manifestations.

Although serum iron levels are useful, toxicity from iron overdose remains a clinical diagnosis. Ill patients require vigorous hydration and support. Children who are completely asymptomatic 6 hours after ingestion are unlikely to develop systemic illness. Among laboratory studies, the presence of metabolic acidosis or acidemia probably best correlates with toxicity. A white blood cell (WBC) count higher than 15000 per mm^3 paired with a serum glucose higher than 150 mg per dL is fairly predictive of elevated serum iron levels (but are not sensitive). Radiopaque material on abdominal radiograph also suggests significant absorption of iron. Measurement of the total iron-binding capacity is no longer believed to be useful in acute management. With these observations in mind, it is possible to construct a protocol for the triage and initial management of the patient who has ingested a possibly toxic amount of iron (Fig. 78.6).

Chelation therapy with parenteral deferoxamine enhances the excretion of iron. The most efficacious route is a continuous i.v. infusion, and the maximum recommended dose is 15 mg per kg per hour (maximum daily dose 360 mg per kg, up to 6 g total). A higher infusion rate has been associated with hypotension but may be necessary (in conjunction with blood pressure support) for severe ingestions. Chelation is continued until the serum iron level returns to normal, metabolic acidosis has resolved, the patient is clinically improved, and the urine color returns to normal. The dose of deferoxamine may be titrated down in concert with the patient's clinical response and fall in iron levels.

Once the patient has been stabilized initially, further problems may include hypotension, profound metabolic acidosis, hypoglycemia or hyperglycemia, anemia and colloid loss

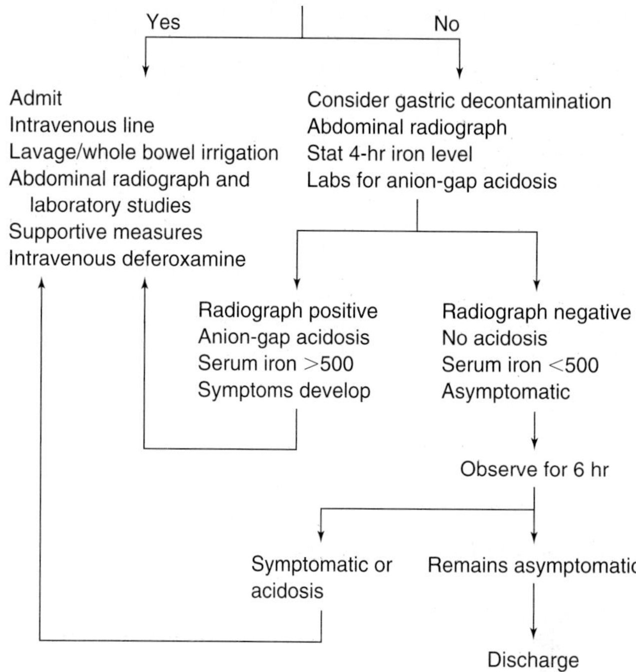

Figure 78.6. The initial approach to the patient who has ingested a possibly toxic dose of iron.

caused by GI hemorrhage (after equilibration), renal shutdown resulting from shock, and hepatic failure with an associated bleeding diathesis. The maintenance of an adequate urine output is critical to prevent renal failure and to foster excretion of the iron–deferoxamine complex. If renal failure supervenes, chelation may be continued with concurrent dialysis because the complex is dialyzable.

Isoniazid

In overdose, the hallmark of isoniazid (INH) poisoning is the triad of seizures, metabolic acidosis, and coma. INH is not usually detected on routine toxin screens, and serum concentrations are of little value. Management of INH intoxication begins with advanced life support. Pharmacologic treatment for INH intoxication includes sodium bicarbonate, anticonvulsants, and pyridoxine. Administration of pyridoxine has been shown to provide specific antidotal therapy for INH poisoning. Pyridoxine is given by i.v. in a dose that equals the estimated dose of INH in milligrams. In cases in which the ingested amount is unknown, a single dose of 5 g (70 mg per kg in children) of pyridoxine is administered. Rarely, repeat administration is necessary.

Lead

CLINICAL FINDINGS

Early signs and symptoms of plumbism are notably vague and nonspecific. Abdominal complaints, including colicky pain, constipation, anorexia, and intermittent vomiting, are common; of course, these same symptoms are often ascribed to relatively normal 2 year olds by their parents. The child with early plumbism may also show listlessness and irritability. When encephalopathy begins, the child develops persistent vomiting and becomes drowsy, clumsy, or frankly ataxic. As encephalopathy worsens, the level of consciousness deteriorates further, and seizures commonly occur. Peripheral neuropathy often occurs in adults with lead poisoning but is rare in children, although it is seen occasionally in those with an underlying hemoglobinopathy. Other organs may be damaged by lead. The kidneys may develop disturbances that range from slight aminoaciduria to a full Fanconi syndrome with glycosuria and phosphaturia (in addition to aminoaciduria). High levels are also associated with a microcytic anemia that results from a defect in hemoglobin synthesis. However, most anemia seen in children with excess lead levels is actually caused by concurrent iron deficiency. A moderately sensitive laboratory measure of lead effect on heme synthesis is the evaluation of erythrocyte protoporphyrin (EP), a heme precursor. Moderately elevated EP levels are seen in iron deficiency, but levels above 250 to 300 μg per dL are almost always the result of chronic lead poisoning.

MANAGEMENT

The asymptomatic child discovered to have a lead level in the 20 to 44 μg per dL range, particularly if the EP is greater than 250 μg per dL, deserves immediate referral to a pediatrician or toxicologist. All symptomatic children and those with lead levels higher than 44 μg per dL need urgent treatment.

RECOGNITION

As stated previously, to recognize mildly symptomatic patients with lead poisoning (or asymptomatic children with high lead levels at great risk to soon become symptomatic) requires a high index of suspicion. All children between 1 and 5 years of age are suspect if they have 1) persistent vomiting, listlessness or irritability, clumsiness, or loss of recently acquired developmental skills; 2) afebrile convulsions; 3) a strong tendency to pica, including a history of acute accidental ingestions or aural or nasal foreign body; 4) a deteriorating pre–World War II house or a parent with industrial exposures; 5) a family history of lead poisoning; 6) iron deficiency anemia; or 7) evidence of child abuse or neglect.

The child between 1 to 5 years of age who comes to the ED with an acute encephalopathy presents a dilemma for the physician: lead intoxication requires urgent diagnosis, but confirmation with a blood level is usually not available on an immediate basis. A constellation of historical features of lead poisoning increases the likelihood of the diagnosis. These features include 1) a prodromal illness of several days' to weeks' duration (suggestive of mild symptomatic plumbism); 2) a history of pica; and 3) a source of exposure to lead. Several nonspecific laboratory findings make lead poisoning likely enough to warrant presumptive chelation therapy until confirmation by lead levels is available. These findings include 1) microcytic anemia; 2) elevated EP level, especially if greater than 250 μg per dL (conversely, a normal or minimally elevated EP level, less than 50 μg per dL, would make lead encephalopathy caused by chronic lead paint exposure unlikely); 3) basophilic stippling of peripheral erythrocytes or, if feasible, of red cell precursors on bone marrow examination; 4) elevated urinary coproporphyrins; 5) glycosuria; 6) aminoaciduria; 7) radiopaque flecks on abdominal radiographs; and 8) dense metaphyseal bands on radiographs of knees and wrists (lead lines).

Abnormalities on examination of cerebrospinal fluid (CSF) are also indicative of lead encephalopathy, including a lymphocytic pleocytosis, elevated protein, and increased pressure. However, a lumbar puncture should not be performed if lead encephalopathy is strongly suspected because the risk of herniation is considerable. If CSF must be examined to rule out bacterial meningitis, the minimal amount (less than 1 mL) necessary should be obtained. Alternatively, one might institute treatment for presumed meningitis, perform a determination of the lead level, and consider a delayed lumbar puncture after several days if the lead level is normal.

TREATMENT

The specific chelating drugs commonly used for symptomatic lead intoxication are edathamil calcium disodium (CaEDTA) and 2,4-dimercaptopropanol (British Anti-Lewisite or BAL) (Table 78.11). Succimer (dimercaptosuccinic acid, or DMSA) has been approved for pediatric use in cases in which lead levels exceed 45 μg per dL (Table 78.11). However, experience with its use in symptomatic patients is limited.

Asymptomatic children found to have lead levels of 45 to 69 μg per dL should have urgent referral and treatment for 5 days with CaEDTA or DMSA alone. If the lead level is above 69 μg per dL, BAL and EDTA are used for at least the first 2 days (Table 78.11). Supportive care includes adequate hydration to promote good urine output. Symptomatic children without frank encephalopathy should receive chelation therapy with a combination of CaEDTA and BAL for 5 days. Supportive care includes close monitoring for signs of encephalopathy and, again, maintenance of urine flow.

Patients with encephalopathy require combination chelation therapy with CaEDTA and BAL, as well as intensive supportive care. Fluid therapy is critical and must be individualized. Adequate urine flow is needed to excrete the lead–chelate complexes; however, fluid overload must be avoided so that cerebral edema is not exacerbated. A reasonable goal is to supply basal water requirements, maintaining urine production at 0.35 to 0.5 mL per kcal per 24 hours. Basal water needs in children av-

TABLE 78.12. Common Nontoxic Plants

Abelis	Echeveria
African daisy	Eugenia
African palm	Gardenia
African violet	Grape ivy
Airplane plant	Hedge apples
Aluminum plant	Hens and chicks
Aralia	Honeysuckle
Asparagus fern (may cause dermatitis)	Hoya
Aspidistra (cash iron plant)	Impatiens
Aster	Jade plant
Baby's teers	Kalanchoe
Bachelor buttons	Lily (day, Easter, or tiger)
Begonia	Lipstick plant
Birds nest fern	Magnolia
Blood leaf plant	Marigold
Boston ferns	Monkey plant
Bougainvillea	Mother-in-law tongue
Cactus—certain varieties	Norfolk island pine
California holly	Peperomia
California poppy	Petunia
Camelia	Prayer plant
Christmas cactus	Purple passion
Coleus	Pyracantha
Corn plant	Rose
Crab apples	Sansevieria
Creeping Charlie	Scheffiera
Creeping Jennie, moneywort, lysima	Sensitive plant
Croton (house variety)	Spider plant
Dahlia	Swedish ivy
Dalsies	Umbrella
Dandelion	Violets
Dogwood	Wandering jew
Donkey tall	Weaping fig
Dracaena	Weeping willow
Easter lily	Wild onion
	Zebra plant

erage 1 mL per kcal and may be calculated as 100 kcal per kg for 0 to 10 kg, plus 50 kcal per kg for 10 to 20 kg, plus 20 kcal per kg for each kilogram above 20 kg.

Organophosphates

CLINICAL FINDINGS

The symptoms of acute organophosphate poisoning usually develop during the first 12 hours of contact. These include findings related to the CNS (dizziness, headache, ataxia, convulsions, and coma); nicotinic signs, including sweating, muscle twitching, tremors, weakness, and paralysis; and muscarinic signs characterized by the SLUDGE mnemonic, including salivation, *l*acrimation, *u*rination, *d*efecation, *g*astrointestinal cramping, and *e*mesis. In addition there may be miosis, bradycardia, bronchorrhea, and wheezing; in severe cases, pulmonary edema develops. Severe intoxications may also cause a toxic psychosis that resembles alcoholism. A depression of plasma or red blood cell cholinesterase activity provides the best laboratory marker of excessive absorption of organophosphates, although it is rarely available on a stat basis; it is important that treatment not be delayed until confirmation of plasma cholinesterase is obtained.

MANAGEMENT

After decontamination, antidotal therapy begins with the administration of atropine sulfate given in a dose of 0.05 to 0.1 mg per kg to children and 2 to 5 mg for adolescents and adults. This dose should be repeated every 10 to 30 minutes or as needed to obtain and maintain full atropinization, as indicated by clearing of bronchial secretions and pulmonary rales. Therapy is continued until all absorbed organophosphate has been metabolized and may require 2 mg to more than 2000 mg of atropine over the course of a few hours to several days. After atropinization has been instituted, severe poisonings should be treated with the addition of pralidoxime. This drug is particularly useful in poisonings characterized by profound weakness and muscle twitching. A dose of 25 to 50 mg per kg should be administered in 250 mL of saline by infusion over approximately 30 minutes; adults may receive 1 to 2 g by i.v. This may be repeated at 1-hour intervals if muscle weakness is not relieved, and then at intervals of 6 to 8 hours for 24 to 48 hours. In patients with severe poisoning, a 2.5% concentration may be infused continuously at the rate of 500 mg per hour in adolescents and adults, or approximately 20 mg per kg per hour in children. Occasionally, patients may require more than 48 hours of therapy; the end-point should be persistent relief of neurologic and cholinergic signs.

Phenothiazines

CLINICAL FINDINGS

With dose-dependent effects, the manifestations of intoxication after acute ingestion vary from mild to severe. In mild intoxication, CNS signs such as sedation, ataxia, and slurred speech occur. The anticholinergic effects of these drugs may cause constipation, urinary retention, and blurred vision. Because phenothiazines have potent actions on the temperature-regulating center of the hypothalamus, temperature disturbances occur in up to 30% of patients and may consist of hypothermia or hyperthermia. Orthostatic hypotension, the probable result of peripheral vasodilation, may also be noted with mild intoxication.

In moderate intoxications, the patients may have significant depression in level of consciousness. Extrapyramidal effects become notable at this level of intoxication with muscle stiffness or "cogwheel" rigidity seen on passive movement of the neck, biceps, or quadriceps. Anticholinergic manifestations are severe and include acute urinary retention and paralytic ileus; hypotension may be profound. Cardiac conduction disturbances may make their appearance and are often heralded by a prolonged Q-T interval.

In severe overdoses, patients are unable to be aroused. Deep tendon reflexes may be hyperactive. Dystonic reactions may occur, involving the head and neck and the cranial nerves (torticollis and opisthotonos). Arrhythmias and shock may result in death.

The dose-independent effect of the phenothiazines is the dystonic reaction. This striking clinical occurrence consists of episodic spasm of voluntary muscles, particularly those of the head and neck. Patients may develop torticollis, bruxism, tongue protrusion, or oculogyric crisis. Dystonic reactions are unrelated to the amount of ingested phenothiazine. They may or may not occur after the first dose. Their onset is 8 to 40 hours after ingestion of a single dose of phenothiazine. This marked delay between ingestion and manifestations often interferes with obtaining an accurate history of ingestion. Fortunately, although painful and distressing, dystonic reactions are rarely life threatening and usually resolve quickly after administration of anticholinergics.

MANAGEMENT

Treatment of acute phenothiazine intoxication hinges on the severity of ingestion. In patients with mild overdose, hospitalization is usually unnecessary. The autonomic signs and symptoms are most often transient and require no treatment. In patients with moderate or severe overdoses, the potential for life-threatening manifestation requires prompt evaluation of vital signs, GI decontamination (if ingestion was within 4 to 6 hours of ED arrival), vascular access, and cardiac monitoring. Pressors such as norepinephrine (see Chapter 3) may be used to correct the hypotension. In those rare instances of hypertension, the use of nitroprusside (see Chapter 28) may be indicated. Severe arrhythmias should be treated aggressively as detailed later under "Tricyclic Antidepressants." Attention should be directed to the treatment of temperature instability and other autonomic disturbances.

Dystonic reactions are effectively controlled by the intramuscular (i.m.) or i.v. administration of diphenhydramine in a dose 1 to 2 mg per kg. This dose may be repeated within 15 to 20 minutes if no effect is noted. An alternative agent is benztropine mesylate (1 to 2 mg for an older child or adolescent). This agent reportedly causes less sedation than diphenhydramine. After resolution of the dystonic reaction, oral treatment should be continued for an additional 24 to 48 hours to prevent recurrences.

Plants/Mushrooms

PLANT TOXICITY

Plants are among the more commonly reported accidental ingestions in children. Most such ingestions involve common house and garden plants. Fortunately, of the many varieties of such plants, only a small fraction pose a serious toxic hazard (Tables 78.13 and 78.14).

MUSHROOMS

Two main groups of mushrooms can be characterized on the basis of the time interval between ingestion and symptom onset: those with the immediate onset of symptoms and those with delayed onset. Regardless of the mushroom, the initial management for all suspected poisonings includes activated charcoal and catharsis.

TABLE 78.13. Common Plant Toxidromes

Gastrointestinal irritants	Atropinic effects
Philodendron	Jimsonweed (thorn apple)
Diffenbachia	Deadly nightshade
Pokeweed	Epileptogenic effects
Wisteria	Water hernlock
Spurge laurel	Cyanogenic effects
Buttercup	Prunus species (chokecherry, wild black cherry, plum, peach, apricot, bitter almond)
Daffodil	Pear (seeds)
Rosary pea	Apple (seeds)
Castor bean	Crab apple (seeds)
Digitalis effects	Hydrangea
Lily-of-the-valley	Elderberry
Foxglove	
Cleander	
Yew	
Nicotinic effects	
Wild tobacco	
Golden chain tree	
Poison hemlock	

Onset of symptoms within 6 hours of ingestion usually confers a benign prognosis, although careful attention to fluid and electrolyte management is critical. Most mushrooms have GI effects. There are five general classes of mushrooms in this group, each possessing a unique toxicologic feature. Some "early-onset" mushrooms cause muscarinic effects, usually within 15 minutes, such as sweating, salivation, colic, and pulmonary edema. This syndrome responds to atropine therapy. Other early-onset mushrooms cause anticholinergic effects, including drowsiness, followed by mania and hallucinations. Another subgroup of early onset mushrooms produces a severe gastroenteritis syndrome. Hallucinogenic mushrooms such as psilocybin make up another class of mushrooms with early-onset symptoms. Finally, some mushrooms precipitate an Antabuse reaction if they are coingested with alcohol. Management for all these agents consists of supportive care and careful monitoring of fluid status.

The second, more important, category of mushrooms that are responsible for 90% of mushroom-related deaths are those associated with onset of symptoms that occur more than 6 hours after ingestion. The most important members of this group are those mushrooms that belong to the *Amanita phalloides* species. With these mushrooms, after a latent period of many hours, GI upset appears. Approximately 24 hours after ingestion, hepatic dysfunction appears, which results in fulminant hepatic failure. Without liver transplantation, such victims generally die.

Treatment of the gastroenteric phase includes fluid and electrolyte replacement. If renal failure develops, dialysis may be necessary. Hepatic damage after *A. phalloides* ingestion may be attenuated by early use of repetitive activated charcoal, which appears to interrupt enterohepatic recirculation of amatoxin.

Tricyclic Antidepressants

CLINICAL FINDINGS

The ingestion of 10 to 20 mg per kg of most tricyclic antidepressants represents a moderate to serious exposure, with coma and cardiovascular symptoms expected. The ingestion of 35 to 50 mg per kg may result in death. Children have been reported to be more sensitive than adults to tricyclic antidepressants and often have symptoms of toxicity at lower dosages.

Cyclic antidepressants have many pharmacologic effects. Anticholinergic activity causes altered sensorium and sinus tachycardia. Alpha-adrenergic blockade may lead to hypotension. However, the more severe cardiovascular effects are pri-

TABLE 78.14. Medications Dangerous to Toddlers in 1–2 Doses[a]

Agent	Minimal potential fatal dose[b]	Maximal dose size	Potential fatal dose	Major toxicity
Benzocaine	<20 mg/kg	10% gel 20% spray	−2 mL Baby Oragel	Methemoglobinemia, seizures
β-blockers (propranolol)	Unclear	160 mg	1–2 tablets	Bradycardia, hypotension, seizures, hypoglycemia
Calcium antagonists (verapamil)	<40 mg/kg	240 mg	1–2 tablets	Bradycardia, hypotension
Camphor	<100 mg/kg	1 g/5 mL	1 tsp camphorated oil 2 tsp Campho-phenique 5 tsp Vicks Vaporub	Seizures, CNS depression
Chloroquine	<30 mg/kg	500 mg	1 tablet	Seizures, arrhythmia
Clonidine	Unclear	0.3 mg tablet 7.5 mg patch	1 tablet 1 patch	Bradycardia, CNS depression
Diphenoxylate (Lomotil)	<1.2 mg/kg	2.5 mg/tablet or tsp	2 tablets/tsp	CNS and respiratory depression
Hypoglycemics, oral (glyburide)	−1 mg/kg	5 mg	2 tablets	Hypoglycemia
Lindane	−mg/kg	1% lotion	2 tsp	Seizures, CNS depression
Methyl salicylate	−200 mg/kg	1.4 g/mL	1/2 tsp oil of wintergreen 2 tsp Icy Hot Balm	Seizures, cardiovascular collapse
Phenothiazines (chlorpromazine)	−20 mg/kg	200 mg	1 tablet	Seizures, arrhythmia
Quinidine	−50 mg/kg	300 mg	2 tablets	Seizures, arrhythmia
Quinine	−80 mg/kg	650 mg	2 tablets	Seizures, arrhythmia
Theophylline	−50 mg/kg	500 mg	1 tablet	Seizures, arrhythmia
TCAs (imipramine)	−20 mg/kg	150 mg	1–2 tablets	Seizures, arrhythmia, hypotension

CNS, central nervous system; TCAs, tricyclic antidepressants.

[a] A long list of commonly encountered, highly toxic, *non*pharmacologic agents can be severely poisonous in 1–2 doses. These are not included here.

[b] For the purposes of this table a "dose" refers to a single pill or roughly a 5-cc swallow. Calculations are based upon a previously healthy toddler of 10-kg body weight.

marily caused by the membrane-depressant or quinidinelike effects that depress myocardial conduction and may lead to multiple focal premature ventricular contractions and ventricular tachycardia. It has been shown that a QRS interval over 0.1 second is associated with a significant morbidity and mortality in these patients; this delay in conduction may progress to complete heart block and cardiac standstill and/or the previously mentioned ventricular arrhythmias. Another typical electrocardiographic finding suggestive of cyclic antidepressant poisoning is the finding of an R wave of greater than 3-mm amplitude in the QRS complex in lead aVR.

Neurologic findings include lethargy, disorientation, ataxia, hallucinations, and with severe overdoses, coma, and seizures. Fever is commonly present initially, but hypothermia may occur later. Additional anticholinergic symptomatology includes decreased GI motility, which delays gastric emptying time, and urinary retention. Muscle twitching has been observed and may be associated with increased deep tendon reflexes. Although the pupils may be dilated, they usually respond to light.

MANAGEMENT

Severe tricyclic antidepressant overdoses require gastric decontamination. Lavage can be considered even for those patients who present as late as 4 to 12 hours after ingestion. Certainly, the administration of activated charcoal should be performed. Significant conduction delays or arrhythmias resulting from tricyclic antidepressants may benefit from alkalinization of the blood. A sodium bicarbonate bolus of 1 to 2 mEq per kg can be given during continuous ECG monitoring. Bicarbonate infusion can then be used to keep the serum pH at 7.45 to 7.55. If arrhythmias persist, appropriate antiarrhythmic therapy should be instituted, perhaps using lidocaine (see Chapters 1 and 72). Quinidine or procainamide should be avoided because each may increase heart block in this situation. Physostigmine, although previously recommended for its antidotal effects on the anticholinergic aspects of these poisonings, has the potential to worsen ventricular conduction defects and to lower the seizure threshold. Its use is currently considered to be contraindicated in cyclic antidepressant overdoses. In the presence of hypotension, many clinicians have advocated the use of norepinephrine infusions (0.1 to 0.3 μg per kg per minute).

Other Antidepressants

Selective serotonin reuptake inhibitors (SSRIs) most commonly produce CNS depression in overdose. Seizures may occur after large ingestions. Life-threatening events from acute overdose of these compounds rarely occur. The serotonin syndrome, manifested by muscular rigidity, myoclonus, flushing, and autonomic instability, more typically occurs as the result of drug interaction and is potentially lethal. Amoxapine has anticholinergic activity but is best known for its convulsant properties and the tendency for victims to present with status epilepticus. Bupropion, prescribed perhaps most commonly in smoking cessation programs, prevents reuptake of biogenic amines and is also seizurogenic. The α-adrenergic antagonism of trazodone may lead to hypotension.

There are three important clinical pictures of monoamine oxidase inhibitor (MAOI) toxicity. First, because GI tract activity of monoamine oxidase is also inhibited by these drugs, patients who take them appropriately and then ingest foods or drugs that contain biogenic amines (eg, tyramine in wines, cheese, or soy sauce and decongestants) may develop severe hypertension with headache, seizures, or stroke. The second picture of MAOI toxicity appears when those who take the drug therapeutically are given certain sympathomimetic or serotonergic agents causing the serotonin syndrome. Important examples of such drugs include common agents in over-the-counter cough and cold preparations such as dextromethorphan, analgesics such as meperidine, and psychotropic medications such as clomipramine and fluoxetine or other SSRIs. In these patients, this drug combination may quickly lead to hyperpyrexia, skeletal muscle rigidity, cardiac arrhythmias, and death. This is one of the few fatal drug interactions known. Finally, those with acute MAOI overdoses develop a clinical syndrome that includes blood pressure instability, hyperpyrexia, skeletal muscle rigidity, seizures, and death.

Because of the toxicity of these agents and the frequent delay in their onset of activity (up to 24 hours), all patients with a history of MAOI ingestion, regardless of symptoms, should be admitted to the hospital for 24 hours. Management of the patient with MAOI toxicity is largely dictated by the specific toxic manifestations. In those with hypertensive reactions, treatment consists of the immediate administration of an antihypertensive. The ideal agent may be nitroprusside because its brief duration of action permits titration of effect. In the treatment of hyperpyrexia, cooling measures are promptly instituted. Because hyperpyrexia is often accompanied by skeletal muscle rigidity and rhabdomyolysis, serum creatine kinase should be measured and close attention should be paid to the urine for any signs of myoglobinuria. Benzodiazepines are often helpful in this situation and neuromuscular blockade may be beneficial in patients who have severe muscle rigidity with hyperthermia. In the patient with acute overdose, treatment is directed to hemodynamic stability. Because blood pressure changes occur quickly and consist of hypotension and hypertension, hypertension should be treated with short-acting agents (see Chapter 28) and hypotension with fluid and vasopressor support (see Chapter 3). Intensive care unit admission is mandatory for these patients because of their clinical instability.

Drugs Dangerous in Small Doses

Toddlers often are brought to EDs for evaluation after possibly having ingested one or two doses of a medication. Most often these children will be fine with little treatment beyond reassurance. There are circumstances, however, when this situation can be life threatening and proper intervention can be lifesaving. It is wise to be familiar with a modest list of pharmaceuticals that may cause dangerous toxicity to young children with just one or two doses (Table 78.14). A systematic approach to these patients includes a careful history, an examination with attention to the presence of toxidromes (Table 78.3), and a guided laboratory assessment. An algorithmic approach to this situation is provided in Fig. 78.7.

Table 78.15 provides a summary of the common drugs of abuse, their typical routes of administration, associated symptoms, toxic levels, and duration of action.

Phencyclidine (Angel Dust)

MANAGEMENT

Phencyclidine (PCP) is easily detected through a qualitative analysis of urine. Serum levels are rarely available and do not correlate with clinical manifestations. Therefore, management must often be based solely on a history of exposure or index of suspicion. Initial treatment is directed at stabilizing vital signs and treating life-threatening events such as seizures. If exposure is the result of ingestion, GI decontamination should be performed by administration of activated charcoal. A quiet room

TABLE 78.15. Drug Abuse Summary of Toxicity

Drug of abuse	Symptoms and signs of drug abuse	Diagnosis	Therapeutic dose	Toxic dose	Toxic serum level	Half-Life
Cannabis Group (marijuana; hashish; Δ9-THC; hash oil)	Pupils unchanged; conjunctiva injected; blood pressure (BP) decreased on standing; heart rate increased; increased appetite, euphoria, anxiety; sensorium often clear; dreamy; fantasy state; time-space distortions; hallucinations rare. Significant airway obstruction with heavy smoking, decreased forced expiratory volume (FEV) and decreased vital capacity. Major psychiatric toxic effects: Panic reaction most common Psychotic reactions (especially in patients with underlying psychopathology) Toxic delirium (disorientation, confusion, memory impairment) in heavy users	*Blood,* urine levels		20 mg Δ9-THC or 1 g cigarette of 2% Δ9-THC produces effects on mood, memory, motor coordination, cognitive ability sensorium, time sense		*1st phase,* minutes, → distribution in lipid-rich tissues; *2nd phase* 1½ days, until mobilized from lipid-rich tissue
Hallucinogens	Pupils dilated (normal or small with PCP); BP elevated, heart rate increased, hyperactive tendon reflexes, increased temperature, flushed face, euphoria, anxiety of panic, paranoid thought disorder, inappropriate effect, time and visual distortions, visual hallucinations, depersonalization.					
LSD	Psychosis with hyperalertness; changes in body image; sense of profound significance, delusions; hallucinations (also with amphetamines), visual perceptual distortions caused by peripheral effects of LSD on visual system.	Blood, urine levels		20–25 μg produce CNS effects; 0.5–2 μg/kg produce somatic symptoms; between 1 and 16 μg/kg intensity of pathophysiologic effects proportional to dose	Variable	3 hr
PCP	Cyclic coma, extreme hyperactivity, violent outbursts, bizarre behavior, amnesia, analgesia, nystagmus, gait ataxia, muscle rigidity. Dystonic reactions, grand mal seizures, tardive dyskinesia, athetosis, bronchospasm, urinary retention, diaphoresis, hypoglycemia. Increased uric acid, increased creatine phosphokinase (CPK), increased creatinine, increased SGOT/SGPT—heralds onset of rhabdomyolysis (risk of renal failure).	Blood, gastric contents, urine (but level dose not correlate with toxicity)		1 cigarette (PCP) = 1–100 mg. Psychosis may last several weeks after 1 dose. Fatal dose = 1 mg/kg: <5 mg = hyperactivity; 5–10 mg = stupor, coma; >10 mg = respiratory depression, convulsions	Individual variability (–0.1 μg/mL)	1–3 days

CNS Stimulants						
Amphetamines	Pupils dilated and reactive, increased BP, pulse, temperature, cardiac arrhythmias; dry mouth; sweating; tremors; sensorium hyperacute or confused; paranoid ideation; impulsivity; hyperactivity; stereotypy; convulsions; exhaustion.	Blood level, urine test	5 mg t.i.d.	1. Variable 2. Rare under 15 mg 3. Severe reactions have occurred at 30 mg 4. 400– 500 mg not uniformly fatal 5. Tolerance is striking; chronic user may take 1,700 mg/day without ill effects	Variable	3 hr
Cocaine	1. Excitement, restlessness, euphoria, garrulousness. 2. Increased motor activity, physical endurance because of decreased sense of fatigue. 3. Increased tremors, convulsive movements. 4. Increased respiration, pulse, blood pressure, temperature, chills.	Urine, serum	Anaesthesia—1 mL of 5% solution for surface anaesthesia (= 50 mg or less)	Fatal dose may be as low as 30 mg; ingested cocaine less toxic than by other routes		1 hr (after PO or nasal route)
CNS Sedatives (barbiturates, chlordiazepoxide, diazepam, flurazepam, glutethimide, meprobamate, methaqualone)	Pupils normal or small (dilated with glutethimide); blood pressure decreased, respirations depressed; drowsy, coma, lateral nystagmus, confusion, ataxia, slurred speech, delirium; convulsions or hyperirritability with methaqualone overdosage; serious poisoning rare with benzodiazepines alone.	Serum level				
Barbiturates (Secobarbital) (Seconal)	As above.	Serum level	30–50 mg, 3–4/d	100 mg per dose	30 µg/mL	19–34 hr
Chlordiazepoxide (Librium)	As above.	Serum level	5–20 mg, 3–4/d	25 mg		
Diazepam (Valium)	As above.	Serum, urine	2–10 mg, 4/d	15 mg or greater	8 µg/mL	8–25 hr
Flurazepam (Dalmane)	As above.	Serum, urine	15–30 mg			20–90 hr
Glutethimide (Doriden)	As above.	Serum level	125–250 mg, 1–3/d	>500 mg (acute intoxication, 3 g)	0.12 µg/mL (fatal)	47–100 hr
					2 mg/100 mL (but even below, full ICU support may be required)	5–22 hr
Meprobamate	As above.	Serum level	400 mg, 4/d	>800 mg		
Methaqualone (Parest, Somnafae)	As above.	Serum level	100 mg, 4/d	200–400 mg	150 µg/mL 10 µg/mL	6–17 hr 20–60 hr
Narcotics	Pupils constricted (may be dilated with meperidine or extreme hypoxia); respiration depressed to absent with cyanosis; BP decreased, sometimes shock; temperature reduced; reflexes diminished to absent, stupor or coma; pulmonary edema; constipation; convulsions with propoxyphene or meperidine; arrhythmia with propoxyphene.	Serum, urine				

continued

TABLE 78.15. (*continued*)

Drug of abuse	Symptoms and signs of drug abuse	Diagnosis	Therapeutic dose	Toxic dose	Toxic serum level	Half-Life
Heroin	As above.	Serum	3 mg[a]	60 mg = toxic[b]		1½ hr[c]
Morphine	As above.	Serum	10 mg[a]	200 mg = fatal dose[b]		3 hr[c]
Codeine	As above.	Serum	120 mg[a]	800 mg = fatal dose[b]	1.1 μg/mL	2 hr[c]
Methadone	As above.	Serum	7.5–10 mg[a]	100 mg = fatal dose[b]	1.6 μg/mL (fatal)	18–97 hr
Propoxyphene	As above.	Serum	65 mg every 4 h[a]	500 mg = fatal dose[b]	2 μg/mL (fatal)	3–12 hr
Anticholinergics (atropine, belladonna, henbane, scopolamine, trihexphenidyl, tricyclic antidepressants, benzotropine mesylate)	Pupils dilated and fixed, heart rate increased, temperature increased, blood pressure increased; drowsy, coma, flushed, dry skin and mucous membranes, erythematous skin, amnesia, disoriented, visual hallucinations, body image alterations.	Urine test				
Atropine	As above.		0.5–1 mg	5 mg		24 hr
Belladonna	As above.		0.6–1 mg	5 mg		24 hr
Scopolamine	As above.		0.6 mg	5 mg		24 hr
Imipramine (Tofranil)	As above.		100–200 mg/d	500 mg		8–16 hr
Amitriptyline (Elavil)	As above.		75–200 mg	>500 mg	5 μg/mL	32–40 hr
Desipramine	As above.			1 g	10 μg/mL	12–54 hr

ICU, Intensive care unit.
[a] Dose is amount given subcutaneously that produces same analgesic effect as morphine 10 mg subcutaneously.
[b] Higher doses given for addicts.
[c] Duration is for subcutaneous dose. Intravenous dose peak is more pronounced and overall effects have shorter duration.
Modified with permission from Dreisbach RH; *Handbook of poisoning.* Los Altos, CA: Lange Medical Publications, 1980.AQ1

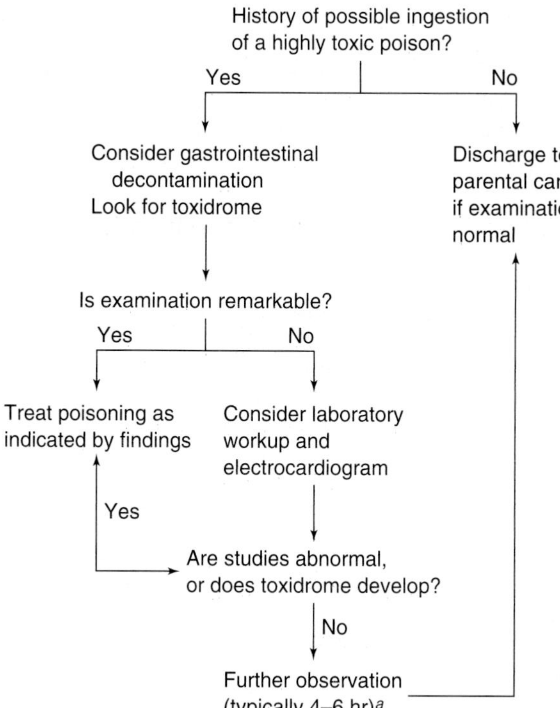
History of possible ingestion
of a highly toxic poison?
Yes
No
Consider gastrointestinal
decontamination
Look for toxidrome
Discharge to
parental care
if examination
normal
Is examination remarkable?
Yes
No
Treat poisoning as
indicated by findings
Consider laboratory
workup and
electrocardiogram
Yes
Are studies abnormal,
or does toxidrome develop?
No
Further observation
(typically 4–6 hr)a

Figure 78.7. Algorithmic approach to a toddler having ingested 1 to 2 doses (1–2 pills or 5–10 cc swallow) of a drug. [a]Medications notorious for their ability to have delayed onset in toxicity, beyond 4 to 6 hours, include oral hypoglycemic agents, sustained-release preparations, monoamine oxidase inhibitors, drugs taken concomitantly with anticholinergic agents, and acetaminophen. (See Table 78.14.)

may be helpful, although the ability to monitor the patient cannot be compromised. Physical restraints should be avoided if possible because they may lead to significant rhabdomyolysis with resulting myoglobinuria and renal injury. For chemical restraint diazepam (0.1 to 0.3 mg per kg i.v.) or lorazepam (0.1 mg per kg i.v.) may be effective, although a major tranquilizer (eg, haloperidol) is often necessary.

Although urine acidification (pH below 5.0) enhances the urinary excretion of PCP, it should never be performed in these patients because it exacerbates metabolic acidosis and may promote deposition of myoglobin in renal tubules. In a review of 27 confirmed cases of PCP poisoning, three patients developed rhabdomyolysis and two progressed to acute renal failure. Both patients had received acidification measures before diagnosis. If tests for muscle enzymes and/or renal function are abnormal and the urine has a positive test for hemoglobin without red blood cells, the patient should be assumed to have rhabdomyolysis and should be treated accordingly (see Chapter 76).

TABLE 78.16. Drugs and Chemicals That May Produce the Central Anticholinergic Syndrome

Antidepressants: amitriptyline (Elavil), imipramine (Tofranil), doxepin (Sinoquan, Adopin)
Antihistamines: chlorpheniramine (Omade, Teidrin), diphenhydramine (Benadryl), orphenadrine (Norflex)
Ophthalmologic preparations: cyclopentolate (Cyclogel), tropicamide (Mydriacyl)
Antispasmodic agents: propantheline (Probanthine), clidinium bromide (Librax)
Antiparkinson agents: trihexyphenidyl (Artane), benztropine (Cogentin), procyclidine (Kemadrin)
Proprietary drugs: Sleep-Eze (scopolamine, methapyrilene), Sominex (scopolamine, methapyrilene), Asthma-Dor (belladonna alkaloids), Excedrin-PM (methapyrilene)
Belladonna alkaloids: Atropine, homatropine, hyoscine, hyoscyamus, scopolamine
Toxic plants: Mushroom (*Amanita muscaria*), bitter-sweet (*Solanum dulcamara*), Jimson weed (*Datura stramonium*), potato leaves and sprouts (*Selenum tuberosum*); deadly nightshade (*Atropa belladonna*)

LSD (Blotter, Acid)

MANAGEMENT

LSD intoxication is rarely associated with life-threatening events. However, vital signs should be assessed to ensure that the patient is stable and in the event there has been drug coingestion. Because LSD is ingested in minuscule doses and onset of symptoms occurs hours after ingestion, GI decontamination is unnecessary, unless coingestion is suspected. Clinical management involves placing the patient in a quiet room. Someone who knows the patient may be able to quietly "talk down" and reassure the patient. The patient's loss of boundaries and fear of fragmentation or self-disintegration create a need for a structuring or a supportive environment. Both benzodiazepines (eg, diazepam 0.1 to 0.3 mg per kg i.v. or midazolam 0.05 to 0.1 mg per kg i.v.) and haloperidol 0.05 mg per kg i.m. are effective tranquilizers in the event that anxiety or agitation persists.

Marijuana (Pot, Reefer, Smoke, Grass, Hemp)

MANAGEMENT

In general, the only treatment required is discontinuation of the drug. In the adolescent patient with a psychotic reaction or acute toxic delirium, a sedative such as diazepam, 5 to 10 mg by mouth or 0.1 mg per kg by i.v., may be necessary. These acute symptoms should improve with drug abstinence over 4 to 6 hours.

Stimulants

AMPHETAMINES (CRANK, SPEED)

Management

Treatment of intoxication after ingestion of these agents should include GI decontamination. For severe agitation, specific treatment consists of administration of a benzodiazepine (eg, diazepam 0.1 to 0.2 mg per kg i.v.) or haloperidol (0.01 to 0.05 mg per kg i.m.). Severe hypertension unresponsive to benzodiazepines may be treated with such agents as phentolamine, hydralazine, or i.v. sodium nitroprusside. Because up to 45% of amphetamines are excreted in the urine unchanged, ample fluids are beneficial.

COCAINE

Management

Immediate attention should be paid to the vital signs, including temperature (which should be obtained rectally). The patient who develops seizures requires immediate airway control as well as anticonvulsant therapy. Benzodiazepines (eg, diazepam 0.1 to 0.3 mg per kg) are considered the anticonvulsants of choice because of their rapid onset of action and because animal data have associated their use with decreased mortality from cocaine intoxication. Benzodiazepines should also be administered liberally to the patient with mild to moderate toxicity (agitation, hypertension, tachycardia) because of their efficacy in reversing many of these clinical manifestations.

Blood pressure instability should be anticipated and treated accordingly. For treatment of hypertensive crises, liberal benzodiazepine use may be combined with a short-acting antihypertensive (eg, nitroprusside). Immediate treatment of hypertension is recommended because it may lead to cerebrovascular or myocardial injury. Cardiac arrhythmias are treated according to advanced cardiac life support protocols (see Chapters 1 and 72).

Hyperthermia must be recognized and treated promptly to prevent its complications. Management is discussed in Chapter 79. Diuresis should be induced if urinalysis is suggestive of myoglobinuria.

Patients with CNS depression or a lateralizing neurologic examination should receive cranial tomography to rule out an intracranial vascular event.

Because cocaine is rarely ingested, the need for GI decontamination is confined to body packers/stuffers or when drug coingestion is suspected. With body stuffers, because bag leakage can lead to abrupt onset of severe intoxication and possibly death, activated charcoal should be administered immediately. Gastric emptying maneuvers and endoscopic removal of cocaine bags are relatively contraindicated because of the risk of bag rupture. Instead, decontamination is confined to administration of activated charcoal and WBI. Multiple-dose activated charcoal is recommended to maximize the opportunity for cocaine to be adsorbed by the charcoal. Because cocaine bags and crack vials are radiopaque in up to 50% of cases, an abdominal radiograph is recommended to determine the location and extent of retained packets after decontamination has been initiated. A contrast study may be considered to improve detection.

Central Anticholinergics

MANAGEMENT

The management of a patient with a known central anticholinergic syndrome is a challenge, particularly because one must also be prepared for the other distinct toxicities of the ingested drug or plant. Also, most plants and many drugs are not detected on toxin screen, so the diagnosis must rely on history and clinical suspicion. Along similar lines, serum drug levels do not predict the degree of anticholinergic symptoms. (See Table 78.16).

GI decontamination is essential after anticholinergic ingestion. Unlike most toxic ingestions, there is clear efficacy to decontamination 12 to 24 hours after ingestion because of the likelihood of drug persistence in the gut lumen for an extended time. Even gastric emptying may be effective for many hours after ingestion and should be considered for patients who present within 4 to 8 hours of ingestion. Activated charcoal with a cathartic is added to enhance fecal expulsion of the drug-charcoal complex in the face of diminished gut motility.

Based on presenting signs and symptoms, the patient may require sedation, and monitoring in an intensive care unit setting to provide ventilatory support for coma, anticonvulsants for seizures, and antiarrhythmic drugs for cardiac arrhythmias. Adequate sedation may be achieved with titrated doses of benzodiazepines. Physostigmine, a potent anticholinesterase, is a recognized antidote for anticholinergic-induced mental status alterations; however, its use is controversial. Physostigmine can produce bronchospasm, bradycardia, hypotension, and seizures. It is therefore reserved for those who have normal ECGs and mental status dysfunction confined to hallucinations or severe agitation. The adult dose is 1 to 2 mg via slow i.v. infusion over 5 minutes. The trial dose can be repeated in 10 to 15 minutes up to a maximum of 4 mg. The pediatric dose is 0.5 mg administered slowly i.v., with repeat every 10 minutes up to a maximum of 2 mg. The smallest effective dose may be repeated every 30 to 60 minutes if symptoms recur over 6 to 8 hours. The muscarinic toxicity of physostigmine may be treated with i.v. atropine at one-half the physostigmine dose given; physostigmine-related seizures may be treated with benzodiazepines.

Central Nervous System Sedative-Hypnotics

CLINICAL SYMPTOMS

After sedative-hypnotic use the adolescent may exhibit sluggishness, difficulty in thinking, dysarthria, poor memory, faulty judgment, emotional lability, and short attention span. Irritability and lability are common. With chronic use, these drugs also lead to dependence so that a picture of abstinence may appear after their disuse, with clinical manifestations of apathy, weakness, tremulousness, agitation, or frank convulsions. In its mildest form, the abstinence syndrome may consist only of rebound increases of rapid eye movement sleep, insomnia, or anxiety.

MANAGEMENT

With victims of acute sedative-hypnotic ingestion, attention should be directed to ensuring a patent airway and an intact gag reflex. Cardiovascular disturbances are rare after sedative use, but because of the possibility of drug coingestion, thorough hemodynamic assessment is necessary. Most sedative-hypnotics are detectable on comprehensive toxin screens so that specimens of serum and urine should be sent for analysis. GI decontamination should be considered and can typically be confined to administration of activated charcoal with a cathartic. Repeated doses of charcoal with cathartic have been shown to enhance clearance of certain barbiturates and benzodiazepines. Urinary alkalinization aids in the excretion of phenobarbital. In extreme cases, charcoal hemoperfusion should be considered.

Optional treatment of sedative overdose includes continuous monitoring in an intensive care unit with intubation and ventilator support as indicated. Flumazenil, a recently released benzodiazepine antagonist, can be administered in cases of suspected benzodiazepine ingestion. Its pediatric dose is 0.01 to 0.02 mg per kg i.v. Indications for flumazenil administration may be 1) to reverse a witnessed, unintentional benzodiazepine overdose in a young child, or 2) to prevent airway intubation after an iatrogenic overdose. Flumazenil must not be given empirically in unknown or intentional overdoses for which induction of seizures may be life threatening.

OPIOIDS (MORPHINE, CODEINE, HEROIN, METHADONE, PROPOXYPHENE)

Clinical Symptoms

Opioids invariably cause miosis, even after development of tolerance. Respiration may be depressed because of decreased responsiveness of brain stem respiratory centers to increases in carbon dioxide tension. Therapeutic doses of morphine have no effect on blood pressure or cardiac rate or rhythm. When blood pressure changes occur, they result from histamine release. Because histamine dilates capacitance blood vessels and decreases the ability of the cardiovascular system to respond to gravitational shifts, sitting or standing may produce orthostatic hypotension.

Many opioids have extensive effects on the GI tract. They decrease secretion of hydrochloric acid, GI motility, and pancreatic secretions while increasing colonic tone to the point of spasm. In addition, the tone of the anal sphincter is augmented. Therapeutic doses of morphine and codeine can also increase biliary tract pressure, producing epigastric distress and biliary colic.

Management

The presence of coma, pinpoint pupils, and depressed respiration should suggest opioid poisoning in the absence of history. The finding of needle marks on the body further suggests this diagnosis. To confirm the diagnosis, toxicologic analysis of urine and serum should be conducted.

The first management step with opioid intoxication is to ensure adequate ventilation of the patient. Endotracheal intubation may be necessary if there is severe respiratory depression or pulmonary edema. If appropriate, GI decontamination should be performed. The narcotic antagonist naloxone (1 to 2 mg) should be given by i.v. If there is no response despite the suspicion of opiate intoxication, the naloxone dose should be repeated (up to 8 to 10 mg), depending on effect and level of suspicion. Naloxone can precipitate an abstinence syndrome in those who have developed physical dependence; in such patients, smaller initial doses of 0.2 to 0.4 μg, with upward titration as needed, are preferable.

When patients who are addicted to opiates are hospitalized, small doses of an opiate may be necessary to prevent severe withdrawal. Methadone substitution is the preferred agent, because in small doses, it is less euphorigenic and its long elimination half-life permits once- or twice-daily dosing. With the patient under observation, 10 to 20 mg of methadone are given, ideally before the appearance of withdrawal symptoms (insomnia, irritability, agitation, piloerection).

Gammahydroxybutyrate and Gammahydroxybutyrolactone

The related agents, gammahydroxybutyrate (GHB) and gammahydroxybutyrolactone (GBL), have become popular substances of abuse among teenagers and young adults. GHB is an endogenous compound with neurotransmitter and/or neuromodulator function, and interacts with dopamine, serotonin, gammaaminobutyric acid (GABA), and endogenous opioid-based neural systems. GHB sales and transportation across state lines is currently restricted by federal law, and possession is illegal in some states. However, it is widely available through the purchase of kits (eg, by mail order, via the Internet) that allow its home synthesis. GBL is actually a precursor to GHB and is the primary ingredient of such kits, and continues to be legally sold in health food stores. However, GBL is rapidly metabolized *in vivo* to GHB, and the clinical effects of ingesting either agent are nearly indistinguishable. These agents are used for a variety of reasons, but primarily as euphoriants and aphrodisiacs at parties or all-night dance clubs ("raves"). GHB has gained a particular notoriety as a date-rape agent. Both agents also have a reputation in the body-builder community as growth hormone stimulants and thus enhancers of muscle development and fat loss.

GHB and GBL are CNS depressants that cause rapid onset of deep sleep that can progress to coma and respiratory depression. Patients who have overdosed may have transient seizure activity, and are often hypothermic and bradycardic. The coma is usually relatively short in duration, on the order of 1 to 2 hours. During emergence, transient delirium and vomiting are often observed. Depressed respiratory effort and airway-protective reflexes are common in the more severe cases, although aspiration pneumonia as a complication has been rare. Many patients are surprisingly responsive to stimulus, and attempts at laryngoscopy to effect endotracheal intubation in a seemingly deeply comatose patient may result in an angry, combative patient who sits up and becomes belligerent toward the endoscopist.

Most patients with acute overdose can be managed with the provision of ambient oxygen, suctioning, and airway and anti-aspiration positioning. A nasal trumpet is helpful in some cases, and endotracheal intubation may be required occasionally, although it may necessitate rapid sequence induction for the reasons previously noted. Atropine has been used for severe bradycardia with success. Blood pressure support is rarely necessary. section iii: medical emergencies.

CHAPTER 79
Environmental Emergencies

Carl R. Baum, M.D.

DROWNING AND NEAR DROWNING

CLINICAL MANIFESTATIONS

In the first moments after rescue, the appearance of the child who has nearly drowned may range from apparently normal to apparently dead. Body temperature is often low, even in temperate, warm-water environments. Respiratory efforts may be absent, irregular, or labored, with pallor or cyanosis, retractions, grunting, and cough productive of pink, frothy material. The lungs may be clear, or there may be rales, rhonchi, and wheezing. Infection may develop as a consequence of aspirated mouth flora or organisms in stagnant water, but this is not usually important in the first 24 hours.

Intense peripheral vasoconstriction and myocardial depression may produce apparent or actual pulselessness. Neurologic assessment may show an alert, normal child or any level of central nervous system (CNS) compromise. A child may display agitation and combative behavior, blunted responsiveness to the environment, or profound coma with stereotypic posturing or flaccid extremities. Superficial evidence of head trauma may be noted in a few children whose submersion episode was a secondary event.

MANAGEMENT

Children should be given the maximum concentration of supplemental oxygen possible (100%) in transport to an emergency facility. Even those rescued with spontaneous ventilation and minimal or no neurologic dysfunction should receive the benefit of supplemental oxygen to minimize the risk of progressive hypoxemia and acidosis with secondary myocardial and cerebral damage. Physical examination is notoriously insensitive to hypoxemia; a seriously hypoxemic child may be alert and talking. Once the child has arrived at an emergency facility (and cardiovascular stability is achieved), pulmonary and neurologic assessment should guide further treatment.

Effective therapy of near drowning depends on the reversal of hypoxemia and metabolic acidosis. The pulmonary status is assessed initially with a chest radiograph and with measurement of arterial oxygen saturation (SaO_2) and arterial blood gas (ABG), as in Table 79.1. If oxygenation is normal on breathing

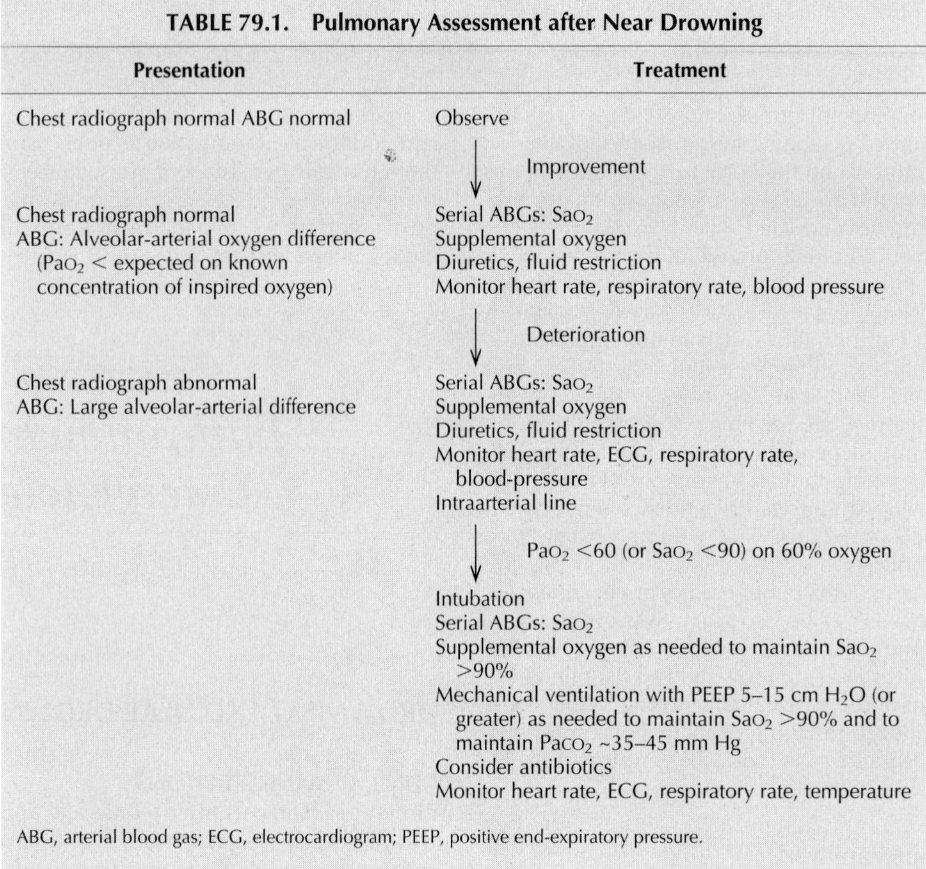

TABLE 79.1. Pulmonary Assessment after Near Drowning

Presentation	Treatment
Chest radiograph normal ABG normal	Observe
	↓ Improvement
Chest radiograph normal ABG: Alveolar-arterial oxygen difference (PaO_2 < expected on known concentration of inspired oxygen)	Serial ABGs: SaO_2 Supplemental oxygen Diuretics, fluid restriction Monitor heart rate, respiratory rate, blood pressure
	↓ Deterioration
Chest radiograph abnormal ABG: Large alveolar-arterial difference	Serial ABGs: SaO_2 Supplemental oxygen Diuretics, fluid restriction Monitor heart rate, ECG, respiratory rate, blood-pressure Intraarterial line
	↓ PaO_2 <60 (or SaO_2 <90) on 60% oxygen
	Intubation Serial ABGs: SaO_2 Supplemental oxygen as needed to maintain SaO_2 >90% Mechanical ventilation with PEEP 5–15 cm H_2O (or greater) as needed to maintain SaO_2 >90% and to maintain $PaCO_2$ ~35–45 mm Hg Consider antibiotics Monitor heart rate, ECG, respiratory rate, temperature

ABG, arterial blood gas; ECG, electrocardiogram; PEEP, positive end-expiratory pressure.

room air, the child can be assumed to have suffered near drowning without aspiration. Observation for 12 to 24 hours with repeat (SaO_2) or ABG determination should be sufficient to assess the possibility of late deterioration in gas exchange. Other initial laboratory evaluation should include complete blood count (CBC), electrolytes, and urinalysis.

Patients with abnormalities of gas exchange and acid-base status (but with normal chest radiographs) can usually be managed with supplemental oxygen, pulmonary physiotherapy, and bicarbonate therapy. Additional blood gas analysis should be performed to document adequate oxygenation and reversal of metabolic acidosis. Any change in mental status or increase in respiratory distress may reflect arterial hypoxemia and should also prompt a repeat ABG determination. Continuous SaO_2 or serial PaO_2 measurements will guide the physician to continue conservative treatment or to intensify ventilatory support.

Patients with obvious respiratory distress, hypoxemia (SaO_2 less than 90% or PaO_2 less than 60% on 60% inspired oxygen), and extensive pulmonary edema or infiltration generally require more vigorous treatment and more extensive monitoring. All should be monitored for heart rate, cardiac rhythm, respiratory rate, and blood pressure. Most will require frequent blood gas analysis and may be more easily monitored through arterial cannulation. Intubation, supplemental oxygen, and mechanical ventilation with positive end-expiratory pressure (PEEP, 5 to 15 cm H_2O) should be provided.

Once blood pressure is stabilized, fluid restriction (to approximately one-half the maintenance rate) and diuretic therapy (eg, furosemide 0.5 to 1 mg per kg i.v.) may improve gas exchange. In the setting of extensive pulmonary damage, pulmonary and cardiovascular components of the disease are intimately entwined. Optimum management requires monitoring of blood gases and systemic arterial pressure.

The risk of pulmonary infection is always present, but retrospective studies have not demonstrated benefit from prophylactic antibiotics, which should be reserved for proven bacterial infection. Exceptions may be made when grossly contaminated water is aspirated and, in the worst cases, when maximal ventilatory support is required to provide any margin for survival. Most studies of bronchoalveolar lavage show no improvement. Steroids have no demonstrated benefit.

Renal function must be maintained. If significant hemoglobinuria exists, forced diuresis is required. Maintenance of an adequate hemoglobin level (more than 10 g per 100 mL) and normal electrolytes is obviously necessary. Specific problems vary from patient to patient in an unpredictable way, and an understanding of the principles outlined in Chapters 76 and 77 is essential.

The patient's clinical condition in the emergency department (ED) dictates further management and may provide prognostic clues. Patients may be assigned to one of three groups (Table 79.2). Those who are awake, alert, and fully responsive have survived the episode, presumably without CNS damage. Conservative observation for only 12 to 24 hours is warranted. The second group includes those who are obtunded but arousable and exhibit a normal respiratory pattern and purposeful responses to pain. These patients have suffered certain but reversible CNS hypoxia; the goal is to prevent further hypoxic damage through intensive management of cardiopulmonary disease. Repeated neurologic evaluation is essential, and fluid restriction and diuretic therapy within the limits of cardiovascular stability may decrease the risk of cerebral edema. There is no demonstrated value in the use of steroids in this setting (see Chapter 110). In both groups, temperature normalization should be prompt. If reversal of coexisting pulmonary damage is effective, neurologic recovery should be complete.

TABLE 79.2. Neurologic Assessment after Near Drowning

Group	Description	Treatment
A (alert)	Alert Fully conscious	Observe
B (blunted)	Obtunded but arousable Purposeful response to pain Normal respiratory pattern	Prevent further hypoxic damage Monitor clinical neurologic status Therapy as required for pulmonary and cardiovascular stability Normalize temperature
C (comatose)	Comatose, not arousable Abnormal response to pain Abnormal respiratory pattern	Prevent further hypoxic damage Therapy as required for pulmonary and cardiovascular stability Maintain normocapnia or mild hyperventilation Monitor core temperature Warm to 32°C (89.6°F) Allow passive warming to 37°C (98.6°F) Avoid hyperthermia
C.1	(Decorticate) Flexion response to pain Chayne-Stokes respiration	
C.2	(Decerebrate) Extension response to pain Central hyperventilation	Monitor temperature
C.3	(Flaccid) No response to pain Apnea, or cluster breathing	Consider withdrawal of support if no protection from hypothermia

There is controversy over patients in a third group—those who have experienced severe CNS asphyxia. These children are not arousable and can be further divided into three subcategories according to neurologic findings: 1) those with decorticate response to pain and Cheyne-Stokes breathing; 2) those with decerebrate response to pain and central hyperventilation; and 3) those who are flaccid with fixed, dilated pupils and apneustic breathing or apnea. Again, reversal of hypoxemia and acidosis is critical. Fluid resuscitation should be designed to prevent hyperglycemia. Avoiding hypercapnia and resultant cerebral hyperemia is generally accepted, but hyperventilation, barbiturate coma, and other measures initially thought to provide cerebral protection and prevent or treat elevated intracranial pressure have not been helpful in these patients.

Hypothermia does appear to have some protective value. Extreme hypothermia should be corrected to at least 32°C (89.6°F) to achieve hemodynamic stability and to minimize the risk of infection. The child should then be allowed to rewarm passively. Although data in humans are limited, animal studies suggest that maintenance of mild brain hypothermia may minimize reperfusion injury. Hyperthermia, a common result of active rewarming, should be avoided.

SMOKE INHALATION

CLINICAL MANIFESTATIONS

A history of exposure in a closed space should heighten concern for smoke inhalation. Need for cardiopulmonary resuscitation at the site implies significant carbon monoxide poisoning and/or hypoxia secondary to decreased ambient oxygen concentration or severe respiratory disease. The physician should also consider the types of material involved to determine the risk of poisoning from carbon monoxide or other toxins.

Physical examination that reveals facial burns, singed nasal hairs, pharyngeal soot, or carbonaceous sputum justifies a presumption of smoke inhalation. Any sign of neurologic dysfunction, including irritability or depression, should be presumed related to tissue hypoxia until proven otherwise. Signs of respiratory distress may be delayed for 12 to 24 hours, but tachypnea, cough, hoarseness, stridor, decreased breath sounds, wheezing, rhonchi, or rales may be detected on presentation. Auscultatory findings often precede chest radiograph abnormalities by 12 to 24 hours. Radiographic changes may include diffuse interstitial infiltration or local areas of atelectasis and edema.

Acute respiratory failure may occur at any point. The cause may be asphyxia or carbon monoxide exposure and subsequent CNS depression initially, or airway obstruction or parenchymal dysfunction later. ABG analysis provides the ultimate assessment of effective respiratory function. Xenon lung scanning may provide evidence for smoke inhalation but does not add significantly to repeated clinical assessment and blood gas determinations in the ED. Bronchoscopy can document the extent of inhalation injury and help remove debris but may worsen airway edema. In general, it is respiratory function, not appearance of lesions that guides supportive care, and therefore most patients can be treated effectively without bronchoscopy.

MANAGEMENT

Initial assessment and resuscitation at the scene of the fire should proceed according to the principles outlined in Chapter 1. Because of the likelihood of carbon monoxide exposure and the difficulty of assessing hypoxemia clinically, all victims should receive the maximum concentration of inspired oxygen possible in transport and in the ED until further evaluation is complete (Table 79.3).

Upon the patient's arrival in the ED, assessment of the airway and respiratory functions must proceed simultaneously with cardiovascular stabilization. Thermal injury to the nose, mouth, or face, or compromise of the upper airway (stridor, hoarseness, barking cough, retractions, delayed inspiration, or difficulty handling secretions) indicates the need for direct laryngoscopy. The presence of significant pharyngeal, supraglottic, or glottic edema mandates elective endotracheal intubation. Although some clinicians may elect to observe closely, worsening edema over 24 hours may lead to respiratory arrest and difficult emergency intubation through a distorted airway. Elective tracheostomy may be considered if placing or securing the endotracheal tube will further traumatize an edematous airway or severe facial burns. However, in the presence of extensive cutaneous burns, tracheostomy dramatically increases the risk of systemic and pulmonary infection.

TABLE 79.3. Management of Smoke Inhalation

Initial management
- Remove from contaminated environment
- Cardiopulmonary resuscitation as needed
- Provide 100% supplemental oxygen
- Ensure patent airway

Laboratory determinations
- Arterial blood gas analysis
- Carboxyhemoglobin level
- Chest radiograph

Monitor
- Heart rate, electrocardiogram, respiratory rate, blood pressure, SaO_2
- Consider central venous pressure
- Consider pulmonary artery catheterization

Fluids
- 5% dextrose in 0.2% saline at maintenance rates or less to maintain urine output 0.5–1.0/mL/kg/h
- Volume expansion in presence of cutaneous burns; normal saline, lactated Ringer solution, or 5% albumin

Respiratory management
- *Intubation for:*
  1. Upper airway obstruction
  2. PaO_2 <60 mm Hg on 60% oxygen
  3. Central nervous system depression with loss of cough and gag reflexes
- Continuous positive airway pressure 5–15 cm H_2O for PaO_2 <60 mm Hg on 60% oxygen
- *Intermittent mandatory ventilation for:*
  1. Hypoxia unresponsive to continuous positive airway pressure or
  2. $PaCO_2$ >50 mm Hg
- Humidification of inspired gases
- Meticulous pulmonary toilette
- Consider inhaled bronchodilators

Cardiovascular stabilization depends on fluid replacement, which is complex when major surface burns have occurred. The details of therapy are elaborated in Chapter 100, but in general, the goals are stabilization of cardiovascular function without fluid overload and compromise of gas exchange. Pulse rate and blood pressure should guide administration of fluid volume. Maintenance of urine output of at least 0.5 mL per kg per hour should provide adequate tissue perfusion. Decreased urine output may respond to diuretics or inotropic agents. Although adequate fluid administration is essential, careful monitoring of renal and cardiovascular systems may prevent or minimize acute pulmonary edema and delayed pulmonary dysfunction secondary to late fluid mobilization and infection.

Oxygen saturation and serial blood gas determinations should be obtained to guide oxygen supplementation and to assess adequacy of ventilation. Intubation is indicated if adequate oxygenation (SaO_2 less than 90 or PaO_2 60 mm Hg or greater) cannot be maintained with an inspired oxygen concentration of 40% to 60%, if $PaCO_2$ rises above 50 mm Hg, or if the work of breathing appears unsustainable. In the presence of small airway edema and disrupted surfactant activity, continuous distending airway pressure may improve oxygenation. Spontaneous ventilation with continuous positive airway pressure (CPAP) causes less cardiovascular interference, but in the patient with severe CNS depression or severe pulmonary parenchymal damage, mechanical ventilation with PEEP will likely be necessary. Maximally humidified oxygen should be delivered by mask or artificial airway to prevent inspissation of debris and occlusion of the airway. The patient with a natural airway should also receive humidified gas mixtures and be encouraged to take deep breaths and cough frequently. If an endotracheal tube is necessary, meticulous pulmonary toilette is essential, with frequent suctioning to remove edema fluid, mucus, and sloughed epithelium that may otherwise occlude the endotracheal tube.

A recent study of lung mechanics in children with inhalation injury compared two modes of ventilation. High-frequency percussive ventilation was superior to conventional mechanical ventilation in reducing work of breathing.

After the first few hours, diuretic therapy (furosemide 0.5 to 1 mg per kg i.v.) within the limits of cardiovascular stability may also improve oxygenation and pulmonary compliance, leading to more effective ventilation. Chemical and particulate irritation of upper airway receptors may cause reflex bronchoconstriction and contribute to lower airway obstruction. Bronchodilators such as nebulized albuterol (2.5 mg in 2.5 mL, 0.9% sodium chloride) or i.v. terbutaline (load 10 μg per kg per dose i.v. or subcutaneously; drip 0.1 to 1.0 μg per kg per minute) may help reverse bronchospasm, but relief depends mostly on removal of secretions and debris from the respiratory tree.

Studies have not demonstrated a role for steroids in reducing airway edema or in decreasing the inflammatory response to smoke inhalation. When steroids are used, there is evidence that sodium and fluid retention increase, healing is delayed and bacterial clearance from the lung is decreased. Little argument remains for their routine use.

Similarly, there is no value in the use of prophylactic antibiotics. Institution of antimicrobial therapy should await specific indications, which rarely occur in the first 24 hours.

CARBON MONOXIDE POISONING

CLINICAL MANIFESTATIONS

History provides the most valuable clue to diagnosis. Carbon monoxide poisoning should be suspected in all fire victims and considered in children exposed to other hazards noted earlier. Presence or absence of the classically described "cherry red" skin color is of no diagnostic value. In fact, patients with thermal injury may appear red, whereas those with vasoconstriction may be quite pale. Both color and respiratory rate may be deceptive and may lead the physician away from recognition of severe tissue hypoxia. PaO_2 and arterial saturation as determined by pulse oximetry (SaO_2) are likely to be normal in carbon-monoxide intoxication; low values reflect coexistent pulmonary dysfunction.

Determination of blood levels of carboxyhemoglobin may help document the diagnosis and may aid prognosis. Spectrophotometric methods are most widely used clinically. Venous blood may be used because of the high affinity of carbon monoxide for hemoglobin, but an arterial sample provides more precise information about acid-base balance and adequacy of ventilation. The level of hemoglobin should also be determined.

Levels of carboxyhemoglobin as low as 5% in nonsmokers may impair judgment and fine motor skills. Mild intoxication (20% carboxyhemoglobin) produces headache, mild dyspnea, visual changes, and confusion. Moderate poisoning (20% to 40%) produces drowsiness, faintness, nausea and vomiting, tachycardia, dulled sensation, and decreased awareness of danger. At lower levels, these symptoms are noted only with exertion, but as the fraction approaches 40%, they are present at rest. At poisoning between 40% and 60% weakness, incoordination, and loss of recent memory occur, and cardiovascular and neurologic collapse is imminent. Above 60%, coma, convulsions, and death are almost certain. Although carboxyhemoglobin levels and symptoms tend to follow the pattern just described, individual patients may be more or less symptomatic than predicted. An important caveat is that blood carboxyhemoglobin levels will fall rapidly with time and may not reflect cellular dysfunction, especially in high-demand tissues of the heart and CNS.

Patients with severe poisoning are peculiarly vulnerable to pressure trauma to skin, subcutaneous tissue, and muscle, especially at sites that support body weight or that are pinned under fallen objects. The history may suggest which sites are most vulnerable, and pain is an early symptom. Muscle breakdown and myoglobin deposition in renal tubular cells may precipitate acute renal failure.

A syndrome of delayed neuropsychological sequelae (DNS) has been described in patients after exposure to carboxyhemoglobin. These patients develop neurologic symptoms acutely, appear to recover with treatment, and then exhibit a broad spectrum of neurologic and psychiatric abnormalities days to weeks after the exposure. Neuropsychiatric testing of children has obvious difficulties. Studies of DNS, many of which are methodologically flawed, have elucidated neither an exact mechanism nor a consensus on prevention and treatment.

MANAGEMENT

Most important and obvious is the immediate need to remove the victim from the contaminated environment (Table 79.4). Resuscitation should proceed according to general principles. As soon as possible, the patient suspected of suffering carbon monoxide poisoning should be provided 100% oxygen. If the patient is breathing spontaneously, this can be accomplished with well-fitting masks supplied with nonrebreathing valves and a reservoir bag. Entrainment of room air precludes simple masks from providing more than 40% oxygen. The half-life of carboxyhemoglobin is approximately 4 hours in a patient breathing room air at sea level and approximately 1 hour if pure oxygen is inspired. The half-life is further reduced to less than 30 minutes if the patient has access to hyperbaric oxygen (HBO) at 2 to 3 atmospheres' pressure. There is no widespread agreement on indications for HBO, and transfer to a hyperbaric chamber should not jeopardize meticulous conventional cardiopulmonary stabilization. However, HBO administration may have effects beyond the mere reduction in carboxyhemoglobin half-life. Some studies in adults suggest a role for HBO in reducing the incidence of mortality and DNS. Well-controlled studies in children would have to be undertaken to answer these questions definitively but would have obvious ethical and methodologic difficulties. In any case, early consultation with an HBO facility should be considered while the patient is receiving 100% oxygen.

TABLE 79.4. Management of Carbon Monoxide Poisoning

Initial management
Remove from contaminated environment
Cardiopulmonary resuscitation as needed
Provide 100% supplemental oxygen
Laboratory determinations
Arterial blood gas analysis
Carboxyhemoglobin level
Complete blood count, electrolytes
Urinalysis for myoglobin
Monitor
Heart rate, electrocardiogram, respiratory rate, blood pressure
Treatment
Correct anemia hemoglobin <10 g/dL
Continue supplemental oxygen until carboxyhemoglobin ≤5%
Decrease oxygen consumption with bed rest, avoid producing anxiety
Maintain urine output >1 mL/kg/h
Consider hyperbaric oxygen

Use of inspired gas mixtures that contain carbon dioxide (5%) to increase minute ventilation may precipitate respiratory failure if used at the scene, as ventilation cannot be well monitored or assisted. It may be considered under closely controlled situations in the hospital but probably is of little benefit.

Metabolic acidosis, if present, should be treated with sodium bicarbonate, although adequacy of ventilation must be assessed to prevent paradoxic intracellular acidosis. The possibility of coexistent cyanide poisoning should be considered in patients involved in closed-space fires (especially where nitrogen-containing synthetic materials have burned) who have a persistent metabolic acidosis in the context of normal carboxyhemoglobin and methemoglobin. Cyanide has high mortality but a short half-life (approximately 1 hour), so empiric cyanide levels on patients who have survived the scene are not recommended generally unless confirmation is needed. If cyanide poisoning is strongly suspected in an early-presenting patient, the cyanide antidote kit (formerly known as the Lilly kit) may be considered. This two-step kit must be used with caution because the nitrite-containing first step induces methemoglobinemia. In case of doubt, the thiosulfate-containing second step, which is able to scavenge cyanide without significant additional toxicity, may be given alone. Anemia (hemoglobin less than 10 g per 100 mL) must be corrected to maximize oxygen-carrying capacity. If myoglobinemia or myoglobinuria is present, vigorous hydration and forced diuresis with furosemide (1 mg per kg i.v.) and/or mannitol (0.25 to 1 g per kg i.v.) with close attention to urine output may preserve renal function. If hydration and diuresis are ineffective, renal failure should be considered and fluids restricted accordingly (see Chapter 76).

The patient should be observed for at least 24 hours to identify other sequelae of smoke inhalation.

ENVIRONMENTAL AND EXERTIONAL

Heat Illness

CLINICAL FINDINGS

Three types of heat illness are recognized and represent different physiologic disturbances (Table 79.5). Heat cramps refer to

TABLE 79.5. Characteristics of Heat Illness

Illness	Who	When	Characteristic	Laboratory
Heat cramp	Highly conditioned Highly acclimatized Adequate water replacement Inadequate salt replacement	After severe work stress Usually when relaxing Triggered by cold	Excruciating cramps in affected muscle occurring in clusters (may simulate acute abdomen)	↓ Serum Na^+ Cl ↓↓ Urine Na^+ BUN nl or slightly ↑
Heat exhaustion				
A. Predominant water depletion	Generally unacclimatized Working in hot environment Inadequate water replacement	During periods of hot weather After physical exertion	T ≤39°C (102.2°F) Progressive lethargy Thirst Inability to work or play Headache Vomiting CNS dysfunction ↓ BP ↑ HR	Na, Cl ↑ Hct ↑ Urine specific gravity ↑
B. Predominant salt depletion	Unacclimatized Inadequate salt replacement Cystic fibrosis	During periods of hot weather After physical exertion	T ≤39°C (102.2°F) Weakness, fatigue Headache GI symptoms prominent Muscle cramp ↑ HR Orthostatic hypotension	Na ↓ Hct ↑ Urine Na ↓↓
Heat stroke	Extremes of age Overdressed infants Infants in closed cars Extreme exertion (young athletes) Drug use (e.g., phenothiazines)	During heat waves After excessive exertion	T ≥41°C (105.8°F) Hot skin Circulatory collapse Severe CNS dysfunction Rhabdomyolysis Renal failure	Na, Cl nl or ↑ CPK ↑ Ca ↓

BUN, blood urea nitrogen; nl, normal; T, temperature; Hct, hematocrit; CNS, central nervous system; BP, blood pressure; HR, heart rate; GI, gastrointestinal; CPK, creatine phosphokinase.

the sudden onset of brief, intermittent, and excruciating cramps in muscles after they have been subjected to severe work stress. Cramps tend to occur after the work is done, on relaxing or on taking a cool shower. Occasionally, abdominal muscle cramps may simulate an acute abdomen. The usual victim is highly conditioned and acclimatized. Typically, these individuals can produce sweat in large quantities and provide themselves with adequate fluid replacement but inadequate salt replacement. Electrolyte depletion is probably the cause of cramps.

Most spasms last less than a minute, but some persist for several minutes, during which a rock-hard mass may be palpated in the affected muscle. Cramps often occur in clusters. Rapid voluntary contraction of a muscle, contact with cold air or water, or passive extension of a flexed limb may reproduce a cramp. Laboratory investigation reveals hyponatremia and hypochloremia and virtually absent urine sodium. The blood urea nitrogen (BUN) level is usually normal but may be mildly elevated.

Heat exhaustion is less clearly demarcated from heat stroke than are heat cramps. In most cases, water depletion predominates because individuals who live and work in a hot environment do not voluntarily replace their total water deficit. Progressive lethargy, intense thirst, and inability to work or play progress to headache, vomiting, CNS dysfunction (including hyperventilation, paresthesias, agitation, incoordination, or actual psychosis), hypotension, and tachycardia. Hemoconcentration, hypernatremia, hyperchloremia, and urinary concentration are typical. Body temperature may rise but rarely over 39°C (102.2°F). If unattended, heat exhaustion may progress to frank heat stroke.

Heat exhaustion may also occur secondary to predominant salt depletion. As in heat cramp, water losses are replaced but without adequate electrolyte supplementation. Symptoms include profound weakness and fatigue, frontal headache, anorexia, nausea, vomiting, diarrhea, and severe muscle cramps. Tachycardia and orthostatic hypotension may be noted.

Unlike heat cramp victims, these patients are typically unacclimatized. Hyponatremia, hemoconcentration and significantly diminished urine sodium are consistent findings. Children with cystic fibrosis, particularly those who are young and unable to meet increased salt requirements, are at risk for electrolyte depletion because salt losses in their sweat apparently do not respond to acclimatization and aldosterone stimulation of the sweat gland.

Heat stroke (Table 79.5) is a life-threatening emergency. Classic signs are hyperpyrexia (41°C [105.8°F] or higher); hot, dry skin that is pink or ashen, depending on the circulatory state; and severe CNS dysfunction. Often, but not invariably, sweating ceases before the onset of heat stroke.

The onset of the CNS disturbance may be abrupt, with sudden loss of consciousness. Often, however, premonitory signs and symptoms exist. These include a sense of impending doom, headache, dizziness, weakness, confusion, euphoria, gait disturbance, and combativeness. Posturing, incontinence, seizures, hemiparesis, and pupillary changes may occur. Any level of coma may be noted. Cerebrospinal fluid findings are usually normal. The extent of damage to the CNS is related to the time and extent of hyperpyrexia and to the adequacy of circulation. Once the body temperature is lowered, consciousness usually is restored quickly, but coma may persist for 24 hours or more.

Patients able to maintain cardiac output adequate to meet the enormously elevated circulatory demand are most likely to survive. Initially, the pulse is rapid and full, with an increased pulse pressure. Total peripheral vascular resistance falls as a result of vasodilation in the skin and muscle beds, and splanchnic flow diminishes. If hyperpyrexia is not corrected, ashen cyanosis and a thin, rapid pulse herald a falling cardiac output. The cause may be either direct thermal damage to the myocardium or significant pulmonary hypertension with secondary right ventricular failure. Even after body temperature is returned to normal, cardiac output remains elevated and peripheral vascular resistance remains low for several hours, resembling the compensatory hyperemia after ischemia noted in posttrauma, postshock, and postseptic states. Persistently circulating vasoactive substances probably account for this phenomenon.

Severe dehydration is not a necessary component of heat stroke but may play a role if prolonged sweating has occurred. Electrolyte abnormalities may occur, especially in the unacclimatized victim, if NaCl has not been replaced. In acclimatized persons, NaCl is conserved but often at the expense of a severe potassium deficit. Polyuria is sometimes noted, often vasopressin-resistant and possibly related to hypokalemia. Acute tubular necrosis may be seen in as many as 35% of cases and probably reflects combined thermal, ischemic, and circulating pigment damage. Hypoglycemia may also be noted.

Nontraumatic rhabdomyolysis and acute renal failure have been described as consequences of various insults, including hyperthermia and strenuous exercise in unconditioned persons. Clinically, there may or may not be musculoskeletal pain, tenderness, swelling, or weakness. Laboratory evidence includes elevated serum creatinine phosphokinase (300 to 120000) and urinalysis that is orthotolidine (Hematest)-positive without red blood cells (RBCs) and shows red–gold granular casts. Typically, serum potassium and creatinine levels rise rapidly relative to BUN. An initial hypocalcemia, possibly a consequence of deposition into damaged muscle, progresses to hypercalcemia during the diuretic phase a few days to two weeks later.

MANAGEMENT

Most cases of heat cramps are mild and do not require specific therapy. Rest and increased salt intake from liberally salted foods are sufficient. In severe cases with prolonged or frequent cramps, i.v. infusion of normal saline is effective. Approximately 5 to 10 mL per kg over 15 to 20 minutes should be adequate to relieve cramping. Oral intake of fluids and salted foods can then complete restoration of salt and water balance.

Heat exhaustion as a result of predominant water depletion is treated with rehydration and rest in a cooled or well-ventilated place. If the child is able to eat, he or she should be encouraged to drink cool liquids and be allowed unrestricted dietary sodium. If weakness or impaired consciousness preclude oral correction, i.v. fluids are given as in any hypernatremic dehydration.

Exhaustion caused by predominant salt depletion also requires rest in a cool environment. Alert, reasonably strong children can be given relatively salty drinks such as consommé or tomato juice and should be encouraged to salt solid foods. Hypotonic fluids (eg, water, Kool-Aid) should be avoided until salt repletion has begun. Patients with CNS symptoms or gastrointestinal dysfunction may be rehydrated with i.v. isotonic saline or Ringer lactate. Initial rapid administration of 20 mL per kg over 20 minutes should improve intravascular volume with return of blood pressure and pulse toward normal. Further correction of salt and water stores should be achieved over 12 to 24 hours. In especially severe cases with intractable seizures or muscle cramps, hypertonic saline solutions may be used. The initial dose of 3% saline solution is 5 mL per kg by i.v. An additional 5 mL per kg should be infused over the next 4 to 6 hours.

Treatment of heat stroke centers on two priorities: 1) immediate elimination of hyperpyrexia and 2) support of the cardiovascular system (Table 79.6). Clothing should be removed and the patient should be cooled actively. Patients should be transported to an emergency facility in open or air-conditioned vehicles. Ice packs may be placed at the neck, groin, and axilla of the patient. Although immersion in ice water may be a more efficient means of lowering body temperature, it may complicate other support and monitoring. Among the most efficient but invasive methods is iced peritoneal lavage. However, a canine model of heat stroke suggested that an evaporative technique in which fans blew room air over subjects sprayed with 15°C (59°F) tap water was equally efficient. Temperature should be monitored continuously with a rectal probe, and active cooling should be discontinued when rectal temperature falls to approximately 38.5°C (101.3°F).

The severity of the patient's presentation determines the degree of cardiovascular support. If the skin is flushed and blood pressure adequate, lowering body temperature with close attention to heart rate and blood pressure may be sufficient. Although severe dehydration and electrolyte disturbances are uncommon, these should be assessed and corrected if necessary. Fluids cooled to 4°C (39.2°F) hasten temperature correction but may precipitate arrhythmias on contact with an already stressed myocardium. Adult patients rarely have required more than 20 mL per kg over the first 4 hours, but determinations of electrolytes, hematocrit, and urine output, and clinical assessment of central vascular volume should guide precise titration of fluids and electrolytes.

Patients with ashen skin, tachycardia, and hypotension demonstrate cardiac output insufficient to meet circulatory demand and are in imminent danger of death. Monitoring of the

TABLE 79.6. Management of Heat Stroke

Initial management
Remove clothing
Begin active cooling
Transport to cool environment
Cardiovascular support
Laboratory determinations
Complete blood count, PT/PTT
Electrolytes, BUN, creatinine, CPK, Ca, P
Urinalysis including myoglobin
Arterial blood gas
Monitor
Temperature
Heart rate, electrocardiogram, blood pressure
Peripheral pulses and perfusion
Urine output
Central nervous system function
Treatment
Active cooling
Fluids
Maintenance: 5% dextrose in 0.2% sodium chloride at maintenance rates
Resuscitation: 20 mg/kg lactated Ringer solution, 0.9% sodium chloride
Additional fluids as determined by lytes, output, and hemodynamic status
Inotropic support
Dobutamine 5–20 μg/kg/min or
Diuresis for myoglobinuria
Maintain urine output >1 mL/kg/h
Consider furosemide 1 mg/kg
Consider mannitol 0.25–1 g/kg

PT, prothrombin time; PTT, partial thromboplastin time; BUN, blood urea nitrogen; CPK, creatine phosphokinase.

electrocardiogram (ECG) and arterial blood pressure (with an indwelling arterial line) should determine support.

Inotropic support may be required after a fluid challenge (see Chapter 3). Dobutamine is probably most appropriate: its β-agonist properties increase myocardial contractility and maintain peripheral vasodilation. Isoproterenol has been used successfully in the past but may cause myocardial oxygen consumption to exceed oxygen delivery. Additional fluid resuscitation may be necessary with the initiation of either dobutamine or isoproterenol to fill the effectively increased vascular space. Normal saline or albumin should be given to maintain the arterial blood pressure in the normal range. Dopamine may also be effective, infused at rates compatible with inotropic support without vasoconstriction. In cases of extreme hemodynamic instability, extracorporeal circulation may provide both circulatory support and a means of rapid temperature correction.

Agents with α-agonist characteristics (epinephrine and norepinephrine) are not recommended for initial management; they cause peripheral vasoconstriction, interfere with heat dissipation, and may compromise hepatic and renal flow further. Atropine and other anticholinergic drugs that inhibit sweating should be avoided.

Renal function should be monitored carefully, especially in patients who have been hypotensive or in whom vigorous exercise precipitated heat stroke. In general, BUN, creatinine, electrolytes, calcium, and urinalysis for protein and myoglobin should be obtained. Once the patient's vascular volume has been restored and arterial pressure normalized, hourly urine output should be monitored. If urine output is inadequate (less than 0.5 mL per kg per hour) in the face of normovolemia and adequate cardiac output, furosemide (1 mg per kg by i.v.) and/or mannitol (0.25 to 1 g per kg by i.v.) should be given. If the response is poor, acute renal failure should be suspected, and fluids should be restricted accordingly. Rapidly rising BUN or potassium (K^+) should prompt consideration of early dialysis.

ACCIDENTAL HYPOTHERMIA

CLINICAL MANIFESTATIONS

The astute clinician must consider the possibility of hypothermia if the diagnosis is to be made in a timely manner. A history of sudden immersion in icy water or prolonged exposure to low environmental temperatures provides the obvious clue, but significantly low core temperatures may occur under much less suggestive circumstances. Examples include trauma victims found unconscious or immobile on a wet, windy, summer day; infants from inadequately heated homes or left exposed during prolonged medical evaluation; adolescents with anorexia nervosa; and patients with sepsis or burns. Severe hypothermia, coma, and cardiac arrest may present as the sudden infant death syndrome. Hypothermia may go undetected if the patient's temperature falls below the lower limit of the thermometer in use or if the thermometer is not shaken down adequately. Low-recording thermometers should be available in EDs and intensive care units. The diagnosis should be borne in mind for any patient with a suggestive history or coma of uncertain cause.

Physical examination reveals a pale or cyanotic patient. At mild levels of hypothermia, mental status may be normal, but CNS function is progressively impaired with falling temperature until frank coma occurs at approximately 27°C (80.6°F). Blood pressure also falls steadily below 33°C (91.4°F) and may be undetectable. Heart rate slows gradually unless atrial or ventricular fibrillation occurs. Intense peripheral vasoconstriction and bradycardia may render the pulse inapparent or absent. Below 32°C (89.6°F), shivering ceases, but muscle rigidity may mimic rigor mortis. Pupils may be dilated and may not react. Deep tendon reflexes are depressed or absent. Evidence of head trauma or other injury, drug ingestion, and frostbite should be sought.

Severe hypothermia mimics death. However, the significant decrease in oxygen consumption may allow life to be sustained for long periods, even after cessation of cardiac function. Signs usually associated with certain death (ie, dilated pupils or rigor mortis) have little prognostic value. If the patient's history suggests that hypothermia is the primary event and not a consequence of death, resuscitation should be attempted and death redefined as failure to revive with rewarming.

Initial laboratory tests should include CBC, platelet count, clotting studies, electrolytes, BUN and creatinine, glucose, serum amylase, and ABGs corrected for temperature. Urine should be sent for drug screening.

MANAGEMENT

Therapy for hypothermia can be divided into two parts: general supportive measures and specific rewarming techniques (Table 79.7). Once hypothermia is diagnosed, temperature must be monitored continuously as treatment progresses.

All patients should be given supplemental oxygen. Patients with profuse secretions, respiratory depression, or impaired mental status should be intubated and mechanically ventilated. Intubation should be performed as gently as possible to minimize the risk of arrhythmias.

A decreased metabolic rate produces less carbon dioxide, and usual minute ventilation would produce respiratory alkalosis, increasing the risk of dangerous arrhythmias. Therefore, ventilation should begin at approximately one-half the normal minute ventilation.

Assessment of acid-base status and ventilation in the hypothermic patient is the subject of considerable confusion. Blood gas machines heat the patient's blood sample to 37°C (98.6°F)

TABLE 79.7. Management of Hypothermia

Initial management
- Provide supplemental oxygen
- Cardiopulmonary resuscitation for asystole, ventricular fibrillation

Laboratory determinations
- Arterial blood gas analysis corrected for temperature
- Complete blood count, platelet count
- Prothrombin time, partial thromboplastin time
- Electrolytes, blood urea nitrogen, creatinine
- Glucose, amylase
- Urine drug screen

Monitor
- Heart rate, electrocardiogram, respiratory rate, blood pressure
- Temperature
- Consider central venous pressure

Treatment
- Correct hypoxemia, hypercarbia
- Correct hypokalemia
- Correct hypoglycemia, 25% dextrose 1 g/kg i.v.
- Tolerate hyperglycemia
- Temperature: ≥32°C (89.6°F): passive rewarming or simple external rewarming
  - <32°C (89.6°F) (acute): external or core rewarming
  - <32°C (89.6°F) (chronic): core rewarming
- Fluid replacement:
  - (acute) 5% dextrose in 0.2% saline at maintenance rates
  - (chronic) Normal saline, 5% albumin, fresh-frozen plasma to maintain blood pressure

before measuring pH and gas partial pressures (thus providing theoretical values if the patient were 37°C [98.6°F]). If the patient's actual temperature is provided with the sample, the machine can correct the values according to the nomogram of Kelman and Nunn. (Table 79.8 shows one set of guidelines for appropriate correction.) However, it is most important to understand two concepts. The first is the ectothermic principle, which relies on the following aspect of physiology: dissociation of ions and partial pressures of gases are decreased in cooled blood. In hypothermia, therefore, neutral pH is higher, whereas "normal" P_{CO_2} is lower than is encountered at 37°C (98.6°F). For example, hypoventilation of the hypothermic patient with a pH of 7.5 would actually induce an undesirable respiratory acidosis. A second, more practical concept is that if the patient's blood volume is restored and oxygenation maintained, acidosis will be corrected spontaneously as the patient is warmed.

Heart rate and rhythm should be monitored continuously and the patient handled gently to avoid precipitation of life-threatening arrhythmias in an exquisitely irritable myocardium. Sinus bradycardia, atrial flutter, and atrial fibrillation are common but rarely of hemodynamic significance. Spontaneous reversion to sinus rhythm is the rule when temperature is corrected. Ventricular fibrillation may occur spontaneously or with trivial stimulation, especially at temperatures below 28°C to 29°C (82.4°F to 84.2°F). Electrical defibrillation is warranted but often is ineffective until core temperature rises. Closed chest massage should be initiated and maintained until the temperature is above 30°C (86°F), when defibrillation is more likely to be effective. Drug therapy is rarely effective and fraught with hazards associated with decreased hepatic and renal metabolism.

Fluid replacement is essential. Relatively little plasma loss occurs in acute hypothermia (as it does after cold-water immersion), but losses may be great in hypothermia of longer duration. Normal saline or lactated Ringer solution, warmed to about 43°C (109.4°F) in a blood warming coil, is appropriate initially. Electrolyte determinations should guide further replacement. If clotting abnormalities occur, fresh-frozen plasma (10 mL per kg) is a useful choice for volume expansion (see Chapter 77). As temperature rises and peripheral vasoconstriction diminishes, hypovolemia is expected. Fluid volume should be sufficient to provide an adequate arterial blood pressure.

Hypoglycemia, if present, is treated with glucose (1 g per kg by i.v.). Hyperglycemia, which may result from impaired insulin release in the hypothermic pancreas, should be tolerated to avoid severe hypoglycemia with rewarming.

A number of rewarming strategies exist. Passive rewarming implies removal of the patient from a cold environment and use of blankets to maximize the effect of basal heat production. For patients with mild hypothermia (temperature over 32°C [89.6°F]), this may be adequate.

Active rewarming is divided into external and core rewarming techniques. Electric blankets, hot water bottles, overhead warmers, and thermal mattresses are simple, easily available sources of external heat. Immersion in warm-water baths is also possible but complicates monitoring or response to arrhythmias. All of these methods, however, cause early warming of the skin and extremities with peripheral vasodilation and shunting of cold, acidemic blood to the core. The well-known "after-drop" of core temperature results. Severe hypotension may also occur in chronic cases as vasodilation increases the effective vascular space. External rewarming techniques limited to the head and trunk may minimize vasodilation and after-drop. In acute hypothermia, active external rewarming is appropriate, but there is some evidence that in chronic cases (more than 24 hours), mortality is higher if active external rewarming is used instead of simple passive techniques.

Core rewarming techniques are almost certainly more rapid and less likely to be associated with after-drop, dangerous arrhythmias, or significant hypotension. These methods are especially valuable in the setting of severe chronic hypothermia (temperature below 32°C [89.6°F]), where fluid shifts are most likely to occur. A nonshivering human model of severe hypothermia indicated that inhalation rewarming offered no rewarming advantage, whereas forced air warming (approximately 200 W) allowed a sixfold to tenfold increase in rewarming rate over controls. A canine study of experimental hypothermia found that heated aerosol inhalation alone contributed less heat than endogenous metabolism, but that peritoneal lavage and pleural lavage had similar effect on rewarming (6°C per hour per m^2). In humans, peritoneal dialysis, with dialysate warmed to 43°C (109.4°F), is effective and requires only equipment routinely available in most hospitals. Limited clinical experience suggests that pleural lavage is a relatively simple and useful measure. Hemodialysis, extracorporeal blood rewarming, and mediastinal irrigation are effective but require mobilization of sophisticated equipment and personnel. Gastric or colonic irrigation has also been advocated, but placement of the intragastric balloon may precipitate dysrhythmias.

Each increment in core temperature produces a "new" patient who requires reassessment and appropriate management, but most children with hypothermia have a good prognosis. In patients with mild temperature depression (above 32°C [89.6°F]), external rewarming techniques, and supportive care based on vital signs, ABGs, and metabolic parameters such as glucose and calcium levels, should result in prompt recovery. Patients with temperatures below 32°C (89.6°F), and especially those in whom hypothermia developed over 24 hours or more, require meticulous attention to continuously changing vital signs and metabolic needs. More elaborate core rewarming techniques are appropriate.

TABLE 79.8. Effect of Body Temperature on Arterial Blood Gases Measured at 37°C (98.6°F)

	For each elevation of 1°C	For each depression of 1°C
pH	−0.015	+0.015
Pa_{CO_2} (mm Hg)	+4.4%	−4.4%
Pa_{O_2} (mm Hg)	+7.2%	−7.2%

ELECTRICAL INJURIES

CLINICAL MANIFESTATIONS

Electrical injury may produce a variety of clinical pictures, ranging from local damage to widespread multisystem disturbances. Typically, deceptively small entry and exit wounds mask extensive damage to subcutaneous tissue, muscle, nerves, and blood vessels. Direct effects on the heart and nervous system are particularly common, and injury to all other symptoms can occur. Much of the injury is revealed immediately, but late complications are often encountered.

Victims of the most severe accidents are commonly pulseless, apneic, and unresponsive. Current that passes directly through the heart may induce ventricular fibrillation. Brainstem (medullary) paralysis or tetanic contractions of thoracic muscles may result in cardiopulmonary collapse. Lightning injury is capable of inducing asystole, from which the heart may recover spontaneously, but the accompanying respiratory failure is commonly prolonged. Unless ventilation is initiated promptly, hypoxia leads to secondary ventricular fibrillation and death.

Other cardiac disorders, including arrhythmias and conduction defects, are common among survivors. Supraventricular tachycardia, atrial and ventricular extrasystoles, right bundle branch block, and complete heart block are most common. Complaints of crushing or stabbing precordial pain may accompany nonspecific ST-T wave changes. Some patients sustain myocardial damage or even ventricular wall perforation. Despite evidence of important cardiac injuries, patients without secondary hypoxic-ischemic injury usually regain good myocardial function.

Nervous system injury is also extremely common and may involve the brain, spinal cord, peripheral motor, and sensory nerves, as well as sympathetic fibers. Loss of consciousness, seizures, amnesia, disorientation, deafness, visual disturbances, sensory deficits, hemiplegia, and quadriparesis occur acutely but may be transient. Vascular damage may produce subdural, epidural, or intraventricular hemorrhage.

Additional problems develop within hours to days after injury. The syndrome of inappropriate antidiuretic hormone secretion may precipitate herniation in rare cases. Electroencephalograms reveal diffuse slowing, epileptiform discharges, or burst suppression patterns, but they may not have prognostic significance. Spinal cord dysfunction yields more motor than sensory deficit. Peripheral neuropathies with patchy distribution may reflect direct thermal injury, vascular compromise, or current flow itself. A variety of autonomic disturbances may resolve spontaneously or persist as reflex sympathetic dystrophy.

Ocular damage is common, particularly after lightning strikes. Direct thermal or electrical injury, intensive light, and confusion contribute to the presentation. Findings include corneal lesions, hyphema, uveitis, iridocyclitis, and vitreous hemorrhage. Choroidal rupture, retinal detachment, and chorioretinitis occur less often. Autonomic disturbances in a lightning victim may cause fixed dilated pupils, which should not serve as a criterion for brain death without extensive investigation of other neurologic and ocular functions. Cataracts and optic atrophy are possible late developments.

Electrical injury may induce direct or indirect complications in other organ systems. Tetanic contractions may cause joint dislocations and fractures, especially of the upper extremity long bones and vertebrae. Fractures of the skull and other long bones may occur when high-tension shock throws the victim from the site of contact. Early cardiopulmonary insufficiency, as well as direct renal effects, may cripple renal function. Damaged muscle releases myoglobin and creatinine phosphokinase (CPK). As in crush injuries, myoglobin may induce renal tubular damage and kidney failure. Pleural damage may cause large effusions, whereas primary lung injury or aspiration of gastric contents may lead to pneumonitis. Gastric dilation, ileus, diffuse gastrointestinal hemorrhage, and visceral perforation may occur immediately or later.

In addition to burns at the site of primary contact, burns are common where current has jumped across flexed joints. Such burns are most common on the volar surface of the forearm and across the elbow and axilla. Arcing current may also ignite clothing and produce typical thermal burns. Entry and exit wounds and arc burns are notoriously poor predictors of internal damage. Tissue that appears viable initially may become edematous and then ischemic or frankly gangrenous over several days. Diminished peripheral pulses may provide immediate evidence of vascular damage, but strong pulses do not guarantee vascular integrity. Blood flow falls to a minimum at about 36 hours, but current or thermal damage may lead to vasospasm, delayed thrombosis, ischemic necrosis, or aneurysm formation and hemorrhage weeks after the injury. Viable major arteries near occluded nutrient arteries may account for apparently adequate circulation and uneven destruction of surrounding tissues.

Young children are vulnerable to orofacial burns, especially of the lips. These full-thickness burns of the upper and lower lips and oral commissure usually involve mucosa, submucosa, muscle, nerves, and blood vessels. The lesion usually has a pale, painless, well-demarcated, depressed center with surrounding pale gray tissue and erythematous border. After a few hours, the wound margin extends and marked edema occurs. Drooling is common. The eschar separates in 2 to 3 weeks and bleeding may occur at this time; granulation tissue gradually fills the wound. Scarring may produce lip eversion, microstomia, and loss of function. Damage to facial or even carotid arteries may result in delayed hemorrhage. Devitalization of deciduous and secondary teeth may occur.

Inadequately debrided burned or gangrenous tissue provides a medium for serious infection. Staphylococcal, pseudomonal, and clostridrial species are common pathogens in the extremities. Streptococci and oral anaerobic organisms may infect mouth wounds.

MANAGEMENT

The first step in emergency management (Table 79.9) is to separate the victim from the current source. The rescuer must be well insulated to avoid becoming an additional casualty. If the current cannot be shut off, wires can be cut with a wood-handled ax or appropriately insulated wire cutters. Contrary to popular myth, a lightning strike victim does not remain "electrified" and presents no risk to another person.

TABLE 79.9. Management of Electrical Injuries

Initial management
- Remove from source of current
- Cardiopulmonary resuscitation as needed
- Provide mechanical ventilation until spontaneous ventilation is adequate
- Immobilize neck and spine

Clinical assessment
- Neurologic examination
- Peripheral pulses and perfusion
- Oral burns/edema
- Chest wall injury
- Abdominal distension
- Eye or ear trauma
- Cutaneous burns or bruises

Laboratory determinations
- Complete blood count
- Blood urea nitrogen, creatinine, urinalysis including myoglobin
- Electrolytes
- Creatine phosphokinase with MB and BB fractions
- Electrocardiogram (ECG)
- Consider skull, spine, chest, long bone radiographs
- Consider computed tomography scan of brain
- Consider electroencephalogram

Monitor
- Heart rate, ECG, respiratory rate, blood pressure

Management
- Maintenance fluids: 5% dextrose in 0.2% sodium chloride
- Volume expansion in presence of thermal burns or extensive deep-tissue injury: 0.9% sodium chloride, lactated Ringer solution or 5% albumin
- Fluid restriction for central nervous system injury
- Maintain urine output >1 mL/kg/h
- Treat arrhythmias
- Treat seizures
- Tetanus toxoid; consider penicillin/other antibiotics
- Consider general, oral, or plastic surgical consultation

Any victim in cardiopulmonary arrest should be resuscitated promptly following the guidelines discussed in Chapter 1. Prolonged efforts to restore adequate cardiopulmonary and cerebral function, especially in the lightning victim, may be appropriate in the context of bizarre neurologic phenomena that inhibit ventilatory efforts, consciousness, or pupillary function. The patient who fails to respond to resuscitative efforts over hours to days and meets standard brain death criteria can be pronounced dead with reasonable certainty.

Any patient who sustains electrical injury deserves a comprehensive physical examination. Bleeding or edema from orofacial burns may compromise the upper airway. The head, particularly eyes, and neck should be examined carefully for evidence of trauma. The skin should be examined carefully for burns and bruises. Limbs should be evaluated for pulses, perfusion, and motor and sensory function, as well as for soft-tissue swelling or evidence of fractures. Burns and deep-tissue injury may progress over hours to days, so repeated examination and monitoring are important.

Neurologic evaluation is especially important in all but the most minor, localized peripheral injuries. Level of consciousness and mental status should be assessed according to the child's developmental level. Cranial nerve, cerebellar, motor, and sensory evaluation are essential.

Children who have sustained minor household electrical injuries and are asymptomatic usually do not require laboratory evaluation, cardiac evaluation, or hospitalization. In one series, investigators were unable to assess the clinical significance of loss of consciousness, tetany, wet skin, or current flow across the heart, and recommended cardiac monitoring if any of these factors is present. If the history is one of a high-tension injury or lightning strike, laboratory evaluation should include ECG, CBC, CPK (with fractionation), BUN, creatinine, and urinalysis, including urine myoglobin. Physical examination that reveals evidence of bruises, bony tenderness, or distorted long bones should prompt appropriate radiographic studies.

Most children who sustain burns of the oral commissure (usually after biting an electrical cord) do not require extensive evaluation or admission. In cases of severe orofacial burns, use of an artificial airway should be considered before progressive edema leads to catastrophe. Mechanical ventilation may be necessary to overcome CNS depression or primary lung involvement.

Patients with persistent coma and loss of protective airway reflexes should be intubated to avoid aspiration. Good oxygenation and ventilation adequate to maintain a normal pH and Pa_{CO_2} of 35 to 40 mm Hg must be ensured. Seizure activity should be treated as indicated (see Chapters 61 and 73).

Care of the CNS is of utmost importance. The neck and back should be immobilized if the patient was thrown from the site of injury. If the mechanism of injury was severe, the cervical collar should be maintained in place despite normal cervical spine radiographs. If a child fails to regain consciousness within a short time or shows signs of neurologic deterioration, a computed tomography (CT) scan will help exclude intracranial hemorrhage.

Any patient who has sustained cardiopulmonary arrest, loss of consciousness, or deep-tissue injury should be admitted to the hospital for evaluation and treatment. Heart rate, respiratory rate, and blood pressure should be monitored regularly. Doppler evaluation may be helpful in cases of vasospasm, which may complicate assessment of blood pressure and subsequent fluid management. True hypotension may require presser support.

Cardiopulmonary support is nonspecific. Most patients resume good circulatory stability unless severe hypoxia and ischemia have weakened the myocardium. Arrhythmias and acidosis should be treated along usual lines (see Chapters 72 and 76).

Patients struck by lightning require only maintenance fluids. Patients with ordinary thermal burns should be treated according to standard recommendations (see Chapter 100), although body surface area calculations may seriously underestimate fluid requirements. Extensive vascular and deep-tissue destruction may lead to extensive fluid sequestration. Isotonic fluid should be given in amounts to maintain normal pulse and blood pressure. In all cases, fluids should be given judiciously to avoid CNS complications.

Cerebral edema may develop over hours to days after injury, especially after a lightning strike. If the child's neurologic status fails to improve or deteriorates, intracranial pressure monitoring and treatment, including hyperventilation, osmotic or loop diuretics, and sedation and neuromuscular blockade, may be necessary. Serum and urine electrolytes and osmolality should be followed closely to recognize promptly the syndrome of inappropriate antidiuretic hormone secretion.

Myoglobin in the urine is consistent with muscle breakdown and sets the stage for renal failure. Hydration and brisk diuresis with furosemide and/or mannitol may prevent renal damage but must be undertaken with caution if there is coexistent CNS injury. Extensive muscle damage after lightning injury is uncommon, however, and major CNS injury is common. Treatment should proceed with these relative risks in mind until definitive information is available.

Most burns associated with lightning injury are superficial. Although they may become more apparent after several hours, most remain first- or second-degree burns. Minor burns on the extremities can be treated with antibiotic ointment and should be allowed to slough and heal. Oral and plastic surgeons should evaluate children who sustain oral burns. In most cases, similar conservative management is recommended, but a removable stent may be necessary to minimize scarring.

High-voltage injuries commonly require more aggressive treatment, and early surgical evaluation is essential. Fasciotomy may be necessary to restore adequate circulation to an injured extremity. The approach to debridement of wounds is controversial, but most surgeons rely on repeated examinations to detect nonviable tissue. Approximately 30% of survivors of high-tension injuries ultimately require amputation of some part of an extremity.

The risk of infection in patients with deep-tissue injury is high. Any patient not clearly immunized against tetanus should be given tetanus toxoid. Prophylactic antibiotics have been recommended for oral injuries, but in general, antimicrobial therapy should be reserved for proven or strongly suspected infection.

CHAPTER 80
Bites and Stings

Dee Hodge III, M.D. and
Frederick W. Tecklenburg, M.D.

MARINE INVERTEBRATES

Phylum Coelenterata (Cnidaria)

CLASS HYDROZOA

Feathered hydroid *(Pennaria tiarelia)* is found from Maine to Florida and along the Texas coast just below the low-tide line.

Portuguese man-of-war *(Physalia physalis)*—commonly considered a jellyfish—is in reality a hydrozoan colony. Local effects include pain and irritation. Systemic reactions include headache, myalgias, fever, abdominal rigidity, arthralgias, nausea and vomiting, pallor, respiratory distress, hemolysis, renal failure, and coma. Death may occur if the area stung is extensive in relation to the size of the victim. Treatment is discussed in the following section, "Class *Scyphozoa*".

CLASS SCYPHOZOA

The common purple jellyfish *(Pelagia noctiluca)* is only mildly toxic. Local skin irritation is the major clinical manifestation. Sea nettle *(Chrysaora guinguecinda)* is a common jellyfish found along the Atlantic coast. Clinical manifestations are the same as those for purple jellyfish. Lion's mane *(Cyanea capillata)* is a highly toxic creature. Contact with the tentacles produces severe burning. Prolonged exposure causes muscle cramps and respiratory failure.

Treatment of hydrozoan and scyphozoan stings is based on the same general principles. It is directed at three objectives: relieving pain, alleviating effects of venom, and controlling shock. The most important step is to remove the tentacles; as long as the tentacle adheres to the skin, the nematocysts continue to discharge. The unexploded nematocysts should be inactivated by topical application for 30 minutes with vinegar (3% acetic acid), a slurry of baking soda, or meat tenderizer (papain). The area should be washed with sea water or normal saline. Any adherent tentacles should be carefully removed with instruments or a gloved hand, and the wound area should be immobilized. There is no antivenin available for *Physalia* or the scyphozoans except for the sea wasp, *Chironex fleckeri,* of Australia. General supportive measures for systemic reactions include oral antihistamines, oral corticosteroids, and codeine or meperidine for pain. Cardiac and respiratory support may be required. Muscle spasms have been treated with 10% solution of calcium gluconate 0.1 mL per kg given intravenously. Local dermatitis should be treated with a topical corticosteroid cream.

CLASS ANTHOZOA

The anemones found within United States tidal zones are only mildly toxic at worst. The clinical picture is one of stinging sensation followed by wheal formation and itching. If the wound is untreated, an ulcer with an erythematous base may form within a few days. Cellulitis, lymphangitis, fever, and malaise commonly occur. Treatment consists of cleaning the wound and irrigation with copious amounts of saline. Removal of foreign particles must be accomplished, and debridement may be necessary. Wounds should be left open. Broad-spectrum antibiotic therapy, particularly tetracycline, at a dosage of 40 mg per kg per day in four divided doses, has been advocated but cannot be used in children younger than 8 years old. For children younger than 8 years, cephalexin (50 mg per kg per day in four divided doses) or trimethoprim–sulfamethoxazole should be used.

Phylum Echinodermata

Phylum Echinodermata includes starfish, sea urchins, and sea cucumbers. Of the three classes, only the *Echinoedae*—sea urchins—have clinical relevance for children in the United States. The spines of these urchins may break off readily and can penetrate wet suits and sneakers. Clinically, penetration is accompanied by intense pain followed by redness, swelling, and aching. Complications include tattooing of the skin, secondary infection, and granuloma formation. In treatment, all spines should be removed as completely as possible. If spines break off in the wound, debridement should be performed with local anesthetic under aseptic conditions, but any spines not reachable will be absorbed in time. Soaking the wound in warm water may be helpful. Systemic antistaphylococcal antibiotics should be used if infection develops.

MARINE VERTEBRATES

Stingrays

CLINICAL MANIFESTATIONS

Because the barb is retropointed, the wound it produces is a combination of puncture and laceration. The sting is followed immediately by pain, which spreads from the site of injury over the next 30 minutes and usually reaches its greatest intensity within 90 minutes. Pain and edema are most often localized to the area of injury; however, syncope, weakness, nausea, and anxiety are common complaints attributed to both the effects of the venom and the vagal response to the pain. Among other generalized symptoms are vomiting, diarrhea, sweating, and muscle fasciculations of the affected extremity. Generalized cramps, paresthesias, hypotension, arrhythmias, and death may occur. The wound often has a jagged edge that bleeds profusely, and the wound edges may be discolored. Discoloration may extend several centimeters from the wound within hours after injury and may subsequently necrose if untreated. Often, parts of the stingray's integumentary sheath contaminate the wound.

MANAGEMENT

Treatment is aimed at 1) preventing complications evoked by the venom, 2) alleviating the pain, and 3) preventing secondary infection. On the patient's arrival in the emergency department (ED), shock, if present, should be treated with intravenous (i.v.) fluids. An attempt should be made to remove any remnants of the integumentary sheath if it can be seen in the wound. The extremity should be placed in hot water (40°C to 45°C [104°F to 113°F]) for 30 to 90 minutes. After soaking, the wound should be reexplored. Further debridement can then be accomplished and the wound can be closed. Pain relief may be achieved with meperidine (1 to 2 mg per kg). Tetanus prophylaxis should always be considered, but antibiotics are reserved for wounds that become secondarily infected.

Sharks

Two types of bite wounds are described: tangential injury and a definitive bite. Tangential injury is caused by the slashing movement of the open mouth as the shark makes a close pass. Severe lacerations, incised wounds, and loss of tissue are seen. Definitive bite wounds vary according to the part of the body seized by the shark. Lacerations, loss of soft tissue, amputations, and comminuted fractures are recorded. Most injuries involve only one or two bites and are confined to the extremities. Hypovolemic shock is the immediate threat to life in shark attacks. Bleeding should be controlled with direct compression, and intravascular volume should be replaced with crystalloid until blood products are available. Tetanus toxoid and tetanus immunoglobulin should be considered, and prophylactic antibiotics with a third-generation cephalosporin or trimethoprim–sulfamethoxazole is suggested.

Scorpaenidae

Severe pain at the site of the wound is the first and primary clinical sign for all species. The wound and surrounding area becomes ischemic and then cyanotic. Paresthesia and paralysis of the extremity may occur. Other clinical signs include nausea, vomiting, hypotension, tachypnea proceeding to apnea, and myocardial ischemia with electrocardiographic (ECG) changes. Treatment involves irrigating the wound with sterile saline. The injured extremity is then immersed in very hot water (40°C to 45°C [104°F to 113°F]) for 30 to 60 minutes or until the agonizing pain is completely relieved. Meperidine hydrochloride (1 to 2 mg per kg) may be required for pain. The patient should be monitored carefully for cardiotoxic effects and respiratory depression. Antivenin is available only for the stings of the stonefish of Australia.

Catfish

The spine of the catfish inflicts a puncture wound or laceration. These spines may become imbedded in the flesh of the victim causing soft-tissue swelling, which may become infected or lead to a foreign body reaction. The venom produces a local inflammatory response—local intense pain, edema, hemorrhage, and tissue necrosis. Treatment involves irrigating the wound with sterile saline. The injured extremity is then immersed in hot water (40°C to 45°C [104°F to 113°F]) for 30 to 60 minutes or until pain is relieved. Meperidine hydrochloride (1 to 2 mg per kg) may be required for analgesia. The wound should be explored to locate any retained spines. Adequate debridement is essential. Systemic antibiotics to cover Gram-negative organisms are recommended. Wounds may be closed using a delayed primary closure.

TERRESTRIAL INVERTEBRATES

Phylum Arthropoda

SCORPIONS

Common symptoms include local pain, restlessness, hyperactivity, roving eye movements, and respiratory distress. Other associated signs may include convulsions, drooling, wheezing, hyperthermia, cyanosis, and respiratory failure. The diagnosis may be difficult because a history of a sting may not be forthcoming. There is no laboratory test for confirmation of envenomation. Treatment modalities have been used in addition to general supportive care. Cryotherapy of the site of sting has been advocated to reduce swelling and local induration. Antivenin should be considered after general supportive care has been instituted only if the following symptoms persist: tachycardia, hyperthermia, severe hypertension, and agitation. Antivenin that is not approved by the Federal Drug Administration (FDA) is available through the Antivenom Production Laboratory at Arizona State University in Tempe, Arizona. Sedative–anticonvulsants, in particular phenobarbital (5 to 10 mg per kg), have been used to treat persistent hyperactivity, convulsions, and/or agitation. Calcium gluconate (0.1 mL per kg of the 10% solution) has been given intravenously to reduce muscular contractions and associated pain, but its benefit has not been proved.

SPIDERS

Loxoscelism (Bite of the Brown Recluse Spider)

The spectrum of reaction ranges from minor local reaction to severe necrotic arachnidism. The local reaction is characterized by mild to moderate pain 2 to 8 hours after the bite. At the site of the bite, erythema develops with a central blister or pustule. Within 24 hours, subcutaneous discoloration appears and spreads over the next 3 to 4 days, reaching a size of 10 to 15 cm. At this time, the pustule drains, producing an ulcerated "crater." The local reaction varies with the amount of venom injected. Scar formation is rare if there is no evidence clinically of necrosis within 72 hours of the bite. Systemic reaction is most commonly noted in small children. Symptoms are noted 24 to 48 hours after the bite and include fever, chills, malaise, weakness, nausea, vomiting, joint pain, morbilliform eruption with petechiae, intravascular hemolysis, hematuria, and renal failure.

Because of the delay in initial diagnosis, treatment varies with the clinical stage of the bite. There is no specific serologic, biochemical, or histologic test to diagnose envenomation accurately. Unless all or part of the spider is brought for identification, definitive diagnosis cannot be made. Table 80.1 lists the spiders found in the United States known to cause necrotic lesions. An algorithm for management of suspected bites is shown in Fig. 80.1. Most victims will heal with supportive care. Large-dose steroids have been advocated in the past; however, recent studies have found no significant alteration of necrosis from the venom by steroids or heparin. Animal studies do not support the use of dapsone, hyperbaric oxygen, or the two in combination in the treatment of these envenomations. However, current recommendations are to limit the use of dapsone to adults with proven brown recluse bites. Dapsone should not be used in children because of methemoglobinemia. Antivenom is not yet commercially available. For systemic manifestations, vigorous supportive care is administered. Platelet count for evidence of hemolysis is needed as well as monitoring of hemoglobin, urine sediment, blood urea nitrogen (BUN), and creatinine for evidence of hemolysis and renal failure.

Latrodectism (Bite of the Black Widow Spider)

Reaction is generalized pain and rigidity of muscles 1 to 8 hours after the bite. No local symptoms are associated with the bite itself. The pain is felt in the abdomen, flanks, thighs, and chest and is described as cramping. Nausea and vomiting are often reported in children. Respiratory distress can occur. Chills, urinary retention, and priapism have been reported. There is a 4% to 5% mortality rate, with death resulting from cardiovascular collapse. The mortality rate in young children may be as high as 50%.

TABLE 80.1. Spiders Known to Cause Necrotic Lesions

Genus names	Common name	Geographic distribution
Argiope	Golden orb weaver	Throughout North America (individual species more restrictive)
Chiracanthium	Running spider	Throughout United States
Loxoscle	Brown recluse	Kansas and Missouri to Texas West to California
Lycosa	Wolf spider	Throughout United States
Phidippus	Black jumping spider	Atlantic Coast to Rocky Mountains

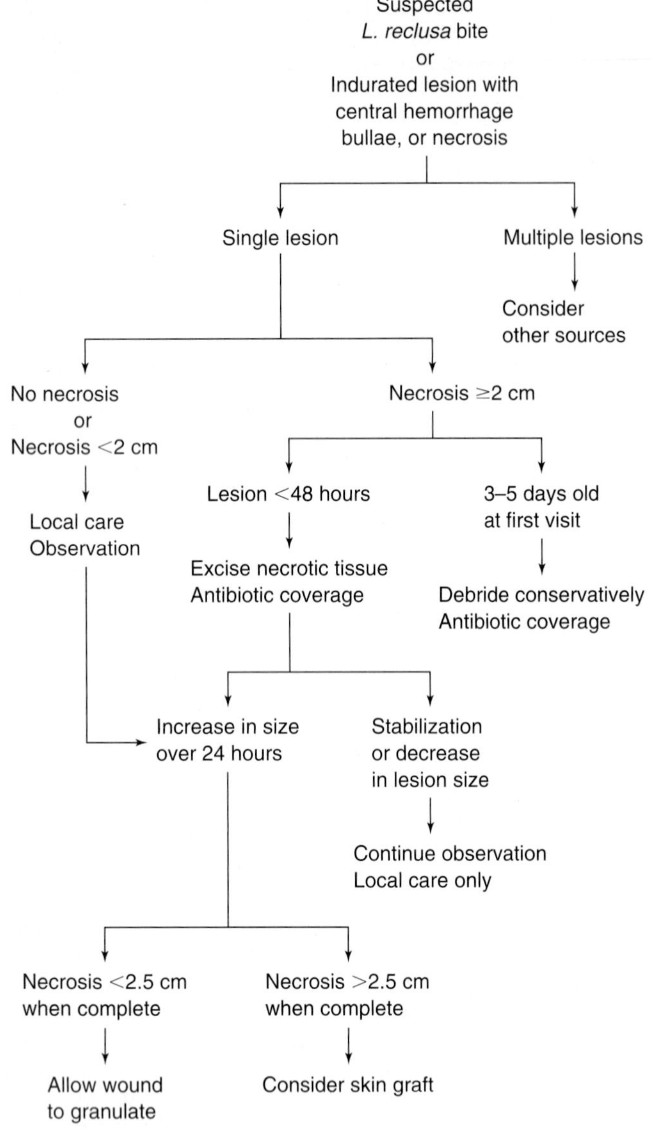

Figure 80.1. Management of suspected brown recluse spider bite.

Because of the size, color, and distinctive markings of this spider, bites are seldom mistaken if the child is old enough to describe the spider. A child who has severe pain and muscle rigidity after a spider bite should be considered a *Latrodectus* bite victim. A clinical grading scale has been developed by Clark (Table 80.2). Treatment with *Latrodectus* antivenin (Lyovac)

TABLE 80.2. Grading Scale for *Latrodectus* Envenomation

Grade	Symptoms
1	Asymptomatic Local pain at bite site Normal vital signs
2	Muscular pain—localized Diaphoresis—localized Normal vital signs
3	Muscular pain—generalized Abnormal vital signs Nausea, vomiting Headaches Diaphoresis

should be instituted as soon as a bite is confirmed in children who weigh less than 40 kg; the usual dose is 2.5 mL (one vial). Antivenin should be administered following the package insert and after skin testing to determine the risk of hypersensitivity to horse serum. For children who weigh more than 40 kg, it is not as urgent to institute antivenin treatment, but indications for its use include patients who are less than 16 years old, who have respiratory difficulty, or who have significant hypertension (grades II and III). Serum sickness is a possible side effect. Because the dosage is low, however, serum sickness is uncommon, with a rate lower than those reported for other types of antivenom. Calcium gluconate 10% solution is often given for control of leg and abdominal cramps. The dosage is 0.1 mL per kg per dose as i.v. push over 5 minutes. Muscle relaxants such as diazepam also have been advocated, but they are variably effective and the effects are short-lived. Analgesia may be achieved with morphine or meperidine.

Tarantulas and Others

Tarantulas, although fearsome in size and appearance, do not bite unless provoked. The venom is mild, and envenomation is not a problem. The wolf spider (*Lycosa* species) and the jumping spider (*Phidippus* species) also have been implicated in bites. Like the tarantula, they have a mild venom that causes only local reactions. Bites from all three of these spiders should be treated with local wound care.

TICK PARALYSIS

Clinical Manifestations

Following tick attachment there is a latent period of 4 to 7 days followed by symptoms of restlessness, irritability, and ascending flaccid paralysis. Laboratory data, including cerebrospinal fluid (CSF) are usually normal, but lymphocytic pleocytosis has been reported. Management is based on general supportive care and a diligent search for the tick. Ticks should be removed using blunt forceps or tweezers. Once the tick is removed, the paralysis is reversible without apparent sequelae.

CENTIPEDES AND MILLIPEDES

Centipedes (class *Myriapode*, order *Chilopoda*) are venomous, biting with jaws that act like stinging pincers. Bites can be extremely painful; however, the toxin is relatively innocuous, causing only local reaction. Treatment consists of injection of local anesthetic at the wound site and local wound care. American millipedes (order *Diplopoda*) are generally harmless.

INSECTS

Bee, Hornet, Yellow Jacket, Wasp

Clinical Manifestations. Clinically, the stings of bees and wasps differ because the barbed stinger of the bee remains in the victim's skin, whereas the wasp may sting multiple times. The allergic reactions may be grouped by severity. Group I consist of a local response at the site of bite or sting. Group II includes the mild systemic reactions typified by generalized pruritus and urticaria. Group III consists of severe systemic reactions, including wheezing, angioneurotic edema, nausea, and vomiting. Group IV consists of life-threatening systemic reactions, including laryngoedema, hypotension, and shock. Anaphylactic reactions secondary to insect stings occur in 0.5% to 5% of the population.

Management. Because the barbed honeybee stinger with venom sac is avulsed and often remains in the victim's skin, it must be removed if seen. Group I reactions can be treated with cold compresses at the site of sting. Group II reactions are treated with diphenhydramine hydrochloride 4 to 5 mg per kg per day (maximum 200 mg) orally in four divided doses for several days. Group III reactions are treated with epinephrine 1:1000 solution 0.01 mL per kg (maximum 0.3 mL) injected subcutaneously followed by diphenhydramine orally. In addition H_2-blockers may provide additional benefit. Ranitidine or cimetidine can be used. These children should be observed in the hospital for 24 hours. Group IV reactions may require intubation if upper airway obstruction is present. Wheezing refractory to epinephrine should be treated with an aminophylline bolus of 6 mg per kg over 20 minutes, followed by a 1.1 mg per kg per hour infusion if needed. Hypotension should be treated with a fluid bolus of saline or lactated Ringer solution 10 to 20 mL per kg given over 20 to 30 minutes. Intravenous epinephrine (1:10000) should be considered if hypotension fails to respond to subcutaneous epinephrine and fluid bolus. Hydrocortisone (2 mg per kg) may be given intravenously every 6 hours for 2 to 4 days. All children in this group should be admitted to an intensive care unit (ICU). Children who have had a group III or IV reaction should be followed by an allergist for hyposensitization. Parents of these children should keep an insect sting emergency kit available in case of future insect stings.

Fire Ants

The clinical picture of fire ant sting is one of immediate wheal and flare at the site. The local reaction varies from 1 to 2 mm up to 10 cm, depending on the amount of venom injected. Within 4 hours, a superficial vesicle appears. After 8 to 10 hours, the fluid in the vesicle changes from clear to cloudy (pustule) and becomes umbilicated. After 24 hours, it is surrounded by a painful erythematous area that persists for 3 to 10 days. Edema, induration, and pruritus at the site occur in up to 50% of patients. Occasionally, systemic reactions occur as with other Hymenoptera. Treatment of fire ant stings is symptomatic.

TERRESTRIAL VERTEBRATES

Venomous Reptiles

CLINICAL MANIFESTATIONS

Pit Viper

Local pain after a *Crotalus* envenomation is typically intense, and a sensation of burning occurs within a couple of minutes. The pain is greater with ensuing edema and presumably increases with larger inocula of venom. Victims of a significant rattlesnake bite often complain within minutes of a perioral numbness, extending to the scalp and periphery. This paresthesia may be accompanied by a metallic taste in the mouth. These patients also may have nausea, vomiting, weakness, chills, sweating, syncope, and other more ominous symptoms of systemic venom absorption. A copperhead or pygmy rattlesnake envenomation produces less local symptoms, and systemic consequences are often minimal or nonexistent unless a small child, multiple bites, or larger than average snake is involved. The water moccasin's effects are more variable.

There is a relative lack of serious pain or swelling with the Mojave rattler bite, although, as in other *Crotalus* bites, the patient may complain of paresthesia in the affected extremity. Within several hours, these patients may develop neuromuscular symptoms such as diplopia, difficulty in swallowing, lethargy, nausea, and progressive weakness from the large portion of neurotoxin in this species.

The wound should be inspected for fang punctures, and if two are present, the distance between them should be noted. An interfang distance of less than 8 mm suggests a small snake; 8 to 12 mm, a medium snake; and more than 12 mm, a larger snake. Fang wounds by small snakes such as the pygmy rattler may be extremely subtle; in larger crotalid snakebites, the fang marks may be hidden within hemorrhagic blebs and edema. Occasionally, only one puncture or two scratches will be present, but both wounds may be potentially venomous. However, not all crotalid bites are envenomated; 10% to 20% of known rattlesnake strikes do *not* inject venom. Other causes of puncture wounds also must be kept in mind—notably rodent bites and thorn wounds. Nonpoisonous snakes sometimes leave an imprint of their two rows of teeth, but the wounds should lack fang puncture marks.

TABLE 80.3. Local Signs of Pit Viper Envenomation

Pain	Ecchymosis
Edema	Vesicles
Erythema	Hemorrhagic blebs

Pit viper envenomations are characterized by intense pain, erythema, and edema at the wound site within 5 to 10 minutes. There may be bloody serosanguinous fluid dripping from the fang punctures. Progressive swelling proportional to the inoculum of venom develops over the next 8 hours and may continue to some degree for an additional 24 hours. Rarely, the venom is deposited predominantly in a muscle compartment, resulting in a deceptively minimal amount of edema. The Mojave rattlesnake bite provides another example of a seemingly innocuous local wound in the setting of a potentially serious envenomation. In a severe diamondback rattlesnake bite, an entire extremity may be swollen within 1 hour.

Local ecchymoses and vesicles usually appear within the first few hours, and hemorrhagic blebs are often present by 24 hours. Lymphadenitis and lymph node enlargement also may become apparent.

Without appropriate therapy, these local manifestations progress to necrosis and may extend throughout the bitten extremity, effectively maiming the victim. Also, as in any animal wound, secondary infection is a risk; the snake's oral flora includes Gram-negative bacteria. Table 80.3 summarizes local characteristics of pit viper bites.

The dramatic signs of crotalid envenomation are derived primarily from the victim's hypovolemic state, hemorrhagic tendencies, and neuromuscular dysfunction. Table 80.4 outlines the more notable physical signs.

Coral Snake

Coral snakes leave unimpressive local signs but can neurologically cripple their prey. The bite may have one or two punctures,

TABLE 80.4. Systemic Signs of Crotalid (Pit Viper) Envenomation

General
  Anxiety, diaphoresis, pallor, unresponsiveness
Cardiovascular
  Tachycardia, decreased capillary perfusion, hypotension, shock
Pulmonary
  Pulmonary edema, respiratory failure
Renal
  Oliguria, hemoglobinuria, hematuria
Neuromuscular
  Fasciculations, weakness, paralysis, convulsions
Hematologic
  Bleeding diathesis

at most 7 to 8 mm apart, as well as other small teeth marks. There is usually only mild pain and little, if any, swelling. Local wound and, eventually, extremity paresthesia and weakness may be reported. Over several hours, generalized malaise and nausea, fasciculations, and weakness develop insidiously. The patient may complain of diplopia and have difficulty talking or swallowing. Physical examination reveals bulbar dysfunction and generalized weakness. Respiratory failure may ensue.

MANAGEMENT

Pit Viper

As in all medical emergencies, the airway, breathing, and circulation (ABCs) of the patient must be addressed before attending to the snakebite (Fig. 80.2). It is important to approach the patient with reassurance and to place him or her at ease. The affected extremity should be stripped of any jewelry or clothing and immobilized in a position of function below the level of the heart. The patient should be kept warm and not allowed anything by mouth.

Incision and suction of the pit viper wound are indicated only if they are started within 5 to 10 minutes of the snake's strike. A constriction band should be placed, then liner incisions, approximately 1× 0.5 cm deep, should be made through the fang marks along the long axis of the extremity, thus avoiding tendons or neurovascular structures. Suction is then applied with a snakebite kit suction cup for the next 30 to 60 minutes. (Note that constriction bands and incision and suction are not recommended in coral snake envenomation.)

A complete blood count (CBC), coagulation studies, platelet count, urinalysis, and blood cross-matching should be obtained on all patients with suspected venomous snakebite. (Blood may be difficult to cross-match after massive hemolysis.) In moderate or severe poisoning, serum electrolytes, BUN, creatinine, fibrinogen, and arterial blood gases also are indicated. Hemolysis, anemia, thrombocytopenia, hypofibrinogenemia, prolonged bleeding times, and metabolic acidosis all may be seen in severe poisoning. Repeat the laboratory studies every 6 hours to ensure no significant changes occur.

Therapy will be based on the clinician's overall grading of

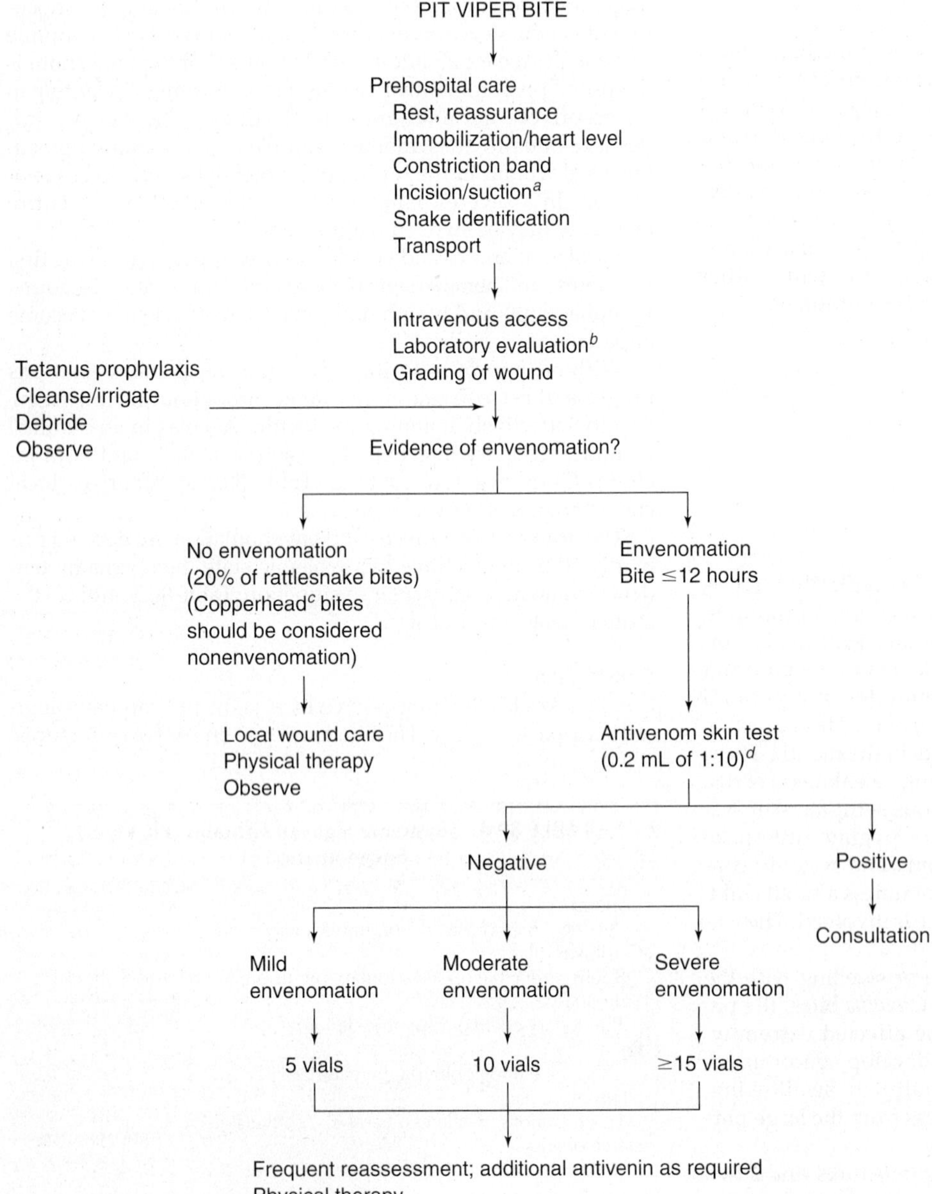

Figure 80.2. Management of pit viper bite. [a]Perform within 5 to 10 minutes of bite; continue suction for 30 to 60 minutes. [b]Complete blood count, platelet count, prothrombin time, partial thromboplastin time, urinalysis, type and hold; in moderate or severe cases, add fibrinogen, arterial blood gases, electrolytes, blood urea nitrogen, and creatinine. [c]Seldom need antivenin; exceptions with large snakes and small children. [d]1:100 dilution if allergy history; saline control; resuscitation medications at hand; antivenin seldom indicated if greater than 12 to 24 hours since bite.

venom toxicity. Local and systemic manifestations, as well as laboratory findings, weigh heavily in this judgment. The clinical pattern may change dramatically as the venom's effects unfold; thus, frequent reassessment is crucial. The physician should measure and record the circumference of the injured extremity at the leading point of edema and 10 cm (4 inches) proximal to this level every 30 minutes for 6 hours then at least every 4 hours for a total of 24 hours. Table 80.5 is derived from a grading system suggested by the Scientific Review Subcommittee of the American Association of Poison Control Centers.

If the history and physical examination on arrival in the ED are consistent with a venomous snakebite, immediate laboratory evaluation and i.v. access are indicated. Aggressive supportive medical care must be available if signs of major system dysfunction are present. Any prehospital care (eg, extremity immobilization) should be rechecked. If an occluding tourniquet is inappropriately present, the physician should place a more proximal constriction band and then cautiously remove the tourniquet, being prepared to respond therapeutically to a systemic release of venom.

One antivenin (antivenin crotalidae polyvalent: Wyeth-Ayerst) is effective for the rattlesnake, water moccasin, and copperhead. For maximal venom binding, the antivenin should be given within 4 hours of the snake strike. Benefits of antivenin administration after 12 hours are questionable, and use is not indicated after 24 hours (an exception may be continued coagulopathy). The initial recommended dosage varies with the severity of the envenomation. The amount of antivenin is not calculated on a weight basis; children require more than adults as a rule. Dosages in the higher range are used when snake or human variables associated with higher morbidity/ mortality are present. For example, a child with two eastern diamondback bites should receive a large dose of antivenin on the basis of potential severity. On the other hand, a copperhead bite is usually mild and often may be observed for progression without any antivenin given.

Antivenin is highly antigenic horse serum; therefore, skin testing is mandatory (read package insert). Resuscitation equipment, including airways and oxygen, i.v. epinephrine (1:10000), antihistamines, and steroids must be kept in close proximity. The standard skin test involves an intradermal injection of 0.02 mL of 1:10 dilution of reconstituted antivenin. If the history suggests a likely reaction, use a more diluted (1:100 or greater) preparation. A saline control in the opposite extremity is useful for judging a positive-reaction wheal, which is usually apparent within 15 minutes.

If the skin test is negative, the reconstituted antivenin (one vial with 10 mL of saline) is diluted with normal saline in a 1:4 dilution. The antivenin should be infused by i.v. slowly (1 to 2 mL per hour). During the first 10 to 20 minutes, the clinician should observe for signs or symptoms of an allergic reaction. If no reaction occurs, the rate of infusion should be increased so that the total volume is completed over 2 hours; extremity edema and vital signs should be measured every 15 minutes for evidence of progressive venom toxicity. The initial dose of antivenin should be repeated every 2 hours until the progression of the swelling has stopped. The number of antivenin vials initially anticipated is a rough estimate; more or less antivenin may be required as the clinical reassessment dictates (as many as 75 vials have been used in a child).

Positive skin tests or allergic signs during antivenin infusion warrant consultation with a medical herpetologist. The absolute threat to life must be reassessed, and if present, plans must be made to continue the antivenin. If mild allergic manifestations develop, the infusion should be stopped and diphenhydramine (1 to 2 mg per kg i.v.) given. Once the allergic symptoms have resolved, a minimum of 5 minutes should pass, then the infusion should be restarted at a slower rate. If symptoms recur, the antivenin should be stopped again; further therapy at this point is controversial. Some authorities recommend an epinephrine drip that is titrated to minimize any allergic phenomena when the antivenin is restarted. If this option is suggested by your consultant, an epinephrine infusion (starting at 0.1 μg per kg per minute) is recommended. Steroids (prednisone 1 to 2 mg per kg per day) are also recommended.

An alternative desensitization method for allergic reactions is described in the product insert but requires at least 3 hours to achieve and thus is not practical in severe envenomations. If life-threatening anaphylaxis occurs, epinephrine 1:10000 (0.01 mL per kg), diphenhydramine (1 to 2 mg), and steroids (methylprednisolone 2 mg per kg every 6 hours) are given by i.v. immediately, and other supportive measures are instituted as needed.

Wound care includes irrigation, cleansing, a loose dressing, and consideration of tetanus prophylaxis. The affected extremity should be maintained just below the level of the heart and in

TABLE 80.5. Grading of Crotalid (Pit Viper) Snakebites

	Mild	Moderate	Severe
Local	Fang mark Intense pain Edema Erythema Ecchymosis ±Vesicles Within 10–15 cm of bite	All local signs extend beyond wound site	Entire extremity involvement
Systemic	None Anxiety-related	Nausea/vomiting Weakness/fainting Perioral, scalp paresthesias Metallic taste Pallor Tachycardia Mild hypotension Fasciculations	As in moderate Hypotension Shock Bleeding diathesis Respiratory distress
Laboratory	No abnormalities	Hemoconcentration Thrombocytopenia Hypofibrinogenemia	Significant anemia Prolonged clotting time Metabolic acidosis

a position of function. Cotton padding between swollen digits is useful. Broad-spectrum prophylactic antibiotics are recommended by most authorities. Analgesics for pain may be offered if the cardiorespiratory status is not in question. Surgical excision of the wound, routine fasciotomy, and application of ice are contraindicated. Excision of the wound does not remove significant venom after 30 minutes, and cryotherapy has been associated with increased extremity necrosis and amputations. Fasciotomy should be reserved for the very rare case of a true compartmental syndrome. Necrosis is usually the result of the proteolytic enzymes or inappropriate therapy and is not caused by compartmental pressure. Superficial debridement will be required at 3 to 6 days; a wound care regimen suggested at this stage includes local oxygen, aluminum acetate (1:20 solution) soaks, and triple dye. Physical therapy is beneficial during the healing phase.

The major thrust of supportive care is correction of the intravascular depletion that results from increased venous capacitance, interstitial third spacing, and hemorrhagic losses. Moderate or severe envenomation mandates two i.v. lines for separate but simultaneous antivenin therapy and volume replacement. Shock usually develops between 6 and 24 hours after the snakebite but may present within the first hour in severe envenomation. Signs of hypovolemia (eg, decreased capillary perfusion, oliguria, tachycardia, anemia, hypotension) deserve aggressive therapy. Central vascular monitoring and accurate urine output measurements are desirable for optimal therapy. Normal saline or lactated Ringer solution (20 mL per kg over 1 hour), followed by fresh whole blood or other blood components, often corrects the hypovolemia (see Chapter 3). Vasopressors are usually needed only transiently in the more severe cases. A bleeding diathesis is best managed with fresh whole blood, or blood component therapy, primarily packed cells (10 mL per kg), and fresh-frozen plasma (10 mL per kg). With life-threatening bleeding, platelets (0.2 units per kg) and a more concentrated fibrinogen source (cryoprecipitate—dose 1 bag per 5 kg body weight) also should be considered. Abnormal clotting parameters, including fibrinogen and platelet and blood counts, should be reevaluated every 4 to 6 hours. Respiratory support also is commonly required when shock has developed. Renal failure is another potential problem in this setting.

Coral Snake

When coral snake wounds are present or the history or specimen is consistent with an eastern coral snakebite, antivenin for *Micrurus* fulvius (Wyeth-Ayerst) is administered before development of further symptoms. This is also an equine serum and requires preliminary skin testing (see package insert). The initial recommended dosage is three to five vials by i.v.; an additional three to five vials may be given as needed for signs of venom toxicity. There is no antivenin available for the Arizona coral snake *(Micruroides euryxanthus)*. Supportive care should provide a satisfactory outcome in these cases. Constriction bands, suction and drainage, and other local measures do not retard coral snake venom absorption and, hence, are not indicated.

Mammalian Bites

CLINICAL MANIFESTATIONS

Mammalian bite wounds cause a spectrum of tissue injuries from trivial to life threatening. Scratches, abrasions, contusions, punctures, lacerations, and their complications are seen commonly in the ED. The complications usually involve secondary infections or damage to structures that underlie the bite. The dog strikes the head and neck in 60% to 70% of victims less than 5 years old and in 50% of those less than 10 years old. These wounds most often involve the lips, nose, and cheek areas, and on rare occasions, they penetrate the skull, with resulting depressed skull fractures and intracranial lesions. The uncommon life-threatening injuries occur almost exclusively in young children and include major vascular injury, visceral penetration, and chest trauma.

Cat bites are located in the infection-prone upper extremities in two-thirds of cases and usually are puncture wounds rather than lacerations or contusions. Infections that complicate these wounds result from the same organisms isolated in dog bites, but a higher incidence of *Pasteurella multocida* is found. *P. multocida* infections characteristically present within 12 to 24 hours of the injury and rapidly display erythema, significant swelling, and intense pain.

Cat scratches are most commonly located on the victim's upper extremities or periorbital region and are more likely to develop secondary bacterial infection than scratches from the other common domesticated species. Corneal abrasions also are occasionally associated with the periorbital wounds. Cat-scratch disease, an uncommon complication of these injuries, is characterized by a papule at the scratch site and a subsequent regional lymphadenitis.

Human bites in older children and adolescents are most commonly incurred when a clenched fist strikes the teeth of an adversary. The wound typically overlies the metacarpal-phalangeal joint, and on relaxation of the fist, the bacterial inoculum penetrates more deeply into the relatively avascular fascial layers. Hand infections, regardless of infection site, usually present with mild swelling over the dorsum of the hand 1 to 2 days after injury. Infected hand bites may be superficial and localized to the wound, but if there is pain with active or passive finger motion, a more serious deep compartmental infection or tendonitis should be suspected. Osteomyelitis occasionally occurs in hand infections. In younger children, human bites are more often on the face or trunk than on the hands. Often, a playmate inflicts the wound, but child abuse must always be considered. Systemic diseases that may be spread by human bites include human immunodeficiency virus, hepatitis B, and syphilis.

Rodent bites have a relatively low incidence of secondary infection (10%). Rat bite fever is a rare disease that may present after a 1- to 3-week incubation period with chills, fever, malaise, headache, and a maculopapular or petechial rash. There are two forms: Haverhill fever *(Streptobacillus moniliformis)* and Sodoku *(Spirullum minus)*, both of which are responsive to i.v. penicillin.

Another uncommon bacterium for which lagomorphs, particularly rabbits, are hosts is *Francisella tularensis*. Tularemia is usually spread to humans by rabbit bites, although contact with or ingestion of contaminated animals or insect vectors is sufficient for transmission. Ulceroglandular tularemia is the most common form of the disease, and streptomycin is the agent of first choice in its treatment.

Serious infections from multiple bacteria, including osteomyelitis, sepsis, endocarditis, and meningitis, have been reported as complications of mammalian bite wounds as well as the more esoteric diseases already mentioned. The risk of rabies or tetanus always must be considered in animal bites.

MANAGEMENT

Meticulous and prompt local care of the bite wound is the most important factor in satisfactory healing and prevention of infection. In more extensive wounds, local anesthesia is achieved before wound hygiene. Then, the skin surrounding the wound should be cleaned with a soft sponge and 1% povidone iodine solution can remove obvious contaminants. The wound itself should be forcefully irrigated with a minimum of 200 mL normal saline. A 19-gauge needle or catheter attached to a 30-mL syringe will supply sufficient pressure for wound decontamination and will decrease the infection rate by twentyfold. Stronger irrigant antiseptics—povidone iodine scrub preparation, 20% hexachlorophene, alcohols, or hydrogen peroxide—may damage wound surfaces and delay healing. Soaking in various preparations has not proved helpful in reducing infections.

Most open lacerations from mammalian bites can be sutured if local care is effected within several hours of the injury and good surgical technique is used. Facial wounds often mandate primary closure for cosmetic reasons and, overall, are low infection risks because of the good vascular supply. The exceptions to suturing are minor hand wounds and other high-risk bites. In large hand wounds, hemorrhage should be carefully controlled. We suggest closing the subcutaneous dead space in these wounds with a minimal amount of absorbable suture material. Cutaneous sutures can be placed after 3 to 5 days if there is no evidence of infection.

Extremities with extensive wounds should be immobilized in a position of function and kept elevated as much as possible. This is especially true of hand wounds, which should have bulky mitten dressings and be supported by an arm sling. All significant wounds should be rechecked in follow-up in 24 to 48 hours.

The following wounds may be considered at high risk for infection: puncture wounds, minor hand or foot wounds, wounds given initial care after 12 hours, cat or human bites, and wounds in immunosuppressed patients. As a rule, these wounds should not be sutured, and prophylactic antibiotics are indicated. No single antibiotic is ideal for all of the most common organisms involved in infected mammalian bite wounds. Amoxicillin–clavulanic acid (Augmentin) comes close. It is effective in *P. multocida, Streptococcus, Staphylococcus,* and anaerobe control, as well as in providing staphylococcus coverage. Combination therapy with phenoxymethyl penicillin (penicillin V) and cephalexin or dicloxacillin has been suggested by some authorities. For high-risk wounds, we recommend amoxicillin–clavulanic acid (30 to 50 mg per kg per day) alone for initial therapy. Erythromycin (40 mg per kg per day) is an alternative for the penicillin-allergic patient. The initial dosage of antibiotic should be given in the ED and continued for the next 3 to 5 days. It must be emphasized that local care ultimately prevents infection more effectively than any prophylactic antibiotics. Studies indicate that prophylactic oral antibiotics for low-risk dog bite wounds are not indicated because the differences in the rate of infection are not significant and the cost–benefit ratio not worth the risks of allergic reactions.

Any bite wound with signs of infection deserves aggressive drainage and debridement and antibiotic therapy after aerobic and anaerobic cultures are obtained. Moderate to severe hand infections or other wounds that involve deep structures usually require debridement and exploration under general anesthesia. Culture swabs should sample the depth of the wound; or, in cases of cellulitis, the specimen can be collected by needle aspiration of the leading edge of erythema. While awaiting cultures, a Gram stain is often helpful in differentiating the probability of staphylococci or streptococci from *P. multocida*.

Parenteral antibiotics and admission to the hospital are indicated if the child has systemic symptoms or has wounds with potential functional or cosmetic morbidity. The choice of parenteral antibiotics should be governed by the same factors considered in selection of prophylactic antibiotics and then modified by culture results.

Tetanus immunization status should be checked in every injury that violates the epidermis, regardless of the cause. Recommendations for tetanus immunoglobulin and immunization are noted elsewhere. Although the incidence of rabies (1 to 5 cases per year) is extremely low, the physician must always assess the possibility of rabies exposure and promptly initiate prophylaxis when indicated.

Rabies prophylaxis is not indicated in bites by a healthy dog or cat with a known owner, assuming the animal's health does not deteriorate over the following 10 to 14 days. Bites by strays and other domesticated mammals should be considered individually and with consultation of the local health department. Scratches, abrasions, and animal saliva contact with the victim's mucous membranes all are capable of rabies spread.

CHAPTER 81
Allergic Emergencies

Roy M. Kulick, M.D., and
Richard M. Ruddy, M.D.

ASTHMA

Clinical Findings

Table 81.1 presents a general guide to several parameters useful for estimating the severity of the episode. The history should include the duration of the current episode and the rapidity of onset, the parent's or patient's subjective assessment of severity, other associated symptoms, and the suspected trigger. The child's current medications should be determined, including details of when the medications were started, the dosage, the route, the timing of the last dose, and a history of missed doses from noncompliance or emesis. A history of previous medications, particularly oral or inhaled steroids in the past 6 months, should be elicited. For children with their first episode of wheezing, the possibility of a foreign-body aspiration or another cause of wheezing should be explored.

The physical examination begins immediately with an overall assessment of the child's degree of respiratory distress. Severe retractions, accessory muscle use, nasal flaring, cyanosis, decreased muscle tone, and altered mental status all are indicative of impending or existing respiratory failure and require immediate intervention. The respiratory rate (RR) and heart rate (HR) should be noted and compared with age-appropriate normals (Table 81.1). The remainder of the respiratory examination includes auscultation for decreased breath sounds, wheezing, rhonchi, and crackles. Crackles can occur and most often are caused by focal areas of atelectasis.

Peak expiratory flow rate (PEFR) can serve as a simple, quantitative, reproducible, and inexpensive measure of airway obstruction in the child with mild to moderate distress. A flow rate of less than 80% of predicted or personal best is considered abnormal, and less than 50% indicates moderate to severe obstruction. Pulse oximetry provides a noninvasive, continuous, and generally valid measure of arterial hemoglobin oxygen saturation (Sa_{O_2}). Confrimation of adequate oxygenation is reassuring and obviates the need for measurements of arterial blood gas (ABG) in most mild to moderate exacerbations. The ABG provides an objective measure of ventilation as well as oxygenation. It is essential in the evaluation of any child in whom impending or existing respiratory failure is suspected clinically, although it should never delay the initiation of therapy. It should be emphasized that a "normal" partial arterial pressure (Pa_{CO_2}) of

TABLE 81.1. Estimation of Severity of Acute Asthma Exacerbation

Sign/symptom	Mild	Moderate	Severe
Respiratory rate[a]	Normal to 30% increase	30–50% increase	>50% increase
Alertness	Normal or agitated	Normal or agitated	Agitated to decreased level of consciousness
Dyspnea	Absent or mild; speech normal	Moderate; speaks in phrases; difficulty feeding	Severe; single words or short phrases; refuses feeding
Accessory muscle use	None to mild intercostal (IC) retractions	Moderate IC with tracheosternal (TS) retraction Use of sternoclaidomastoid muscle Chest hyperinflation	Severe IC and TS retraction Nasal flaring Chest hyperinflation
Color	Normal	Pale	Possibly cyanotic
Wheeze	Often end expiratory only	Throughout exhalation	Throughout inhalation and exhalation; breath sounds markedly decreased
Oxygen saturation (in room air)	>95%	91–95%	<91%
Peak expiratory flow rate[b] (% predicted or personal best)	>80%	50–80%	<50%
P_{aCO_2}	<42 mm Hg	<42 mm Hg	≥42 mm Hg

Adapted from Expert Panel Report of the National Heart, Lung, and Blood Institute, 1991 and 1997.
Note: Within each category, the presence of several parameters, but not necessarily all, indicate general classification of exacerbation. Many of these parameters have not been systematically studied, so they serve only as general guides.

[a] Normal rates of breathing in awake children

Age	Normal rate (per min)
<2 mo	<60
2–12 mo	<50
1–5 yr	<40
6–8 yr	<30

Normal pulse rates in children

Age	Normal rate (per min)
2–12 mo	<160
1–2 yr	<120
2–8 yr	<110

[b] For children at least 5 years of age or older.

40 mm Hg in a child with tachypnea or significant respiratory distress may be a sign of impending respiratory failure and requires aggressive management and close monitoring. The role of chest radiographs in the emergency management of acute asthma is not well defined. Typical findings on routine films such as hyperinflation, atelectasis, and peribronchial thickening do not correlate with severity and rarely alter management. Patients for whom a chest radiograph may be of a higher yield include those with failure to respond to therapy, persistence of focal findings after bronchodilator therapy, reduced oxygen saturation after therapy, or clinical suspicion of a complication or a cause for wheezing other than asthma. Radiographic evaluation of the sinuses may be helpful for the child with chronic, persistent wheezing in whom sinusitis is suspected.

The uncommon child taking theophylline may benefit from a theophylline level to help determine further management. The level should be obtained early in the course of therapy. Serum potassium measurement should be considered in children at risk for hypokalemia secondary to receiving frequent β-agonist therapy.

Complications

The most common pulmonary complication is atelectasis secondary to mucous plugging. Air leaks that lead to a pneumomediastinum or a pneumothorax are potentially life threatening. A pneumothorax should be suspected in any child with a sudden deterioration associated with chest pain, asymmetry of breath sounds, or a shift of the trachea. Cardiac arrhythmias are associated with adrenergic agents and with theophylline alike. Frequent β-agonist therapy can cause hypokalemia. The syndrome of inappropriate antidiuretic hormone secretion (SIADH) also is a potential, although rare, complication of acute asthma.

Management

INITIAL APPROACH

The primary goals in the acute management phase of an asthma exacerbation are to correct hypoxemia and rapidly to reverse airflow obstruction. Supplemental oxygen, repetitive β_2-agonists, and the early addition of systemic corticosteroids achieve this. For children who are discharged, the emergency physician should prescribe an intensified regimen for a minimum of 3 to 5 days and should recommend appropriate follow-up so that chronic management issues can be addressed. This section of the chapter presents a stepwise approach that is summarized in algorithm form in Figure 81.1, with specific dosage recommendations in Table 81.2.

All children with acute asthma can be assumed to be hypoxemic unless oxygen saturation is measured immediately and indicates otherwise. Hence, unless SaO_2 is greater than 90%, humidified oxygen should be administered immediately It should be delivered at a flow rate sufficient to eliminate cyanosis and, ideally, to maintain SaO_2 levels greater than 90% (95% in infants).

Repetitive, inhaled β_2-agonists are the mainstay of initial bronchodilator therapy in children. Frequent (every 15–30 minutes) doses of nebulized albuterol appear to be effective in reversing airway obstruction. Although the ideal dose of albuterol (0.5%) has not been determined, the Expert Panel 2 of the National Institutes (NIH) recommends 0.15 mg per kilogram of body weight per dose. From a practical standpoint, patients older than 1 year who weigh less than 30 kg should be given 2.5 mg (0.5 mL) and those who weigh more than 30 kg should be given 5 mg (1 mL). A minimum dose of 1.25 mg (0.25 mL) is used for infants less than 1 year old. Recent evidence suggests that an albuterol metered-dose inhaler (MDI) and chamber may be just as effective as nebulized treatments.

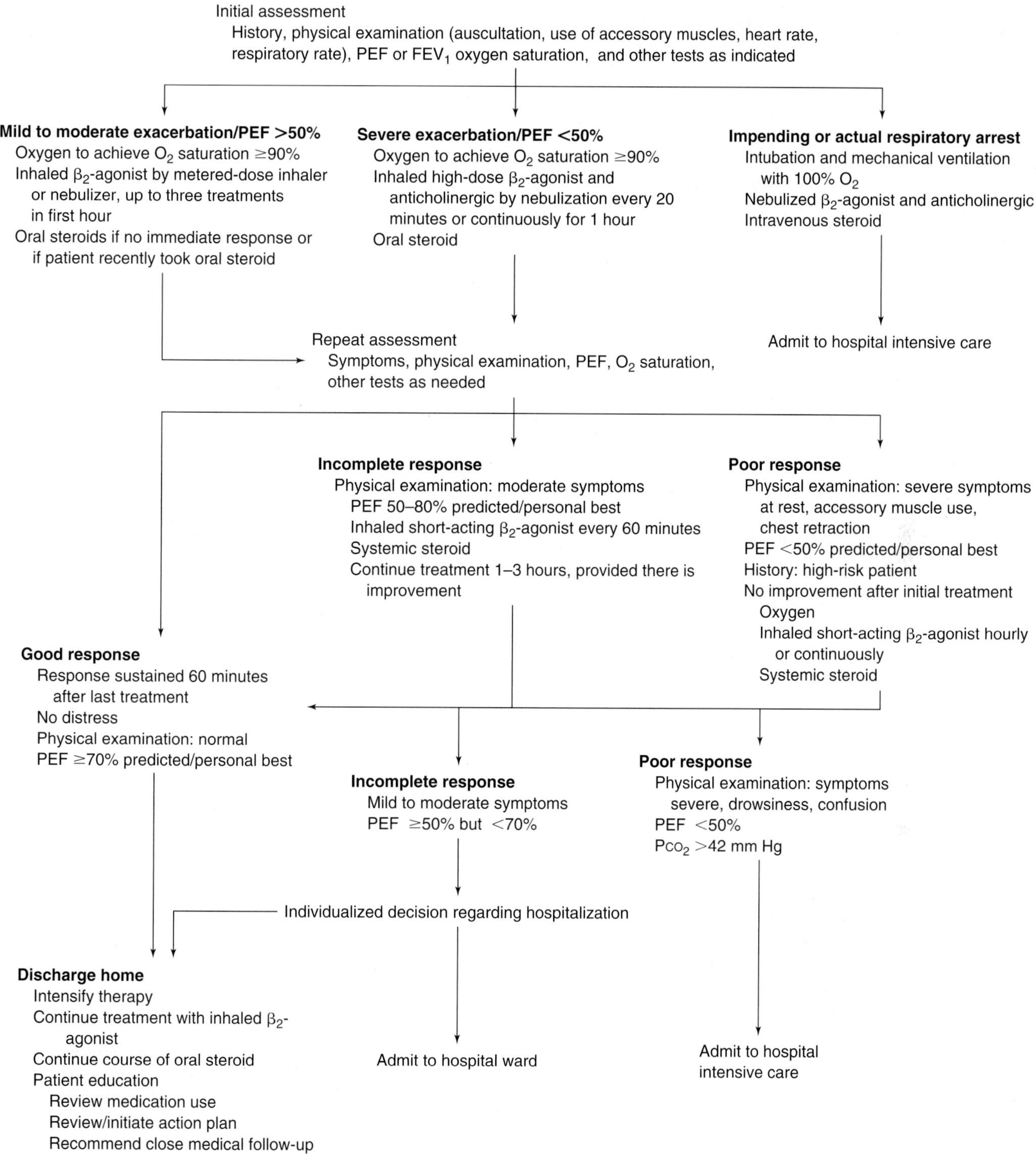

Figure 81.1. Approach to acute asthma in children. *PEF,* peak expiratory flow; *FEV$_1$*, forced expiratory volume in 1 second. (Modified with permission from Expert Panel 2 Report, NIH, 1997.)

Subcutaneous injection of epinephrine or terbutaline remains an acceptable alternative in settings where nebulized therapy is unavailable or delayed or for the toddler resisting an inhalation treatment. It also may be indicated as initial therapy for the child with severe obstruction, hypoventilation, or apnea in whom the delivery of nebulized medication to the airways is believed to be inadequate. Under these circumstances, the injection can be given simultaneously with the initial aerosol and, if indicated, by mask ventilation during preparation for intubation.

Early treatment of asthma exacerbations with steroids has been shown to prevent progression of airway obstruction, to decrease the need for emergency treatment and hospitalization, and to reduce morbidity. As a rule, almost all children who have had a significant exacerbation ultimately receive steroids. An exception is made for children with mild symptoms who require either no nebulizer treatments or, at worst, one treatment that immediately produces adequate resolution. Exposure to chickenpox in the unprotected host is one of the rare instances in

TABLE 81.2. Emergency Department Acute Asthma Therapy

Therapy	Dose	Maximum	Comments
Oxygen	Maintain S_{aO2} >90% (>95% in infants)		
Adrenergic agents			
Aerosolized			
Albuterol (0.5%) Nebulizer solution	Intermittent: 0.15 mg/kg q15–20min in 2 mL normal saline solution ×3, then 0.15–0.3 mg/kg q1–4hr	5 mg/dose	2.5 mg minimum Usual dose: <30 kg 2.5 mg ≥30 kg 5 mg
	Continuous: 0.5 mg/kg/hr	15 mg/hr	
Metered-dose inhaler	4–8 puffs q20min ×3, then q1–4hr as needed		Use spacer/holding chamber
Subcutaneous			
Epinephrine 1:1000	0.01 mL/kg s.c. q15–20min	0.3–0.5 mL	See text for indications
Terbutaline (0.1%)	0.01 mL/kg s.c. q15–20min	0.25 mL	See text for indications
Intravenous			
Terbutaline (0.1%)	Loading dose: 10 μg/kg over 10 min Initial maintenance: 0.4 μg/kg/min		Titrate up by 0.2 μg/kg/min Usual effective range 3–6 μg/kg/min
Anticholinergics			
Ipratropium bromide			
Nebulizer solution (0.25 mg/mL)	0.25 mg q20min ×3, then q2–4hr as needed	0.5 mg	May mix with same nebulizer as albuterol; should not be used as first-line therapy, should be added to β_2-agonist
Corticosteroids			
Methylprednisolone	2 mg/kg i.v. bolus	125 mg	
Prednisone	2 mg/kg p.o.	80 mg	

s.c., subcutaneously; i.v., intravenously; p.o., orally.

which steroids may need to be avoided acutely. Depending on the level of distress and the child's ability to tolerate oral medications, the dose of corticosteroid is given either intravenously (methylprednisolone 2 mg/kg or equivalent; maximum 125 mg) or by mouth (prednisone or prednisolone 2 mg per kilogram; maximum, 80 mg). Studies suggest that nebulized steroids may have a role in the management of acute asthma exacerbations. Children taking inhaled steroids with minor exacerbations may sometimes be adequately managed by doubling their inhaled steroid dose.

Ipatropium may be mixed with albuterol and delivered simultaneously. Recommendations vary, but the NIH guidelines suggest 0.25 mg for children (0.5 mg in adolescents and adults) every 20 to 30 minutes mixed with the first three albuterol treatments and then every 2 to 4 hours as needed.

After 2 to 4 hours of frequent bronchodilator treatments and the initiation of corticosteroid therapy, the limit of emergency department (ED) management has been reached and a disposition decision should be made. If appropriate resources are available, continued management of the patient in an "observation unit" or "clinical decision unit" for up to 24 hours may avoid the need for hospital admission.

APPROACH TO THE CHILD WITH RESPIRATORY FAILURE

The options include continuous nebulized albuterol, intravenous β_2-agonist therapy, and mechanical ventilation. The use of continuous nebulized therapy is well established in the intensive care unit (ICU) unit setting and currently is under study in EDs. Continuous terbutaline and albuterol have been demonstrated to reverse respiratory failure and to eliminate the need for mechanical ventilation. Albuterol is administered as 0.5 mg per kilogram each hour (maximum, 15 mg per hour). Intravenous β_2-agonist therapy is an option for children for whom continuous nebulized therapy fails. In the United States, terbutaline is administered as a 10 μg per kilogram loading dose over 10 minutes followed by an initial infusion of 0.4 μg per kilogram per minute. The infusion is titrated in increments of 0.2 μg per kilogram of body weight per minute up to effect while the child is monitored for unacceptable tachycardia. The usual effective range is 3 to 6 μg per kilogram per minute. If the child continues to deteriorate, intubation and mechanical ventilation should be considered. Many authorities consider ketamine (1–2 mg per kilogram administered intravenously) to be the induction agent of choice because of its bronchodilating effects. Agents that may increase bronchospasm through histamine release, such as meperidine, morphine, D-tubocurare, and atracurium, are best avoided. Volume-controlled ventilation is preferred using larger-than-average tidal volumes (10–20 mL per kilogram), normal respiratory rates for age, and high flow rates to ensure long expiratory times.

Although intravenous magnesium sulfate has been studied extensively in adults and appears to improve pulmonary function, there is no consensus regarding its role in the management of asthma exacerbations. A recent study of children with moderate to severe exacerbations showed that patients treated with magnesium (25 mg per kilogram administered intravenously; maximum, 2 g) had greater improvement in forced expiratory volume in 1 second(FEV_1), were less likely to require admission, and had no significant adverse effects compared with the group treated with placebo. This study suggests that intravenous magnesium may have a role as an adjunct in the treatment of children with moderate to severe acute asthma exacerbations.

Disposition

Admission should be considered for children who meet any of the following criteria: (1) persistent respiratory distress; (2) SaO_2 of 91% or less in room air; (3) PEFR less than 50% of predicted levels; (4) inability to tolerate oral medications (ie, vomiting); (5) previous emergency treatment in last 24 hours; (6) underlying high-risk factors, including congenital heart disease, bronchopulmonary dysplasia, cystic fibrosis, and neuromuscular disease; and (7) evidence of air leak. Children who also meet

TABLE 81.3. Criteria for Admission to the Intensive Care Unit

Severe respiratory distress
  Estimate in severe range after therapy[a]
  P_{aO_2} <60 mm Hg or S_{aO_2} <90% in 40% O_2
  P_{aCO_2} <42 mm Hg
Significant complications
  Pneumothorax
  Arrhythmia
  Theophylline toxicity

[a] See Table 81.1.

the criteria listed in Table 81.3 should be admitted to an ICU setting.

Discharge Management

In general, if a child already on a regimen of medication has had an exacerbation that requires emergency management, this regimen must be intensified, at least for the next 3 to 5 days. Short-course, high-dose oral steroids (ie, prednisone, 2 mg per kilogram daily up to 80 mg daily for 3–5 days) should be prescribed and administered for essentially all children who arrive at the ED with a significant exacerbation. In addition, all patients currently taking or who have recently been taking oral or inhaled corticosteroids must be given steroids as part of the acute management of their exacerbation. Children who experience frequent acute exacerbations, nocturnal symptoms, or multiple absences from school also may benefit from the addition of a systematic or inhaled corticosteroid to their regular regimen.

For children who experience their first episode of wheezing or who are not receiving long-term therapy, an inhaled albuterol is generally well tolerated in the subacute phase following the acute episodes. Children younger than 5 years should use an MDI with a spacer and mask or a nebulizer. The use of a spacer device in all children will improve delivery of medications in MDIs. If the child is receiving other long-term therapy, such as cromolyn sodium or inhaled steroids, it is important to continue it during acute exacerbations. Table 81.4 lists outpatient treatment options.

ANAPHYLAXIS

Clinical Findings

The time between exposure to the inciting agent and onset of symptoms can vary from minutes to hours, although most reactions occur within 1 hour. Some patients experience a biphasic reaction in which symptoms may recur up to 12 hours after the initial reaction, although this is an uncommon occurrence. The signs and symptoms of anaphylaxis vary in both the spectrum and severity of involvement. Reactions may be limited to the skin, as in a mild urticarial reaction, or catastrophically involve multiple systems, leading to shock and death.

In general, systemic reactions include cutaneous involvement such as pruritus, flushing, erythema, urticaria, and, in more severe cases, angioedema. A more detailed discussion of

TABLE 81.4. Outpatient Asthma Therapy

Medication	Dose	Maximum	Comments
Quick-Relief β_2-agonists			
Metered-dose inhaler (MDI)			
Albuterol	2 puffs q4–6hr	q4hr	Use spacer May double dose for mild exacerbations Encourage to consult physician if more frequent use required
Nebulized			
Albuterol	0.05–0.1 mg/kg q4–6hr in 2 mL normal saline solution	5.0 mg	1.25-mg minimum May mix with cromolyn or ipratropium solutions May double dose for exacerbations
Long-acting β_2-agonists			
Salmeterol			Should not be used for symptom relief or for exacerbations
MDI	1–2 puffs q12hr		
DPI 50 μg/blister	1 blister q12hr		
Corticosteroids			
Oral			
Prednisone Prednisolone	2 mg/kg/day ×3–5 d	60–80 mg/day	May require taper
MDI			
Beclomethasone Budesonide Flunisolide Fluticasone Triamcinolone	Doses vary greatly depending on severity of chronic asthma Consult with primary care physician or asthma specialist		May consider doubling usual daily dose for minor exacerbation in lieu of systemic steroids; long-term use has adrenal suppressive effect Use spacer to limit local adverse effects
Cromolyn sodium			
MDI	2 puffs q6–12hr		
Nebulized	20 mg q6–12hr		
Leukotriene modifiers			
Zafirlukast 20-mg tablet	20 mg p.o. b.i.d.		Age ≥12 yr
Zileuton 300- or 600-mg tablet	600 mg q.i.d.		Age ≥12 yr

p.o., orally; b.i.d., twice daily; q.i.d., four times daily.

urticaria is found at the end of this section (see also Chapter 57). Mucous membrane involvement may be limited to pruritus and congestion of the eyes, nose, and mouth. Swelling of the lips or tongue can potentially impair swallowing and ventilation.

An immediate life-threatening feature of anaphylaxis is upper airway obstruction that results from edema of the larynx, epiglottis, and other surrounding structures. This may be experienced as subtle discomfort of the throat or as obvious stridor and respiratory distress. Anaphylaxis also can cause lower airway disease secondary to bronchospasm, which leads to findings similar to acute asthma, such as a sense of chest tightness, cough, dyspnea, wheezing, and retractions.

Another potential life-threatening feature of anaphylaxis is cardiovascular collapse and hypotensive shock. Although the mechanisms are not fully understood, these cardiopulmonary manifestations are thought to result from profound vasodilation, increased vascular permeability, capillary leak, and intravascular volume depletion, as well as a possible direct toxic effect of circulating mediators. Arrhythmias and electrocardiographic evidence of myocardial ischemia also may be seen. Gastrointestinal symptoms are relatively common and include nausea, vomiting, diarrhea, and crampy abdominal pain.

Urticaria is a common manifestation of immediate hypersensitivity reactions as well as a number of other disease processes. In the patient with acute urticaria from an immunoglobulin E-mediated process, the urticaria may be localized to the area of exposure, such as the area around a sting. In addition to the localized urticaria, there may be a systemic reaction. Urticaria may be associated with *angioedema*, or swelling of the lower dermis and subcutaneous tissues. The angioedema associated with urticaria is pruritic. Angioedema without pruritus usually is secondary to processes other than immediate hypersensitivity. The physical urticarial reactions may be life threatening, and they should be included in the differential diagnosis of anaphylaxis.

Management

MAINTENANCE OF THE AIRWAY AND OXYGENATION

The physician should administer 100% oxygen with bag-valve-mask ventilation, as indicated, to assist ventilation. If there is complete airway obstruction, immediate endotracheal intubation should be attempted. If intubation is unsuccessful, cricothyrotomy is indicated. Rapid administration of epinephrine may lessen the difficulty of airway management release. Epinephrine can be administered subcutaneously in the patient with reasonable perfusion (epinephrine 1:1000, 0.01 mL per kilogram to a maximum of 0.5 mL). If the patient is hypotensive or hypoperfused or if the initial subcutaneous dose is ineffective, the epinephrine should be administered intravenously or through an intraosseous needle as a 1:10000 solution, 10 μg per kilogram (0.1 mL per kilogram) over 1 to 2 minutes. In severe cases, this may need to be followed by a continuous epinephrine infusion of 0.1 μg per kilogram per minute, which can be titrated to effect up to a maximum of 1.0 μg per kilogram per minute (6 mg epinephrine should be added to 100 mL of D5W normal saline solution; 1 μg/kg per minute = 1 mL per kilogram per hour). Bronchospasm should be treated aggressively with supplemental oxygen, β_2-agonists such as albuterol or epinephrine, and corticosteroids, as outlined in the previous section on asthma.

Maintenance of the Circulation

Hypotensive patients should be placed in the Trendelenburg position, and a rapid bolus of 20 mL per kilogram of body weight of a crystalloid solution should be administered immediately and repeated as necessary. Because plasma volume may fall precipitously by 20% to 40%, large amounts of fluid may be necessary. If hypotension persists after epinephrine, normal saline bolus, and positioning, a continuous infusion of epinephrine should be started as previously described.

Other Therapy

The H_1-receptor antihistamines such as diphenhydramine (1–2 mg per kilogram administered either intramuscularly or intravenously; maximum, 50 mg) are indicated in histamine- mediated allergic reactions. They work synergistically with the epinephrine therapy. Corticosteroids do not take effect during the initial resuscitative phase of anaphylaxis. In significant reactions, however, their early administration may block or reduce the late-phase reactions over the next several hours or days. They can be administered as methylprednisolone 1 to 2 mg/kg by IV (maximum, 125 mg) or prednisone 1 to 2 mg/kg by mouth (maximum, 80 mg). Many authorities recommend H_2-blocking antihistamines such as cimetidine (5 mg per kilogram; maximum, 300 mg) or ranitidine (1 to 2 mg per kilogram; maximum, 50 mg) in addition to H_1-blocking antihistamines, particularly for more severe reactions.

MANAGEMENT OF LIMITED REACTIONS

Most children with allergic reactions present with involvement limited to a diffuse, pruritic rash, localized swelling, or benign involvement of the mucous membranes. Appropriate management of these children varies according to the specific presentation. Options include subcutaneous epinephrine (eg, for evolving urticaria), antihistamines, and corticosteroids. Diphenhydramine (5 mg per kilogram daily divided every 4 to 6 hours, with a maximum of 300 mg every 24 hours) and hydroxyzine (2 mg per kilogram daily divided every 4 to 6 hours, with a maximum of 200 mg daily) are the antihistamines most commonly prescribed for urticaria. In the case of cold urticaria, cyproheptadine (0.25–0.5 mg per kilogram daily divided every 12 hours, with a maximum of 32 mg daily) is the drug of choice, whereas hydroxyzine is preferred for cholinergic urticaria or most other cases of chronic urticaria.

Disposition

Patients with severe reactions that involve upper airway obstruction or shock generally should be monitored for a minimum of 8 to 24 hours. Children with a history of asthma appear to be at increased risk for delayed and severe reactions and also may require prolonged monitoring. Those with less severe manifestations can be discharged home on a course of antihistamines and, in selected cases, corticosteroids. As a rule, therapy initiated in the ED should be continued for a minimum of 48 hours. Follow-up with the child's primary care physician also is advised. All children with a history of significant anaphylaxis with an antigen that cannot be avoided totally (eg, *Hymenoptera* venom or food) should be instructed to carry a preloaded syringe of epinephrine to be used in emergencies (EpiPen).

SERUM SICKNESS

Clinical Findings

The reaction is characterized by fever, malaise, and a rash that is most commonly urticarial but also may appear as maculopapular or vasculitic. Other manifestations include arthralgias or arthritis, lymphadenopathy, angioedema, and nephritis. Other less common problems include abdominal pain, carditis, anemia, and neuritis. Characteristically, the onset of symptoms occurs 7 to 14 days after the primary exposure. If there has been

TABLE 81.5. Possible Laboratory Evaluation of Serum Sickness[a]

Blood tests	Hepatitis B screen
Erythrocyte sedimentation rate	Heterophil antibody
Complete blood count with differential CH50, C3, C4	Immune complex assay
	Other laboratory tests
Blood urea nitrogen, creatinine	Urinalysis
Antinuclear antibody	Electrocardiogram
Rheumatoid factor	Stool Hematest
Hepatic enzymes	Computed tomography scan

[a] Laboratory evaluation should be tailored for each individual patient as noted in text.

prior sensitization, however, reexposure can result in onset of a few days.

Examination of the skin may reveal a maculopapular eruption, urticaria, or the palpable purpura of a cutaneous vasculitis. Painful angioedema is commonly present. Generalized lymphadenopathy often occurs. In more severe reactions, the joints show erythema, warmth, and effusion. Wheezes may be appreciated on auscultation of the lungs, and a pericardial friction rub may be audible if pericarditis is present. The liver and spleen often enlarge. Rarely, neurologic deficits will occur secondary to a vasculitis of the central nervous system.

A list of other studies that may be indicated for individual patients with immune complex–mediated disease is outlined in Table 81.5. The erythrocyte sedimentation rate (ESR) may be elevated. A CBC and differential may reveal leukopenia or leukocytosis. The C3, C4, and CH_{50} may decrease because of complement activation. Stool Hematest should be performed, and an ultrasound should be considered for patients with abdominal pain or other symptoms involving the gastrointestinal tract. If carditis is suspected, a screening electrocardiogram should be performed. Severe headache or focal neurologic deficits are indications for a computed tomography scan.

Management

If possible, the offending antigen should be eliminated. Pharmacologic management usually involves one or more of the following: antihistamines, nonsteroidal antiinflammatory drugs (NSAIDs), and corticosteroids. Pruritus, rash, and angioedema can be managed with an antihistamine such as hydroxyzine (2 mg per kilogram per 24 hours divided every 6 to 8 hours, with a maximum of 200 mg every 24 hours). Although experience in the treatment of serum sickness is limited, use of the second-generation nonsedating antihistamines also may be considered (Table 81.6). Urticarial lesions and angioedema that evolves rapidly may respond acutely to subcutaneous epinephrine (1:1000, 0.01 mL per kilogram subcutaneously, with a maximum 0.30 mL) or longer-acting Sus-Phrine (0.005 mL per kilogram administered subcutaneously, with a maximum of 0.15 mL). Mild joint involvement or fever or both will often improve with use of an NSAID such as ibuprofen (30–50 mg per kilogram every 24 hours divided every 6 to 8 hours up to a maximum 2.4 g per 24 hours). In more severe disease or after failure to respond to these measures, a burst of corticosteroids may be indicated. This involves the use of 1 to 2 mg per kilogram daily of prednisone in divided doses for 7 to 10 days, followed by a taper for 3 to 4 weeks (maximum, 80 mg daily). In life-threatening serum sickness with significant circulating immune complexes, plasmapheresis may play a role, but this procedure has not been used extensively for treatment of this disease. Most children with serum sickness can be managed as outpatients with close follow-up by their primary care physicians. Children with more severe involvement may benefit from hospitalization.

ALLERGIC RHINITIS

Clinical Findings

The classic symptoms of allergic rhinitis include nasal congestion, paroxysmal sneezing, pruritus of the nose and eyes, and watery, profuse rhinorrhea. Other complaints may include

TABLE 81.6. Emergency Department Management of Allergic Rhinitis

Medication	Dose	Comments
Antihistamines		
First-generation		
Chlorpheniramine maleate	0.35 mg/kg q6–12hr depending on formulation	Sedation, anticholinergic effects
Brompheniramine maleate		Maximum: 24 mg/day
Second-generation (nonsedating)		
Claritin (loratadine)	<30 kg 5 mg q.d.	≥3 yr
10-mg tab or 10 mg/10 mL syrup	>30 kg 10 mg q.d.	
Claritin D	1 tablet b.i.d.	≥12 yr
12-hr (loratadine 5 mg/pseudoephedrine 120 mg)	1 tablet q.d.	
24 hr (loratadine 10 mg/pseudoephedrine 240 mg)		
Allegra (Fexofenadine)	1 cap b.i.d.	≥12 yr
60-mg caps		
Zyrtec (Cetirizine)	2–6 yr: 5 mg/d	± sedating
5- or 10-mg tablet	6–12 yr: 5–10 mg/d	FDA approved ≥2 yr
5 mg/5 mL syrup		
Decongestants		
Oral		
Pseudoephedrine	4 mg/kg/day q6–8hr	Maximum: 180 mg/d
Topical		
Oxymetazoline	Age 2–5: 0.025% Age >6: 0.05% 2–3 drops each nostril b.i.d.	Limit use to <5 d to avoid rebound congestion

q.d., daily; b.i.d., twice daily; FDA, Food and Drug Administration.

TABLE 81.7. Topical Treatment for Allergic Rhinitis

Trade name	Generic name	Dosage	Ages (yr)
Corticosteroids			
Vancenase AQ 84 μg	Beclomethasone (aqueous: 84 μg/spray)	1–2 sprays each nostril q.d.	≥6
Vancenase AQ	Beclomethasone (aqueous: 42 μg/spray)	1–2 sprays each nostril b.i.d.	≥6
Vancenase pocket inhaler	Beclomethasone (42 μg/puff)	1 spray each nostril t.i.d.	≥6
Beconase	Beclomethasone (42 μg/spray)	1 spray each nostril t.i.d.	≥6
Beconase AQ	Beclomethasone (aqueous: 42 μg/spray)	1–2 sprays each nostril b.i.d	≥6
Rhinocort	Budesonide (32 μg/actuation)	2 sprays each nostril b.i.d. or 2–4 sprays each nostril q.d.	≥6
Flonase	Fluticasone (50 μg/spray)	1–2 sprays each nostril q.d.	≥12
Nasacort	Triamcinolone (55 μg/puff)	2 sprays each nostril q.d.	≥6
Nasacort AQ	Triamcinolone (55 μg/spray)	2 sprays each nostril q.d.	≥12
Nasarel	Flunisolide	2 sprays each nosril b.i.d.	≥6
Nasonex	Mometasonefuroate (50 μg/spray)	2 sprays each nostril q.d.	≥12
Others			
Nasalcrom	Cromolyn (mast-cell stabilizer)	1 spray each nostril q4–8hr	≥6
Astelin	Azelastine (137 μg/spray) (antihistamine)	2 sprays each nostril b.i.d.	≥12

q.d., every day; q.i.d., four times daily; b.i.d., twice daily.

noisy breathing, snoring, repeated throat clearing or cough, itching of the palate and throat, "popping" of the ears, and ocular complaints such as redness, itching, and tearing. The physical examination is variable but may reveal the "gaping" look of a mouth breather, dark discoloration of the infraorbital ridge caused by venous congestion (allergic shiners), and a transverse external nasal wrinkle secondary to chronic rubbing of the nose (allergic salute). Intranasal findings are variable. The mucosa often is edematous and may appear pale or violaceous. The nasal secretions may be clear, mucoid, or opaque.

Management

Recognizing that long-term therapy must be highly individualized, the emergency physician generally will limit interventions to those that safely provide rapid, symptomatic relief and then refer the child to the primary care physician for long-term therapy. In addition, topical corticosteroids, first-line therapy for chronic allergic rhinitis, may require as long as 2 weeks to achieve maximal relief. Generally, rapid relief can be achieved by prescribing an antihistamine (Table 81.6). The first-line approach for patients who require long-term therapy is topical corticosteroids (Table 81.7), with or without a second-generation oral antihistamine. For completeness, other categories of topical treatment are also listed in Table 81.7. Children with significant ocular symptoms also may benefit from topical ophthalmic treatment (Table 81.8).

TABLE 81.8. Ophthalmic Drops

Trade name	Generic name	Category	Dosage	Ages (yr)
Naphcon-A	Nephazoline and Pheniramine	Antihistamine–decongestant	1–2 gtt q.d.	>6
Livostin	Levocabastine	Antihistamine	1–2 gtt q.d.	>12
Alomide	Lodoxamide Tromethamine	Mast-cell stabilizer	1–2 gtt q.d.	>2
Patanol	Olopatadine	Mast-cell stabilizer and antihistamine	1–2 gtt q.d.	>3
Acular	Ketotifen	NSAID	1–2 gtt q.d.	>12

b.i.d., twice daily; q.i.d., four times daily; NSAID, nonsteroidal antiinflammatory drug.

CHAPTER 82
Gastrointestinal Emergencies

Dennis R. Durbin, M.D., M.S.C.E., and Chris A. Liacouras, M.D.

GASTROINTESTINAL BLEEDING

Upper Gastrointestinal Bleeding

BACKGROUND

Upper gastrointestinal (GI) bleeding generally is regarded as originating proximal to the ligament of Treitz. Hematemesis or bloody gastric aspirates from a nasogastric tube may originate from the mouth, nasopharynx, esophagus, stomach, biliary tree, or duodenum. The most common causes of upper GI bleeding in children are mucosal lesions, including esophagitis, gastritis, Mallory–Weiss tear, peptic ulcer disease, and duodenitis. Less common but important causes include bleeding esophageal varices and vascular lesions. The profile of common diagnoses has changed recently because increasing use of endoscopy enables specific, often microscopic, diagnoses to be substituted for previously documented "bleeding of unknown origin." Endoscopy, when performed by a well-trained physician, is the most sensitive and specific diagnostic procedure for determining the cause and site of upper GI bleeding. Specific diagnosis should be pursued in patients who have (1) active bleeding documented by nasogastric lavage; (2) evidence of severe hemorrhage (hemodynamic instability or equilibrated hemoglobin level <10 g per deciliter); (3) conditions that affect healing or clotting, such as catabolic state or serious chronic disease; (4) a history of previous unexplained gross or occult bleeding or unexplained iron deficiency anemia; or (5) a history of chronic dyspepsia (vomiting, abdominal pain, nausea, oral regurgitation, heartburn, dysphagia).

The pathophysiology, clinical manifestations, and specific management issues related to each of the most common causes of upper GI bleeding in children are discussed. As noted in Chapter 23, an upper tract source for GI bleeding often is indicated by a history of hematemesis or by obtaining fresh (red) or old (coffee ground) blood via gastric lavage after placement of a nasogastric tube.

GENERAL PRINCIPLES OF NASOGASTRIC LAVAGE

Not every child with a history of possible upper GI bleeding requires nasogastric lavage. Patients who have a history of acute self-limited hematemesis of streaks of blood or a small amount of coffee-ground material in the context of forceful emesis, recurrent gastroesophageal reflux, symptoms of infectious gastroenteritis, or epistaxis often can be managed presumptively without gastric lavage; however, nasogastric lavage should be performed in all patients suspected of having significant GI bleeding that is indicated by either history or physical examination (eg, pallor, unexplained tachycardia, poor perfusion). The purpose of gastric lavage is to confirm the level of bleeding and to estimate the rate of bleeding. There is no evidence that gastric lavage has any therapeutic role in controlling hemorrhage. It is important to realize that a clear nasogastric aspirate does not exclude major bleeding from the upper GI tract.

Most patients can be effectively lavaged with a nasogastric sump tube (12 F in small children; 14–16 F in older children). Verification of the location of the tube in the stomach by injection of air and auscultation over the stomach is essential. The recommended volume for each saline infusion depends on age: 50 mL for infants, 100 to 200 mL for older children. With the patient's head elevated 30 degrees, the solution, at room temperature, is rapidly infused into the stomach, allowed to stand for 2 to 3 minutes, and then aspirated by gentle suction. Return volumes should approximate input volumes, and discrepancies should be recorded. If aspiration meets with significant resistance, the physician should reposition the tube, reposition the patient, or increase the amount of solution introduced. Saline lavage of the stomach should be performed by two people. One person fills and empties the stomach while the other person empties and fills the syringes.

Blood-flecked gastric aspirate or coffee-ground material indicates a low rate of bleeding. In contrast, bright red blood, especially if it does not clear with repeated lavage for 5 to 10 minutes, suggests a significant or ongoing hemorrhage. No benefit is derived from continuous lavage longer than 10 minutes if return is not clearing. The tube can be left to gravity or low suction and irrigated every 15 to 30 minutes to assess the activity of the bleeding. The presumed lesion causing the bleeding determines the subsequent management of the patient.

NONSPECIFIC MUCOSAL LESIONS

Background

Gastrointestinal bleeding may be a complication of all acute and chronic nonspecific upper GI mucosal lesions (esophagitis, gastritis, Mallory–Weiss tears, and duodenitis). Regardless of the cause, upper GI bleeding usually stops spontaneously, often by the time the patient arrives in the emergency department (ED). Esophagitis as a result of gastroesophageal reflux (GER) is being diagnosed more often with improved pediatric fiberoptic endoscopes. Increasing use of endoscopic biopsy has documented esophagitis in 60% of patients with clinically significant GER. Exposure to aspirin and nonsteroidal antiinflammatory drugs (NSAIDs) (eg, ibuprofen, naproxen sodium) has been associated with gastritis and mucosal ulceration. A large randomized clinical trial designed to assess the risk of serious GI bleeding (requiring hospitalization) in febrile children after the use of ibuprofen demonstrated no greater risk than with acetaminophen. The study was not able to assess less serious (and clinically inapparent) occurrences of GI bleeding. Mallory–Weiss tears are mucosal lacerations of the gastric cardia or gastroesophageal junction induced by retching or vomiting. These lesions are relatively rare in children, accounting for approximately 5% of cases of upper GI bleeding.

Pathophysiology

The upper GI mucosa bleeds when an ulcerating process erodes into a blood vessel, usually an artery in the base of the ulcer. In most cases, normal mechanisms of thrombosis and healing stop the bleeding and prevent recurrent bleeding. Erosion of larger arteries, however, in which blood flow exceeds the capacity of normal hemostasis results in continuous hemorrhage. A more common scenario is that thrombosis temporarily stops the bleeding, but aneurysmal dilation of the artery in the recanalization process or continuing arteritis from the chemical irritation of acid digestion facilitate recurrent hemorrhage. Acid and pepsin also produce profound adverse effects on platelet aggregation and plasma coagulation. The pathogenesis of Mallory–Weiss tears involves the production of transient large gradients between the intragastric and intrathoracic pressures at the gastroesophageal junction as a result of forceful retching. The gradient results in dilation of the gastroesophageal junction and, thus, tears.

Clinical Manifestations

Diagnosis usually is suspected by an antecedent history of vomiting or abdominal pain and an absence of physical findings suggestive of chronic liver disease or portal hypertension. Reflux esophagitis is suspected in infants, usually younger than 1 year, who have a history of recurrent nonprojectile emesis, "wet burps" after feeding, or a documented diagnosis of GER and who present with emesis that is blood streaked or contains a small amount of coffee-ground material. Infants may be fussy but consolable and may have been diagnosed with colic. Reflux esophagitis also should be suspected in infants with guaiac-positive stools or iron deficiency anemia. A history of repeated aspirin or NSAID use for the control of fever or pain should prompt suspicion for gastric mucosal lesions as the cause of upper GI bleeding. Mallory–Weiss tears should be suspected in older children with a history of protracted forceful vomiting and streaks of hematemesis appearing after several episodes of nonbloody emesis.

Management

For patients who have significant bleeding and for whom nasogastric lavage was initiated, if gastric contents clear following initial saline lavage and immediate endoscopy is not planned, gastric irrigation is performed every 15 minutes for 1 hour and then every hour for 2 to 3 hours. Antacid (eg, Maalox 7, 15 mL, infants; 30 mL, preschool-age children; 60 mL, school-age children) is infused into the tube after every lavage. The dosage of antacid is titrated during the hourly monitoring so that gastric pH 1 hour after antacid infusion is greater than 3.5. If the patient is hemodynamically stable and gastric return remains clear for the aforementioned period, the tube is electively removed. Persistent nausea or vomiting or the presence of ileus points to the need for continued drainage.

Patients with nonspecific mucosal lesions theoretically should benefit from neutralization of intragastric acidity by antacids and reduction of gastric acid and pepsin secretion by H_2-receptor antagonists. For patients with significant symptoms or blood loss, H_2-antagonists may be given initially by the intravenous route, switching to the oral route when the nasogastric tube is removed. Either ranitidine (1.0–1.5 mg per kilogram of body weight per dose administered intravenously every 6 hours or 2 mg per kilogram per dose administered orally two times a day) or cimetidine (6.0–7.5 mg per kilogram per dose administered intravenously every 6 hours or 10 mg per kilogram per dose orally four times a day) is appropriate. For patients who have acute self-limited bleeding and who are not considered candidates for endoscopy, oral H_2-antagonists are continued for 2 to 4 weeks, at which time they are empirically discontinued if the patient is asymptomatic.

In general, all patients with a history suggestive of significant upper GI bleeding should be admitted to the hospital for observation. A clear nasogastric aspirate should never be used as an indication to discharge a patient from the ED if the history suggests significant bleeding. The main reason for admission is the unknown incidence of rebleeding from these lesions in children. Unremitting or recurrent mucosal bleeding requires therapeutic endoscopy, therapeutic angiography, or surgery. In the hands of a qualified endoscopist, therapeutic endoscopy using either a heater probe or multipolar electrocoagulation is the treatment of choice.

ESOPHAGEAL VARICES

Background

Portal hypertension may result from either extrahepatic presinusoidal obstruction (50%–65% of cases in children) or from hepatic parenchymal disorders. Extrahepatic obstruction (eg, portal or splenic vein obstruction) is associated with omphalitis, dehydration, sepsis, and umbilical vein catheterization. Hepatic parenchymal disease may result from biliary cirrhosis associated with biliary atresia, cystic fibrosis, hepatitis, α_1-antitrypsin deficiency, or congenital hepatic fibrosis. Patients with both types of portal hypertension are susceptible to GI hemorrhage from bleeding esophageal varices and from congestive or hemorrhagic gastritis. After development of portal hypertension, the onset of esophageal varices can be variable, from a few months to many years.

Pathophysiology

Portal hypertension results from relative obstruction of portal venous blood flow, leading to the development of portal systemic collateral veins, or *varices*. Portal–systemic collaterals will develop in any area where veins draining the portal venous system are in close approximation to veins draining into the caval system (ie, submucosa of the esophagus, submucosa of the rectum, and anterior abdominal wall). Esophageal and gastric fundal varices, connecting branches of the coronary veins with branches of the azygous vein, are the most likely to be the site of spontaneous hemorrhage (Fig. 82.1).

Clinical Manifestations

Patients with portal hypertension may have occult bleeding, but more commonly, the bleeding is brisk, and patients will have melena or hematemesis. The possibility of bleeding esophageal varices should be considered in any patient with a history of jaundice (beyond the newborn period), hepatitis, blood transfusion, chronic right-sided heart failure, pulmonary hypertension, omphalitis, umbilical vein catheterization, or one of the hepatic parenchymal diseases previously noted. Accordingly, the physical examination may reveal stigmata of the underlying disease leading to portal hypertension, including jaundice, ascites, rectal hemorrhoids, and hepatosplenomegaly.

Management

The initial management of suspected variceal hemorrhage is identical to that of massive upper GI bleeding from any source. Overexpansion of the intravascular volume should be avoided because it contributes to rebleeding. Coagulation abnormalities should be managed aggressively with intravenous vitamin K, fresh-frozen plasma, and platelets. Bleeding varices may be the initial sign of sepsis in patients who have cirrhosis; therefore, any patient who has fever should be started on broad-spectrum antibiotics such as ampicillin 200 mg per kilogram daily and gentamicin 5 to 7.5 mg per kilogram of body weight daily pending the results of blood cultures.

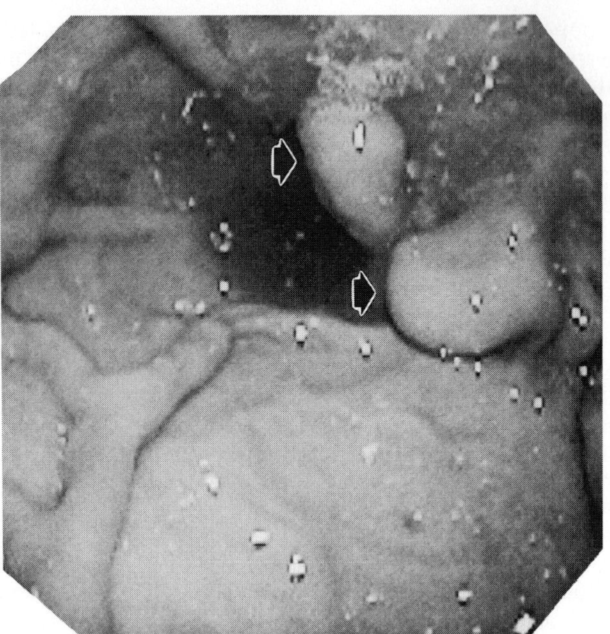

Figure 82.1. Gastric varices. The arrows represent two large blood-filled varices in the gastric cardia.

Suspicion of variceal bleeding is not a contraindication to pass a nasogastric tube. If bleeding ceases during the initial gastric lavage, the tube should be managed as previously described. Antacids and H_2-antagonists are given in the doses used for mucosal lesions. Pharmacologic therapy of acute variceal hemorrhage uses the splanchnic arterial constrictor vasopressin and the prokinetic agent metoclopramide. Vasopressin administration has been well documented to decrease blood flow and pressure through the portal circulation. Infusion may be initiated before diagnostic endoscopy if variceal bleeding is suspected. The physician should begin infusing 0.1 U per minute and increase the dosage by 0.05 U per minute hourly up to a maximum of 0.2 U per minute in children younger than 5 years, 0.3 U per minute in children aged 5 to 12 years, and 0.4 U per minute in adolescents aged more than 12 years. Side effects can be significant; thus, the child must be monitored carefully. Major complications include myocardial ischemia, life-threatening arrhythmias, and limb vasoconstriction or ischemia. Minor complications include water retention with sodium depletion, benign arrhythmias, and acrocyanosis. The vasopressin is usually given in 5% dextrose in water; the exact dilution is based on overall volumes of fluids being infused. Infusing vasopressin through a large-bore, preferably central venous, line is the safest method. The reported success rate of vasopressin infusion in adults is 50% to 70%. Because of the high rate of rebleeding, once begun, the drug should be continued at the dosage that controls bleeding for a minimum of 12 to 24 hours after all bleeding has stopped. This management plan stems from studies showing sustained vasoconstrictive effects of vasopressin on splanchnic vessels in dogs for more than 24 hours. This point is controversial because tachyphylaxis reportedly also develops with prolonged use of vasopressin.

If bleeding continues after the use of vasopressin, emergency flexible endoscopy should be performed as soon as the patient's vital signs have been stabilized. Actively bleeding esophageal varices or an overlying clot on a varix confirms variceal bleeding. The endoscopist may choose to perform emergency sclerotherapy at that point. Alternatively, sclerotherapy may be delayed until hemorrhaging has been controlled by pharmacologic agents or balloon tamponade, especially if the endoscopist has difficulty obtaining a clear field of vision. Sclerotherapy should not be considered a therapeutic option to control bleeding gastric varices.

Gastroesophageal balloon tamponade is a high-risk procedure. It should be considered only for endoscopically proven gastric or esophageal varices. Indications of these varices include massive life-threatening hemorrhage or continued bleeding despite 2 to 6 hours of intravenous vasopressin. Either a Sengstaken–Blakemore (S-B) (Fig. 82.2) or a Linton tube may be used. The S-B tube has both gastric and esophageal balloon tubes, whereas the Linton tube has a single lavage gastric balloon. Gastroesophageal tamponade is reported to arrest bleeding initially in 50% to 80% of cases; however, the reported incidence of major complications from use of the S-B tube ranges from 9% to 35%. Death directly attributed to the use of the tube has been reported in 5% to 20% of patients on whom the tube was used. Other major complications include rupture or erosion of the esophageal or gastric fundal mucosa, occlusion of the airway by the balloon, and aspiration of secretions resulting from inadequate drainage of the occluded esophagus.

When a hemostatic tube is used, it should be inserted only by a physician who is skilled in its use. The S-B tube is preferred (Fig. 82.2). A pediatric tube is used for children younger than 11 to 13 years old; the adult tube is used in adolescents. Passage through the nose is the procedure of choice, but in small children, passage through the mouth may be necessary. Intranasal oxymetazoline hydrochloride (0.05%) is used for local vasoconstriction. Each balloon is pretested for air leaks before insertion. The tube is heavily lubricated and passed through the nose to its full length; 50 to 100 mL of air is instilled into the gastric balloon and the balloon is pulled up until the resistance of the gastroesophageal junction is encountered. An emergency radiograph is performed to ensure correct balloon position immediately below the diaphragm. Additional air is then instilled into the gastric balloon, up to 150 mL in the pediatric balloon and 250 mL in the adult balloon; the tube is pulled taut and is taped at the nose. In many cases, the gastric balloon alone will stop bleeding by preventing flow of blood from the stomach into the esophagus or by directly occluding a gastric varix. It is absolutely essential to pass a second nasoesophageal tube to aspirate saliva and blood from ongoing esophageal hemorrhage. If esophageal bleeding continues, the esophageal balloon is inflated with air. The volume in the esophageal balloon is determined by the pressure within the balloon, which is measured by connecting its inflow tube to a sphygmomanometer. The pressure is maintained at the minimum required to control bleeding, with the maximum being no more than 40 mm Hg.

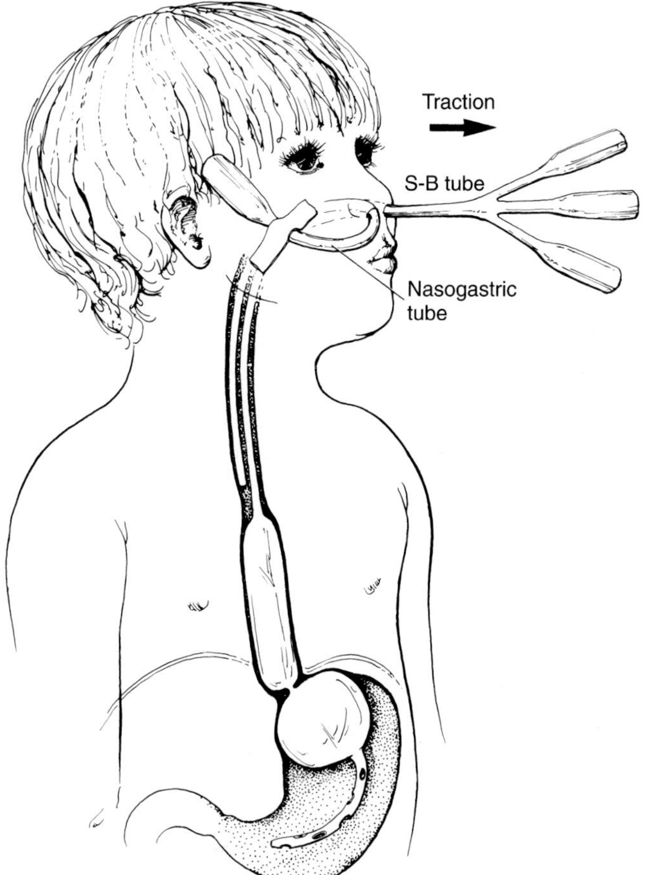

Figure 82.2. Gastroesophageal tamponade using a Sengstaken–Blakemore tube.

If bleeding is controlled, the balloons are kept inflated for 24 hours. The esophageal balloon is deflated first, then the gastric balloon approximately 1 hour later. The gastric tube is irrigated every 30 minutes for 1 to 2 hours more, and then the tube is removed.

A patient with an indwelling S-B tube must be transferred to an intensive care unit. A pair of scissors should be kept at the bedside; if any respiratory embarrassment occurs, the tube should be cut immediately, thereby deflating the balloons.

Endoscopic sclerotherapy should be performed on an elective basis within 6 to 24 hours after active bleeding has been controlled by pharmacologic therapy or balloon tamponade. Recent reports have noted success with endoscopic variceal ligation (EVL) using an elastic band ligature device in children. Randomized studies of endoscopic variceal sclerotherapy (EVS) versus EVL in adults have demonstrated that EVL has a lower complication rate, less recurrent bleeding, and better variceal eradication than EVS. In a recent case series of EVL in children, 55% of children achieved variceal eradication with EVL after an average of four treatment sessions. Urgent shunt surgery is indicated only if two attempts at sclerotherapy fail to control active or recurrent bleeding. An alternative to shunt surgery in patients with cirrhotic portal hypertension is esophageal transection with or without devascularization.

MISCELLANEOUS CAUSES OF UPPER GASTROINTESTINAL BLEEDING

In the first few days of life, or in breast-fed infants, *swallowed maternal blood* may be the cause of hematemesis or melena in an infant who otherwise appears healthy. Performing a guaiac test on expressed breast milk may suggest the diagnosis. An Apt–Downey test should be performed on a sample of emesis or nasogastric aspirate to diagnose the condition definitively. Blood from the aspirate is placed on filter paper and mixed with 1% NaOH. Adult hemoglobin will be reduced to form a rusty brown or yellow color. Fetal hemoglobin is resistant to denaturation and will retain a bright pink or red color.

Dieulafoy lesion is an unusual cause of GI bleeding in which massive hemorrhage occurs from a pinpoint nonulcerated arterial lesion, usually high in the fundus of the stomach. The bleeding results from an unusually large submucosal artery that travels a tortuous course through the submucosa and may erode through a mucosal defect. Its characteristic presentation is one of recurrent, massive hematemesis, usually without any prodromal symptoms. This diagnosis is made primarily in adults, but patients as young as 20 months have been diagnosed with a Dieulafoy lesion, and most series contain a number of teenagers. Management is similar to that for any patient with a significant GI hemorrhage. Diagnosis can be made by endoscopy, during which the Dieulafoy lesion can usually be located.

Finally, swallowed foreign bodies can cause significant trauma and GI bleeding. Most swallowed foreign bodies, even those with a sharp edge, will pass spontaneously and require no specific therapy. On occasion, however, a sharp foreign body may be the cause of GI bleeding. Removal by endoscopy is indicated if significant bleeding occurs.

Lower Gastrointestinal Bleeding

BACKGROUND

Rectal bleeding is a relatively uncommon but worrisome complaint in the ambulatory or ED setting. A recent case series of children presenting with rectal bleeding to the ED at Boston Children's Hospital indicated that rectal bleeding was involved in the chief complaint of 0.3% of all ED visits during a 1-year period. The average age of patients was approximately 5 years, with nearly half of the patients younger than 1 year. No patient in the series was judged hemodynamically unstable in the ED, nor did any patient require a blood transfusion. The most common presentation was for hematochezia (98% of patients), with 10% of patients presenting with melena (some patients presented with both complaints). Diarrhea (37% of patients), abdominal pain (43%), and constipation (22%) were the most common associated symptoms, with only 2% of patients presenting with fever. Presumptive diagnoses were made in two-thirds of patients, most of which (81%) did not change with follow- up. Potentially life-threatening disorders (intussusception and Meckel diverticulum) were found in 4% of cases.

The cause of lower GI bleeding varies with age. Among infants less than 6 months of age, the most common diagnoses are milk-protein sensitivity (allergic colitis), anorectal fissures, and infectious gastroenteritis. Children aged 1 to 5 years are most likely to have infectious gastroenteritis, intussusception, Meckel diverticulum, colonic polyps, and anorectal fissures. Older children typically have infectious gastroenteritis, inflammatory bowel disease (IBD), and hemorrhoids or rectal varices. The pathophysiology, clinical manifestations, and specific management indicated for the most common conditions causing lower GI bleeding in children are discussed in the following sections.

ANORECTAL FISSURES AND HEMORRHOIDS

Anal fissures are the most common proctologic disorder during infancy and childhood. Most occur in infants less than 1 year of age. Anal fissure may result from diarrhea, which causes perineal irritation, but it is more commonly associated with constipation. The fissure usually starts when passage of a hard stool tears the sensitive squamous lining of the anal canal. Subsequent bowel movements are associated with pain or bleeding. Bright red blood is seen coating the stool. The infant begins to withhold stool, leading to increasing constipation and a vicious cycle of hard stools, bleeding, and pain. Anal fissure can be seen by spreading the perineal skin to evert the anal canal. Simply spreading the buttocks to view the anal opening is not sufficient. Treatment consists of local skin care combined with stool softeners. Malt extract (Maltsupex 1–3 tablespoons per day) or mineral oil (1–3 tablespoons per day) can be given to soften the stool. Local care involves sitz baths four times a day, a perianal cleansing lotion (Balneol) after each bowel movements, and an emollient protective ointment (Balmex) after each bowel movement.

Small varicosities of the external hemorrhoidal plexus (ie, hemorrhoids) may occur in the healing process associated with anal fissure. They rarely cause pain or bleeding. Therapy is directed at treatment of the anal fissure. The presence of external hemorrhoids does not imply associated internal hemorrhoids. The latter may develop in response to portal hypertension and may be a cause of painless rectal bleeding.

All patients with perianal excoriation, multiple anal fissures, recurrent anal fissure, or fissure resistant to conservative management should have perianal cultures for β-hemolytic streptococcus. If this organism is recovered, the patient should receive a 7-day course of oral penicillin.

POLYPS

Two major types of polyps may be diagnosed in infancy or childhood: hamartomatous and adenomatous. Hamartomatous polyps are generally benign and are the usual type of polyp found in juvenile polyps, juvenile polyposis coli, and Peutz–Jeghers syndrome. Adenomatous polyps are potentially premalignant and are found in a number of syndromes, including familial adenomatous polyposis and Gardner syndrome.

Juvenile polyps are the most common of the polyp syndromes in children, found in 15% of patients in one series who had colonoscopy for rectal bleeding. More than one polyp may be found in more than 50% of cases of juvenile polyps. Most (75%) of the polyps are rectosigmoid or in the descending colon, 15% are found in the transverse colon, and 10% in the ascending colon. Autoamputation of juvenile polyps, especially in the rectum, occurs spontaneously in most cases. In juvenile polyposis coli, multiple juvenile polyps are found throughout the colon. Peutz–Jeghers syndrome is the association of mucocutaneous pigmented lesions and hamartomatous polyps. It has autosomal-dominant inheritance with a high degree of penetrance. The macular, melanin-containing pigmented lesions characteristically occur on the buccal mucosa, lips, face, arms, palms and soles, and perianal region. The polyps are typically located in the small intestine but can be found throughout the GI tract.

Familial adenomatous polyposis is an autosomal-dominant inherited syndrome consisting of multiple adenomatous polyps that are generally confined to the colon but that can be found throughout the GI tract.

A 6% incidence of malignant transformation of these lesions is present by age 15 years, prompting recommendations for total proctocolectomy by age 18. Gardner syndrome is an autosomal-dominant inherited syndrome that consists of hereditary adenomatous polyps of the small and large intestine and soft-tissue and bony tumors. The tumors are often epidermoid cysts, fibromas, or osteomas of the skull and mandible and are often the initial manifestation of the disease.

Pathophysiology

Juvenile polyps are proliferations of mature colonic epithelium with aggregates of lymphoid tissue and cystic dilation of normal glandular elements. This histopathology has prompted the use of other terms such as *retention, inflammatory,* or *hyperplastic polyps.* The surface epithelium is often ulcerated, with a loss of mucosal surface. Adenomatous polyps may appear grossly similar to juvenile polyps, although on microscopic examination, adenomatous polyps are distinguished by the amount of cellular atypia seen within colonic epithelial cells.

Clinical Manifestations

The most common presentation for juvenile polyps is painless rectal bleeding, often with blood streaking the outside of the stools. The peak incidence for presentation is between 4 and 5 years of age. Prolapse of the polyp through the rectum may occur. The polyp also may form the "lead point" of an intussusception. All patients with rectal bleeding should have a careful rectal examination because 30% to 40% of polyps are palpable by rectal examination.

Polyps may be part of various inherited syndromes; therefore, a complete physical examination should be performed on any patient with rectal bleeding. A careful search for pigmented lesions or soft-tissue and bony tumors may aid in the diagnosis of inherited polyposis syndromes as previously described.

Management

The initial ED management of patients who have suspected polyps is aimed at assessing the amount of blood loss and arranging the appropriate diagnostic study. Blood loss is rarely life threatening, but significant losses may be noted from chronic intermittent bleeding. All patients should have a complete blood count (CBC) performed, and if the history of blood loss is significant, a type and crossmatch may also be indicated. Patients with palpable polyps on rectal examination should have elective flexible colonoscopy. Endoscopic removal of a polyp is safe and effective therapy even in a young child. For patients with painless hematochezia and for whom rectal examination is negative, a Meckel diverticulum also must be considered. This possibility may prompt a decision to perform a technetium-99 (^{99m}Tc) radionucleotide scan before colonoscopy in an effort to identify the possible location of bleeding.

DIETARY PROTEIN SENSITIVITY SYNDROMES ("ALLERGIC COLITIS")

Dietary proteins are capable of inducing significant bowel injury and may be the cause of several different types of enterocolitis presenting throughout childhood. Each condition, by definition, is induced by a dietary protein and resolves completely after the protein is eliminated from the diet. Immunologic responses may vary from classic allergic mast cell activation to immune complex formation. The development of proctocolitis in response to cow's milk protein exposure was among the first to be described. Subsequently, a similar condition has been described in response to soybean-based formula and among exclusively breast- fed infants, presumably in response to maternal dietary protein intake.

Pathophysiology

The appearance of the rectum and colon on colonoscopic examination characteristically consists of diffuse inflammation, friability, edema, and frequent focal ulcerations. Rectal biopsies demonstrate both acute and chronic inflammatory changes and eosinophilic infiltration is often present.

Clinical Manifestations

The typical presentation of milk-protein sensitivity colitis is that of acute onset of blood-streaked, mucoid diarrheal stools in an otherwise well-appearing infant younger than 6 months. Mean age of onset among 35 infants in one series was 4.3 + 4.1 weeks. It is unusual to present within the first week of life. Blood loss is typically limited, infants do not appear acutely dehydrated and are afebrile, and weight gain has typically been within normal limits since birth. The differential diagnosis includes anal fissures and infectious enterocolitis. External anal fissures can be ruled out by careful physical examination. Appropriate viral and bacterial cultures of stool may be indicated to rule out infectious causes.

Management

These patients are rarely hemodynamically unstable or seriously ill; therefore, initial ED management is focused on making a presumptive diagnosis based on initial laboratory testing, initiation of appropriate dietary therapy, and arranging adequate follow-up with the patient's primary care physician or a pediatric gastroenterologist. Initial laboratory testing should consist of a CBC with white blood cell (WBC) differential, assessing the hemoglobin as well as assessing for leukocytosis and eosinophilia. Patients with histologically proven milk-protein sensitivity colitis have higher mean peripheral eosinophil counts compared with age-appropriate normal values. In the individual patient, however, a higher-than-normal eosinophil count is actually an insensitive marker (sensitivity = 10%) for histologically proven colitis. In addition, a serum albumin level should be obtained because hypoalbuminemia has been demonstrated to have a sensitivity of approximately 80% for histologic colitis. Examination of stool for blood, fecal leukocytes, and routine bacterial culture should be performed on all infants. Infants who have milk-protein sensitivity colitis characteristically have leukocytes seen on fecal smear, although eosinophils may not be present in the stool.

Treatment consists of the elimination of the offending protein from the infant's diet. The diagnosis typically is confirmed by the rapid resolution of symptoms within 72 hours of the dietary change. Infants receiving cow's milk–based or soy protein formulas should be changed to a formula containing casein hydrolysate as the protein source. (Nutramigen, Pregestimil, and Alimentum are currently available in the United States.) Gross symptoms of allergic colitis respond within a few days to elimination diet therapy, although guaiac-positive stools may persist for several weeks. In exclusively breast-fed infants, elimination of the offending protein from the mother's diet also leads to clinical improvement, and breast-feeding usually can be continued. Persistent evidence of gross bleeding for 5 to 7 days following formula change is indication for flexible proctosigmoidoscopy. Most infants who come to endoscopy are found to have nodular lymphoid hyperplasia. Infants who do respond to dietary elimination should be rechallenged with the original formula in 4 to 6 weeks. Parents should be counseled that symptoms of allergy may change with increasing age such that a positive challenge may evoke vomiting, diarrhea, or GI signs of allergy rather than recurrent rectal bleeding.

INFECTIOUS ENTEROCOLITIS

Infectious causes of GI bleeding are predominantly a result of bacterial pathogens, including *Campylobacter*, pathogenic *Escherichia coli*, *Salmonella*, and *Shigella*. Less commonly, infection with *Giardia* or rotavirus is associated with heme-positive stools. A detailed discussion of the pathophysiology, clinical manifestations, and management of bacterial gastroenteritis can be found in Chapter 74.

Pseudomembranous colitis is a form of inflammatory colitis characterized by the pathologic presence of pseudomembranes consisting of mucin, fibrin, necrotic cells, and polymorphonuclear leukocytes. The entity develops as a result of colonic colonization and toxin production by the gram-positive obligate anaerobe *Clostridium difficile*, in most cases after normal bowel microflora have been altered by antibiotic therapy. All classes of antibiotics have been associated with pseudomembranous colitis. Patients usually present with profuse diarrhea, tenesmus, and crampy abdominal pain, usually beginning during the first week of antibiotic therapy. Frank hematochezia is rare. The diagnosis and management of pseudomembranous colitis are discussed more fully in Chapter 74.

MISCELLANEOUS CAUSES OF LOWER GASTROINTESTINAL BLEEDING

Henoch–Schönlein purpura (HSP) (see Chapter 76) is a systemic vasculitis that may cause edema and hemorrhage in the intestinal wall. Peak age of onset is between 3 and 7 years and the male-to-female ratio is 2:1. The presentation consists of the onset of a purpuric rash, typically confined to the buttocks and lower extremities, followed by arthralgias, angioedema, and diffuse abdominal pain. GI symptoms may precede the usual cutaneous symptoms and include abdominal pain (60%–70%), occult bleeding (50%), gross bleeding (30%), massive hemorrhage (5%–10%), and intussusception (3%). In a recent series, thickening of the duodenal wall was noted by ultrasonography in 82% of children who had HSP, with multiple hemorrhagic duodenal erosions noted by endoscopy in two patients. All children with suspected HSP and GI symptoms should have a stool guaiac test performed as well as a urinalysis to monitor for the onset of renal involvement (nephritis). Children with HSP limited to involvement of the skin and joints often can be managed as outpatients; however, severe abdominal pain or GI hemorrhage would be indications for admission.

Hemolytic uremic syndrome (HUS) (see Chapter 76) is a disorder characterized by the triad of acute microangiopathic hemolytic anemia, thrombocytopenia, and oliguric renal failure. The disease is heralded by a prodrome of intestinal symptoms ranging from diarrhea (in 100% of patients) to hemorrhagic colitis (80%). Fever (20%–30%), vomiting (75%–80%), and abdominal pain (60%) are also commonly seen. Acute infectious gastroenteritis or colitis secondary to infection with *E. coli* O157:H7 is now considered the most important initial causative event in both sporadic and epidemic cases of HUS.

All children with HUS require admission to the hospital. Laboratory studies should be obtained, including a CBC, platelet count, prothrombin time (PT), partial thromboplastin time (PTT), electrolytes, blood urea nitrogen (BUN), and creatinine. Intravenous access needs to be secured immediately for the correction of dehydration and the administration of blood products. As with HSP, the GI manifestations of HUS resolve, usually without sequelae or the need for antibiotic treatment of the initial intestinal infection.

Gastrointestinal *vascular malformations*, including hemangiomas, angiodysplasia, and arteriovenous malformations (AVMs), are rare causes of GI bleeding in children and often are seen as part of congenital syndromes. GI hemangiomas may be part of the Klippel–Trenaunay–Weber syndrome, which consists of a capillary or large vessel hemangioma on an extremity with hypertrophy of that limb. Diffuse visceral hemangiomatosis is rare, often fatal, and always is associated with cutaneous vascular lesions. GI hemangiomatosis should be suspected in any child with unexplained anemia and a syndrome of cutaneous hemangiomata.

Intestinal AVMs are rare in the pediatric age group, may occur as both solitary and multiple AVMs, and are typically part of a congenital syndrome (eg, Osler–Weber–Rendu disease). Many GI vascular malformations, particularly cavernous hemangiomas and AVMs, can be detected using computed tomographic scans with intravenous contrast. Intestinal angiography or tagged red blood cell scans often are used to identify the source of bleeding during an acute hemorrhage. ED management of patients with GI bleeding from vascular malformations is the same as for any patient with potentially significant blood loss. After initial stabilization, referral to an appropriate subspecialist for diagnosis and definitive treatment is warranted.

INFLAMMATORY BOWEL DISEASE

Clinical Manifestations

Clinical manifestations of IBD can be varied and related to either GI inflammation or the development of either GI tract or extraintestinal complications. Severe abdominal pain is among the most common complaints prompting a visit to the ED by the patient with IBD. Abdominal pain and diarrhea with or without occult blood are the most common symptoms at presentation. The pain is often colicky and, in Crohn disease, may localize to the right lower quadrant or periumbilical area, prompting a consideration of acute appendicitis in the differential diagnosis. The abdominal examination may elicit guarding and rebound tenderness. Frank rectal bleeding occurs in fewer than 25% of all cases but is more common in ulcerative colitis. Perianal disease, including fissures, skin tags, fistulae, and abscesses, occurs in 15% of children with Crohn disease. Perianal disease may precede the appearance of the intestinal manifestations of Crohn disease by several years.

A low-grade fever and mild leukocytosis commonly occur. Approximately 10% of children with ulcerative colitis and a lesser percentage of those with Crohn disease present with a fulminant onset of fever, abdominal cramps, and severe diarrhea with blood, mucus, and pus in the stools. A fulminant episode also may occur in the patient who has a known disease. There may be associated anemia and dehydration. IBD occasionally causes massive lower GI bleeding. Rarely, Crohn disease causes complete intestinal obstruction. The patient always gives a history of antecedent abdominal pain, diarrhea, and weight loss. The presence of abdominal distention, accompanied by diminished or absent bowel sounds, should raise the suspicion of actual or impending perforation, even in the absence of severe pain. Perforation may occur after even minor abdominal trauma and must be ruled out when patients with known IBD complain of abdominal pain after trauma.

The development of massive colonic distension is a rare complication of both ulcerative colitis and Crohn disease. Toxic megacolon represents a life-threatening emergency that has a reported mortality rate as high as 25%. Approximately 40% of the cases occur with the first attack of IBD; another 40% of cases are seen in patients receiving high-dose steroid therapy for fulminant colitis. Toxic megacolon almost always involves the transverse colon. The pathophysiology is believed to be an extension of the inflammatory process through all layers of the bowel wall with resulting microperforation, localized ileus, and loss of colonic tone. The result is imminent major perforation, peritonitis, and overwhelming sepsis. Antecedent barium enema, opiates, or anticholinergics may all precipitate toxic megacolon. Clinical features include (1) a rapidly worsening clinical course usually associated with fever, malaise, and even lethargy; (2) abdominal distension and tenderness usually developing over a few hours or days; (3) a temperature of 38.5°C (101.3°F) or higher and a neutrophilic leukocytosis; and (4) an abdominal radiograph showing distension of the transverse colon of more than 5 to 7 cm. The differential diagnosis of acute fulminant colitis includes acute bacterial enteritis, amebic dysentery, ischemic bowel disease, and radiation colitis.

Other potential clinical manifestations of IBD related to extraintestinal complications include thrombosis of cerebral, retinal, or peripheral vessels that may lead to coma, seizures, or focal visual or motor deficits; renal calculi leading to hematuria; and pancreatitis.

Management

The initial ED management of IBD is determined primarily by whether the patient is known to have been previously diagnosed with ulcerative colitis or Crohn disease and by an assessment of the severity of GI symptoms and systemic toxicity. Several clinical classification systems are used, but in general, mild disease is associated with less than six stools per day and an absence of systemic signs such as fever and severe anemia. Moderate disease is characterized by more than six stools per day, fever (>38°C [100.4°F]), hypoalbuminemia (serum protein <3.2 g per deciliter), and anemia (hemoglobin concentration <10 g/dL). Severe disease is indicated by more than eight stools per day, marked abdominal cramping and tenderness, high fever, significant anemia (hemoglobin concentration <8 g per deciliter), leukocytosis (WBC count >15000), and occasionally toxic megacolon.

Initial blood studies most commonly needed to evaluate patients who have known or suspected IBD include a CBC, serum electrolytes, BUN, serum albumin and total protein, transaminases [alanine aminotransferase (ALT) and aspartate aminotransferase (AST)], and, depending on the amount of suspected blood loss, a blood type and crossmatch. The erythrocyte sedimentation rate can be a useful marker of inflammation; it is elevated in up to 90% of patients with Crohn disease and in more than 50% of those with ulcerative colitis. The diagnostic yield of plain supine and upright or decubitus abdominal radiographs is relatively low (10% or less) in terms of positive findings of clinical relevance. Nevertheless, plain films can be useful in establishing the diagnosis of toxic megacolon, bowel obstruction, or perforation and should be strongly considered in the initial management of any patient with known or suspected IBD and who presents to the ED with abdominal pain or tenderness.

Stool examination for occult blood and fecal leukocytes may indicate the presence of active inflammation. For patients who have not been previously diagnosed with IBD, as well as during flare-ups in patients with a known diagnosis, stool should be obtained for culture to rule out infectious colitis, which may often either mimic IBD or complicate a known case. Noninfectious causes of rectal bleeding, including polyps, Meckel diverticulum, HSP, and HUS, as discussed further in this and other chapters (see Chapters 76 and 103) also may be considered in some instances, with appropriate diagnostic evaluation tailored accordingly.

Patients with known or previously undiagnosed IBD, who have mild manifestations of disease, and whose initial laboratory and radiographic studies do not reveal significant abnormality can be discharged from the ED after arranging follow-up with an appropriate specialist (pediatric or general gastroenterologist). Further diagnostic studies such as sigmoidoscopy, colonoscopy, or air-contrast barium enema, as well as the institution of medical management with corticosteroids and/or sulfasalazine, can be arranged on an outpatient basis.

The goal of initial management of patients with moderately severe disease is supportive, and intravenous hydration with crystalloid solutions is often necessary to correct acute dehydration. Normal saline may be given as a 20 mL per kilogram of body weight bolus infusion and repeated as necessary to achieve hemodynamic stability. An infusion of a dextrose-containing electrolyte solution then can be initiated based on the initial serum electrolytes. When severe abdominal pain occurs in a patient who is not known to have IBD, surgical consultation is indicated if diagnoses such as acute appendicitis or bowel obstruction are possibilities. Hospitalization of patients with moderately severe disease often is indicated to initiate or modify specific therapy such as systemic corticosteroids or immunosuppressive agents such as azathioprine or 6-mercaptopurine. In addition, improved nutritional intake, either via enteral or parenteral means, is often necessary.

All patients with acute fulminant colitis should be admitted to the hospital. Oral intake should be discontinued and an intravenous infusion begun with normal saline until electrolyte and BUN levels are known. Opiate or anticholinergic drugs should be avoided because they may precipitate toxic megacolon. If toxic megacolon is suspected, arrangements should be made for admission to an intensive care unit. The patient should discontinue all antidiarrheal and anticholinergic medicines. The first priority in the management of children with toxic megacolon is the treatment of intravascular dehydration and shock. Intensive intravenous therapy with normal saline, albumin, or blood must be sufficient to correct hypotension and to ensure adequate urine flow. A nasogastric tube, or preferably a Miller–Abbott tube for small bowel decompression, should be placed. Patients should be started on broad-spectrum antibiotics such as ampicillin (200 mg per kilogram daily), gentamicin (5–7.5 mg per kilogram daily), and clindamycin (40 mg per kilogram daily) in combination. Suitable alternative therapies include either ampicillin/sulbactam or cefoxitin in combination with gentamicin.

Management of significant GI bleeding should be performed as described earlier in this chapter. Emergency management of suspected intestinal obstruction includes gastric decompression with nasogastric drainage and intravenous rehydration, initially with normal saline. Patients with fulminant colitis, suspected toxic megacolon, significant GI bleeding, or suspected intestinal obstruction all should receive prompt surgical consultation as part of their initial ED evaluation.

PEPTIC ULCER DISEASE

CLINICAL MANIFESTATIONS

Symptoms of peptic ulcer disease vary with the patient's age. Nonspecific signs and symptoms predominate among infants and preschool-aged children, with boys and girls affected equally. The older the child, the more specific (and similar to adult patterns of presentation) the signs and symptoms become. Among teenagers with peptic ulcer disease, a male predominance is seen, with boys outnumbering girls nearly 4:1. Infants with peptic ulcer disease (usually secondary to some other condition) may present either with nonspecific feeding difficulties and vomiting, or more fulminantly with upper GI bleeding or perforation. Preschool-aged children often complain of poorly localized abdominal pain, vomiting, or GI hemorrhage and either manifest as hematemesis or melena. Older children and adolescents present almost invariably with abdominal pain, which is described as waxing and waning, sharp or gnawing, and localized to the epigastrium. It may awaken the child at night or in the early hours of the morning. The presence of nocturnal pain may assist in distinguishing recurrent abdominal pain as a result of peptic ulcer disease from functional abdominal pain, which rarely occurs at night. A careful history of the pain as well as a family history of peptic ulcer disease will often suggest the diagnosis of peptic ulcer disease in the older child. History also should be obtained regarding the presence of predisposing factors such as smoking or regular use of NSAIDs.

Physical examination may reveal abdominal tenderness, poorly localized in young children and more commonly localized to the epigastrium or to the right of the midline in older children and adolescents. Stool should be tested for occult blood, and the remainder of the physical examination should be directed toward assessment of the hemodynamic stability of the patient and, in younger children, to identifying the underlying condition (eg, sepsis) that may have predisposed them to the development of peptic ulcer disease. Weight loss may be noted.

Differential Diagnosis

Numerous conditions may mimic the presentation of peptic ulcer disease. Abdominal pain is a common symptom during childhood, occurring in 10% to 15% of school-aged children. Most children with recurrent abdominal pain have a "functional" cause. These patients typically do not have any weight loss or vomiting and report that their pain is localized to the umbilical area. Further discussion regarding the differential diagnosis of abdominal pain can be found in Chapter 42. It should be noted that the prevalence of *H. pylori* infection in children who have recurrent abdominal pain varies widely in the literature, with most patients studied selected from among those presenting to tertiary hospital gastroenterology clinics. Children with *H. pylori* infection characteristically are asymptomatic. In fact, a recent population-based study found fewer GI symptoms among children infected with *H. pylori* than in those without infection.

Gastritis, distal esophagitis, *Giardiasis,* and pancreatitis all can cause epigastric pain and tenderness. Biliary tract disease and a ureteropelvic junction obstruction may cause right upper quadrant tenderness. Children who have IBD, HSP, or diabetes mellitus may also present with abdominal pain, tenderness, or GI bleeding.

Diagnosis

Radiologic examination, with either single- or double-contrast (with air) barium upper GI series, is not an effective diagnostic tool to either confirm or rule out the presence of peptic ulcer disease in children. These studies often do not detect superficial ulcers, and, conversely, barium trapped in a gastric or duodenal fold may give a false impression of an ulcer. Radiologic examination may be used to rule out other conditions, however, such as malrotation with volvulus or other structural anomalies of the GI tract.

Flexible fiberoptic esophagogastroduodenoscopy with mucosal biopsy is the most accurate method of diagnosing peptic ulcer disease in children. In most tertiary care referral centers, this procedure can be performed safely even on infants. It is typically not performed in the presence of active hemorrhage, although some centers are gathering experience with the use of therapeutic endoscopy to control significant bleeding. When performed, biopsy specimens should routinely be obtained from any area of endoscopic abnormality as well as from the distal esophagus, antrum, and second part of the duodenum. No clear guidelines exist to indicate which pediatric patients should undergo endoscopy for evaluation of peptic ulcer disease. Suggested guidelines include any child with chronic abdominal pain (>3 months) associated with any of the following signs and symptoms: (1) hematemesis, (2) a history of peptic ulcer disease in a first-degree relative, (3) nocturnal pain, (4) pain occurring within 1 hour of eating or relieved by eating, (5) recurrent vomiting, (6) weight loss, or (7) abdominal tenderness localized to the epigastrium (particularly in older children). In addition, endoscopy should be strongly considered in any patient presenting acutely with significant upper GI bleeding.

All patients for whom an obvious cause of secondary gastric or duodenal ulceration (eg, stress, sepsis, burns) does not exist should undergo diagnostic evaluation for the presence of *H. pylori* infection. *H. pylori* infection can be confirmed in a variety of ways in patients with primary peptic ulcer disease. Histologic examination of biopsy specimens obtained during endoscopy should be performed routinely because *H. pylori* is readily seen using a variety of staining techniques. In centers with appropriate facilities for culturing the organism, biopsy specimens also may yield growth of the organism, which can assist in the choice of appropriate antibiotic therapy, particularly in recalcitrant infections. A variety of commercially available assays take advantage of the urease activity of the organism for diagnostic purposes. A biopsy specimen is mixed with the assay, which typically contains urea and an indicator dye that changes color when the urea is converted to ammonia by the organism. The urease activity also can be detected through the use of breath tests in which radiolabeled (^{13}C or ^{14}C) urea is ingested by the patient. Degradation of the urea by *H. pylori* results in the release of the radiolabeled carbon, which can be detected in the expired air. Finally, enzyme-linked immunosorbent assays are available for the detection of immunoglobulin G (IgG) antibodies to *H. pylori* in serum. Noninvasive tests such as serology and breath tests are useful but should not be promoted as the sole method of diagnosing *H. pylori*–associated peptic ulcer disease in children because they cannot distinguish between incidental infection and the presence of peptic ulceration. At this time, therefore, the presence of suspected peptic ulcer disease should be confirmed by endoscopy using the guidelines for performance of endoscopy previously suggested.

Management

The focus of ED management of patients with suspected peptic ulcer disease is on the detection and stabilization of life-threatening complications such as perforation and major GI hemorrhage and on ruling out other potential serious or life-threatening conditions that may require urgent intervention. Depending on the suspected amount of blood loss, all patients with GI bleeding should have a CBC and blood type and screen obtained. If vomiting has been prominent, electrolytes, BUN, creatinine, serum amylase, and lipase also should be obtained. If physical examination findings suggest significant abdominal tenderness with guarding or rebound tenderness, plain radiographs of the abdomen should be obtained to rule out a perforation or bowel obstruction. Intravenous access should be obtained in all patients who have significant emesis, dehydration, weight loss, or concerning abdominal examination findings. An initial bolus of normal saline (20 mL per kilogram) should be given and vital signs monitored frequently, with additional boluses given as needed to achieve hemodynamic stability.

Numerous approaches are available for treatment of peptic ulcer disease in children. Therapies can be categorized as those that neutralize acid, block acid secretion, are cytoprotective, or are antiinfective. Antacids are a low-cost, safe, and effective means of treating peptic ulcer disease in children and can be used in patients of any age. Side effects of antacids are related to the cation present in the preparation: magnesium-containing products cause diarrhea, whereas aluminum-containing products cause constipation. Some products are available combining the two to minimize these effects. The usual dosage for children is 0.5 mL per kilogram, given 1 hour after eating and before bed. Patients with food-related or nocturnal abdominal pain without associated signs of serious illness can be started on empirical therapy with antacids, assuming good follow-up with a primary care physician. Referral to a pediatric gastroenterologist can then be made if the patient fails to respond to 2 weeks of therapy.

H_2-receptor antagonists are the most common agents used to treat peptic ulcer disease. Patients with significant GI bleeding, vomiting, or abdominal tenderness should be admitted to the hospital and begun on intravenous therapy with an H_2-receptor antagonist. Currently, more physicians have pediatric experience with the use of cimetidine and ranitidine than with famotidine. All three agents are competitive H_2-receptor antagonists that reduce gastric acid output, thereby raising gastric pH. Structural differences among the three agents render famotidine the most potent and longest acting, followed by ranitidine and then cimetidine. In addition, ranitidine and famotidine generally have fewer side effects than cimetidine. The recommended oral dosage for cimetidine is 7 mg per kilogram of body weight given every 6 to 8 hours. The dosage of ranitidine commonly used to treat peptic ulcer disease is 1 to 2 mg per kilogram of body weight given every 8 hours in infants and younger children, every 12 hours in older children. Less published experience exists with the use of famotidine in pediatrics. Available data suggest a starting dosage for children older than 1 year of 0.5 mg per kilogram given intravenously every 8 to 12 hours. Patients for whom initial outpatient therapy is appropriate can be started on an H_2-receptor antagonist following an ED visit, but this therapy is best done in consultation with either the patient's primary care physician or pediatric gastroenterologist, who will establish appropriate follow-up for the patient.

Sucralfate is an aluminum salt that "coats" damaged gastric mucosa, effectively insulating it from further damage by acid, pepsin, or bile. It is typically given as a slurry and can be used with H_2-receptor antagonists, provided the drugs are given at least 1 hour apart. The usual adult dosage is 1 g four times a day; this can be titrated down for pediatric patients, although firm dosage guidelines for pediatric use are currently unavailable.

Results of a national consensus conference on *H. pylori* in peptic ulcer disease recommend that ulcer patients with *H. pylori* infection receive antimicrobial treatment as well as antisecretory drugs, both at first presentation as well as for recurrent disease. Eradication of *H. pylori* infection has been shown to reduce the recurrence of primary duodenal ulcers in children. Most children with *H. pylori* infection are asymptomatic, and no convincing evidence that *H. pylori* causes symptoms in the absence of ulceration has been presented; therefore, antimicrobial therapy is currently not recommended for children without ulcers or gastritis who harbor the organism. Several antimicrobial agents, either alone or in combination, have been studied. Although optimal treatment guidelines have not been established for children, several studies have demonstrated that omeprazole in combination with clarithromycin and amoxicillin or metronidazole is an effective regimen for clearance of the organism in those infected. Optimal length of therapy has not been clearly established. Most authorities currently recommend a 2- to 3-week course of therapy.

ACUTE BILIARY TRACT DISEASE

Clinical Manifestations

The pain of biliary colic is acute in onset, often follows a meal, and is usually localized to the epigastrium or right upper quadrant. Some children may localize the pain to the periumbilical area. Characteristically, the pain increases to a plateau of intensity over 5 to 20 minutes, typically after meals, and persists for a variable duration, usually less than 4 hours (although <1 hour in 50% of patients). In contrast to the colicky pain of intestinal or ureteral origin, biliary colic does not worsen in relatively short cyclic paroxysms or bursts but instead is characterized by its sustained, intense quality. Unlike pancreatitis, the patient tends to move about restlessly, and the pain is not improved by changes in position. In addition, referred pain is common, particularly to the dorsal lumbar back near the tip of the right scapula. Nausea and vomiting are commonly associated with biliary colic but are not severe and protracted as seen with pancreatitis. Mild jaundice occurs in 25% of patients, but the serum bilirubin rarely exceeds 4 mg per deciliter. An attack of acute cholecystitis begins with biliary colic, which increases progressively in severity or duration. Pain lasting longer than 4 hours suggests cholecystitis. As the inflammation worsens, the pain changes character, becoming more generalized in the upper abdomen and increased by deep respiration and jarring motions. The temperature usually is mildly elevated, ranging from 37.5° to 38.5°C (99.5°–101.3°F).

In contrast, acute cholangitis should be suspected in the patient who has right upper quadrant abdominal pain, shaking chills, and spiking fever (temperature >39°C [102.2°F]) with jaundice (Charcot triad). These patients usually have a history of abdominal surgery. The danger of this disorder is that overwhelming sepsis can develop rapidly. Listlessness and shock are characteristic of advanced or severe cholangitis and usually reflect gram-negative septicemia. Cholangitis can evolve rapidly before development of significant jaundice. Clinically apparent jaundice may be absent even in postsurgical biliary atresia patients. Hydrops of the gallbladder is associated with a palpable right upper quadrant mass and pain. Fever and jaundice generally do not occur.

In addition to scleral icterus, nonspecific physical findings that suggest gallbladder disease include right upper quadrant guarding, Murphy's sign (production of pain by deep inspiration or cough when the physician's fingers are depressing the abdomen below the right costal margin in the midclavicular line and abrupt cessation of inspiration because of pain), and production of pain or tenderness by a light blow applied with the ulnar surface of the hand to the subcostal area. In about one-third of patients with cholecystitis, the gallbladder is palpable as a sausage-shaped mass lateral to the midclavicular line. A rigid abdomen or rebound tenderness suggests local perforation or gangrene of the gallbladder.

Laboratory tests are typically nonspecific. A CBC and blood smear may show evidence of hemolysis. The leukocyte count averages 12000 to 15000/mm^3 with a neutrophilic leukocytosis. Leukocyte counts greater than 15000^3 suggest cholangitis. The serum bilirubin may be elevated but rarely exceeds 4 mg per deciliter. Higher values are more compatible with either complete common duct obstruction or cholangitis. Serum transaminases, ALT and AST, and alkaline phosphatase may be mildly elevated but are often normal. Marked elevation of transaminases may occur with acute, complete common duct obstruction. Serum amylase may be mildly elevated without other evidence of pancreatitis. Abdominal flat and upright radiographs may show right upper quadrant calcification of gallstones, particularly in patients with hemolytic anemia (pigment stones) or a right upper quadrant mass. Abdominal radiographs are particularly important to rule out perforation. The erythrocyte sedimentation rate is often elevated in children with cholangitis, and organisms may be recovered by blood culture.

Abdominal ultrasound is the most commonly used test to confirm gallbladder disease. This test is noninvasive, easily performed, and provides information on the surrounding organs such as the liver, pancreas, and kidneys. Ultrasound can determine the presence of most gallstones, dilated bile ducts, a thickened gallbladder wall or hydropic gallbladder, sludge, and hepatic abscesses. Other radiographic tests, such as cholecystograph or radionuclide testing, are not typically used in the emergency setting.

Other conditions to be considered in the differential diagnosis of biliary tract disease include perforated peptic ulcer, pneumonia, intercostal neuritis, pancreatitis, hepatitis, and hepatic and abdominal sickle cell crisis. Therefore, evaluation should also include stool guaiac, chest radiograph, amylase-to-creatinine ratio, and a peripheral blood smear.

Management

All patients with suspected acute biliary tract disease and acute symptoms should be admitted to the hospital. The exception is the patient with biliary colic that has resolved spontaneously, in which case an urgent outpatient evaluation by ultrasound can be pursued. Conditions associated with acalculous cholecystitis should be evaluated and treated if identified. General ED management includes discontinuation of oral intake, support with intravenous fluids, and surgical consultation. Cholecystitis and cholangitis associated with gallstones are general indications for surgery. The patient should be made NPO (nothing by mouth) and given intravenous fluids, pain medication, and antibiotics, if cholangitis is considered. Antibiotic coverage should include gram-negative organisms as well as enterococcus. Ampicillin (200 mg per kilogram per dose) and gentamicin (5 to 7.5 mg per kilogram daily) provide good coverage; ampicillin and sulbactam (ampicillin 200 mg per kilogram daily) also can be used. Narcotics are useful to alleviate the pain and to reduce gallbladder mucosal secretion; however, pain medication should be withheld until a tentative decision regarding early surgery is reached. When given, a dose of meperidine, 1 to 2 mg per kilogram of body weight, is the treatment of choice.

In all patients with suspected cholangitis, blood cultures should be drawn before antibiotics are administered. When possible, antibiotics should be withheld pending a liver biopsy for definitive culture; however, the exception is the clinically septic child in whom antibiotic coverage should be immediately instituted with ampicillin (200 mg per kilogram of body weight daily) or a cephalosporin, such as cefazolin (100 mg per kilogram daily), and gentamicin (5–7.5 mg per kilogram daily). In these cases, a liver biopsy performed after the institution of antibiotics may still show histologic evidence of cholangitis.

ACUTE PANCREATITIS

Clinical Manifestations

Epigastric abdominal pain is the most consistent symptom of pancreatitis and may vary from tolerable distress to severe incapacitating pain. Symptoms may be chronic and insidious, but they typically progress rapidly, building to a crescendo over several hours. The pain usually is localized to the epigastrium and may radiate to the back (left or right scapula) or the right or left upper quadrants. The pain usually is described as knifelike and boring in quality and is aggravated when the patient lies supine. Classically, the pain of pancreatitis is constant, as opposed to colicky pain, which waxes and wanes. Nausea and vomiting are the most common associated symptoms. Vomiting may be severe and protracted. Low-grade fever [temperature <38.5°C (101.3°F)] is present in 50% to 60% of cases. In cases of severe necrotic pancreatitis, patients may complain of dizziness. Mental aberrations are common in necrotic pancreatitis; patients may act overtly psychotic or present in coma.

Early in the course of the disease, there may be a discrepancy between the severity of the patient's subjective pain and the objective physical findings. During the examination, patients are usually quiet and prefer sitting or lying on their side with knees flexed. The abdomen may be distended but is usually not rigid. There may be mild to moderate voluntary guarding in the epigastrium. A palpable epigastric mass suggests pseudocyst. Ascites is rare. Bowel sounds may be decreased or absent. Associated physical findings may include signs of parotitis, mild hepatosplenomegaly, epigastric mass, pleural effusions, and mild icterus. Although rare, rebound tenderness or a rigid abdomen are poor prognostic signs if present. A bluish discoloration around the umbilicus (Cullen sign) or flanks (Grey Turner sign) is also a poor prognostic sign and evidence of hemorrhagic pancreatitis. Signs of overt hemodynamic instability are rarely evident at initial presentation. It is particularly important to evaluate patients for clinical signs of hypocalcemia (Trousseau and Chvostek signs).

The clinical diagnosis is often tentative because the same constellation of symptoms (abdominal pain, vomiting, and low-grade fever) and signs (abdominal tenderness and guarding) may be mimicked by several other conditions, including penetrating peptic ulcer, gastritis, esophagitis, biliary colic, acute cholecystitis, intestinal obstruction, and appendicitis.

Currently, two easily attainable laboratory tests are used to make a diagnosis of pancreatitis: serum amylase and serum lipase. The combination of the aforementioned clinical symptoms and an elevation of the level of one or both of these enzymes strongly point to pancreatitis. In acute pancreatitis, the serum amylase increases hours after the onset of the autodigestive process and returns to normal within 3 to 5 days; elevated serum triglycerides may interfere with the assay and result in false-normal values. The degree of serum amylase elevation rarely corresponds to the severity of pancreatic inflammation. Although controversial in the past, lipase assays are now accurate and are commonly used to diagnose pancreatitis. Serum lipase may remain elevated for up to 14 days after the onset of acute pancreatitis. Generally, because amylase is rapidly cleared by the kidneys, serum amylase may return to normal after several days even though pain persists. In these cases, following the serum lipase may be more beneficial. Normalization of serum amylase typically indicates resolution of disease, but occasionally hemorrhagic or necrotizing pancreatitis may develop in patients with normal amylase.

Serum amylase and lipase are not pathognomonic for pancreatitis. Many situations, including penetrating or perforated ulcer, intestinal obstruction or infarction, Crohn disease, pneumonia, hepatitis, liver trauma, acute biliary tract disease, salpingitis, salivary adenitis, renal failure, diabetic ketoacidosis, and benign macroamylasemia, can cause an amylase elevation. Causes for an elevated serum lipase include perforated peptic ulcer and bone fracture with pulmonary fat embolism.

Radiographically, the abdominal ultrasound provides a noninvasive, direct view of the pancreas and is probably the most useful test in diagnosing pancreatitis. Ultrasound can assess pancreatic size, contour, and the presence of calcifications and pseudocyst formation. Ultrasound should be considered in all cases of suspected pancreatitis. Abdominal computed tomography and endoscopic retrograde cholangiopancreatography (ERCP) are being used more often to assess the severity of pancreatitis and pseudocyst formation and to determine possible causes of pancreatitis. ERCP should not be performed in the acute phase, however, or in patients with acute pseudocyst formation or pancreatic abscess formation but should be reserved for patients with chronic, recurrent pancreatitis. Rarely, ERCP may be indicated in acute pancreatitis if an obstructing gallstone is present in the common bile duct.

Management

All patients with evidence of pancreatitis or suspected pancreatitis should be admitted to the hospital. Treatment, however, should begin in the ED. The goals of medical treatment include suppression of pancreatic secretion and relief of pain. Morbidity and mortality in pancreatitis are directly related to complications that may already be present at the time of initial presentation. Therefore, aggressive early maintenance of intravascular volume and treatment of hypocalcemia, respiratory distress, and suspected infection are mandatory.

Intravenous fluids should be started immediately, and the patient's oral intake should be discontinued. The patient should be assessed for hypotension. When the patient is judged stable, intravenous fluids should be given at 1.5 times the maintenance rate. Vital signs and urine output should be monitored frequently. Continuous nasogastric suction should be started; aspiration of gastric contents is based on the premise that prevention of delivery of gastric acid into the duodenum will diminish hormonal stimulation of the pancreas. Nasogastric suction also relieves pain and prevents development of ileus. Use of anticholinergics or cimetidine to reduce gastric secretions is controversial and is not recommended in the initial management of patients. A crucial part of management is the treatment of abdominal pain. Pain should be treated with Nubain (0.1 mg per kilogram of body weight per dose intravenously; maximum, 20 mg) or meperidine (1–2 mg per kilogram of body weight administered intravenously; maximum, 100 mg). Morphine or codeine should not be used because they increase spasm at the sphincter of Oddi.

Blood studies that should be performed in the ED include amylase, lipase, CBC, electrolytes, BUN, calcium, glucose, SGOT, SGPT, bilirubin, alkaline phosphatase, triglyceride, PT, and PTT. Arterial blood gases should be obtained in patients with tachypnea. A chest radiograph should be obtained and evaluated for pleural effusion, interstitial pneumonic infiltrates, and basilar atelectasis. A flat and upright abdominal radiograph is needed to rule out perforation, ascites, and pancreatic calcifications. In severe cases or in those cases of questionable diagnosis, an abdominal ultrasound should be obtained.

In most cases, maintenance of intravascular volume and relief of pain will result in rapid resolution of symptoms. Prognostic indicators of necrotizing or hemorrhagic pancreatitis include hypocalcemia ($<$8.0 mg per deciliter), hyperglycemia ($>$200 mg per deciliter), clinical shock, elevated hematocrit or BUN, ascites, and oxygen partial pressure less than 60 mm Hg. Such patients should be admitted to an intensive care unit, given sufficient colloid (albumin 0.25 g per kilogram) to maintain normal intravascular volume, and have more extensive monitoring with an arterial line and urinary catheter. A P_aO_2 lower than 60 mm Hg is an indication for elective intubation. Early peritoneal dialysis should be started if rapid clinical deterioration occurs.

Antibiotics are not indicated in the initial management of pancreatitis. Pancreatic abscess should be considered if the patient's temperature is higher than 38.5°C (101.3°F). In those cases, broad-spectrum antibiotic coverage with ampicillin (200 mg per kilogram daily) and gentamicin (5–7.5 mg per kilogram daily) is indicated pending the results of blood cultures and diagnostic ultrasound. Emergency surgery is rarely necessary in acute pancreatitis; however, indications for surgery include active intraperitoneal bleeding, suspected abscess, biliary duct obstruction, and suspected traumatic transection. Therapeutic surgery for acute, necrotizing pancreatitis has been reported in adults, but this approach has not been accepted in pediatrics.

FULMINANT LIVER FAILURE

Clinical Manifestations

Many patients do not exhibit serious clinical features of acute liver failure. Typically, pediatric patients who develop acute liver failure were previously healthy and had no prior medical problems. Initially, patients may complain of fatigue, nausea, vomiting, and diffuse abdominal pain. Occasionally, right upper quadrant pain may be severe. Commonly, a history of a prodromal viral illness can be elicited. The presence of jaundice usually initiates the first visit to the physician. As liver failure progresses, patients become more jaundiced and lethargic and begin to develop tremors. In a short time, they become confused or somnolent and may begin to have problems with easy bruising or bleeding.

The onset of encephalopathy occurs in conjunction with the severity and progression of liver failure. Encephalopathy is graded on a scale from I to IV. Grade I is manifested by a coherent individual who shows mild or episodic drowsiness, poor concentration, and impaired intellect. In grade II, the patient continues to be coherent and conversant but also becomes disoriented and fatigued. Agitation and aggressive behavior in conjunction with extreme drowsiness is manifested in grade III encephalopathy. Unresponsive patients who respond only to painful stimuli and who have evidence of cerebral edema are labeled as having grade IV encephalopathy. The clinical features of increased intracranial pressure include systemic hypertension, "decerebrate posturing," hyperventilation, abnormal pupillary responses, and impairment of brainstem reflexes. Cerebral edema is associated with increased mortality and requires aggressive supportive management. Finally, bleeding esophageal and gastric varices as well as ascites may rapidly develop secondary to increased portal hypertension.

Laboratory Findings

Because it may be difficult to diagnose patients clinically, biochemical evidence may be collected that provides evidence of liver failure. The liver plays an important role in hemostasis because the liver synthesizes a number of coagulation factors. An uncorrectable coagulopathy is usually the first laboratory manifestation of liver failure. Other factors may have a shorter half-life, but the PT is the most commonly used marker of the severity of liver disease. A prolonged PT despite intravenous supplementation of vitamin K should alert the physician to impending liver failure. Other laboratory markers suggestive of liver failure include evidence of increasing cholestasis manifested by a rising serum bilirubin, hypoalbuminemia, and hypoglycemia.

It is also important to monitor serum transaminases. Falling transaminases usually indicate resolving liver disease, whereas a decrease in transaminases in association with increasing jaundice and coagulopathy indicates hepatocyte death rather than hepatocyte repair. Monitoring for hypoglycemia is extremely important because the liver is the primary organ for gluconeogenesis. Serum fibrinogen is usually decreased in patients with liver failure. In cases in which the patient has splenomegaly, thrombocytopenia and leukocytopenia may be present.

Hypoglycemia almost always accompanies acute liver failure and may complicate the signs of encephalopathy. Portal hypertension may cause bleeding from esophageal varices or ascites. Hepatorenal syndrome occurs in approximately 75% of patients who reach grade IV encephalopathy. The cause of hepatorenal syndrome is unclear; however, the result is oliguria in the presence of near normal intravascular pressures. Metabolic acidosis occurs in approximately 30% of patients who have liver failure, and the risk of sepsis is increased secondary to the patient's compromised immune function.

Management

All patients in whom liver failure is suspected should undergo a complete physical examination, including a thorough neurologic evaluation. Laboratory testing should include serum glucose, transaminases, total and direct bilirubin, albumin, PT, GGTP, CBC with differential, electrolytes, blood culture, and fibrinogen. Patients with hypoglycemia should be given intravenous fluids with 10% dextrose and should undergo frequent blood glucose monitoring (every 1 hour) until their blood sugar stabilizes. Metabolic acidosis should be corrected; however, correction of hyponatremia should be gradual in patients with ascites. Patients who have a coagulopathy should be given intravenous vitamin K (2.5 mg in infants; 5 mg in older children and adolescents). A repeat PT should be performed 6 to 8 hours after administration. An uncorrectable PT is suggestive of severe hepatocyte damage. The management of bleeding esophageal varices has been previously discussed in this chapter. Therapeutic management of ascites should occur only in the face of respiratory distress or renal failure; otherwise, the introduction of a diuretic (Aldactone) to achieve a slow, gradual change in ascites is all that is initially required.

Patients with encephalopathy should be monitored frequently for changes in neurologic function. In cases in which the patient has developed cerebral edema, management consists of an intensive care setting, insertion of a subdural transducer, mechanical ventilation (hyperventilation), and administration of mannitol (0.3–0.4 mg per kilogram of body weight) to maintain near-normal levels of intracranial pressure.

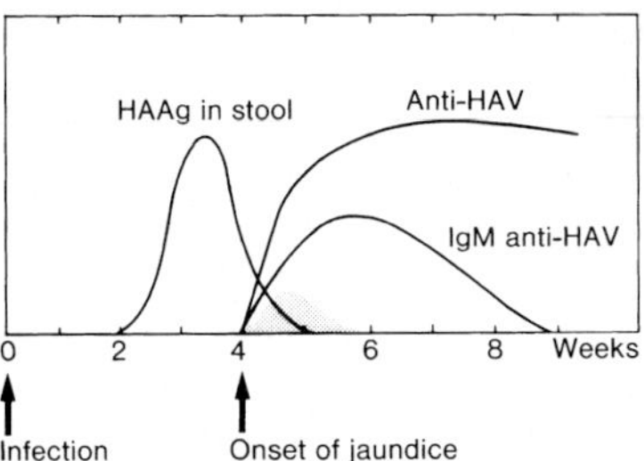

Figure 82.3. Serologic changes in hepatitis A. HAAg, hepatitis-associated antigen; HAV, hepatitis A virus.

ACUTE VIRAL HEPATITIS

Clinical Manifestations

Most childhood cases of acute hepatitis produce minimal symptoms, are anicteric, and—unless suspected by palpation of tender hepatomegaly—usually are confused with a GI flulike illness. Clinical hepatitis classically consists of a 5- to 7-day prodrome of variable constitutional symptoms (low-grade fever, anorexia, nausea, vomiting, malaise, fatigue, and epigastric or right upper quadrant abdominal pain), followed by acute onset of scleral icterus, jaundice, and passage of dark urine. Pruritus and diarrhea are rare. Physical examination after the onset of jaundice may reveal tender hepatomegaly. Mild splenomegaly is present in 25% to 50% of patients. Hepatitis B virus patients also may present with extrahepatic signs and symptoms, such as arthralgia, arthritis, or papular acrodermatitis (on face, buttocks, and extensor surfaces of arms and legs). When the rash is associated with lymphadenopathy and fever, it is called the *Gianotti–Crosti syndrome*. Onset of the icteric phase of acute hepatitis most commonly is temporarily associated with improvement in the constitutional symptoms. In up to 15% of cases, severe fatigue, anorexia, nausea, and vomiting persist. The icteric period usually lasts 1 to 4 weeks. Occasionally, the jaundice is prolonged for 4 to 6 weeks with increasing pruritus at 2 to 3 weeks.

Differential Diagnosis

Numerous infectious agents may mimic a viral hepatitis-like illness. The most common are Epstein–Barr virus (EBV, infectious mononucleosis) and cytomegalovirus (CMV). Both agents rarely produce clinical jaundice, and high fever and diffuse adenopathy are more characteristic. Less common agents include herpes, adenovirus, coxsackievirus, reovirus, echovirus, rubella, arbovirus, leptospirosis, toxoplasmosis, and tuberculosis.

Diagnostic Evaluation

The following laboratory tests are usually performed in all cases of suspected viral hepatitis: serum transaminases (AST and ALT), alkaline phosphatase, total and direct bilirubin, CBC, PT, electrolytes, BUN, glucose, total protein, albumin, globulin; these tests also are performed in patients older than 5 years, ceruloplasmin. AST and ALT are the best indicators of ongoing hepatocellular injury. Alkaline phosphatase levels are usually less than two times the upper limit of normal for age. Levels greater than three times normal should raise suspicions of EBV or CMV hepatitis or biliary tract disease. Hepatitis classically produces direct fractions of serum bilirubin in excess of 30% of total, indicating definite liver disease. Hyperbilirubinemia may be present in the absence of scleral icterus or jaundice because these signs usually cannot be appreciated until levels of total bilirubin exceed 3 to 4 mg per deciliter. Serum bilirubin levels peak 5 to 7 days after the onset of jaundice. The initial biochemical screen may reveal several indicators of severe hepatocellular injury, including (1) total bilirubin greater than 20 mg per deciliter, (2) serum transaminases that exceed 3000 U per liter, (3) WBC count greater than 25000/mm^3, (4) elevated PT, and (5) hypoglycemia.

Serum albumin and globulin are usually normal. Decreased albumin or increased globulin should suggest an acute flare of chronic liver disease. Serum ceruloplasmin level should be drawn in all patients older than 5 years of age who have suspected hepatitis to rule out Wilson disease. A chest radiograph may reveal cardiomegaly if any suspicion of low cardiac output states exists. Figures 82.3 and 82.4 contrast the sequence of clinical, biochemical, and serologic events in typical hepatitis A virus (HAV) and HBV infection. The serodiagnosis of acute hepatitis is approached best by first testing for anti-HAV IgM, HB surface antigen, HB e antigen, HB serum DNA, anti-HB core Ab, anti-HCV, anti-CMV, and EBV serology. The finding of serum IgM anti-HAV is diagnostic of acute HAV infection because the antibody is present at the time of clinical symptoms. A positive HB surface antigen suggests the diagnosis of HBV in a symptomatic patient. A positive HB e antigen or anti-HB core Ab is helpful in the rare patient who rapidly clears HB surface antigen from the serum. It is also important to note that in chronic HB surface antigen carriers who have HDV superinfection, the suppression of HBV replication may lead to a transient absence of HBV markers in the serum; unless HDV markers in the serum are sought, the diagnosis may be missed. Anti-HCV does not appear in the patient's circulation until 1 to 3 months after onset of acute illness. In rare cases, detectable levels may not be demonstrated for up to 1 year. Thus, unless the acute presentation is ac-

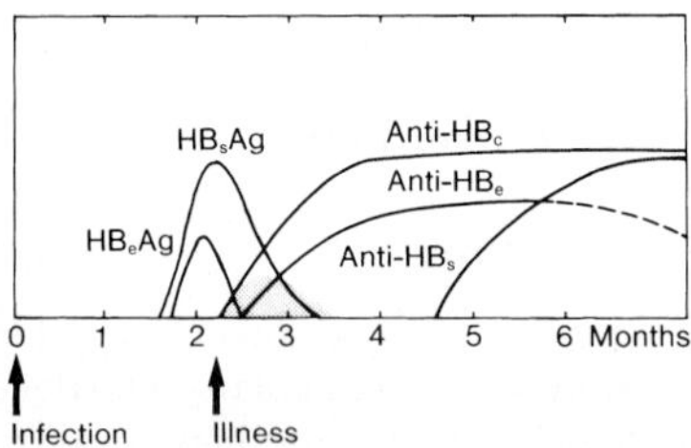

Figure 82.4. Serologic changes in hepatitis B. HBsd>sAg, hepatitis B$_s$ antigen; HB$_c$, hepatitis B$_c$; HB$_e$, hepatitis B$_e$; HB$_e$Ag, hepatitis B$_e$ antigen.

tually a flare of chronic HCV, serodiagnosis will await long-term follow-up.

Management

No specific treatment is available for acute viral hepatitis. Most patients can be managed at home.

No restrictions in diet or ambulation are necessary. The traditional recommendations of a low-fat, high-carbohydrate diet and bed rest are now recognized to have no effect on the symptoms or duration of the disease. Parents should be told that anorexia and fatigue are common symptoms. Small, frequent feedings may be helpful. Drugs should be strictly avoided. The key for both the patient and other household contacts is personal hygiene. Infants and children should avoid contact with the patient even after they have received immunoprophylaxis. In HAV, shedding of the virus may occur for up to 2 weeks after the onset of jaundice. Patients should be kept at home during this time. After this, they may return to school. Indications for hospitalization of a patient who has acute hepatitis include the following:

1. Dehydration secondary to anorexia and vomiting
2. Bilirubin level greater than 20 mg per deciliter
3. Abnormal PT
4. WBC count greater than 25000/mm^3
5. Level of transaminases greater than 3000 U per liter

Patients who have acute hepatitis and who are hospitalized should be isolated. Follow-up studies of all patients with acute hepatitis should be performed to document biochemical resolution. Follow-up serology may also establish a specific cause in cases of apparent non-A, non-B hepatitis (fourfold increase in CMV serology, development of anti-HCV). Reevaluation of patients with HBV is especially important to ensure clearance of HB surface antigen or to recognize the development of the HB surface antigen carrier state.

Postexposure Prophylaxis

HEPATITIS A

The mean incubation period for HAV infection is about 4 weeks (range, 15–45 days). Conventional immune serum globulin (ISG 0.02 mL per kilogram intramuscularly) confers passive protection against clinical HAV infection if given during the incubation period up until 6 days before the onset of symptoms. Individuals exposed during the late incubation period or early acute phase of illness should also be promptly immunized. Seventy-five percent of this group will develop detectable levels of anti-HAV IgM, suggesting passive–active immunity. Postexposure immunoprophylaxis is suggested for (1) household and close personal contacts, (2) institutionalized contacts, and (3) contacts within a daycare facility. Grade-school classroom contacts of an isolated case and routine play contacts do not require ISG. A second case within a class is indication for immunoprophylaxis of the rest of the class. An alternative method for determining who should receive ISG is to test high-risk contacts for anti-HAV IgG.

Hepatitis B

Prophylactic treatment to prevent infection after exposure to HBV should be considered in the following situations seen in the ED: (1) sexual exposure to the HBV surface antigen–positive patient; (2) inadvertent percutaneous or permucosal exposure to HBV surface antigen–positive blood; and (3) household exposure of an infant less than 12 months of age to a primary caregiver who has acute HBV. Before treatment in the first two situations, testing for susceptibility is recommended if it does not delay treatment beyond 14 days after exposure. Testing for anti-HBV core antibody is the most efficient prescreening procedure. All susceptible persons should receive a single dose of hepatitis B immunoglobulin (0.06 mL per kilogram) administered intramuscularly and hepatitis B vaccine in recommended doses.

CHAPTER 83
Pediatric and Adolescent Gynecology

Jan E. Paradise, M.D.

GYNECOLOGIC DISORDERS OF CHILDHOOD

Congenital Vaginal Obstruction

CLINICAL MANIFESTATIONS

The two most common anomalies with these features are transverse vaginal septum (sometimes called *vaginal atresia*) and imperforate hymen.

Infancy

Although vaginal obstruction should properly be identified during the initial examination of the newborn female, infants with hydrocolpos often go unrecognized until days or weeks later, when they develop the three hallmarks of this condition: (1) a lower abdominal mass, (2) difficulty with urination, and (3) a visible bulging membrane at the introitus. Except in mild cases, the lower abdominal mass consists of the bladder as well as the hydrocolpos itself. The infant strains to micturate or has urinary retention because the urethra is obstructed extrinsically. In more severe cases, infants also may have constipation, hydronephrosis, edema of the lower extremities, and hypoventilation. Inspection of the perineum should immediately indicate the proper diagnosis.

Adolescence

The girl with congenital vaginal obstruction who escapes notice during infancy will not come to attention until late in puberty when she presents with either primary amenorrhea or lower abdominal pain. She will have had satisfactory pubertal development until her menarche apparently fails to occur. Accumulating menstrual blood then eventually will produce vague lower abdominal pain that is not necessarily cyclic. As the hematocolpos grows, it will finally interfere with comfortable micturition, producing symptoms of urgency, frequency, or dysuria. The history of amenorrhea and the finding of a lower abdominal mass may lead the physician to suspect a tumor or even pregnancy, but the characteristic appearance of the introitus covered by a bluish bulging membrane is diagnostic of hematocolpos with imperforate hymen. Patients with a high transverse vaginal septum will not be diagnosed so easily because the introitus will appear normal; however, palpation of the vagina will promptly show that it is obstructed and that the cervix cannot be felt.

The complication of congenital vaginal obstruction most likely to require urgent attention among both infants and adolescents is acute urinary retention. Rarely, an infant may have respiratory insufficiency or inferior vena caval obstruction because of the large mass.

MANAGEMENT

Patients with congenital vaginal obstruction need surgical treatment. Hydrocolpos or hematocolpos complicated by respiratory insufficiency, compression of the inferior vena cava, or hydronephrosis must be corrected without delay. The management of simple imperforate hymen can be modified according to the patient's age. Surgery should be scheduled promptly for adolescents but can be performed electively for asymptomatic infants and children.

Labial Adhesions

CLINICAL MANIFESTATIONS

The parent who notices a daughter's labial adhesions at home usually brings her to the emergency department (ED) with a chief complaint that the child's vagina is "closing up." Alternatively, a physician may notice the adhesions during the child's routine physical examination. The situation is much more difficult when, as occasionally happens, the child is brought to the ED for evaluation because another clinician has mistakenly informed the parents that their daughter has congenital absence of the vagina or ambiguous genitalia. Imperforate hymen is another notable misdiagnosis.

The diagnosis of labial adhesions can be made promptly and confidently by simple inspection of the child's genitalia. When the labia majora are gently retracted laterally, a flat plane of tissue marked by a central vertical line of adhesion obstructs the view of the introitus within. This thin vertical raphe is pathognomonic of labial adhesions. Even when adhesions appear to have closed the vulva completely, a pinpoint opening generally permits the egress of urine. Most girls with labial adhesions are asymptomatic. A few have associated dysuria, frequency, or refusal to void that may be a result of either the obvious mechanical obstruction or concurrent urinary tract infection. Whether associated urinary tract infections are a cause or an effect of adhesions is uncertain, but they are a recognized complication of the condition.

MANAGEMENT

Treatment is not indicated for asymptomatic girls with labial adhesions because the condition spontaneously remits early in puberty as a result of increasing endogenous estrogen. Some parents, however, prefer that their daughters be treated. Of girls with labial adhesions, 90% can be treated successfully with a small amount of estrogen cream (Premarin or Dienestrol) dabbed onto the adhesions at bedtime for 2 to 4 weeks. After the labia have separated, an inert cream (zinc oxide, Vaseline, Desitin) is applied nightly for an additional 2 weeks to keep the labia apart while healing is completed.

Urethral Prolapse

CLINICAL MANIFESTATIONS

Vaginal bleeding or spotting is the chief complaint of 90% of children with significant urethral prolapses. The bleeding is painless, occasionally misinterpreted as hematuria or menstruation, and accompanied by urinary frequency or dysuria in about one-fourth of cases. Only a minority of girls or their parents are aware of the presence of a vulvar mass. On the other hand, it is not rare for the physician simply to note a small prolapse during the routine examination of an asymptomatic child.

On examination of the child's vulva, a red or purplish, soft, doughnut-shaped mass is seen. Most prolapses are not tender and measure 1 to 2 cm in diameter. By retracting the labia majora posterolaterally, the examiner often demonstrates that the mass is separate from and anterior to the vaginal introitus, but this process may be difficult if the prolapse is large. A small central dimple in the mass indicates the urethral lumen. This dimple can be missed if lighting is inadequate, bleeding is active, or mucosal edema is significant. In most cases, the appearance of the prolapse is diagnostic. If the diagnosis is in doubt, however, sterile straight catheterization of the bladder through the mass can be performed to demonstrate the anatomic relationships safely and rapidly. No other test is needed.

MANAGEMENT

For the symptomatic patient with a small segment of prolapsed mucosa that is not necrotic, warm moist compresses or sitz baths, combined with a 2-week course of topical estrogen cream, may be prescribed. Most patients treated in this way have improved within 10 to 14 days and remained normal thereafter, thus avoiding surgery. Patients with dark red or necrotic mucosa should be treated surgically within several days by reduction of the prolapse and/or excision of necrotic tissue.

GYNECOLOGIC DISORDERS OF ADOLESCENCE

Dysmenorrhea

CLINICAL MANIFESTATIONS

Typical primary dysmenorrhea consists of cramping, dull, midline, or generalized lower abdominal pain at the onset of a menstrual period. The pain may coincide with the start of bleeding, or it may precede the bleeding by several hours. Many women have associated symptoms, including backache, thigh pain, diarrhea, nausea or vomiting, and headache. The discomfort usually abates within 48 hours. Because dysmenorrhea is a hallmark of ovulation, adolescents characteristically do not experience dysmenorrhea until after several months of painless, anovulatory cycles. Menstrual pain that begins either at menarche or more than 4 years after regular cycles have been established is less common. The patient with such early or late dysmenorrhea should be assessed carefully for a possible underlying disorder, but she is still more likely to be having simply a particularly early or late onset of fertile cycles. Because they inhibit ovulation, both combined oral contraceptive pills and contraceptive progestins almost uniformly abolish dysmenorrhea. Patients with straightforward dysmenorrhea have normal physical examinations and no associated abnormalities on routine laboratory evaluation.

MANAGEMENT

The virginal adolescent with a typical history of dysmenorrhea should undergo a routine physical examination, but a pelvic examination is unnecessary; however, virginal patients with atypical or severe pain should undergo rectoabdominal or one-finger vaginoabdominal palpation. Sexually experienced adolescents with pelvic pain cannot be evaluated adequately without a complete pelvic examination to screen for pelvic infection and unsuspected pregnancy.

Nonsteroidal antiinflammatory drugs (NSAIDs) are the treatment of choice for patients with moderate or severe dysmenorrhea, providing pain relief for 60% to 80% of symptomatic women. Aspirin (650 mg four times a day) can be recommended for patients with mild discomfort but is several hundred times less potent an inhibitor of prostaglandin synthesis. Like aspirin, but to a lesser extent, NSAIDs cause gastrointestinal irritation, inhibit platelet aggregation, and prolong the bleeding time. NSAIDs also may reduce the volume of menstrual blood loss, a little recognized but potentially beneficial side effect. Both NSAIDs and aspirin are contraindicated for patients with aspirin hypersensitivity, gastrointestinal ulcers, and bleeding disorders. Examples of commonly used NSAID treatment regimens are as follows:

Mefenamic acid: 500 mg once orally, followed by 250 mg four times a day
Ibuprofen: 400 to 600 mg orally four times a day
Naproxen: 500 mg once orally, followed by 250 mg four times a day
Naproxen sodium: 550 mg once orally, followed by 275 mg four times a day

For sexually active adolescents with dysmenorrhea, birth control pills are an attractive and effective alternative to NSAIDs because they provide both contraception and pain relief. Other agents commonly recommended in the past for the treatment of dysmenorrhea—acetaminophen, caffeine, propoxyphene—lack specific antiprostaglandin action and have only limited effectiveness.

Dysfunctional Uterine Bleeding

CLINICAL MANIFESTATIONS

Dysfunctional uterine bleeding (DUB) has a substantial capacity to disrupt the everyday activities of adolescent patients discomfited by an unpredictable, urgent need for bathroom facilities and the risk of visible bloodstains. Large amounts of bleeding often provoke considerable fear in both patients and their parents. These concerns can overshadow the history of the bleeding itself, but the details of the problem's chronology and an estimate of blood loss (in pads per day) will help the physician assess the severity of the bleeding, follow the patient's clinical course, and gauge her prognosis. The symptoms that characteristically accompany only ovulatory menstrual cycles—mittelschmerz, premenstrual breast tenderness, bloating, mood changes, and dysmenorrhea—should be absent. DUB is classically painless, but occasionally a patient with active bleeding may experience crampy pain if a large quantity of blood is passed rapidly. Weakness or fainting should alert the examiner to the possibility of significant blood loss. Pertinent questions should include whether the patient is pregnant, whether she uses contraception if she has been sexually active, and whether she has an underlying platelet disorder (eg, thrombocytopenia, von Willebrand disease).

The physical examination starts with measurement of the patient's vital signs, including a check for orthostatic changes in the pulse and blood pressure. Pertinent signs, including pallor, petechiae or bruises that might indicate a bleeding disorder, and hirsutism or obesity consistent with the polycystic ovary syndrome, should be sought and noted. The pelvic examination is likely to be normal except for the presence of bleeding but should be performed to evaluate the patient for pelvic infections, previously unrecognized pregnancy, and functional ovarian cysts. If necessary, rectoabdominal palpation can be substituted for the standard bimanual examination. Ovarian enlargement is an uncommon finding even among adolescent patients with clear polycystic ovary syndrome. The differential diagnosis of DUB is discussed at greater length in Chapter 67.

MANAGEMENT

A determination of the hemoglobin or hematocrit is essential for the emergency evaluation of patients with DUB because historical estimates of blood loss are imprecise. A platelet count also should be obtained because thrombocytopenia is the most common hematologic disorder that produces menorrhagia. The history and physical examination should be used to guide the choice of additional laboratory tests. Sexually active adolescents should receive a pregnancy test, a cervical culture for gonorrhea, and an antigen-detection test for chlamydial infection because sexually transmitted disease (STD)-associated endometritis is a common cause of otherwise unexplained uterine bleeding. Patients with menorrhagia beginning at menarche, severe hemorrhage, or a history of bleeding problems should undergo further evaluation for possible disorders of platelet number or function.

In order of decreasing urgency, management of DUB includes the identification and treatment of the following problems: shock or acute hemorrhage, moderate bleeding usually accompanied by anemia, and minor bleeding that produces distress but no imminent danger for the patient (Table 83.1). For patients with brisk hemorrhage or hypotension, prompt hospitalization and volume resuscitation as necessary (see Chapter 3) are the first order of business.

Control of the bleeding itself is accomplished with hormonal treatment. (Pregnancy must be excluded in every case before hormonal treatment is begun.) Estrogen is used to support the endometrium acutely and to stop the bleeding. A progestational agent must be administered simultaneously to produce a secretory endometrium; otherwise, the problem will recur predictably whenever the estrogen is stopped. Any of the oral contraceptive pills with 35 or 50 g of either ethinyl estradiol or mestranol and a progestin provides a convenient means of administering the two hormones together. The dosage for patients with active bleeding and anemia is one estrogen–progestin tablet orally four times a day for 5 days. In almost every case, bleeding will decrease substantially within 24 hours and stop within 2 to 3 days. A rarely needed alternative treatment for hospitalized patients consists of conjugated estrogens 20 to 25 mg administered intravenously every 4 hours until the bleeding stops, with a maximum of six doses. This treatment must be accompanied by a progestational agent (medroxyprogesterone, 10–20 mg orally per day for 5–12 days). If hormonal treatment

TABLE 83.1. Management of Dysfunctional Uterine Bleeding

Clinical situation	Treatment	Comments
Shock, acute hemorrhage	Volume resuscitation Conjugated estrogens 20–25 mg i.v. every 4 hr with maximum of 6 doses Curettage if estrogen unsuccessful	Add progestin promptly Prescribe iron
Moderate bleeding	Oral estrogen plus progestin, q.i.d. regimen Intravenous estrogen if oral treatment unsuccessful	Anemia common Prescribe iron
Minor bleeding	Oral estrogen plus progestin, b.i.d. regimen Observation without treatment acceptable	

q.i.d., four times daily; b.i.d., twice daily.

fails to arrest the bleeding, dilation and curettage should be performed, but the procedure is almost never necessary.

For patients with light but prolonged bleeding and a normal hemoglobin level, the oral regimen can be reduced to one estrogen–progestin tablet twice a day for 5 days. Nausea is a common side effect of estrogen in each of these regimens and can be treated symptomatically. Vomiting rarely precludes oral therapy. A progestin alone in higher dosages (norethindrone acetate 10–20 mg daily for 5–12 days) can be used if estrogen is contraindicated or not tolerated, but the resulting hemostasis is less prompt and less predictable.

Treatment with combined estrogen–progestin pills is stopped at the end of 5 days; progestin-only treatment is stopped after 5 to 12 days. After the cessation of treatment, a self-limited, heavy menstrual period will follow within 2 to 3 days. The family must be forewarned so that they anticipate this episode and do not misinterpret it as a recurrence of the DUB. This withdrawal bleeding will stop spontaneously within several days. Subsequent therapy must be tailored to the individual patient. A course of medroxyprogesterone (10 mg orally, daily for 10–12 days) can be used every 6 to 8 weeks to produce a secretory endometrium and a controlled withdrawal flow if spontaneous menstruation has not intervened. For sexually active adolescents and those with chronic or recurrent DUB, long-term combined oral contraceptive pills are an excellent therapeutic choice.

Iron supplementation is prudent for all patients with DUB; those without frank anemia are likely to have depleted marrow stores of iron. Finally, outpatient follow-up is an essential component of management because treatment may be needed for months or years and because chronic anovulation is a risk factor for both infertility and the late development of endometrial carcinoma.

Sexual Abuse and Assault

The four major gynecologic aspects of treating a girl who has been sexually abused or assaulted are (1) collection of evidence from the genital area, (2) screening and treatment for STDs, (3) management of injury, and (4) prevention of pregnancy. The overall management of sexually abused children is discussed in Chapter 111.

Police and prosecutors ask physicians to document observations and to collect evidence that might corroborate a patient's history of sexual assault or abuse. This evidence may consist of a child's exact statement concerning the abuse; the finding of prostatic acid phosphatase in vaginal secretions, indicating the presence of seminal fluid; a small bruise on the labia majora; or the discovery of leaf or grass fragments in the underwear of a child who states that she was assaulted in a park. As a rule, any material that might be helpful should be collected if the child has had sexual contact within 72 hours of evaluation in the ED. Numerous commercially available "rape kits" contain swabs, tubes, and evidence tape to simplify this process; however, the clinician should not feel compelled to follow rape kit instructions slavishly because many of the specimens called for (eg, pubic hair sample, fingernail scrapings) are rarely relevant to the circumstances of victimized children. If material is collected that may be used in court, its movement from physician's possession to locked storage or police officer's custody should be documented with signatures, times, and dates to preserve the chain of evidence that will allow the material's origin to be verified in court. When, as is often the case, a sexually abused child is not examined until several weeks after the most recent episode of sexual contact, the likelihood of the physician's finding physical evidence is low.

Sexually transmitted diseases are seen in about 5% of abused children, generally mirroring their relative prevalence in the adult population. Although trichomoniasis is among the most common STDs in adults, it is not seen in prepubertal abused girls because trichomonads do not proliferate in the absence of an estrogenic milieu. Syphilis certainly can be transmitted by sexual assault and abuse, but it occurs only rarely. Sexual abuse has been reported as the suspected mode of transmission for some children infected with human immunodeficiency virus (HIV).

In the past, most authorities recommended universal screening of sexually abused children for syphilis and for gonorrhea and *Chlamydia trachomatis* from three sites (pharynx, vagina or urethra, and rectum). The yield of infections from such surveillance is low, however, and the cost is substantial. An alternative strategy accepted as appropriate by most experts is to restrict STD screening to high-risk children (ie, children victimized by more than one assailant or by an assailant with a known or suspected STD) and to adolescents. All adolescents are screened because they are at higher risk than younger children of acquiring STDs and especially of subsequently developing pelvic inflammatory disease (PID) if cervicitis is present. Serologic screening for syphilis and HIV infection should be offered to all children. Before a child is screened for HIV, the parent must be advised that a positive test may indicate vertical transmission and parental infection rather than acquisition via the assault. Screening for hepatitis B infection can be limited to adolescents who have not received hepatitis B vaccine.

As is true for STD screening, antibiotic prophylaxis after sexual abuse is best limited to children victimized in high-risk situations and to adolescents. The antibiotic regimen should include coverage for both chlamydia and gonorrhea. For adolescents, coverage for trichomonas and bacterial vaginosis (and for hepatitis B if the patient is unvaccinated) should be added. Giving the first vaccine dose (followed in 1 and 6 months by the subsequent doses) is adequate prophylaxis for hepatitis B. Consideration should be given to offering antiretroviral prophylaxis to children and adolescents when the circumstances of an assault seem to pose a high risk of HIV infection.

For sexually abused children with symptoms or signs of an STD, the question of screening is irrelevant; diagnostic tests should be directed at identifying all suspected infections. The diagnosis and treatment of STDs are reviewed elsewhere in this chapter and in Chapters 74 and 75. When sexual abuse is involved, for the diagnosis of gonorrhea, chlamydial infection, and herpes simplex virus infection, cultures should be used either in place of or as confirmation of indirect diagnostic methods (eg, Gram stain, DNA probe, other immunologic tests) because the risk of false-positive presumptive tests is substantial and because test results that may be presented in legal proceedings should be definitive.

Few girls sustain serious physical injuries as a result of sexual abuse or assault. Any sexually abused girl who has vaginal bleeding that cannot be attributed to a clearly visible injury or infection must be examined carefully to determine the source of the bleeding. This usually requires the use of sedation or general anesthesia in premenarchal girls. The management of girls with vaginal bleeding is discussed at greater length in Chapter 67.

The emergency physician must consider the possibility of pregnancy in every postmenarchal girl who has been sexually abused or assaulted. A pregnancy test should be conducted in the ED to ascertain whether the patient is pregnant when she is first evaluated. If an adolescent is not pregnant and is not using hormonal contraception, her risk of becoming pregnant as a result of rape must be assessed. The risk of pregnancy from a single unprotected coitus at midcycle is estimated to be 15%. The risk from coitus occurring more than 6 days before or after ovulation is negligible. Postcoital contraception—100 g ethinyl estradiol and 1 mg dl-norgestrel (2 Ovral tablets) given once immediately and a second time 12 hours later—reduces the likelihood of pregnancy by about 50% and should be offered to patients seen within 72 hours of a rape. An antiemetic also should be prescribed because the estrogen often produces nausea. The effectiveness of this regimen for preventing pregnancy decreases as the time from coitus to treatment increases. The patient can expect to have her next menstrual period within 21 days after treatment and should be given an appointment for follow-up about 3 weeks after the ED visit.

GENITAL TRACT INFECTIONS

Vaginitis

TRICHOMONAL VAGINITIS

Clinical Manifestations

A small proportion of vaginally delivered female neonates acquire trichomonal vaginitis from their infected mothers. Infants harboring only a few trichomonads may never develop clinical disease, but the remainder will have a thin whitish or yellowish vaginal discharge that appears within 10 days after birth and may persist for several months if untreated. Infected babies may be irritable but are otherwise well.

The classic vaginal discharge of trichomonal vaginitis after puberty is pruritic, frothy, and yellowish; however, many infected women do not complain of excessive discharge, and the discharge may be scant or nondescript. The so-called strawberry cervix with multiple punctate areas of hemorrhage is pathognomonic for trichomoniasis but is visible without colposcopy in only about 2% of infected patients.

For patients of all ages, the diagnosis is made easily and rapidly if characteristically motile, flagellated trichomonads are seen in a saline suspension of discharge examined microscopically within about 15 minutes after the specimen has been obtained. If a longer delay occurs, the organisms will gradually lose their mobility and normal shape, making them much more difficult to identify. The false-negative rate for wet mount examinations can be as high as 40%. More sensitive methods for detecting trichomonal infection are culture and colorimetric probes for trichomonal DNA.

Management

Metronidazole is effective for the treatment of vaginal trichomoniasis. The dosage for infants is 15 mg per kilogram of body weight daily administered orally in three divided doses for 7 days. A single oral dose (2 g) is prescribed for adolescents. Because trichomoniasis is sexually transmitted, the adolescent patient's partner(s) also must be referred for treatment. Recent data indicate that metronidazole is not a teratogen, but many clinicians prefer to postpone treatment of pregnant patients until the second trimester. Intravaginal clotrimazole (two intravaginal tablets at bedtime for 7 days) can provide symptomatic relief for pregnant patients but will cure only 10% to 20%.

SHIGELLA VAGINITIS

Clinical Manifestations

Shigella flexneri, *S. sonnei*, *S. boydii*, and *S. dysenteriae* can produce vaginal infections in infants and children but do not appear to cause genital disease after puberty. The vaginitis is characterized by a white to yellow discharge that is bloody in three-quarters of cases. Associated pruritus and dysuria are uncommon. One-third of patients have diarrhea that precedes, accompanies, or follows the vaginal discharge. On inspection, the vulvar mucosa is often inflamed or ulcerated. The diagnosis is established by culture of a specimen of vaginal discharge. Rectal cultures are positive in some cases.

Management

Patients with *Shigella* vaginitis should be treated with oral antibiotics chosen on the basis of sensitivity testing. If the antibiotic sensitivity is unknown, trimethoprim–sulfamethoxazole (8 mg of trimethoprim per kilogram daily administered orally in two doses for 5 days) should be used.

STREPTOCOCCAL VAGINITIS

Clinical Manifestations

Streptococcal pyogenes can be identified in cultures of vaginal specimens taken from about 14% of prepubertal girls with scarlet fever. Most of these vaginal infections produce either no symptoms or minor discomfort, but a few patients develop outright vaginitis with a purulent discharge. Streptococcal vaginitis can accompany or follow symptomatic pharyngitis and occurs uncommonly in girls with neither symptomatic pharyngitis nor scarlet fever. Most of these latter patients are pharyngeal carriers of the organism. Streptococcal vaginitis causes genital pain or pruritus and can mimic candidal or gonococcal vaginitis. A swab of the patient's discharge should be cultured to verify the clinical diagnosis, as well as to exclude gonococcal infection.

Management

As for any other infection with group A β-hemolytic streptococci, penicillin is the preferred antibiotic. Intramuscular benzathine penicillin G is an alternative if poor compliance with oral treatment is anticipated. Oral erythromycin ethylsuccinate or azithromycin can be prescribed for children who are allergic to penicillin (see Table 83.2 for dosages).

CANDIDA VULVOVAGINITIS

Clinical Manifestations

Candida albicans frequently colonizes the vagina after the onset of puberty, when estrogen stimulates local *increases in glycogen stores and acidity that both appear to enhance its growth. If the ecologic balance of the vagina is changed either by inhibition of the normal bacterial flora, by impaired host immunity, or by an increase in the availability of nutrients (broad-spectrum antibiotics, immunodeficiency states, corticosteroids, diabetes mellitus, pregnancy), the resulting proliferation of Candida* will produce symptoms in a fraction of affected patients. Most patients with candidiasis, however, have no identifiable predisposing risk factor for infection. Because of the importance of estrogen in promoting fungal growth, candidal vulvovaginitis is rare among prepubertal girls.

The most common clinical manifestation of vulvovaginal candidiasis is vulvar pruritus. In severe infections, vulvar edema and erythema can occur. "External" dysuria is produced when urine comes in contact with the inflamed vulva. Vaginal discharge is variable in quantity and appearance. In severe cases, the vaginal vault is red, dry, and has a whitish, watery, or curdlike discharge that may be relatively scanty. Patients with mild disease may have only intermittent itching and an unimpressive discharge.

Microscopic examination of a sample of vaginal discharge suspended in 10% potassium hydroxide solution to clear the field of cellular debris can provide a rapid diagnosis of candidiasis if hyphae are seen. In as many as 50% of cases, however, wet mounts are falsely negative. Gram-stained smears of discharge

TABLE 83.2. Treatment of Vaginal Infections

Infection	Drug	Dose, Route	Comments
Bacterial vaginosis	Metronidazole	500 mg, p.o. b.i.d. for 7 days[a]	
Candida vaginitis	Butoconazole 2% cream	1 full applicator HS for 3 nights	All these are nonprescription regimens
	Clotrimazole	500-mg tablet per vaginum as single dose	
	Miconazole	200-mg suppository HS for 3 nights	
	Tioconazole 6.5% ointment	1 full applicator HS as single dose	
Shigella vaginitis	Trimethoprim-sulfamethoxazole	8 mg/kg/day of trimethoprim p.o. in 2 divided doses for 5 days	If susceptibility unknown; otherwise, use susceptibility profile to select antibiotic
Streptococcal vaginitis	Penicillin V	*Patients <40 kg:* 250 mg p.o. t.i.d. for 10 days *Patients ≥40 kg:* 500 mg p.o. b.i.d. for 10 days	
	Benzathine penicillin	*Patients <27 kg:* 600,000 U i.m. *Patients ≥27 kg:* 1.2 million U i.m.	
	Erythromycin estolate	20–40 mg/kg/day in 2–4 divided doses	For penicillin allergy
	Azithromycin	12 mg/kg/day in single dose for 5 days	For penicillin allergy
Trichomonal vaginitis	Metronidazole	*Infants:* 15 mg/kg/day p.o. in 3 divided doses for 7 days *Adolescents:* 2 g p.o. as single dose[a]	

b.i.d., twice daily; HS, at bedtime; PO, orally; IM, intramuscularly.
[a]See text for information about treatment regimens during pregnancy.

are somewhat more sensitive because hyphae and yeast cells are Gram positive and more easily visible. Culture can only corroborate or fail to corroborate the clinical impression of candidiasis because the vaginal flora includes *C. albicans* in up to 25% of young women who have no symptoms or signs of infection. Similarly, cultures from patients with classic signs of candidal infection may yield only a light growth of the organism, making heavy growth an inadequate criterion for diagnosis. From these considerations, it is apparent that although the presence of *C. albicans* can be confirmed by laboratory tests, the diagnosis and subsequent treatment of this infection should be guided by the presence or absence of clinical disease.

Management

Topical imidazoles will promptly cure 80% to 90% of patients with candidal infections. Most are available without prescription. The creams are packaged with intravaginal applicators, but many premenarchal and virginal girls can be treated adequately and more comfortably by applying cream to the vulva alone. Effective, nonprescription, short-course treatments for patients with mild to moderate candidal vulvovaginitis include butoconazole 2% cream (one full applicator at bedtime for three nights), clotrimazole 500-mg tablets (one tablet intravaginally as a single dose), miconazole 200-mg suppositories (one suppository at bedtime for three nights), and tioconazole 6.5% ointment (one full applicator as a single dose). For patients with severe discomfort, one of the 5- or 7-day formulations of a topical agent is likely to be more effective. Fluconazole, an oral fungicide, treats candidal vulvovaginitis as effectively as the topical preparations, and many patients prefer oral to topical treatment; however, the potential for promoting fungal resistance and the risks, albeit low, of systemic toxicity and allergy are important disadvantages of oral antifungal agents.

NONSPECIFIC VAGINITIS IN CHILDREN

Clinical Manifestations

The term *nonspecific vaginitis,* referring to a disorder of prepubertal girls, encompasses a variety of genitourinary symptoms and signs that are sometimes caused by poor perineal hygiene but that in other cases have no readily identifiable cause. Genital discomfort, discharge, itchiness, and dysuria are relatively common childhood complaints. When a girl with such symptoms has either a normal vulva and vagina or only mild vulvar inflammation on physical examination, a specific vaginal infection is unlikely, and other possible explanations for the complaint—smegma, pinworms, urinary tract infection, a local chemical irritant, or sexual abuse, for example—should be sought with appropriate questions and laboratory tests. (It should be noted that commercially available bubble bath is not often the culprit.) If, on the other hand, a vaginal discharge *is* present on physical examination, the specific vaginal infections discussed in this chapter are diagnostic possibilities, and cultures should therefore be obtained. In reported series of premenarchal girls with vaginitis who have been systematically evaluated, between 25% and 75% ultimately are categorized as having nonspecific vaginitis. The diagnosis should not be made until other entities have been excluded. (A more comprehensive discussion of the differential diagnosis of genital complaints is presented in Chapters 67 and 68.)

Management

General measures to promote cleanliness and comfort should be initiated for the girl with nonspecific vaginitis. Daily soaking in a bath of warm water, either plain or with some baking soda added, gentle perineal cleaning with a soft washcloth, and the use of cotton underwear can be recommended. The girl should be taught to wipe toilet paper anteroposteriorly after having a bowel movement. Using these suggestions, most girls with perineal irritation will be improved within 2 weeks. The remaining patients should be reevaluated to exclude any specific but previously unrecognized disorder. If none is found, these girls may benefit from a brief course of topical estrogen cream (a small amount dabbed onto the vulva nightly for 2–4 weeks) to stimulate thickening of the vaginal mucosa so that it is more resistant to local irritation. Parents should be cautioned that estrogen cream is capable of producing breast growth if it is used for a prolonged period.

Bacterial Vaginosis

CLINICAL MANIFESTATIONS

The symptoms of bacterial vaginosis—malodor and discharge—are not distinctive and can resemble those of trichomonal infection. A complaint of dysuria or pruritus goes against the diagnosis. As many as half of women who have signs of vaginosis are asymptomatic. The vaginal discharge is moderate or copious, grayish-white, and homogeneous. On examination, the vulva, vagina, and cervix are not inflamed, but concomitant infection with trichomonas or gonorrhea can complicates this picture.

Compared with the composite Amsel criteria, use of single tests (eg, pH, clue cells, or whiff test alone) produces lower positive and negative predictive values for the diagnosis of bacterial vaginosis. When a wet mount of vaginal discharge is examined, epithelial cells are seen to be studded with large numbers of small bacteria and have a granular appearance with shaggy borders. The ratio of epithelial cells to polymorphonuclear leukocytes in the discharge is 1 or higher. Lactobacilli (long rods) are sparse. Gram stain can be used to confirm the presence of clue cells and the scarcity of long gram-positive rods (lactobacilli). Because 35% to 55% of women without bacterial vaginosis have positive cultures for *Gardnerella vaginalis,* culture is not a useful diagnostic test. Trichomonal infection is the major diagnostic alternative for patients suspected of having bacterial vaginosis.

MANAGEMENT

The standard treatment for bacterial vaginosis is oral metronidazole. Regimens are 500 mg twice daily for 7 days in nonpregnant women and 250 mg three times daily for 7 days in pregnant women. These regimens are moderately effective, yielding a recurrence rate of up to 30% within 3 months. Treatment of patients' sexual partners does not reduce the recurrence rate and is not recommended. Common side effects of metronidazole include gastrointestinal upset, headache, and a metallic taste. A recent meta-analysis indicated that metronidazole in standard doses is not a human teratogen. Some clinicians, however, prefer to postpone treatment of pregnant women until the second trimester. Intravaginal clindamycin cream and metronidazole gel are alternative treatments for nonpregnant women but are not recommended during pregnancy. Oral clindamycin (300 mg twice daily for 7 days) is an alternative treatment regimen for pregnant patients with bacterial vaginosis.

Gonococcal Infections

CLINICAL MANIFESTATIONS

Prepubertal girls with vaginal gonorrhea uniformly have an obvious whitish to greenish purulent discharge that can be pruritic. Because the child's vaginal flora is normally fairly sparse, a Gram-stained smear of the vaginal discharge can provide a rapid presumptive positive diagnosis if, on microscopic examination, at least eight pairs of typical gonococci can be seen in each of at least two polymorphonuclear leukocytes. Because the social and legal implications of the diagnosis are major and because this fastidious microorganism can fail to grow in the laboratory, *all management decisions about gonorrhea in a child, including informing the parents of the diagnosis, reporting the case to the state child protective services agency, and instituting antibiotic treatment, should be delayed until after the suspected diagnosis has been confirmed by bacterial culture.*

After puberty, higher estrogen levels stimulate the growth of a thick vaginal mucosa that is relatively resistant to infection by gonococci, and lower genital tract infection is localized to the cervix or urethra. A vaginal discharge, excessive menstrual bleeding, or symptoms of cystitis may prompt an infected patient's ED visit, but most infections will produce no symptoms at all. On examination of the cervix, there may be marked central erythema, a purulent discharge, or no abnormality. A culture of a single specimen taken from the endocervical canal with a cotton-tipped swab, plated on a selective medium, and incubated properly will identify about 85% of women with uncomplicated gonorrhea. The remaining 15% includes patients with urethral, rectal, and pharyngeal infections without cervicitis and those with cervicitis not detected with a single culture.

MANAGEMENT (TABLE 83.3)

Girls with culture-proven gonococcal vaginitis should be treated with a single intramuscular dose of ceftriaxone.

TABLE 83.3. Summary of Treatment Regimens for Lower Genital Tract Gonorrhea and Chlamydial Infection

Patient circumstance	Drug	Dose, route	Comments
Treatment for gonorrhea			
In children <45 kg	Ceftriaxone	125 mg i.m.	
In children >45 kg and adolescents	Ceftriaxone or	125 mg i.m.	Regimens other than ceftriaxone may not treat incubating syphilis
	Cefixime or	400 mg p.o.	
	Ciprofloxacin or	500 mg p.o.	
	Ofloxacin	400 mg p.o.	
Penicillin allergy			
In children	Spectinomycin	40 mg/kg i.m.	Maximum dose 2 g
In adolescents	Spectinomycin	2 g, i.m.	May not treat incubating syphilis
Treatment for chlamydial infection			
In children <45 kg	Erythromycin base	50 mg/kg/day p.o. in 4 doses for 10–14 d	Effectiveness about 80%
In children ≥45 kg and in adolescents	Azithromycin	1 g, p.o.	Single-dose regimen obviates compliance problems
In children ≥8 yr old and in adolescents	Doxycycline	100 mg, p.o. b.i.d. for 7 d	
During pregnancy	Erythromycin base or	500 mg p.o. o.d. 7 d	
	Erythromycin ethylsuccinate	800 mg p.o. o.d. for 7 d	

Adapted from Centers for Disease Control and Prevention. 1998 Guidelines for treatment of sexually transmitted diseases. *MMWR* 1998;47(RR-1), with permission.
i.m., intramuscularly; p.o., orally.

Treatment for *C. trachomatis* should not be given presumptively for children but rather should be withheld pending the results of screening chlamydial cultures. Pharyngeal and rectal swabs for culture of *N. gonorrhoeae* should be obtained from every child in whom gonococcal vaginitis is confirmed by culture. The finding of gonorrhea in a child mandates detailed psychosocial evaluation and a report to the state child protective services agency for suspected sexual abuse in every case. All household contacts of the child, both children and adults, should be cultured because epidemiologic studies indicate that about 25% of them are likely to have gonorrhea also. Hospitalization of the child may facilitate this investigation in some cases.

Adolescents with uncomplicated genital gonorrhea should receive one of the treatments listed in Table 83.3. The oral treatment regimens have the advantages of easy administration and avoiding both a painful intramuscular injection and the risk of accidental needle stick. Since 1982, the Centers for Disease Control and Prevention (CDC) have suggested that every adolescent patient treated for lower genital tract gonorrhea also be treated presumptively for coexisting chlamydial infection because of the substantial likelihood of dual infection.

Every patient with gonorrhea should receive a screening serologic test for syphilis and should be offered screening for HIV infection. None of the treatment regimens for gonorrhea will cure established syphilis, but ceftriaxone is likely to eradicate incubating syphilis. The management of a case of gonorrhea is never complete until the patient's sexual partner(s) has been notified and treated presumptively. Test-of-cure cultures are not indicated because the treatment regimens for gonorrhea are efficacious. Follow-up remains desirable for adolescents with gonorrhea to review their contraceptive behavior, to counsel them about risk reduction, to identify reinfections, and to obtain Papanicolaou smears.

Chlamydial Infections

Clinical Manifestations

Most prepubertal children with urethral, vaginal, and rectal infections are asymptomatic, although a few complain of dysuria, enuresis, or vaginal discharge. The diagnosis should be suspected in prepubertal girls with vaginal discharge that persists after therapy for a prior gonococcal infection and in girls with urethritis or vaginitis who have had sexual contact. Culture of a urethral or vaginal sample is advisable to confirm the diagnosis in children because the rapid antigen-detection tests can yield false-positive results and because the social and legal implications of a positive test are serious.

In adolescents, *C. trachomatis* can cause dysuria-pyuria syndrome and mucopurulent cervicitis but is often asymptomatic. Untreated lower genital tract infection can result in bartholinitis, perihepatitis, PID, and infertility (see the following section). On speculum examination, the cervix may be erythematous and friable when swabbed. Infected secretions collected from the cervical os may appear yellowish on a cotton swab. The diagnosis in an adolescent should be confirmed by an antigen or DNA detection test of the cervix or urine. These tests have good sensitivity and specificity.

Management

Antibiotic treatment regimens for children and adolescents with lower genital tract chlamydial infections are summarized in Table 83.3. Children should be treated despite the absence of symptoms because complications of the infection may develop after puberty. Adolescents with chlamydial infections should be counseled about the importance of treatment for their sexual partner(s), abstinence until 1 week after all sexual partners have completed treatment, and barrier methods of contraception. Patients should receive follow-up examinations 4 to 6 weeks after treatment to screen for reinfection, coexisting STDs, and cervical dysplasia.

BARTHOLIN GLAND ABSCESS AND CYST

Clinical Manifestations

The patient with a Bartholin gland abscess presents with a painful, tender, fluctuant mass bulging on the involved side of the vestibule inferior to the labium minus. Pus sometimes can be milked upward from the gland to the duct orifice. The patient with a cyst complains of vulvar discomfort; the unilateral mass is typically 1 to 3 cm in diameter and mildly tender. Cyst fluid is usually sterile.

Management

Abscesses and symptomatic cysts are treated similarly, generally with incision, drainage, and placement of a Word catheter. Each of these procedures opens the cyst cavity widely and facilitates prolonged drainage.

PELVIC INFLAMMATORY DISEASE

Clinical Manifestations

Although the constellation of symptoms and signs associated with PID—abdominal pain, irregular uterine bleeding, abnormal vaginal discharge, and lower abdominal and pelvic tenderness—is well known, no single symptom or sign or combination of symptoms and signs is both sensitive and specific. Clinical findings that improve the specificity of the diagnosis of PID (ie, increase the likelihood that the diagnosis is correct) do so only at the expense of sensitivity (ie, exclude patients who do in fact have PID). Minimum, additional, and definitive criteria for the diagnosis of PID suggested by the CDC are shown in Table 83.4. It is noteworthy, however, that approximately one-fourth of women who have pelvic pain but who do not meet the CDC's minimum criteria have been shown nevertheless to have PID on laparoscopy or endometrial biopsy.

In patients with suspicious symptoms and signs, a fever higher than 38°C (100.4°F) is about 80% specific for PID but will incorrectly exclude the diagnosis in about 60% to 75% of patients who do have it (25%–40% sensitivity). A peripheral white blood cell count of more than 10000/mm^3 is approximately 90% specific but will incorrectly exclude the diagnosis of PID in about 40% of patients with PID (60% sensitivity). A C-reactive protein greater than 5 mg per deciliter and an erythrocyte sedimentation rate greater than 15 mm per hour are each approximately 50% to 80% specific for PID but will each incorrectly exclude the diagnosis in about 10% to 30% of patients who have it. Perihepatitis (Fitz-Hugh–Curtis syndrome), consisting of right upper quadrant pain and tenderness produced by inflammation of the liver capsule in association with PID, occurs in 5% to 10% of patients with either chlamydial or gonococcal PID. On transvaginal ultrasonography, about one-third of patients with PID will have visible fallopian tubes, and about one-fifth will have a demonstrable tuboovarian abscess.

A complication of PID that warrants prompt diagnosis is ruptured tuboovarian abscess. About 15% of tuboovarian abscesses rupture spontaneously. The symptoms and signs of a ruptured abscess may be mild if only a small amount of pus has

TABLE 83.4. Minimum, Additional, and Definitive Criteria for the Diagnosis of Pelvic Inflammatory Disease

Minimum criteria	Lower abdominal tenderness Tenderness produced by motion of the cervix Bilateral adnexal tenderness
Additional criteria	Oral temperature >38°C (100.4°F) Abnormal vaginal discharge on examination Erythrocyte sedimentation rate >15 mm/hr Elevated C-reactive protein Documented gonococcal or chlamydial cervical infection
Definitive criteria	Fallopian tube visible or fluid-filled on ultrasonography Tubo-ovarian abscess on ultrasonography Laparoscopic abnormalities consistent with pelvic inflammatory disease Endometritis on endometrial biopsy

Adapted from Centers for Disease Control and Prevention. 1998 Guidelines for treatment of sexually transmitted diseases. *MMWR* 1998;4(RR-1):80; and Case definitions for infectious conditions under public health surveillance. *MMWR* 1997;46(RR-10):52, with permission.

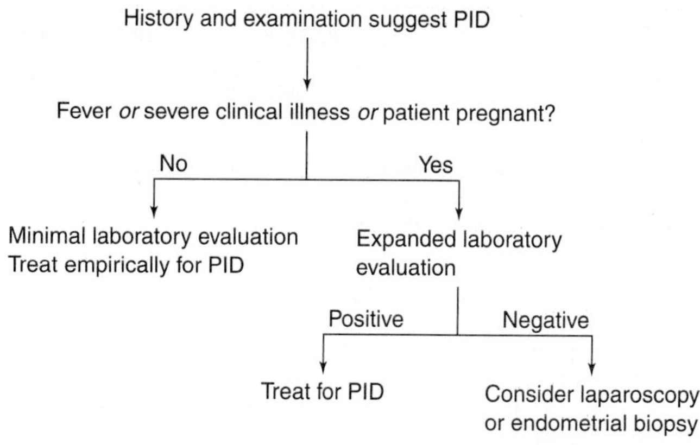

Figure 83.1. Strategy for diagnosis of pelvic inflammatory disease. Minimal laboratory evaluation should include tests for gonococcal and chlamydial cervicitis. Expanded laboratory investigation may include, in addition to the minimal evaluation, complete blood count, C-reactive protein or erythrocyte sedimentation rate, and pelvic or transvaginal ultrasonography. (Adapted from Kahn JG, Walker CK, Washington E, et al. Diagnosing pelvic inflammatory disease. *JAMA* 1991;266:2594–2604, with permission.)

leaked out, but the usual clinical picture includes peritonitis and shock. A pelvic mass is palpable in fewer than one-half of cases. Prompt surgical intervention can be lifesaving.

Laparoscopy confirms the diagnosis of PID in only about 60% of all patients who are suspected to have it, either by gynecologists or by primary care physicians, on clinical grounds of having the disease. Conditions most often mistaken for PID are acute appendicitis, endometriosis, hemorrhagic and nonhemorrhagic ovarian cysts, and ectopic pregnancy. In up to 25% of women judged clinically to have PID, no abnormality can be identified laparoscopically.

The emergency physician must consider the possibility of pregnancy in adolescents with presumed PID for two reasons. First, ascending genital tract infection is rare during pregnancy. As a result, alternative diagnoses to PID, including ectopic pregnancy, should be considered, and hospitalization of the patient is recommended (see the following sections). Second, treatment with fluoroquinolones should be avoided during the first trimester of pregnancy. (Pregnant patients may receive metronidazole for PID because, in a recent meta-analysis, first-trimester exposure was not associated with an increase in the rate of major congenital malformations among live-born infants.)

An important pathophysiologic irony is the observation that tubal occlusion is associated more often with a relatively unimpressive clinical presentation of PID (ie, long duration of symptoms, no signs of peritonitis, normal peripheral leukocyte count) than with "hot" clinical disease (ie, short duration of symptoms, fever, peritoneal signs, leukocytosis). Similarly, chlamydial PID is associated with both a longer duration of pain at patient presentation and a higher risk of infertility than is gonococcal PID. Thus, if the diagnosis of PID is allowed to depend substantially on patients' appearance—as either "well" or "sick"—clinicians may be tempted to reject the diagnosis of PID and to withhold antibiotic treatment from those patients at highest risk of subsequent ectopic pregnancy and infertility.

The Kahn approach to the clinical diagnosis of PID is recommended for the emergency physician (Fig 83.1). This strategy emphasizes diagnostic sensitivity for women with relatively mild illness, encouraging clinicians to err on the side of providing rather than withholding antibiotic treatment, and diagnostic specificity for women with relatively severe illness, focusing on the consideration of major competing diagnoses.

Management

The CDC guidelines for the treatment of PID (1998) are summarized in Table 83.5. The antibiotics listed were selected for their effectiveness in combination against *N. gonorrhoeae*, *C. trachomatis*, and the aerobes and anaerobes responsible for polymicrobial PID. Principal differences between the 1998 treatment guidelines and previous versions of these guidelines are (1) ultrasonographic findings of fallopian tube fluid and thickening are included as definitive criteria for the diagnosis of PID; (2) the previous recommendation that all adolescents with PID be hospitalized is eliminated; (3) 24 hours, rather than 48 hours, of parenteral treatment is recommended after clinical improvement; (4) clindamycin is omitted as an alternative to metronidazole in the oral ofloxacin/metronidazole treatment regimen; and (5) repeat evaluation for *N. gonorrhoeae* and *C. trachomatis* 4 to 6 weeks after completion of therapy is presented as optional.

Hospitalization is recommended for any patient with PID whose diagnosis is uncertain, particularly if ectopic pregnancy or appendicitis seems likely; for patients with severe clinical illness, including those with fever or suspected pelvic abscess; and for patients who are either immunodeficient or pregnant. Parenteral treatment, on either an outpatient or an inpatient basis, is recommended for patients likely to fail a course of oral antibiotics because of either poor compliance or vomiting and for those whose illnesses have not responded to prior oral antibiotics.

The follow-up of outpatients should include a return visit after about 3 days of treatment. The average duration of symptoms among women with gonococcal salpingitis treated with oral antibiotics is 3 to 4 days; the corresponding interval for nongonococcal salpingitis is 4 to 6 days. A poor response to therapy should alert the physician to the possibilities of inadequate compliance, abscess formation, or an alternative diagnosis.

Follow-up for all patients should include reexamination at the end of antibiotic therapy to check for residual pelvic tenderness and adnexal masses. To identify patients with persistent or repeated infection resulting from noncompliance with antibiotics or an untreated sexual partner, follow-up tests for gonococcal or chlamydial cervicitis should be scheduled 3 to 4 weeks after the end of treatment. The importance of identifying and treating sexual partners of women with PID cannot be overem-

TABLE 83.5. Treatment Regimens for Pelvic Inflammatory Disease

	Initial therapy	Subsequent therapy	Comments
Regimen A Extended parenteral treatment	Cefotetan 2 g i.v. every 12 hr *or* Cefoxitin 2 g i.v. every 6 hr *with* Doxycycline 100 mg p.o. or i.v. every 12 hr	Doxycycline 100 mg p.o. b.i.d. to complete 14 days of therapy	Oral doxycycline is preferred to avoid infusion pain. Parenteral treatment may be stopped 24 hr after clinical improvement.
Regimen B[a] Extended parenteral treatment	Clindamycin 900 mg i.v. every 8 hr *with* Gentamicin 2 mg/kg, then 1.5 mg/kg i.v. or i.m. every 8 hr	Doxycycline 100 mg p.o. b.i.d. *or* Clindamycin 450 mg p.o. b.i.d. to complete 14 d of therapy	Clindamycin is preferred for oral treatment of tubo-ovarian abscess. Parenteral treatment may be stopped 24 hr after clinical improvement.
Regimen C Combined parenteral/oral treatment	Ceftriaxone 250 mg i.m. *or* Cefoxitin 2 mg i.m. with probenecid 1 g p.o.	Doxycycline 100 mg p.o. b.i.d. for 14 d	Ceftriaxone has better coverage than cefoxitin against *N. gonorrhoeae.* Adding metronidazole to this regimen will enhance anaerobic coverage.
Regimen D Oral treatment	Ofloxacin 400 mg p.o. b.i.d. for 14 days *with* Metronidazole 500 mg p.o. b.i.d. for 14 d		Ofloxacin is not approved during pregnancy or lactation or for patients less than 18 yr of age.

Adapted from Centers for Disease Control and Prevention. 1998 Guidelines for treatment of sexually transmitted diseases, *MMWR* 1998;47(RR-1):79 86, with permission.
i.v., intravenously; i.m., intramuscularly; p.o., orally.
[a] Alternative parenteral treatment combinations include ofloxacin with metronidazole, ampicillin/sulbactam with doxycycline, and ciprofloxacin with doxycycline and metronidazole. Ciprofloxacin has poor coverage against *C. trachomatis.*

phasized. About 25% of such men have asymptomatic urethritis and are unlikely to seek treatment on their own. If contact tracing fails, these men become part of the reservoir of undetected carriers of STDs. All patients with gonococcal and chlamydial infections should be counseled about HIV and offered serologic screening for both syphilis and HIV infection.

GENITAL WARTS

Clinical Manifestations

Most patients with genital warts either have no complaint or report noticing "bumps" in the genital area. Uncommonly, large perianal warts can be painful and interfere with defecation. Prepubertal girls with vulvovaginal warts may have a bloody vaginal discharge. Because human papillomavirus (HPV) infection in males is so consistently asymptomatic, most female patients are not aware of their exposure to an infected partner.

Warts can occur anywhere on the perineum, but their growth seems to be encouraged by moisture. The most common locations in females are the posterior fourchette, adjacent areas of the labia minora and majora, and the lower vagina. Single warts 1 cm or larger in diameter and clusters of seedlings, each a few millimeters across, are both common. Warts can be velvety and flat or papillomatous. Large warts often contain distinct cauliflower-like lobulations. On the cervix, acetowhite infected areas are usually seen only with the use of colposcopy. Most visible lesions in men involve the penile frenulum or coronal sulcus. Immunodeficient patients are particularly susceptible to extensive or severe disease with an increased risk of malignant change. Genital warts must be differentiated from condylomata lata, a contagious manifestation of secondary syphilis, molluscum contagiosum, and, in men, from pearly penile papules.

Management

The diagnosis of genital warts is easy to make in patients with obvious lesions but can be more difficult in patients with flat warts or "microwarts" of the vulva. A magnifying lens or colposcope can be used to inspect suspicious areas that have been soaked in 5% acetic acid for 5 minutes. Infected skin, areas of nonspecific inflammation, and skin treated with podophyllin will turn white after soaking. To exclude syphilis, patients should also receive serologic screening.

Although anogenital warts in young children can result from vertical transmission or nonsexual contact with common warts, sexual abuse is another possible source of infection. The management of a child with genital warts should include either consultation with an expert in child abuse and neglect or a report to the state child protective service agency (see Chapter 111). Parents of children with genital warts should be examined for both common and genital warts. Excisional biopsy is preferred to ablative treatment for warts in children because histologic examination of the biopsied tissue can confirm the clinical diagnosis. Viral typing of anogenital warts in children may suggest abuse if a condylomatous HPV type is identified but cannot exclude sexual contact if a cutaneous type is found because fondling is a common manifestation of child sexual abuse.

The goal of treatment is removal of bothersome tissue. Eradicating visible lesions does not end the viral infection. Whether it reduces contagiousness is uncertain. Spontaneous improvement or resolution of genital warts occurs in a minority of patients. Each of the several available treatment methods has advantages and disadvantages, but none is more than about 50% to 60% effective, and recurrences are common. Podophyllin resin and trichloroacetic acid (TCA) are destructive agents that are applied topically. Podophyllin resin, in solutions of up to 25% concentration in tincture of benzoin, and TCA 80% solution are applied by the clinician. Podofilox in a 0.5% gel or solution and 5% imiquimod cream, an immune response modifier that induces cytokines, are available for self-application by patients.

Systemic absorption of podophyllin can produce bone marrow suppression, peripheral neuropathy, coma, and death. It is a teratogen and has been associated with stillbirths. Podophyllin should not be used during pregnancy or on warts that are large, bleeding, or located on mucosal surfaces. Safe maximum doses of 10% podophyllin solution are 4 mL for patients weighing more than 40 kg and 0.1 mg per kilogram of body weight for children. TCA can be applied to mucosal surfaces and can be administered to pregnant patients; however, TCA has a viscosity lower than water and can spread to unaffected skin rapidly, producing patient discomfort during application more often than does podophyllin. Imiquimod commonly produces local itching, erythema, and burning but is generally tolerated well by patients.

For extensive or recurrent disease or when repeated applications of podophyllin, TCA, or imiquimod are not successful, alternative treatments include surgical removal, cryotherapy, and intralesional interferon. All women with genital warts should be referred to a primary care clinician for gynecologic care, including Papanicolaou screening.

CHAPTER 84 *Pulmonary Emergencies*

M. Douglas Baker, M.D., and
Richard M. Ruddy, M.D.

ACUTE RESPIRATORY FAILURE

Pathophysiology

CLINICAL MANIFESTATIONS

Acute respiratory failure represents the severe end of the spectrum of respiratory distress; it signifies an imbalance of O_2 consumption and CO_2 production. Table 84.1 describes the causes of acute respiratory failure by anatomic location, and Table 84.2 outlines the clinical findings and laboratory abnormalities. Few clinical manifestations appear early in the progression of respiratory failure. It is important to remember that prevention of the "blood gas"–proven respiratory failure should be the goal of the emergency physician. Therefore, in many cases, therapy should be initiated before the laboratory criteria have been fulfilled.

Management

Treatment of respiratory failure is divided into three categories (Table 84.3). First, the physician always should assume that hypoxemia is present and should give sufficient supplemental oxygen [starting at 1.00 fraction of inspired oxygen (FiO_2) in severe situations] to improve arteriolar oxygen levels. The goal of this procedure should be to achieve a minimal acceptable P_aO_2 of 60 mm Hg (SaO_2 >90%) in newborns and 70 mm Hg (SaO_2 >93%–95%) in older children. If hypoxemia persists after adequate supplemental oxygen is administered, assisted positive-pressure ventilation should be initiated (mask bag reservoir, then proceeding to endotracheal intubation) to improve the efficiency of gas exchange. In general, pressure-cycle or pressure-limited ventilators are used for children who weigh less than 10 kg (most children with acute respiratory failure) and are at significant risk of the complications of ventilation.

Intravenous fluids should be titrated to maintain normal vascular volume as determined by observation of heart rate, blood pressure, peripheral perfusion, and urine output. In severely ill children who require more prolonged therapy in the emergency department, the measurement of central venous pressure may provide a more exact guide.

BRONCHOPULMONARY DYSPLASIA

Clinical Manifestations

Bronchopulmonary dysplasia (BPD) is a chronic lung disorder that may follow moderate to severe hyaline membrane disease or other acute lung insults around birth. Typically, infants with BPD are discharged from the nursery initially at 3 to 6 months of age for home therapy, although more severely affected patients may require assisted ventilation for much longer intervals. These children have tachypnea and retractions at rest or during the mildest respiratory infections or fever. Their lungs are hyperinflated (increased anteroposterior chest diameter), and they may have crackles, wheezes, or decreased breath sounds in areas of the thorax. Some patients will manifest dyspnea and moderate to severe failure to thrive. Arterial blood gas (ABG) tensions show P_aO_2 <60 mm Hg (SaO_2 <90%–92%) or P_aCO_2 more than 45 mm Hg in room air, often despite respiratory rates of greater than 60 to 80 breaths per minute. Chest roentgenograms demonstrate varying amounts of hyperinflation; several patterns occur, including cystic areas with signs of fibrosis, which are often confused with congenital lobar emphysema; severe cystic fibrosis; and new infiltrates when previous radiographs are not available for comparison.

Management

Emergency physicians most often will evaluate children with BPD accompanied by acute respiratory infections. Management is limited to primarily supportive care: ensuring oral or intravenous intake, providing relief of hypoxemia, and, when necessary, providing assisted ventilation for hypercarbia and acidosis. Pulse oximetry can be beneficial in assessing the degree of oxygen saturation and may obviate the immediate need for arterial puncture in mild illness. ABG is always necessary when signs and symptoms may be the result of hypercapnia or when cyanosis, respiratory distress or deterioration from baseline cannot be easily reversed. A chest radiograph is helpful in most episodes but often merely corroborates clinical changes. Indications for admission include a respiratory rate above 70 to 80 breaths per minute (or significant change from baseline), increasing hypoxia or hypercarbia, poor feeding associated with respiratory symptoms, apnea, or new pulmonary infiltrates. If the acute exacerbation is mild, outpatient therapy may be indicated. Home therapy may include supplemental oxygen, bronchodilators, and corticosteroids. Most children with BPD have had trials of β-agonists. Nebulizer delivery is favored because it may be easier to use during the infant's sleep time. Some children benefit from diuretic therapy and have a need for increased oxygen supplementation during the acute illness. Antibiotic therapy should be considered when the risk of bacterial infection appears higher.

TABLE 84.1 Causes of Acute Respiratory Failure in Children

Neurologic disease	
Central nervous system	Status epilepticus
	Severe static encephalopathy
	Acute meningoencephalitis
	Brain abscess, hematoma, tumor
	Brainstem insult
	Central nervous system
	Arnold–Chiari malformation
	Drug intoxication
	General anesthesia
Spinal/anterior horn cell	Transverse myelitis
	Poliomyelitis
	Polyradiculitis (Guillain–Barré)
	Werdnig–Hoffmann syndrome
Neuromuscular junction	Myasthenia gravis
	Botulism—infant, food, wound
	Tetanus
	Myopathy
	Neuropathy
	General anesthesia, drugs succinylcholine, curare, pancuronium organophosphates
Airway obstruction	
Upper	Acute epiglottitis
	Laryngotracheobronchitis (croup), bacterial tracheitis
	Foreign body aspiration
	Adenotonsillar hypertrophy
	Retropharyngeal abscess
	Subglottic stenosis, web, hemangioma
	Tracheomalacia
	Laryngoedema
	Congenital anomalies
	Static encephalopathy
Lower	Reactive airway disease (asthma)
	Foreign body aspiration
	Cystic fibrosis
	Bronchiectasis
	Tracheobronchomalacia
	Bronchopulmonary dysplasia
	α1-Antitrypsin deficiency
	Hydrocarbon aspiration, aspiration syndromes
	Congenital lobar emphysema bronchiolitis
Chest wall deformity disorders	Diaphragmatic hernia
	Pneumothorax, hemothorax, chylothorax
	Kyphoscoliosis (severe)
	Restrictive lung disease associated with chest deformity
Pulmonary diseases	Infectious pneumonias
	Tuberculosis (often large airway extrinsic obstruction)
	Pertussis, parapertussis syndrome
	Cystic fibrosis
	Drug-induced pulmonary disease
	Vasculitis, collagen vascular disease
	Pulmonary dysgenesis
	Pulmonary edema
	Near drowning
Other diseases	Cardiac disease
	Anemia (severe)
	Acidemia (severe—i.e., sepsis, renal failure, diabetic ketoacidosis, hepatic disease)
	Oxygen dissociation—methemoglobinemia, carbon monoxide, or cyanide poisoning
	Hypothermia, hyperthermia
	Sepsis
	Obstructive sleep apnea syndrome (e.g., Pickwickian syndrome)

TABLE 84.2. Diagnosis of Acute Respiratory Failure from Pulmonary Causes in Children

Clinical findings
- Vital signs: tachycardia, tachypnea
- General appearance: cyanosis, diaphoresis, confusion, restlessness, fatigue, shortness of breath, apnea, grunting, stridor, retractions, decreased air entry, wheezing

Blood gas abnormalities
- $Paco_2$ ≥50 with acidosis (pH <7.25)
- $Paco_2$ ≥40 with severe distress
- Pao_2 <60 (or Sao_2 <90%) on 0.4 Fio_2

Pulmonary function abnormalities
- Vital capacity (<15 mL/kg)
- Inspiratory pressure (<25–30 cm H_2O)

ASPIRATION PNEUMONIA

Clinical Manifestations

Aspiration pneumonia should be suspected in any at-risk child who has signs of respiratory distress. Most often, after the aspiration of gastric contents, a brief latent period occurs before the onset of respiratory signs and symptoms. More than 90% of patients are symptomatic within 1 hour, and almost all patients have symptoms within 2 hours. Fever, tachypnea, and cough usually are seen. Hypoxia is common. Apnea and hypotensive shock are seen less commonly. Sputum production is usually minimal. Diffuse crackles and wheezing are common; cyanosis appears with progression of the diseases. Chest roentgenograms may show either localized or diffuse infiltrates, which are often bilateral. The chest roentgenogram of a patient who has aspirated stomach contents may evolve suddenly from normal to complete bilateral opacification within 8 to 24 hours.

Management

The suspicion of aspiration should be confirmed with a chest radiograph. Children with a significant aspiration pneumonia (lobar infiltrates, moderate to severe respiratory distress) require admission to the hospital. Table 84.4 outlines therapeutic modalities that may be useful.

TABLE 84.4. Initial Treatment of Aspiration Pneumonia

Proven measures	Optional modalities
Suction	Corticosteroids
Airway protection	Antibiotics
Oxygen	

In the acute-care setting, children who aspirate stomach contents require primarily supportive care. Supplemental oxygen should be administered as determined by pulse oximetry or direct measurement of oxygenation with an ABG. The management of subsequent bacterial infection is addressed in the following section. The use of corticosteroids in the treatment of aspiration pneumonia is controversial; administration in the emergency department is not indicated. Another consideration in the therapy of aspiration pneumonias is the role of prophylactic antibiotic administration, which is often given to children with fever and leukocytosis. Community-acquired pneumonias generally involve anaerobes and are adequately treated with penicillin, whereas nosocomial infections require antibiotics effective against both aerobes (including *Staphylococcus aureus* and gram-negative bacilli) and anaerobes, such as a combination, for example, clindamycin and gentamicin.

PULMONARY EMBOLISM

Clinical Manifestations

The classic presentation of massive pulmonary embolism with severe circulatory compromise is easily recognized; however, most patients have nonspecific signs and symptoms and no pathognomonic laboratory abnormalities (Table 84.5). The most common presenting abnormalities in children and adolescents are pleuritic pain (which may radiate to the shoulders), dysp-

TABLE 84.3. Management of Acute Respiratory Failure

Treatment	
Primary hypoxemia	1. Supplemental oxygen (titrate for cyanosis; use arterial blood gases or pulse oximetry) 2. Consider endotracheal intubation when Fio_2 ≥0.6 or when decreased lung compliance and Fio_2 >0.4 3. Use CPAP or PEEP to improve oxygenation 4. Use assisted ventilation to improve gas exchange (increased inspiratory time, normal respiratory rates, tidal volume: 10–15 mL/kg; pressure cycle ventilation if wt <10 kg, volume cycle ventilation if wt >10 kg) 5. Treat underlying cause
Primary alveolar hypoventilation	1. Supplemental oxygen (as above) 2. Support ventilation a. Oral/nasal pharyngeal tube or endotracheal intubation b. Mask-bag ventilation with high-flow oxygen c. Use assisted ventilation (normal to increased respiratory rates; increased expired time, increased flow rates) d. Use increased tidal volume (pressure) with obstructive airway disease or with atelectasis e. Monitor carefully for side effects of ventilation
Adjunctive therapy	1. Intravenous fluid to achieve normal vascular volume (less fluid for child with interstitial lung disease) 2. Diuretics such as furosemide (1 mg/kg) for acute pulmonary edema or fluid overload 3. Sedatives/analgesics—morphine sulfate (0.1–0.2 mg/kg) every 1–2 hr intravenously; midazolam (0.1–0.2 mg/kg every 2–4 hr intravenously) 4. Muscle relaxants—vecuronium bromide (Pavulon), starting at 0.1 mg/kg every 1–2 hr or alternative 0.1–0.2

CPAP, constant positive airway pressure; PEEP, positive end-expiratory pressure.

TABLE 84.5. Clinical Manifestation of Pulmonary Embolism

	Nonspecific	Suggestive	Diagnostic
Symptoms	Syncope Sweating Pleuritic pain Dyspnea Cough Apprehension	Dyspnea out of proportion to degree of abnormal findings Hemoptysis	
Signs	Tachypnea Tachycardia Distant or absent breath sounds Rales Fever	Pleural friction rub Unexplained cyanosis Accentuated S_2	
Laboratory/radiography	Decreased PaO_2 ECG abnormalities: R/L axis deviations ST-T wave changes Ectopic (A & V) beats Right bundle branch block	Wedged infiltrate with ipsilateral elevated hemidiaphragm Abnormal ventilation-perfusion scan ECG abnormality: S_1-Q_3-T_3 pattern	Abnormal pulmonary angiography

ECG, electrocardiogram; *R/L*, right/left; *A & V*, atrial and ventricular.

nea, cough, and hemoptysis. Additional findings may include apprehension, nonproductive cough, fever, sweats, and palpitations.

Aside from tachycardia, abnormalities on physical examination are often lacking. If a sufficiently large associated infarction is identified, there may be decreased resonance over the lung fields and a pleural friction rub. Breath sounds may be distant or absent, and rales may be heard. The presence of hypoxemia not completely explained by the underlying disease process or clinical state should suggest the possibility of pulmonary embolism.

The diagnosis of pulmonary embolism can be established with high probability based on ventilation–perfusion lung scan findings. The characteristic pattern is normal ventilation of poorly perfused areas of lung. Many physicians consider pulmonary angiography to be the preferred diagnostic method in previously healthy individuals. The reliability of this method diminishes with time after the acute embolism, however. The electrocardiogram (ECG) is neither a specific nor a sensitive indicator of pulmonary embolism. The S_1-Q_3-T_3 pattern that has been described with pulmonary embolus may be seen in other conditions, including a pneumothorax. Although the presence of a pulmonary infiltrate with an ipsilateral elevated hemidiaphragm is suggestive of a pulmonary embolism, there are no pathognomonic radiographic signs in the acute-care setting. ABGs generally indicate a decreased partial pressure of oxygen. About 15% of patients have a P_{aO_2} greater than 80 mm Hg, however, and 5% have greater than 90 mm Hg. In one series, all patients had a decreased A-a gradient, if it was measured.

Management

In all patients strongly suspected of having a pulmonary embolism, a chest radiograph, ECG, and ABG should be obtained. If the clinical suspicion is high, regardless of the results, the patient should be admitted for initiation of definitive treatment. When the patient is vaguely suspected of having pulmonary embolism, all the aforementioned tests are normal, the patient's clinical condition permits, and the likelihood of pulmonary embolism appears low, the patient may be discharged with close follow-up. When abnormalities are uncovered, further diagnostic workup (ie, ventilation–perfusion scan) and admission to the hospital should be considered.

Initial therapy includes supplemental oxygen, ventilatory support as indicated, and achievement of venous access. Intravenous heparin remains the mainstay of definitive therapy for pulmonary embolism because its onset of action is immediate and it is rapidly metabolized. It should be kept in mind, however, that heparin is a common cause of in-hospital drug-related deaths in reasonably healthy adults, and it has been cited as a source of in-hospital complications in adolescents. The initial dosage is 500 U per kilogram daily given as a continuous intravenous infusion, which is adjusted to maintain the partial thromboplastin time at 1.5 to 2 times the baseline value. Warfarin sodium is the orally administered anticoagulant usually used to maintain long-term anticoagulation. This drug may be initiated either at initial treatment with heparin or 1 to 2 days thereafter. The required daily dose varies, depending on concomitant medical illness and other drug ingestion. In adults, the dose is adjusted to maintain the prothrombin time at twice normal. Warfarin is usually continued for 2 months beyond the time of diagnosis; however, the role of fibrinolytic agents in the treatment of children has not been established.

PULMONARY EDEMA

Clinical Manifestations

Pulmonary edema refers to the abnormal accumulation of fluid within the alveolar spaces and bronchioles. The onset of pulmonary edema is variable but may be rapid. Tachypnea, cough (often producing frothy, pink-tinged sputum), dyspnea, shortness of breath, and chest pain are commonly seen. Grunting often occurs in an effort to prevent lung collapse. On physical examination, the child may appear pale or cyanotic and have a rapid pulse. Decreased breath sounds and moist ("bubbly") rales are the most common auscultatory findings; however, these are generally absent with small increases in lung fluid. Indeed, auscultatory and roentgenographic findings may not manifest until the interstitial and extravascular fluid has doubled or tripled in volume.

Unless it is massive, acute fluid accumulation may not be detectable by chest roentgenogram. Lymphatic and interstitial fluid accumulations may be visible as Kerley A and B lines (septal lines). Flattening of the diaphragm on radiograph also may

TABLE 84.6. Treatment of Pulmonary Edema

Oxygen	Venodilation
Diuresis	Morphine 0.1 mg/kg i.v.
Furosemide 1 mg/kg i.v.	Digitalis (see Table 72.2 for dosage)

i.v., intravenous.

be a finding with pulmonary edema, which presumably is caused by air trapping that results from airway narrowing as a result of bronchiolar fluid collections. It should be kept in mind that if pulmonary edema is superimposed on another pulmonary process, the clinical and roentgenologic findings can be obscured by those of the primary illness. Similarly, once pulmonary edema is severe enough, it may be difficult to separate edema, atelectasis, and inflammation on the roentgenogram.

Management

The management of patients with pulmonary edema ultimately should be directed toward treatment of the primary disorder. Initial efforts (Table 84.6) should be directed toward reversal of hypoxemia by the administration of oxygen and by mechanical ventilation if necessary. Continuous positive airway pressure (CPAP) therapy delivered via face mask also has been effective in some patients. In addition to satisfying the patient's oxygen demands, reversal of hypoxemia is often useful in relieving chest pain and is important to the metabolism of vasoactive mediators that affect microvascular permeability.

Other therapeutic measures should be tailored somewhat to fit the patient's individual needs. When heart failure is the cause of pulmonary edema, in addition to oxygen and ventilation, diuretics (to decrease plasma volume), digitalis (to improve contractility), and bronchodilators (to improve contractility and afterload and to produce bronchodilation) are useful. Morphine dilates the venous system and may be helpful in relieving anxiety and dyspnea. In patients with ARDS, clinical studies have shown that the use of methylprednisolone does not improve outcome and may in fact increase the mortality and incidence of secondary infections.

Alveolar fluid clearance can be augmented with β-adrenergic agonists, which enhance sodium transport. When decreased plasma colloid osmotic pressure is an issue, albumin administration may be helpful. To minimize initial rises in vascular pressures, colloids should be infused slowly, usually in conjunction with diuretics.

PULMONARY HEMORRHAGE

Clinical Manifestations

The hallmark of pulmonary hemorrhage is recurrent intrapulmonary bleeding with lung injury and secondary depletion of body iron stores. Therefore, the symptoms and signs include hemoptysis, recurrent pneumonias (manifest by fever, tachypnea, tachycardia, and coarse or fine crackles), and pallor. Emesis of blood arising in the pulmonary tree may mislead the clinician to investigate the gastrointestinal tract. Associated symptoms of fatigue and poor weight gain are common.

Laboratory findings after recurrent hemorrhage most characteristically include a microcytic, hypochromic anemia with low serum iron. Leukocytosis and eosinophilia may be present, and the stool usually tests positive for blood. Roentgenograms may show alveolar infiltrates that may be transient, localized processes or that may be diffuse and chronic. Cardiorespiratory embarrassment ensues in children with severe anemia. Severely affected patients may develop secondary restrictive lung disease with retention of CO_2. A presumptive diagnosis can be made by finding siderophages (iron-laden microphages) in nasogastric washings.

Management

Most children with pulmonary hemorrhage have a chronic disease requiring supportive therapy for hypoxia and anemia in the form of blood transfusions and supplemental O_2. Occasionally, pulmonary hemorrhage is so severe that it causes respiratory insufficiency or hypotension. Positive-pressure ventilation with PEEP is the preferred treatment in this situation; bleeding is usually not rapid or well enough localized to be identified and controlled by bronchoscopy. In allergic, vasculitic, and idiopathic hemorrhage, the use of corticosteroids is indicated as either methylprednisolone (2 mg per kilogram daily) or hydrocortisone (8 mg per kilogram daily) administered intravenously in three to four divided doses. When hemorrhage is caused by infection, especially tuberculosis, antimicrobial therapy should be instituted and steroids avoided. Admission is necessary to support the child until the cause of the process has been determined or acutely until the hemorrhage has been controlled. Bronchoscopy can be useful diagnostically to determine infectious causes and may localize bleeding sites. Occasionally, when the bleeding is brisk as in bronchiectasis with erosion to a bronchial vessel as in cystic fibrosis, embolization of vessels may be needed to stop the bleeding.

PLEURITIS

Clinical Manifestations

The causes of pleural inflammation are varied. The determination of the nature of pleural fluid may be helpful from a diagnostic standpoint (Table 84.7). The hallmarks of pleural disease are pain, shortness of breath, fever, and an abnormal chest roentgenogram. Inspiratory chest pain from pleural inflammation is the most characteristic symptom.

In "dry" pleurisy, which is caused by a minor pulmonary infection, the patient is febrile with an irritating, nonproductive cough. The symptoms often follow an upper respiratory infection and often last only a few days. Patients are acutely ill appearing, with grunting respirations as a result of pain. Pressure over the involved area elicits tenderness. Upon palpation, a coarse vibration may be felt.

A pleural friction rub is most apt to be heard in pleural inflammation that is associated with little or no effusion. Although symptoms of pleural effusion are varied and relate to the primary cause of the effusion, most patients complain of some degree of dyspnea. Pleuritic chest pain is also a common complaint and can occur before the accumulation of fluid. Characteristic physical findings include restriction of movement of the chest wall on the affected side, flatness to percussion, diminished to absent tactile and vocal fremitus, and decreased to absent breath sounds.

Pleural effusion is the most common radiographic manifestation of pleural disease. The first roentgenographic sign of a pleural effusion is usually blunting of the costophrenic angles, producing wedge-like menisci that extend upward along the lateral chest wall. Similar collections are seen in the posterior costophrenic angles on lateral views. Larger effusions

TABLE 84.7. Differential Diagnosis of Pleural Effusion

Transudative pleural effusions	Gastrointestinal diseases
Congestive heart failure	Pancreatitis
Cirrhosis	Esophageal rupture
Nephrotic syndrome	Subphrenic abscess
Acute glomerulonephritis	Hepatic abscess
Myxedema	Whipple disease
Peritoneal dialysis	Diaphragmatic hernia
Hypoproteinemia	Peritonitis
Meigs syndrome	Trauma
Sarcoidosis	Hemothorax
Vascular obstruction	Chylothorax
Ex vacuo effusion	Drug hypersensitivity
Exudative pleural effusions	Nitrofurantoin
Infectious diseases	Methysergide
Tuberculosis	Miscellaneous diseases
Bacterial infections	Asbestos exposure
Viral infections	Pulmonary and lymph node myomatosis
Fungal infections	Uremia
Parasitic infections	Postmyocardial infarction syndrome
Neoplastic diseases	Trapped lung
Mesotheliomas	Congenital abnormalities of the lymphatics
Metastatic disease	Postradiation therapy
Collagen vascular diseases	Drug reactions
Systemic lupus erythematosus	
Rheumatoid pleuritis	
Pulmonary infarction/embolization	

From Light RW. Pleural effusions. *Med Clin North Am* 1977;61:1339, with permission.

may be seen to extend up the entire lateral chest wall or retrosternally.

Management

The management of pleural disease is aimed at determining the cause, treating the primary disorder, and relieving associated functional disturbances. When no effusion is present, relief of chest pain is one of the most pressing issues. Analgesics, bed rest, or mild sedatives may be indicated. It should be kept in mind that irritability and restlessness could be a result of pain, which, in dry pleurisy, can occur with every phase of respiration.

The accumulation of pleural fluid usually provides relief from pain. Thoracentesis is indicated when fluid accumulation is extensive enough to cause dyspnea or for diagnostic purposes (Fig. 84.1). Sonographic guidance can simplify and enhance the success of this procedure with small effusions. The complications of thoracentesis include pneumothorax, hemothorax, reexpansion pulmonary edema, and, rarely, air embolism. Thoracostomy tube placement (often performed using the Seldinger technique) provides an alternative when reaccumulation of the fluid is likely.

Diagnostic tests of pleural fluid should include gross and microscopic examination; Gram stain; and protein, glucose, lactate dehydrogenase (LDH), and pH determinations. Cytology should also be performed if malignancy is known or suspected. On gross examination, empyema fluid is opaque and viscous, fluid high in cholesterol has a characteristic satin-like sheen, and chylous effusions are milky white. A clear or slightly yellow pleural fluid is generally a transudate; however, exudates may also appear clear.

Pleural fluid pH values greater than 7.2 to 7.3 generally are found in sterile fluids that do not require drainage. In adults, a pleural fluid pH of less than 7.3 limits the differential diagnosis to empyema, malignancy, collagen vascular disease, tuberculosis, hemothorax, or esophageal rupture; a pH of less than 7.0 is seen only in empyema, collagen vascular disease, or esophageal rupture. One notable exception to the previous statement is empyema caused by *Proteus mirabilis,* which causes an elevated pleural fluid pH. It is also important to remember that pleural fluid pH will be lowered in the face of systemic acidosis. Therapeutically, in adults, a pleural fluid pH of less than 7.2 suggests that the effusion will not resolve spontaneously and will require chest tube drainage. Pleural fluid should be collected anaerobically in a heparinized syringe and transported to the laboratory on ice to ensure proper pH measurement.

Most commonly performed, but least helpful, is the white blood cell count. Although counts are generally higher (>10000 per milliliter) in children with purulent effusions and lower (<1000 per milliliter) in clear transudates, values overlap considerably. In large series of both adult and pediatric patients, pleural fluid white blood cell counts have not been helpful in narrowing the differential diagnosis or in determining the need for or duration of closed chest tube drainage.

OBSTRUCTIVE SLEEP APNEA

Clinical Manifestations

Most young children with obstructive sleep apnea (OSA) have abnormal daytime sleepiness. Other commonly associated behavioral abnormalities included hyperactivity, continuous fighting with peers, crying easily (especially in younger children), short attention span, and quick shifts from hyperactivity to excessive somnolence and withdrawal behavior.

Older children complain of sleepiness, tiredness, and fatigue. Decreased school performance, especially with regard to language acquisition, is seen in some children. One-fourth of patients report morning headaches, and more than half demonstrated signs of failure to thrive. Severe symptoms included massive obesity in 11%, hypertension in 8%, and acute cardiac or cardiorespiratory failure in 17%.

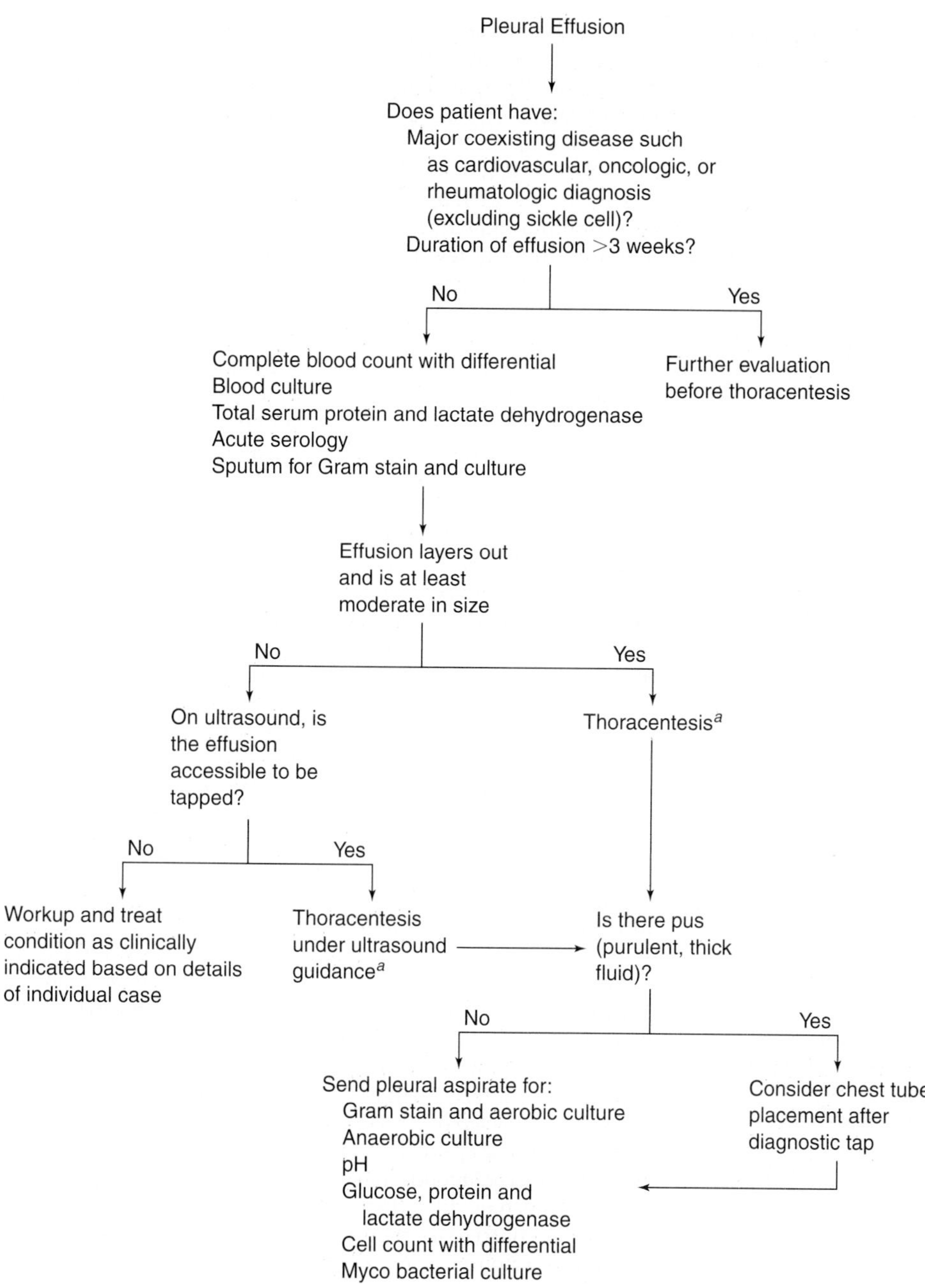

Figure 84.1. Approach to pleural effusion. [a]Consider simultaneous placement of small gauge (8–10 F) chest tube by Seldinger technique for large, free-flowing effusions.

Disordered sleep is the most common symptom of obstructive sleep apnea. All children have continuous snoring, which is interspersed with pauses and snorts. More than 80% have disrupted nocturnal sleep (eg, nightmares, night terrors, sleepwalking), and 90% sweat profusely during the night. Intermittent or nightly enuresis is also commonly noted (26%). Chronic nighttime cough may also be observed as a result of intermittent aspiration of small amounts of pharyngeal secretions and may aggravate other chronic conditions such as asthma.

Teenagers generally complain of daytime tiredness, fatigue, and sleepiness. Other common symptoms include deterioration of memory and judgment, nausea, headaches, mood swings, and neurotic behavior. Polycythemia, hypertension, cardiac arrhythmias, anoxic seizures, gastroesophageal reflux, and esophagitis are less common associated serious consequences. Two-thirds of one group of adult patients were reported to be overweight (>20% over estimates of ideal weight). This presentation occasionally is seen in children, but most are not obese. Because it is difficult for affected children to eat and breathe at the same time, they are often in the lower 25th percentile by weight and appear to have failure to thrive.

Management

Any child with a definite history of apnea must be managed with caution and concern. Hospitalization in a monitored setting is the rule. At presentation, children might not appear in extremis, by definition, during wakeful periods; however, these children run the risk of repeated apnea and the related complication of subsequent hypoxemia. Many children with OSA have preexisting anatomic airway abnormalities (eg, facial dysmorphia syndromes or enlarged lymphoid tissue) that require the expertise of an otolaryngologist.

Polysomnography is an accepted method for evaluating apnea; however, it is inconvenient and expensive. This method of evaluation is generally reserved for the most severely obstructed patients. Roentgenograms of the neck taken with the child lying on his or her back can be helpful but are not a definitive method of diagnosis. Both radiographs and physical examination of the pharynx have similar limitations in that the dynamics of the tissues at night cannot be observed.

Numerous methods of management of OSA have been suggested and studied. Patients with obesity–hypoventilation syndrome (Pickwickian syndrome) may benefit from maintained weight reduction. For some such patients, nasally administered CPAP successfully alleviates hypoventilation. Trials of progesterone and protriptyline have also been reported to have some degree of success. Occasionally, patients require artificial airway placement or supplemental ventilation.

Patients with hyperplasia of the tonsils and adenoids as their only cause for obstruction often have dramatic relief of symptoms following tonsillectomy and adenoidectomy. Patients with craniofacial anomalies and with neuromuscular disorders also usually have significant improvement after adenotonsillectomy. Other surgical procedures can be helpful in relieving obstruction in children with craniofacial anomalies or neuromuscular degenerative disorders.

CHAPTER 85
Cystic Fibrosis

Thomas F. Scanlin, M.D.

Cystic fibrosis (CF) is the most common lethal inherited disease among whites in the United States. Most homozygotes for the disease have the "classic triad" of clinical findings: (1) chronic pulmonary disease, (2) malabsorption secondary to pancreatic insufficiency, and (3) elevated concentration of sweat electrolytes. Some of the more common and severe symptoms of CF that are likely to be seen by a physician in an emergency department are listed in Table 85.1. If any of these conditions are present in a patient not previously diagnosed as having CF, the patient should be referred for a sweat.

CLINICAL MANIFESTATIONS

Presentation

Failure to thrive and a history of chronic respiratory or gastrointestinal symptoms are fairly typical. The respiratory symptoms may vary from a mild but persistent cough to recurrent pneumonia and atelectasis. The atypical asthmatic patient who has digital clubbing, bronchiectasis, or a cough productive of purulent sputum may also have CF. Frequent passage of pale, bulky, loose, and excessively foul-smelling stools is characteristic of CF. Edema and hypoproteinemia may develop in children with CF, especially in those who are receiving a soy protein formula. In addition, a hemorrhagic diathesis resulting from vitamin K malabsorption has been reported.

TABLE 85.1. Common Manifestations of Cystic Fibrosis Requiring Emergency Interventions

Meconium ileus	Pneumothorax
Rectal prolapse	Hemoptysis
Intestinal obstruction	Pulmonary exacerbation
Hypoelectrolytemia with metabolic alkalosis	Cor pulmonale
	Respiratory failure

MECONIUM ILEUS

Cystic fibrosis often presents as intestinal obstruction secondary to meconium ileus in the neonatal period. A typical history is that after the first few feedings the infant develops abdominal distension and begins vomiting. The child usually has a history of passing little or no meconium stool. In addition to the obvious abdominal distension, peristaltic waves may be seen on the abdomen, and a mass may be palpable. Three-view radiographic examination may show dilated loops of bowel and a bubbly, granular density in the lower abdomen. In cases of uncomplicated meconium ileus, an enema with diatrizoate methylglucamine (Gastrografin) can be used to clear the obstructing meconium, and surgery may not be necessary.

RECTAL PROLAPSE

Rectal prolapse occurs most commonly in children younger than 3 years old. Although several other conditions may cause a rectal prolapse, the association with CF is common and a sweat test should be performed on a child who has had rectal prolapse. In a child who is known to have CF, rectal prolapse usually results when pancreatic enzyme therapy has been inadequate. Although it may be frightening in appearance, the prolapse can easily be reduced by placing the infant in a comfortable position and using a lubricated glove for manual reduction. It is only in the unusual situation when an intussusception is responsible for the prolapse that bowel strangulation may occur.

INTESTINAL OBSTRUCTION

Acute or chronic crampy abdominal pain is common in CF patients, and an associated fecal mass in the right lower quadrant is often present. Intestinal obstruction occurring beyond the neonatal period in patients with CF is often referred to as *meconium ileus equivalent*. In its mildest form, this situation may be responsible for intermittent abdominal pain. Eventually the fecal mass may cause an obstruction or serve as a leading edge for either an intussusception or a volvulus.

When the roentgenogram of the abdomen shows signs of obstruction, such as dilated loops of bowel and air–fluid levels, a barium or diatrizoate methylglucamine enema must be performed. If a nonreducible volvulus or intussusception is seen, emergency surgery is necessary. In some cases, an associated intussusception may be reduced by using diatrizoate methylglucamine as the contrast agent. If only a fecal mass is present without an associated volvulus or intussusception, medical management using diatrizoate methylglucamine and saline enemas usually results in dissolution of the impacted feces. Because diatrizoate methylglucamine has a very high osmolarity, the infant must be well hydrated before, during, and after the procedure. In cases of fecal impaction without complete obstruction, enemas and oral administration of mineral oil and *N*-acetylcysteine (30 mL in 30 mL of cola) have been reported to be effective.

HYPOELECTROLYTEMIA AND METABOLIC ALKALOSIS

Especially during periods of hot weather, the increased loss of sodium and chloride in the sweat of patients with CF may lead to severe and symptomatic electrolyte depletion. Examples of the electrolyte abnormalities that were seen in two infants are shown in Table 85.2. In these patients, prompt fluid replacement with isotonic saline is critical; 20 to 30 mL per kilogram of body weight should be given within 15 minutes if signs of shock are present or within 1 hour in less severely ill patients. Potassium

TABLE 85.2. Hypoelectrolytemia with Metabolic Alkalosis in Cystic Fibrosis Patients

		Serum electrolytes (mEq/L)				
Patient	Age (mo)	Na	K	Cl	CO_2	Serum pH
1	9	123	2.2	49	48	7.60
2	6	125	2.4	55	41	7.63

chloride should be administered as soon as urine output is established; however, the concentration of potassium should not exceed 40 mEq per liter.

PNEUMOTHORAX

Sudden onset of chest pain often referred to the shoulder and sometimes associated with the acute onset of increasing dyspnea and cyanosis is most likely the result of a pneumothorax. CF patients with a pneumothorax of larger than 10% of the area of the hemithorax should be treated with tube thoracostomy. Needle aspiration of the pneumothorax should be avoided unless the patient's condition is rapidly deteriorating as the result of developing a tension pneumothorax.

HEMOPTYSIS

The expectoration of a small amount of blood, usually seen as blood streaking of the sputum, is a fairly common. The patient's usual home-care regimen does not need to be altered other than considering an appropriate course of antibiotic therapy to treat any intercurrent pulmonary infection. Significant hemoptysis has been arbitrarily defined as the expectoration of at least 30 to 60 mL of fresh blood. Hospitalization for observation is indicated for significant hemoptysis. Blood should be sent for a type and crossmatch in addition to hematocrit and prothrombin time determinations. Intravenous antibiotics against *Staphylococcus* and *Pseudomonas* usually are started. If the patient is dyspneic, oxygen should be administered. If the prothrombin time is prolonged, vitamin K (5 mg initially) should be given. CF patients occasionally present with an episode of massive hemoptysis with volumes of blood loss ranging from 300 to 2500 mL. Massive hemoptysis represents a life-threatening situation, and in addition to instituting the measures already described, the skilled intervention of a team, including a bronchoscopist, anesthesiologist, and thoracic surgeon, may be necessary to maintain an airway and to locate and ligate the bleeding vessel. Bronchial artery embolization has been described for CF patients, and although potentially serious complications may result, this procedure may be valuable when conservative measures fail and surgery is not feasible.

PULMONARY EXACERBATION

Cystic fibrosis patients who experience an increase in respiratory symptoms, such as cough and the rate and effort of breathing, require careful evaluation. On physical examination, the patient will be tachypneic with intercostal retractions and may be cyanotic. Auscultation may reveal areas of coarse rales. A chest roentgenogram should be taken to determine whether pneumothorax, effusion, or local consolidation or atelectasis is present. In many cases, however, the roentgenogram will show only diffuse peribronchial thickening with a varying amount of fluffy infiltrates and hyperinflation. If lobar atelectasis, significant respiratory distress, or hypoxia (PaO_2 <60 mm Hg) is present, the patient should be treated in a hospital setting with vigorous chest physiotherapy and antibiotics effective against *S. aureus* and *P. aeruginosa* (until results of sputum culture are available). Oxygen therapy should be guided by arterial blood gas determination or pulse oximetry. Diffuse expiratory wheezing and prolonged expiration in a patient with CF suggest the possibility of coexisting asthma. A history of respiratory allergy with a good response to bronchodilators provides further support for this diagnosis. If these findings are present, therapy should be administered as outlined under "Asthma" in addition to treating for CF.

COR PULMONALE

Patients with CF who have moderately severe pulmonary insufficiency and some degree of hypoxia eventually develop right ventricular hypertrophy secondary to pulmonary hypertension. In addition to cyanosis, tachypnea, and tachycardia, other associated signs are an enlarged, tender liver and in some patients a gallop rhythm, peripheral edema, and ascites. Most of these patients will have pronounced digital clubbing, which reflects the severity of their pulmonary disease. Rather than the elongated, narrow cardiac silhouette usually seen in the patient with CF, the chest roentgenogram will now show some cardiac enlargement with a prominence of the pulmonary vasculature. Oxygen and diuretics (furosemide 1 mg per kilogram of body weight given intravenously as an initial dose) have been most helpful in addition to starting treatment for the underlying pulmonary disease. Digitalis and pulmonary vasodilators have not been shown to be of proven benefit; however, many CF centers use digitalis during an acute episode of congestive failure and in selected CF patients.

RESPIRATORY FAILURE

When a CF patient presents with respiratory failure (ie, hypercarbia—$PaCO_2$ >60 mm Hg) in addition to hypoxia, the management decisions become extremely difficult. If an acute episode such as viral pneumonia or status asthmaticus precipitates respiratory failure in a CF patient who had a history of good pulmonary function before the episode, mechanical ventilation should be considered. When respiratory failure with increasing hypercarbia occurs in a CF patient after a course of progressive pulmonary insufficiency despite adequate medical therapy, mechanical ventilation is not indicated; however, consultation with the physicians providing long-term care for the patient is important before choosing this course.

CHAPTER 86
Endocrine Emergencies

Daniel E. Hale, M.D.

Table 86.1 summarizes the major clinical features, recommended investigations, and treatments of pediatric endocrine emergencies.

DIABETIC KETOACIDOSIS

Clinical Manifestations

In cases of new-onset diabetes, the child usually has a history of polyuria and polydipsia for a few days or weeks before the acute

TABLE 86.1. Summary of Clinical Features, Investigations, and Initial Treatment of Pediatric Endocrine Emergencies

Condition	Major clinical features	Urgent investigations	Initial treatment
Diabetic ketoacidosis	Polyuria; polydipsia, dehydration, ketotic breath, hyperpnea, nausea, vomiting, abdominal pain, coma	Blood glucose, pH	0.9% saline 20 mL/kg in first hour i.v.; insulin infusion 0.1 U/kg/hr; later, may need KCl 20–30 mEq/L + KPhos; 20–30 mEq/L
Hypoglycemia	*Older child:* hunger, sweatiness, dizziness, convulsions, coma *Neonate:* apnea, hypotonia, hypothermia, irritability, tremor, convulsions	Blood glucose Serum for growth hormone, cortisol, insulin; first voided urine for organic acids and toxin screen	25% dextrose 1–2 mL/kg i.v. bolus or 10% dextrose 5–10 mg/kg/min i.v. infusion, glucagon 0.5–1 mg i.m. stat (if hyperinsulinism)
Congenital adrenal hyperplasia	Ambiguous genitalia in females; poor feeding, weight loss, irritability, vomiting, dehydration	Plasma sodium, potassium, glucose, 17-hydroxyprogesterone; karyotype and pelvic ultrasound	0.9% saline 20 mL/kg in first hour i.v.; deoxycorticosterone acetate 0.5–1 mg i.m. stat; hydrocortisone 25 mg i.v. stat
Adrenal insufficiency	Nausea, vomiting, abdominal pain, weakness, malaise, hypotension, dehydration, hyperpigmentation	Plasma sodium, potassium, glucose, cortisol, and ACTH (for retrospective confirmation of diagnosis)	Hydrocortisone 100 mg i.v. stat; 10% dextrose in 0.9% saline 20 mL/kg in first hour
Hypercalcemia (hyperparathyroidism)	Headache, irritability, anorexia, constipation, polyuria, polydipsia, dehydration, band keratopathy	Plasma calcium, phosphate	0.9% saline at 2–3 times maintenance rate; furosemide 1 mg/kg
Hypocalcemia (hypoparathyroidism)	Cramps, carpopedal spasms, paresthesias, lethargy, apathy, convulsions	Plasma calcium, phosphate, alkaline phosphatase	10% calcium gluconate 0.6% mg/kg (or 5 mg Ca/kg) i.v. over 15 min
Diabetes insipidus	Polyuria, polydipsia, dehydration, irritability, fever, drowsiness, coma	Paired plasma and urine osmolality and sodium	*Central:* 1.5 times maintenance rate; DDAVP 0.4 μg/kg nasally *Nephrogenic:* 5% dextrose at 1.5 times maintenance
Syndrome of inappropriate antidiuretic hormone secretion	Anorexia, headache, nausea, vomiting, irritability, seizures, coma	Paired plasma and urine osmolality and sodium	*Seizures:* 3% saline at 1–3 mL/kg ± furosemide 1 mg/kg i.v. stat *Otherwise:* fluid restriction
Thyroid storm	Goiter, exophthalmos, high fever, tachycardia, congestive cardiac failure, delirium, stupor	Serum T_4, or free T_4, TSH	Propranolol 10 μg/kg i.v. over 15 min; Lugol iodine 15 drops/day orally; propylthiouracil 2–3 mg/kg t.i.d. orally; tepid sponging
Neonatal thyrotoxicosis	Goiter, failure to gain weight, irritability, tachycardia, congestive cardiac Failure	Serum T_4, or free T_4, TSH	Propranolol 1 mg/kg t.i.d. orally; potassium iodide 2 drops/day orally; propylthiouracil 2–3 mg/kg t.i.d. orally
Congenital hypothyroidism	Asymptomatic: hypothermia, hypoactivity, poor feeding, constipation, prolonged jaundice, large posterior fontanelle	Serum T_4, TSH	L-Thyroxine 37.5 μg orally if weight ≥3 kg; 25 μg if <3 kg
Hypopituitarism	See features listed for adrenal insufficiency and hypoglycemia		

i.v., intravenously; i.m., intramuscularly; t.i.d., three times daily; ACTH, adrenocorticotropic hormone; TSH, thyroid-stimulating hormone.

decompensation. Significant weight loss often occurs despite a vigorous appetite. In children known to have diabetes, the prodrome may be less than 24 hours and precipitated by an intercurrent illness, inappropriate sick-day management, or omission of insulin doses. Patients may complain of nausea, vomiting, and abdominal pain, and the parents may have noticed increasing listlessness. On physical examination, particular attention should be paid to the degree of dehydration, including skin turgor and dryness of mucous membranes. In severe cases, the child may exhibit signs of shock, including a thready pulse, cold extremities, and hypotension. The smell of ketones on the breath and the presence of deep sighing (Kussmaul) respirations reflect the ketoacidosis. The patient's consciousness level, which may range from full alertness to deep coma, should be noted. The child may have exquisite abdominal tenderness with guarding and rigidity, which can mimic an acute abdomen. The ears, throat, chest, and urine should be examined because infection is often a precipitating factor.

Typical laboratory findings include a serum glucose greater than 200 mg per deciliter (usually 400–800 mg per deciliter), the presence of glucose and ketones in the urine, acidosis (venous pH <7.3 and HCO <15 mEq per liter), high or normal plasma potassium, and a slightly elevated blood urea nitrogen. Occasionally, diabetic ketoacidosis (DKA) occurs with normoglycemia when persistent vomiting and decreased intake of carbohydrates are accompanied by continued administration of insulin. The serum sodium is usually low or in the low-normal

TABLE 86.2. Principles of Management of Diabetic Ketoacidosis

Life-threatening complications
- Immediate (within the first hours after admission):
  - Cardiovascular collapse
  - Profound metabolic acidosis
- Short-term (within 8–24 hr after start of therapy)
  - Hypokalemia
  - Cerebral edema

Areas of Management Decisions:
- Fluids. Treat hypovolemia with extracellular fluid expander. Use normal saline (154 mEq/L) and infuse 20 mL/kg in the first hour. (Avoid hypotonic solutions initially because they are inefficient volume expanders and may contribute toward cerebral edema.) Continue infusion at this rate until the blood pressure is normal. After first 1–2 hr, start half-normal saline. Total fluid administration in first 24 hr = maintenance + fluid deficit (10% body weight). If calculated serum osmolality is >320 mOsm/L, replace fluid deficit over 36–48 hr.
- Alkali. Consider administering $NaHCO_3$ if blood pH 7.10 or lower. Usual dosage, 2 mEq/kg $NaHCO_3$ infused over 1–2 hr. Then recheck pH, Pco_2 and HCO_3^-. (Avoid bolus infusion of HCO_3 because this may acutely lower serum potassium.)
- Potassium. Start potassium therapy after the patient urinates (usually 1–2 hr after start of fluid therapy). Potassium replacement should be 40 mEq/L as a combination of potassium chloride and potassium phosphate. If the patient is hypokalemic (<4 mEq/L), a higher concentration of potassium, 60 mEq/L, may be necessary. Administer high concentrations of potassium only with electrocardiographic monitoring.
- Insulin. Low-dose insulin is safe and effective. May be given as either a continuous i.v. infusion (0.1 U/kg/hr) or an IM injection (0.25 U/kg initially, followed by 0.1 U/kg/hr).
- Glucose. Add 5% glucose to solutions when serum glucose is approximately 300 mg/dL. This may be given as 5% dextrose in half-normal saline solution.

Monitoring
- Clinical monitoring. Blood pressure, pulse, respirations, neurologic status, and fluid intake and output.
- Laboratory monitoring. Obtain initial glucose, electrolytes, blood gases, and blood urea nitrogen. Measure blood glucose every hour initially as guide to insulin dosage. Repeat electrolytes and pH measurements as necessary.
- Use flow sheet.

range. Leukocytosis may be noted but does not necessarily signify an underlying infection.

Management

This section focuses primarily on the child who is significantly dehydrated, acidotic, and unable to take oral fluids because of vomiting or altered level of consciousness. Many cases of mild DKA can be managed with rehydration, either oral or intravenous, and with supplemental insulin either at home or in the emergency department (ED). This possibility is addressed at the end of this section. For the severely dehydrated child, initial treatment is directed toward rapid expansion of intravascular volume and correction of the acidosis because these are life-threatening conditions. Subsequent treatment is directed at the normalization of all biochemical parameters by the use of insulin. Medical intervention carries significant risks of hypokalemia and cerebral edema (Tables 86.2 and 86.3).

TABLE 86.3. Guide to Treatment of Severe Diabetic Ketoacidosis

			Approximate hourly infusion amount by age (and body weight)[a]						
Calculated osmolality	Time (hr)	Type of fluid	1 (10 g)	5 (18 kg)	10 (30 kg)	15 (50 kg)	Potassium replacement	Bicarbonate replacement	Insulin Infusion Rate (units/kg/hr)
Not relevant	Initial hour[b]	0.9% saline	200	360 mL	600 mL	1000 mL	None	Consider if pH <7.1 or inadequate respiratory compensation	0.1
<320 mOsm/L	1–8[c,d]	0.45% saline	105	170	260	400	If K^+ >4 mEq/L 20 mEq/L KCl+ 20 mEq/L K phosphate	If acidosis does not begin to resolve within the first 8-hr period, suspect either inadequate hydration, inadequate insulin, or underlying illness (e.g., pneumonia)	0.1 adjust to maintain rate of fall of glucose to ~100 mg/dL/hr
>320 mOsm/L[e]	1–16	0.45% saline[f]	75	120	160	250			
<320 mOsm/L	9–24	0.45% saline	75	120	160	250	If K^+ <4 mEq/L 30 mEq/L KCl+ 30 mEq/L K phosphate		
>320 mOsm/L	16–48	0.45% saline	60	90	110	170			

[a] Suggested rate does not include ongoing fluid losses secondary to osmotic diuresis. Urine output in excess of 5 mL/kg/hr should be replaced milliliter for milliliter.
[b] If the child is severely volume depleted, an additional bolus of normal saline (20 mL/kg) may be required. The adequacy of the initial bolus can be evaluated by improving capillary refill and by declining pulse rate.
[c] Rates are based on 10% dehydration and replacement of of deficit in the first 8 hr along with maintenance fluids. Some clinicians now simply distribute the deficit replacement over the entire 23-hr period. The initial bolus of fluids to establish vascular sufficiency is not included in these calculations.
[d] Glucose will need to be added to infusion when glucose is <300 mg/dL. Because the rate of fall in glucose is predictable, the appropriate fluid can be ordered well in advance of this time to avoid the possibility of hypoglycemia.
[e] Rates are based on 10% dehydration and replacement of of deficit in the first 16 hr along with maintenance fluids. The initial bolus of fluids to establish vascular sufficiency is not included in these calculations.
[f] More concentrated saline may be required to prevent excessively rapid fall of osmolality.

FLUID AND ELECTROLYTE REPLACEMENT

In the first hour, isotonic (0.9%) saline should be infused intravenously at 20 mL per kilogram of body weight each hour to establish an adequate vascular volume and to improve tissue perfusion. This procedure may need to be repeated if the pulse rate and capillary refill rate do not decrease. Once adequate intravascular volume is established, the fluid deficit can be replaced over the next 24 to 48 hours, depending on the degree of hyperosmolality; however, once the child is able to drink, rehydration may occur enterally. It can be assumed that the fluid deficit is 10% of the body weight in children with DKA. Dehydration actually may be greater than that estimated on clinical appearance because of the hyperosmolar state. The volume of fluid given should replace the deficit (100 mL per kilogram), provide daily maintenance fluids (see Chapters 14 and 76), and replace ongoing urinary losses in excess of 5 mL per kilogram per hour (osmotic diuresis). For the child whose calculated osmolality is less than 320 mOsm per liter, the deficit can be replaced over 24 hours, but a longer period (36–48 hours) should be used for children with higher osmolalities. From a practical point of view, half-normal (0.45%) saline can be started after the initial bolus of normal saline. If the initial serum K^+ is greater than 4 mEq per liter, 40 mEq per liter of potassium is added to the infusion after vascular competency has been established and the child has urinated. Generally, K^+ is provided as potassium chloride (or acetate) and potassium phosphate in equal amounts. If the initial serum K^+ is less than 4 mEq per ltier, potassium replacement should be initiated promptly; doses of K^+ of 60 mEq per liter or greater may be necessary. If the K^+ initial concentration is low, electrocardiographic (ECG) monitoring is indicated.

ALKALI

The use of sodium bicarbonate for correction of acidosis remains controversial because of the potential for paradoxical acidosis of the central nervous system (CNS) and resultant cerebral depression. Most children's acidosis will correct during rehydration and initiation of insulin therapy without recourse to alkali. Bicarbonate therapy is generally reserved for children with an initial arterial pH of less than 7.1 and for those who are unable to compensate for their acidosis by hyperventilation. The adequacy of compensation can be evaluated if a P_{CO2} and the serum [HCO] are known. If the P_{CO2} is in excess of (1.5 HCO) +8, respiratory effort is inadequate for the degree of acidosis, and bicarbonate is required. The amount of bicarbonate needed may be calculated using the formula:

Amount of bicarbonate (mEq) = Base deficit (mEq/L) × Body weight (kg) × 0.6 (distribution factor for bicarbonate)

Half of this amount is given intravenously over 2 hours. Biochemical studies then are repeated; the need for continued bicarbonate is reevaluated, and, if necessary, a new dose of bicarbonate is calculated and administered. Alternatively, 1 to 2 mEq per kilogram may be given intravenously every hour until the pH is more than 7.25 and the HCO is more than 15 mEq per liter.

INSULIN

Regular insulin is used for the treatment of ketoacidosis. Insulin should be started at the same time as initial fluid expansion to correct the acidosis and either may be infused intravenously or injected intramuscularly at hourly intervals. Subcutaneous injections of insulin should be avoided because of the uncertainties of absorption in a dehydrated patient. The starting dose of insulin for continuous infusion is 0.1 U per kilogram per hour, which is normally infused by a regulated pump. The rate of insulin infusion should be adjusted to sustain a fall in the blood glucose of about 100 mg per deciliter per hour. Failure of the glucose to decrease in response to insulin suggests improper insulin preparation, inadequate hydration, or serious underlying disease (eg, appendicitis with resultant significant increases in counterregulatory hormones). It is unnecessary to give an initial bolus of insulin. The dose for the hourly intramuscular injection is 0.25 U per kilogram as a priming dose followed by 0.1 U per kilogram per hour. Once the blood sugar is less than 300 mg per deciliter, glucose should be added to the intravenous fluids. As long as the child remains acidotic, insulin infusion should never be stopped; instead, the amount of glucose in the IV infusion should be increased and the insulin infusion adjusted to maintain the blood sugar between 100 and 200 mg per deciliter. When the child is able to eat and is no longer significantly acidotic, intravenous infusion of insulin can be discontinued. Because intravenous insulin is metabolized rapidly, subcutaneous insulin must be given promptly after the infusion is stopped. The initial dose of regular insulin should be about 0.25 U per kilogram.

The serum glucose should be measured hourly until the blood glucose is stable and below 300 mg per deciliter and as long as the child is on an insulin infusion. Glucose measurement may be less frequent once the patient has been changed to subcutaneous insulin. Serum K^+ needs to be measured every 3 to 4 hours until the acidosis and hyperglycemia are normalized or more frequently if hypokalemia is encountered or bicarbonate therapy is used. An arterial pH should be obtained before treatment and repeated if bicarbonate therapy is used or contemplated.

Mild Ketoacidosis

Some children with new-onset diabetes also may have hyperglycemia without ketoacidosis or with only mild acidosis. Generally, these patients are hospitalized for at least 12 to 24 hours to allow time to educate the family and stabilize the insulin dosage. These children require rehydration (as described in the next section), similar to patients with known diabetes and mild ketoacidosis. Insulin therapy can be initiated subcutaneously, at a total daily dose of 0.25 to 0.5 U per kilogram daily for the prepubertal child and 0.5 to 0.75 U per kilogram daily for the adolescent. Two-thirds of the total daily dose is administered in the morning and one-third before dinner; two-thirds of the morning dose and one-half of the evening dose should be as an intermediate duration insulin (NPH, Lente).

Children with known diabetes often develop mild ketoacidosis during the course of intercurrent illness, especially gastroenteritis, or secondary to omission of insulin doses. Even the mildly dehydrated (5%) child with slight acidosis who presents to the ED benefits from a fluid bolus (20 mL per kilogram of normal saline); furthermore, this bolus will be given while awaiting laboratory test results. Once the laboratory results are available, the physician must decide whether to hospitalize the child, continue treatment in the ED, or send the child home. For purposes of definition, *mild DKA* is defined as a pH of more than 7.3, a bicarbonate of more than 15 mEq/L, and a calculated osmolality of less than 320 mOsm/L. Children who are significantly acidotic or hyperosmolar should be hospitalized and managed as outlined in the earlier section of this chapter. Several factors must be considered before sending a child home:

1. Is the child conscious and alert?
2. Can the child drink and retain oral fluids?
3. Can home glucose monitoring be done, and are all related supplies available in the home?
4. Will the child have competent supervision at home?
5. Does the family have access to both a telephone and transportation?

6. Is there a physician available with whom the family can communicate by telephone?
7. Is the family comfortable with managing the mild acidosis at home?

If all these questions can be answered in the affirmative, the child may be sent home.

Oral intake should be about the same as would be given intravenously to resolve the deficit and provide maintenance (eg, the 10-year-old child would normally get about 260 mL per hour during the first 8 hours, administered intravenously, if he or she was hospitalized; therefore, the physician should suggest that the family try to get in about 8 ounces of liquid every hour for the next 6 to 8 hours). It is best if this liquid is taken in as sips. Additional insulin will be required. In the ED, two decisions will need to be made regarding insulin: First, how much should be given to the child before dismissal? Usually, an amount equal to 10% of the child's usual daily dose will be adequate (eg, a child normally takes 12 U R and 6 U N in the morning and 6 U R and 6 U N in the evening). The total daily dose is 30 U. Ten percent of 30 = 3 U. Therefore, 3 U of regular insulin would be given to the child before discharge. Second, how much should be given at home and with what frequency? Once home, the preceding 10% rule is generally applicable. If the blood glucose has not come down within 1 to 2 hours, consultation with the child's physician is recommended. If the blood glucose has decreased but is still more than 250 mg per deciliter, a second dose of similar size is indicated. If a third home dose is contemplated, consultation with the child's physician is required. Many children have insulin adjustment algorithms for premeal adjustments from their endocrinologist. The family can begin using this algorithm once the child is able to return to a normal intake. Last, hourly monitoring of blood glucose, urine output, and ketones is recommended with the expectation that the blood glucose should decline, the urine output should fall, and the urine ketones should begin to clear.

HYPOGLYCEMIA

Clinical Manifestations

A differential diagnosis of hypoglycemia, as it may present in the ED, is provided in Table 86.4. The acutely ill child warrants a glucose determination if the level of consciousness is altered because hypoglycemia may accompany an illness that interferes with oral intake. Historical evidence may aid in establishing the cause of hypoglycemia. The possibility of ingestion should be considered because ethanol, propranolol, and oral hypoglycemic agents are in common use. The clinical findings of hypoglycemia reflect both the decreased availability of glucose to the CNS and the adrenergic stimulation caused by a decreasing or low blood sugar. Adrenergic symptoms and signs include palpitations, anxiety, tremulousness, hunger, and sweating. Irritability, headache, fatigue, confusion, seizure, and unconsciousness are neuroglycopenic symptoms. Any combination of these symptoms should lead to a consideration of hypoglycemia. Any child presenting with a seizure or unconsciousness should have a serum glucose determination.

Management

If hypoglycemia is suspected, blood should be obtained, if at all possible, before treatment is initiated. An extra tube (3 mL, red top) should be obtained and refrigerated until the laboratory glucose is known. Rapid screening should be performed using a portable glucose monitor while awaiting definitive laboratory results. Therapy should be instituted if this screen is suggestive of hypoglycemia. If the laboratory glucose confirms that the blood glucose was less than 50 mg per deciliter, the reserved serum can be used for chemical (β-hydroxybutyrate, acetoacetate, free fatty acids, carnitine), toxicologic, and hormonal (insulin, growth hormone, cortisol) studies and may provide the correct diagnosis without extensive additional testing. The first voided urine after the hypoglycemic episode should be saved for toxicologic and organic acid evaluation.

The preferred treatment for hypoglycemia is 0.25 g of dextrose per kilogram of body weight (2.5 mL per kilogram of 10% dextrose per kilogram, 1.0 mL per kilogram of 25% dextrose per kilogram) rapidly. The serum glucose should then be maintained by an infusion of dextrose at a rate of 6 to 8 mg per kilogram per minute. Generally, this goal can be accomplished by providing 10% dextrose at 1.5 times maintenance rates. Glucagon (1 mg administered intramuscularly) may be used to treat hypoglycemia that is known to be caused by hyperinsulinism but is not indicated as part of the routine therapy of hypoglycemia. Cortisol should not be used because it has minimal

TABLE 86.4. Causes of Childhood Hypoglycemia

Decreased availability of glucose
Decreased intake—fasting, malnutrition, illness
Decreased absorption—acute diarrhea
Inadequate glycogen reserves—defects in enzymes of glycogen synthetic pathways
Ineffective glycogenolysis—defects in enzymes of glycogenolytic pathway
Inability to mobilize glycogen—glucagon deficiency
Ineffective gluconeogenesis—defects in enzymes of gluconeogenic pathway
Increased use of glucose
Hyperinsulinism—islet cell adenoma or hyperplasia, nesidioblastosis, ingestion of oral hypoglycemic agents, insulin therapy
Large tumors—Wilms tumor
Diminished availability of alternative fuels
Decreased or absent fat stones
Inability to oxidize fats—enzymatic defects in fatty acid oxidation
Unknown or complex mechanisms
Sepsis/shock
Reye syndrome
Salicylate ingestion
Ethanol ingestion
Adrenal insufficiency
Hypothyroidism
Hypopituitarism

acute benefit and may delay identification of the cause of hypoglycemia. Any child with documented hypoglycemia not secondary to insulin therapy should be hospitalized for careful monitoring and diagnostic testing.

ACUTE ADRENAL INSUFFICIENCY

Clinical Manifestations

The historical information suggestive of adrenal insufficiency depends on the cause. Children with a primary adrenal defect are more likely to have had a gradual onset of symptoms, such as general malaise, anorexia, fatigue, and weight loss. Salt craving and postural hypotension also may have been noted. A child with secondary adrenal insufficiency is more likely to have a history of neurosurgical procedures, head trauma, CNS pathology, or chronic disease necessitating the prolonged use of glucocorticoids. Findings on physical examination are more likely to be characteristic of the precipitating illness or trauma rather than specifically suggestive of adrenal insufficiency. Although a lack of glucocorticoid and aldosterone can be associated with hypotension and dehydration, a better clue to the possibility of adrenal insufficiency is inappropriately rapid decompensation in the face of metabolic stress. Hyperpigmentation may be present in primary adrenal insufficiency, especially of long duration. Biochemical evidence suggestive of adrenal insufficiency includes hyponatremia, hyperkalemia, hypoglycemia, and hemoconcentration. Mild metabolic acidosis and hypercalcemia may be present. The definitive diagnosis depends on the demonstration of an inappropriately low level of cortisol in the serum.

Management

Treatment of adrenal crisis is based on rapid volume expansion and the administration of glucocorticoids. Immediate management consists of 50 to 100 mg of hydrocortisone administered intravenously. Subsequent management is hydrocortisone 50 mg/m^2 per 24 hours given continuously intravenously or methylprednisolone (Solu-Medrol) 7.5 mg/m^2 per 24 hours divided and administered every 8 hours intravenously. Volume expansion is accomplished with normal saline (20 mL per kilogram) in the first hour, followed by fluids appropriate for maintenance and replacement. Additional Na^+ may be needed in primary adrenal insufficiency because of ongoing urinary Na^+ losses. These fluids should contain 10% dextrose and should not contain potassium until the serum potassium is within the normal range. Mineralocorticoid therapy is rarely important in the acute phase, provided fluid therapy is adequate; however, patients with primary adrenal insufficiency may need replacement with a mineralocorticoid for long-term management. Specific therapy directed toward correction of the hyperkalemia is rarely required unless cardiac arrhythmias are present. Hypoglycemia is remedied by the use of dextrose and by the hyperglycemic effects of glucocorticoids. The precipitating factor, such as infection, also requires appropriate therapy.

CONGENITAL ADRENAL HYPERPLASIA

Clinical Manifestations

Initial evidence of congenital adrenal hyperplasia (CAH) may be acquired at birth with the discovery of ambiguous genitalia, between 2 to 5 weeks of age when the infant presents with acute salt-losing crisis, or during childhood with the onset of precocious puberty. The subsequent discussion deals primarily with the recognition and management of the acute salt-losing crisis, which is life threatening. Salt wasting is present shortly after birth, but acute crisis usually does not occur until the second week of life. The appearance of symptoms can be insidious, with a history of poor feeding, lack of weight gain, lethargy, irritability, and vomiting. The nonspecificity of symptoms may lead to consideration of diagnoses far removed from CAH and delay initiation of treatment.

In severe cases, there may be shock and metabolic acidosis. The genitalia should be examined carefully because the degree of ambiguity of the genitalia varies considerably. Virilized females may have an enlarged clitoris and fusion of the labial folds. An undervirilized male may have a small phallus or hypospadias. The presence of gonads in the inguinal canals or labioscrotal fold is suggestive of a male karyotype. Hyperpigmentation of the labioscrotal folds and the nipples is occasionally present in the neonatal period; however, it is rarely prominent enough to alert the examiner to the possibility of CAH.

In the ED, the most urgent investigations are plasma electrolytes and blood glucose. The combination of hyperkalemia and hyponatremia is often the first clue to the diagnosis of CAH, especially in male infants. The plasma potassium is elevated, but in the presence of vomiting and diarrhea, the rise may be blunted. Levels between 6 and 12 mEq per liter are commonly encountered, often without any clinical cardiac dysfunction or ECG changes. The plasma bicarbonate level is usually low, reflecting the metabolic acidosis that results from the retention of hydrogen ions in exchange for sodium loss. The blood glucose is usually normal; however, hypoglycemia may occur secondary to the lack of cortisol and the reduced caloric intake during the acute illness. Serum should be drawn for determination of an adrenal steroid profile to include 17-hydroxyprogesterone, dehydroepiandrosterone, androstenedione, and testosterone.

Management

If the child is dehydrated, fluid replacement is urgent. Volume expansion should be effected by the rapid infusion of 20 mL per kilogram of normal saline in the first hour or more rapidly, if needed. Because the dehydration in salt-losing CAH represents urinary losses of isosmotic fluid, replacement should consist of normal saline (0.9%). The volume to be replaced should constitute the child's daily requirements as well as the estimated fluid loss. Principal management of the mineralocorticoid deficit is by the provision of sodium. In addition, hydrocortisone has some mineralocorticoid effect, particularly at high dosages. For long-term management, the child will require mineralocorticoid replacement (fludrocortisone 0.1 mg daily). Most infants also require oral Na^+ supplements for the first several months of life. Hydrocortisone (25 mg) should be given in an intravenous bolus, followed by hydrocortisone 50 mg/m^2 per 24 hours as a constant infusion. Alternatively, cortisone acetate 25 mg intramuscularly immediately, followed by 25 mg every 24 hours, may be used.

Infants with CAH tolerate hyperkalemia far better than do other children and adults, with potassium levels as high as 12 mEq per liter reported without clinical signs. Volume restoration with normal saline is the major, and usually the only, measure needed to lower the potassium. In the presence of arrhythmias, intravenous 10% calcium gluconate can be given for its membrane-stabilizing properties. Therapy with glucose and insulin is contraindicated because of the danger of precipitating hypoglycemia. If hypoglycemia is found at presentation, it should be treated acutely by the administration of dextrose (0.25 g per kilogram) intravenously and by the subsequent inclusion of 10% dextrose in the infusion. Acidosis generally does not require specific treatment; however, the low serum bicarbonate may take days to fully correct.

PHEOCHROMOCYTOMA

Clinical Manifestations

The most common symptoms are headache, palpitations, and excessive or inappropriate sweating. The headache, characteristically, is pounding and may be severe. The palpitations may be accompanied by tachycardia. Almost all patients will have one of the three symptoms listed, and most will have at least two. Other symptoms may include nervousness, tremor, fatigue, chest or abdominal pains, and flushing. The most useful screening tool for pheochromocytoma is the blood pressure cuff because most pheochromocytomas are associated with hypertension. Because this hypertension may be continuous or paroxysmal, frequent and repeated blood pressure determinations may be necessary. Hypertension is most likely to be found when the patient is symptomatic. A hypertensive patient who is asymptomatic is unlikely to have a pheochromocytoma.

The diagnosis of a pheochromocytoma also should be considered in patients with malignant hypertension, in those who fail to respond or respond inappropriately to antihypertensive medications, and in those who develop hypertension during the induction of anesthesia or during surgery. Incidence of pheochromocytomas is increased among patients with neurofibromatosis and in those with multiple endocrine neoplasia syndromes type II and type III. Documentation of excess catecholamine in either the urine or serum confirms the diagnosis of pheochromocytoma. The most readily available and widely used test for this purpose is the measurement of urinary catecholamines or their metabolites (3-methoxy-4-hydroxymandelic acid and total metanephrines) in a 24-hour urine collection.

Management

The focus of ED management should be on controlling hypertension and hypertensive crisis that may occur before the surgical procedure. α-Adrenergic blocking agents are useful in controlling hypertension and in minimizing blood pressure fluctuations during the surgical procedure. Preferred drugs for controlling hypertension are phenoxybenzamine (Dibenzyline) and prazosin (Minipress). Dosage schedules and quantity must be tailored to the individual for adequate control of hypertension. Hypertensive crisis may be appropriately managed with intravenous phentolamine (Regitine 1 mg intravenously for children; 5 mg for adolescents) or sodium nitroprusside (0.5–8.0 μg per kilogram per minute).

DIABETES INSIPIDUS

Clinical Manifestations

Either a deficiency of ADH secretion from the hypothalamus and posterior pituitary gland or renal unresponsiveness to ADH can cause this diabetes insipidus (DI) (Table 86.5). Urine excretion is increased in both volume and frequency in the child with DI. This condition may manifest as enuresis in the younger child. Provided the thirst mechanism is intact and fluids are accessible, the child can compensate for the water loss by drinking more. A history may be elicited of the child's awakening in the middle of the night to drink. If fluids are not available or if fluid intake is interrupted because of a viral illness, dehydration rapidly ensues. In the young infant who is not provided with adequate fluids and consequently is chronically dehydrated, the child may fail to thrive or may have a history of intermittent low-grade fevers. On the other hand, if the cries of the infant are interpreted as hunger rather than thirst, the infant with DI may be obese.

Physical examination may be normal, or signs of dehydration, such as dryness of mucous membranes, decreased skin turgor, sunken eyes, and in an infant, a depressed anterior fontanel, may be present. Because of the hyperosmolarity, the degree of dehydration may be underestimated on physical examination. Hypothalamic or pituitary lesions can lead to other endocrine abnormalities such as secondary hypothyroidism and growth failure. A craniopharyngioma or optic nerve glioma may affect the visual fields or cause raised intracranial pressure, which is indicated by papilledema.

TABLE 86.5. Causes of Diabetes Insipidus in Children

- Antidiuretic hormone deficiency
  - Head injury
  - Meningitis
  - Idiopathic
  - Suprasellar tumors and their treatment by surgery or radiotherapy
    - Craniopharyngioma
    - Optic nerve glioma
    - Dysgerminoma
  - Septooptic dysplasia
  - Association with midline cleft palate
  - Familial (dominant or sex-linked recessive)
  - Wolfram syndrome (diabetes insipidus, diabetes mellitus, optic atrophy, deafness)
  - Histiocytosis X (Hand-Schuller-Christian disease)
- Nephrogenic diabetes insipidus
  - Sex-linked recessive
  - Renal disease
    - Polycystic kidneys
    - Hydronephrosis
    - Chronic pyelonephritis
  - Hypercalcemia
  - Hypokalemia
  - Toxins:
    - Demeclocyclin
    - Lithium
  - Sickle cell disease
  - Idiopathic

Diagnosis of DI is achieved by demonstrating that the kidneys fail to concentrate urine when fluid intake is restricted. This condition can be difficult to prove in children. Nonetheless, an adequate working diagnosis usually is obtained by finding an elevated serum osmolality (normal, <290 mOsm/L) and an elevated serum [Na] (normal, <145 mmol per liter) in the presence of dilute urine (normal osmolality >150 mOsm per liter). Blood glucose and serum creatinine levels are normal. The definitive diagnosis is made by a formal water deprivation test.

Management

In most cases, a diagnosis of DI is not known at presentation; therefore, the acute management is directed toward correction of the dehydration and the hyperosmolar state. The treatment of DI is similar to that described for hypernatremic dehydration (see Chapter 14) with the notable addition that the fluid required for the replacement of urinary fluid losses will be far greater. In fact, the high urinary output, despite significant dehydration, often provides the first and most convincing evidence for DI. If the child is hypotensive or if the serum Na^+ is greater than 160 mmol per liter, initial volume expansion is necessary, using 20 mL per kilogram of normal saline during the first hour or more rapidly, if needed. Once an adequate intravascular volume has been achieved, further fluid replacement is accomplished slowly because overly rapid volume correction can cause cerebral edema, seizures, and death. If the child is not hypotensive, or once the hypotension has been corrected, free water replacement is done over 48 hours. Calculations of appropriate fluids must include maintenance requirements, replacement needs, and ongoing urinary losses (see Chapter 14).

If DI is strongly suspected on the basis of discrepant serum and urine osmolality, desmopressin (DDAVP; 5–20 μg intranasally or 0.2–0.4 μg per kilogram administered subcutaneously) may be a useful adjunct to intravenous fluid therapy. If DDAVP is not available or cannot be used for some reason, other antidiuretic agents are available (aqueous pitressin 1–5 U administered intramuscularly or 2–3 μU per kilogram per minute as a constant intravenous drip). DDAVP acts rapidly to promote tubular resorption of free H_2O; clinically, this reaction is apparent as decreased urinary output with increased osmolality within an hour of administration. Failure to respond to DDAVP suggests the possibility of tubular unresponsiveness to ADH (nephrogenic DI); however, more commonly, failure to respond results from improper administration of the medication or use of DDAVP that has lost its potency. Because of these factors, if cessation of diuresis is not noted within 2 hours of administration of the first dose, a second dose from a different bottle of DDAVP should be tried. Paradoxically, the thiazide diuretics have proven useful in the chronic control of nephrogenic DI.

SYNDROME OF INAPPROPRIATE ANTIDIURETIC HORMONE SECRETION

Clinical Manifestations

Most patients with the syndrome of inappropriate antidiuretic hormone secretion (SIADH) (Table 86.6) are asymptomatic until the plasma [Na] falls below 120 mmol per liter.. Symptoms associated with hyponatremia range from anorexia, headache, nausea, vomiting, irritability, disorientation, and weakness to seizures and coma, leading ultimately to death. Absence of edema and dehydration are significant clinical findings. Laboratory investigations for diagnostic purposes must include concomitant serum and urine samples (Table 86.7). Hyponatremia, hypoosmolality (serum), and low blood urea nitrogen will be present. In contrast, the urinary osmolality and [Na] are inappropriately elevated for the hypotonicity of the serum. Radioimmunoassay for ADH is now available and has been helpful in defining this syndrome; however, the results of this test are unlikely to be available on an emergency basis. The underlying cause of the syndrome should be investigated according to the physician's' clinical judgment. In the presence of hyperglycemia, hyperlipidemia, or hyperproteinemia, the serum sodium may be falsely low. Renal salt wasting, secondary to adrenal insufficiency, should be accompanied by hyperkalemia and dehydration. The urine osmolality in water intoxication states is usually low compared with that found in SIADH.

Management

SEVERELY SYMPTOMATIC CHILDREN

Patients with a persistent seizure attributable to severe hyponatremia and those who are lethargic or comatose need urgent treatment. Hypertonic (3%) saline is the preferred treatment. Infusing small amounts of 3% saline in the range of 3 mL per kilogram of body weight every 10 to 20 minutes until symptoms remit is probably the safest course of treatment. A single dose of furosemide (1 mg per kilogram) also can be administered intra-

TABLE 86.6. Some Causes of Syndrome of Inappropriate Antidiuretic Hormone Secretion (SIADH) in Children

Disorders of central nervous system	Miscellaneous
Infection (meningitis, encephalitis)	Pain (e.g., after abdominal surgery)
Trauma, postneurosurgery	Severe hypothyroidism
Hypoxic insults, especially in the perinatal period	Congenital deficiency
Brain tumor	Tumors (e.g. neuroblastoma)
Intraventricular hemorrhage	Idiopathic deficiency
Guillain-Barré syndrome	Drug-induced
Psychosis	Increased antidiuretic hormone secretion
Intrathoracic disorders	Vincristine
Infection (tuberculosis, pneumonia, empyema)	Cyclophosphamide
Positive-pressure ventilation	Carbamazepine
Asthma	Adenine arabinoside
Cystic fibrosis	Phenothiazines
Pneumothorax	Morphine
Patent ductus arteriosus ligation	Potentiation of antidiuretic hormone effect
	Acetaminophen
	indomethacin

TABLE 86.7. Criteria for Diagnosis of Syndrome of Inappropriate Antidiuretic Hormone Secretion (SIADH)

Hyponatremia, reduced serum osmolality
Urine osmolality that is inappropriately elevated (a urine osmolality <100 mOsm/kg usually excludes the diagnosis)
Urinary Na concentration that is excessive in comparison to the degree of hyponatremia (usually >18 mEq/L)
Normal renal, adrenal, and thyroid function
Absence of volume depletion

venously. Close monitoring of fluid balance, plasma and urinary sodium, potassium, and osmolality is essential. Phenytoin (Dilantin) intravenously (5–10 mg per kilogram) inhibits ADH release and may be helpful in the patient with seizures secondary to CNS causes of SIADH. The underlying cause of SIADH, such as meningitis, should be treated when possible; successful treatment is usually accompanied by remission of inappropriate antidiuresis.

ASYMPTOMATIC OR MILDLY SYMPTOMATIC CHILDREN

Asymptomatic or mildly symptomatic patients are treated by rigorous fluid restriction. If the patient is not vascularly compromised, fluid input should be sharply limited, often below insensible loss, until the [Na] and osmolality begin to rise. If the initial [Na] is less than 125 mmol per liter, all fluids must be withheld. The child with chronic or recurrent episodes of SIADH may require treatment with demeclocycline 10 mg per kilogram of body weight. The underlying cause should be identified, treated, and eliminated, if possible.

HYPERPARATHYROIDISM

Clinical Manifestations

Hyperparathyroidism has two common presentations in children. The first presentation is the critically ill infant who is found to have severe hypercalcemia during the course of diagnostic investigations. The second presentation is a child in the early to midteens with nonspecific symptoms including nausea, constipation, unexplained weight loss, personality changes, and headaches. Diffuse bone pain or renal colic may be reported, although these symptoms are less common in children than in adults. The physical findings of hypercalcemia are hypotonia, weakness, and listlessness. Rarely, a palpable mass is located in the parathyroid region. Radiologic findings consistent with hyperparathyroidism include evidence of demineralization and bone resorption.

Hypercalcemia is usually present but may be subtle or intermittent in mild cases. The serum inorganic phosphate level is usually low but may be normal, especially in patients with decreased renal function. Mild hyperchloremic acidosis may be present. Alkaline phosphates level and urinary hydroxyproline excretion may be elevated secondary to increased osteoclast activity. Because parathyroid hormone (PTH) causes a significant increase in cyclic adenosine monophosphate (cAMP) in the kidney tubule, the presence of excess cAMP in the urine is strongly suggestive of excess PTH production. The determination of PTH levels is critical for diagnostic purposes, and elevated levels of PTH, when the patient is hypercalcemic, is a definitive laboratory finding.

Management

Acute management of hyperparathyroidism is essentially the same as management of hypercalcemia (see Chapter 76). The specific management of hyperparathyroidism depends on the level of calcium and on the presence of signs and symptoms. In the asymptomatic patient with a serum calcium level below 12 mg per deciliter, careful follow-up with close attention to both bone mass and renal function is recommended. If the child is persistently hypercalcemic, parathyroid surgery is the preferred treatment.

HYPOPARATHYROIDISM

Clinical Manifestations

The predominant historical features and clinical manifestations of hypoparathyroidism are the same as those of hypocalcemia (see Chapter 76). The particular symptoms and signs found depend on the age at onset of the disease, the chronicity of the disease, and the presence of other autoimmune or syndromic phenomena. Papilledema without hemorrhage may be seen during the initial examination and tends to resolve within several days after the initiation of therapy. Lenticular cataracts are common in hypoparathyroidism and are associated with long-standing hypocalcemia of any cause. Psychiatric and neurologic disorders occur in association with hypoparathyroidism. Subnormal intelligence occurs in about 20% of children with the idiopathic form of hypoparathyroidism, and the severity correlates closely with the period of untreated hypocalcemia. Dry, scaly skin is a common finding, as is patchy alopecia. Psoriasis or mucocutaneous candidiasis may be found on occasion. Unusually brittle fingernails and hair are often found. Hypoplasia of tooth enamel may be seen if hypoparathyroidism was present at the time of dental development. Intestinal malabsorption and steatorrhea have been reported in association with hypoparathyroidism.

In most cases, the diagnosis of hypoparathyroidism is first considered when low serum calcium is found. If an elevated phosphate accompanies low calcium, a low or normal serum alkaline phosphate, and normal blood urea nitrogen, hypoparathyroidism is a likely possibility. Finding a low or unmeasurable level of PTH in the presence of hypocalcemia and hyperphosphatemia makes the definitive diagnosis. Because PTH increases cAMP levels in the urine, the excreted amount of cAMP in the urine is low in patients with hypoparathyroidism and rises briskly with the administration of exogenous PTH.

Management

The acute management of hypoparathyroidism is essentially the management of the hypocalcemia (see Chapter 76). Long-term management consists of treatment with vitamin D, usually with one of its more active analogs—1,25-$(OH)_2D_3$. Supplemental oral calcium is almost always necessary.

RICKETS

Clinical Manifestations

Children with rickets may come to medical attention because of specific physical abnormalities (bowed legs), limb pain and swelling, seizures, failure to thrive (renal tubular acidosis), biochemical abnormalities (hypocalcemia), or radiographic findings (broadened, frayed metaphysis). A thorough social and dietary history is helpful in delineating the probable cause and in sparing the patient an extensive and expensive evaluation. A family history may be useful in identifying the 1-hydroxylase deficiency or renal phosphate wasting.

The clinical findings in rickets may vary considerably depending on the underlying disorder, the duration of the problem, and the child's age. Most features are related to skeletal deformity, skeletal pain, slippage of epiphyses, bony fractures, and growth disturbances. Muscular weakness, hypotonia, and lethargy are often noted. Failure of calcification affects those parts of the skeleton that are growing most rapidly or that are under stress. For example, the skull grows rapidly in the perinatal period; therefore, craniotabes is a manifestation of congenital rickets. On the other hand, the upper limbs and rib cage grow rapidly during the first year of life, and abnormalities at these sites are more common at this age (ie, rachitic rosary, flaring of the wrist). Bowing of the legs is unlikely to be noted until the child is ambulatory. Dental eruption may be delayed, and enamel defects are common.

Radiography is the optimal way to confirm the clinical diagnosis because the radiologic features reflect the histopathology. Characteristic findings include widening and irregularity of the epiphyseal plates, cupped metaphyses, fractures, and bowing of the weight-bearing limbs. The clinical laboratory is often helpful in correctly identifying the cause of rickets. Frank hypocalcemia (<7 mg/dL) is unusual in rickets. Calcium levels in the range of 7 to 9 mg per deciliter range are common and warrant careful attention because the initiation of vitamin D treatment increases bony deposition of calcium and may lead to a fall in serum calcium. Phosphate levels are often low. An amino aciduria is often present and may lead to some confusion of simple vitamin D deficiency with Fanconi syndrome. Alkaline phosphatase levels are significantly increased, reflecting extremely active bony metabolism.

Management

Treatment depends on the nature of the underlying disease. The response to treatment may be helpful in differentiating simple dietary vitamin D deficiency from more complex causes of rickets. In the absence of chronic disease, dietary rickets may be adequately treated with daily doses of 1000 to 2000 IU of vitamin D until healing occurs. If the initial serum calcium is borderline low or low, supplemental calcium should be initiated 48 hours before the institution of vitamin D, especially in the young child. Otherwise, the institution of vitamin D may cause a further decrease in serum calcium and elicit frank hypocalcemia. Children with symptomatic hypocalcemia or an initial serum calcium level of less than 7 mg per deciliter on presentation warrant hospitalization and frequent calcium determinations.

CHAPTER 87

Metabolic Emergencies (Inborn Errors Of Metabolism)

Marc Yudkoff, M.D.

UREA CYCLE DEFECTS

CLINICAL MANIFESTATIONS

Neonatal Catastrophe

The disorder usually manifests during the first few days of life, after the baby ingests protein in infant formula or breast milk. Vomiting is a common early finding, followed by poor feeding, a loss of muscle tone, and a progressive diminution of consciousness culminating in frank coma. Convulsions occur in many cases. Hepatomegaly without liver failure is often observed.

Recurrent Coma in the Older Infant and Child with Retarded Psychomotor Development

Urea cycle defects may be the true cause of developmental delay in the older infant or child who is thought to have cerebral palsy. Careful questioning of the parents may elicit a history of vomiting and/or lethargy after ingestion of protein-rich foods.

Recurrent Vomiting and Ataxia

Frank psychomotor retardation does not occur, but physical development is poor because of inadequate dietary intake. Vomiting, dizziness, ataxia, and obtundation may result in repeated hospitalizations.

Progressive Neurologic Deterioration

These patients seem normal for years, after which intellectual performance and overall neurologic function decline progressively.

LABORATORY FINDINGS

Blood ammonia levels are usually elevated in the acutely ill child. The blood urea may be low, as would be anticipated in a disorder of ureagenesis, but a normal blood urea does not exclude a congenital hyperammonemia syndrome. The blood electrolytes, including pH, are usually normal. Extreme hyperammonemia may be accompanied by elevation of the blood transaminases and other enzymes marking liver dysfunction. Indeed, the urea cycle defects have been confused with Reye syndrome.

MANAGEMENT (SEE TABLE 87.1)

Blood ammonia must be lowered as quickly as possible because the long-term prognosis depends on the severity and duration of hyperammonemia. Effective management should include: 1) minimization of ammonia production and 2) facilitation of ammonia removal. The administration of 10% glucose and 45 mEq

TABLE 87.1. Summary of Clinical Features, Investigations, and Initial Treatment of Inborn Errors of Metabolism

Condition	Major clinical features	Urgent investigations	Initial treatment
Urea cycle defects	Neonate: obtundation, vomiting, seizures, apnea, hypotonia, irritability, hepatomegaly Older child: mental retardation, growth failure, recurrent ataxia, headache, personality changes, inappropriate reaction to infection, neurodegeneration Argininemia: presents as progressive spastic diplegia	Measure blood NH_3, amino acids, electrolytes, glucose Ascertain whether the child has increased intracranial pressure	Sodium benzoate 500 mg/kg/d if NH_3 >200 mM; 250 mg/kg/d if NH_3 <200 mM Sodium phenylbutyrate 500 mg/kg/d if NH_3 >200 mM; 250 mg/kg/d if NH_3 <200 mM I.V.: 10% glucose and 40 mEq/L NaCl, 20 mEq/L KCl at 2× maintenance
Organic acidemias	Neonate: obtundation, poor feeding, vomiting, seizures, hypothermia, apnea, irritability, unusual odors, peeling skin, increased intracranial pressure	Measure blood for pH, P_{CO_2}, amino acids, glucose, electrolytes, NH_3, lactate, pyruvate Measure urine for organic acids, ketones, pH Ascertain whether the child has increased intracranial pressure	Acidemia: 1–3 mEq/kg $NaHCO_3$ (severe acidemia requires higher dosages) Hypoglycemia: 1 g glucose/kg (4 mL/kg of 25% solution); follow with 10% infusion I.V.: 10% glucose and 20 mEq/L NaCl + 20 mEq/L $NaHCO_3$ + 20 mEq/L KCl at 2× maintenance
Galactosemia	Neonate: jaundice, hepatomegaly, diarrhea, vomiting, emaciation, cataracts, irritability, seizures, hemolysis, *Escherichia coli,* sepsis Older child: mental retardation, growth failure, cataracts, pseudotumor cerebri, milk intolerance	Urine for reducing substances (Clintest) If positive, do carbohydrate chromatography of urine and screening test for galactose-1-phosphate uridyl transferase in erythrocytes	I.V.: 10% glucose and 40 mEq/L NaCl, 20 mEq/L KCl at 2× maintenance Withhold all galactose-containing foods

per liter sodium chloride at twice the maintenance fluid rate should be adequate. Unless the patient has acidemia, bicarbonate should not be given because alkalinization of the blood favors conversion of NH_4^+ to NH_3, which more readily traverses the blood–brain barrier than does the ionized species.

In the emergency department (ED), it is preferable to administer benzoate (250 to 500 mg per kg per day) as a parenteral (10%) solution. Benzoate treatment can be supplemented with enteral (oral or nasogastric) sodium phenylbutyrate (250 to 500 mg per kg per day), which the liver converts to phenylacetate. For defects involving either of the next two steps of the urea cycle (ie, citrullinemia or argininosuccinicaciduria), treatment with arginine (1 to 3 mmol per kg per day) is indicated. If parenteral solutions are unavailable, benzoate, phenylbutyrate, and arginine can be administered by a nasogastric tube. A 10% solution in water is usually convenient. A therapeutic effect, that is, a lowering of blood ammonia, should be noted in about 2 hours. In addition to the treatments already described, gut sterilization may minimize ammonia formation by enteric urea-splitting bacteria. Absorption of ammonia from the gut can be lowered by giving lactulose (5 mL for infants, 10 to 20 mL for children).

ORGANIC ACIDURIAS

CLINICAL MANIFESTATIONS

Acute Catastrophe in the Newborn Period

This clinical presentation has been noted in association with almost all the disorders listed in Table 87.2. The infant seems well for the first few days or weeks of life, after which he or she becomes increasingly apathetic and irritable. Progression to frank coma can occur abruptly. Vomiting, mild hepatomegaly, hypothermia, hypotonia, and convulsions occur often. An unusual symptom may be a bizarre odor in the urine, breath, perspiration, saliva, or ear cerumen (Table 87.3).

Recurrent Coma in a Child with Mental Retardation and Growth Failure

A subset of patients come to attention because of delayed psychomotor and physical development. Cerebral palsy may have been misdiagnosed. An otherwise trivial infection may cause sudden clinical decompensation, including vomiting, obtundation, and frank coma. Physical examination discloses a comatose, hyperventilating child whose weight and height are often below average. Both urine and breath should be scrutinized

TABLE 87.2. Inherited Organic Acidurias

I. Disorders of Amino Acid Metabolism
   A. Maple syrup urine disease
   B. Isovaleric acidemia
   C. Propionic acidemia
   D. Methylmalonic acidemia
   E. β-Ketothiotase deficiency
   F. β-Methylcrotonic aciduria
   G. Holocarboxylase synthetase deficiency
   H. Biotinidase deficiency
   I. Glutaric aciduria (types I and II)
   J. β-Methylglutaconic aciduria
II. Disorders of Carbohydrate and Energy Metabolism
   A. Primary lactic acidosis
      1. Pyruvate dehydrogenase deficiency
      2. Pyruvate carboxylase deficiency
      3. Inherited defects of the tricarboxylic acid cycle
      4. Disorders of the electron transport chain
   B. Glyceric aciduria
III. Disorders of Fatty Acid Oxidation
   A. Medium-chain acyl-CoA dehydrogenase deficiency
   B. Long-chain acyl-CoA dehydrogenase deficiency
   C. Very-long-chain acyl-CoA dehydrogenase deficiency
   D. Carnitine palmitoyltransferase II deficiency
   E. Type II glutaric aciduria
   F. 3-Hydroxy-acyl-CoA dehydrogenase deficiency
   G. Primary carnitine deficiency

TABLE 87.3. Odors Associated with Organic Acidurias

Disorder	Odor
Maple syrup urine disease	Burnt sugar or maple syrup
Isovaleric acidemia	Sweaty socks or cheeselike
Methylmalonic acidemia	Fruity (from ketosis), ammoniacal
Phenylketonuria	Mouse urine, musty
Tyrosinemia	Cabbagelike
Methionine malabsorption	Malt or hops
3-Methylcrotonic aciduria	Tomcat urine
3-Hydroxy-3-methylglutaric aciduria	Tomcat urine
Propionic acidemia	Fruity (ketosis), ammoniacal

for unusual odors. Convulsions and focal neurologic findings may be present.

Older Infant or Child with Acute Decompensation and Liver Failure

These children may have mild to moderate mental retardation and/or growth failure. Some may be asymptomatic until severe vomiting and dehydration develop in association with a stress, usually a viral illness. The progression to altered consciousness and coma may be very rapid. A careful history often reveals that these children have been hospitalized previously with vomiting and loss of consciousness.

A subset of these children have defects of fatty acid oxidation, such as medium-chain acyl-CoA dehydrogenase deficiency or primary carnitine deficiency. The primary clinical findings are coma, hypoglycemia, hyperammonemia, and hepatomegaly. Muscle weakness and cardiomyopathy may occur. Analysis of the urine organic acids usually discloses a typical pattern of metabolite excretion.

LABORATORY FINDINGS

Metabolic acidosis may occur during the acute illness when an anionic gap develops. The alkali requirement may be very high, perhaps 10 to 15 mEq per kg per day of HCO_3^-, to maintain the blood bicarbonate in the low-normal range. Patients may occasionally demonstrate hyperchloremic metabolic acidosis. Ketonuria is common and probably reflects an inhibition of ketone body oxidation by accumulated organic acids. Hypoglycemia is common. Hyperammonemia occurs because high levels of organic acids may inhibit ureagenesis.

Neutropenia and thrombocytopenia are common findings. Analysis of urine organic acids usually points to a specific syndrome.

The emergency physician will often lack access to specialized laboratory tests such as gas–liquid chromatography. An alternative approach to diagnosis is the use of simple liquid screening tests that can be performed in any ED. Thus, the ferric chloride reaction is grayish green in the urine of children with maple syrup urine disease. The 2,4-dinitrophenol reaction is positive (ie, a yellowish precipitate forms), in the same disorder. The para-nitroaniline reaction gives a bright emerald green reaction in the urine of patients with methylmalonic aciduria.

MANAGEMENT

The treatment of a child with primary organic aciduria should be directed to three primary goals: 1) correction of abnormalities (eg, acidosis) that are consequences of the primary metabolic insult; 2) reduction of organic acid production; and 3) if possible, enhancement of organic acid disposal. The urine pH should be kept at 6 or higher. The initial dose of bicarbonate should be 1 to 2 mEq per kg, or based on arterial blood gases.

TABLE 87.4. Specific Treatments for Organic Acidurias

Thiamine (25–100 mg/d, orally or parenterally)
- Maple syrup urine disease
- Primary lactic acidosis with megaloblastic anemia

Biotin (10–40 mg/d, orally or parenterally)
- Holocarboxylase synthetase deficiency
- Biotinidase deficiency

Vitamin B_{12} (2 mg intramuscularly)
- Methylmalonic acidemia with homocystinuria

Folic acid (1–5 mg/d, orally or parenterally)
- Methylmaloric acidemia with homocystinuria

Lipoic acid (25–50 mg/kg/d, orally)
- Primary lactic acidosis secondary to lipoamide dehydrogenase deficiency

Vitamin C (50 mg/kg/d) and Vitamin K (0.6 mg/kg/d as menadione)
- Primary lactic acidosis secondary to electron transport defect

Glycine (250 mg/kg/d, orally or parenterally)
- Isovaleric acidemia

Carnitine (50 mg/kg/d, orally)
- Carnitine deficiency

Dichloroacetate (experimental, dose not established)
- Primary lactic acidosis

In addition to metabolic acidosis, hypoglycemia is common during the acute presentation. Therefore, clinicians should carefully monitor the blood glucose. Emergency treatment consists of intravenous administrations of 1 g (4 mL) per kg of 25% glucose followed by a 10% glucose infusion.

Organic acid production must be minimized by avoiding the administration of compounds that are precursors to the organic acid in question. Most clinically relevant organic acids are derived from amino acids; therefore, protein intake should be restricted. In the ED, the patient should receive adequate glucose (ie, a 10% glucose infusion) to provide a source of calories and to minimize endogenous protein catabolism.

The organic acidurias are best conceptualized as toxicity syndromes, and a specific antidote is often available, as indicated in Table 87.4. Another therapeutic approach is the administration of L-carnitine. Exogenous carnitine may favor esterification and thereby alleviate the toxicity associated with high free organic acid concentrations. Recent evidence indicates that dialysis, which efficiently removes ammonia from the body (see previous section), can dramatically reduce organic acid levels in the acutely affected child.

GALACTOSEMIA

CLINICAL MANIFESTATIONS

Failure to thrive is characteristic and may be the reason for referral. Most affected children also have gastrointestinal problems, particularly vomiting and diarrhea, a few days after exposure to dietary lactose. By the end of the first week of life, the classic patient shows signs of liver disease. Hyperbilirubinemia, which may be intense, is caused by both hepatic dysfunction and hemolysis. Cataracts are present in almost all babies at birth, although a slitlamp examination may be necessary to visualize an embryonic cataract. Neurologic deterioration with coma ensues in severe cases. The risk of infection is also increased, and death from *Escherichia coli* septicemia is not unusual, often as the initial manifestation of the disorder.

LABORATORY FINDINGS

A presumptive diagnosis is made by the presence of galactosuria in a symptomatic individual. This diagnosis is accomplished most simply by testing the urine for the presence of a reducing agent. Clinitest tablets are commonly used for this purpose. If a reducing substance is present, the urine should be tested with a paper strip impregnated with glucose oxidase to rule out glycosuria. Precise quantitation of galactose in the urine or blood requires either enzymatic assay or isolation of the galactose with gas–liquid chromatography. Most patients have abnormal liver function tests. Jaundice is common, especially in babies who initially develop indirect hyperbilirubinemia followed by direct hyperbilirubinemia 1 to 2 weeks later.

Urine may disclose bicarbonaturia and generalized aminoaciduria. The most important clinical counterpart of the renal tubular dysfunction is hyperchloremic metabolic acidosis.

In some patients, particularly during the newborn period, hemolysis may be prominent and may be so severe that it is confused with erythroblastosis.

MANAGEMENT

Complete exclusion of dietary galactose is the mainstay of treatment. In the newborn period, this treatment is accomplished by feeding the child a lactose-free formula, such as Nutramigen or Pregestimil. The goal of diet therapy should be to maintain erythrocyte galactose-1-phosphate levels as close to normal as possible. Because defective bactericidal activity seems to be an intrinsic feature of the syndrome, appropriate cultures should be obtained and antibiotic therapy instituted quickly in the newly diagnosed infant.

CHAPTER 88
Dermatology

Paul J. Honig, M.D.

ATOPIC DERMATITIS

CLINICAL MANIFESTATIONS

During infancy, the itch–scratch cycle, which usually begins at 2 to 3 months of age, produces the erythematous, exudative lesions that appear on the cheeks and extensor surfaces. At times, the process becomes generalized. Near the age of 2 years, the more characteristic flexural involvement occurs. Also indicative of atopic dermatitis are 1) patches of hypopigmentation of various sizes, especially prominent on the cheeks (pityriasis alba); 2) patchy or diffuse, fine papules (follicular accentuation); 3) scaling in the scalp with or without hair loss; and 4) hyperlinear palms and soles, which may show desquamation. Involvement of the feet in such a manner often leads to the misdiagnosis of tinea pedis, which occurs less often in the pediatric population before adolescence. During adolescence, the distribution remains the same; however, a greater incidence of involvement of the face, neck, posterior auricular areas, and the hands and feet occurs. The major physical findings of chronicity, hyperpigmentation, and lichenification are often present. Other possible features are listed in Table 88.1. Many immune and metabolic disorders are also associated with a rash that is similar in appearance to atopic dermatitis. These disorders are listed in Table 88.2.

Complications

Infection of the existing dermatosis is the principle complication in atopic dermatitis. Colonization and infection with *Staphylococcus aureus* is common among atopic children and may account for flare-ups or failure to respond to therapy. Group A β-hemolytic streptococci are also cultured from many individuals with secondarily infected skin. The common cause for what is termed Kaposi varicelliform eruption is herpes simplex virus (eczema herpeticum) infection. Groups of umbilicated vesicles or areas of increased crusting and ulceration should be cultured for herpes simplex.

TABLE 88.1. Diagnostic Features of Atopic Dermatitis

Major	Ichthyosis
Typical morphology and distribution	Tendency toward nonspecific hand and foot dermatitis (pseudotinea pedis)
Pruritus	Tendency toward repeated cutaneous infections
Chronically relapsing course	White dermographism
Personal or family history of atopic disease	Elevated serum immunoglobulin E
Additional features	*Minor*
Xerosis	Cataracts
Hyperlinear palms and soles	Keratoconus
Follicular accentuation	Dennie-Morgan (infraorbital) fold
Pityriasis alba	
Scaling of the scalp	

MANAGEMENT (TABLE 88.3)

The four main objectives in the treatment of uncomplicated atopic dermatitis are 1) reduction of pruritus, 2) reduction of inflammation, 3) protection of the skin from unknown irritants, and 4) removal of known irritants. Reduction of pruritus can be accomplished in numerous ways. Most important of these methods is limitation of bathing (at times, to only once per week) and the use of a mild soap (eg, Dove, Tone, Caress). Lubrication of the skin with Nivea cream, Eucerin cream, or Moisturel (which contains no lanolin or perfumes) in order to ameliorate dryness, which may be a factor in producing pruritus. Antihistamines can be helpful, although, during infancy, the necessity for soporific doses results in their being less helpful therapeutically. Newer preparations include topical doxepin and oral cetirizine. Control of inflammation is accomplished with the use of topical steroids (Table 88.4). During the acute phase, potent steroids should be used to bring the situation under control. (At times, systemic steroids are used to bring an acute flare-up under control. Fortunately, this measure is rarely necessary.) Once control is achieved, steroids of mild potency should be used and applied less often. (Note: Steroids should not be used on the face for prolonged periods.)

Appropriate antibiotics are important in the treatment of secondary bacterial infections; erythromycin (40 mg per kg per day) or dicloxacillin (50 mg per kg per day) provide suitable

TABLE 88.2. Immune and Metabolic Disorders Causing Rash That Resembles Atopic Dermatitis

Metabolic disorders	Immunologic disorders
Phenylketonuria	Ataxia-telangiectasia
Acrodermatitis enteropathica	Letterer-Siwe disease
Histidinemia	Wiskott-Aldrich syndrome
Gluten-sensitive enteropathy	X-linked agammaglobulinemia
Hartnup syndrome	Hyperimmunoglobulin E syndrome
Hurler syndrome	Selective immunoglobulin A deficiency
	Severe combined immunodeficiency

TABLE 88.3. Acute Treatment of Atopic Dermatitis

Reduction of pruritus	*Reduction of inflammation*
Mild soaps } skin care	Skin care
Infrequent washing } skin care	Topical steroids (high potency)
Skin lubrication } skin care	Systemic steroids (rarely necessary)
Topical steroids (high potency)	*Control of infection*
Systemic steroids (rarely necessary)	Penicillinase-resistant antibiotics
Antihistamines (children >4 yr old)	

coverage. Eczema herpeticum that is localized and that has not produced toxicity in a child can be treated symptomatically and will usually clear in 2 to 3 weeks. With severe infection, especially in young infants, more aggressive therapy may be necessary. A daily dosage of 700 mg per m^2 per 24 hours of acyclovir, given in a 1-hour intravenous (i.v.) infusion every 8 hours, is advised. More localized primary or secondary infections can be treated orally at a dosage of 15 to 30 mg per kg per 24 hours in four to five divided doses for 10 days.

SEBORRHEIC DERMATITIS

CLINICAL MANIFESTATIONS

The two common locations of skin involvement during infancy are the scalp ("cradle cap") and diaper area. Most commonly, yellow, greasy scales are found over the anterior fontanel. Occasionally, the scaling is spread to the forehead, eyebrows, nose, ears, and neck. The intertriginous and flexural areas may also become involved. This reaction is especially seen in the diaper area. The child is not irritable, and pruritus is not present. Between the periods of infancy and adolescence, scaling of the scalp usually indicates causes other than seborrheic dermatitis (atopic dermatitis or tinea capitis). In fact, true seborrheic dandruff does not appear until puberty, when excessive production of sebum occurs. Seborrheic dermatitis of the scalp during the adolescent period is similar in nature to the condition in adults. Scaling in the scalp appears, and the seborrheic areas are variably involved. Erythema and scaling occur between the eyebrows, on the eyelid margins, and in the nasolabial creases, sideburns, beards, mustache, posterior auricular areas, and aural canals.

TABLE 88.4. Potency of Topical Steroids[a]

Mild
Hydrocortisone 1%
Moderate
Aristocort ointment 0.1% (triamcinolone acetonide)
Cordran ointment 0.05% (flurandrenolide)
Synalar cream 0.025% (fluocinolone acetonide)
Synalar ointment 0.025% (fluocinolone acetonide)
Valisone cream 0.1% (betamethasone valerate)
Potent
Diprosone ointment 0.05% (betamethasone dipropionate)
Florone ointment 0.05% (diflorasone diacetate)
Lidex cream or ointment 0.05% (fluocinonide)
Topicort ointment 0.25% (desoximetasone)

[a] All the synthetic preparations are fluorinated. Hydrocortisone is not.

MANAGEMENT

Seborrheic dermatitis of the scalp responds readily to antiseborrheic shampoos (ie, selenium sulfide) and topical steroids such as fluocinolone acetonide or betamethasone valerate (Table 88.4). Secondary infection with bacteria can be treated with appropriate antibiotics. If *Candida albicans* secondarily invades the lesions, topical clotrimazole cream, applied twice a day, is useful.

ALLERGIC CONTACT DERMATITIS

CLINICAL MANIFESTATIONS

The acute onset of linear or geometric areas of erythema, edema, eczematization, and papulovesiculation usually indicates the presence of allergic contact dermatitis. Because skin involvement is limited to areas of contact, the distribution, pattern, and shape of the dermatitis provide important clues for the clinician (Table 88.5). Therefore, a round lesion on the back of the wrist would incriminate a wristwatch; a linear pattern encircling the waist points to the rubber in the waistband of a garment; linear lesions on exposed portions of the body indicate brushing against the leaves of a poison ivy plant; and extensive involvement of exposed areas of skin suggests an airborne allergen, as with ragweed or vaporized oil transmitted in the smoke of burning poison ivy. The most common causes of contact dermatitis in order of frequency are rhus (poison ivy, oak, sumac), nickel, and rubber compounds.

MANAGEMENT

Rhus

Avoidance of exposure is the best prophylaxis in treatment. Once the oil has been removed, spread does not occur, even from vesicular fluid. Antipruritic lotions such as calamine are useful. Topical steroids are minimally effective, and topical antihistamines and anesthetics should be avoided because they can be sensitizers. Antihistamines can be helpful. With generalized reactions, oral prednisone 1 to 2 mg per kg once daily for 1 week, then tapered over the next week, is advisable.

Nickel Contact Dermatitis

Treatment consists of removing the offending object, avoiding further contact with nickel-containing jewelry, and applying topical steroids to the affected areas of skin.

TABLE 88.5. Regional Predilection of Various Substances That Cause Contact Dermatitis

Head and neck
Scalp—hair dye, hair spray, shampoo
Ear canal—neomycin
Forehead—hat band
Eyelids—nail polish, volatile gases, false eyelash cement, mascara, eye shadow/cosmetics
Perioral—dentrifices, bubble gum, chewing gum
Ears—earrings, perfume
Trunk
Axilla—deodorant, clothing dye
Breasts—metal, elastic in bra
Arms
Wrist—cosmetic jewelry (nickel), leather (*p*-phenylenediamine, chrome)
Abdomen
Waistline—rubber dermatitis from elastic in pants, jockstrap (lower)
Lower extremities
Feet—shoe dermatitis

Shoe Contact Dermatitis

Control is achieved by avoiding shoes when possible, treating secondary infection with appropriate antibiotics, and using topical steroids. All antihistamines are helpful for reducing pruritus. An "id" reaction consisting of huge bullae on the hands and feet can occur. If the child is often unable to walk, hospitalization and/or the use of systemic steroids are necessary.

DIAPER DERMATITIS

CLINICAL MANIFESTATIONS

Occlusion Dermatitis

Occlusion dermatitis contains two components. The first, friction, occurs mainly on those portions of the diaper area where contact with the diaper is greatest (inner thighs, lower abdomen, and prominent surfaces of the genitalia and buttocks). The rash waxes and wanes and often has a shiny, glazed surface appearance. Occasionally, papules are associated with the rash. The second component, trapped moisture, causes the erythema and maceration that occurs in the intertriginous parts of the diaper area (inguinal, genital, intergluteal, and folds of the thighs).

Atopic Dermatitis

The appearance of this rash in the diaper area is not different from occlusion dermatitis. It is, however, more chronic and difficult to treat. Examination may disclose lesions on other body surfaces (cheeks, antecubital and popliteal spaces) typical of atopic involvement, and a family history of atopy often exists.

Seborrheic Dermatitis

Generally, this rash has an erythematous, salmon-colored base that is covered with yellow, greasy scaling. Similar involvement of other seborrheic locations such as the scalp, postauricular area, or other flexures helps to establish the diagnosis. At times, a family history of seborrheic dermatitis exists.

Moniliasis

Moniliasis is the most characteristic of the diaper rashes. The skin in the diaper area has clusters of erythematous papules and pustules that go on to coalesce into an intensely red confluent rash with sharp borders. Beyond these borders are satellite papules and pustules. At times, the infant has concomitant oral thrush.

Mixed or Undiagnosable Rashes

Mixtures of the above categories of diaper dermatitis are often found on infants. A diagnosis is often difficult to make. Secondary invasion with *C. albicans* is common as mentioned. The potential for secondary bacterial infection exists. If blistering occurs, *S. aureus* infection should be considered.

MANAGEMENT

Treatment is determined by the cause of the dermatitis. In general, proper skin care, which includes decreased frequency of washing, use of mild soaps, and keeping the diaper off as much as possible, will help resolve diaper dermatitis resulting from any cause. With occlusive dermatitis, avoidance of tightly fitting diapers, plastic-covered paper diapers, and rubber pants is important. When atopic dermatitis is present, the use of topical steroids is necessary. It is important to avoid fluorinated or other potent steroids in the diaper area because occlusion by the diaper enhances the steroid effect and is more likely to produce skin atrophy and striae. The newer antifungal–steroid combinations should also be avoided for these same reasons. Therefore, 1% hydrocortisone cream no more than twice daily over a short period is recommended. Hydrocortisone (1%) is also effective for seborrheic diaper dermatitis and can be used intermittently.

With monilial diaper dermatitis, the use of preparations such as econazole twice a day is effective. If thrush is also present, oral nystatin 200000 units (2 mL) four times a day for 7 days, is advisable. Patients with id reactions, as described before, require oral nystatin, econazole on the diaper and intertriginous areas, and 1% hydrocortisone applied to the plaques. Secondarily infected dermatitis, such as bullous impetigo, should be treated with the appropriate systemic antibiotics. Whether traditional diaper creams and ointments are effective is still unproven.

DRUG REACTIONS IN THE SKIN

CLINICAL MANIFESTATIONS

Urticaria

Urticaria constitutes the most common expression of drug sensitivity. Most commonly, reactions occur within 1 week of drug exposure. When an individual is on multiple agents and has a reaction, the clinician should suspect those agents that were most recently introduced or those medications that are known to be commonly associated with drug reactions (Table 88.6).

Maculopapular Eruptions Similar to Those of a Viral Exanthem

Maculopapular eruptions are the second most common of all drug-induced rashes and may be caused by many different agents. These eruptions are symmetric and consist of erythematous macules and papules with areas of confluence. Variable involvement of the palms, soles, and mucous membranes, as well as purpura may occur. The presence and severity of pruritus is variable. Ampicillin is a medication often associated with this type of skin reaction, particularly in patients with infectious mononucleosis.

Erythema Multiforme

Erythema multiforme is an acute and often recurrent inflammatory syndrome often secondary to drugs (eg, penicillins, sulfonamides, hydantoins, barbiturates) or infections. Recent observations suggest that a significant portion of idiopathic erythema multiforme cases may be caused by herpes simplex virus. The skin findings include macules, papules, vesicles, and pathognomonic target or iris lesions that tend to be more or less symmetrically distributed. Bullous lesions may also be present. In the more severe cases, constitutional symptoms occur; when mucous membranes are involved, the term *Stevens-Johnson syndrome* is used. Erythema multiforme consists of two lesion types: macular-urticarial and vesicular-bullous. There is a predilection for the backs of the hands, palms, soles, and extensor surfaces of

TABLE 88.6. Drugs Most Commonly Associated with Allergic Skin Reactions

Trimethoprim–sulfamethoxazole	Cephalosporins
Ampicillin	Dipyrone
Semisynthetic penicillins (carbenicillin, cloxacillin, dicloxacillin, methicillin, nafcillin, oxacillin)	Nitrazepam
	Barbiturates
	Nitrofurantoin
Sulfisoxazole	Glutethimide
Penicillin G	Indomethacin
Gentamicin	

the limbs. The lesions may begin at these sites and then spread diffusely or they may begin generalized. In 25% of the patients, the mucous membranes are involved and, in fact, can be the sole site of involvement. The usual sites of mucous membrane involvement are the lips, buccal mucosa, palate, conjunctivae, urethra, and vagina. With severe involvement, the pharyngeal, tracheobronchial, and esophageal mucous membranes are also affected. Less common sites are the anal and nasal mucosa. When the eyes are involved, there may be simple conjunctivitis, severe keratitis, or panophthalmitis. These changes may lead to blindness in 3% to 10% of these patients. Therefore, close attention to involvement of the eyes is necessary. Lesions may continue to erupt in crops for as long as 2 to 3 weeks. Death occurs in 3% to 15% of patients.

Vasculitis

The classic lesions of vasculitis are palpable purpura. Although these lesions are characteristic, vasculitis may be manifest by erythematous macules, papules, urticaria, and hemorrhagic vesicles and bullae. The diagnosis is made by a skin biopsy, which shows leukocytoclasis, endothelial cell necrosis, and destruction of dermal vessels.

Erythema Nodosum

The lesions of erythema nodosum appear as deep, tender, erythematous nodules or plaques of the extensor surfaces of the extremities. They are thought to be hypersensitivity phenomena secondary to infections (eg, streptococcal pharyngitis, tuberculosis, coccidioidomycosis, histoplasmosis), inflammatory bowel disease, sarcoidosis, malignancies, and occasionally, drugs. The exact immunologic mechanism has not been clarified.

Toxic Epidermal Necrolysis

Drug-induced toxic epidermal necrolysis (TEN) must be differentiated from an illness caused by a circulating staphylococcal exotoxin. If a child who has TEN has been taking medication for a prolonged period of time or shortly before onset of the rash, is over 6 years of age, or has a mixed rash (ie, areas with the appearance of erythema multiforme as well as toxic epidermal necrolysis), a biopsy must be performed to distinguish between the two disorders. With drug-induced TEN, dermal–epidermal separation is visible on histologic examination. If epidermolytic toxin has been released by staphylococci, epidermal cleavage occurs in the granular layer. With extensive exfoliation of skin, fluid and electrolyte disturbances may occur, and the potential for bacterial sepsis is present.

MANAGEMENT

Vital to the management of any suspected drug reaction is the identification and removal of the offending drug. Pruritus can be controlled with antihistamines, and open lesions are responsive to compressing with Burow solution and topical silver sulfadiazine. When extensive exfoliation occurs, attention to fluid and electrolyte balance and secondary infection is essential. Any patient with mucous membrane involvement should have an ophthalmologic examination to rule out the presence of corneal involvement. Hospitalization should be considered in any patient who has severe involvement of the skin, is toxic, or has extensive exfoliation.

The literature suggests that steroid therapy of Stevens-Johnson syndrome and drug-induced toxic epidermal necrolysis is of no value, will prolong hospital stays, and may in fact be harmful. If denudation progresses to greater than 25% of body surface area the child should be transferred to a burn unit.

STAPHYLOCOCCAL SCALDED SKIN SYNDROME

CLINICAL MANIFESTATIONS

Staphylococcal scalded skin syndrome (SSSS) begins with malaise, fever, and irritability. The irritability is often caused by significant tenderness of the skin when touched. A "sunburn" erythema follows, which first begins and is most intense around the neck, the intertriginous areas, and periorificially (especially the eyes and mouth). The erythema spreads to varying portions of the skin surface, and the child may be very toxic. With mild involvement of the skin, superficial desquamation (flaking) then follows similar to the reaction that occurs after an ordinary sunburn. With severe involvement, large sheets of skin shear away, leaving a denuded, oozing surface similar to the reaction that occurs after a burn. The skin can often be rubbed off (Nikolsky sign). Vesicles, pustules, and bullae can also occur during the exfoliative phase. Often, a purulent discharge emits from the eyes, but no conjunctival injection is present. Mucous membranes are not involved. Most children do well, and clearing of the skin occurs in 12 to 14 days, leaving no residua. Causes other than *S. aureus* or drugs may produce a similar clinical picture (Table 88.7).

MANAGEMENT

Most of the time, SSSS is a self-limited disorder. Antibiotics probably ameliorate the course of the disease, but steroids have no beneficial effects. Neonates and children less than 1 year of age should be admitted to the hospital and started on i.v. antistaphylococcal antibiotics (cefazolin, oxacillin) after blood cultures are obtained. In addition, any older child who is toxic or who has severe skin involvement with significant denudation should be admitted.

BITES AND INFESTATIONS (SEE ALSO CHAPTER 80)

Mosquitoes and Fleas

Mosquito bites are generally limited to the warm months of the year. On the other hand, flea bites, which predominate from spring to fall, can also occur during the winter months as a result of cats and dogs living indoors. The distribution of lesions is a valuable clue in making the diagnosis of mosquito or flea bites. Insect bites generally involve the exposed surfaces of the head, face, and extremities. The lesions are usually urticarial wheals that occur in groups or along a line on which the insect was crawling. On occasion, both mosquito bites and flea bites can cause blistering lesions. These lesions are not caused by secondary infection but rather by a violent immune response to the bite. Certainly, excoriation with resulting secondary infection with *S. aureus* or group A streptococci can complicate a simple bite. A recurrent papular eruption called papular urticaria can occur in young children who become sensitized to insect bites. Although the lesions tend to occur on exposed parts of the body, with sensitization they may appear at sites distant from the pri-

TABLE 88.7. Toxic Shock Syndrome

Fever	Sterile pyuria
Toxic epidermal necrolysislike rash	Elevated bilirubin and enzymes
Desquamation (after 10 days)	Low platelets
Hypotension	Disorientation or alteration in consciousness
Vomiting/diarrhea	
Hyperemia of the mucous membranes	

mary bite. Unfortunately, no specific treatment exists for insect bites. Antihistamines, calamine lotion, or topical steroids have a limited or temporary effect.

Tick Bites

Tick bites may cause local reactions. Various methods have been recommended for removal of ticks from the skin. The only safe method is to use a blunt curved forceps, tweezers, or fingers protected by rubber gloves. The tick is grasped close to the skin surface and pulled upward with a steady even force. The tick must not be squeezed, crushed, or punctured. If mouth parts are left in the skin, they should be removed.

Scabies Infestation

The cardinal symptom of any infestation with scabies is pruritus. Infants and children excoriate themselves to the point of bleeding. Two clues should be considered when attempting to make this diagnosis: 1) distribution (concentration on the hands, feet, and folds of the body, especially the finger webs) and 2) involvement of other family members. It is important not only to ask other family members if they have pruritus but also to examine their skin. In contrast to adults, infants may develop blisters and also exhibit lesions on the head and face. The diagnosis is made by scraping involved skin and looking for mites under the ×10 microscope objective. The introduction of 5% permethrin cream (Elimite) has obviated the need for lindane and its potential risks. This cream should be applied from head to toe and left on for 8 to 14 hours. The preparation is then washed off with soap and water. Its safety for use in pregnant females has not been proven. All family members and close contacts (eg, babysitters, grandparents) should be treated.

Louse Infestation

Three forms of lice infest humans: 1) the head louse, 2) the body louse, and 3) the pubic or crab louse. The major louse infestation in children involves the scalp and causes pruritus. The female attaches her eggs to the hair shaft. The egg then hatches, leaving behind numerous nits that resemble dandruff. Secondary infection can occur from vigorous scratching. Body lice generally reside in the seams of clothing and lay their eggs there. They go to the body to feed, particularly the interscapular, shoulder, and waist areas. Red pruritic puncta that become papular and wheal-like then occur. Pubic lice occur in the genital area, lower abdomen, axillae, and eyelashes. Transmission is usually venereal. Blue macules (maculae ceruleae) that are 3 to 15 mm in diameter can be seen on the thighs, abdomen, or thorax of infested persons. These macules are secondary to bites.

Because the body louse resides in clothing, therapy consists mainly of disinfecting the clothing with steam under pressure. Pediculosis capitis is most effectively treated with 1% permethrin cream rinse (Nix). Any nits are removed with a fine-toothed comb. The safest treatment for lice in the eyelashes is the application of white petrolatum (Vaseline) twice daily for 8 days. The lice stick to this substance, cannot feed, and die.

SUPERFICIAL FUNGAL INFECTIONS OF THE SKIN

Tinea Corporis

Tinea corporis is characterized by one or more sharply circumscribed scaly patches. The center of the circular patch generally clears as the leading edge spreads out. The leading edge may be composed of papules, vesicles, or pustules. The lesions are most commonly confused with nummular eczema. These lesions do not fluoresce under the Wood's light. Treatment with topical antifungal agents such as clotrimazole, miconazole, or econazole produces clearing in 7 to 10 days. Therapy should be maintained for 2 weeks. If improvement does not occur, treatment with griseofulvin (15 mg per kg per day in two divided doses) will usually resolve the problem.

Tinea Capitis

The *Microsporum* species generally causes round patches of scaling alopecia. Illumination of a lesion with a Wood's lamp gives a blue–green fluorescence. Kerion formation can occur as a swollen, boggy abscess. The *Trichophyton* species usually causes scattered alopecia, not always oval or rounded; the alopecia is irregular in outline with indistinct margins. Normal hairs grow within the patches of alopecia. At times, the hairs break off at the surface of the scalp, leaving a "black dot" appearance. Diffuse scaling may simulate dandruff, and although minimal hair loss is present, it is not perceived. Wood's light examination of the lesion does not produce fluorescence. The organism can cause a folliculitis, suppuration, and kerion formation. The clinician should consider the presence of tinea capitis when a nonresponsive seborrheic or atopic dermatitis of the scalp is present, black dots are seen, or increased scaling follows the use of topical steroids. With the use of dermatophyte test media (DTM), a color change occurs in the media (yellow to red) in the presence of a growing dermatophyte. If a kerion is present, the swelling (allergic reaction to the fungus) can be controlled by a combination of prednisone and griseofulvin.

Treatment for tinea capitis consists of orally administered griseofulvin 15 to 20 mg per kg per day in two divided doses with a glass of milk for 6 weeks. Adjunctive therapy includes the use of 2.5% selenium sulfide shampoo twice weekly. With the use of this shampoo, shedding of spores is decreased within 1 to 2 weeks. Two newer oral medications, itraconazole and terbinafine, are currently under study and may eventually replace griseofulvin as the preferred medication.

Tinea Versicolor

Tinea versicolor refers to a superficial infection of the skin caused by *Pityrosporum orbiculare,* which produces color changes of the skin, hypopigmentation, hyperpigmentation, and redness. Wood's light examination usually shows yellowish–brown fluorescence. Because moisture promotes growth of the organism, exacerbations occur in warm weather or in athletes who sweat excessively. The infection is difficult to eradicate and recurs frequently. A KOH preparation shows large clusters of spores and short, stubby hyphae, often called meatballs and spaghetti. Treatment consists of lathering the entire body with selenium sulfide shampoo (2.5% concentration) after wetting the skin surface in a shower. The lather is left on for 20 minutes and is then showered off. This procedure is carried out multiple times during the first week, with decreasing frequency over the ensuing weeks. Maintenance therapy is advisable because of the high incidence of recurrence. Localized areas of involvement can be treated with topical antifungal agents (eg, econazole, ketoconazole topically). Adolescents can be treated with 400 mg of oral ketoconazole initially and then 200 mg at monthly intervals during the warm summer months or during a sports season when the child sweats frequently.

URTICARIA

Urticaria can be localized or generalized. At times, the lesions are giant with serpiginous borders. Individual wheals rarely last more than 12 to 24 hours. Most commonly, the lesions appear in one area for 20 minutes to 3 hours, disappear, and then reappear in another location. The total duration of an episode is usually 24 to 48 hours; however, the course can last 3 to 6 weeks. Acute relief can be accomplished with subcutaneous epinephrine (1:1000) 0.01 mL per kg and intramuscular diphenhydramine 1 mg per kg. Oral antihistamines are useful for maintenance therapy for transient urticaria.

PITYRIASIS ROSEA

Pityriasis rosea can occur in all age groups but is seen predominantly after 10 years of age and only rarely under 5 years of age. In 80% of children, a large, oval, solitary lesion known as the herald patch appears on the trunk before the eruption of subsequent lesions. Individual lesions are oval and slightly raised, pink to brown, with peripheral scaling. Because the lesions follow the cleavage lines of the skin, the backs of patients have a "Christmas tree" appearance. Generally, the face, the scalp, and distal extremities are spared. On occasion, an inverse distribution occurs (lesions on the face and extremities with truncal sparing). The rash is pruritic early in the course but then becomes asymptomatic. It lasts 4 to 8 weeks. When pityriasis rosea appears in adolescence, it must be differentiated from secondary syphilis. Clinical clues are helpful (Table 88.8), but serologic testing is necessary. Antihistamines and topical emollients can help the pruritus.

ERYTHEMA NODOSUM

Erythema nodosum seems to be a hypersensitivity reaction to infection (streptococci, tuberculosis, coccidioidomycosis, histoplasmosis), inflammatory bowel disease, sarcoidosis, and drugs. The exact immunologic mechanism has not been clarified. The entity occurs predominantly in adolescents during the spring and fall. Females are affected more often than males. Ibuprofen helps with lesions that are painful.

WARTS

The common wart resembles a tiny cauliflower. The shape of the wart varies with its location on the skin. They may be long and slender (filiform) on the face and neck or flat (verruca plana) on the face, arms, and knees. When located on the soles, they are called plantar warts, and when in the anogenital area, they are referred to as condyloma acuminata. Because most warts disappear spontaneously with time, procedures that are least traumatic for the child should be attempted first (Table 88.9). The simple, nontraumatic method of airtight occlusion with plain adhesive tape for 1 month has been shown to be successful on many occasions. Topical application of salicylic acid in flexible collodion (Duofilm; Table 88.10) is good for home use, as are some of the over-the-counter preparations (eg, Compound W). When simple methods are unsuccessful, touching the warts with liquid nitrogen for 20 to 30 seconds or surgical removal can be attempted. Plantar warts can be treated with 40% salicylic acid plaster. Anogenital warts are treated with 20% podophyllin.

TABLE 88.8. Differential Diagnosis

	Pityriasis rosea	Syphilis
Herald patch	+	–
Ovals follow dermatomes	+	–
Lymphadenopathy	–	+
Mucous membrane lesion	–	+

TABLE 88.9. Management of Warts

Decrease irritation—cover with tape (1–2 mo)
Over-the-counter preparations such as Compound W (1 mo)
Salicylic in collodion (Duofilm) (1 mo)
Refer to dermatologist

Molluscum Contagiosum

The lesion, produced by the common poxvirus, is a papule with a white center. It occurs at any age during childhood. Most lesions resolve in 6 to 9 months, but some may persist for more than 3 years. Spread is by autoinoculation. Lesions can be single or numerous and favor intertriginous areas such as the groin. They are usually 2 to 5 mm in diameter, but several can coalesce and form a lesion 1.5 cm in diameter. They may become inflamed, which sometimes heralds spontaneous disappearance. At times, an eczematous reaction occurs around some lesions, and they can become secondarily infected.

Treatment should be gentle. Removal of the white core will cure the lesion. This treatment can be performed by applying eutectic mixture of local anesthetics (EMLA) cream under occlusion to the lesion 1 to 2 hours before treatment. This procedure will anesthetize the area and allow the physician to prick the skin open over the core with a 26-gauge needle, and squeeze the core out with a comedome extractor. Multiple light touches with liquid nitrogen can also be effective. With widespread lesions, nonpainful procedures are preferable. Application of 0.1% retinoic acid one to two times daily may induce enough inflammation to hasten the host's immune response or cause extrusion of the central core.

CONGENITAL HERPES SIMPLEX VIRUS

Congenital herpes simplex virus (HSV) infection encompasses a broad clinical spectrum ranging from localized cutaneous and mucosal lesions to life-threatening central nervous system and internal organ involvement. The incubation period of congenital HSV infections ranges from 2 to 30 days after exposure. Lesions present at birth or shortly thereafter have been explained by transplacental passage of the virus. The clinical manifestations of congenital HSV infection are diverse, but more than 50% of infected neonates present with external involvement. In vertex deliveries, the scalp is a common site for the vesicles. Conversely, infants delivered by breech often develop

TABLE 88.10. Use of Duofilm

1. Soak wart for 5 min.
2. Dry.
3. Surround with petroleum jelly.
4. Apply Duofilm (let dry for few minutes).
5. Cover with tape.
6. Repeat twice a day.
7. Pare dead skin.

lesions of the buttocks and perianal area initially. The lesions are not unlike those seen in older children or adults in that they are grouped tense vesicles arising on an erythematous base. However, the infection may present on the skin as individual vesicles, pustules, bullae, or denuded skin. Unfortunately, when infants have disease limited to the integument, HSV infection is often not considered as a possibility. Instead, these children are treated for "impetigo." The correct diagnosis may not be considered until constitutional symptoms such as fever, hypothermia, poor feeding, irritability, lethargy, and vomiting have appeared. By then, dissemination of the disease has occurred.

Diagnosis of congenital HSV infection should be suspected in any infant less than 1 month of age who has a vesicular eruption on an erythematous base. Rapid slide tests, using monoclonal antibodies, are available for rapid diagnosis. Viral culture still remains the gold standard for proving that HSV is present. All infants with suspected congenital HSV should be treated with i.v. acyclovir, which is the preferred drug. Acyclovir is should be given at a dosage of 30 mg per kg per day, divided every 8 hours (10 mg per kg per dose), in a 1- to 2-hour i.v. infusion.

CHAPTER 89
Oncologic Emergencies

Michael D. Hogarty, M.D. and
Beverly Lange, M.D.

LEUKEMIA

Table 89.1 outlines the initial care of patients with acute leukemia. Fortunately, most patients require only general supportive care. However, some patients require immediate intervention for specific life-threatening problems. All patients and their families require emotional support and sensitivity to deal with the fear and disorientation they feel when confronted with the diagnosis of cancer.

Hematologic Complications

ANEMIA

At the time of diagnosis, most children with leukemia are anemic. If the hemoglobin is less than 8 g per dL, administration of packed blood cells is advisable because the child is unlikely to have the ability to produce erythrocytes for several weeks; however, if the child is not having symptoms or showing signs of severe anemia, transfusion does not need to take place in the emergency department (ED). If, in the absence of hemorrhage, the child has profound anemia (ie, hemoglobin, 1 to 4 g per dL), transfusions at the usual rate can precipitate heart failure. Blood should be replaced slowly, at 3 to 5 mL per kg over 4 hours, and supplemental oxygen should be given to enhance oxygen delivery to tissues. Furosemide (1 mg per kg) can help avoid fluid overload or heart failure; however, if the white blood cell (WBC) count is greater than 100000 per mm^3, diuretics should be withheld because intravascular dehydration encourages sludging and thrombosis. Exchange transfusion has been advocated by some physicians in these exceptional circumstances. When hemorrhage is the cause of a low hemoglobin, transfusion therapy should be carried out quickly to replace losses.

HEMORRHAGE

In most newly diagnosed leukemic children, bleeding problems can be controlled with local measures alone (ie, pressure and topical thrombin for epistaxis), or in conjunction with platelet transfusions (0.2 unit per kg platelets). Epistaxis is sometimes a serious problem that may last for hours and may fail to respond to pressure. If local measures (see Chapter 18) and platelets fail, packing is a necessary but uncomfortable therapy.

In some patients with acute myelogenous leukemia (AML), especially those with hypergranular promyelocytic leukemia and some with monoblastic leukemia, a bleeding diathesis may occur at presentation or upon initiation of therapy. Bleeding is generally refractory to platelet transfusion.

Patients show prolonged prothrombin and partial thromboplastin times, elevated fibrin split products, and drastically shortened fibrinogen half-life. The most common form of bleeding in this situation is in the central nervous system (CNS); it may be fatal in the first few days of illness. Fresh-frozen plasma (10 mL per kg) and cryoprecipitate can help maintain levels of fibrinogen and clotting factors. Platelet transfusions (0.2 unit per kg) are given to correct thrombocytopenia. Heparinization (loading dose, 50 units per kg; then 5 to 10 units per kg per hour to maintain the partial thromboplastin time at approximately 1.5 times normal) is often given to patients who show no improvement with aggressive blood product support.

EXTREME LEUKOCYTOSIS

In acute leukemia, extreme leukocytosis predisposes patients to early bleeding and thrombosis in the CNS. Hydration and alkalinization often result in a substantially lower WBC count (Table 89.1).

Infectious Complications

Although fever is a symptom of leukemia in 25% of patients, more often it indicates infection. Management of fever begins with a thorough physical examination to search for localizing signs of infection. Even an apparently minor swelling or a tear in the skin or a mucosal surface can be a source of disseminated infection. Blood and urine cultures should be obtained. All leukemic patients should have baseline chest radiograph films taken. Thereafter, chest radiograph is needed only if the child has respiratory symptoms or signs. Bacterial meningitis is rare in leukemia, but if symptoms of meningitis are found, spinal fluid should be sent for bacterial, fungal, and viral culture and for cytology to rule out CNS leukemia.

After the appropriate cultures are obtained, intravenous (i.v.) broad-spectrum antibiotics should be started in a patient with leukemia and fever.

Metabolic Complications

URIC ACID NEPHROPATHY

To prevent urate nephropathy, all children with leukemia should receive the xanthine oxidase inhibitor allopurinol (150 mg per day orally in three daily doses for those 6 years old or younger; 300 mg per day orally in three daily doses for those older than 6 years) for at least 24 hours before starting therapy. Hydration at the rate of twice maintenance and alkalinization of urine to pH between 6.5 and 7.5 with sodium bicarbonate (40 mEq per L) facilitates dissolution of uric acid crystals.

TABLE 89.1. Emergency Department Care of the Patient with Probable or Certain Acute Leukemia

Communication
1. Call referring physician to obtain medical and social history.
2. Call consulting pediatric hematologist/oncologist.
3. Review possible diagnoses with family and be available to answer questions.
4. Contact support staff—social worker or psychologist—who can assist the family with psychological stress.

Initial Diagnostic Studies
1. Complete blood count with manual differential
2. Electrolytes—include K^+, Ca^{2+}, phosphorus
3. Blood urea nitrogen, creatinine, and uric acid
4. Coagulation studies—PT and PTT
5. Blood group, type, antibody screen, complete red blood cell antigen typing
6. Liver function tests to include lactate dehydrogenase
7. Chest radiograph to assess for infection or mediastinal mass
8. Blood cultures if patient is febrile
9. Do not perform bone marrow aspirate

General Supportive Care
1. In patients with high WBC count, large liver and/or spleen, mediastinal mass or electrolytes suggesting tumor lysis, obtain intravenous access and start D_5W/0.25 NS + 40 mEq/L $NaHCO_2$ at 1.5–2 times maintenance (*no KCl*); stop $NaHCO_2$ after 24 h.
2. Allopurinol 150 mg/day t.i.d. if ≤6 yrs old or 300 mg/d t.i.d. if >6 yrs old for 3–4 d.
3. Transfuse if symptomatic from hemorrhage, heart failure, shock. Write order for blood products: "All blood products should be irradiated, cytomegalovirus-negative (or frozen and reconstituted), and given with an in-line leukocyte-depletion filter until further notice."
4. Begin broad-spectrum antibiotics if patient is febrile and appears toxic or has foci of infection.
5. Do not begin corticosteroid.

Specific Problems That Require Immediate Intervention

Problem	*Laboratory data*	*Therapy*
1. Anemia	Hgb 8–10 g/dL	Transfuse 10 mL/kg PRBC over 4 h, if symptomatic and no contraindications (e.g., WBC count >100,000)
	4–6 g/dL	Transfusions of 5 mL/kg PRBC until Hgb 8–10
	<4 g/dL	Transfusion of PRBC = mL/kg Hgb level over 4 h (e.g., Hgb = 3, then 3 mL/kg initial transfusion) Consider supplemental oxygen
2. Thrombocytopenia	Platelet count	
	≥20,000/mm³	No therapy unless signs of hemorrhage
	<20,000/mm³	Platelet transfusion 0.1–0.2 U/kg up to 6 U
3. Hemorrhage	PT, PTT, fibrinogen, and fibrin split products	Give Vitamin K 5 mg intravenously Fresh-frozen plasma 10 mL/kg
	Platelet count <50,000/mm³	Platelet transfusion 0.1–0.2 U/kg up to 6 U
4. Hyperleukocytosis	WBC count > 200,000/mm³ or massive tumor burden (i.e., liver or spleen below umbilicus, multiple nodes > 5 cm², anterior mediastinal mass)	Increase intravenous fluids to 2–4× maintenance Allopurinol, as above; follow lytes, blood urea nitrogen, creatinine, and uric acid at least every 6 h, until stable Consider radiation therapy for superior vena cava syndrome (p. 458) Therapy for acute renal failure as needed (see Chapter 76) Consideration of leukocytopheresis
5. Fever	Blood and urine culture Additional cultures from site of local symptoms; chest radiograph; no lumbar puncture unless meningeal signs present	At diagnosis, consider all patients to be neutropenic despite actual WBC count, empiric broad-spectrum antibiotics; observe closely for signs of poor perfusion and treat for shock as needed
6. Metabolic	Electrolytes, blood urea nitrogen, uric acid, every 6 h, until stable	See under hyperleukocytosis; correct specific abnormality (see Chapter 76)
7. Pain	Search for specific cause (i.e., pathologic fracture) with examination and radiographs	Specific antineoplastic therapy; no aspirin; acetaminophen, codeine, or other narcotics, as needed

PT, prothrombin time; PTT, partial thromboplastin time; WBC, white blood cell; D_5W, 5% dextrose in water; Hgb, hemoglobin; PRBC, packed red blood cell.

HYPERCALCEMIA

Interim supportive management consists of hydration with normal saline (200 mL per m^2 per hour), followed by diuresis with furosemide (1 to 2 mg per kg i.v. every 4 to 6 hours). Corticosteroids, calcitonin, gallium nitrate, or dialysis may be indicated in symptomatic hypercalcemia (usually greater than 12 to 15 mg per dL).

TUMOR LYSIS SYNDROME

Antineoplastic therapy can cause a potentially fatal tumor lysis syndrome that consists of a rapid rise in serum potassium and phosphorus, a precipitous fall in serum calcium, and elevations of the serum uric acid, blood urea nitrogen (BUN), and creatinine. Hyperkalemia, the most dangerous abnormality, demands prompt treatment with Kayexalate, insulin and glucose infusion, or dialysis.

Other Complications

SPINAL CORD COMPRESSION

Symptoms include radicular pain, back pain, difficulty with urination, paresis, and paralysis. Therapy consists of immediate corticosteroid administration (dexamethasone 0.25 to 0.5 mg per kg every 6 hours), prompt irradiation, or both. Leukemia and lymphoma of the spinal cord respond to steroids or radiation therapy and do not require laminectomy.

THORACIC TUMORS

Anterior Mediastinum

Hodgkin disease and non-Hodgkin lymphoma (NHL) are the most common malignant tumors of the anterior mediastinum. Other tumors include thymoma, thymic cyst, thymic hyperplasia, teratoma, ectopic thyroid, thyroid carcinoma, sarcomas, neuroblastoma (rarely), lymphangiomas, and inflammatory processes such as sarcoid. Half of anterior mediastinal masses are benign. However, almost all large tumors and masses that cause compromise to the great vessels or cause pleural effusions are malignant.

Large tumors in the anterior mediastinum can cause tracheal narrowing, superior vena cava (SVC) syndrome, or both. Tracheal compression causes tracheal deviation, stridor, cough, dyspnea, and orthopnea. Compression of the vena cava by tumor may cause headache, dyspnea, orthopnea, syncope, or cardiovascular collapse. Physical examination may be unremarkable or may show venous distension, plethora, cyanosis, and edema anatomically confined to the head, neck, thorax, and arms. When the arm is involved, the veins will remain full when the arm is raised. Conjunctival and retinal vessels may be engorged. Children with SVC syndrome are often anxious and diaphoretic and will resist efforts to place them in a supine position. When these findings are present, narcotics, sedatives, and any drugs that interfere with venous return are contraindicated. Chest radiograph reveals a mass in the anterior mediastinum (Fig. 89.1). If a tumor is causing SVC syndrome in a child or adolescent, the diagnosis is almost certain to be NHL or Hodgkin disease.

SVC syndrome is life-threatening. It may be ill-advised to try to obtain a histologic diagnosis under general anesthesia because these patients tolerate procedures poorly. Even placing the patient in the computed tomography (CT) scanner can cause cardiorespiratory decompensation. If both arms are involved, i.v. infusions should be started in the feet, provided that venous return is good in the lower extremities. Infusions in an affected arm can cause respiratory distress, thrombosis, or phlebitis. In the unstable patient with SVC syndrome, empiric therapy with radiation (50 to 100 cGy to the midplane for 2 or 3 days), corticosteroids (hydrocortisone 2 mg per kg every 6 hours), or both may alleviate symptoms. If the patient can tolerate procedures, effusions should be drained, a bone marrow aspirate should be taken as early as possible (to rule out NHL), and a biopsy should be performed on an accessible peripheral node under local anesthesia.

NEUROBLASTOMA

Treatment of neuroblastoma is directed toward both the tumor itself and complications of the tumor. Emergency physicians need to recognize special conditions in neuroblastoma.

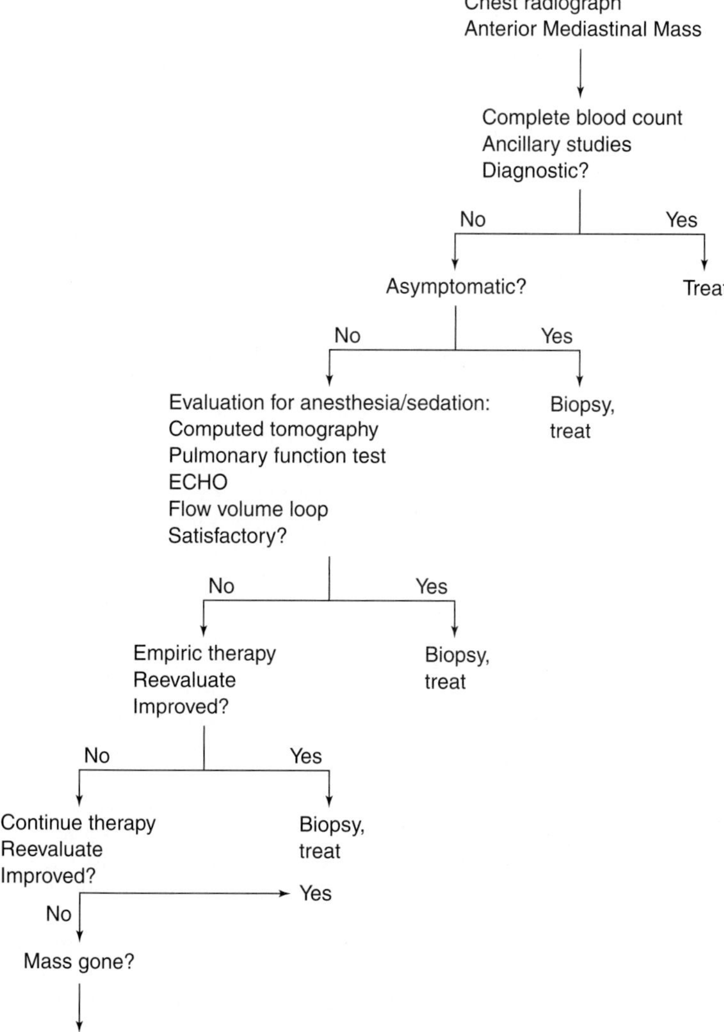

Figure 89.1. Management guidelines for children with an anterior mediastinal mass who are at risk for superior vena cava syndrome. (Modified with permission from Kelly KM, Lange B. Oncologic emergencies. *Pediatr Clin North Am* 1997;44:809–831.)

1. Massive hepatomegaly in a neonate or infant can cause hepatic failure or respiratory embarrassment. These children need to be admitted for supportive care.
2. Dumbbell tumors can cause cord compression. Treatment may consist of chemotherapy, laminectomy, surgical removal, and irradiation.
3. Children with neuroblastoma and fever and neutropenia need to be managed similarly to children with leukemia.

CENTRAL NERVOUS SYSTEM TUMORS

The role of the emergency physician in the management of CNS tumors is one of recognizing CNS lesions, performing the initial diagnostic procedures to establish the presence of the lesion, and stabilizing the patient who has a life-threatening increase in intracranial pressure or spinal cord compression. Lumbar puncture is rarely useful in the initial evaluation of a child with a CNS tumor. If focal neurologic signs or signs of increased intracranial pressure are present, a CT scan should precede any attempt to perform a lumbar puncture. Increased intracranial pressure may be treated with the administration of dexamethasone (0.5 to 1.0 mg per kg per day in four divided doses) and diuretics such as mannitol (1 to 2 g per kg over 30 to 60 minutes). Depending on the severity of the neurologic findings, intubation and hyperventilation may be indicated.

COMPLICATIONS OF THERAPY AND PROGRESSIVE DISEASE

Children with cancer have many problems that are no different from those of normal children. However, the effects of their disease and of the surgery, chemotherapy, and radiation used to treat their disease create problems unique to these patients. These problems generally arise from 1) bone marrow suppression, 2) metabolic derangements caused by the primary disease or chemotherapy, and 3) major organ damage caused by treatment or progressive disease.

The evaluation of a patient with cancer who presents to the ED begins with establishing the patient's history. Table 89.2 lists the basic data needed to evaluate a cancer patient. Knowledge of the most recent course of therapy is important because it establishes the potential for bone marrow suppression at the time of the visit.

TABLE 89.2. Basic Historical Data Needed for Evaluation of a Cancer Patient in the Emergency Department

I. Primary diagnosis	IV. Central venous access device
A. Disease	A. Type
B. Primary and metastatic sites	B. Previous infections
C. Date of diagnosis	V. Current medications
D. Status of disease (remission, relapse, completed therapy)	A. Corticosteroids
II. Surgical history	B. Chemotherapy
A. Date	C. Trimethoprim–sulfamethoxazole prophylaxis
B. Extent of resection	D. Growth factors (e.g., g-CSF, erythropoeitin)
III. Last treatment	VI. How is the child acting?
A. Chemotherapy	VII. Has the problem occurred before?
1. Drugs	VIII. What does the parent believe to be the problem or the cause of the problem?
2. Date	
B. Radiation therapy	
1. Dosage	
2. Fields	
3. Date	

Hematologic Complications

ANEMIA

Anemia is common in children being treated for cancer and is usually well tolerated.

Guidelines for the use of packed red blood cells (RBCs) are reviewed in Table 89.1. If there is a question about the need for cytomegalovirus-negative blood, the child's oncologist or the blood bank director should be consulted. RBC products should be irradiated to 1500 cGy before transfusion. Leukodepletion filters should be used.

HEMORRHAGE

After infection, hemorrhage is the second most common serious complication of cancer therapy. Often the hemorrhage is minor (mild epistaxis, gum bleeding), but when the platelet count is below 10000 to 20000 per mm^3, spontaneous intracranial hemorrhage or gastrointestinal bleeding becomes more likely. See the previous section on "Hemorrhage" in the discussion of "Leukemia" and Table 89.1 for treatment guidelines.

For epistaxis or bleeding of the oral mucosa, local measures to control the bleeding should be tried before blood products are used. Local pressure should be applied to the bleeding site or to the nasal bridge; the use of 2 to 3 drops of phenylephrine (0.25% or 0.5%) is often helpful in epistaxis. One or two vials of topical thrombin (1000 units per vial, as the powder) may be applied after the large unstable clot is removed. Desmopressin (DDAVP, 10 μg per m^2 i.v.) has been used successfully in thrombocytopenic patients with mucosal bleeding that is unresponsive to local measures and platelet transfusion.

LEUKOCYTOSIS/LEUKOPENIA

Leukocytosis is discussed in the previous section on "Leukemia."

Infectious Complications

FEBRILE NEUTROPENIC PATIENT

Children tolerate neutropenia better than adults, and most can remain free of infection with counts of more than 500 neutrophils per mm^3. A thorough physical examination sometimes uncovers the source of fever. In addition to examining the common sites of infection in children (the buccal mucosa, perianal area, and nail beds), muscles, joints, bones, and former sites of i.v. infusions should be evaluated. In a patient undergoing treatment for cancer, just as in the patient with newly diagnosed leukemia, an apparently minor swelling or a tear in a mucosal surface or the skin can be a source of disseminated infection. Perirectal abscesses, commonly seen in patients with AML, may cause pain and discoloration but no edema. Seemingly insignificant paronychia may be the source of significant bacteremia. Blood and urine cultures should be obtained and a chest radiograph should be taken in patients with respiratory symptoms, but a lumbar puncture is not indicated unless signs of meningitis are present; for unknown reasons, infectious meningitis is rare in children with cancer.

The accepted practice in treating a febrile neutropenic patient is to begin empiric antibiotic therapy with combinations of i.v. broad-spectrum antibiotics. The choice of antibiotic combination depends on the prevailing patterns of infection and antimicrobial resistance in the area.

VARICELLA AND HERPES VIRUS INFECTION

Up to half the children with Hodgkin disease develop varicella–zoster during or after therapy. About 1% develop lethal visceral dissemination. In patients with acute lymphocytic leukemia (ALL), varicella has replaced *Pneumocystis carinii* pneumonia as the most common cause of death during remission. Acyclovir 1500 mg per m^2 per day i.v. divided every 8 hours can shorten the course of the illness and lessen the risk of dissemination in the immunocompromised patient.

Any immunocompromised patient who has a vesicular rash should be admitted for i.v. treatment with acyclovir. Oral treatment is inadequate. All chemotherapy should be discontinued. On admission, an appropriate diagnostic test (viral culture or rapid detection test) should be done because herpes simplex virus (HSV) can present as a vesicular skin eruption in the immunocompromised host; for HSV, a lower dosage of acyclovir is used (750 mg per m^2 per day divided every 8 hours).

COMMON CHILDHOOD INFECTIONS

Children with cancer acquire common pediatric viral and bacterial infections. For the child who is receiving maintenance therapy for ALL, or who is not neutropenic from therapy for other malignancies, diseases such as otitis media, urinary tract infection, streptococcal pharyngitis, impetigo, infectious mononucleosis, mumps, influenza, and the ubiquitous upper respiratory tract infections may be managed as they would be in an otherwise healthy child. However, varicella and measles (rubeola) infections are dangerous in oncology patients regardless of the status of their disease. Varicella should be treated as described in the previous section on "Varicella and Herpes Virus Infection."

Neurologic Complications

SEIZURES

Seizures in a child with cancer should be evaluated and treated in much the same way as outlined in Chapter 61. Metabolic abnormalities account for 7% of seizures in children with cancer. Cisplatin, ifosfamide, and amphotericin B can all cause renal wasting of electrolytes, especially potassium, phosphorus, magnesium, and calcium. A rapid assessment of potassium, calcium, and magnesium levels is essential in patients who have received these drugs. Vincristine, intrathecal methotrexate, and cytosine arabinoside may directly cause seizures. L-Asparaginase predisposes cancer patients to CNS thrombosis, which may result in seizures. A child in whom a shunt malfunction or primary or metastatic tumor in the CNS is a possibility must have imaging studies performed to localize the problem. Infectious meningitis is rarely a problem except in the child who has a CNS foreign body or who has had a recent lumbar puncture.

CEREBROVASCULAR ACCIDENTS

In children with cancer, a cerebrovascular accident (CVA) may result from direct or metastatic spread of tumor, the effects of chemotherapy or radiation, or as a result of a bleeding diathesis associated with thrombocytopenia or disseminated intravascular coagulation (secondary to leukemia or sepsis). CT scan with contrast should be taken for all oncology patients suspected of having a CVA.

SPINAL CORD COMPRESSION

Spinal cord compression is almost always a result of direct invasion of tumor into the spinal canal. Occasionally, a patient taking high-dose corticosteroids may develop nerve root compression after the collapse of an osteopenic vertebral body. Radiation-induced spinal cord injury is rare but should be considered in the differential diagnosis if the patient received more than 4500 cGy to the cord. Spinal cord compression is treated with surgery, radiotherapy, or chemotherapy. The choice of treatment is determined by the type of tumor and the duration and severity of symptoms. Dexamethasone should be given to all patients at an initial dose of 1 to 2 mg per kg i.v. The restoration of bowel and bladder continence can have a profound impact on quality of life. Therefore, even in a terminally ill patient, spinal cord compression should be considered an emergency.

SECTION IV

Trauma

CHAPTER 90

An Approach to the Injured Child

Richard M. Ruddy, M.D. and
Gary R. Fleisher, M.D.

Physicians delivering care in an emergency department (ED) must be prepared to treat injured children. Although pediatric trauma victims have needs distinguishing them from adults, it is only in the past decade that investigators have begun to systematically look at the care of the injured child. It is the intent of this chapter to help prepare physicians in the ED for the triage, assessment, and initial care of children with the spectrum of injury from minimal to life threatening.

The approach discussed here provides a framework to decrease morbidity and mortality and is aimed at secondary prevention—after the "impact" has occurred. Secondary prevention is performed in the field by emergency medical services (EMS) providers or after arrival at the hospital. Injury severity scales have been developed to assist in the care of the trauma patient. The two most commonly quoted are the Revised Trauma Score and the Pediatric Trauma Score. These scales have served as useful tools to assess the appropriateness of care provided to injured children. Because both scales are similarly predictive of severity, many recommend use of the Revised Trauma Score because it is suitable for both children and adults. However, the approach to the injured child requires more than the use of a scale for retrospective evaluation.

GENERAL PRINCIPLES OF MANAGEMENT

The child who has sustained more than a trivial injury must be considered at risk of dying; thus, an immediate decision must be made regarding the severity of the trauma (Table 90.1). The clinical approach includes primary assessment, resuscitation (initial treatment), secondary assessment, and definitive care. This approach provides a set of principles for efficiently diagnosing and treating life-threatening conditions without neglecting less severe but important injuries. The primary assessment includes the vital signs and a quick review of the essential functions of all organs; the emphasis is on uncovering treatable injuries and preventing complications (eg, paralysis from an unstable cervical spine fracture). Concomitantly, resuscitation (initial treatment) attempts to normalize vital functions and prevent further deterioration such as hypoxia or blood loss. Primary assessment and resuscitation occupy the first 5 to 10 minutes of the encounter in most cases. As soon as possible, reassessment of the entire patient (secondary assessment) should take place to fine-tune the details of management. The secondary assessment includes the use of radiographs and laboratory tests. To be effective, physical examinations must be repeated serially and then compared. Although resuscitation of unstable patients is critical and requires a strong team approach, the close surveillance of the apparently stable patient at risk of single or multiorgan trauma may be even more demanding. Definitive care includes stabilization of specific local injuries, preparation of the patient for the operating room, and surgery, as indicated. At the completion of care for trauma patients, a tertiary survey is performed. This is a last thorough check for occult injuries. It is done upon discharge, when a patient goes home after assessment, or in the light of day for admissions.

MULTIPLE TRAUMA

CLASSIFICATION

Multiple trauma (see Chapter 91), as defined for the emergency physician, may vary from mild to severe (Table 90.2). The child with a history of an injury caused by minimal force and a physical examination that shows only superficial lesions in two or more areas of the body would be assigned to the mild category—for example, a 7-year-old child who fell while running and is found to have an abrasion on the forehead and right elbow and tenderness of the right flank. The discovery on examination of signs suggestive of deeper injury places the child in at

TABLE 90.1. Classification and Disposition of Trauma by Severity

		Physical examination			
Category	History	Vital signs	Local findings	Lab radiographic studies	Probable disposition
Mild	Minimal force	Normal	Superficial only	Few	Discharge
Moderate	Significant force	Normal	Suspicious for internal injury	Intermediate	Evaluate
Severe	Critical force	Abnormal	Indicative of internal injury	Many	Immediate therapy; admit

TABLE 90.2. Severity of Multiple Trauma

Category	History	Physical examination	
		Vital signs	Local findings
Mild	Minimal force	Normal	Abrasions/contusions
Moderate	Significant force	Normal	Refer to Tables 90.6 to 90.8 by anatomic region
Severe	Critical force	Abnormal	Refer to Tables 90.6 to 90.8 by anatomic region

least the moderate category. Detection of a serious injury or abnormal vital signs (unrelated to anxiety alone) make for classification as severe. Unfortunately, classification of injury by mechanism alone is not a uniformly useful predictor in blunt trauma in children or adults.

MANAGEMENT

Mild Multiple Trauma

The major goal in the management of a child with apparent mild multiple trauma is to confirm the initial impression of lack of severity. If there is any question of more severe injury, a large-bore peripheral intravenous line should be inserted and blood studies obtained, including a complete blood count (CBC) and type and cross-match. However, in cases that obviously seem to involve minimal trauma, the physician can proceed directly to the examination. Initially, the vital signs should be obtained. Subsequent examination includes a complete assessment with special attention to the level of consciousness; tenderness or limitation of motion of the cervical spine; auscultation of the heart and lungs; palpation of the abdomen, back, and pelvis; and extremities tenderness. The complete physical examination should include vital signs with capillary refill; Glasgow Coma Scale score; inspection and palpation of the head for injuries, pupillary reactions, extraocular muscle function, nasal tenderness, and dental/oral trauma; cervical spine motion (if the child is alert, not in a cervical collar, and without complaint and tenderness); neck vein distension; auscultation of the breath and heart sounds; inspection and palpation of the chest; evaluation of bowel sounds; inspection and palpation of the abdomen; palpation and inspection of the back, flank, and pelvis; rectal and genital examination; evaluation of extremities for deformity or tenderness; palpation of peripheral pulses; neurologic evaluation; and careful survey of the skin and soft tissues.

Laboratory evaluation of a child with a history of minimal multiple trauma and a normal examination may require no studies. If there is any concern, a CBC and urinalysis should be obtained. No other laboratory or radiographic studies are routine.

Moderate Multiple Trauma

The child with multiple trauma categorized as moderate requires immediate intervention, as well as a thorough diagnostic evaluation. A child in this category has an obvious history of involvement of several areas of the body, but initially may have only evidence of musculoskeletal or several superficial local injuries. A 3-year-old child who has been hit by an automobile and has a significantly deformed femur and a few ecchymoses on the upper extremities, or an older child who fell off a second-story roof but appears well, may fit this group. As a first step, a minimum of one large-bore peripheral intravenous catheter should be placed. If the child is in respiratory distress, supplemental oxygen should be administered. Any suggestion of cervical spine injury mandates immobilization of the neck with a semirigid collar or sandbags. If the vital signs and primary survey are normal for age, the physician then should proceed with a thorough examination, as outlined in mild multiple trauma.

Most patients with moderate multiple trauma require ancillary studies in addition to a urinalysis. These might include a CBC and radiographs of the chest and cervical spine or abdomen. A type and screen for red blood cells is indicated. In fully awake patients, a completely normal examination may be relied upon to exclude the need for all screening studies. Many patients in this category require admission to the hospital. However, an older child with a history of a moderately severe impact, who has an unremarkable examination and normal studies, may be discharged from the ED after observation for several hours.

Severe Multiple Trauma

The management of the child with severe multiple trauma demands immediate action. The initial approach assumes either obvious life-threatening injury or a reasonable likelihood that such an injury exists. An alteration of vital signs (hypotension, tachycardia), diaphoresis, or depressed consciousness automatically categorizes the injury as severe. Although helpful as an initial guide, mechanism alone (eg, a fall from a two-story building) is not a highly accurate predictor of risk. To adequately manage the child with severe multiple trauma, the physician must understand the need to institute treatment before completing a full examination and to continually intersperse detailed reassessments into an intensive treatment protocol. Table 90.3 provides an outline for organizing the initial approach to severe multiple trauma in the ED. It uses a four-pronged strategy: assessment, treatment, monitoring, and diagnostic testing.

LOCALIZED HEAD TRAUMA

CLASSIFICATION

Head trauma (see Chapters 31 and 92) can be divided into penetrating and nonpenetrating. Cases that involve penetration of the cranial vault entail severe injuries and often require operative intervention. Nonpenetrating head trauma can be classified as mild, moderate, or severe (Table 90.4).

MANAGEMENT

Penetrating Trauma

Wounds limited to the scalp and not entering the cranial vault are appropriate for primary repair in the ED. Minor wounds from sharp objects, when the likelihood of penetration is high, should have radiologic evaluation and local exploration before

TABLE 90.3. Management of Severe Multiple Trauma

Time (min)			Phase
0	1.	A	Pulse, respiration, active hemorrhage, capillary refill, level of consciousness (AVPU or Glasgow)
		T	Airway management with stabilization of cervical spine (bag-valve-mask, endotracheal intubation)
			(Surgical airway p.r.n.)
			Ventilation with FiO_2 1.00, hyperventilation as needed
			Tamponade major hemorrhage
			Intravenous access/volume infusion
			Cardiac compression (CPR) as needed
			Decompress pneumothorax/thoracostomy tube placement as needed
			Assess disability
			Exposure—remove all clothing
		M	Heart rate (electrocardiogram)
			Blood pressure (mercury or Doppler)
		D	Pulse oximeter, complete blood count, type and cross-match, chemistries (amylase, ALT, AST)
5	2.	A	Adequacy of ventilation and circulation
			Penetrating wound assessment
			Level of consciousness (AVPU or Glasgow), temperature
		T	Nasogastric tube (orogastric if suspected midface fracture)
			Thoracotomy or thoracostomy tube as needed
			Pericardiocentesis as needed
			Central line or cutdown as needed
			Drug therapy (e.g., epinephrine, bicarbonate)
			Blood transfusion/volume
		M	$ETCO_2$ (end-tidal carbon dioxide)
			Temperature (especially infants)
		D	Arterial blood gases (ABGs)
			Chemistries (as above, electrolytes, glucose), ultrasound, if available, prothrombin time, partial thromboplastin time
10	3.	A	Adequacy of ventilation and circulation
			Head, neck, chest, abdomen, pelvis, extremities
		T	Additional venous access p.r.n./volume
			Thoracotomy as needed
			Drug therapy
			Operating suite as needed
		M	Urinary catheter (except in suspected urethral disruption)
			Arterial access as needed
		D	Chest and spine radiographs
20	4.	A	Adequacy of ventilation and circulation, Glasgow, neurologic assessment, repeat full examination
		T	Cervical traction as needed
			Splint fractures
			Drug therapy (e.g., tetanus toxoid or tetanus immune globulin, antibiotics)
			Treat increased intracranial pressure (ICP)
		M	ICP bolt as needed
		D	Repeat ABGs
			Further imaging studies: computed tomography, ultrasound, intravenous pyelogram, etc.

A, assessment; AVPU, alert, verbal stimuli response, painful stimuli response, unresponsive; T, treatment; M, monitoring; D, diagnostics.

TABLE 90.4. Severity of Blunt Head Trauma

		Physical examination	
Category	History	Vital signs	Local findings
Mild	Minimal force No/momentary LOC	Normal	Glasgow = 15 Abrasions/contusions
Moderate	Significant force LOC 15 min	Normal	Glasgow ≥13 Drowsiness
Severe	Critical force LOC >5 min	Abnormal	Glasgow ≤12 Focal neurologic abnormalities

LOC, loss of consciousness.

primary closure. All other penetrating injuries require initial stabilization and neurosurgical consultation, as discussed under severe blunt head trauma. Protruding objects should be left in place until definitive management.

Blunt Trauma—Mild

Most children seen in the ED have sustained mild head trauma and have at most momentary loss of consciousness (less than 1 minute), arrive awake, and primarily need a thorough physical examination. The head should be palpated for evidence of local injury, assessing for evidence of a depressed fracture. Bruises around the eyes or behind the ear or a hemotympanum suggest a basilar fracture. The pupils will be equal and reactive and the extraocular muscle function intact, unless the severity of injury has been misjudged. Ideally, the fundi should be visualized; however, this is not essential in most cases. Almost never will an alert child have any significant funduscopic pathology from trauma, nor will visualization of the fundi always be possible in uncooperative infants and young children. In general, papilledema is a late sign of increased intracranial pressure. Although the finding of focal neurologic abnormalities is unlikely, a careful neurologic examination is mandatory. Skull radiographs and computed tomography (CT) are generally unnecessary, but either may be indicated in selected situations, such as palpation of a potentially depressed fracture (see Chapter 31).

Patients with minor head trauma may be discharged from the ED with specific instructions to watch for changes indicative of increased intracranial pressure or hemorrhage.

Blunt Trauma—Moderate

The child with moderate head trauma has sustained a concussion or, perhaps, a cerebral contusion. Moderate head injury includes any clear-cut prolonged loss of consciousness (1 to 5 minutes) or a history suggesting a severe injury, even without specific physical findings to confirm it. Once again, a thorough examination is required to search for signs of intracranial hemorrhage. The most important feature of the examination is a serial evaluation such as the Glasgow Coma Scale. The initial score serves as the baseline for the detection of subsequent deterioration. Radiographs are reserved for the same indications as for mild trauma; CT scanning is often but not necessarily performed in awake patients upon arrival, but it becomes mandatory upon deterioration in mental status or in the presence of focal abnormalities. Because of the small chance of subsequent intracranial hemorrhage or worsening cerebral edema, prolonged observation in the ED or admission is warranted in many cases with moderate injury.

Blunt Trauma—Severe

The child with severe head trauma is at risk for sudden intracranial catastrophe, acute respiratory insufficiency, or a secondary insult (eg, brain swelling) to the central nervous system. After initial steps to assess the adequacy of respiration and circulation, these functions should be supported as necessary. The cervical spine should be stabilized with a semirigid collar or sandbags. At times, gentle opening of the airway with maintenance of the head in the neutral position will allow adequate ventilation. If intubation is required immediately, extension of the neck should be avoided, and an assistant should stabilize the cervical spine during the procedure. In less urgent situations, intubation may be deferred until a cross-table lateral radiograph of the cervical spine is obtained. In all cases, supplemental oxygen should be administered and two intravenous cannulas inserted. Most children with serious head injury will hyperventilate spontaneously if their airway is patent and decrease their cerebral blood flow, which will help maintain normal intracranial pressure. Intubated, apneic children should be hyperventilated manually to achieve a $Pa{CO_2}$ of 30 to 35 mm Hg. Ideally, continuous noninvasive end-tidal CO_2 monitoring with an arterial blood gas to maximize accuracy should be the goal in the ED. An arterial catheter can be placed as needed. If the patient has an isolated head injury, parenteral fluid administration should be no greater than two-thirds of the daily maintenance rate unless there is evidence of hypovolemia. Corticosteroids are not recommended by most authorities. Osmotic agents are not used prophylactically, but mannitol (0.5 to 1.0 g per kg of a 20% solution) occasionally is necessary to decrease intracranial pressure when acute herniation is suspected or proved.

Standard skull radiographs are time consuming and provide little useful information in the patient with serious head injury. More efficient management calls for an immediate CT to evaluate the intracranial space. Rarely, neurosurgical intervention must precede imaging of the cranial contents. See Chapter 92 for more specific management.

LOCALIZED NECK TRAUMA

CLASSIFICATION

Within the confined anatomic space of the neck pass the larynx and trachea, the carotid arteries, the jugular veins, the spinal cord, and the esophagus. Thus, both penetrating and nonpenetrating insults can cause devastating injuries. All penetrating trauma, with the exception of tangential wounds superficial to the platysma muscle, should be considered serious and be referred promptly for surgical evaluation and possible exploration. Weapons or objects protruding from the neck should be left in place. Children with neck trauma (see Chapter 93) should be carefully examined in the ED for thoracic injuries, such as pneumothorax.

Isolated blunt trauma to the neck does not occur often in children. However, the potential for major disruptions of the airway or large vessels demands a thorough evaluation. Particularly, the examiner should palpate for crepitus, unequal carotid pulses, expanding hematomas, and cervical spine tenderness. Based on the history and physical findings, an estimate of the severity of the injury can be made (Table 90.5). A thorough neurologic examination, with particular emphasis on spinal cord disruption, is essential.

MANAGEMENT

Penetrating Trauma

Wounds clearly superficial to the platysma muscle are appropriate for repair in the ED. Children with penetrating injuries deep to the platysma require stabilization and subsequent surgical evaluation. Initial measures are directed at establishing a patent airway, providing adequate ventilation, tamponading hemorrhage, and restoring the circulation. Protruding objects should be left in place by the physician in the ED.

Blunt Trauma—Mild

If the history is one of a minimal force and no physical findings are indicative of trauma to the deeper structures, the child is symptomatically treated and discharged from the ED. Exceptions might be patients with underlying illnesses such as hemophilia, who are at risk for delayed complications. Follow-up after discharge should be defined clearly to ensure that intervention occurs before compromise to internal structures.

Blunt Trauma—Moderate

The child with an apparent moderate injury to the neck by definition has no evidence of respiratory or vascular compromise. However, either the history of the amount of force involved or the local findings may raise the possibility of cervical spine or other injuries. Such patients require immobilization of the cervical spine with a semirigid collar or sandbags and a meticulous neurologic examination. As a first step, a cross-table lateral radiograph of the cervical spine should be obtained with the child immobilized, usually in the ED. If this first radiograph shows all seven cervical vertebrae to be intact and properly aligned, a complete radiologic evaluation of the cervical spine can be performed, which may include anteroposterior, oblique, and open-mouth views. The discovery of a bony or ligamentous injury requires consultation with appropriate specialists. Spinal cord injury without radiographic abnormality may be present and should be pursued, when symptoms or signs are suggestive. The neurologically intact child with a normal cervical spine

TABLE 90.5. Severity of Blunt Neck Trauma

		Physical examination	
Category	**History**	**Vital signs**	**Local findings**
Mild	Minimal force	Normal	Abrasions/contusions
Moderate	Significant force	Normal	Refusal to move head Cervical spine tenderness
Severe	Critical force	Abnormal	Crepitus Expanding hematoma Unequal carotid pulse Paralysis or sensory loss

evaluation and no other neck trauma who remains well on repeat physical examination may be discharged after observation.

Moderate trauma to the anterior neck requires careful evaluation for possible disruption of the major vessels, trachea, and esophagus. Cervical spine radiographs may outline the airway adequately. However, it is important to pay attention to the alignment of the larynx and trachea and to check for air in the soft tissues from a tear in the airway or esophagus. The carotid triangle must be palpated carefully. If there is a hematoma or abnormality of the pulse, referral for possible arteriogram should be made.

Blunt Trauma—Severe

Classification of blunt neck trauma as severe indicates concern for overt injury to the airway, the major vessels, or the spinal cord. The initial goals of management are establishment of a patent airway, stabilization of the cervical spine, and intravenous access. The first choice for establishment of the airway is orotracheal intubation, with maintenance of the head in the neutral position. The inability to intubate a critical airway requires an immediate surgical approach to the trachea. Blood should be sent for a type and cross-match; if vascular injury is suspected, multiple units of blood should be available. A surgical consultant should decide whether to proceed with an exploration in the operating room or to rely on further diagnostic studies such as bronchoscopy, arteriography, or esophagoscopy.

LOCALIZED THORACIC TRAUMA

CLASSIFICATION

Penetrating chest injuries (see Chapter 94) are extremely relevant to physicians in the ED because they may be rapidly life threatening if untreated, yet usually respond to fairly straightforward therapeutic maneuvers. Any object that enters the thoracic cavity will result in significant injury. Patients with large open wounds or instability of vital signs should be considered to have sustained life-threatening trauma.

Blunt chest trauma is seen more often than penetrating injury in civilian practice in general and in children in particular. As with trauma to other anatomic regions, blunt thoracic trauma can be divided into mild, moderate, and severe categories (Table 90.6).

MANAGEMENT

Penetrating Trauma

Patients with mild injury, in which the wound clearly entered only the superficial tissues and not the thoracic cavity, may need only ED management. However, for any knife or gunshot injuries, it is advisable to have an experienced physician explore the wound and to obtain radiographs to determine the extent of injury.

Patients with deeper wounds require chest radiography, CBC, and type and cross-match. An arteriogram may be necessary in the stable patient with a suspected aortic injury. Tube thoracostomy should be performed to drain a hemothorax or pneumothorax. Hemorrhage can be managed starting with crystalloid, followed by blood replacement. For the child sustaining a cardiopulmonary arrest in the ED after a penetrating thoracic injury, immediate resuscitative thoracotomy may be lifesaving.

Blunt Trauma—Mild

The child with a history of a minimal blow to the chest, normal vital signs, and no local signs of trauma other than abrasions or contusions has sustained a mild injury. The absence of bony tenderness, tachypnea, or decreased breath sounds obviates the need for radiologic evaluation of the thoracic cage or its contents.

Blunt Trauma—Moderate

If the history indicates significant force, bony tenderness is elicited, or there is a question of decreased breath sounds, a chest radiograph, electrocardiogram (ECG), and CBC are often helpful. Particularly in children, a pneumothorax may follow blunt injury with or without a rib fracture. Widening of the mediastinum on chest radiograph suggests disruption of the aorta. The detection of a solitary rib fracture is not important per se because no specific treatment is necessary. However, it raises the suspicion of visceral or vascular disruption. In particular, fracture of the first rib is correlated in adults with injuries to the great vessels. Although the data are scant in pediatrics, an injury to the first rib may require arteriography. The chest radiograph may provide a clue to the diagnosis of pericardial hemorrhage (by showing a slightly enlarged cardiac silhouette), but it is more often normal in this condition. Bleeding into the pericardial space leading to tamponade will invariably manifest on the physical examination at some point; findings include tachycardia, followed by hypotension, distended neck veins, and muffled heart tones. A pulmonary contusion or aspiration may produce a consolidation on chest radiograph. The ECG is obtained as an aid in the diagnosis of myocardial contusion; elevated ST segments are characteristic of this entity.

In the setting of moderate blunt chest injury, it is advisable to achieve venous access and order a type and cross-match. Sophisticated diagnostic studies, such as CT scan and arteriography, are reserved for children with abnormal findings on the preliminary evaluation. Admission for observation is often warranted; however, the child who shows improvement on examination over the observation interval and does not have an abnormal chest radiograph, ECG, or CBC may often be discharged.

TABLE 90.6. Severity of Blunt Chest Trauma

		Physical examination	
Category	History	Vital signs	Local findings
Mild	Minimal force	Normal	Abrasions/contusions
Moderate	Significant force	Tachypnea Normal pulse and blood	Splinting Bony tenderness Decreased breath sounds
Severe	Critical force	Abnormal pulse or blood pressure	Flail chest Distant heart tones Absent breath sounds

Blunt Trauma—Severe

The child with abnormal vital signs or local findings indicative of internal injuries has sustained an immediate life-threatening injury. Initial therapy includes airway management, the institution of two large-bore intravenous lines, and the administration of supplemental oxygen. Depending on the condition of the child, chest tube insertion may be necessary for treatment of hemopneumothorax before radiographic studies are obtained. In selected circumstances, resuscitative thoracotomy in the ED may be beneficial, although in blunt trauma to the chest the outcome is almost uniformly poor if there has been cardiopulmonary arrest. Admission to the hospital is mandatory, and a full diagnostic evaluation should be performed to ascertain the need for surgery.

LOCALIZED ABDOMINAL TRAUMA

CLASSIFICATION

Penetrating abdominal injuries (see Chapters 95 and 96) often cause moderate to severe trauma. However, the physician may cautiously define a small category of mild injuries, depending on the weapon involved.

All gunshot wounds must be considered at least moderate because almost all penetrate the peritoneum. Of those that penetrate the peritoneum, most cause visceral injury. If the vital signs are abnormal after a gunshot, the trauma should be considered severe.

Stab wounds, on the other hand, may be superficial to the peritoneum. The patient with stable vital signs and an apparent superficial stab wound may be judged to have a mild injury if local exploration confirms the clinical impression. Stab wounds that violate the peritoneum should be considered moderately serious and the patient should be referred for surgical consultation. By definition, stab wounds that lead to unstable vital signs have produced severe trauma.

MANAGEMENT

Penetrating Trauma

All gunshot wounds are of at least moderate severity. Thus, these children require two large-bore intravenous lines (preferably inserted above the diaphragm), a nasogastric tube; radiographs of the abdomen and chest; and laboratory studies, including CBC, urinalysis, amylase, aspartate transaminase (AST), alanine transaminase (ALT), and type and cross-match. In the child with unstable vital signs, appropriate resuscitation should be initiated and laparotomy urgently considered. Otherwise, an initial CT scan may be preferable to delineate the extent and location of internal injury. All patients will require hospitalization.

Stab wounds produce variable degrees of internal injury, and the approach to management differs among institutions. Patients with abnormal vital signs require stabilization in the ED, including appropriate resuscitative measures, intravenous access, a nasogastric tube, radiographs, and laboratory studies. Transfer to the operating room may be necessary on an urgent basis. Patients whose vital signs are stable are evaluated further by local exploration, lavage, or laparotomy.

Blunt Trauma—Mild

Mild blunt abdominal injuries often occur when there is contusion of the abdominal wall from local trauma (eg, a fist, a fall). After a careful history and physical examination, including rectal palpation and testing of the stool for blood, usually only a urinalysis for red blood cells is required.

Blunt Trauma—Moderate

Moderate blunt abdominal trauma is often seen in patients with multiple injuries or those in whom there has been an isolated but forceful blow to the abdomen. These patients should have a CBC, amylase, AST, ALT, radiographs, and type and cross-match. At least one intravenous catheter should be inserted, preferably above the diaphragm. A CT scan is often warranted. A diagnostic ultrasound may be useful to reduce the need for immediate CT in some settings. In many cases, hospitalization or prolonged observation in the ED is indicated. Other imaging studies, such as intravenous pyelography, are obtained in selected situations (see Chapters 95 and 96).

Blunt Trauma—Severe

Severe blunt abdominal trauma usually warrants prompt surgery after an initial stabilization of the vital signs. The issue of whether to perform peritoneal lavage before exploratory laparotomy or whether to do a CT scan is discussed at length in Chapter 95.

In general, patients who have stable vital signs after initial fluid resuscitation may be evaluated with CT scanning to define intraabdominal bleeding. The scans help define the need for surgery, especially if a hepatic or splenic injury producing limited hemorrhage is identified. Peritoneal lavage is usually reserved for children with a decreased level of consciousness, requiring CT scanning of the brain, who experience hemodynamic instability or deterioration in the ED.

In the presence of significant hematuria or strong suggestion of renal injury, a CT scan should be performed (see Chapter 96). In symptomatic patients with severe blunt trauma, the absence of red blood cells in the urine is not by itself sufficient evidence of an intact genitourinary tract. Avulsion of the renal pedicle may occur without hematuria.

TABLE 90.7. Severity of Penetrating Extremity Trauma

Category	History	Physical examination: Vital signs	Physical examination: Local findings
Mild	Minimal force	Normal	Laceration
Moderate	Significant force (e.g., stab)	Normal	Laceration of tendon or nerve Significant venous hemorrhage
Severe	Critical force (e.g., gunshot)	Abnormal	Partial/complete amputation of arm of leg Arterial hemorrhage Open fracture

TABLE 90.8. Severity of Blunt Extremity Trauma

Category	History	Physical examination	
		Vital signs	Local findings
Mild	Minimal force	Normal	Contusions/point tenderness
Moderate	Significant force	Normal	Obvious dislocation of major joint
	Crush injury		Displaced fracture
Severe	Critical force	Abnormal	Decreased or absent pulses

EXTREMITY TRAUMA

CLASSIFICATION

Most injuries to the extremities of children (see Chapter 101) seen in the ED are mild. A few injuries are of moderate extent, and occasionally, extremity trauma may be life- or limb-threatening. Both penetrating (Table 90.7) and nonpenetrating trauma (Table 90.8) run the gamut in terms of severity. With penetrating wounds, the major immediate concern is hemorrhage, although impairment of neurovascular or musculoskeletal integrity with concomitant loss of long-term function is also a consideration. On the other hand, nonpenetrating trauma may cause vascular insufficiency without external bleeding.

MANAGEMENT

Penetrating Trauma

The child with mild penetrating trauma requires appropriate wound care and tetanus prophylaxis in the ED. A radiograph is indicated if a radiopaque foreign body (including glass) is suspected in the wound. Moderate injuries require careful physical examination and often local exploration to define the extent of the trauma and the degree of functional impairment. At times, prompt surgical consultation or follow-up with a specialist is indicated. Some injuries require repair in the operating room; however, others—even extensive lacerations or extensor tendon disruptions—may be handled, time permitting, in the ED by an experienced physician. Surgical referral is mandatory for children in the severe category, and it is important to proceed as rapidly as possible when vascular damage is suspected.

Blunt Trauma—Mild

Children with mild nonpenetrating injuries often require a radiograph to detect underlying fractures. Particularly when there is tenderness at the end of long bones, careful consideration should be given to radiologic evaluation for growth plate (epiphyseal) injuries, keeping in mind that a normal radiograph does not exclude a nondisplaced Salter-Harris type I fracture.

Blunt Trauma—Moderate

Obvious dislocations should be repositioned as expeditiously as possible, usually after radiographs confirm the diagnosis. Depending on the joint involved, discharge is acceptable after reduction and radiologic reevaluation (eg, shoulder, patella, metacarpal, phalangeal, or interphalangeal joints). Crush-type injuries may initially manifest with pain and swelling. Of particular concern is the possibility that crush injury may lead to a compartment syndrome over the ensuing 6 to 24 hours.

Blunt Trauma—Severe

Extremity injury associated with hemodynamic disturbances or disruption of the vascular supply are severe. These include de-gloving and crush (ie, wringer-type) injuries, as well as some long-bone fractures with high-energy transfer. Patients with severe extremity injuries should receive a rapid but thorough overall assessment, followed by prompt surgical consultation.

CHAPTER 91
Major Trauma

Moritz M. Ziegler, M.D. and
Javier A. Gonzalez Del Rey, M.D.

Accidents continue to account for close to half of all deaths in children from the ages of 1 to 14 years, exceeding all other causes of childhood mortality and accounting for more than 20000 deaths per year in children less than 19 years of age in the United States. More than half of these deaths are related to motor vehicle injury. Nearly 22 million children are injured each year in the United States, surpassing all major diseases in children and young adults. Two of three childhood accidents occur in boys. The peak accidental age range is between 4 and 12 years, with the highest frequency at 8 years of age. Accidental injury also accounts for approximately 30% of infant deaths. The societal impact of years of life lost from childhood mortal accidental injury is staggering.

The mortality rate for children hospitalized after an accident is reported to be low, but that is because 80% of all trauma deaths occur either at the accident scene or in the hospital emergency department (ED). The most common preventable cause of death in injured children is failure to secure the airway. As much as 18% of hospital trauma deaths are avoidable if a correct diagnosis is made and a treatment regimen is instituted. The most common single injury associated with death in injured children is head trauma, which alone or in association with other injuries is responsible for 80% of trauma deaths. Combined thoracoabdominal injuries produce an 82% mortality or condition of extremis upon arrival at the hospital ED.

ORGANIZATION OF THE TRAUMA SERVICE

The regionalization of trauma care in the United States is still in its evolutionary stage. Hospitals have been designated as Level I, II, or III institutions based both on their capability and on their desire to care for the multiply injured patient. Under the guidance of the American College of Surgeons' Committee on Trauma, the eventual benefit of such a designation plan is to triage Category I–, Category II–, or Category III–injured patients to appropriate, qualified facilities. Because no one hospital can be expected to have in its immediate geographic area the childhood trauma volume necessary to be an independent and freestanding trauma center, regionalization becomes a necessity, using rapid transportation to transport children over distances.

Each institution must develop its own in-house organizational tree for a trauma service. Such a service needs a well-established chain of command with an appropriately designated leader, a responsibility that may change hands as additional personnel arrive at a resuscitation in the ED. The role of this leadership position in a hospital trauma service is to accept responsibility for patient care and organize the multisystem specialists needed to care for the patient with multisystem injury. Such organization begins at the scene of an accident, includes transport, and involves patient triage after initial evaluation and care once the patient arrives in the hospital ED. Subsequently, a decision to transfer the patient to another hospital, admit him or her to an intensive care unit, or take him or her straight to the operating room will be made by the team leader after consultation with the other varied specialists involved. If at this time it is clear that the predominant injury is to a single body system, it is appropriate for the team leader to transfer patient care responsibility to the designated head of a given subspecialty. Figure 91.1 demonstrates a flow diagram of a response to the traumatized child, an example of organizational schema put into action when or before a victim of serious trauma arrives in the ED.

ASSESSMENT AND MANAGEMENT

Initial Evaluation

A rapid and reproducible schema of immediate, simultaneous, and subsequent evaluation and treatment principles should be applied to every child with major multiple trauma admitted to the ED (Table 91.1). This initial assessment includes a primary survey, resuscitation, a secondary survey, and eventual triage. Two key principles must be followed in the initial assessment of the trauma patient. First, if any physiologic threat to the patient is identified, that threat must be treated immediately. The order of priority is airway, breathing, and circulation (ABCs). For example, relief of a tension pneumothorax takes precedence over intravenous (i.v.) access. Second, if at any point in the patient's secondary survey or subsequent care there is an unexpected physiologic deterioration, rapidly repeat the primary survey in order of priority (A, B, C). A "trauma stat," alerting appropriate personnel, should be called upon notification of an impending arrival or simultaneously with an unexpected arrival of a child with multiple injuries in the ED, and all participants of the trauma care team should participate in this initial evaluation and treatment of the patient (Fig. 91.1). The indication for declaring a trauma stat is any one of the criteria listed in Table 91.2.

TABLE 91.1. Initial Assessment and Management Guidelines for the Injured Child

- I. Primary survey
  - A. Airway maintenance, cervical spine control
  - B. Breathing
  - C. Circulation
  - D. Disability
  - E. Exposure
- II. Resuscitation
  - A. Oxygenation, airway management, and ventilation
  - B. Shock management
  - C. Intubations—urinary tract, gastrointestinal tract
- III. Secondary survey
  - A. Head
  - B. Neck
  - C. Chest
  - D. Abdomen
  - E. Extremities
  - F. Neurologic
- IV. Triage

Primary Survey

The first priority in assessment and management is to secure an adequate airway while concomitantly stabilizing the neck to protect the cervical spinal cord from a yet-to-be-diagnosed cervical spine injury. The chin-lift or jaw-thrust maneuver and cleaning the oropharynx of accumulated foreign debris and secretions are the initial steps in establishing an airway. A cervical spine injury should be assumed to be present in all patients with major trauma, especially those injured above the clavicle. Adequate cervical spine radiographs and a normal clinical ex-

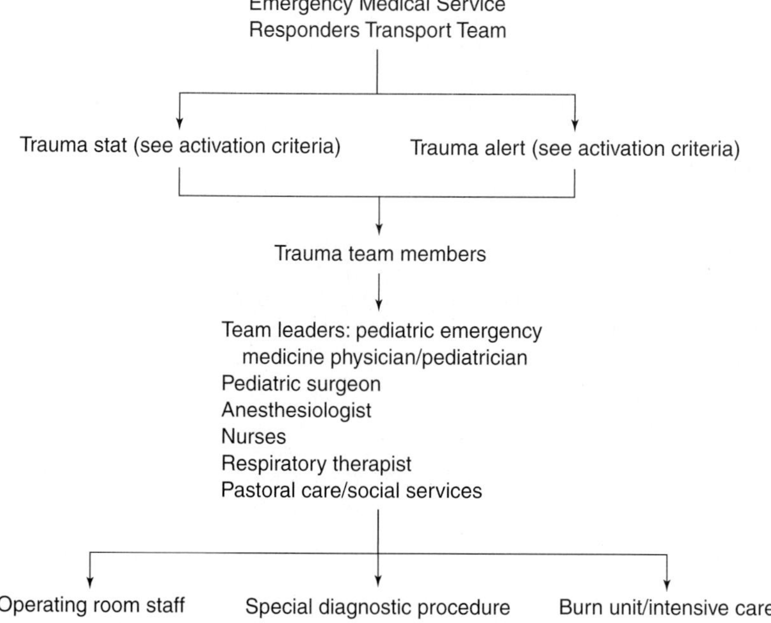

Figure 91.1. Sample flow diagram of a response to a traumatized child that is placed into action when or before a victim of serious trauma arrives in the emergency department.

TABLE 91.2. Declaration of Trauma Stat and Alert

Trauma Stat
I. Physiologic
1. Cardiopulmonary arrest
2. Shock
3. Respiratory distress
4. Neurologic failure (Glasgow Coma Scale score ≤8)
5. Trauma score <12
II. Anatomic
1. Penetrating (gunshot or stab) wound to head, chest, or abdomen
2. Facial/tracheal injury with potential airway compromise
3. Burn >30% body surface area; inhalation airway burn
4. Major electrical injury
Trauma Alert
I. Mechanism
1. Ejected from motor vehicle
2. Extrication time of ≥20 min
3. Fatality of another passenger in motor vehicle accident
4. Intrusion of vehicle ≥20 inches by collision
5. Vehicle traveling ≥20 mph in pedestrian accident or passenger unrestrained in motor vehicle accident (≥35 mph restrained)
6. Fall ≥20 feet
7. Run over by vehicle
8. Lightning
II. Anatomic
1. Significant injuries both above and below the diaphragm
2. Two or more proximal long bone fractures
3. Burn of 15%–30% body surface area (second/third degree)
4. Traumatic amputation of limb proximal to wrist or ankle
5. Crush injury of torso
6. Spinal injury with paralysis

amination are required to exclude this problem. Therefore, until such films are taken, the head and neck should be neither hyperextended nor hyperflexed during maneuvers to secure the airway. Before any effort at intubation, artificial ventilation may need to be established using a bag-valve-mask device (see Chapter 1).

Breathing is deemed acceptable only in the face of a patent airway and adequate air exchange with normal oxygen saturation and carbon dioxide excretion. Early monitoring with pulse oximetry is important. Compromise of ventilatory function in an injured child can occur with a depressed sensorium, airway occlusion, restriction of lung expansion, and direct pulmonary injury (see Chapter 84). Compromise of diaphragmatic excursion is a special hazard because of the increased importance of the diaphragm in ventilation in children. Gastric distension, a common event in an injured child, can significantly limit diaphragmatic excursion. In these situations, cricoid pressure should be performed while preparations are made for an artificial airway. This maneuver prevents possible aspiration of gastric content caused by passive regurgitation and/or increased intragastric pressure. Therefore, the early use of a nasogastric or an orogastric tube to decompress the stomach may need to be considered. If the child is obtunded or comatose, ventilation may require use of a bag-valve device that is connected to a mask or endotracheal tube delivering sufficient oxygen-enriched air (approximately 12 to 15 mL per kg) to produce an appropriate rise in the chest and an adequate oxygen saturation. Prompt attention to a hemopneumothorax, especially with mediastinal shift secondary to tension, is essential to the assessment of breathing (see "Secondary Survey" later in this chapter).

Circulation is initially assessed by examining the pulse, skin color, and capillary refilling time; from this information the peripheral perfusion and oxygenation may be estimated. A palpable peripheral pulse will generally correlate with a pressure greater than 80 mm Hg; a palpable central pulse indicates a pressure greater than 50 to 60 mm Hg, and a normovolemic patient capillary refilling time, as assessed by color return after blanching, will be within 2 seconds. External hemorrhage should be controlled by direct pressure or pneumatic splints, but the application of extremity tourniquets or hemostats to bleeding vessels is less useful. A mild Trendelenburg position may be of benefit in mild low-perfusion states to restore the central circulation.

To assess patient disability, a rapid neurologic examination is completed to establish the level of consciousness, as well as pupillary size and reaction. Table 91.3 lists the AVPU (alert, verbal stimuli response, painful stimuli response, unresponsive) method of assessing level of consciousness, in addition to pupillary assessment as previously mentioned. The Glasgow Coma Scale (Table 91.4) provides a quantitative measure of the level of consciousness.

To facilitate both assessment and treatment, the patient should be undressed and exposed, while careful attention is paid to the maintenance of body heat. Radiant warmers, air shields, and i.v. fluid warmers are useful tools in maintaining adequate temperature control in the pediatric patient.

Resuscitation

All patients with major trauma should receive supplemental oxygen therapy. Vascular access is another early necessity in resuscitation, and percutaneous or cut-down cannulation of upper or lower extremity veins should be of first priority, establishing two i.v. lines to facilitate resuscitation. Although large-bore cannulas are ideal, the size of the available veins should guide the choice of which cannulas to use. In a hypotensive child, the visible veins may be small. Successful placement of a 22- or 20-gauge cannula is preferable to a failed attempt to place a larger cannula. In a small child, one can give large volumes of fluids and blood through a small cannula. Improvement in vascular volume may then permit placement of a larger cannula at an alternative site. Early resuscitation also may be begun by intraosseous infusion into the tibial marrow space by a transtibial needle. We prefer percutaneous cannulation of an antecubital vein plus a saphenous vein at the ankle. In a hypotensive child in whom peripheral access is quickly found to be unsuccessful, the femoral vein provides a safe site for insertion of a central line, often accomplished rapidly using a guidewire technique. Rapid cut-down access is best done on an antecubital vein or the saphenous vein at either the ankle or in the groin just below the saphenofemoral junction.

At cannulation, blood should be sent for a type and crossmatch and for baseline hematologic and chemical parameters (Table 91.5). Central vein cannulation above the diaphragm is not a preferred primary access route, and in children, such access should be done only by experienced personnel.

The presence of shock must be assessed by appreciating whether or not inadequate organ perfusion exists. Shock after trauma is usually hypovolemic but may be cardiogenic or neurogenic. As a rule, isolated head trauma is not a cause of shock. Any injured patient who is cool and tachycardic is in shock until proved otherwise.

Hypovolemic shock is most common after major trauma and

TABLE 91.3. AVPU Method for Assessing Level of Consciousness

A—*A*lert	P—Responds to *p*ainful stimuli
V—Responds to *v*ocal stimuli	U—*U*nresponsive

TABLE 91.4. Pediatric Coma

	Glasgow coma scale	Modified infant coma score	
Eye opening	Spontaneous	Spontaneous	4
	To voice	To voice	3
	To pain	To pain	2
	None	None	1
Verbal response	Oriented	Coos, babbles	5
	Confused	Irritable cry, consolable	4
	Inappropriate	Cries to pain	3
	Garbled	Moans to pain	2
	None	None	1
Motor response	Obeys commands	Normal movements	6
	Localizes pain	Withdraws to touch	5
	Withdraws to pain	Withdraws to pain	4
	Flexion	Flexion	3
	Extension	Extension	2
	Flaccid	Flaccid	1

TABLE 91.5. Rapid Approach to the Pediatric Trauma Patient

Time interval patient priority	System assessment	Initial therapy	System monitor	Diagnostic study
First 5 min Primary survey	Respiration	C-spine stabilization (sand bags, collar) Airway (mask, intubate) Ventilation with O_2		
	Pulse	Cardiac compression	Heart rate (electrocardiogram) Blood pressure	
	Ventilation	Needle/tube thoracostomy—tension pneumothorax Dressing to sucking chest wound	Pulse oxymetry	
	External hemorrhage	Tamponade		
Second 5 min Resuscitation	Perfusion	Intravenous/intraosseus needle access; 20 mL/kg crystalloid; uncross-matched blood Needle pericardiocentesis Thoracotomy, aortic clamping	Perfusion Pulse Blood pressure PO_2, PCO_2, pH	Type and cross-match Complete blood count Amylase Liver function Blood urea nitrogen, glucose Electrolytes
	Level of consciousness	Nasogastric tube Urinary catheter Drugs	Temperature	Blood gas Urinalysis
Third 5 min Secondary survey	Ventilation	Venous access/central line	Perfusion	
	Perfusion	Type specific blood	Pulse	
	Head	Crystalloid	Blood pressure	Lateral neck film
	Neck		Arterial line	Chest radiograph
	Chest	Tube thoracotomy—pneumothorax, hemothorax		
	Abdomen	Drugs		Plan for abdominal or head computed tomography scan Peritoneal lavage
	Pelvis	Operating room		Urgent intravenous pyelogram
	Neurologic			
	Extremities			
Fourth 5 min Triage	Ventilation			
	Perfusion			
	Neurologic status	Splint fractures Drugs for intracranial pressure Type specific blood Intensive care unit Radiograph Operating room	Perfusion Pulse Blood pressure Temperature	Blood gas Intracranial pressure bolt

is usually secondary to a significant acute loss of the 8% to 9% of body weight made up by the child's blood volume. To quantify the extent of the problem and decide on treatment priorities, hemorrhagic shock can be classified according to severity (Table 91.6). Reliance on the hematocrit alone may prove unreliable because a near-normal hematocrit level does not exclude the possibility of significant blood loss. Class I hemorrhage occurs with up to 15% acute blood volume loss (approximately a 250-mL blood loss in a 20-kg child), and physiologic changes will be minimal. Primary fluid replacement will stabilize the circulation. Class II hemorrhage, 15% to 30% blood loss (approximately 250- to 500-mL blood loss in a 20-kg child), is associated with a mild tachycardia and tachypnea along with a fall in pulse pressure as catecholamine release produces elevation of peripheral vascular resistance. Such patients may have impaired capillary refilling, and they may be either frightened or belligerent. These patients initially may be stabilized with crystalloid infusion, although blood transfusion eventually may be necessary. Class III hemorrhage is physiologically more significant, the 30% to 40% blood loss corresponding to 500 to 650 mL of blood in a 20-kg child. These patients have obvious signs of shock with altered mental status, tachycardia, tachypnea, and a measurable diminution in systolic pressure. Crystalloid resuscitation should be begun promptly, and most patients also will require blood products. Class IV hemorrhagic shock is immediately life-threatening. Patients are mentally depressed, cold, and pale; they have profound tachycardia and tachypnea, the pulse pressure is narrow, and there is no urine output. After rapid transfusion, such patients usually require prompt operative intervention.

Cardiogenic shock after major childhood injury is rare, but it could be a result of cardiac tamponade or a direct cardiac contusion. Dilated neck veins in a patient with a decelerating injury, sternal contusion, or a penetrating thoracic injury should arouse such suspicion (see Chapters 72 and 94). Neurogenic shock classically presents with hypotension without tachycardia or vasoconstriction; however, isolated head injuries do not produce shock, and causes of hypovolemia should always be sought in such patients. Septic shock rarely occurs immediately after injury, even in the face of abdominal content contamination.

Crystalloid isotonic solution, preferably Ringer lactate or normal saline solution, is the initial resuscitative fluid of choice. The initial infusion is given as rapidly as possible in a dose of 20 mL per kg with careful monitoring of patient physiologic response to the fluid. Table 91.6 emphasizes the anticipated fluid needs, depending on the degree of shock, and the formulation is based on the premise that the patient will require 300 mL of crystalloid for each 100 mL of blood loss—the 3:1 rule. The restoration of perfusion may be clinically assessed, and at times invasive monitoring with elective placement of a central venous line or a pulmonary artery catheter facilitates this assessment. A most useful practical guide is the monitoring of urinary output; 1 mL per kg per hour is optimum, although for children less than 1 year of age, preferred output should approach 2 mL per kg per hour.

Blood transfusion preferably is done with fully cross-matched warmed blood passed through a 160-μm macropore filter. In the face of a transient or absent benefit from a rapid crystalloid infusion, fully cross-matched, type-specific, or type O negative blood should be given as a whole-blood transfusion. In summary, fluid and blood are given rapidly enough to maintain stable vital signs and adequate urine output. Vasopressors, steroids, and sodium bicarbonate do not play a role in the initial treatment of hypovolemic shock.

After perfusion has been restored, if not already accomplished, placement of urinary and gastric catheters should be done. Urinary catheterization should not be attempted before a retrograde urethrogram has proved urethral integrity if blood has been noted at the urethral meatus or in the scrotum, or if there is abnormal prostate placement on rectal examination. The urinary specimen should be immediately analyzed. In the presence of blunt head trauma with blood coming from the ears, nose, or mouth, care must be taken in inserting a nasogastric tube to avoid passage into the brain through a cribriform plate fracture. Such patients are better intubated through the mouth or through a soft nasopharyngeal airway.

Secondary Survey

A systematic assessment of organ systems must be done after securing the airway, breathing, and circulation. A pertinent history includes allergies, medications, past illnesses, time of the last meal, and the events preceding the injury.

A head examination includes reevaluation of pupillary size and reactivity, a conjunctival and fundic examination for hemorrhage or penetrating injury, and a quick assessment of visual acuity. A thorough palpation of skull and mandible will detect fracture-dislocations, but if the airway is secure, maxillofacial bony trauma is of low priority in the total treatment plan.

Injury to the cervical spine is uncommon in children (see Chapter 93), but risk of injury must still be considered. This is especially true for any child with injury above the clavicles. It is also true for young children who fall one or more floors, are hit by a motor vehicle at 30 mph or more, and who are unrestrained or poorly restrained occupants of a motor vehicle involved in a crash. In older children, sports injuries are the second most common cause of cervical spine injury. In a child with a low risk for cervical spine injury (eg, a fall when running), the neck can be cleared with a normal lateral cervical spine film, showing all seven cervical spine vertebrae. Also, a normal clinical examina-

TABLE 91.6. Therapeutic Classification of Hemorrhagic Shock in the Pediatric Patient

	Class I	Class II	Class III	Class IV
Blood loss %				
Blood volume[a]	Up to 15%	15%–30%	30%–40%	40% or more
Pulse rate	Normal	Mild tachycardia	Moderate tachycardia	Severe tachycardia
Blood pressure	Normal/increased	Normal/decreased	Decreased	Decreased
Capillary blanch test	Normal	Positive	Positive	Positive
Respiratory rate	Normal	Mild tachypnea	Moderate tachypnea	Severe tachypnea
Urine output	1–2 mL/kg/h	0.5–1.0 mL/kg/h	0.25–0.5 mL/kg/h	Negligible
Mental status	Slightly anxious	Mildly anxious	Anxious/confused	Confused/lethargic
Fluid replacement (3:1 rule)	Crystalloid	Crystalloid	Crystalloid + blood	Crystalloid + blood

[a] Assume blood volume to be 8%–9% of body weight (80–90 mL/kg)

tion in an awake, cooperative child (active but controlled flexion and extension and rotatory motion with no symptoms or signs of spasm, guarding pain, or tenderness) is the most important part of the assessment in ruling out neck injury. Ligamentous disruption and dislocation injuries of the cervical spine without radiographic evidence of bony injury are not uncommon in children because of the weakness of the soft tissue of the neck and the incomplete development of the bony spine. In approximately 40% of children with spinal cord injury, injury occurs without radiologic abnormality (SCIWORA). In children with a high-risk mechanism of trauma, it is best to obtain anteroposterior, odontoid, and lateral views. If the patient has an altered sensorium, a cervical collar should be left in place even if the three survey films are negative. When the patient recovers sufficiently to permit a fuller evaluation of the neck, the collar can be removed.

Three situations require a special approach. First, if a seriously injured child has had an endotracheal intubation placed, one can get a computed tomographic (CT) scan of C1–C2 when getting a head CT scan. Second, if the patient is brought to the hospital with a helmet on (eg, football or motorcycle) and if there is no respiratory distress or other problem requiring immediate intubation, an initial cervical spine series can be done before helmet removal. If it is necessary to remove the helmet before the neck is cleared, a two-person technique ensuring neck immobilization should be used. Third, in the case of penetrating injuries to the neck, wounds deep to the platysma usually warrant operative exploration. In the case of missile injuries, the entry site should be denoted with an opaque marker, and anteroposterior and lateral spine films should be obtained.

Visual inspection of the chest will identify a sucking chest wound, best treated by immediate application of a sterile occlusive dressing; a major flail component, treated by splinting or endotracheal intubation; or a penetrating wound (see Chapter 94). Palpation of all thoracic bony parts must be done quickly, and auscultation may reveal a pneumothorax, hemothorax, or cardiac tamponade. The former two should be treated by tube thoracostomy. The latter may best be detected by muffled heart sounds, distended neck veins, and a narrow pulse pressure, and should be relieved by prompt pericardiocentesis. A diagnosis of tension pneumothorax is supported by observing a contralateral tracheal shift and distended neck veins in addition to diminished breath sounds. Needle thoracentesis should provide relief, but tube thoracostomy should follow, with placement of the tube to water seal drainage plus suction. If an impaled object is protruding from the chest or any part of a patient, it is best debrided from surrounding clothing and left in place until definitive operation. If the history suggests a severe deceleration injury and the chest radiograph demonstrates a widened mediastinum with or without a fractured first rib, a thoracic aortic injury is suggested, and aortography is promptly indicated. If the chest radiograph reveals air lucencies suggesting intestine, a ruptured diaphragm is a possibility.

The purpose of the secondary abdominal examination is to establish whether an injury exists (see Chapters 91 and 95); it is not to give an exact diagnosis. Injury should be suspected in the presence of abdominal wall contusion, distension, abdominal or shoulder pain, signs of parietal peritoneal irritation, and/or shock. Hence, in most patients a baseline imaging study such as an abdominal CT scan should be done as soon as possible. Diagnostic peritoneal lavage (DPL) should be considered in the ED to expedite the decision about whether a patient needs an immediate laparotomy. In children, this is primarily of benefit in a patient who is unstable despite appropriate resuscitation; who has penetrating trauma that does not clearly involve the abdomen (eg, gunshot wound of the lower chest); or who requires urgent, nonabdominal operative intervention (eg, decompression of an epidural hematoma). In fact, most children with documented intraabdominal or retroperitoneal injury who remain stable or rapidly become so do not require surgery. A positive DPL with greater than 100000 red blood cells (RBCs) per cubic millimeter may correlate with a laceration of the spleen or liver but is not necessarily an indication for surgery in a stable patient. Of such patients, 80% will stop bleeding without surgical intervention. However, diagnosis of injury is important in planning for care. Table 91.7 summarizes the indications and contraindications for this procedure. After emptying the urinary bladder, a midline approach above or below the umbilicus is used. If the initial aspirate is grossly bloody or if the aspirate after instilling 10 mL per kg of Ringer lactate reveals greater than 100000 RBCs per mm^3; greater than 500 white blood cells (WBCs) per cubic millimeter; a spun effluent hematocrit greater than 2%; or the presence of bile, bacteria, or fecal material, the paracentesis is positive. Lavage is most commonly falsely positive in the face of a pelvic fracture, or it may be falsely negative despite injuries to pancreas, duodenum, genitourinary tract, aorta, vena cava, and diaphragm.

A rectal examination is essential to assess sphincter tone, rectal integrity, prostatic position, pelvic fracture, and presence of blood in the stool.

A thorough extremity examination should assess deformity, contusions, abrasions, penetration, and perfusion, including pulse palpation. The presence of a distal extremity pulse does not exclude a concomitant proximal arterial injury. Soft-tissue injuries should be thoroughly inspected for both wound foreign bodies and the presence of devitalized tissue. Long bones should be palpated with rotational or three-point pressure for tenderness, crepitation, or abnormal movement, and pressure must be applied to the pubis and anterior iliac spines to assess for the presence of a pelvic fracture. Severe extremity angulations should be straightened, joints should be immobilized, and traction splints should be applied. Compound fracture sites should be covered with sterile dressings. Generous irrigation and debridement of open wounds is beneficial in early wound care to minimize contamination before considering primary or delayed wound closure (see Chapter 108).

Supplemental studies (including regular and contrast imaging studies; biochemical analyses of liver, pancreatic, and renal function; and electrocardiographic analysis of cardiac function) may now be done. Tetanus prophylaxis should be considered (see Chapter 90), and antibiotics should be administered if specifically indicated.

Imaging the Pediatric Trauma Patient

In any child with major trauma caused by a blunt mechanism, a basic radiographic survey series should be considered. Traditionally, these included cervical spine, chest, and pelvic ra-

TABLE 91.7. Peritoneal Lavage in the Evaluation of Abdominal Trauma in Childhood

Indications
- Potential false-negative examination—head injury, medication overlay, spinal cord trauma
- Potential false-positive examination—rib, pelvic, or spine fractures
- Unexplained hypovolemia
- Anesthetic need for unrelated injury
- Selected penetrating injury

Absolute contraindications
- Multiple previous operations by history
- Already determined need for laparotomy

Relative contraindications
- Pregnancy

TABLE 91.8. Emergency Department Assessment and Management Plan for the Injured Child

Assessment	Diagnosis	Management	Laboratory study
Airway/breathing ↓		Clear airway Intubate Ventilate	
Cardiac function ↓		External cardiac massage	Cardiorespiratory monitor
Shock ↓	External hemorrhage →	Direct pressure	Complete blood count (CBC)
	Internal hemorrhage →	Trendelenburg position Establish intravenous/intraosseous access	Cross-match for one blood volume
Head/neck injury ↓	Closed head injury Possible cervical spine fracture	Sand bag splint of neck Hyperventilation	Computed tomography (CT) scan, head Lateral neck film
Chest injury ↓	Cardiac contusion →	Electrocardiographic monitor Pericardiocentesis	Chest radiograph Electrocardiogram Cardiac ultrasound Arterial blood gas Chest CT
	Hemopneumothorax →	Tube thoracostomy	
	Flail chest →	Intubation/ventilation	
	Sucking wound →	Sterile dressing	
Abdominal injury ↓	Penetrating injury →	Nasogastric tube Serial examination	Plain/upright radiograph
	Blunt injury →	Serial examination Paracentesis with lavage	Tilt table test Abdominal CT Amylase Liver function tests Serial CBC
Renal/urinary injury ↓	Renal contusion/laceration →	Bladder catheterization	Urinalysis Plain abdominal radiograph Intravenous pyelogram
	Bladder/urethral injury →	Delayed catheterization	Voiding cystourethrogram
Musculoskeletal injury ↓	Dismembered part →	Salvage, irrigate, and cool	Extremity radiographs Angiography
	Compound fracture →	Sterile dressing; splint	
	Bony injury →	Splint, traction	
Soft-tissue injury		Irrigate, debride Primary versus delayed repair	Radiograph to exclude foreign body

diographs. Recent studies have demonstrated that patients with a Glasgow Coma Scale score of 15, no distracting injury, and no pain in the pelvic region have a low incidence for pelvic fractures. In these patients, the routine use of pelvic radiographs is not necessary but also rarely helpful in the acute initial management of the traumatized child. In a stable, cooperative patient, the clinician should review the lateral cervical spine film first and then proceed with the other films. In a less stable or neurologically compromised patient, it is best to obtain all films at once while continuing to protect the cervical spine. In patients with trauma to the torso, a pelvic film is important as a clinical indicator; 80% of children with multiple fractures of the pelvis have concomitant abdominal or genitourinary injuries. Additional survey films of the thoracolumbar spine and extremities depend on clinical findings and the mechanism of trauma.

The primary and secondary survey may then suggest the need for more definitive imaging studies.

SUMMARY

Tables 91.5 and 91.8 describe a rapid approach to the patient. Over a 20-minute interval, the patient may be sequentially and simultaneously assessed, treated, monitored, and subjected to further diagnostic study while the format of primary survey, resuscitation, secondary survey, and triage is followed. Each physician dealing with the injured child should have such a format within his or her armamentarium. In addition, one should be able to recognize the need for and be able to perform an emergency resuscitative thoracotomy in a patient with chest trauma who is deteriorating despite maximum fluid resuscitation (see Chapter 94). With these treatment formats well in hand, the clinician can optimize the subsequent care of the patient after admission or can provide for successful transfer of the patient to a tertiary care trauma center.

CHAPTER 92
Neurotrauma

David S. Greenes, M.D. and
Joseph R. Madsen, M.D.

HEAD TRAUMA

Head trauma accounts for approximately 250,000 hospital admissions and nearly 5 million visits to emergency departments (EDs) for pediatric patients each year. Brain injury is the leading cause of death and disability among pediatric trauma patients. Because morbidity and mortality after head trauma can be lessened by prompt stabilization, emergency physicians need to be thoroughly familiar with the manifestations of significant head injury and the necessary diagnostic and therapeutic maneuvers.

The approach to the child with a head injury is outlined in Chapter 31. This chapter focuses on the clinical anatomy, pathophysiology, clinical manifestations, diagnosis, and management of specific traumatic lesions to the head.

Pathophysiology

PRIMARY VERSUS SECONDARY BRAIN INJURY

Discussions of traumatic brain injury typically divide the injury into two main components: primary and secondary brain injury. Primary brain injury refers to neural damage that is attributed directly to the traumatic insult itself. Shearing of neuronal axons, contusion or laceration of cerebral tissue, or direct penetration of the brain by a missile, for instance, all constitute primary brain injury.

Secondary brain injury refers to subsequent injury, after a trauma has occurred, to brain cells not injured by the initial traumatic event. Secondary brain injury may result from numerous causes, including hypoxia, hypoperfusion, excitotoxic damage, free radical damage, or metabolic derangements. In some cases, the effect of secondary brain injury is far more devastating than was the primary brain injury itself. Because many of the causes of secondary brain injury are at least theoretically preventable, most of the efforts in neurotrauma care are directed at monitoring for, and attempting to prevent, these complications.

CEREBRAL ISCHEMIA

Probably the most important cause of secondary brain injury is brain ischemia, resulting from inadequate cerebral blood flow (CBF). Adequate CBF depends first on the presence of patent cerebral vessels to deliver blood to the brain. Rarely, severe head injury can be associated with shear, dissection, compression, or thrombosis of the major cerebral vessels, leading to tissue infarction. Vasospasm of the cerebral vasculature can also contribute to secondary brain injury. Vasospasm is not uncommon in cases of severe head injury, especially in those cases associated with subarachnoid hemorrhage.

Adequate CBF depends not only on patent vessels but also on adequate cerebral perfusion pressure (CPP). The cerebral perfusion pressure reflects a balance between the mean arterial pressure (MAP) of blood flowing to the brain, and the intracranial pressure (ICP), which acts as a counterforce, limiting blood flow to the brain. The relationship between these forces can be described mathematically: CPP = MAP − ICP.

In healthy children, the ICP is less than 20 mm Hg, and MAP is 70 to 80 mm Hg or greater (depending on the patient's age), yielding a CPP of 50 to 60 mm Hg or greater. The CPP fluctuates, but the healthy body maintains constant CBF in the face of minor fluctuations in CPP through autoregulation. Autoregulation is a process of reflex vasoconstriction or vasodilation in response to changes in CPP, thereby modulating resistance to blood flow in the cerebral vasculature to maintain a constant CBF. However, if the CPP drops too low (ie, less than 40 or 50 mm Hg), the body will not be able to maintain adequate CBF despite maximal vasodilation. At this point, cerebral ischemia ensues.

INCREASED INTRACRANIAL PRESSURE

Severe drops in CPP can result from systemic hypotension (as in the multiply traumatized patient with exsanguinating injuries) or from significant increases in ICP. Increases in ICP are common in patients with serious head injuries, and they account for much of secondary brain injury.

Increased ICP may result from any process that increases the volume of the intracranial contents. Because the cranium has a fixed size and is relatively noncompliant, it can only accommodate a certain volume of intracranial contents at low pressure. An idealized pressure-volume curve (as seen in Fig. 92.1) represents the relationship between intracranial volume and ICP. In the normal state, small increments in intracranial volume can be made without significant change in the ICP (point 1 on the curve in Fig. 92.1). At this point, the intracranial contents are not particularly "tightly" packed into the cranium, and there is room for additional volume. After a certain critical point is reached, however (as indicated by point 2 on the curve), additional volume begins to lead to increases in ICP. At some point soon thereafter, the compliance of the intracranial space is exhausted (point 3 on Fig. 92.1), and the pressure-volume curve becomes steep, with even tiny increments in intracranial volume leading to massive increases in ICP. For patients on this steep part of the curve, the addition or removal of even 1 mL of intracranial volume may cause significant changes in the clinical status.

CEREBRAL HERNIATION SYNDROMES

Cerebral herniation refers to the abnormal passage of brain tissue into an anatomic space in which it does not normally reside. Cerebral herniation occurs when the brain tissue is displaced by a large intracranial hematoma and/or massive brain swelling. Several distinct herniation syndromes exist, each correlated with distinct anatomic sites of herniation.

The best known herniation syndrome is tentorial herniation, which refers to the herniation of the parahippocampal gyrus and often the uncus of the temporal lobe through the tentorial notch, from the middle into the posterior fossa. Tentorial herniation most typically results from a focal mass lesion in or overlying the ipsilateral cerebral hemisphere, although it may also result from massive diffuse brain swelling. As the mass lesion or swelling expands, it pushes the brain tissue down, until a portion of the temporal lobe begins to slide through the tentorial notch. As the temporal cortex passes through, it becomes pressed against the brainstem structures and against cranial nerve III, which runs along the edge of the tentorial notch. In addition, the feeding vessels (branches of the basilar artery system) in this region may be stretched and distorted.

Most discussions of tentorial herniation describe a stereotyped sequence of clinical events that follows from the anatomic

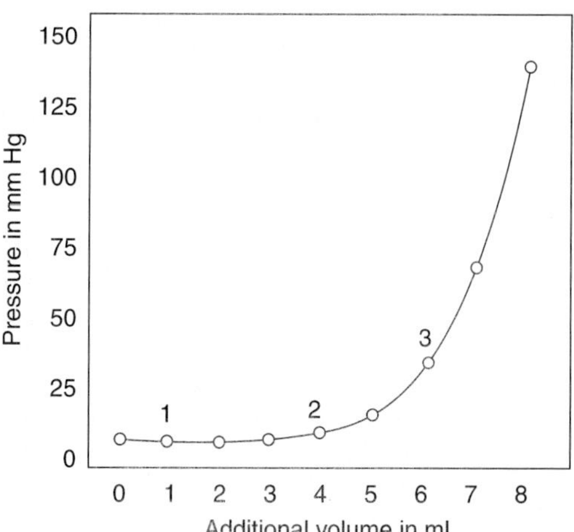

Figure 92.1. Effect of additional intracranial volume on intracranial pressure.

progression described previously. In many patients, however, the constellation of clinical findings varies considerably from this "classic" presentation. Classically, the patient first complains of headache, which may reflect stretching of the dura or the basal blood vessels. Next, a depression in the level of consciousness occurs, as the reticular activating system is compressed. The ipsilateral third nerve is compressed next, with resulting pupillary dilation ("blown pupil") and eventually loss of third nerve motor function (ptosis, and loss of medial gaze). As the process continues and the cerebral peduncle is compressed, hemiparesis or decerebrate posturing develops (usually contralateral to the herniating cortex, but sometimes ipsilateral). Brainstem control of vital signs is also affected, with the development of bradycardia, hypertension, and irregular respirations (Cushing triad). As herniation and brainstem compression continue to progress, the patient typically loses function of both pupils and develops decerebrate posturing or flaccid paresis bilaterally. Ultimately, respiratory arrest ensues. Even if the cause of the herniation is relieved before cardiorespiratory arrest occurs, prolonged compression of brainstem structures may be associated with hyperemia of the brainstem and fatal brainstem hemorrhages after the compression is relieved.

Some other brain herniation syndromes should also be recognized. One site of herniation is the foramen magnum, through which the cerebellar tonsils may herniate. This form of herniation is usually a result of the progression of a posterior fossa mass lesion. The herniation process produces compression of the cervicomedullary junction. As the brainstem and aqueduct of Sylvius are compressed, ventricular outflow obstruction may occur, with the acute onset of hydrocephalus, which will severely worsen the increased ICP, exacerbating the herniation process. Patients with herniation at the foramen magnum may present with symptoms of neck pain, vomiting, depressed mental status, bradycardia, or hypertension. In other cases, the patient may be relatively asymptomatic until sudden cardiorespiratory arrest occurs.

Another herniation syndrome is subfalcine herniation, which occurs when one cerebral hemisphere herniates beneath the falx cerebri to the opposite side. This form of herniation typically results from the progression of a unilateral supratentorial mass lesion. It is associated with symptoms of unilateral or bilateral leg weakness, and disturbances of bladder control, which result from compression and ischemia in the territory of the anterior cerebral artery.

Finally, the clinician should consider the retroalar herniation syndrome, which results from herniation of frontal lobe tissue posteriorly across the lesser wing of the sphenoid bone, usually as a result of frontal lobe mass lesions, or of swelling of the frontal lobes. The herniation may lead to distortion or compression of one or both intracranial carotid arteries, with resultant ischemia and infarction in the territories of the anterior and middle cerebral arteries.

METABOLIC DERANGEMENTS

Other physiologic mechanisms of secondary brain injury are important as well. Hypoxia, resulting from thoracic injuries, airway obstruction, or inadequate respiratory effort can be an important cause of brain injury. Hyperthermia increases cerebral metabolism and magnifies the severity of ischemia to an already compromised brain. There is increasing evidence that hyperglycemia also contributes to cerebral injury in the compromised brain.

The role of other substances in contributing to secondary brain injury has been carefully evaluated by investigators in the past decade. It appears that excess concentrations of the neurotransmitter glutamate, released from injured neurons into the synaptic cleft, can lead to injury through excess excitation of otherwise healthy postsynaptic neurons. Oxidizing agents and oxygen free radicals, released from injured neurons or elaborated as part of the brain's inflammatory response to injury, also appear to play a role in causing secondary brain injury.

MANAGEMENT AND GENERAL PRINCIPLES

Initial Resuscitation

Management of the patient with a head injury focuses on the prevention of secondary brain injury. As with all emergency care, management begins with the ABCs (airway, breathing, and circulation) of resuscitation. A patient with a head injury who has altered sensorium may require assistance with positioning of the airway or suctioning of oral and pharyngeal secretions. The clinician must recognize the potential for cervical spine injury in all patients with head injuries, and cervical spine precautions must be taken during airway management. Immobilization of the cervical spine with a semirigid cervical collar or with in-line manual stabilization must be maintained until the clinician can be certain that no cervical spine injury has occurred.

Breathing may be impaired if the patient's neural control of respiratory function is compromised or if traumatic injuries involve the thorax. All seriously traumatized patients require 100% inspired oxygen until it is certain that supplemental oxygen is not needed. Positive-pressure ventilation with a bag-valve-mask apparatus should be provided for any patient with inadequate respiratory effort. Unless there is increased ICP, the clinician should aim to achieve normocarbia (P_{CO_2} 35 to 40), and oxygen saturations of 100%. If there is evidence of increased ICP, therapeutic hyperventilation may be indicated (see the following).

Endotracheal intubation should be performed for any patient making inadequate or labored respiratory effort, or for patients who have a blunted gag reflex, cannot manage their oral secretions, or are comatose. Orotracheal intubation is generally safer than nasotracheal intubation if there is any concern about injuries to the midface. Care must be taken to minimize manipulation of the cervical spine during the process of intubation. Rapid sequence intubation is indicated for most patients with head injuries to ensure that the patients are comfortable and that intubation can be safely achieved. However, adequate oxygenation, ventilation, and protection of the airway are always the first priority. If intravenous (i.v.) access cannot be rapidly achieved, attempts at intubation may need to proceed without the use of adjunct medications.

Premedication for rapid sequence intubation begins with atropine 0.02 mg per kg (maximum dose 0.5 mg) for children less than 8 years of age, to lessen the vagal response to intubation. Lidocaine may also be useful, at a dosage of 1 to 2 mg per kg, as premedication to blunt the airway reflexes, thereby reducing the risk of coughing or choking, which may increase ICP.

If possible, a sedative drug should be used, both to make the patient comfortable, and to decrease the patient's responsiveness to airway manipulation. Thiopental at a dosage of 4 to 7 mg per kg is an ideal drug for patients with head injuries who have increased ICP because it decreases cerebral metabolism, thereby reducing the risk of ischemia. It must be used cautiously, however, in patients with any hemodynamic instability because it may reduce vasomotor tone and cardiac contractility, thereby leading to a decrease in blood pressure. If thiopental cannot be used, an alternative regimen is fentanyl (2 to 3 μg per kg) and midazolam (0.1 mg per kg), which provide sedation and analgesia with minimal effect on cardiac contractility or vasomotor tone. In cases in which intubation must proceed but i.v. access cannot be achieved, midazolam may be given intramuscularly (0.1 mg per kg), with onset of action in about 3 minutes. Ketamine should be avoided in patients with head injuries because it can increase ICP.

For neuromuscular blockade, succinylcholine (1 to 1.5 mg per kg i.v.) offers the advantage of rapid action, with intubating conditions developing within 45 to 60 seconds. In theory, the diffuse fasciculations caused by succinylcholine may serve to increase resistance to venous drainage from the head and increase ICP. This potential risk can be avoided with the use of nondepolarizing agents, such as vecuronium (0.1 mg per kg i.v.) or rocuronium (0.6 to 1.2 mg per kg i.v.), which do not cause fasciculations. Although the onset of action for these agents is slower than for succinylcholine, rocuronium, at the higher end of its dosage range, can be expected to provide intubating conditions in approximately 60 to 90 seconds.

The circulatory status of patients with isolated head trauma is generally not compromised, although the potential for other organ system trauma, with associated hemodynamic compromise, must be immediately recognized. Intravenous access should be obtained immediately in all patients with moderate or severe head injuries.

Isotonic crystalloid solutions—normal saline or lactated Ringer solution—should be given as needed to restore normal intravascular volume (see Chapter 91). The clinician should remember that the patient will only have an adequate cerebral perfusion pressure if the MAP is maintained in a normal range. On the other hand, for patients with adequate intravascular volume, excess fluid administration should be avoided. These patients can be treated with normal saline or lactated Ringer solution, running at one-half to two-thirds the maintenance fluid rate, while evaluation and treatment of the head injuries are being performed.

Brain-Specific Therapies

Once the ABCs of resuscitation have been addressed and the patient has been stabilized, attention can be given to the neurologic status. The neurologic assessment of the patient with a head injury, and the criteria for deciding which patients need neuroimaging are described in detail in Chapter 31.

Medical treatment for increased ICP should be undertaken immediately when increased ICP is suspected. This treatment includes elevation of the head of the bed to an angle of 30 degrees, which promotes venous drainage from the head (thereby decreasing the volume of the intracranial vasculature). The head should be maintained in a midline position, which helps maintain venous outflow through the jugular system as well. Furthermore, sedating medications may be needed to prevent the patient from coughing and choking or from becoming agitated, both of which might be associated with increased intrathoracic pressure and, therefore, impaired venous drainage. Sedation should be used as sparingly as possible, however, so that the neurologic status can be monitored. Paralytic agents should be used only when sedating agents cannot be tolerated or when maximal therapy with sedation fails to control the patient's behavior.

Hyperventilation also decreases ICP by decreasing the volume of the intracranial vasculature. The cerebral arteriolar circulation responds to hypocarbia with reflex vasoconstriction. The therapeutic use of hyperventilation requires a delicate balance: too little ventilation leads to vasodilation and increased ICP, but too much ventilation leads to excess vasoconstriction and decreased CBF. The optimal balance for therapeutic hyperventilation appears to be achieved at a P_{CO_2} of 30 to 35 mm Hg. The gold standard for monitoring P_{CO_2} is the arterial blood gas. Therefore, an arterial line is invaluable in monitoring the progress of hyperventilation in the patient with a head injury. In the short run, however, useful information about trends in P_{CO_2} can be obtained readily with the use of end-tidal CO_2 monitoring.

Mannitol can also be given to lower the ICP, at an i.v. dose of 0.5 to 1 g per kg, which increases the serum osmolarity. The increased serum osmolarity draws free water into the vasculature, thereby leading to a decrease in the viscosity of blood. Because of the lower viscosity of blood, CBF is improved. The improvement in CBF leads to improved cerebral oxygenation, which helps prevent cerebral ischemia. Furthermore, the autoregulatory system responds to the improved cerebral oxygenation with reflex vasoconstriction, thereby lowering intracerebral volume (and ICP) without compromising CBF. The effect of mannitol on ICP is seen within a few minutes of administration. Over the ensuing hour or so, mannitol also leads to some degree of intravascular volume depletion because of its action as an osmotic diuretic. Clinicians should be cautious about the use of mannitol in any patient with possible hemodynamic compromise because the administration of a diuretic may exacerbate hypovolemia and worsen perfusion.

There is disagreement in the literature about the optimal use of hyperventilation and mannitol in the management of the patient with a head injury. The clearest indication for these maneuvers is to "buy time" for several minutes in a patient with clinical signs of impending herniation. Stabilization of the patient with impending herniation by using hyperventilation and/or mannitol may allow enough time for the patient to be safely transferred to the radiology suite, for emergency head computed tomography (CT) imaging. If an evacuable hematoma is discovered on CT, these maneuvers can be used to stabilize the patient en route to the operating suite, where the increased ICP will be more definitively relieved.

It is less clear that sustained hyperventilation or repeated doses of mannitol are useful in patients who have diffuse brain swelling but who do not have surgical mass lesions. In particular, numerous studies in recent years have documented a clear relationship between even mild degrees of hyperventilation (P_{CO_2} 30 to 35) and decreased CBF. Because the overall goal of resuscitation in the patient with a head injury is to optimize CBF, prolonged hyperventilation may be counterprotective in that it may actually worsen cerebral ischemia. Therefore, hyperventilation is most useful as a transient therapy for acute changes in neurologic condition or as a second-line therapy after other methods of managing ICP have failed.

Some concern has also been raised that repeated doses of mannitol may be counterproductive in the ongoing care of patients with brain swelling because mannitol can leak across the injured blood–brain barrier, with its osmotic pull serving to worsen cerebral edema. Although some experimental models have documented this phenomenon, most data from clinical studies indicate lasting improvements in CBF with repeated doses of mannitol. Therefore, many authors consider mannitol to be a useful adjunct in the management of increased ICP in patients with brain swelling.

Anticonvulsant medications are clearly indicated for patients who are having ongoing seizure activity. Short-acting benzodiazepines (lorazepam or diazepam) may be used acutely in the management of ongoing seizures, and phenytoin or fosphenytoin may be used for maintenance anticonvulsant effect.

Phenytoin is also commonly used as prophylaxis for patients who have intracranial lesions associated with an increased risk of seizure activity, such as cerebral contusion, intraparenchymal hemorrhage, subarachnoid hemorrhage, or subdural hemorrhage. Patients who have epidural hematoma but no associated parenchymal injuries usually are not treated prophylactically.

Disposition

Generally, all patients with intracranial hematomas or brain injuries noted on head CT imaging should be hospitalized, no matter how mild or severe their symptoms. In addition, any patient with an abnormal mental status or neurologic examination should be hospitalized, even if head CT findings are normal. Patients with neurologic compromise and sizable intracranial hematomas require emergency operative intervention, and they are monitored postoperatively in the intensive care unit (ICU) for development of cerebral edema or recurrence of bleeding. Patients with neurologic compromise but no surgical lesions also need intensive care monitoring, often with the placement of a device for the measurement of ICP. In general, ICP monitors are indicated for any patient with a head injury who is comatose and who has an abnormal head CT. Although numerous different types of ICP monitors have been used, the intraventricular catheter has the advantage of being useful both for monitoring and for therapy because cerebrospinal fluid (CSF) can be drained through the catheter if needed to lower the ICP acutely. The goal of ICU management for patients with ICP monitors is to maintain an adequate CPP, which generally entails maintaining ICP at 20 mm Hg or less. More mildly symptomatic patients with a normal neurologic status and small cerebral contusions or intracranial hematomas may be candidates for observation in a ward setting.

Well-appearing patients with head injuries who either required no head CT scan (see Chapter 31) or who have no intracranial lesions on head CT imaging may be suitable for discharge to home with careful instructions. A discussion of the management of these patients follows.

BLUNT TRAUMA: SPECIFIC LESIONS

Concussion

Concussion is defined by the Centers for Disease Control and Prevention as a head-trauma–induced alteration in mental status that may or may not involve loss of consciousness. Most clinicians use the term concussion to refer to mild head injuries, with no or minor depression in the level of consciousness (Glasgow Coma Scale scores of 13 to 15), and with no associated focal neurologic deficits. Concussion most commonly results from falls in infants and toddlers and from motor vehicle collisions or sports-related injuries in older children and adolescents.

Common symptoms of concussion include initial loss of consciousness, amnesia, confusion, headache, nausea, vomiting, and dizziness. For the most part, clinicians diagnose concussion in those patients with minor head trauma who have no brain imaging performed, or as a diagnosis of exclusion for patients with minor head injury who have no evidence of intracranial pathology on a head CT scan.

Increasingly in recent years, it has been recognized that many concussed patients with normal head CT findings do have subtle evidence of brain contusion or diffuse axonal injury noted on magnetic resonance imaging (MRI) of the brain. Researchers have also found abnormalities in cerebrovascular autoregulation in some patients with concussion who have normal CT scans.

In general, patients with concussion can be expected to do well, and no specific therapy is required. A number of large studies have shown that patients with minor head injury who have normal head CT scans are at low risk for clinical deterioration. In general, these patients may be safely discharged to home if no other issues require inpatient care.

There are several case reports in the literature of the second impact syndrome, in which patients have experienced an initial minor head injury during a sporting event, with some associated concussive symptoms, and then have had serious neurologic deterioration or died after a second seemingly minor head impact occurred. It is presumed that in these cases, the athletes had a relatively asymptomatic contusion or diffuse axonal injury, perhaps associated with impaired autoregulation, exacerbated by the second impact. Based on these frightening reports, the American Academy of Neurology has published recommendations for the management of athletes who have sustained a concussion. A summary of the recommendations has been published in *Morbidity and Mortality Weekly Report* and is presented in Table 92.1.

In addition to these recommendations, the patient should be instructed to rest until symptoms improve. Acetaminophen may be prescribed for headache, but more potent analgesics should probably be avoided so that any progression of symptoms can be detected. The warning signs of progressing intracranial injury should be reviewed with the patient before discharge, with instructions to return immediately if any of these new symptoms or signs appear.

Symptoms after a concussion generally resolve quickly, often within minutes or hours after the injury. However, some patients develop the postconcussion syndrome, in which symptoms of confusion, amnesia, headaches, or dizziness may persist for days or even weeks after the injury.

Skull Fracture

CLINICAL FINDINGS AND DIAGNOSIS

Infants are clearly at a higher risk for skull fracture than older children, probably because their skulls are thinner. Many skull fractures in infants result from short distance falls; generally,

TABLE 92.1. Recommendations for Return to Sports Activity after Concussion

Grade I concussion
- Definition: transient confusion, no loss of consciousness, mental status abnormalities for ≤15 minutes.
- Management: return to sports activities same day only if all symptoms resolve within 15 minutes; if a second grade 1 concussion occurs, no sports activity until asymptomatic for 1 week

Grade 2 concussion
- Definition: transient confusion, no loss of consciousness, mental status abnormalities for >15 minutes.
- Management: no sports activity until asymptomatic for 1 week; if a grade 2 concussion occurs on the same day as a previous grade 1 concussion, no sports activity for 2 weeks

Grade 3 concussion
- Definition: concussion involving loss of consciousness
- Management: no sports activity until asymptomatic for 1 week if loss of consciousness was brief (seconds), or for 2 weeks if loss of consciousness was prolonged (minutes or longer)
- Second grade 3 concussion, no sports activity until asymptomatic for 1 month
- Any abnormality on computed tomography or magnetic resonance imaging, no sports activity for remainder of season; patient should be discouraged from any future return to contact sports

Modified from *Morbidity and Mortality Weekly Report*, Centers for Disease Control and Prevention.

about 50% of infants with skull fracture have fallen less than 4 or 5 feet. As the child matures beyond the first year of life, the propensity to sustain skull fracture disappears quickly.

Fractures may occur in any bone of the skull, although fractures of the parietal bone constitute about 70% of cases. The occipital and temporal bones are the next most commonly involved, with the frontal bone least likely to fracture. Basilar skull fractures commonly occur in pediatrics as well, although less commonly in infants, and more often in older children and adolescents.

Most cases of skull fracture are associated with soft-tissue swelling or hematoma overlying the fracture site. Skull fracture may occur in the absence of recognized soft-tissue findings as well, perhaps because subtle swelling is missed beneath the patient's hair, or because it may take several hours after the injury before the swelling becomes clinically evident. Palpable bony abnormalities are rarely detected in cases of linear or minimally depressed skull fracture but may be evident in cases with more severe depression. Other symptoms and signs of head injury, such as loss of consciousness, vomiting, lethargy, seizures, or irritability, may be present, especially if intracranial lesions are associated, but they are often absent in cases of isolated skull fracture.

Signs of basilar skull fracture may include hemotympanum, Battle sign (hematoma or discoloration overlying the mastoid bone), "raccoon eyes" (blue or purple discoloration of the periorbital tissue), or CSF rhinorrhea or otorrhea. There may be no abnormalities on examination of the scalp, and there may be no signs or symptoms of intracranial injury.

Skull fracture may be diagnosed by plain radiographs of the skull or by head CT imaging. A head CT scan is usually the preferred imaging modality for evaluating children with head injuries because it provides information not only about the skull but also about the intracranial contents. Skull radiographs are somewhat more sensitive for detecting skull fracture, especially for those horizontal fractures that run parallel to and between adjacent "cuts" on the CT scan. Head CT imaging is better than skull radiography, however, for detecting subtle degrees of depression of the bony fragments. Head CT imaging is also preferred in cases in which a diagnosis of basilar skull fracture is considered because it allows better imaging of the basilar skull and for visualization of pneumocephaly or fluid in the mastoid air cells, which are common associated findings.

MANAGEMENT

Linear Skull Fracture

The main significance of linear skull fractures is that they indicate that the risk of intracranial injury is increased by as much as tenfold to twentyfold. In cases in which acute linear skull fracture is diagnosed, therefore, a head CT scan is essential to evaluate for possible intracranial injury. In addition, any diagnosis of skull fracture should lead the clinician to consider the possibility of child abuse. If the history provided is not a plausible explanation for the injuries observed, further evaluation for possible child abuse should be initiated.

Many clinicians routinely admit children with skull fracture to the hospital for a period (eg, 24 hours) of observation to exclude the small possibility of late complications. For well-appearing children with a linear skull fracture and no associated intracranial injuries, however, the risk of late complications is low. Therefore, if a child with skull fracture but no intracranial lesions remains well over a short period of observation in the ED and child abuse is not suspected, the child may be considered for discharge to home. The warning signs of advancing intracranial injury should be carefully reviewed, with advice to return immediately if any of these signs are noticed. The family should also be counseled to expect the possible development of a subgaleal hematoma, which becomes more evident as the clotted blood overlying the fracture site begins to liquefy, and which presents as a large boggy swelling of the scalp, usually between 5 and 7 days after the injury. Unless the hematoma develops signs of infection, it will resolve gradually on its own and should not be aspirated.

Linear skull fractures generally heal well, with no specific therapy required. Fewer than 1% of patients will develop a growing skull fracture; that is, a fracture that fails to heal and becomes wider over time. All patients should have a follow-up examination 1 month after the initial injury to ensure that there is no evidence of development of a growing fracture.

Depressed Skull Fracture

Skull fractures may be associated with depression of the fracture fragments, which may range from barely detectable depressions to more obvious, palpable deformities in the skull. If there are no other complicating features, isolated skull fractures with minimal depressions can be managed in a fashion similar to that previously described for linear skull fractures.

More significant depressions of the skull, however, are more serious because they may be associated with contusion or laceration to underlying brain. In cases in which injury to underlying brain is noted on head CT imaging, especially if there are seizures or focal neurologic findings referable to the brain injury, prompt surgical elevation of the fracture fragments may be required. Surgical intervention is also usually necessary for compound, or open, depressed skull fractures, in which early debridement and closure is performed, especially for those patients who have lacerations of the dura mater. Penetrating injuries of the skull are a special case of open, depressed skull fracture and are discussed later in this chapter.

Surgical elevation is generally necessary (although not necessarily emergently) for patients with depressed skull fracture who have associated compression to underlying brain parenchyma or intraparenchymal bone fragments. Patients with significant cosmetic deformity are candidates for surgical repair as well. Most neurosurgeons would recommend surgical repair for any skull fracture with a 1-cm or greater depression, or for depressions with a depth greater than the thickness of the skull.

Basilar Skull Fracture

Fractures through the skull base are unique in that they may involve disruption of the mastoid air cells or the paranasal sinuses, raising the possibility of intracranial infection. Most recent studies suggest that the risk of meningitis after basilar skull fracture is low, with rates between 0.4% and 5%. The highest risk is in patients with evident CSF rhinorrhea or otorrhea. Although some controversy exists in the literature, it appears that prophylactic antibiotics reduce the risk of meningitis in high-risk patients. Many would recommend, therefore, that patients with basilar skull fracture and CSF leak be admitted to the hospital for i.v. antibiotics. Neurosurgical management of CSF leaks may also include several maneuvers, such as external CSF drainage to lower pressure and allow the leak to heal, packing of the sinuses, or surgical repair of dural lacerations.

Although it has been traditional management for all patients with basilar skull fracture to be admitted to the hospital for observation, recent authors have suggested that if patients with basilar skull fracture are neurologically normal, have no intracranial pathology on head CT, and have no CSF leak, they may be safely discharged to home. If they are to be discharged, instructions about the management of head injury, as previously described for linear skull fractures, should be discussed in detail. Furthermore, the family should be warned to watch closely for fever, stiff neck, photophobia, or any other signs of developing intracranial infection.

Parenchymal Injuries

CEREBRAL CONTUSION AND INTRAPARENCHYMAL HEMATOMA

Cerebral contusion refers to bruising of the cerebral cortex. On a microscopic level, there is focal injury to neurons, glial cells, and blood vessels, with some extravasation of blood noted, and some swelling of neural cells.

The presence of cerebral contusion indicates primary brain injury to the tissue involved. Focal neurologic deficits associated with dysfunction of the contused tissue should be expected. In addition, cerebral contusion leads to a risk for secondary brain injury because the contusion may exert some mass effect on surrounding tissue, with resulting cerebral dysfunction and risk for further ischemia. Finally, contusions are associated with a risk of late intraparenchymal hematoma.

Intraparenchymal hematoma may occur as a late complication of an initially nonhemorrhagic contusion, or it may be evident from the initial time of injury. These hemorrhages usually result from severe traumatic forces. The presence of hemorrhage may cause impaired blood flow to the adjacent parenchyma. If the hemorrhage becomes large enough, it may exert mass effect and even lead to cerebral herniation.

Clinical Manifestations

The severity of the clinical manifestations associated with cerebral contusion can vary widely. Often, there is history of loss of consciousness and/or some disturbance in the mental status. Focal neurologic deficits related to the contusion may be noted. Frontal contusions, for instance, may be associated with behavioral alterations, and temporal contusions may be associated with disturbances of memory. Seizures are relatively common as well.

With the increasing use of CT and MRI for patients with mild head trauma, an increasing number of contusions are being discovered in patients with no or mild symptoms (headache, nausea and vomiting, lethargy).

Most patients with intraparenchymal hematomas are comatose, and they may have focal neurologic deficits. Rare patients with intraparenchymal hematoma may initially be alert, but they have a high risk for deterioration over the ensuing hours.

Diagnosis

Cerebral contusions are generally evident on a head CT scan as hypodense areas of edema, sometimes intermingled with hyperdense areas of hemorrhage. Intraparenchymal hematomas are more uniformly hyperdense, although areas of active bleeding may be isodense.

Management

All patients with acute cerebral contusion and intraparenchymal hematoma should be admitted to the hospital for observation. Patients with a smaller contusion, a normal neurologic status, and no other lesions noted on head CT imaging may be appropriately managed on the inpatient ward. More seriously ill patients with an abnormal neurologic status generally require ICU monitoring. Patients with intraparenchymal hemorrhage should be admitted to the ICU as well.

Management of cerebral contusions focuses on efforts to prevent secondary brain injury, with the recognition that the contused tissue and surrounding areas are at especially high risk for ischemia. For patients in coma, ICP monitoring is generally indicated, and maneuvers for managing increased ICP may be required. The clinician must be especially alert for the possibility that an initially nonhemorrhagic contusion will undergo late hemorrhage, which would manifest as a sudden increase in ICP and/or deterioration in clinical status.

The prognosis for patients with cerebral contusion can vary widely, depending mainly on the patient's neurologic status on presentation, and on the presence or absence of other lesions. Patients with more significant cerebral contusion often have some residual neurologic disability. Follow-up CT scans on such patients show areas of encephalomalacia at the site of injury. Other patients may have essentially full recovery, with no residual neurologic deficits evident. Patients with intraparenchymal hematomas tend to have incurred severe brain injury, and they often have a poor outcome.

Diffuse Axonal Injury

Diffuse axonal injury (DAI) is characterized pathologically by injury to the white matter tracts of the brain, often at the junction of gray and white matter or sometimes deeper at the level of the corpus callosum, brainstem, or cerebellum. Pathologically, degeneration of the axons themselves is noted, with the presence of axonal retraction balls, microglial proliferation, and demyelination. In addition, there is usually accompanying endothelial damage to the capillaries, with some punctate areas of hemorrhage. Edema is sometimes, but not always, associated.

DAI results from the application of severe acceleration/deceleration or angular rotational forces to the brain, which lead to shear injuries of the axons and associated vasculature.

DAI reflects diffuse primary injury to the white matter. In addition, DAI is often associated with other focal lesions, or with global brain swelling.

CLINICAL MANIFESTATIONS

The clinical manifestations of DAI can vary greatly, ranging from those patients who have symptoms of concussion to those who present in coma. Loss of consciousness is common. In one study of patients with DAI, 82% developed coma. In general, patients with more diffuse areas of DAI noted on radiographic imaging (especially if involving the brainstem) have more severe symptoms.

DIAGNOSIS

DAI is evident on CT scan as small nonexpansive hemorrhagic lesions of the white matter, most typically seen at the gray–white junction of the cerebral hemispheres, or in the corpus callosum, brainstem, or cerebellum. Cerebral swelling sometimes accompanies DAI, but it need not be present for a diagnosis of DAI to be made. Intraventricular hemorrhage is sometimes noted. Intraparenchymal hemorrhages and cerebral contusions are commonly noted in patients with DAI as well.

MANAGEMENT

Patients with a radiographic diagnosis of DAI should be admitted to the hospital for observation. Patients with DAI who have a normal neurologic examination and no other lesions evident on CT scan may be able to be managed on a general inpatient unit. Those with an abnormal neurologic status require ICU level monitoring. Management of patients with DAI is supportive, with efforts directed mainly at preventing secondary brain injury. ICP monitoring is generally indicated for patients who present in coma. Specific therapies may be required for the management of increased ICP, as outlined previously.

In some large series of patients with DAI, mortality rates

range from 10% to 15%. Of those who survive, persistent neurologic dysfunction is common, occurring in 30% to 40% of patients. In general, however, children with DAI have a better prognosis than adults. A good functional outcome can be expected for patients with DAI who have mild symptoms of head injury (Glasgow Coma Scale score of 13 to 15).

DIFFUSE BRAIN SWELLING

Diffuse brain swelling (DBS) is a common manifestation of head trauma, especially in pediatrics. In one large series of children with severe brain injury, 41% had DBS. The origin of DBS is probably multifactorial. One component of DBS appears to be an increase in intracerebral vascular volume, probably caused by a loss of normal autoregulatory reflexes and diffuse vasodilation.

Many authors argue that the time course of DBS, occurring within minutes after a traumatic insult, is most consistent with this process of vasodilation, rather than the development of edema, which might be expected to take longer. Nonetheless the development of edema likely plays at least some role in many, if not all, cases of DBS as well. Edema may be vasogenic (extravasated from injured or inflamed blood vessels), cytotoxic (representing intracellular swelling of injured brain cells), or interstitial (from inadequate drainage of CSF).

DBS is probably a final common manifestation of brain injury caused by a number of different mechanisms. It may, in some cases, be a manifestation of primary brain injury, as when it accompanies large areas of brain contusion or DAI. In other cases, it probably represents secondary brain injury, caused by hypoxia or hypoperfusion. If left unchecked, the development of DBS can lead to a vicious cycle. That is, the presence of DBS causes an increase in ICP, and then the resulting ischemia leads to the development of more DBS.

CLINICAL MANIFESTATIONS

Most patients with DBS are comatose on initial evaluation, sometimes with associated focal neurologic deficits. Rarely, patients with DBS have less impressive symptoms, with more minor neurologic deficits. These patients often experience neurologic deterioration over the ensuing several hours.

DIAGNOSIS

DBS is diagnosed by a head CT scan when there is evidence of smaller ventricles, effacement of the sulci, or obliterated basal cisterns, in the absence of other intracranial pathology that may be exerting significant mass effect. Signs of cerebral edema per se, such as loss of gray–white differentiation, may be present. Other accompanying intracranial lesions, such as diffuse axonal injury, subdural hemorrhage, cerebral contusion, or subarachnoid hemorrhage are often diagnosed as well. In one large study of children with DBS, however, 60% had no other intracranial lesions identified.

MANAGEMENT

Patients with DBS need to be admitted to the hospital. Generally, admission to the ICU is required for careful monitoring of hemodynamics, oxygenation and ventilation, and ICP. ICP monitors are indicated for any patient with DBS in coma.

Management of the patient with DBS focuses on optimizing cerebral perfusion and minimizing any stressors that may lead to worsening of the DBS. If the ICP is elevated, measures to control the ICP are required. DBS is often worse between 1 and 3 days after the primary injury occurred, so patients who initially have well-controlled ICP may have more serious difficulties later.

Numerous studies have shown that the outcome of DBS after head trauma is better for children than it is for adults. In one large study, 78% of children with DBS had a functional outcome. Patients with more severe neurologic symptoms on presentation clearly have worse outcomes, as do those with accompanying intracranial lesions, especially subarachnoid hemorrhage or intraventricular hemorrhage. Patients who experience secondary systemic insults (eg, hypotension, hypoxia) clearly have a worse prognosis as well.

Epidural Hematoma

Most epidural hematomas (EDHs) result from blunt impact to the cranium. In most cases of EDH, the skull is fractured, with an associated laceration to the epidural vessels underlying the fracture site. In other cases, there is no fracture, but the deformation of the skull and associated linear deceleration from impact leads to shearing of the epidural arteries or veins.

Many patients with EDH have experienced relatively low-energy mechanisms of injury. In pediatrics, most cases of EDH result from falls, although a minority result from motor vehicle collisions, child abuse, or other mechanisms. About half of pediatric cases of EDH result from falls from heights of 6 feet or less.

Other mechanisms of injury, such as the shaking often implicated in cases of child abuse, are less likely to be associated with EDH because they do not lead to deformation of the skull. On the other hand, because the low impact falls that lead to EDH rarely involve high energy being applied to the brain itself, about 90% of cases EDH have no associated parenchymal injuries.

A small EDH may be asymptomatic. As the EDH expands, however, it begins to occupy an increasingly large intracranial volume. This increasing mass effect leads to an increase in ICP and, if left unchecked, may result in diffuse secondary brain injury. If the EDH continues to expand, it may lead ultimately to cerebral herniation.

CLINICAL SYMPTOMS/SIGNS

The classic presentation of EDH involves an initial loss of consciousness at the moment of impact, the "lucid interval" of several hours after the trauma when the patient is awake and relatively asymptomatic, and then neurologic deterioration as the enlarging hematoma begins to exert its mass effect.

In fact, however, pediatric patients with EDH rarely present with these classic symptoms. In one large series of pediatric patients with EDH, only 20% had an initial loss of consciousness, and 38% were alert with normal neurologic examinations at the time of diagnosis. The most common symptoms of EDH in pediatrics are headache, vomiting, and lethargy. In addition, ataxia may be noted in cases of posterior fossa EDH. Seizures are relatively rare, occurring in less than 10% of cases.

A small number of patients with EDH may not have any symptoms indicative of brain injury. Skull fracture may be a particularly important indicator of the risk of EDH, especially in patients with few other symptoms because skull fracture is noted in 70% to 80% of cases of EDH. Temporal or parietal skull fractures are particularly associated with a risk of EDH.

DIAGNOSIS

EDH can be readily diagnosed by noncontrast CT of the head. The classic appearance on CT is that of a high-density biconvex lesion just subjacent to the skull. The EDH is usually bounded by suture lines but may rarely cross these lines if diastasis of the suture has occurred. EDH is most commonly noted in the parietal, temporal, or temporoparietal regions (approximately 78%), and rarely in the frontal (16%) or occipital (6%) regions. The classic high-density appearance on CT indicates clotted blood. Occasionally, an adjacent or intermixed, swirled isodense lesion is noted, which represents ongoing acute bleeding that has yet to clot.

On CT midline shift, small ventricles, and loss of patency of the basal cisterns indicate a mass effect from the EDH. Signs of herniation may be seen. A careful survey for other associated intradural hematomas or parenchymal injuries should also be undertaken.

MANAGEMENT

The mainstay of treatment for EDH is craniotomy, with drainage of the hematoma and repair of the lacerated epidural vessels. Patients with EDH who have any depression in their level of consciousness, focal neurologic findings, pupillary abnormalities, and/or signs of increased ICP should proceed immediately to surgical intervention.

Increasingly in recent years, however, neurosurgeons have recognized that some patients with EDH may safely be managed with observation. Conservative management is only acceptable for patients with a small EDH (generally less than 30 mL in volume, and with a thickness of less than 2 cm), no focal neurologic deficits, and a normal level of consciousness.

Mortality rates in EDH range from 0 to 10%. Approximately 85% of surviving children with EDH have a good neurologic outcome.

The most important predictor of outcome is the patient's neurologic status on presentation. Patients who present with coma and pupillary abnormalities are much more likely to have sustained secondary brain injury. But even among these patients, a significant percentage will have a good outcome. In one series, 64% of children presenting with an initial Glasgow Coma Scale score of 5 or less had a good neurologic outcome. In another study, 82% of patients with EDH who presented with bilateral nonreactive pupils survived, and 55% had either a good outcome or moderate disability. In general, those patients with EDH who are able to be managed conservatively do well, with a normal neurologic outcome in approximately 95% of cases.

Subdural Hematoma

Subdural hematomas (SDHs) result from tearing of the bridging veins that traverse the subdural space. Mechanisms of injury that are associated with shear forces being applied to these veins are especially likely to lead to SDHs. In particular, SDHs result from injuries associated with significant acceleration/deceleration forces.

In older children and adolescents, SDHs most commonly result from motor vehicle collisions. In infants, SDHs are commonly a result of the shaking impact syndrome of child abuse. SDHs may result from falls as well, especially if the fall is from a significant height. Because of the more significant forces applied to the brain in most injuries leading to SDHs, the SDH is often associated with other intracranial lesions. However, infants appear to be prone to the development of small SDHs even after more minor head injury, perhaps because they have wider subarachnoid spaces, which cause the bridging veins to be under more tension and more prone to shear injury.

CLINICAL MANIFESTATIONS

SDHs are often associated with an initial loss of consciousness and with a depressed mental status. Approximately 50% of patients with SDH present in coma. Pupillary abnormalities may be noted as well, indicating impending herniation. In less severely ill patients, headaches, vomiting, lethargy, irritability, visual difficulties, or seizures may be noted. In patients with SDHs involving the posterior fossa, cerebellar signs such as ataxia or nystagmus may be noted. Because CT scanning is being used more routinely in cases of minor head injuries, many cases of asymptomatic SDH are being discovered as well.

Although most cases of SDH present within hours after the trauma, occasional cases of chronic SDH are diagnosed, days or even weeks after a head trauma. In pediatrics, chronic traumatic SDH is most commonly seen in infants, usually as a consequence of child abuse. Presenting symptoms in these infants may include tense fontanel, macrocephaly, psychomotor retardation, depressed level of consciousness, seizures, vomiting, irritability, or focal neurologic deficits.

DIAGNOSIS

On head CT, acute SDH is seen as a hyperdense crescentic collection of extraaxial fluid. There may be areas of hypodense fluid intermingled, which represent active bleeding, sometimes termed a hyperacute SDH. Because the subdural space is continuous around each hemisphere, subdural blood flows freely through this space, while respecting the midline and tentorial margins. SDH is usually noted unilaterally, although cases of child abuse are often associated with bilateral SDH. The CT should be evaluated for evidence of mass effect, and for associated intracranial lesions, such as brain swelling, cerebral contusions, or subarachnoid hemorrhage.

The density of the subdural fluid collection varies over time. With older chronic hematomas, the collection may be almost isodense with CSF.

MANAGEMENT

In the early 1980s a number of researchers were able to show remarkable decreases in mortality from SDH if patients underwent timely surgical drainage. Not surprisingly, this effect was most evident in those patients with large SDHs associated with midline shift and coma. In this subgroup, the neurologic prognosis is optimized when surgery is performed within 4 hours of the trauma. It appears that early relief of the mass effect in these patients prevents secondary brain injury.

Many patients with SDH who are not so severely ill can be managed nonoperatively. Some authors have proposed nonoperative management for patients with SDH who are not comatose, who have small SDHs with no mass effect, and who have patent basal cisterns. Generally, even well-appearing patients with posterior fossa SDHs are not candidates for nonoperative management because of the high risk of brainstem compression if the lesion expands. Even if a patient appears to be a candidate for nonoperative management, however, immediate consultation with a neurosurgeon is essential because of the potential for rapid clinical deterioration over the first several hours of observation.

The clinician must recognize the strong association of SDH with child abuse, especially in infants with no clear mechanism of injury reported, and in those patients with associated retinal hemorrhages. If the circumstances of the injury cannot be clearly explained, further evaluation for nonaccidental trauma should be pursued.

In several studies, mortality rates for children with acute SDH range from 10% to 20%. Of those who survive, persistent neurologic sequelae are common. Those patients who are comatose on admission or who have pupillary abnormalities clearly have poorer prognoses. In addition, those patients with CT evidence of more significant brain injury or increased ICP have a worse prognosis. Even the patients who appear to be at high risk, however, may do relatively well. In one study, 14 of 21 patients with a Glasgow Coma Scale score of 8 or less who were less than 40 years of age were functional survivors.

Subarachnoid Hemorrhage

Subarachnoid hemorrhage (SAH) is a common complication of head trauma, especially in more severely injured patients. In one large study SAH occurred in approximately 25% of patients who were comatose on initial evaluation.

SAH results from tearing of the small vessels of the pia mater. SAH generally occurs after relatively severe blunt trauma to the head, or as a result of significant shear forces.

Because the cerebral subarachnoid space is large and freely communicates with the basal cisterns and the spinal subarachnoid space, the blood in an SAH can be distributed widely. As a consequence of this wide distribution and because it is generally smaller pial vessels that bleed, SAH rarely accumulates to the extent that it causes clinically important mass effect.

SAH appears to exert its main pathophysiologic effect by causing cerebral vasospasm. A number of studies have shown that SAH is associated with increased cerebrovascular resistance, and consequently, with an increased risk of cerebral ischemia or infarction. In general, SAH is seen in association with other intracranial injuries, especially SDH, cerebral contusion, and intraparenchymal hemorrhage. Because SAH is often seen in association with other intracranial injuries, its presence may be most important as a marker for severe primary brain injury, rather than as a cause of secondary injury in itself.

CLINICAL MANIFESTATIONS

Patients with posttraumatic SAH often have other intracranial hemorrhage or parenchymal injuries as well, so they may present with a wide range of symptoms, from those who have minimal if any symptoms to those who are comatose with signs of impending cerebral herniation. As an isolated intracranial lesion, SAH most commonly causes headache and other signs of meningeal irritation, such as nausea and vomiting, nuchal rigidity, and photophobia. Patients with isolated SAH often have a history of loss of consciousness, and sometimes present with depressed mental status or even coma. Seizures are reported in 2% to 10% of cases. Subhyaloid or preretinal hemorrhages, located just adjacent to the optic nerve head, may be seen with SAH as well.

DIAGNOSIS

SAH can usually be detected on noncontrast head CT as a collection of hyperdense fluid in the CSF spaces, either in the subarachnoid space overlying the cerebral convexity or in the basal cisterns. Subarachnoid blood overlying the cerebral hemisphere can be distinguished from SDH in that the subarachnoid blood may flow into the depths of the brain sulci, fissures, and cisterns, whereas the subdural space does not penetrate into these depths. Head CT imaging has a sensitivity of only about 90% for detecting SAH, with a lower sensitivity for patients seen later than 24 hours after the SAH began. However, lumbar puncture is not recommended and may be dangerous in the setting of focal intracranial pathology or brain swelling because it may increase the risk of cerebral herniation.

MANAGEMENT

All patients with traumatic SAH should be admitted to the hospital for observation. In most cases, specific therapy directed at the SAH is not required. The general principles of management for patients with head injuries should, of course, be followed. Prophylactic anticonvulsants are often used for patients with SAH.

In one study, 24% of patients with traumatic SAH died, and another 24% had a poor neurologic outcome. Patients with associated intracranial injuries and those with a larger SAH (especially if it involves both the hemispheric convexities and the basal cisterns) have the worst outcome. Patients with minor or no symptoms and small SAH generally do well.

PENETRATING TRAUMA

Penetrating trauma includes injury from sharp objects, such as knives, darts, or animal bites, and from missiles, usually bullets. Penetrating head trauma is far less common than blunt head trauma in pediatrics, but the incidence of penetrating injuries, especially from gun shots, has increased at an alarming rate in the past decade. Several urban hospitals have reported that the rate of hospital admissions for teenagers shot in the head increased by as much as tenfold between the 1980s and 1990s.

Penetrating head trauma leads to brain injury by several mechanisms. First, there is direct injury along the path of the penetrating object, with laceration or contusion of neural tissue, and hemorrhage from injured vessels. For low-velocity penetrating injuries (eg, knife wounds), this may be the primary source of brain injury.

Higher-velocity injuries (from bullets) also cause significant damage because of the shock waves created by the impact of the penetrating object. These shock waves can cause contusions or vascular injury at sites that had no contact with the penetrating object itself.

Vascular injury may result from direct laceration, or from percussion-related damage. Dissection of an intimal flap, thrombosis of the vessel lumen, or aneurysm formation may result. Ischemia or infarction resulting from these vascular injuries may occur immediately after impact, or they may occur days or even weeks later.

Because the skull and dura are violated by the penetrating object, there is direct communication from the CSF spaces or brain to the outside world, and consequently, a risk for intracranial infection. Penetrating objects that pass through the paranasal sinuses or mastoid air cells particularly increase the risk of intracranial infection.

CLINICAL MANIFESTATIONS

The local signs of penetrating injury can sometimes be subtle, especially if the penetrated area is covered by hair or by a dressing. Without careful exploration, the entrance wound might be mistaken for a superficial scalp laceration. In more obvious cases of penetrating injury, meningeal or parenchymal tissue may be visualized in the wound, or CSF may be oozing.

Signs of neurologic injury are often severe for patients with high-velocity injuries, but they may be more subtle in patients with low-velocity injuries. Patients with progressively enlarging intracranial hematomas or worsening brain swelling may deteriorate quickly over the several hours after presentation.

MANAGEMENT

The initial management of the patient who has sustained penetrating head trauma focuses on the ABCs of resuscitation, as outlined previously. Once the ABCs have been addressed, attention can be focused on the possible need for brain-specific therapies, as described.

In addition to the management priorities already outlined, some unique aspects of caring for the patient with penetrating head trauma should be discussed. The patient should be examined carefully for evidence of entrance or exit wounds. The clinician should recognize the potential for multiple penetrating wounds, or for exit wounds in unpredicted locations because of a complicated migratory path of the penetrating object.

Patients with penetrating head injuries generally require prophylactic antibiotic therapy. A first-generation cephalosporin such as cefazolin (30 mg per kg i.v.; maximum dose 2 g) is usually appropriate.

Most patients with penetrating head injuries are started on prophylactic anticonvulsant therapy (usually with phenytoin), especially if there is any concern about parenchymal injury or subarachnoid hemorrhage.

Patients with penetrating injuries to the head require immediate head CT to delineate the extent of brain injury and to assess for associated intracranial hematomas, brain swelling, and/or mass effect. The head CT is also able to demonstrate the presence of intracranial foreign material.

In addition, most patients with penetrating injuries to the head require prompt operation to debride the infected or contused brain tissue at the entry site. Controversy exists about the need for extensive debridement of deeper tissues along the path of the penetrating object. Increasingly, published reports have shown equally high success rates with more limited debridement. After debridement, the dura must be repaired to achieve a watertight seal.

Most patients with penetrating head injuries need to have angiography performed (either conventional or MRI angiography) to exclude the possibility of traumatic injuries to the cerebral vasculature. Although some controversy exists about the optimal timing of angiography, most authors recommend angiography as soon as it can safely be performed.

The prognosis after penetrating head injury depends most on the level of neurologic function at the time of presentation. For patients with severe neurologic dysfunction (Glasgow Coma Scale scores in the range of 3 to 5), the likelihood of a good functional outcome is low, although occasional patients will do well. Most neurosurgeons will not operate on patients who present with an absence of neurologic function (Glasgow Coma Scale score of 3 and nonreactive pupils) because the prognosis is so dismal for this subgroup.

SPINAL CORD TRAUMA

Spinal cord injury is rare in pediatrics. Most case series in the literature from pediatric trauma centers report only 1 to 2 patients with spinal cord injuries each year. Nonetheless, spinal cord injuries, when they do occur, are associated with significant morbidity and mortality, and the consequences of missing patients with early signs of spinal cord injury can be devastating. Furthermore, recent clinical evidence suggests that prompt diagnosis and therapy for spinal cord injuries may improve the prognosis.

CLINICAL MANIFESTATIONS

Spinal cord injuries are generally associated with significant mechanisms of injury, such as motor vehicle collisions, falls from significant heights, or child abuse. Patients with injuries to the spinal cord often have evidence of injuries to other organ systems. In particular, there is a high association between head injuries and injuries to the cervical spine and/or spinal cord. Injuries to the thoracic or lumbar spine may also be associated with head injuries, but they are seen more often in the setting of chest or abdominal trauma.

Patients with high cervical cord injuries may sometimes have abnormal vital signs, reflecting an interruption of autonomic impulses to the heart and the vasculature. These patients demonstrate bradycardia and hypotension, along with peripheral vasodilation, a syndrome known as spinal shock. They may also have abnormal or absent respiratory effort. Because most trauma patients with hypotension are hypovolemic and have a reflex tachycardia, those with bradycardia should be strongly suspected of having spinal shock.

Spinal cord injuries should also be suspected in any traumatized patient who complains of decreased motor strength, or in whom focal deficits in strength or tone are noted on examination. In the acute setting, severe spinal cord injuries are usually associated with decreased or absent reflexes. Partial injuries to the cord, on the other hand, may be associated with initial hypertonia and hyperreflexia. Abnormalities of bladder control and rectal tone may also be noted.

Motor deficits correspond to the spinal roots whose neural impulses are compromised by the spinal cord injury. Most typically, all motor impulses that originate from spinal nerve roots at or below the level of the spinal cord injury are affected. An understanding of the motor deficits after spinal cord injury requires knowledge of the innervation of the important muscle groups of the body. A list of the important muscle groups and the spinal roots that serve them is presented in Table 92.2.

Sensory deficits may be noted as well, and these may range from paresthesias to complete loss of sensation. Because sensory impulses are carried in both the dorsal columns and the lateral compartments of the spinal cord, injuries to one of these compartments may lead to partial sensory deficits (eg, loss of pain and temperature sense from the lateral compartment or loss of joint position sense and vibration sense from the dorsal column), but with other forms of sensation intact for the same body part. Often, a well-demarcated sensory "level" of the spinal cord can be identified, below which sensory impulses are absent, and above which sensation is intact.

Many injuries to the spinal cord involve solely or predominantly one of the two lateral sides of the cord. Because of the distribution of sensory and motor neurons in the spinal cord, a lesion to the left spinal cord affects left-sided motor strength but right-sided sensation. This classic crossed pattern of sensory and motor deficits is known as the Brown-Séquard syndrome.

Other patterns of neurologic deficits may also be noted. Partial injuries to the spinal cord may result in partial deficits. In some cases of ventral cord injury, for instance, only motor deficits may be observed. Cases of hyperextension injury may cause more severe injury to the central, or deep regions of the cord (the gray matter) while sparing the more superficial white matter. This leads to a "paradoxic" pattern of symptoms known as the central cord syndrome, in which the more distal function (served by the white matter) is spared, but more proximal function (served by gray matter) is compromised. Finally, occasional patients with more minor injuries to the spinal cord report transient symptoms of paresthesias, numbness, or weakness that may have resolved by the time of evaluation.

MANAGEMENT

As with all trauma patients, care for the patient with spinal cord injury begins with the ABCs of resuscitation. This initial resuscitation must be accomplished with meticulous attention to the stabilization of the spine. For older children and adolescents, a semirigid cervical collar or manual in-line stabilization should be used. For infants, a semirigid cervical collar might actually be too large and may lead to distraction or hyperextension, which could be deleterious. For some infants, therefore, it may be preferable to immobilize with sandbags on the sides of the head, without using a cervical collar. In addition, the patient should be maintained in a supine position on a backboard so that no undue manipulation of the spine occurs. Because infants have a relatively large occiput, supine positioning on a flat surface may result in flexion of the neck. Proper neutral positioning for these young patients may require that the occiput be allowed to rest at a level slightly lower than the shoulders. Any transfers of the pa-

TABLE 92.2. Major Muscle Groups, Listed with the Spinal Roots and Peripheral Nerves That Supply Them

Muscle	Segmental innervation	Peripheral nerve
Diaphragm	C3–C5	Phrenic nerve
Trapezius	C3–C4	Spinal accessory nerve
Deltoid	C5–C6	Axillary nerve
Supraspinatus	C5–C6	Suprascapular nerve
Biceps brachii	C5–C6	Musculocutaneous nerve
Triceps brachii	C6–C8	Radial nerve
Wrist extensors	C6–C7	Radial nerve
Finger extensors	C6–C8	Radial nerve
Wrist flexors	C6, C7–T1	Ulnar, median nerve
Intrinsic hand muscles	C8–T1	Ulnar nerve
Psoas	L1–L2	Psoas nerve
Quadriceps femoris	L2–L4	Femoral nerve
Gastrocnemius	L5–S1	Deep peroneal nerve
Urinary bladder	S2–S4	

tient from one bed to another or "log-rolling" of the patient to examine the back should be done with careful attention to maintaining neutral positioning at all times.

The patient with spinal cord injury requires adequate oxygenation, ventilation, and perfusion.

As soon as possible after an injury, the patient's neurologic status should be assessed and recorded so that any early progression of neurologic symptoms can be noted and so that no undue concerns are raised that the injuries were a result of the emergency care provided. For conscious, cooperative patients, the neurologic examination should include a test of motor strength in all four extremities, tone in all extremities, and deep tendon reflexes. Rectal tone should also be assessed. The sensory examination, assessing for light touch, pain sensation (as from a pinprick), and joint position sense (of fingers and toes) should be assessed as well. For patients with depressed consciousness, an assessment of tone and reflexes may be all that is possible.

Patients with suspected spinal cord injury should have plain radiographs of the spine to evaluate for fractures or subluxations. However, the absence of abnormalities on radiographic imaging does not eliminate the possibility of spinal cord injury. The syndrome of spinal cord injury without radiographic abnormalities (SCIWORA) is well reported in the literature. Several series of children with spinal cord injury report that 15% to 20% of cases may be classified as SCIWORA. Children have an especially high risk for SCIWORA because of the flexibility of the pediatric spinal column, which allows the spinal cord to withstand shear or compressive forces without necessarily causing a fracture. In some cases, the flexible and lax spinal column may sublux transiently, causing a compressive injury to the cord and then reduce back into normal position before radiographs are obtained.

In recent years, MRI has become a mainstay for the diagnostic evaluation of patients with suspected spinal cord injury. MRI offers the advantage of providing good detail of the soft tissue of the spinal cord itself, which cannot be well imaged by plain radiographs or by CT. A number of studies in the literature have reported evidence of spinal cord contusion, transection, or hemorrhage seen on MRI in most patients with spinal cord injury, and especially in those with more severe and lasting deficits. Increasingly, MRI has been used to document spinal cord abnormalities in cases that would be classified as SCIWORA by plain radiographs and CT.

Specific therapy directed at the spinal cord focuses on the prevention of secondary cord injury. The mainstay of this therapy is careful immobilization, as outlined previously. In all cases of spinal cord injury, a neurosurgeon should be consulted immediately. If compressive spinal cord lesions are noted, especially with incomplete but progressing neurologic injury, emergent laminectomy with surgical evacuation of the lesion may be necessary. Displaced fractures or subluxations of the spinal column require immobilization and generally some form of traction (eg, a halo brace, skull tongs) to reduce them and maintain stability (see Chapter 93 for more details). Some patients with irreducible subluxations or unstable fractures require urgent surgery to achieve reduction. Patients with SCIWORA usually require long-term immobilization as well because they should be presumed to have some ligamentous instability of the spine, even if the initial radiographic studies show normal alignment.

High-dose corticosteroid therapy is widely used in the setting of spinal cord injury. It is believed that corticosteroid therapy decreases the extent of secondary cord injury by interfering with the lipid peroxidation pathway. The use of corticosteroids is based on the results of a multicenter prospective, randomized trial known as NASCIS (the National Acute Spinal Cord Injury Study). The NASCIS found that high-dose corticosteroid therapy significantly improved the outcome for those patients treated within 8 hours of injury, but not in those patients treated later. On the basis of these findings, the following regimen is recommended for patients with neurologic deficits attributable to spinal cord injury who are seen within 8 hours of injury: methylprednisolone at an initial i.v. bolus dose of 30 mg per kg followed by an infusion of methylprednisolone at 5.4 mg per kg per hour for the subsequent 23 hours.

Penetrating Spinal Cord Trauma

Penetrating spinal cord trauma is an especially rare phenomenon in pediatrics. It may occur as a result of violent injuries, from stabbing or from gunshot wounds. Accidental injuries may occur, most commonly from shards of glass that penetrate into the spinal column.

Stab wounds or penetrating sharp foreign bodies usually involve penetration from the posterolateral aspects of the neck. These injuries generally lead to hemisection of the cord, with only one side of the cord affected. This predilection for unilateral injury probably reflects the fact that the posterior spinous processes and lateral transverse processes form an anatomic "gutter" through which the penetrating object is guided, thereby offering some protection to the opposite side of the cord. Bullets, on the other hand, propelled by high energy forces, may penetrate the bones of the spinal column and cause less predictable patterns of injury.

When penetrating spinal cord injury is suspected, the principles of management, as outlined previously, should be followed. Plain radiographs demonstrate the presence of many radiopaque foreign bodies; in some cases, CT may be required to demonstrate less radiodense materials. In cases in which no foreign body is left in the wound, plain radiographs and CT may be normal. MRI is the best imaging modality for delineating injury to the cord itself.

PERIPHERAL NERVE INJURIES

Pathophysiology

Peripheral nerve injuries in pediatrics usually involve the extremities, most commonly the hand and upper extremity. Most peripheral nerve injuries in pediatrics result from acute traumatic insults. Transection of the nerve may result from deep soft-tissue lacerations or from severe crush injuries. Rarely, transection of a nerve may also result from a fracture, with laceration of the nerve by a displaced bony fragment.

More commonly, however, displaced fractures or dislocations lead to reversible compression injuries to the nerve. Nerve compression may also occur in the absence of acute trauma, usually because of tight anatomic compartments that exert constant pressure on the nerve (carpal tunnel syndrome is one common example).

Peripheral nerve injuries may be graded in terms of the severity of the clinical course. The mildest form of nerve injury is known as neurapraxia, which refers to nerve conduction impairment without structural injury to the axon itself. Neurapraxia commonly results from a situation of transient compression or ischemia, as when a patient complains that a limb has "fallen asleep." The numbness and paresthesias reflect a rapidly reversible physiologic conduction block. If biopsy of the nerve were performed in this situation, no histologic abnormalities would be expected.

More severe cases of neurapraxia may be associated with symptoms that persist for as long as several months. In these cases, histologic examination reveals focal demyelination in the injured area of the nerve, but with no injury to the axon itself. In general, as long as the axon itself is not injured, full recovery can be expected.

Axonotmesis is a more severe injury to peripheral nerve, involving injury to the axon itself, but with preservation of the surrounding connective tissue of the nerve sheath. Axonotmesis generally results from crush injuries to the nerve. Good recovery of peripheral nerve function is likely to occur, although it will progress slowly, with lengthening of the nerve axon from its proximal stump progressing at a rate of approximately 1 to 4 mm per day. Distal nerve lesions, in close proximity to the target muscles or sensory regions, are associated with earlier and more complete recovery of function than in more proximal lesions.

The most severe form of nerve injury is known as neurotmesis, which involves injury both to the nerve axon and to the surrounding connective tissue. Neurotmesis usually results from direct laceration to the nerve or, rarely, from severe crush injuries. Because there is no intact nerve sheath to guide the development of the regenerating proximal nerve, spontaneous recovery of function is unlikely, and surgical repair is required.

CLINICAL MANIFESTATIONS

Significant peripheral nerve injuries usually are seen in association with other obvious signs of traumatic injury, such as a soft-tissue laceration, crush injuries to the extremity, or fracture. In some cases, however, such as with repetitive microtrauma or with anatomic compressive lesions (as seen in carpal tunnel syndrome), the symptoms of peripheral nerve injury may be the primary complaint.

The cardinal symptoms of peripheral nerve injury are disturbances of sensory or motor function in the distribution of the nerve. Appropriate diagnosis of peripheral nerve injury requires an understanding of the anatomic distribution of sensory and motor function of the major peripheral nerves. A full description of this clinical anatomy is beyond the scope of this discussion, but a summary of the motor functions of the major peripheral nerves is presented in Table 92.2.

Disturbances of sensation may include paresthesias, pain (which may be described as sharp, burning, or stabbing), or numbness. In some cases, the patient may not report a sensory deficit, but sensory abnormalities are noted on examination. A gross assessment of sensory function can be obtained simply by testing the patient's ability to recognize light touch stimuli in the distribution of the nerve in question.

A more sensitive test for identifying disturbances in sensory function is two-point discrimination. Although instruments for assessing two-point discrimination are commercially available, in common practice, a paper clip is often used. The paper clip should be unfolded so that the two ends are in close proximity, with a distance of approximately 1 cm in between. The patient should then be briefly trained on an uninjured part of the body to differentiate between being touched with one or two points of the paper clip simultaneously. Once it is determined that the patient can reliably perform the task, the injured area should be assessed.

The two points must touch the skin simultaneously, and they must occur in the same axial line. If the patient is able to successfully discriminate one- and two-point stimuli, the distance between the two ends of the paper clip can be decreased successively to find the patient's threshold for discrimination. A hand with normal sensation should be able to distinguish between two points that are 2 to 5 mm apart at the fingertips, 7 to 10 mm at the base of the palm, and 7 to 12 mm on the dorsum of the hand. More proximal parts of the upper extremity may have even less sensitive discriminatory abilities.

A problem occasionally arises in trying to assess sensory function in a patient who is unresponsive or who cannot communicate with the examiner. In these cases, a test of sympathetic innervation, such as the O'Riain wrinkle test, may be useful. To perform this test, the patient's hand is immersed in a warm water bath for approximately 20 minutes. Normal digital pulps will wrinkle; fingers with disrupted sympathetic innervation will not wrinkle.

Appropriate motor testing of the peripheral nerves depends on careful isolation of muscle activity that reflects the peripheral nerve in question. The clinician must be careful to recognize that a patient will compensate for a motor deficit by using other motor groups to accomplish the same task. Motor function can be assessed by examining not only active motor strength but also resting tone and, for more chronic injuries, muscle bulk.

MANAGEMENT

Clean lacerations to a primary nerve are often repaired primarily. There is some evidence to indicate that recovery of function is better if the nerve is repaired within 48 hours of injury. Crush injuries to peripheral nerves are often repaired secondarily, several days or weeks after the injury. For these cases, many surgeons believe that delayed repair allows better debridement of devitalized tissue and easier identification of injured nerve tissue that needs to be resected. In all cases in which transection of a peripheral nerve is suspected, prompt consultation with an appropriate surgical consultant is indicated so that a decision can be made about the appropriate timing of repair.

Injuries to peripheral nerve associated with fracture or dislocation generally improve after the orthopedic injury is reduced. If there is any question about the recovery after reduction, nerve function should be carefully followed.

Nerve compression syndromes not associated with acute traumatic injuries can generally be treated with rest and nonsteroidal antiinflammatory medications. Splinting may be indicated for some syndromes as well. In all cases, appropriate follow-up should be arranged so that the patient can be referred for further interventions if necessary.

CHAPTER 93
Neck Trauma

George A. Woodward, M.D.

Pediatric neck injuries, fortunately, are uncommon. Many children will be evaluated for cervical spine injuries secondary to trauma, but few will have injuries identified. Even fewer children will need to be evaluated for penetrating or direct blunt trauma to the neck. However, neck injuries can be life threatening and need to be assessed in a timely and orderly manner. It is imperative to appreciate how apparently minor or innocuous neck injuries can progress rapidly to more serious and life-threatening events. Subtle neck injuries can be easily overlooked in a patient with obvious head or chest trauma.

When considering injuries to the neck in a child, initial management must include immediate assessment of airway, breathing, circulation (ABCs) and treatment of abnormalities with care not to allow an injury to progress to a more significant event. Airway abnormality may be subtle but progressive, with the precipitating injury not obvious on initial examination. Patients should be monitored closely and physically observed during their emergency department (ED) stay. A listing of common mechanisms of neck injury is given in Table 93.1.

The neck can be divided into three anatomic zones (Figs. 93.1 through 93.3). Zone I encompasses the area between the thoracic inlet and the cricoid (the lower boundary of zone I is the thoracic inlet, the upper boundary is most often classified as the cricoid; most authors use the clavicle or sternal notch as the upper boundary as well). Zone II is the area between the cricoid (clavicle or sternal notch) and the angle of the mandible. Zone III is the area above the angle of the mandible. Knowledge of the divisions and structures they contain is useful in evaluation and management of neck trauma (Fig. 93.1 through 93.3). Lesions in zones I and III are often occult and difficult to diagnose by physical examination alone. Operative exploration is more difficult in zones I and III than in zone II, where injury presentation and surgical exploration are often more straightforward. The neck can also be divided into anterior and posterior elements, with the dividing line being the palpable transverse processes of the cervical spine. The posterior neck contains muscles with their individual nerve supplies and the posterior elements of the cervical spine, and the anterior neck houses most vital organs and structures. No major vascular components are contained in the posterior area of the neck.

TABLE 93.1. Common Mechanisms of Blunt and Penetrating Neck Injuries

Penetrating trauma	Blunt trauma
High-velocity missiles	Motor vehicle accidents
Low-velocity missiles	Sports
Knives	Fights
Windshields	Falls
Sharp objects	Clothesline injuries
Explosions	Handlebars
Iatrogenic (intubation, endoscopy, gastric tubes)	Barotrauma (bottlecap under pressure or compressed air source)
	Nonaccidental (abuse)
	Exposures (fires, caustics)

PENETRATING TRAUMA

Penetrating neck trauma is uncommon in children. Penetrating trauma may be associated with extracervical injuries and may involve multiple organ systems within the neck. Most pediatric penetrating trauma is the result of a wound from a gunshot (usually low velocity), knife, broken windshield, other sharp object, or explosion (Table 93.1). The history is important in evaluation of penetrating neck trauma.

Many gunshot wounds seen in pediatric patients involve low-velocity weapons, including handguns (90 meters per second) or shotguns (300 meters per second) at ranges of greater than 5 meters as opposed to shotguns at close range or military-style weapons (760 meters per second).

Unlike high-velocity missiles, low-velocity missiles tend to be redirected when they encounter vascular or other structures. Visceral injuries may be anticipated but not completely predicted by the path of the missile. Internal injuries may be more predictable with an isolated knife wound. Low-velocity neck wounds are associated with major pathology in approximately 50% of cases compared with more than 90% with high-velocity missiles.

Vascular injury is the most common complication of penetrating trauma and is the second most common cause of death. History of large blood loss, pulsatile lesion, rapidly expanding hematoma, hypovolemic shock, or neurologic deficits (paresis, visual loss or aphasia, altered level of consciousness) indicates the possibility of cervical arterial injury. Injury to the vessels can be dramatic, with exsanguination, rapidly expanding hematoma causing airway compromise, acute neurologic deficits from ischemia or hypoperfusion, or venous air embolism, or it may be subtle with an initially normal examination. Approximately one-third of arterial injuries present with neurologic deficits, whereas the remaining two-thirds are often more challenging to diagnose. The symptoms and signs suggestive of vascular and other neck injuries are presented in Table 93.2. Completely transected arteries often retract and contract with minimal bleeding.

Direct nervous system injury (brachial plexus, spinal cord, cervical nerves, cervical sympathetics) is possible with penetrating neck trauma, and evaluation of the patient should assess these structures. Symptoms will correspond to the injured structure, which may or may not require primary surgical repair (Fig. 93.4). Primary injury to the cervical cord often results from bony or foreign body penetration or impingement or cord distraction. Secondary cord injury can occur from vascular compromise, edema, lipid peroxidation, ischemia, and ligamentous damage. When assessing neurologic findings or predicting location of

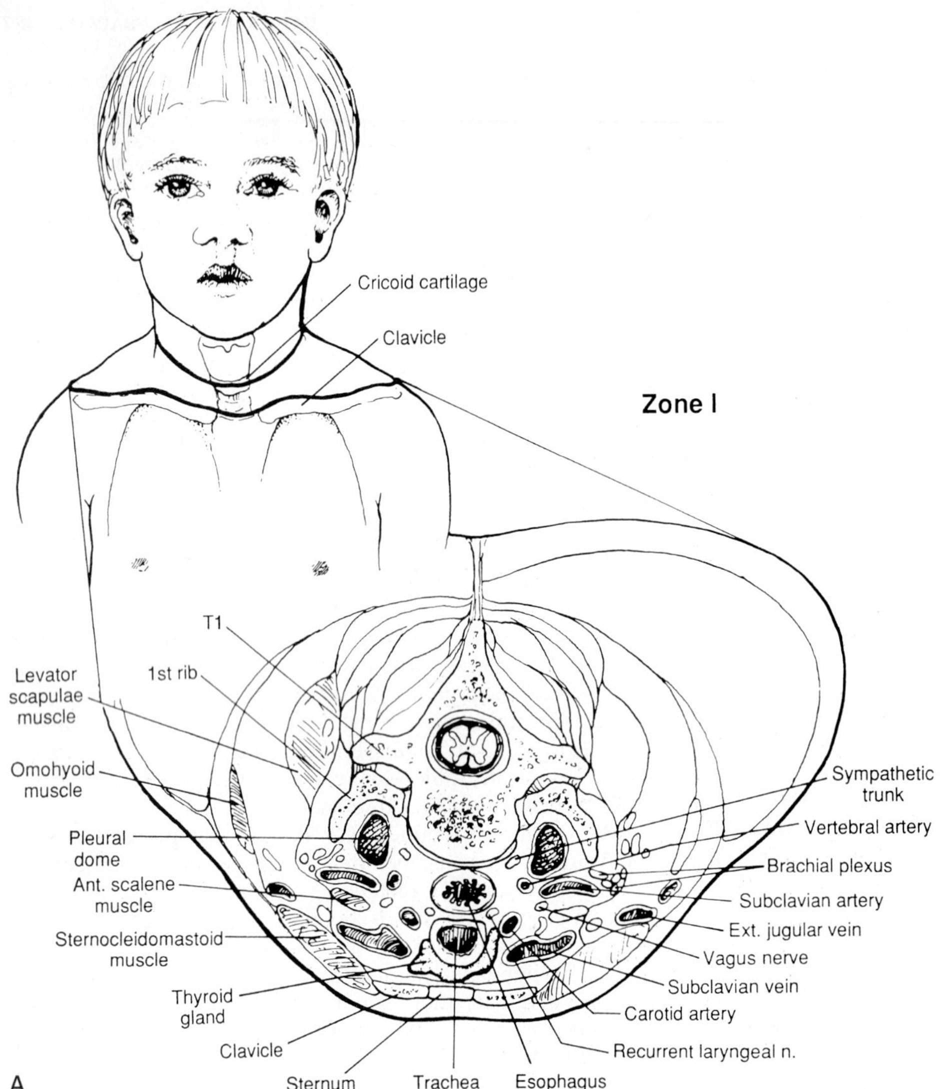

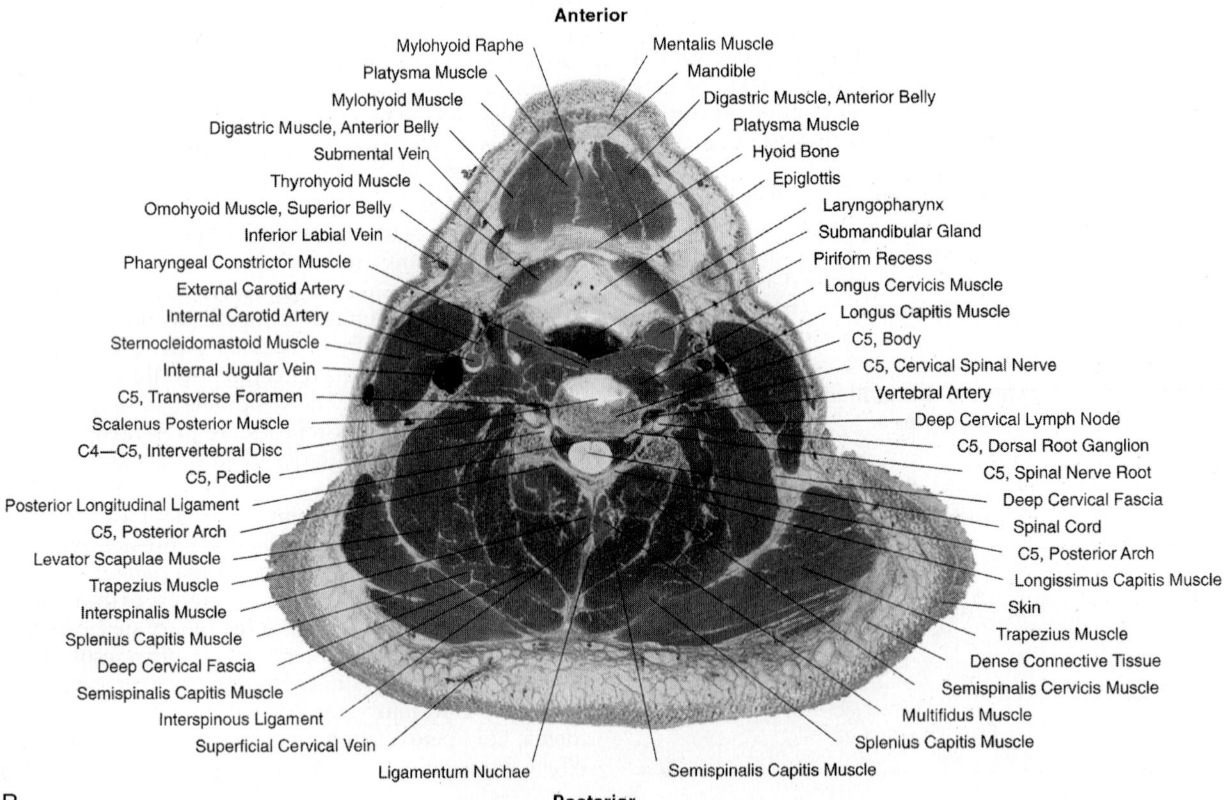

Figure 93.1. A: Anatomic neck divisions and contents of zone I. Zone I encompasses the area between the thoracic inlet and the cricoid (some authors use the clavicle or sternal notch as the upper boundary). **B:** Anatomic specimen demonstrating zone I relationships. (93.1B reprinted with permission from Spitzer VM, Whitlock DG. *National library of medicine atlas of the visible human male. Reverse engineering of the human body*. Sudbury, MA: Jones & Bartlett, 1997.)

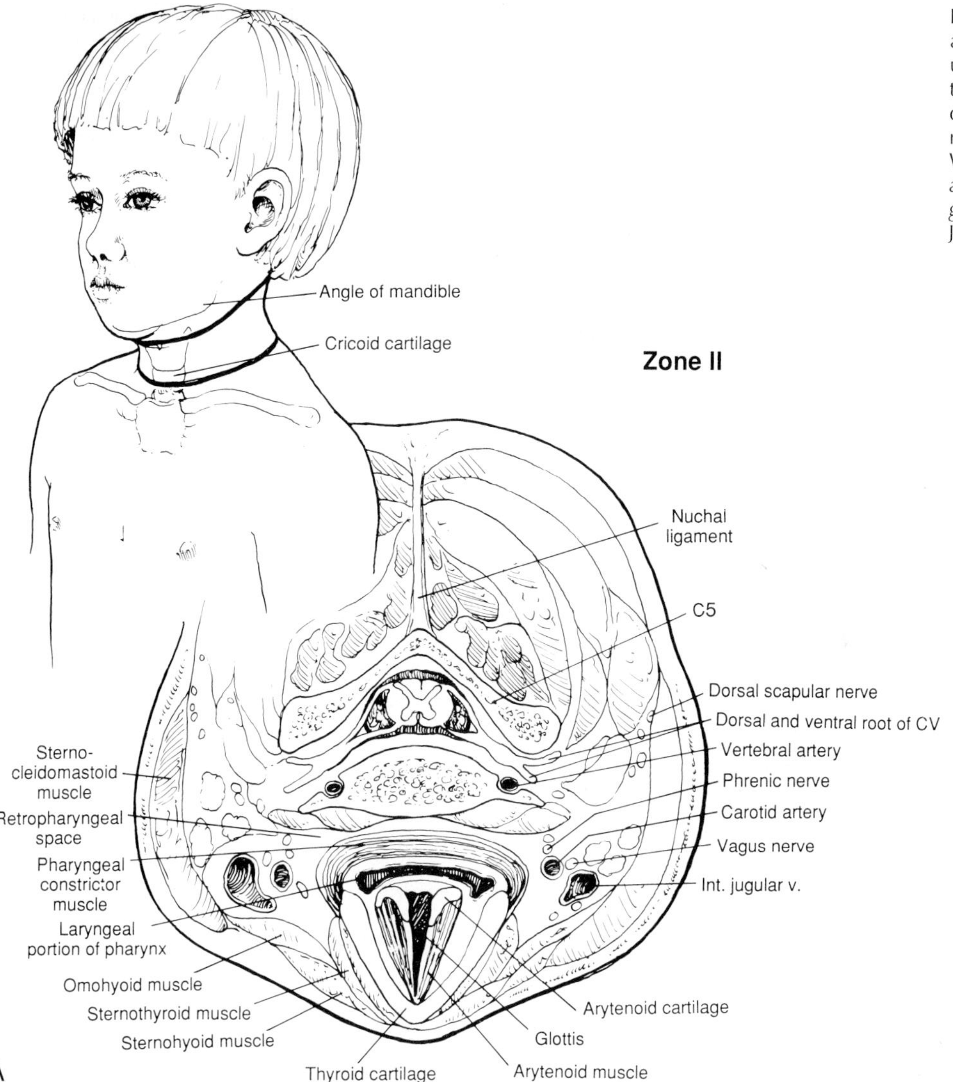

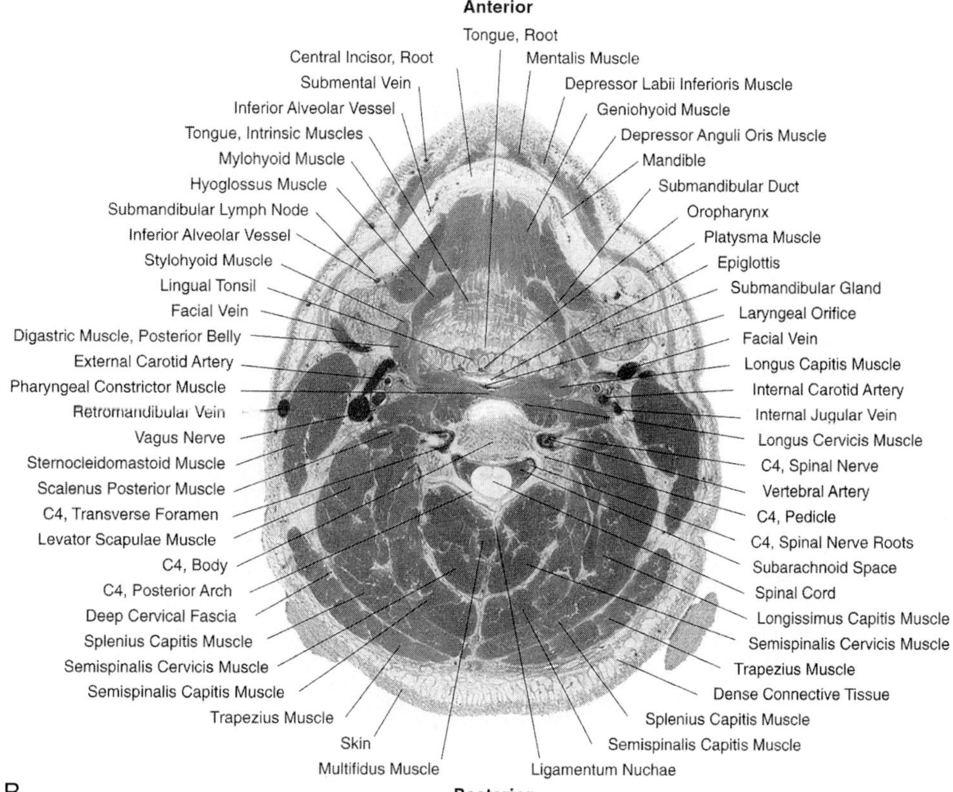

Figure 93.2. **A:** Anatomic neck divisions and contents of zone II located between the upper boundary of zone I and the angle of the mandible. **B:** Anatomic specimen demonstrating zone II relationships. (93.2B reprinted with permission from Spitzer VM, Whitlock DG. *National library of medicine atlas of the visible human male. Reverse engineering of the human body*. Sudbury, MA: Jones & Bartlett, 1997.)

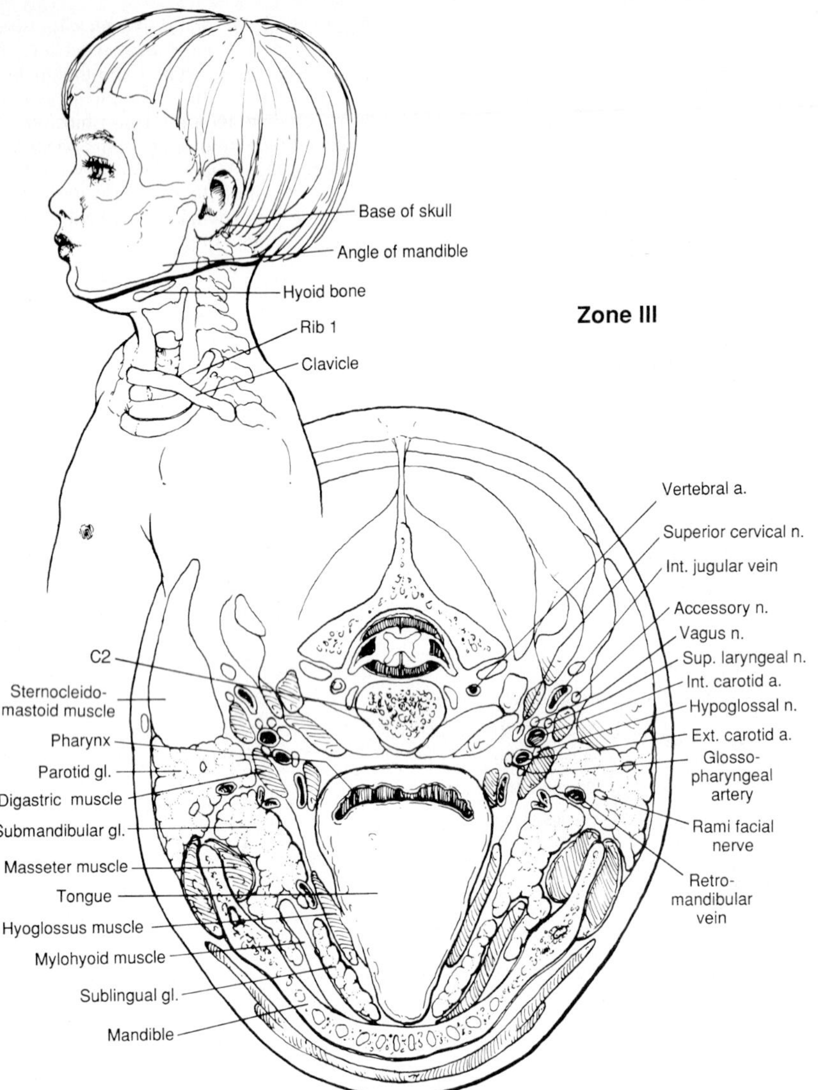

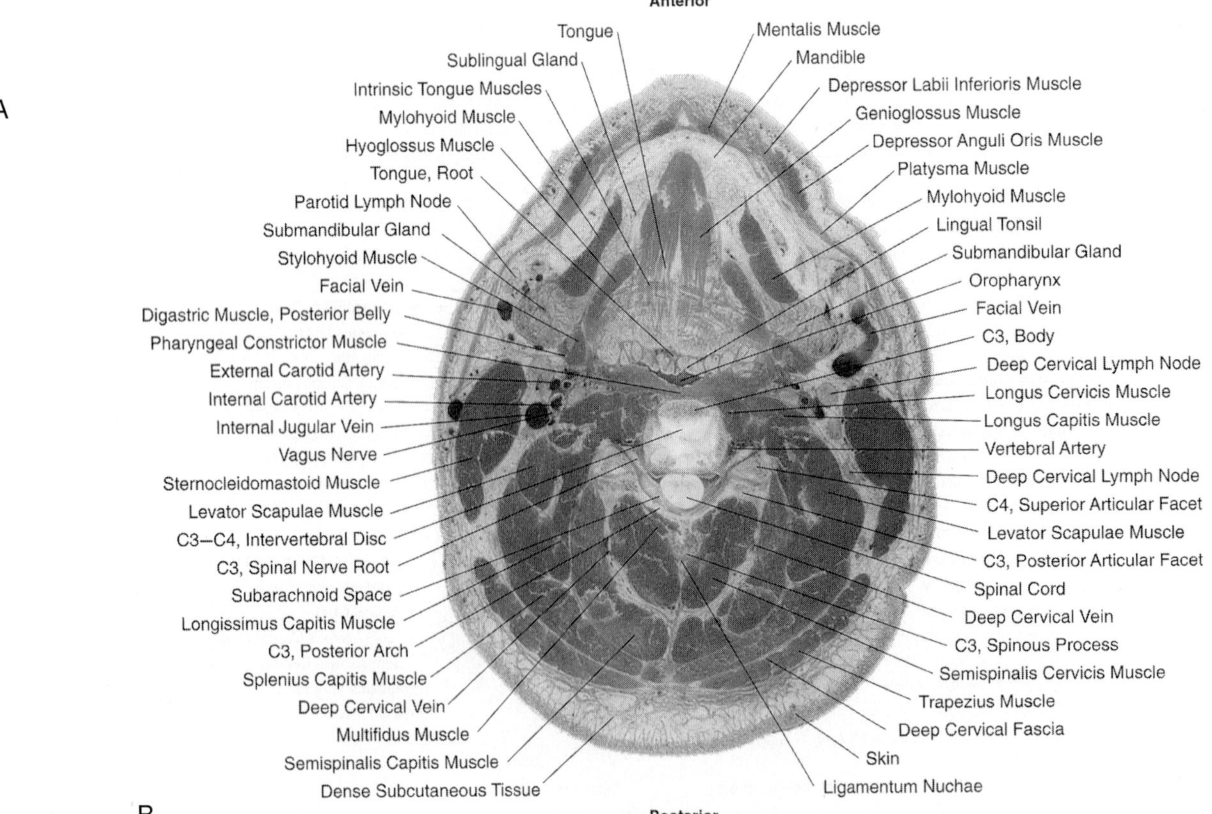

Figure 93.3. **A:** Anatomic neck divisions and contents of zone III. Zone III includes the area above the upper boundary of zone II. **B:** Anatomic specimen demonstrating zone III relationships. (93.3B reprinted with permission from Spitzer VM, Whitlock DG. *National library of medicine atlas of the visible human male. Reverse engineering of the human body*. Sudbury, MA: Jones & Bartlett, 1997.)

TABLE 93.2. Symptoms and Signs of Neck Injuries

Laryngotracheal	Digestive	Vascular	Neurologic
Airway obstruction	Crepitus	Vigorous bleeding, internal or external	Altered consciousness
Dyspnea	Retropharyngeal air	Expansile or pulsatile hematoma	Generalized weakness
Stridor	Subcutaneous emphysema	Bruit	Hemiparesis
Retractions	Pneumomediastinum	Absent pulsations (carotid, superficial temporal, or ophthalmic artery)	Hemiplegia
Cough	Hematemesis	Unexplained hypotension	Quadriplegia
Aspiration	Chest or neck pain	Hemothorax	Seizures
Pneumomediastinum	Neck tenderness	Cardiac tamponade	Bruit
Pneumothorax	Dysphagia	Hemiplegia	Cervicosensory deficits
Crepitus	Odynophagia	Hemiparesis	Aphasia
Subcutaneous emphysema	Saliva in wound	Aphasia	Horner syndrome (Ipsilateral cervical sympathetics)
Tracheal deviation	Drooling	Monocular blindness	Cranial nerve IX–XII dysfunction
Endobronchial bleeding	Fever	Loss of consciousness	Tongue deviation (hypoglossal)
Hemoptysis	Mediastinitis	Neck asymmetry, swelling, or discoloration	Drooping of corner of mouth (mandibular branch of facial nerve)
Epistaxis		Wide mediastinum	Hoarseness (vagus/recurrent laryngeal)
Hematemesis		Cranial nerve abnormality	Immobile vocal cords (vagus/recurrent laryngeal)
Hemothorax		Clavicle/first rib fracture	Trapezius weakness (spinal accessory)
Dysphagia			Brachial palsy (arm paresthesias)
Odynophagia			Monocular blindness (vertebral artery)
Bubbling, sucking, or hissing wound			Diaphragm paralysis (phrenic)
Neck deformity			
Asymmetry			
Loss of landmarks			
Flat thyroid prominence			
Laryngotracheal tenderness			
Dysphonia			
Aphonia			
Voice changes			
Hoarseness			
Drooling			
Neck pain, tenderness (with coughing or swallowing)			

injury, it is important to remember that spinal cord and vertebral levels are not the same. In the cervical area, the cord level lies one segment higher than the corresponding vertebral level (C4 cord level lies opposite the C3 vertebral body). In the lower cervical area, a disparity of up to two levels may be present.

BLUNT TRAUMA

Blunt trauma is often the result of a motor vehicle accident, although it can also be seen from sports; clothesline-type and handlebar injuries from bicycles, motorcycles, all-terrain vehicles, and snowmobiles; strangulation; hanging; blows from fists or feet; and the battered child syndrome (Table 93.1). Blunt trauma is often associated with extracervical injuries, especially maxillofacial, head, and chest, but is less likely than penetrating trauma to involve multiple structures within the neck. Blunt trauma is less likely than penetrating trauma to cause vascular damage, but the incidence of aerodigestive tract injuries is increased. The airway is often injured with direct blunt trauma in part as a result of the anterior and relatively fixed position of the larynx and trachea. A prime target for airway fracture is the cricoid ring, which is the only complete tracheal ring. The triad of dyspnea, stridor, and hemoptysis suggests laryngeal injury, although any or all of the symptoms and signs listed in Table 93.2 may be present.

CERVICAL SPINE EVALUATION

Cervical spine injuries are also uncommon in children, occurring in an estimated 1% to 2% of patients with multiple trauma. However, the clinician must assume that all children who sustain multiple trauma, have head or neck injuries, or have symptoms of neurologic impairment, including altered level of consciousness, have a cervical spine injury until proven otherwise. Goals in the care of these children include effectively stabilizing the primary injury that has occurred and preventing progression to a more severe or significant injury. The devastating nature of a cervical cord injury makes it imperative to not inadvertently miss a potentially unstable cervical spine injury. While attending to the basic ABCs of trauma resuscitation, the clinician should stabilize the cervical spine. Caution must be exercised when applying airway maneuvers to a child with a possible cervical spine injury. Airway interventions, however, often cannot wait until the cervical spine is "cleared." The clinician must prioritize and proceed with lifesaving airway maneuvers, while minimizing motion of the potentially unstable cervical spine.

Hyperextension of the neck to facilitate intubation should be avoided. A vigorous chin lift or jaw thrust may also inadvertently hyperextend the unstable cervical spine. Gentle cricoid pressure should not cause excessive movement to the cervical spine; however, if applied vigorously, it may cause flexion of the spine. When in-line neck immobilization is used to assist with airway maneuvers, the clinician should be careful to avoid applying significant traction to the spine as this pressure can also stress the unstable cervical column. Tracheal intubation in a patient with a potential cervical spine injury ideally requires at least two participants to perform the procedure safely and efficiently. One provider should maintain in-line immobilization of the neck, while another performs the intubation. The immobilization is often best accomplished from below, allowing the intubator as much room as possible to maneuver (Fig. 93.5). The hard cervical collar should be opened anteriorly, or removed,

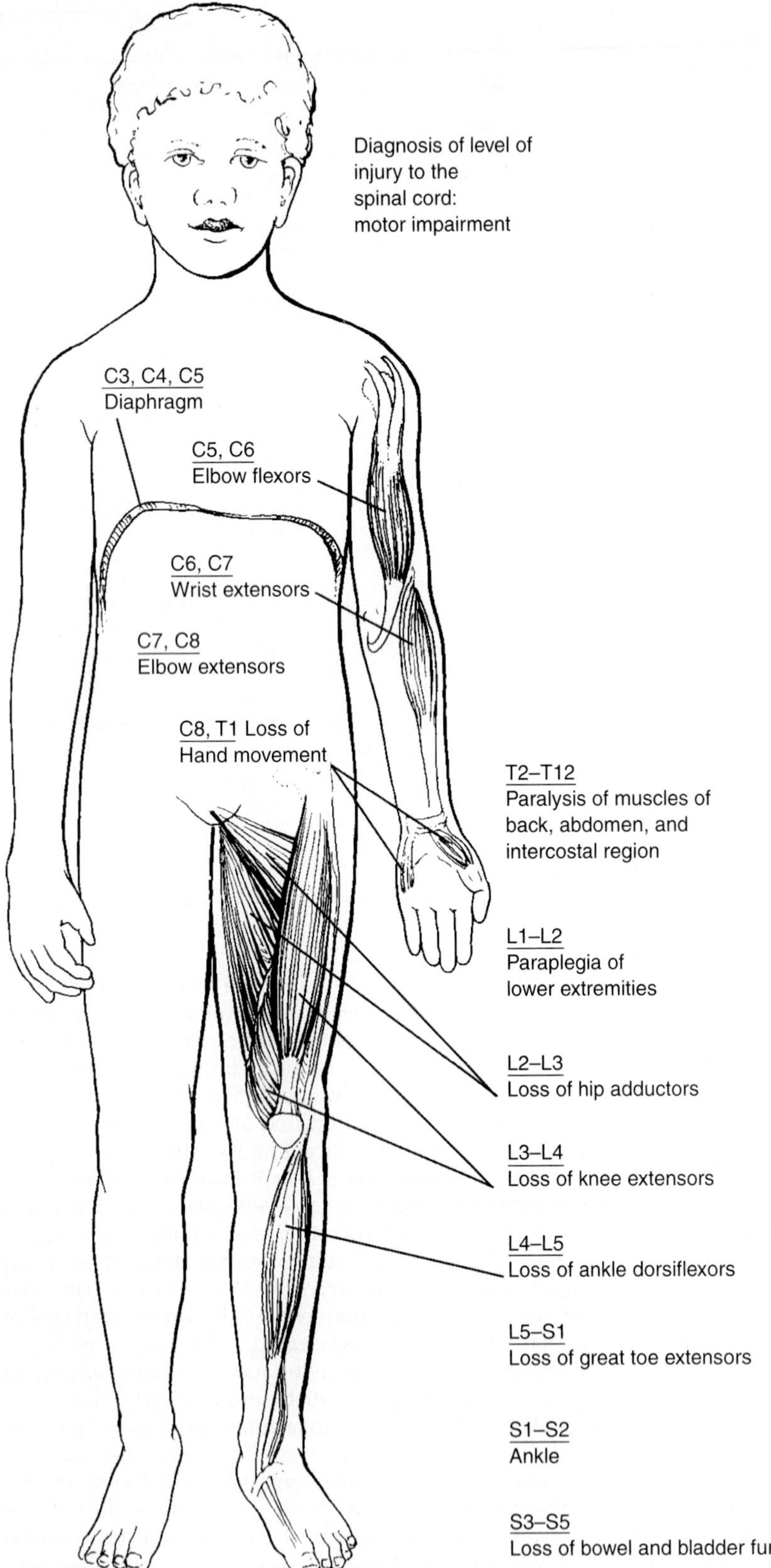

Figure 93.4. Motor dermatomes. Knowledge of sensory and motor dermatomes can be invaluable in description of neurologic findings during initial and subsequent evaluations.

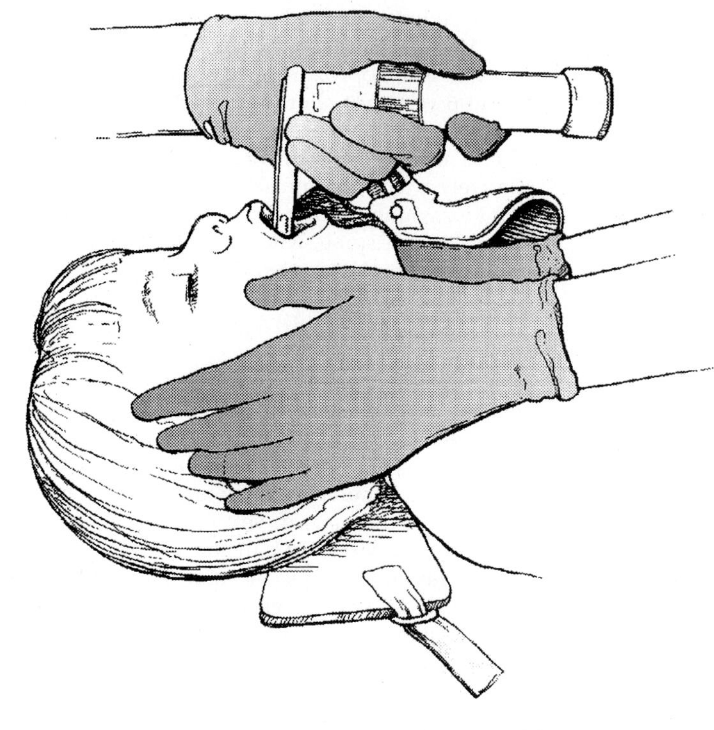

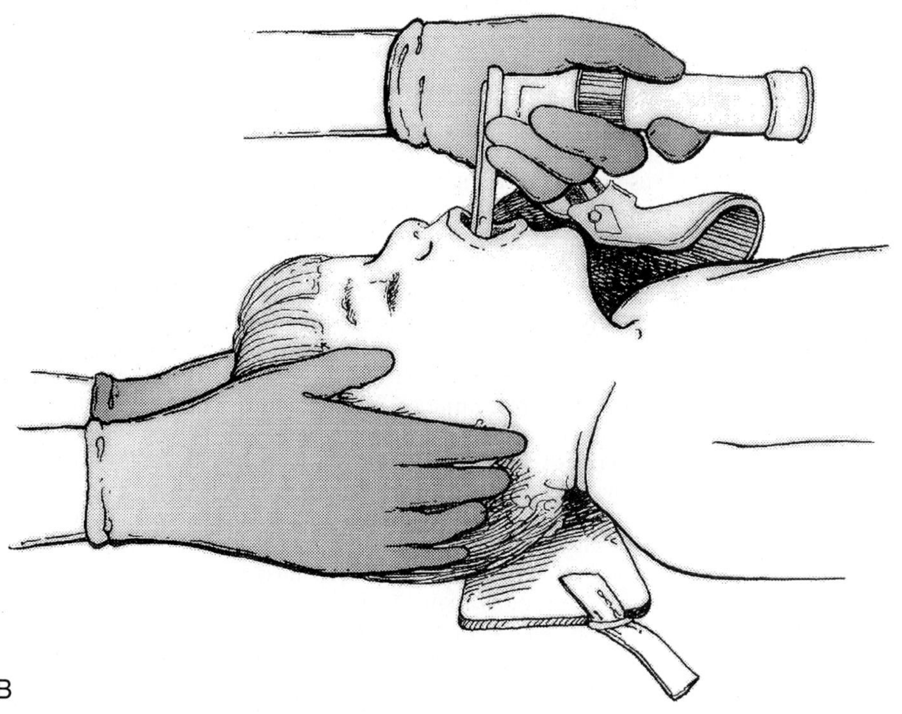

Figure 93.5. **A:** Manual immobilization from below. **B:** Manual immobilization from above. Adequate and expert manual cervical spine immobilization is required during airway maneuvers. The head and neck can be adequately secured from above or below. Immobilization by the second provider from below allows the airway maneuver to be accomplished without requiring a change in preferred positioning of the professional performing the maneuver.

while this process in being performed. It is difficult to intubate a child with the anterior trachea unless the jaw immobilization afforded by the collar is temporarily removed. As usual, oral intubation is often the preferred method because of the child's anterior airway and the usual experience of providers. The collar should be resecured after the airway intervention is complete.

Several concepts should be kept in mind concerning cervical immobilization in children. Soft cervical collars offer no protection to an unstable spine and hard (Philadelphia, Stifneck) collars alone still allow a fair amount of flexion, extension, and lateral movement of the cervical spine. Ideal immobilization involves a hard cervical collar in conjunction with a full spine board, soft spacing devices, and securing straps. An appropriately sized hard cervical collar should be chosen. The tallest collar that does not hyperextend the neck is the correct choice. The choice between a one-piece (Stifneck) or two-piece (Philadelphia) collar is important only in that correct fit must be ensured and the provider must understand how to apply the specific brand of collar. It is helpful to fold over the Velcro connectors on the collar before sliding it under the patient's neck to avoid Velcro attachment to the child's hair or clothing. If a patient is seated and needs to have a collar placed, this maneuver should be accomplished by positioning the collar's chin portion first, followed by placement of the posterior portion. If the patient is wearing a helmet, it should be carefully removed. Helmet removal, if possible, should involve at least two people to avoid potential neck motion. In-line stabilization is ensured by one provider while the helmet is spread and gently removed. Occasionally, mechanical bivalving of the helmet may be required for safe removal.

The clinician must be prepared to log-roll the patient if vomiting occurs. This reaction may happen at any stage of the immobilization process and should be anticipated. Adequate personnel to safely log-roll the vomiting patient are required to avoid potential gagging, aspiration, or secondary spinal or cord injury. The patient should be secured to a long spine board by tape or straps that cross the forehead, chin area of the cervical collar, and bony prominences of the shoulders and pelvis. Incorrect immobilization may impede respiration by obstructing chest rise or contributing to secondary spinal injury by hyperextending the neck. The securing straps should be assessed periodically to ensure adequate and safe attachment of the patient to the spine board. When a child is immobilized on a spine board, the clinician must consider that the child's head is disproportionately large compared with the adult's. A child's head reaches 50% of postnatal growth by approximately age 2 years, whereas chest circumference reaches 50% of postnatal growth by about age 8 years. This disparate growth of the head and trunk causes the neck to be forced into relative kyphotic position when a child is placed on a hard spine board (Fig. 93.6). This is distinctly different from the adult patient whose neck is in 30 degrees of lordosis, the neutral position, when immobilized on a hard spine board. Suggestions have been made to allow a recess in the head area of the spine board to accommodate the child's large occiput or to place a spacing device such as a blanket underneath the torso to allow the neck to rest in a neutral position (Fig. 93.6).

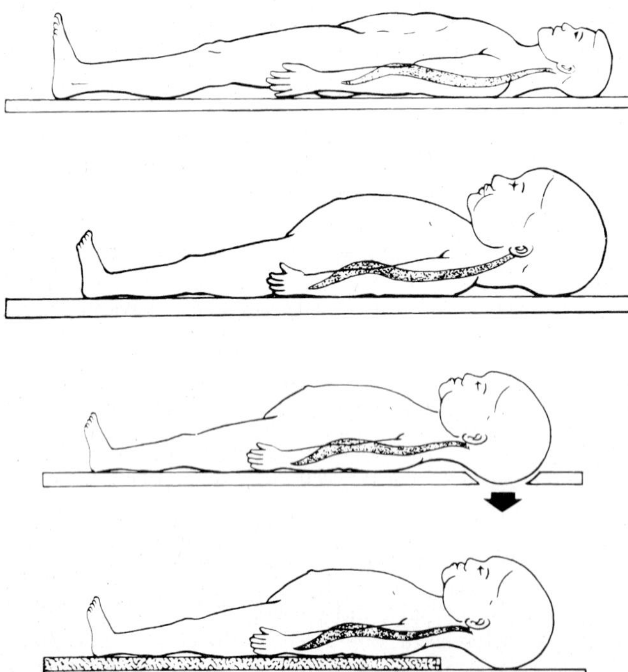

Figure 93.6. Effects of backboard on cervical spine position. **A:** Adult and child immobilized on standard backboard. **B:** Backboards modified with occipital recess and mattress pad to allow neutral positioning of the cervical spine in a young child. (Reprinted with permission from Herzenberg J, Hensinger R, Dedrick D, et al. Emergency transport and positioning of young children who have an injury of the cervical spine: the standard backboard may be hazardous. *J Bone Joint Surg* 1989;71-A:15–21.)

The pediatric cervical spine and its evaluation differ in many ways from the adult spine. The fulcrum of the cervical spine of an infant is at approximately C2-3 and reaches C3-4 by the age of 5 to 6 years. At about the age of 8, the fulcrum (C5-6) and other characteristics of the cervical spine approximate that of an adult. The higher fulcrum of a child's spine in combination with relatively weak neck muscles and poor protective reflexes account for young children often having fractures that involve the upper cervical spine, whereas older children and adults have fractures that more often involve the lower cervical spine. Neurologic disability can occur from cervical lesions at all levels, but high cervical cord injuries are more likely to be fatal than are lower cervical cord injuries.

A neurologic history is imperative to assess whether there was any evidence of abnormal findings such as paresthesias, paralysis, or paresis at any time after the injury. These symptoms may have been transient and may not be present at the time of the examination or volunteered by the patient during gathering of the history, yet they are important because they may suggest a cervical contusion, a concussion, or a spinal cord injury without radiographic abnormality (SCIWORA).

Consideration of cervical spine radiographic evaluation is the next step in assessment. Radiographic options include radiographs, computed tomography (CT), and magnetic resonance imaging (MRI). MRI scans are more appropriate when evaluating the subacute or chronic stages of injury or when looking for an acute problem with cord impingement by blood or soft tissues such as tumors or intervertebral discs. MRI does not image cortical bone well and should not be used to evaluate the cervical spine for fractures, whereas the CT scan demonstrates fractures clearly. A CT scan is often used as a secondary screen when adequate plain radiographs cannot be obtained or to substantiate suspected fractures. A common scenario is the use of CT to supplement viewing the C1/C2 region in young, traumatized children. The CT scan images soft tissue well; however, it does not demonstrate the intrathecal, ligamentous, disc, or vascular detail that can be obtained with an MRI scan.

The plain radiograph remains the preferred initial test for acutely traumatized patients. Several authors have attempted to devise criteria to limit the use of cervical spine radiographs because the number of positive studies constitutes a small proportion of the total number of radiograph studies completed. The perception of unnecessary tests should be balanced against the severity of consequences that may occur with a missed cervical spine injury. The literature suggests that if the patient does not have a high-risk mechanism of injury (motor vehicle accident, fall, dive, or sports injury), is awake and alert, can have an interactive conversation (not inebriated, no altered level of consciousness, older than 4 to 5 years of age), does not complain of cervical spine pain, has no tenderness on palpation (especially in the midline), has normal neck mobility, has a completely normal neurologic examination without history of abnormal neurologic symptoms or signs at any time after the injury, and has no other painful injuries (which may distract the patient and mask neck pain), the patient probably does not need radiographic evaluation of the cervical spine. The clinician must be sure, however, to never "clear" the cervical spine, regardless of studies performed, in an unconscious patient in the ED.

When radiographs are obtained, a normal lateral radiograph does not "clear" the cervical spine. The sensitivity of a lateral cervical spine radiograph varies between 82% and 98% in the literature. When evaluating a lateral cervical spine radiograph, the clinician must ensure that C-1 through C-7 are included as well as the C7–T1 junction. Additional films, which include an anteroposterior (AP) view of C-3 through C-7, and an AP openmouth (odontoid) view of C1-2, increase the sensitivity of initial radiographic evaluation to more than 95%. An adequate open-mouth (odontoid) view is often technically difficult to obtain in young children and those who are intubated. If further information is required, a CT scan of C-1/C-2 can be useful to augment or replace the open-mouth view. A CT scan is more expensive than a plain film of C-1/ C-2, but it is easier to obtain, offers better and more consistent information, and avoids the risk of missing a subtle injury in that critical area. The advent of the spiral CT scan allows this study to be completed in 1 to 2 minutes and to be reconstructed by the computer to demonstrate vivid detail of the region. An algorithm for considering radiographic evaluation is presented in Fig. 93.7. An approach to ordering cervical spine imaging studies is shown in Fig. 93.8.

The cervical spine has anterior (vertebral bodies, intervertebral discs, ligaments) and posterior (lamina, pedicles, neural foramen, spinous processes, ligaments) components. The initial three-view series evaluates the anterior cervical spine well; however, it is not ideal for evaluating the posterior cervical spine. Oblique (pillar) views are helpful in imaging those posterior elements. In practice, however, oblique films rarely add significant information to the initial radiographic assessment. Flexion and extension films are accomplished in an awake patient by having the patient flex and extend the neck as far as possible without discomfort. As the end-point involves the sensation of pain, flexion/extension films should not be performed in a patient who has preexisting neck pain. Dynamic fluoroscopy could be substituted in specific instances for flexion/extension films. These studies can help evaluate underlying soft-tissue or ligamentous injury that was not evident on the initial films. If a question remains concerning the integrity of the cervical spine after following this radiographic scheme, a CT scan should be considered. An MRI should be considered to detect ligamentous, soft-tissue, or subtle cord injuries.

A systematic approach should be used when evaluating radiographs of the cervical spine. The ABC method is a useful approach (Fig. 93.9). Alignment is assessed, keeping in mind that the spinal cord lies between the posterior spinal line and the spinolaminal line. These lordotic curves may not be present in children less than 6 years of age, those on hard spine boards or in cervical collars, or those with cervical neck muscle spasm. Gross malalignment should be detectable with this assessment.

Soft-tissue evaluation is extremely important. Abnormal soft-tissue spaces may be the only clue to the underlying ligament, cartilage, or subtle bone injury, which may not be obvious on the radiograph. The soft-tissue widening may represent blood or edema, which suggests an underlying injury. The prevertebral space at C-3 should be less than one-half to two-thirds of the AP width of the adjacent vertebral body. This space will

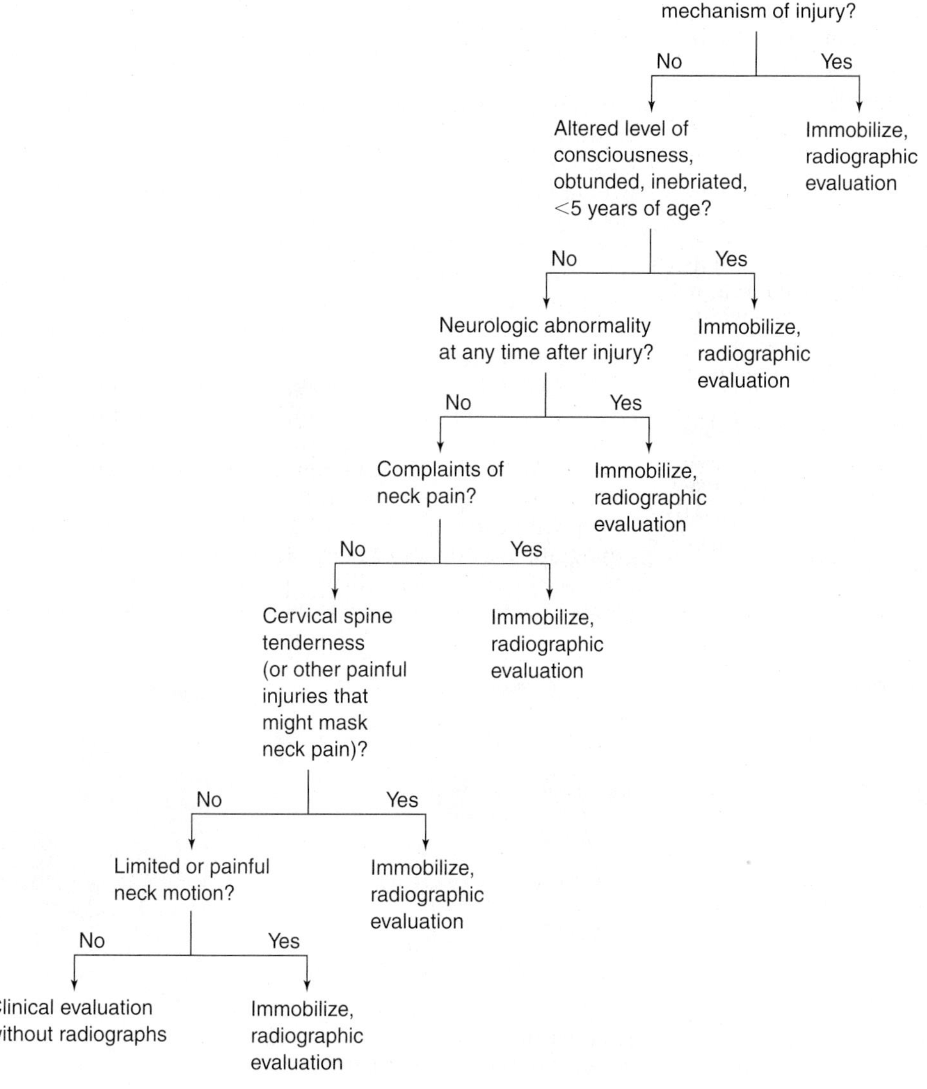

Figure 93.7. Decision tree for radiographic and clinical evaluation of patient with possible neck injury.

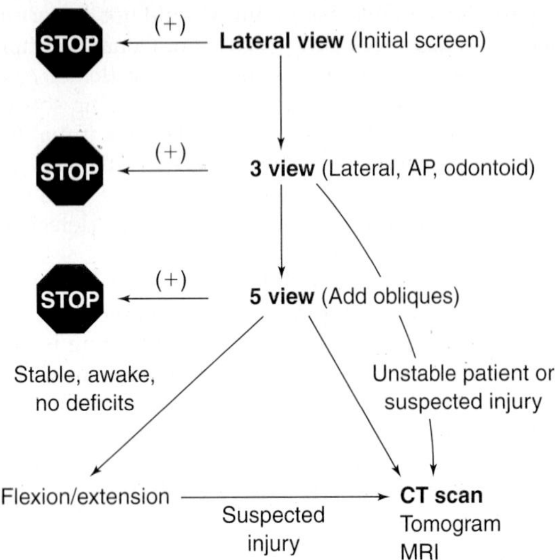

Figure 93.8. Approach to ordering cervical spine radiographs. Additional films may not be needed in the acute situation if a fracture or other abnormality is identified. If an abnormality is suspected, but not demonstrated, continue with algorithm as presented.

double, to approximately the width of the adjacent vertebral body, below C-4 (the level of the glottis) as the usually non–air-filled esophagus is present at this area. Care must be taken when evaluating the prevertebral soft-tissue space because crying, neck flexion, or the expiratory phase of respiration may produce a pseudothickening in the prevertebral space. Soft-tissue abnormality should be reproducible on repeated radiographs if an actual underlying injury exists.

SPECIFIC INJURIES

The Jefferson fracture is a bursting fracture of the ring of C-1 as a result of an axial load. The axial force compresses the ring of C-1 between the occipital condyles of the skull and the lateral masses of C-2. This reaction can cause an outward burst of C-2, but it rarely causes immediate neurologic impairment because the fracture does not physically impinge on the spinal cord. The radiographic criteria for diagnosis of a Jefferson fracture is lateral offset of the lateral mass of C-1 of greater than 1 mm from the vertebral body of C-2. Neck rotation may give a false-positive radiograph.

The hangman's fracture is a traumatic spondylolisthesis of C-2. This injury occurs as a result of hyperextension, which fractures the posterior elements of C-2. Hyperflexion, with resultant ligamentous damage, may follow the hyperextension or may lead to anterior subluxation of C-2 on C-3 and subsequent damage of the cervical cord. The subluxation associated with a hangman's fracture can sometimes be mistaken for the normal or physiologic subluxation that exists in the C2-3 or C3-4 region in approximately 25% of children less than the age of 8 years; it also may be seen up to the age of 16.

Atlantoaxial (AA) subluxation is a result of movement between C-1 and C-2 secondary to transverse ligament rupture or a fractured dens (Fig. 93.10). Ligament instability may be precipitated by tonsillitis, cervical adenitis, pharyngitis, arthritis, or connective tissue disorders. It is also well described in patients with Down syndrome. Approximately 15% of patients with Down syndrome have radiographically demonstrated AA subluxation and therefore should be discouraged from contact sports. The presence or absence of AA subluxation in patients with Down syndrome, once thought to be a static phenomenon, may actually be transient and/or progressive. Neurologic symptoms often are not seen until the predental space exceeds 7 to 10 mm. A dens fracture is the cause of AA subluxation more often than ligamentous disruption in a young child because the weakest part of the musculoskeletal system in a child is the osseous component (Fig. 93.10).

Cervical distraction injuries may result from rapid acceleration- or deceleration-type incidents, such as high-speed motor vehicle or pedestrian accidents. This is an injury usually incompatible with long-term survival, but for which initial cardiopulmonary resuscitation may be successful.

Vertebral compression injuries are suggested by isolated anterior wedging, teardrop fractures, or burst vertebral bodies. The vertebral bodies should be regular, cuboid, and consistent between adjacent cervical levels. A flexion/rotation stress can lead to anterior subluxation of one vertebral body on another with facet dislocation ("locked" or "jumped" facet). If the anterior displacement is less than 50% of the vertebral body width, it is consistent with a unilateral facet dislocation. More than a 50% anterior subluxation suggests a bilateral facet dislocation. These injuries are often accompanied by widened interspinous and interlaminar spaces, anterior soft-tissue swelling, and a narrowed disc space.

SCIWORA has been described as occurring in up to 67% of children with cervical cord injuries. SCIWORA probably accounts for about 25% of cervical cord injuries in children less than 8 years of age. These injuries mainly occur in children less than 8 years of age who present with or develop symptoms consistent with cervical cord injuries without any radiographic or tomographic evidence of bony abnormality. SCIWORA is not often seen in the older pediatric population (older than age 8) because the forces necessary to injure the spinal cord also cause

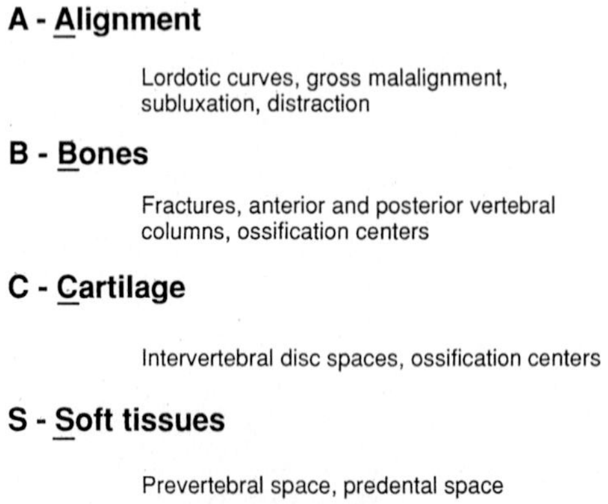

A - Alignment

Lordotic curves, gross malalignment, subluxation, distraction

B - Bones

Fractures, anterior and posterior vertebral columns, ossification centers

C - Cartilage

Intervertebral disc spaces, ossification centers

S - Soft tissues

Prevertebral space, predental space

Figure 93.9. The airway, breathing, circulation (ABCs) of radiographic cervical spine interpretation.

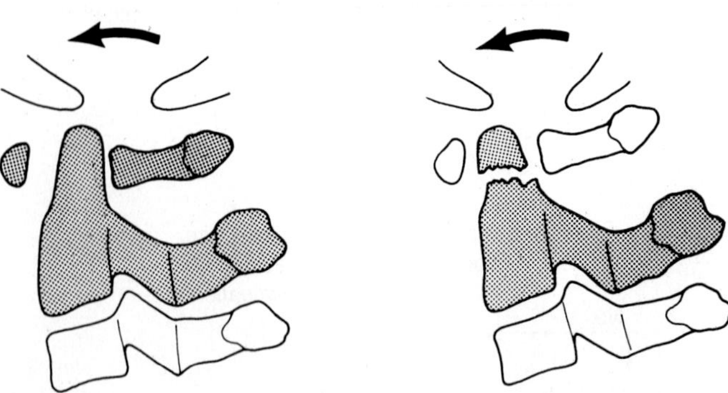

Figure 93.10. Diagrammatic representation of transverse ligament disruption **(left)** and dens fracture **(right)**.

persistent spinal abnormalities. Therefore, many clinicians recommend hospitalization and immobilization for young patients who have a history of transient neurologic symptoms. At the least, neurologic consultation is recommended if the history suggests a SCIWORA-type injury in a child less than 8 years of age.

Torticollis (wry neck) is a common complaint in the pediatric ED. The clinician should always inquire about traumatic causes because an underlying bone injury may be present. Often, however, torticollis is caused by spasm of the sternocleidomastoid (SCM) muscle. The patient with muscular torticollis has muscle spasm of the SCM on the opposite side that the chin points because the cause of torticollis is muscular spasm. This condition is opposite from rotary subluxation. Rotary subluxation is a cervical spine injury that is often misdiagnosed or undiagnosed because of difficulty in interpreting these patient's radiographs. Rotary subluxation or displacement may be spontaneous or may follow an upper respiratory infection or minor or major trauma. These patients rarely present with abnormal neurologic findings. They will assume the typical (cockrobin) position with the muscle spasm of the SCM on the same side as the chin points. Rotary subluxation should be suspected if, on an open-mouth radiograph, one of the lateral masses of C-1 appears forward and closer to the midline, while the opposite lateral mass appears narrow and away from the midline (lateral offset), although a normal film does not rule out rotary subluxation. Cineradiography can demonstrate that C1-2 moves as a unit; however, the CT scan appears to be the most useful diagnostic tool in rotary subluxation. Patients with mild rotary subluxation should be treated with a cervical collar and analgesia for comfort, whereas those with moderate or resilient rotary displacement may need immobilization and traction. If anterior displacement of C-2 on C-1 is present, longer immobilization may be needed to allow injured ligaments to heal.

CHAPTER 94
Thoracic Trauma

Howard Kadish, M.D.

Thoracic trauma in the pediatric population is relatively uncommon, and only in the last two decades has it received careful scrutiny. Included in thoracic trauma are injuries to the chest wall, trachea, bronchi, lungs, heart, thoracic aorta and great vessels, esophagus, and diaphragm. The report of the National Pediatric Trauma Registry contains a detailed analysis of major thoracic trauma in children. In the United States, only 4% to 6% of children admitted to pediatric trauma centers have thoracic injuries, but because severe injuries to vital thoracic organs produce profound physiologic disturbances, many patients die at the scene and never reach a hospital. For patients who reach the hospital, most thoracic injuries do not require operative intervention other than tube thoracostomy.

INITIAL MANAGEMENT

The ABCs (airway, breathing, and circulation) of trauma management apply regardless of the organ system injured. A top priority in any patient with respiratory or circulatory failure should be airway stabilization (see Chapter 5) and identification and treatment of shock (see Chapter 3). The injured child should be evaluated according to the primary survey of trauma management. The first priority in trauma patients with or without thoracic injury is establishing a secure, patent airway. Indications for endotracheal intubation in the thoracic trauma patient include depressed neurologic status, inadequate oxygenation or ventilation, compromised circulatory status, or an unstable airway including burns.

After the airway is secured, breathing is assessed. Inspection (symmetry, adequate chest rise, neck veins, displaced trachea) and auscultation (equal breath sounds, heart tones) of the chest provide information about ventilation. The ideal site for auscultation of the lungs is in the midaxillary line. Measurement of oxygen saturation by oximetry provides information on oxygenation.

If a patient has an abnormal examination but appears to be oxygenating and ventilating well and is not in shock, chest radiography is indicated. If breathing is inadequate after endotracheal intubation and breath sounds are asymmetric, intervention is required before a chest radiograph. The patient with absent breath sounds on one side and tracheal shift to the opposite side requires immediate needle decompression and subsequent tube thoracostomy. Only after the patient is stabilized should a chest radiograph be obtained.

The patient's circulatory status is evaluated after airway and breathing are stabilized. Pericardial tamponade and a tension pneumothorax or hemothorax should be considered in the poorly perfused, shocky patient, especially when sources of blood loss have been excluded and volume resuscitation has not improved the patient's status. Physical examination may reveal muffled heart or breath sounds with decreased or absent pulses. Pericardiocentesis or thoracentesis and subsequent tube thoracostomy are lifesaving procedures that usually need to be performed in the unstable trauma patient before going to the operating room for definitive treatment.

Once the patient is stabilized and the immediate life-threatening injuries, such as airway obstruction, tension pneumothorax, hemothorax, and pericardial tamponade, are treated, a chest radiograph and thoracic computed tomography (CT) scan should be obtained to provide valuable information regarding other potentially life-threatening and operative injuries. Thoracic injuries requiring operative intervention are described in Table 94.1 and in Figure 94.1. The use of ultrasound is rapidly

TABLE 94.1. Thoracic Trauma Injuries Requiring Operative Intervention

Injury	Signs and symptoms
Tracheal/bronchial rupture	Active chest tube air leak
Lung parenchyma, internal mammary artery laceration, intercostal artery laceration	Chest tube bleeding >2–3 mL/kg/hr or hypotension unresponsive to transfusions
Esophageal disruption	Abnormal esophagogram (leak) or esophagoscopy; gastric contents in the chest tube
Diaphragmatic hernia	Abnormal gas pattern in the hemithorax; displaced nasogastric tube in the hemithorax
Pericardial tamponade	Positive pericardiocentesis
Great vessel laceration	Widened mediastinum
	Tracheal or nasogastric tube deviation; blurred aortic knob; abnormal aortogram ("gold standard")

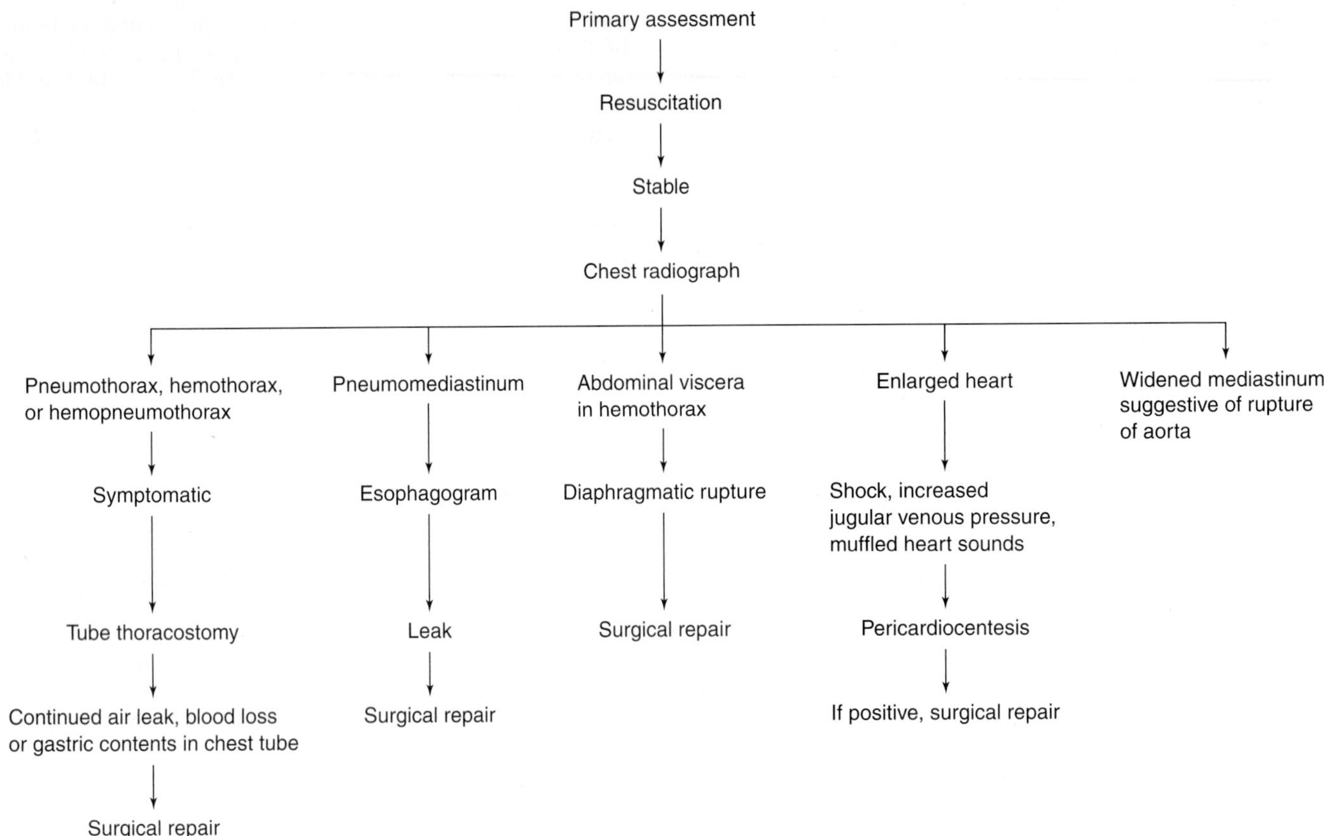

Figure 94.1. Indications for surgery in thoracic trauma.

becoming a standard diagnostic modality in the evaluation of the adult trauma patient. One adult study demonstrated that thoracic ultrasound was as sensitive and specific in identifying a hemothorax as a chest radiograph. The utility of ultrasound in the pediatric trauma patient has yet to be determined. No study has been conducted to ascertain specifically its usefulness except in the evaluation of cardiac injuries. Numerous studies have shown thoracic CT to be superior to routine chest radiograph in identifying pulmonary contusions, pneumothoraces, and hemothoraces. Thoracic CT should be part of the initial evaluation of pediatric trauma patients if a lung contusion, pneumothorax, or a hemothorax is suspected or if the cause of the patient's respiratory distress is unknown. Thoracic CT is also useful in the asymptomatic patient with chest radiograph findings suggestive of a traumatic rupture of the thoracic aorta.

CHEST WALL INJURIES

The elasticity and flexibility of a child's thoracic cage make chest wall injuries less common than internal organ injuries, such as a pulmonary contusion. When chest wall injuries occur, the patient is at increased risk for intrathoracic injuries. Included in chest wall injuries are rib, sternal, and scapular fractures and flail chest.

Rib Fractures

Rib fractures can occur from either a direct blow to the rib or compression of the chest in an anterior–posterior direction. With a direct blow, the rib will fracture inward and may puncture the pleural cavity, causing a pneumothorax. A hemothorax is caused by a rib lacerating an intercostal artery, an internal mammary artery, or the lung parenchyma. Compression of the chest wall can cause the lateral portions of the ribs to fracture outward. Intrathoracic injury is seen less commonly with this type of fracture.

In one study, rib fractures occurred in 32% of all children admitted to the hospital with thoracic trauma. Motor-vehicle accidents were the most common mechanism of injury, similar to adult studies. Single rib fractures did not correlate with the severity of injury, but as the number of fractures increased, so did the likelihood of multisystem and intrathoracic injuries. Children with rib fractures and both head and thoracic injuries had a doubled mortality rate compared with children with rib fractures and an isolated thoracic injury.

Because of the relatively protected nature of the first rib and the amount of force required to fracture it, first rib fractures should be approached with a high index of suspicion for other serious injuries, such as vascular disruption or tracheal laceration. Patients with these lesions are usually symptomatic (hypotension, anuria, pulse differences or deficits). In one study, all patients with a first rib fracture and injury to the great vessels exhibited physical examination abnormalities, such as loss of the radial pulse on the involved side, discrepancy in blood pressure between the upper extremities, a flail chest, or hypotension. No patients with an isolated first rib fracture and a completely normal physical examination had an injury to a great vessel. In this and other studies, no correlation existed between the level of rib fracture and associated vascular injury in the otherwise asymptomatic patient.

The pediatric patient with a rib fracture may splint and hypoventilate secondary to pain. Physical examination may reveal point tenderness and, if the pleura has been involved, crepitus. If the patient has any respiratory or circulatory compromise, a tube thoracotomy is indicated for a pneumothorax or hemothorax. The tube should be placed at a separate site from the area of the fracture. If the patient is stable, relief of pain, monitoring the respiratory status, and further evaluation (chest radiography, thoracic CT) for underlying injury is indicated. Wrapping or binding the chest wall are contraindicated because these measures can impair ventilatory function. Analgesics are helpful but should be used with caution because they also can cause respiratory depression. Epidural analgesia is helpful, especially for lower rib fracture. Intercostal nerve block is also useful but should be performed carefully to avoid puncturing the pleura.

Patients with multiple rib fractures should be admitted to the hospital for pain control, pulmonary physiotherapy, and observation for worsening respiratory status. Prognosis for isolated rib fractures is excellent, with most healing within 6 weeks. The chest wall will remodel, leaving no permanent disability.

Sternal and Scapular Fractures

Sternal and scapular fractures are uncommon in children, secondary to the marked compliance of the chest wall. Although they require a thorough evaluation for other thoracic injuries because of the significant force required to fracture these bones, sternal and scapular fractures are rarely associated with vascular or brachial plexus injuries. In one adult study, scapular fracture alone was not a significant marker for mortality or neurovascular injury. In another study that evaluated patients with blunt cardiac injury, only 2% had an associated sternal fracture.

Flail Chest

Fracturing two or more ribs on the same side may result in that particular chest wall segment losing continuity with the thoracic cage. This condition is called a *flail chest*. Direct impact to the rib, as in a crush injury, is the most common mechanism for a flail chest. Flail chest is uncommon in children because of the significant compliance of the chest wall. In adult thoracic trauma series, flail chest occurred in approximately 10% of patients, compared with fewer than 1% in the pediatric population. When a flail chest occurs, it is usually associated with an intrathoracic injury, most often pulmonary contusion, because of the force involved.

The pediatric patient may develop respiratory distress and failure as a result of a flail chest caused by numerous mechanisms. In the early 1900s, Bauer described the pendelluft theory, which attributes inefficient ventilation and oxygenation to a pendulum-like movement of air from the injured lung to the uninjured lung. The harder and faster a patient works to breathe, the more shifting of air from one side to the other occurs. The paradoxic movement of the chest also impairs the normal inspiratory–expiratory function of the lung (Fig. 94.2). Another mechanism for respiratory distress is the association of underlying pulmonary injury with a flail chest. Edema within the airways alters alveolar ventilation–perfusion ratios and produces pulmonary arteriovenous shunting with hypoxemia and subsequent respiratory distress. Finally, the pain associated with rib fractures causes voluntary and involuntary splinting. These patients are at increased risk for atelectasis and pneumonia secondary to poor pulmonary function.

The goal of treatment should be to stabilize the involved portion of the thoracic cage. At the scene of an accident, the patient can be placed with the injured side down, thus improving tidal volume and ventilation. Any patient with respiratory distress should be intubated and placed on positive-pressure ventilation. For patients with an underlying pulmonary contusion, fluids must be carefully monitored. Fluid may leak out of the injured capillary bed, worsening the pulmonary contusion.

PULMONARY CONTUSIONS AND LACERATIONS

Pulmonary contusion is the most common thoracic injury in children. Pulmonary contusion occurs when a blunt force, such as a crush injury, is applied to the lung parenchyma. As in any contusion or bruise, the capillary network becomes damaged, leaking fluid into the surrounding tissues. A ventilation–perfusion mismatch occurs because of the extravasation of fluid, interfering with oxygenation. As the edema and swelling worsen, the patient's respiratory status also deteriorates. Initially, a pulmonary contusion may be invisible on a chest radiograph. Chest CT is more sensitive in detecting pulmonary contusion. Lung parenchymal injuries often are noted when a few cuts of the thoracic cavity are imaged while obtaining an abdominal CT.

In one study, tachypnea, abnormal breath sounds, external thoracic wall contusion, and fracture of the bony thorax each were absent in more than 50% of patients with a pulmonary contusion. Interestingly, the chest radiograph in these patients did not dramatically worsen from time of admission. Nonetheless, mild contusions require close observation in the hospital for worsening respiratory status and supportive care.

Patients with moderate to severe pulmonary contusions may be tachypneic and may have an oxygen requirement secondary to shunting within the lung. If the patient can no longer maintain oxygenation, endotracheal intubation and mechanical ventilation with positive pressure are the preferred treatment. Fluid restriction is helpful to avoid exacerbation of pulmonary edema. Many of these patients have associated injuries, making fluid restriction difficult; intensive care management with measurement of central venous and pulmonary arterial pressure may be helpful for those patients with major multisystem trauma. Double-lumen endotracheal–endobronchial tubes can be used

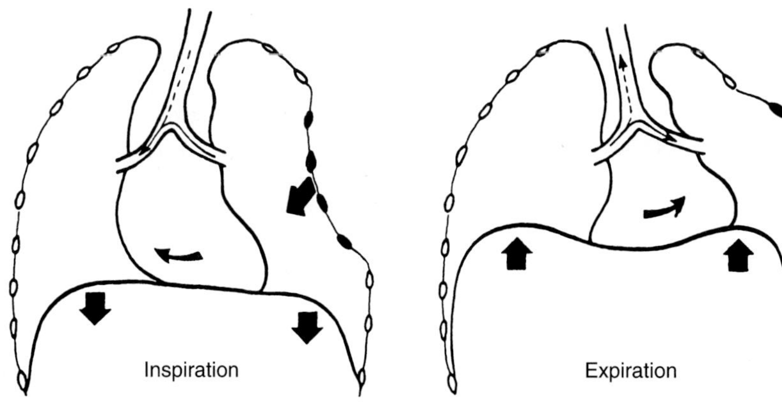

Figure 94.2. Pathophysiologic consequence of flail chest with paradoxical motion.

in patients with severe lung contusions refractory to normal ventilatory management.

Pulmonary lacerations occur more often in penetrating trauma but can occur in rapid deceleration injuries. Rib fractures secondary to blunt trauma also can puncture the lung. Patients are usually tachypneic and have abnormal breath sounds. Large lacerations may cause hemoptysis. Chest radiograph shows pneumothorax or hemothorax. Treatment includes endotracheal intubation for patients in respiratory distress and tube thoracotomy for pneumothorax or hemothorax. Adequate intravenous access and blood for transfusion should be available before chest tube placement. Insertion of the chest tube can disrupt hemostasis in the chest cavity, and the patient may exsanguinate. Indications for surgery include continuous hemorrhage or air leak through the chest tube, massive hemoptysis, or air embolism.

Air embolism is usually fatal, but it should be considered when a patient deteriorates suddenly after endotracheal intubation, when focal neurologic findings develop without evidence of a craniospinal injury, or when frothy blood is withdrawn from an arterial puncture. Treatment includes open thoracotomy with either occlusion of the hilar structure on the affected side or direct aspiration of the air. Neither treatment option is usually successful.

INTRAPLEURAL INJURIES

In one study, intrapleural injury occurred in 40% of children with a thoracic injury. Hemopneumothorax, hemothorax, and pneumothorax were evenly distributed. Pneumothorax was associated with the lowest mortality rate (15%), and hemothorax had the highest incidence (57%). Auscultation is helpful but not 100% accurate in diagnosing a hemothorax, pneumothorax, or hemopneumothorax. A recent report found that auscultation to detect hemothorax, pneumothorax, or hemopneumothorax had a sensitivity of 58% and a specificity of 98%. Most intrapleural injuries do not need surgical intervention and can be managed either by hospital observation or tube thoracostomy (Fig. 94.3).

PNEUMOTHORAX

Pneumothorax is the second most commonly encountered entity in blunt thoracic trauma and the most common in penetrating thoracic trauma. Air within the pleural cavity can arise from chest wall penetration, lung parenchyma disruption, a tear of the tracheobronchial structures, or esophageal rupture.

Patients may be asymptomatic, complain of pleuritic chest pain, have tachypnea, or be in severe respiratory distress. Physical examination may be normal, or it may reveal diminished or absent breath sounds, crepitus, or hyperresonance to percussion on the side of the pneumothorax. In the asymptomatic or mildly symptomatic patient, a chest radiograph is helpful in diagnosing and determining the type of treatment necessary. If the pneumothorax is small and the patient asymptomatic, observation in the hospital and administration of 100% oxygen is all that is necessary. A small pneumothorax is classically described as being less than 15%, although it is common to underestimate the size of a pneumothorax on plain films, only

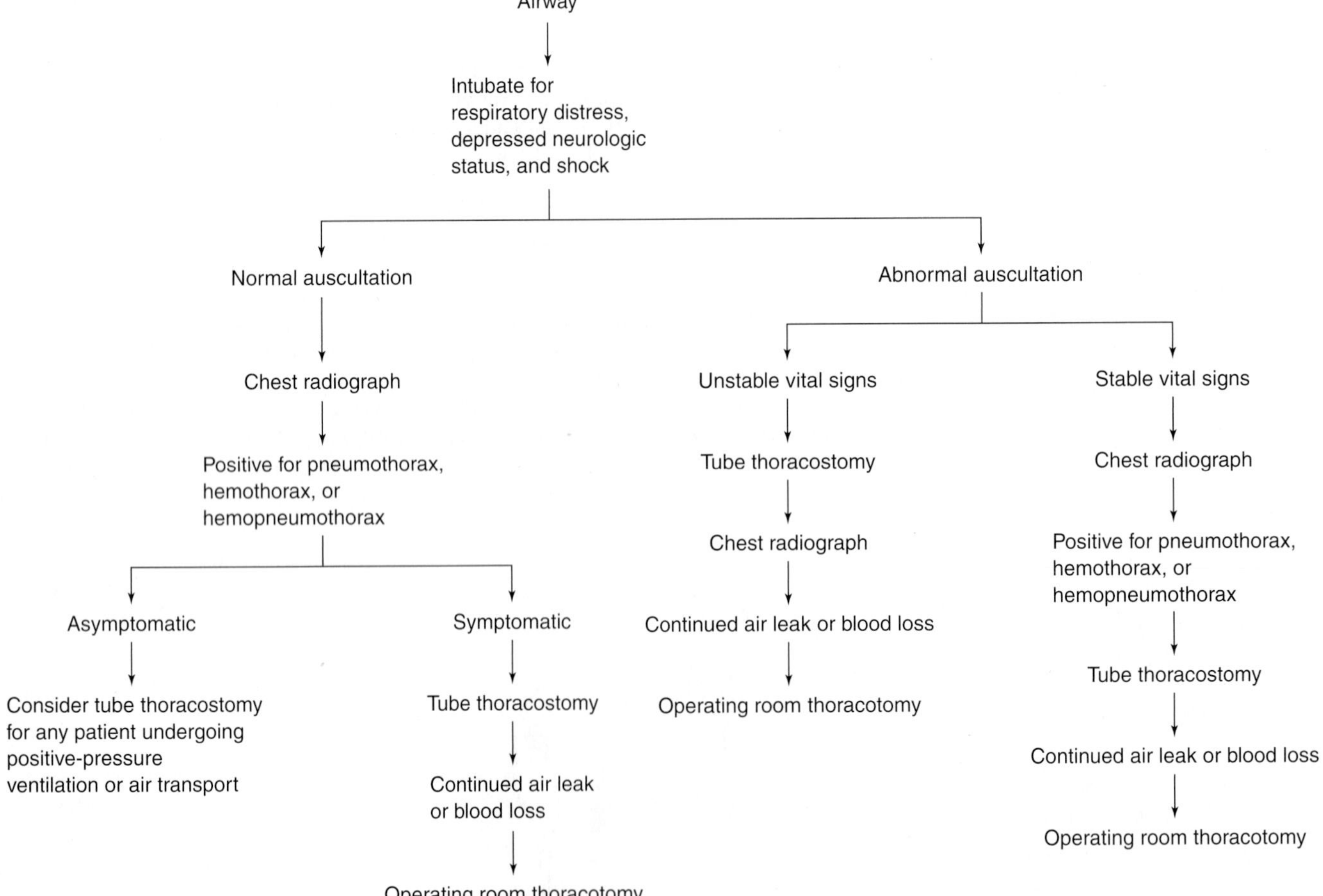

Figure 94.3. Algorithm for the management of intrapleural injuries.

to find a much more extensive lesion on CT scan. Tube thoracostomy is indicated in symptomatic patients, patients undergoing positive-pressure ventilation, and those requiring air transport. An asymptomatic patient can become symptomatic rapidly if a small, simple pneumothorax progresses to a tension pneumothorax; therefore, even asymptomatic children with a traumatic pneumothorax should be admitted to the hospital for observation.

Tension Pneumothorax

A tension pneumothorax is the most common complicated intrapleural injury. Tension pneumothorax develops in up to 20% of children after simple pneumothorax. A tension pneumothorax occurs when air progressively accumulates within the pleural cavity. A laceration to the chest wall, pulmonary parenchyma, or bronchial wall may function as a one-way valve, allowing air to enter but not leave the pleural space. The progressive accumulation of air within the pleural cavity not only collapses the ipsilateral lung but compresses the contralateral lung as well. These patients may present in severe respiratory distress with decreased breath sounds on the side of the pneumothorax. The mediastinal structures also shift to the contralateral side. Two-thirds of the blood supply to the body is returned to the heart via the inferior vena cava. Because the inferior vena cava is relatively fixed and cannot shift as much as the superior vena cava, venous return to the heart is reduced and the patient may appear tachycardic, peripherally vasoconstricted, and in hypotensive shock. This underscores the importance that whenever a trauma patient suddenly deteriorates, the treating physician must return to airway and breathing, before jumping to circulation.

Initial treatment consists of needle decompression performed in the midclavicular second intercostal space of the ipsilateral side. If a tension pneumothorax is present, an immediate release of air should be noted. If positive, the needle decompression is only a temporizing measure and must be followed by tube thoracotomy. Tube thoracotomy is usually done in the midaxillary line at the level of the fifth intercostal space (nipple level). Chest radiograph is performed only after the insertion of the chest tube and should not be used to diagnose a tension pneumothorax in the symptomatic patient. If a significant air leak continues after chest tube placement, a tracheobronchial rupture must be considered.

Open Pneumothorax

An open pneumothorax is the result of penetrating trauma. A direct connection exists between the pleural space and the outside atmosphere. As in a bronchial tear or lung parenchymal injury, air may enter but not leave the pleural space.

Initial treatment includes placement of an occlusive dressing at the wound site. This is best done when the patient is in full expiration. A chest tube should be placed immediately to prevent development of a tension pneumothorax. The chest tube should be inserted at a site different from the open wound. Larger open wounds may need surgical closure. Any patient in respiratory distress should be intubated and receive positive-pressure ventilation.

HEMOTHORAX

Hemothorax is much more common in penetrating than in blunt thoracic trauma. In blunt thoracic trauma, a hemothorax can occur from rib fractures lacerating the lung, pulmonary parenchymal injuries without rib fractures, lacerations of the internal mammary arteries or intercostal arteries, or disruption of the major vascular structures in the mediastinum or hilum. A hemothorax secondary to a major injury of the great vessels usually results in death. Liver and spleen injuries also can cause a hemothorax with disruption of the diaphragm. The most common cause of a hemothorax is injury to the intercostal or internal mammary arteries, whereas injuries to the lung or great vessels causing a hemothorax are much less common but more serious.

Patients may present in respiratory distress or in profound shock secondary to obstruction of venous return or massive blood loss. Decreased breath sounds are noted on the affected side and tracheal or mediastinal deviation may occur. Thirty to forty percent of the patient's blood volume may be rapidly lost into the pleural cavity. This reaction usually occurs with major vessel lacerations. Bleeding from the intercostal or internal mammary arteries stops secondary to low systemic pressures. Also, when the lung is reexpanded, effective tamponade of the bleeding occurs. A chest radiograph should be obtained to confirm the diagnosis. If a hemothorax is suspected clinically and the patient is in severe respiratory or circulatory distress, immediate tube thoracostomy should be performed before a chest radiograph is taken.

Treatment of a major hemothorax should include aggressive airway and circulatory management and evacuation of the pleural blood. Endotracheal intubation and positive-pressure ventilation should be initiated in any unstable airway. Patients should be typed and cross-matched for packed red blood cells and adequately volume resuscitated, preferably with two large intravenous lines in place. O-negative blood, if type-specific blood is not available, should be available at the patient's bedside as soon as possible.

Tube thoracotomy is performed to evacuate blood within the pleural cavity, reexpand the lung, and prevent or treat any mediastinal shift. The chest tube is placed in the midaxillary line at the level of the fifth intercostal space (nipple level). This location is the same as in a pneumothorax. Many hemothoraxes actually represent hemopneumothoraxes. After placement of a chest tube, blood should be slowly evacuated from the pleural space. Blood within the pleural cavity may tamponade a significant bleeding source within the chest, and evacuating that blood may cause new bleeding to occur. Patients can exsanguinate rapidly; therefore, intravenous access, adequate volume resuscitation, and blood available for transfusion should be a priority. Blood removed by thoracostomy can be administered to the patient as an autotransfusion. Thoracostomy drainage needs to be closely monitored. Large ongoing blood loss from a chest tube should be collected in a system that allows autotransfusion. Thoracotomy is indicated for continued bleeding (>1–2 mL per kilogram of body weight per hour), an inability to expand the lung, or retained blood within the pleural cavity. Failing to drain a hemothorax adequately can result in restrictive lung disease from a fibrothorax or an empyema from the clotted material becoming infected.

CHYLOTHORAX

Chylothorax is rare in thoracic trauma, occurring most commonly secondary to iatrogenic complications. Chylothorax can result from penetrating injuries or from a hyperextension injury to the spine. Disruption of the thoracic duct will lead to chyle draining into the mediastinum and pleural space. Diagnosis is confirmed when chyle is aspirated from the pleural cavity. Infection is rare because chyle is bacteriostatic, and treatment consists of tube thoracostomy, dietary manipulation, and, if all else fails, thoracic duct ligation.

TRACHEOBRONCHIAL INJURIES

Injury to the tracheobronchial tree in children occurs rarely, with an incidence of less than 1%. In most cases, this injury results from acceleration or deceleration forces. Major vessels or pulmonary parenchyma are more likely to be injured in penetrating trauma than are the tracheobronchial tree or esophagus. A cervical tracheal rupture can be caused by a direct blow to the trachea, or it can result from the patient's head violently traveling forward and backward. This whiplash effect can cause a tear between two cartilaginous rings. Lower tracheobronchial injury usually occurs from a sudden increase in intrabronchial pressure. Because the child's chest wall is elastic, the trachea and main bronchi can be compressed between the chest wall and the vertebral spine. Compression of the chest with a closed glottis can cause a sudden increase in intrabronchial pressure, resulting in a tracheobronchial tear. Shear forces, traction, and crushing the airway between the chest and vertebral column also can cause a tracheobronchial injury. About 80% of tracheobronchial injuries occur near the origin of the main stem bronchus.

The diagnosis of tracheobronchial injury may be difficult to make in the pediatric population. Mechanism of injury (eg, fall, crush, a direct blow) provides an important clue. Symptoms such as chest pain and dyspnea are common but nonspecific.

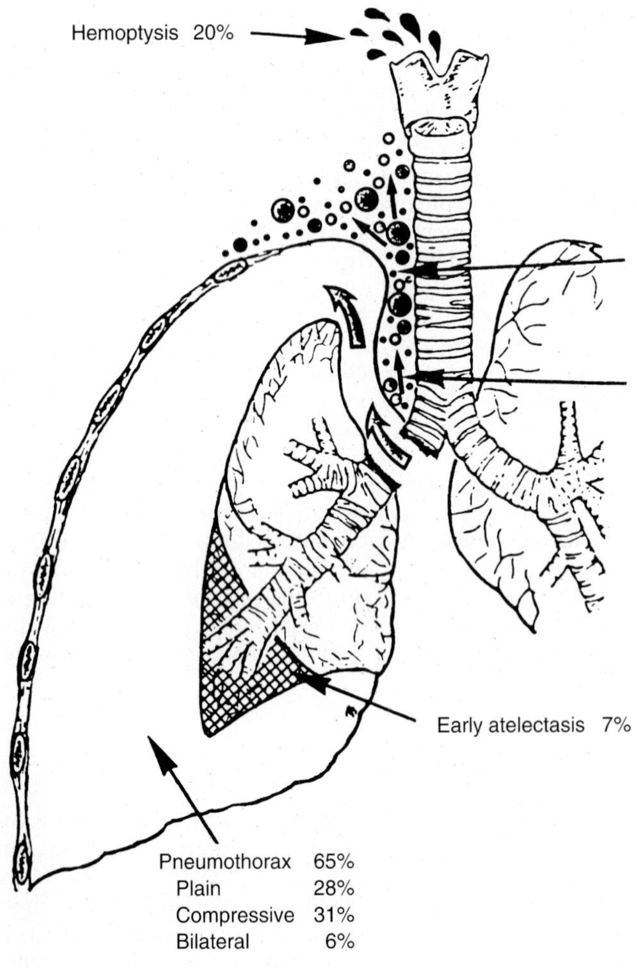

Figure 94.4. Initial signs of bronchial rupture.

Unlike the adult population, rib fractures are rare because of the elastic nature of the child's chest. Clinical signs include cyanosis, hemoptysis, tachypnea, and subcutaneous emphysema (cervical, mediastinal, or both). Pneumomediastinum and cervical emphysema are seen commonly in airway rupture (Fig. 94.4). If a pneumothorax is present with these findings, a bronchial rupture should be suspected. A continued air leak after insertion of a thoracostomy tube also should alert the physician to the possibility of a bronchial tear. Because of anatomic differences, ruptures of the bronchi occur on the right side more often than on the left. In the absence of a pneumothorax, tracheal rupture should be suspected if a pneumomediastinum or cervical emphysema is present.

Treatment includes initial airway stabilization and then bronchoscopic evaluation of the airway. Numerous reports in the literature record a partial tracheal tear becoming complete after endotracheal intubation. Therefore, if the airway is stable, oral tracheal intubation should be performed in the operating room under bronchoscopic guidance. This procedure prevents further trauma to the airway, and if a complication arises, emergency surgical access to the airway is readily available. If the airway is unstable and emergent endotracheal intubation needs to be performed, efforts should be made to prepare for backup measures such as cricothyroidotomy, tracheostomy, or fiberoptic bronchoscopy. An advantage of early bronchoscopy is exact identification and location of the lesion. The best surgical results are achieved when operative exploration is performed early. In the stable patient, CT of the chest also can help confirm the diagnosis and identify other injuries.

ESOPHAGEAL INJURIES

Esophageal injury is rare in children but presents a diagnostic challenge when it does occur. Timely and accurate diagnosis of an esophageal injury is paramount. The complications include mediastinal sepsis and death. The most common cause for esophageal perforation in the pediatric population is iatrogenic, followed by penetrating trauma (eg, gunshot wound, stab wound). Esophageal perforation can occur in blunt trauma if a significant amount of chest compression occurs. The cervical and thoracic regions are more commonly affected, with the thoracic region having the highest mortality rate (35%).

The patient's signs and symptoms depend on which region is injured. Patients with an esophageal rupture in the cervical region may complain of neck stiffness or neck pain. They may regurgitate bloody material and have cervical subcutaneous emphysema or odynophagia. A lateral neck radiograph may show retroesophageal emphysema. In the thoracic region, patients may present with abdominal pain and guarding, chest pain, subcutaneous emphysema, tachycardia, or dyspnea. A chest radiograph may show a pneumothorax, pneumomediastinum, or an air–fluid level in the mediastinum. Perforation of the intraabdominal esophagus may cause retrosternal, epigastric, or shoulder pain.

Patients with suspected esophageal perforation should be adequately volume resuscitated, have a nasogastric tube placed, and receive antibiotics covering gram-positive, gram-negative, and anaerobic organisms. The diagnosis of an esophageal perforation can be made by esophagography, esophagoscopy, or both. In one study, flexible esophagoscopy had a sensitivity of 100% and a specificity of 96%. Depending on the expertise at each institution and the patient's stability, these studies may be paired to lessen the chance of a misdiagnosis. Once the diagnosis is made, prompt surgical correction is mandatory. If the diagnosis is made within 24 hours, the mortality rate is approximately 5%. Delayed diagnosis for more than 24 hours after injury is associated with a mortality rate of 70%.

DIAPHRAGMATIC INJURIES

Diaphragmatic injuries are more common in blunt trauma. A crushing force will produce a sudden increase in the intrathoracic and intraabdominal pressure against the fixed diaphragm. Because of the flexible nature of the child's chest wall, rib fractures are rare. Even though penetrating thoracoabdominal trauma is uncommon in children, a diaphragmatic injury should be suspected in any thoracic or abdominal penetrating injury. The level of the diaphragm fluctuates greatly with respirations, and injuries of the diaphragm have been reported with penetrating wounds as high as the third and as low as the twelfth rib. Early reports of blunt traumatic diaphragmatic rupture were mostly left-sided injuries. Because of a greater awareness of diaphragmatic injuries, right and bilateral diaphragmatic injuries have been reported more recently. About 80% of diaphragmatic injuries still occur on the left, and 20% occur on the right.

Patients may present in respiratory distress and may have a scaphoid abdomen, although they are more likely to be symptomatic from associated injuries than from the diaphragmatic rupture. The verbal child may complain of chest pain or ipsilateral shoulder pain. The presence of bowel sounds within the thoracic cavity is nonspecific because in children bowel sounds can be transmitted from the abdominal cavity. More commonly, bowel sounds are absent because of an associated ileus. A nasogastric tube may be difficult to pass for patients with a diaphragmatic injury and gastric herniation. Even though usually the diagnosis is made on initial review of the chest radiograph, some series reported that up to 30% to 50% of initial chest radiographs were normal with a diaphragmatic injury. This finding emphasizes the importance of serial evaluations and chest radiographs in patients suspected of having a diaphragmatic injury. Other diagnostic studies, such as chest and abdominal CT with contrast or upper and lower gastrointestinal tract series, can help confirm the diagnosis.

TRAUMATIC ASPHYXIA

Traumatic asphyxia results from direct compression of the chest or abdomen. The most common mechanism is a child being hit by a motor vehicle or being pinned underneath a heavy object. In anticipation of impending injury, the child may inspire, tensing the thoracoabdominal muscles and closing the glottis. Traumatic asphyxia also occurs in patients with asthma, seizures, persistent vomiting, and pertussis.

Positive pressure is transmitted to the mediastinum, and blood is forced out of the right atrium into the valveless venous and capillary system. The clinical manifestations occur because the increase in pressure dilates the capillary and venous system. Areas drained by the superior vena cava are particularly affected, explaining the significant difference between the patient's head and neck as opposed to the lower body. Patients with traumatic asphyxia usually present with the clinical picture of subconjunctival and upper body petechial hemorrhages, cyanosis, periorbital edema, respiratory distress, altered mental status, and associated injuries.

The primary goal of treatment is to stabilize the patient and identify associated injuries. The external appearance of a patient with traumatic asphyxia is impressive, but initial attention should be paid to the airway, breathing, and circulatory status. Pulmonary contusions and hepatic injuries are commonly seen with traumatic asphyxia, and CT is helpful in identifying head, chest, and abdominal injuries.

AORTIC AND OTHER VASCULAR INJURIES

Traumatic rupture of the thoracic aorta (TRA) is uncommon in children but carries a high mortality rate (75%–95%). TRA is associated with sudden deceleration forces, commonly from automobile accidents, causing a sheering stress. The aortic arch remains fixed, but the descending aorta is mobile. With deceleration, bending or sheering takes place at the level of the ligamentum arteriosum, which is the most common site of aortic tears in adults and children.

In adults, TRA occurs in about 10% to 30% of adults sustaining blunt trauma, but it is much less common in the pediatric population. In one study, TRA occurred in only 2.1% of pediatric patients with thoracic trauma. The overall mortality rate was 93%. Why pediatric patients have a lower incidence of TRA than adults is unclear. One reason may be the mechanism of injury. In adults, most TRAs occur when the driver of an automobile forcibly strikes the steering wheel. The sudden deceleration force is isolated to the chest. Children who are passengers in a motor vehicle are less likely to strike an object that can deliver deceleration forces centrally to the chest. In children, one of the most common causes of blunt trauma is automobile–pedestrian accidents, which produce forces distributed over a much wider area.

Children are usually symptomatic from associated injuries, and TRA can be missed easily. Clinical signs may include difference in pulses between the arms or arms and legs, thoracic ecchymosis, thoracic and back tenderness, paraplegia, and anuria. Patients with paraplegia and back pain may be diagnosed initially as having a spinal cord injury. Unfortunately, 50% of patients may have no signs pertaining directly to TRA. More than 90% of patients have an abnormal chest radiograph. Widened mediastinum, loss of the aortic knob, left-sided pleural cap, tracheal deviation, and nasogastric tube deviation all may be seen on a chest radiograph. Much has been written in the adult literature about the association of TRA with first rib fractures. More recent studies have shown that isolated first rib fractures without any other signs or symptoms do not correlate with TRA.

Early diagnosis is imperative in patients with TRA (Fig. 94.5). Morbidity and mortality rates increase threefold if operative intervention is delayed more than 12 hours. The preferred method for diagnosing TRA is aortography. Thoracic CT is only 55% to 65% accurate but is helpful in diagnosing associated injuries. If the patient is stable and TRA is suspected, aortography should be performed. Life-threatening intracranial, thoracic, or intraabdominal injuries must first be evaluated and stabilized before aortography. If the patient is unstable, a transesophageal echocardiography can be performed while the patient's other life-threatening injuries are being treated.

PERICARDIAL TAMPONADE

Pericardial tamponade occurs when the myocardium is injured and blood accumulates in the pericardial sac. Because of the nondistendible pericardium, pressure is exerted on the heart. Cardiac output decreases secondary to a decrease in venous return and stroke volume. The body initially tries to compensate with an increase in the pulse rate and peripheral vascular resistance. As the pressure within the pericardial sac increases, the systolic blood pressure decreases, causing a narrowing of the

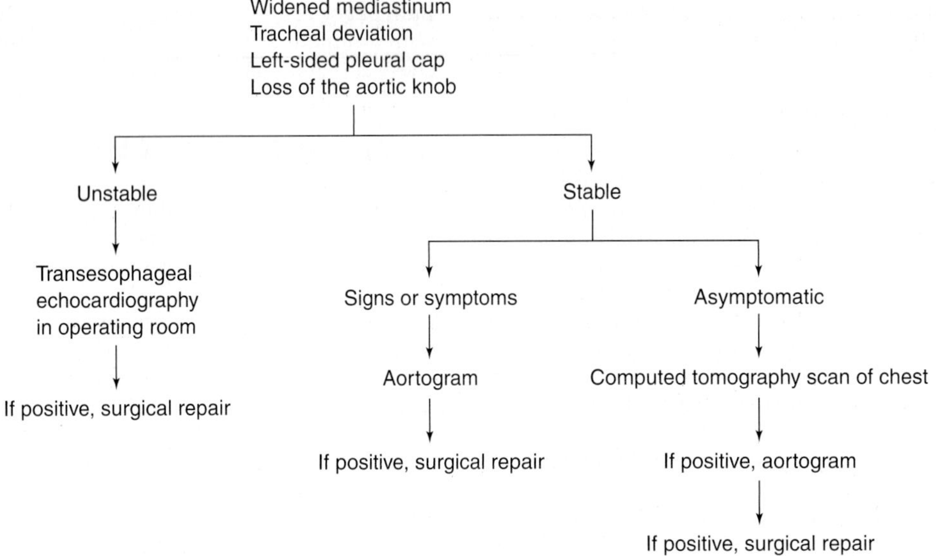

Figure 94.5. Algorithm for the evaluation and diagnosis of traumatic rupture of the thoracic aorta.

pulse pressure and subsequent hypotension and cardiogenic shock.

Pericardial tamponade may be difficult to diagnose initially because of associated injuries obscuring the clinical signs and symptoms. Patients may present with distant heart sounds, low blood pressure, poor perfusion, a narrow pulse pressure, or electromechanical dissociation (Fig. 94.6). Pulsus paradoxus, blood pressure falling more than 10 mm Hg during inspiration, occurs in fewer than one-half of patients with pericardial tamponade and should not be relied on to make the diagnosis of pericardial tamponade. Chest radiograph may show an enlarged heart and electrocardiography (ECG) may show low-voltage QRS waves. Neither of these tests is diagnostic for pericardial tamponade, and performing these tests should not delay treatment in the unstable patient. In the stable patient, an echocardiogram can demonstrate fluid within the pericardial sac.

In the unstable patient in whom pericardial tamponade is suspected, treatment includes control of the airway, intravascular volume resuscitation, and pericardiocentesis (Fig. 94.7). Pericardiocentesis is performed by inserting a 20-gauge spinal needle below the xiphoid process at a 45-degree angle toward the left shoulder. If time permits, an ECG monitor can be attached to the spinal needle. If the needle touches the heart, a current will be noted on the ECG monitor. Blood aspirated from the pericardial sac can be differentiated from intracardiac blood because pericardial blood is defibrinated and does not clot. Even though patients may show transient improvement after removal of blood from the pericardial sac, the patient should be taken to the operating room immediately for a pericardial window or other surgical intervention. A catheter should be placed in the pericardial sac over a wire guide for continual drainage of blood until surgical correction can be performed.

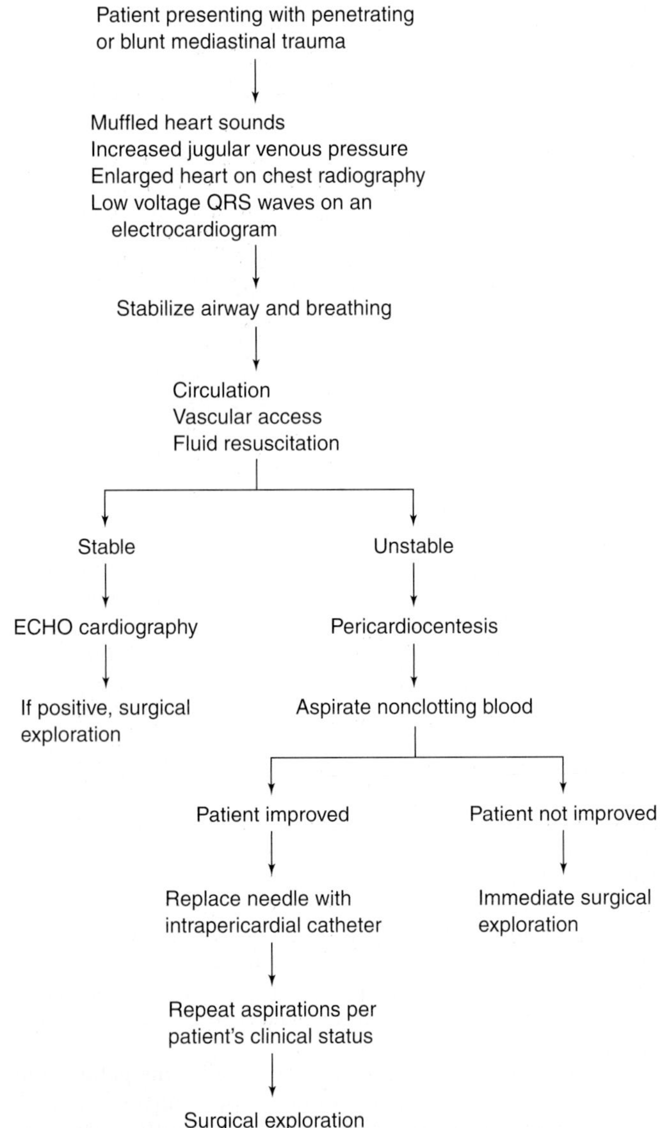

Figure 94.6. Algorithm for the evaluation and diagnosis of pericardial tamponade.

BLUNT CARDIAC INJURIES

Blunt cardiac injury (BCI) occurs more commonly with associated injuries than in isolation and represents a spectrum of injuries. Myocardial contusion, ventricular or atrial rupture, and valvular disruption are all considered BCIs. Myocardial contusion is the most common and ventricular rupture the most lethal of injuries. In one study of 1288 patients with blunt thoracic

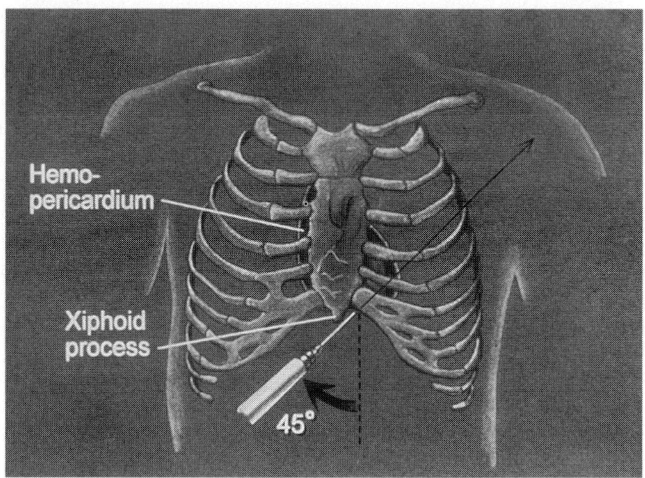

Figure 94.7. Pericardiocentesis is performed by inserting a 20-gauge spinal needle below the xiphoid process at a 45-degree angle toward the left shoulder.

trauma, 60 (4.6%) had a diagnosis of BCI. Other series reported the incidence of BCI to range from 0% to 43%. Complications of BCI include arrhythmias, pump failure, congestive heart failure, and shock.

Cardiac rupture is the most common cause of death in blunt cardiac trauma. The right ventricle is the chamber most commonly ruptured because of its location directly beneath the sternum. Septal rupture can also occur, with the condition of the patient correlating with the size of the rupture. Patients with valvar injury may present in congestive heart failure with a new regurgitation murmur. Coronary artery injury is rare but should be considered in patients with persistent ECG changes consistent with ischemia following blunt thoracic trauma.

Unlike adults, pediatric patients with BCI often have few presenting signs or symptoms. Approximately 70% of adults with BCI complain of chest pain, whereas in one pediatric study fewer than half of the awake patients with BCI complained of chest pain, and external evidence of thoracic injury was present in only 60% of these patients. In the same study, cardiac examination was abnormal in fewer than one-quarter of the patients. BCI should be considered in any patient with thoracic trauma who develops a cardiac arrhythmia or a new murmur or who is in congestive heart failure.

Evaluation of suspected BCI remains controversial. In one study, all children who developed heart failure or serious cardiac arrhythmias during their hospital course initially presented to the emergency department (ED) either in shock or with a serious arrhythmia. Patients with suspected BCI can be monitored in the ED or hospital and, if no arrhythmias develop on ECG, can be safely sent home. CPK-MB ratios have a high false-positive rate and are not a helpful screening tool. Transesophageal echocardiography should be performed in thoracic trauma patients with an abnormal ECG or arrhythmia, or a new heart murmur. Transesophageal echocardiography is more sensitive than transthoracic echocardiography in detecting myocardial injury.

Some general guidelines regarding patients with suspected BCI include the following: (1) If a pediatric patient with suspected BCI is hemodynamically stable and has not experienced any arrhythmias, a serious life-threatening arrhythmia or pump failure is unlikely. (2) Any patient with suspected BCI who is hemodynamically unstable or has arrhythmias should undergo a thorough evaluation, such as with transesophageal echocardiography, and should be admitted to the intensive care unit. (3) All patients with suspected BCI need close follow-up.

PENETRATING THORACIC TRAUMA

Although not as common as blunt thoracic trauma, penetrating thoracic trauma is becoming more common in the pediatric population. In one study, penetrating thoracic trauma occurred in 20% of pediatric patients evaluated for a thoracic injury. The most common mechanism of injury was gunshot wounds followed by stab wounds. Pediatric patients with blunt thoracic trauma are more likely to die from associated intracranial and intraabdominal injuries. In contrast, penetrating thoracic trauma is usually a single-system disease, and more than 95% of deaths are caused by the thoracic wound.

The most common penetrating thoracic injuries are hemothorax and pneumothorax, which almost always require tube thoracostomy. Intraabdominal injuries always should be suspected because of the close proximity of abdominal contents to the thoracic cavity. In one study, intra-abdominal injuries occurred in 20% of patients with penetrating thoracic injury. More than half of children with penetrating thoracic injury require operative intervention. This percentage is higher than the 15% reported in the adult literature. Why children have this higher rate of operative intervention is unclear, but it may be a result of the close proximity of the vital organs in the thoracic cavity compared with adults.

Evaluation and treatment include airway stabilization, fluid resuscitation, and management of the chest wound. Radiopaque markers (paperclips) can be placed at the entry and exit sites to help determine the course of the missile. Penetrating injuries near the mediastinum may be critical, especially if the patient is hemodynamically unstable. Pericardial tamponade should be considered and treated in the unstable patient. In the stable patient, transesophageal or transthoracic echocardiogram is helpful in evaluating the heart and determining whether fluid has entered the pericardial sac. Diaphragmatic lacerations are difficult to diagnose and sometimes require exploratory laparotomy or laparoscopy for diagnosis and treatment.

CHAPTER 95
Abdominal Trauma

Richard A. Saladino, M.D., and
Dennis P. Lund, M.D.

Recognition of intraabdominal injuries may be difficult, especially in the context of multisystem trauma. The physician should approach any child with a high index of suspicion for intraabdominal injury. In addition, intraabdominal injury may be occult in cases of child battering, and the examining physician must exclude abdominal trauma in these instances.

INITIAL MANAGEMENT PRINCIPLES

Basic Principles of Management

Treatment of the seriously injured patient requires a team approach, which includes a designated leader who directs team members who have specific responsibilities during the initial

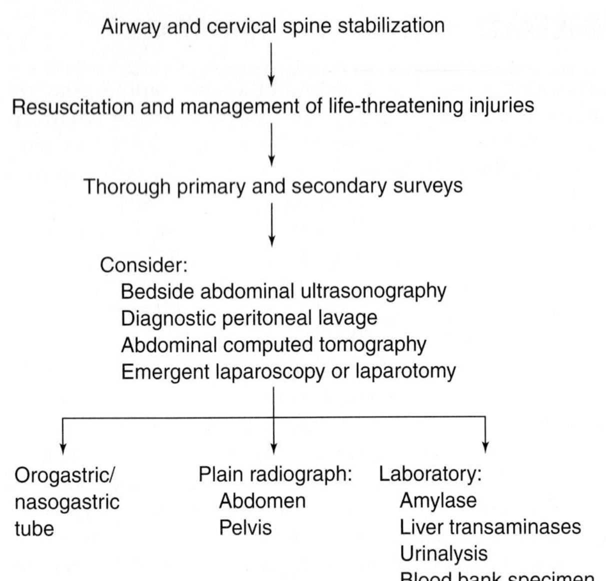

Figure 95.1. Initial evaluation and treatment of the child with abdominal trauma.

evaluation and management. Airway management and cervical spine stabilization are first priorities (Fig. 95.1). Any child with significant injuries should receive supplemental oxygen, especially if signs of shock are present. Intravenous or intraosseous access should be obtained.

The current recommendation by the American College of Surgeons remains that aggressive fluid resuscitation be pursued. Although data from animal studies suggest that limited (hypotensive) fluid resuscitation may improve survival by limiting hemorrhage into the peritoneal space, application to the management of children is still controversial.

As the initial evaluation proceeds, the priorities of management depend on the extent of multisystem injuries and the stability of the patient (Fig. 95.2). Patients who are unstable as a result of ongoing blood loss or an expanding intracranial hemorrhage require intervention early in the evaluation phase.

The Unstable Patient

Immediate life-threatening injuries, such as airway obstruction, tension pneumothorax, pericardial tamponade, and obvious sources of external blood loss, must be treated promptly. The role of emergency department (ED) thoracotomy is controversial in children; its use should be confined to situations in which control of intrathoracic bleeding is needed (eg, with lung or heart lacerations) or in situations in which previously detected vital signs are lost. If emergent thoracotomy is performed in the latter instance for presumptive intraabdominal hemorrhage, the aorta is cross-clamped at a level just above the diaphragm.

If significant head trauma has occurred, a determination must be made with regard to the need for immediate neurosurgical intervention. A rapidly performed computed tomography (CT) scan of the head is usually sufficient to determine the presence of a hematoma, which can be drained by the neurosurgeon. If hemodynamic instability or the need for immediate cran-

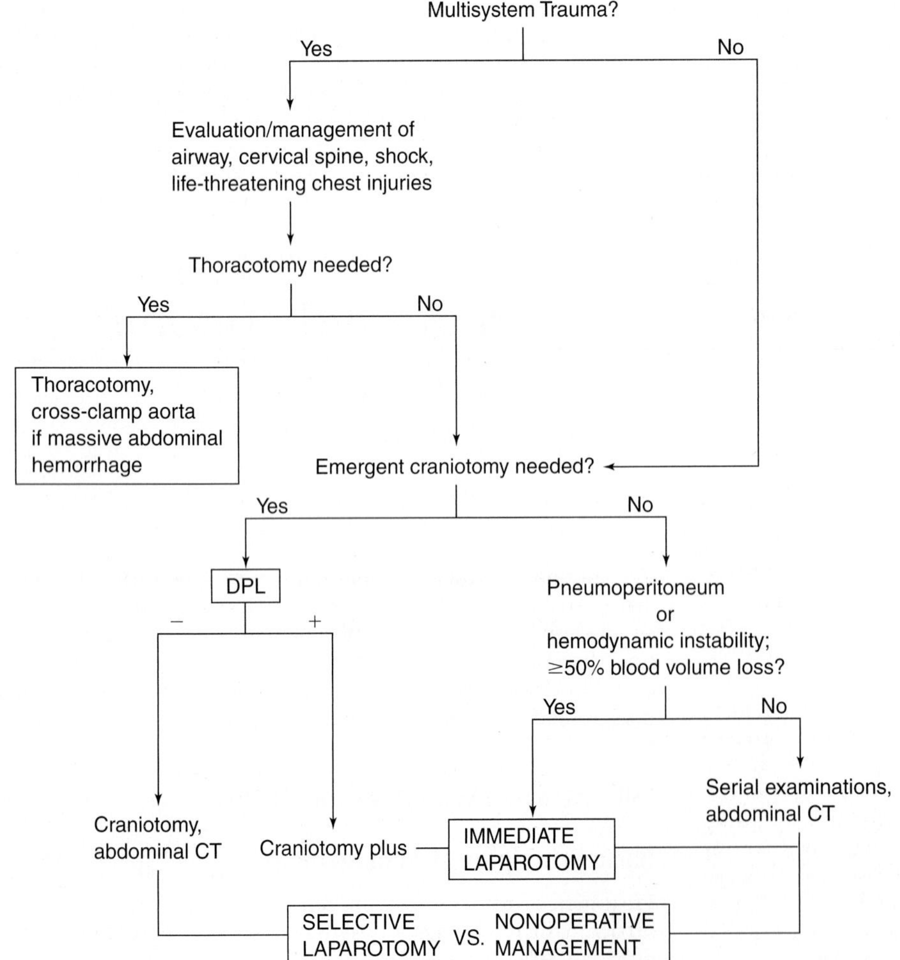

Figure 95.2. Management of blunt abdominal trauma. DPL, diagnostic peritoneal lavage; CT, computed tomography (see Table 95.2).

TABLE 95.1. Indications for Abdominal Computed Tomography Scan in the Pediatric Trauma Patient

Mechanism of injury suggesting abdominal trauma
Slowly declining hematocrit
Unaccountable fluid or blood requirements
Neurologic injury precluding accurate abdominal examination
Hematuria
Acute "need to know" (e.g., before general anesthesia)

iotomy exists and does not allow for CT evaluation of the abdomen (Table 95.1), a diagnostic peritoneal lavage (DPL) should be performed either in the ED or in the operating suite. If the peritoneal lavage is positive (Table 95.2), laparotomy and craniotomy proceed simultaneously. Finally, if neither thoracotomy nor craniotomy is indicated, emergent laparotomy is performed when pneumoperitoneum is noted on a plain radiograph or when the patient remains hemodynamically unstable in the face of historical or physical evidence of abdominal trauma (Fig. 95.2).

The Stable Patient

Commonly, the injured child can be stabilized in the ED with proper airway and cervical spine management and with intravenous fluid therapy and blood transfusion. A careful secondary survey should then be performed. Based on history and careful and serial abdominal examinations, CT is indicated when intraabdominal injuries are suspected (Table 95.1). Children who have had even minor injuries should be examined serially and monitored in the ED. At times, an abdominal CT scan is merited based solely on severe force inherent in a particular mechanism of injury despite an unremarkable physical examination.

DIAGNOSTIC IMAGING

Radiographic evaluation of children with abdominal trauma includes plain radiographs, contrast studies, radionuclide scans, ultrasound, and CT. The stable child with abdominal trauma is best evaluated with abdominal CT using intravenous contrast. If a nasogastric or orogastric tube is in place, it should be withdrawn temporarily into the esophagus to avoid an artifact from its radiopaque marker. Abdominal CT has its lowest sensitivity for small gastrointestinal perforations and pancreatic injury. Although CT is the most common technique used in childhood trauma, the surgeon's decision to proceed to laparotomy may be based more on the clinical status of the child than on the radiologic findings. Although abdominal CT is considered the most sensitive diagnostic tool, abdominal ultrasonography may provide important data early in the course of the management of a child with suspected intraabdominal injuries. Data from the adult literature show that the sensitivity for the detection of intraperitoneal fluid ranges from 85% to 98%. Although currently not a universal component of the evaluation of the child with blunt abdominal trauma, the value of ultrasound as a rapid diagnostic tool is evident and will become a part of trauma evaluation protocols.

TABLE 95.2. Positive Diagnostic Peritoneal Lavage Criteria

>5 mL of gross blood
Obvious enteric contents (e.g., bile)
Peritoneal lavage fluid exiting from chest tube, urinary bladder catheter
Positive laboratory analysis of peritoneal lavage fluid:
1. >100,000 RBC/mm^3
2. >500 WBC/mm^3
Elevated amylase in effluent

RBC, red blood cells; WBC, white blood cells.

TABLE 95.3. Indications for Immediate Laparotomy for Children with Abdominal Trauma

Multisystem injuries with indications for craniotomy in the presence of a positive diagnostic peritoneal lavage, free peritoneal fluid on ultrasonography, or strong historical, physical, or radiographic evidence of abdominal injury
Persistent and significant hemodynamic instability with evidence of abdominal injury in the absence of extraabdominal injury
Penetrating wounds to the abdomen
Pneumoperitoneum
Significant abdominal distension associated with hypotension

DIAGNOSTIC PERITONEAL LAVAGE

Occasionally, DPL is a helpful adjunct to the management of children with abdominal trauma. The disadvantages of DPL include the introduction of air and fluid into the abdomen (subsequent radiologic evaluations are less helpful) and peritoneal irritation caused by the procedure (subsequent physical examinations are less reliable).

It is rarely necessary to perform laparotomy on children with free intraperitoneal blood; thus, DPL, which effectively detects small volumes of blood, is often too sensitive in children. The primary indication for DPL in children is an urgent "need to know" with regard to the status of the peritoneal cavity, such as in the child who is hemodynamically unstable or requires immediate craniotomy and cannot delay for abdominal CT.

EMERGENT VERSUS SELECTIVE LAPAROTOMY

The indications for immediate laparotomy are limited in blunt abdominal trauma (Table 95.3). In most cases of childhood trauma (Fig. 95.2), emergency laparotomy is not necessary, and further diagnostic studies direct either elective (selective) laparotomy or observation and monitoring.

The indications for emergent laparotomy in children with penetrating trauma are illustrated in Figure 95.3. Any gunshot wound to the abdomen mandates immediate exploration. Other types of penetrating wounds in the presence of unexplained hemodynamic compromise, evisceration, pneumoperitoneum, or any evidence of violation of the peritoneum require prompt laparotomy.

BLUNT ABDOMINAL TRAUMA

Abdominal Wall Contusions

Many children have minor trauma to their abdomen in the course of play and as a result of minor accidental events. Balls, bats, swings, toys, and rough play may cause contusions of the abdominal wall.

Children without signs of intraabdominal pathology can be sent home. Those with a troubling history or any worrisome

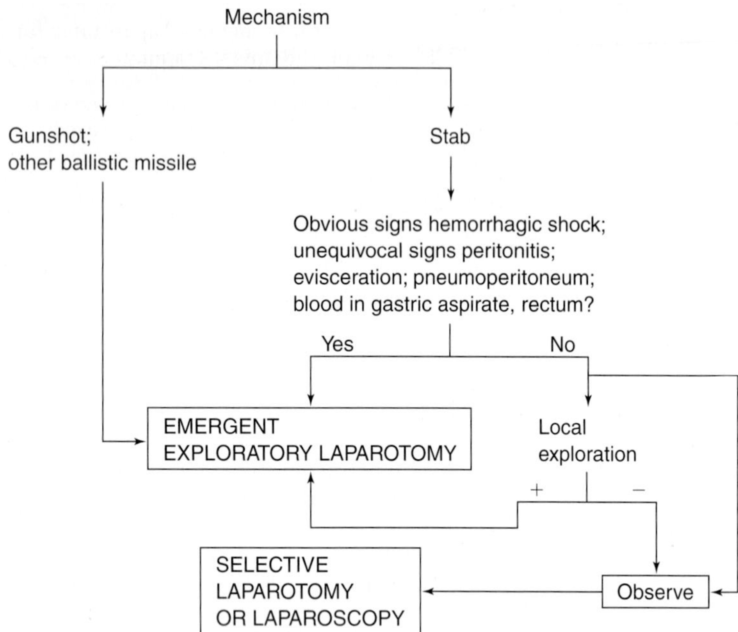

Figure 95.3. Management of penetrating abdominal trauma.

signs should receive a diagnostic laboratory evaluation and be observed in consultation with a surgeon.

Solid-organ Injuries

Patients who have splenic injuries may present with either diffuse abdominal pain or localized tenderness. Subphrenic blood may cause referred left shoulder pain. Percussion and palpation tenderness are usually of greatest magnitude in the left upper quadrant of the abdomen. Abdominal radiographs occasionally reveal a medially displaced gastric bubble. CT or a radionuclide splenic scan will identify the extent of injury.

Management of splenic injuries has evolved over the last three decades since the recognition of the postsplenectomy sepsis syndrome, resulting from the influence of both clinical and diagnostic advances. Nonoperative management of splenic injuries has largely replaced the traditional treatment, which included splenectomy or splenorrhaphy. The safety of nonoperative management for most childhood spleen injuries has been well documented, and postsplenectomy sepsis has declined. The availability of noninvasive diagnostic CT also has allowed greater confidence in the nonoperative approach to splenic trauma.

Blunt liver trauma is the most common fatal abdominal injury. Mechanisms of injury are those that are common with splenic trauma. Diffuse abdominal tenderness may be a result of hemoperitoneum, but maximal tenderness is elicited in the right upper quadrant of the abdomen. As with trauma to the spleen, nonoperative management of blunt hepatic injuries has become more common and is now the rule rather than the exception.

Blood transfusion therapy was necessary in 5.5% of patients in the National Pediatric Trauma Registry in 1997, and fewer than 1% of patients with blunt trauma admitted to Children's Hospital in Boston over the last year required transfusion therapy. The need for blood transfusion is based on careful monitoring of vital signs, clinical status, serial abdominal examinations, and analysis of hematocrit and fluid balance.

Pancreatic Injuries

Blunt abdominal injuries, particularly from bicycle handlebars, are the most common cause of pancreatic pseudocyst formation in children, although this injury is uncommon. Diagnosis is often delayed because of the nonspecific nature of subjective complaints and physical examination findings. The classic triad of epigastric pain, a palpable abdominal mass, and hyperamylasemia are detected only rarely in children and may develop slowly. The pancreas is relatively well protected, and associated trauma such as hepatic and intestinal injuries commonly are present when injury to the pancreas has occurred. Abdominal ultrasound and contrast CT (often serial examinations) are used to make the diagnosis; however, acute pancreatic injuries may not be apparent on the initial CT scan.

Severe injury of the pancreas is rare, but blood loss and leakage of enzyme-laden secretions may result in hypovolemia and peritonitis. Blunt abdominal trauma also may injure the ductal elements of the pancreas, and diagnosis depends on a high index of suspicion, consideration of the mechanism of injury, physical examination, serum amylase determination, and diagnostic imaging. Of note, however, is that the absence of hyperamylasemia does not preclude pancreatic trauma because elevated serum amylase is detected in 16% to 80% of cases of blunt injury. Elevated serum amylase should suggest the possibility of pancreatic injury, but the absolute value does not correlate with the degree of injury.

Nasogastric decompression and bowel rest are indicated when pancreatic injury is suspected. Normally, nonoperative therapy is used initially for children with isolated pancreatic pseudocyst caused by blunt trauma.

Hollow Abdominal Viscera Injuries

Intestinal perforation caused by blunt abdominal trauma is rare in the pediatric age group, but the most common causes of these injuries are automobile–pedestrian trauma, automobile lap belt injuries, and child abuse. The mechanisms of injury usually involve rapid acceleration or deceleration of a structure near a point of anatomic fixation (eg, ligament of Treitz) or trapping of a piece of bowel between two unyielding structures, such as a lap belt and the spine. Hollow viscera injury may be difficult to diagnose because physical findings may be minimal or nonspecific for the first few hours, and abdominal CT is not particularly sensitive for this injury. Succus entericus, bile, and activated pancreatic enzymes are extremely irritating to the peritoneum over time; the development of fever or worsening peritonitis on serial physical examinations should alert the examining physician to the possibility of bowel perforation.

Plain radiographs of the abdomen demonstrate free intraabdominal air in only 30% to 50% of cases. Similarly, pneumoperitoneum or leakage of gastrointestinal contrast is only rarely seen on the CT scan. DPL may demonstrate bile or amylase in the effluent and is sensitive for bowel perforations. Most perforations or transections of bowel are found through laparotomy, which the surgeon has chosen to perform because of advancing peritonitis or unexplained persistent fever. Management depends on the site and extent of structural injury.

Late Presentations of Intraabdominal Trauma

Some children with abdominal trauma do not have evidence of intraabdominal pathology on the initial evaluation but may return days or weeks later with abdominal distension or pain, persistent emesis, or hematochezia. In particular, three injuries are characterized by late presentations: (1) pancreatic pseudocyst (previously discussed), (2) duodenal hematoma, and (3) hematobilia.

Intramural duodenal hematoma is an uncommon injury that results from a direct blow to the epigastrium (blunt force delivered by a small-diameter instrument such as a broom handle or the toe of a boot) or from rapid deceleration and may cause partial or complete gastric outlet obstruction. Bleeding into the wall of the duodenum causes compression and therefore symptoms of intestinal obstruction, including pain, bilious vomiting, and gastric distension. Diagnosis is made by ultrasonography or a contrast upper gastrointestinal study, which will reveal the "coiled spring sign." Injury of the pancreas must be suspected when duodenal hematoma is considered. Nonoperative management includes nasogastric decompression and parenteral nutrition for up to 3 weeks.

Rupture of the gallbladder is rare and almost always is associated with severe blunt trauma to the liver. Likewise, hematobilia is associated with hepatic trauma and is a result of pressure necrosis from an intrahepatic hematoma or direct injury to the biliary tree. Children with hematobilia present several days after a blunt abdominal trauma with abdominal pain and upper gastrointestinal bleeding. Cholangiography confirms the diagnosis. Embolization is used to achieve hemostasis, but hepatic resection is necessary when this treatment fails.

PENETRATING ABDOMINAL TRAUMA

The high morbidity and mortality rates associated with penetrating trauma to the abdomen are results of the destructive force of ballistic missiles and fragments, rapid hemorrhage of vascular structures and solid organs after missile and stab injuries, difficulty of surgical repair of grossly injured intraabdominal organs, and postoperative complications. Intraabdominal organs are at risk for penetrating trauma, depending on their size and location. The colon and small bowel are large in volume and are the most commonly injured structures, followed by the liver, spleen, and major vessels. Hypovolemia or signs of peritonitis are then the result of brisk hemorrhage and spillage of enteric contents into the peritoneal space.

Gunshot Wounds

The destructive energy of ballistic missiles and fragments is related to mass and velocity (kinetic energy = $\frac{1}{2}MV^2$, where M is the mass, and V is the velocity), and more than 90% of gunshot wounds to the abdomen are associated with significant injuries. Hollow viscera and large vessels are often involved, and solid organs such as the liver and spleen may demonstrate burst injuries. Therefore, laparotomy is mandated in all gunshot wounds to the abdomen.

Stab Wounds

Stab wounds to the abdomen carry potential for devastating injury, depending on which intraabdominal structures are involved. The extent of the injury also depends on the type, size, and length of the weapon and on the trajectory. Major vascular injuries pose the greatest threat; commonly injured vessels include the intraabdominal aorta, the inferior vena cava, the portal vein, and the hepatic veins.

Anterior stab wounds are explored via laparotomy if hemodynamic instability or signs of peritonitis are present, if blood is noted in the gastric aspirate or on rectal examination, or if pneumoperitoneum or evisceration is noted (Fig. 95.3). Local exploration is needed to rule out penetration of the peritoneum even in minor stab wounds.

Stab wounds to the flank or back are less readily and less quickly diagnosed than anterior wounds; the retroperitoneal structures are more protected by paraspinal musculature, and bleeding is often tamponaded in this area. Dorsal stab wounds sometimes are managed nonoperatively unless hemodynamic instability or signs of peritonitis are present, although selective laparotomy is a common surgical strategy.

LAP AND SHOULDER BELT AND AIR-BAG INJURIES

Children who are too large for child safety seats but too small for adult seat belts are at increased risk for injuries. In particular, children restrained only by lap belts in motor vehicles involved in rapid deceleration crashes are at risk of sustaining Chance fractures (compression or flexion–distraction fractures of the lumbar spine) in association with intraabdominal injuries (the lap-belt complex). As many as half of the children with Chance fractures have intraabdominal injuries; therefore, a high index of suspicion must be maintained to detect such injuries. The hallmark indicator of the lap-belt complex is abdominal or flank ecchymosis in the pattern of a strap or belt. A normal abdominal CT does not rule out ruptured viscous, and laparoscopy or laparotomy should be considered for children in whom the lap belt complex is suspected. Carotid injuries caused by high-riding shoulder restraints in motor-vehicle collisions are much less common.

CHILD ABUSE

At least 1.6 million children are abused or neglected every year in the United States. Major blunt abdominal trauma resulting from physical child abuse is uncommon but highly fatal; mortality rates are as high as 50%. This high fatality rate is the result of the unfortunate but typical delay with which parents or caretakers who abuse children seek treatment.

CHAPTER 96
Genitourinary Trauma

Carmen Teresa Garcia, M.D.

The clinical approach to the injured child should strictly follow advanced trauma life-support guidelines. Figure 96.1 provides an algorithm for diagnostic evaluation of the pediatric patient with genitourinary trauma.

KIDNEY

The most common urinary tract injury encountered in children is injury to the kidney. More than 47% of genitourinary injuries involve the kidney. Blunt trauma accounts for up to 90% of renal injuries. Most pediatric renal trauma is sustained in motor-vehicle accidents. Falls, sports incidents, and direct blows are also common mechanisms of injury.

Children are more likely than adults to sustain renal injuries. In the child, the kidney is larger in proportion to the size of the abdomen than in the adult. The child's kidney may retain fetal lobations, which allow for easier parenchymal disruption. Weaker abdominal musculature, a thoracic cage that is less well ossified, and less developed perirenal fat and fascia fail to provide adequate protection for the kidney.

Coincidental congenital renal anomalies and intrarenal tumors have been documented in up to 10% of injuries. Symptoms and signs of a significant renal injury sustained with only minimal trauma should alert the clinician to the presence of preexisting anomalies, such as ureteropelvic junction obstruction, horseshoe kidney, pelvic kidney, or Wilms tumor.

Clinical Presentation

Children who sustain significant renal injuries usually present with localized signs such as flank tenderness, flank hematoma, or a palpable flank mass. Findings also include nonspecific symptoms and signs often associated with injury to other intraabdominal organs. Generalized abdominal tenderness, rigidity of the abdominal wall, paralytic ileus, and hypovolemic shock may all be part of the clinical picture. Penetrating injuries to the chest, abdomen, flank, and lumbar

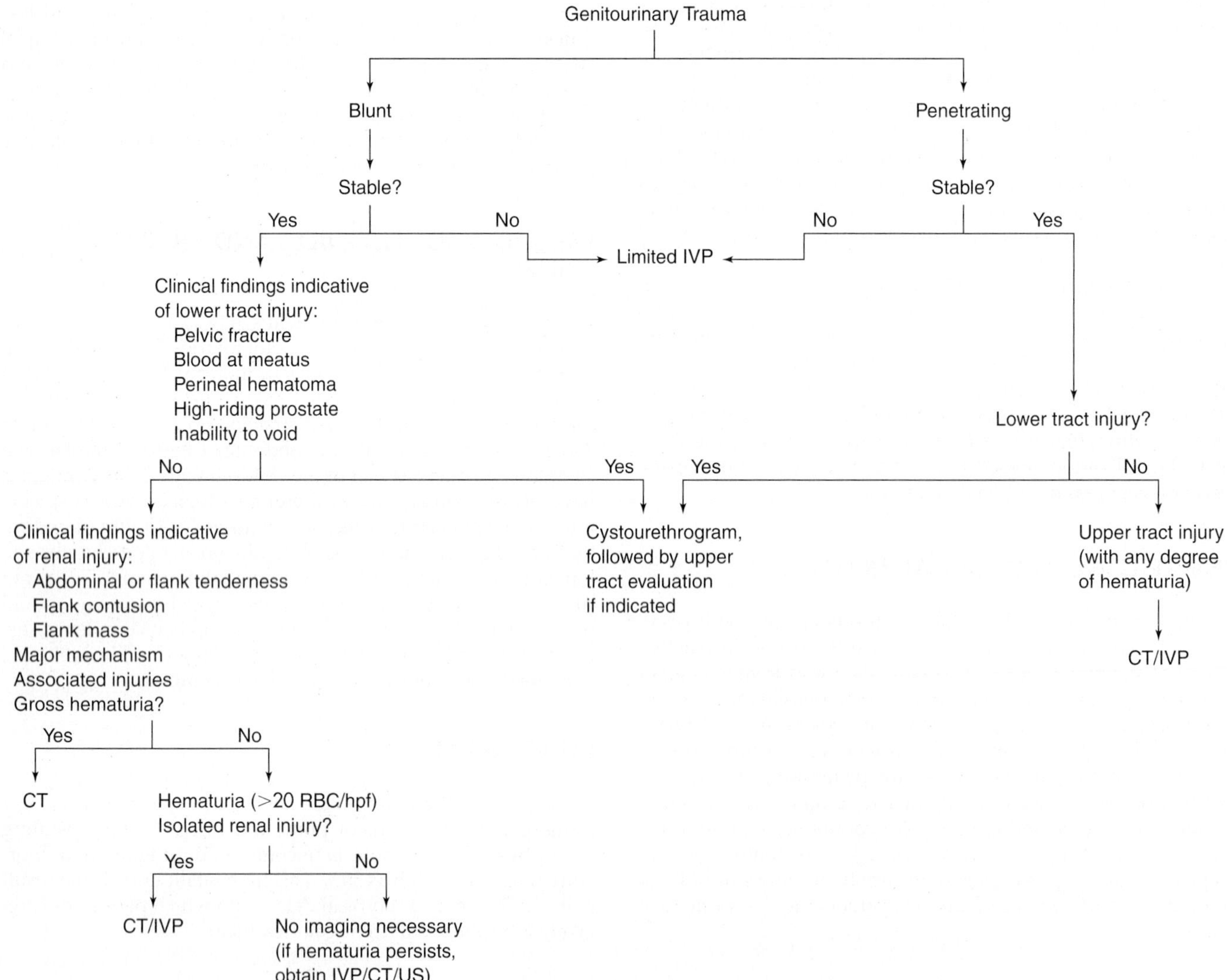

Figure 96.1. Algorithm for evaluation of the pediatric patient with genitourinary trauma. IVP, intravenous pyelogram; CT, computed tomography; RBC, red blood cells; hpf, high-powered field; US, ultrasound.

regions should alert the clinician to the possibility of renal injury.

Hematuria has long been considered the cardinal marker of renal injury. Although controversy exists about the correlation between the degree of hematuria and the severity of the injury, the presence of any degree of hematuria should be regarded as a potential indication of underlying renal injury or anomaly. It should be emphasized that hematuria may be absent in up to 50% of patients with vascular pedicle injuries and in 29% of patients with penetrating injuries. Hematuria out of proportion to the mechanism of injury should suggest a congenital anomaly or neoplasm.

Diagnostic Evaluation

Radiographic evaluation of the genitourinary tract is necessary in patients with gross hematuria or microscopic hematuria associated with a major mechanism, clinical findings indicative of renal injury, or other significant injuries (Fig. 96.1). Hematuria of more than 20 red blood cells per high-powered field in patients without associated clinical findings has been recommended as a threshold for radiographic workup. Microscopic hematuria with shock is one of the clinical criteria used to guide radiographic evaluation in the adult population. Hypotension is an uncommon event in children with renal injuries and therefore is not a reliable indication of renal injury in the pediatric population.

Initial evaluation of suspected pediatric renal trauma should include radiographs of the chest, abdomen, and pelvis. Plain films may show obliterated renal and psoas shadows, scoliosis with the concavity toward the injured site, intraabdominal mass effect, or a coincident rib, spinous process, or pelvic fracture.

Traditionally, the intravenous pyelogram (IVP) has been the cornerstone of evaluation in renal trauma. IVP is available in most institutions and provides information about both kidneys. It can be obtained on an unstable patient urgently in the emergency department (ED) or in the operating room before surgery. A scout radiograph should be made before the contrast study. IVP is performed by administering 1 to 4 mL per kilogram of body weight (maximum 100 mL) of nonionic contrast agent administered intravenously, followed by abdominal films in 1, 5, and 15 minutes. A one-shot IVP may be indicated for the unstable patient and is completed by obtaining a single film 3 to 5 minutes after injection of contrast material. Indications of renal injury include delayed excretion of contrast by the injured kidney, nonvisualization of the caliceal system, or extravasation of contrast into the perinephric tissues. The presence of a normally functioning kidney contralateral to the injured kidney should be specifically noted.

Even under optimal conditions, the IVP cannot always reliably identify and stage renal trauma. In one review, Cass reported the urogram to be definite in 5% of contusions, 50% of lacerations, and 29% of pedicle injuries. The importance of the IVP, however, lies in rapidly assessing the overall functional and anatomic integrity of the kidney as well as the presence of urinary extravasation and a congenital anomaly. More recently, contrast-enhanced computed tomography (CT) has become the preferred study for evaluation of major abdominal injury, including renal injury. The CT scan has certain advantages over the IVP, the most important of which is the detection of associated injuries. In addition, CT provides three-dimensional views and imaging independent of the vascularity of the kidney.

Computed tomography imaging can be used to determine the degree of renal parenchymal injury, to evaluate the presence of nonviable tissue, to demonstrate extravasation and perirenal collections, and to diagnose most pedicle injuries. The diagnostic accuracy of the CT scan has been reported to be as high as 98%, and CT scanning has become the standard imaging modality for renal trauma. CT scanning also has proved to be a useful tool for following patients after trauma.

Management

The principle underlying the management of pediatric renal trauma is preservation of renal tissue and function with minimal morbidity and mortality. Once the patient's general condition has been assessed and the presence of associated injuries established, treatment of renal trauma should proceed based on staging of the traumatic lesion.

In cases of blunt trauma, minor injuries, such as contusions and lacerations without urinary extravasation (grades I, II, and III), are treated conservatively. Current therapy involves strict bed rest, analgesia, and prophylactic antibiotics. Once gross hematuria has cleared, limited activity is instituted until microscopic hematuria resolves. Management of the remaining patients (grades IV and V) evokes significant controversy and should be guided by an urologist.

URETER

Ureteral injuries are uncommon in the child, accounting for fewer than 1% of all urologic trauma. These injuries can be caused by blunt, penetrating, or iatrogenic trauma.

Blunt trauma usually involves the ureteropelvic junction. Disruption of the ureter from the pelvis results from stretching of the ureter by sudden hyperextension of the trunk. Traditionally, this injury has been described more often in children. The degree of hyperextension necessary to cause avulsion of the ureter was thought to be fatal in adults; however, an increased number of ureteropelvic junction injuries recently was reported in adults. In the past, many of the injuries in adults may have been misdiagnosed as parenchymal lacerations involving the collecting system.

Trauma to the ureter should be suspected in patients presenting with fracture of the transverse process of a lumbar vertebra. Pelvic fracture, hip fracture, lower-rib fracture, splenic laceration, liver laceration, and diaphragmatic rupture also have been reported in association with ureteral injuries.

Early diagnosis of blunt ureteral injuries is critical. The injury is often overlooked. Fewer than 50% of patients are diagnosed within 24 hours of presentation. The physical examination may be unremarkable; however, an enlarging flank mass in the absence of signs of retroperitoneal bleeding suggests urinary extravasation. Hematuria is an unreliable sign. The urinalysis may be normal in 30% of confirmed cases. When the diagnosis has been delayed, ureteral injury may manifest with fever, chills, lethargy, leukocytosis, pyuria, bacteriuria, flank mass or pain, fistulas, and ureteral strictures.

The management of complete transection of the ureter depends on the level of the injury. Important elements include debridement of devitalized tissue and a watertight, tension-free anastomosis.

If the ureteral lesion is identified within 5 to 10 days of the injury, prompt repair of the ureter is indicated. If diagnosis is delayed for more than 10 days, urinary diversion above the lesion should be performed with subsequent definitive repair 4 to 6 months later. The incidence of nephrectomy is approximately 5% when the injury is detected early, but it is as high as 32% when recognition is delayed.

BLADDER

Bladder injuries may occur after blunt or penetrating trauma. Blunt trauma secondary to motor-vehicle accidents is the leading cause of bladder injuries. About 80% of bladder injuries are associated with pelvic fractures and penetration of the bladder by a bony fragment; however, only 10% of patients with pelvic fractures sustain lower urinary tract injury. The probability of having an associated bladder injury increases proportionally with the number of fractured pubic rami. The mortality rate associated with bladder rupture may be as high as 40%. Death usually is caused by associated head injuries rather than by bladder injuries themselves.

Hematuria and dysuria are symptoms commonly seen at presentation. More than 90% of patients with rupture of the bladder have hematuria. Microscopic hematuria is associated with less severe injuries such as contusions. Inability to void may be associated with large tears. Patients with intraperitoneal ruptures may develop a palpable fluid wave from extravasation of urine into the peritoneal cavity and peritoneal irritation. Elevated levels of blood urea nitrogen out of proportion to creatinine result from more rapid peritoneal reabsorption of urea.

Diagnostic evaluation is indicated for patients who sustain pelvic or lower abdominal trauma with hematuria and inability to void. Evaluation begins with a radiograph to exclude a pelvic fracture. If no pelvic fracture, no blood at the meatus, and no dislocation of the prostate on rectal examination are present, the urethra can be catheterized gently, and a retrograde cystogram can be performed.

Cystography of a contused bladder may show a teardrop shape or elevation of the bladder out of the pelvis. No evidence of extravasation of contrast material will be apparent. Extraperitoneal perforation is demonstrated by the presence of extravasated medium in the area of the pubic symphysis and pelvic outlet. In cases of intraperitoneal rupture, contrast may outline intraabdominal organs or paracolic gutters. Contrast-enhanced CT scan and CT cystography also can be used in the evaluation of bladder injuries.

Conservative management with or without urethral catheter drainage is the standard of care for patients with contusion. Extraperitoneal vesical rupture can be managed by urethral catheter or suprapubic drainage for 7 to 10 days. Treatment of large extraperitoneal tears or intraperitoneal tears involves transperitoneal exploration and repair with placement of a suprapubic cystostomy tube.

URETHRA

Motor-vehicle accidents, straddle injuries, and instrumentation account for most urethral injuries sustained during childhood. Urethral injuries occur primarily in male patients. In boys, the urethra is divided by the urogenital diaphragm into an anterior (pendulous and bulbous) and posterior (membranous and prostatic) urethra (Fig. 96.2). Anterior and posterior urethral injuries differ from each other by mechanism of injury, clinical presentation, and treatment.

Anterior urethral injuries result from direct trauma, are often isolated, and are associated with a low mortality rate. The pendulous urethra may be damaged by blunt or penetrating forces. Bulbar injuries are commonly caused by straddle injuries as the urethra is compressed between the symphysis pubis and a solid object. The major sign of acute anterior injury is bleeding from the urethra. Blood at the meatus has been reported in up to 90% of patients sustaining anterior urethral injuries. Other findings include hematuria, inability or difficulty voiding, and periurethral or perineal edema and ecchymosis. Perineal ecchymosis in the shape of a butterfly is typical for these injuries. Blind placement of a urethral catheter may convert a partial tear into a complete transection and therefore should be discouraged.

Anterior urethral injuries can be managed by 7 to 10 days of urethral catheterization and antibacterial therapy. More severe injuries require urinary diversion by suprapubic cystostomy. Penetrating wounds demand surgical repair with exploration, debridement of devitalized tissue, and copious irrigation.

Posterior urethral injuries occur with severe trauma to the body and usually are associated with other injuries, particularly pelvic fractures. The mortality rate with fractured pelvis has been reported to be as high as 30%. The high death rate in these patients is attributed primarily to associated injuries.

Initial management of posterior urethral injuries remains

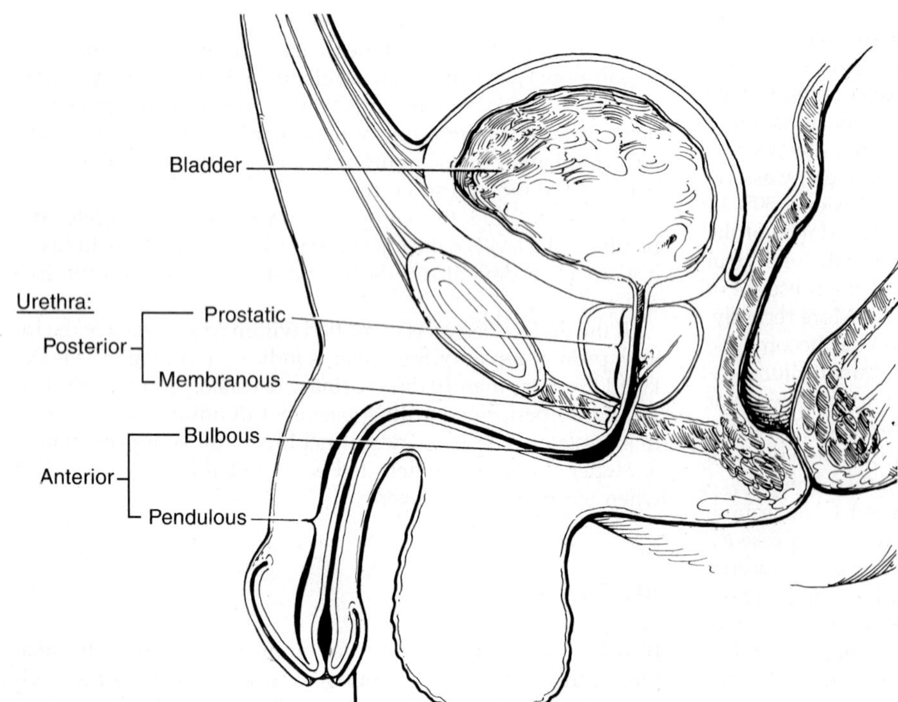

Figure 96.2. Sagittal section of male lower urinary tract illustrating levels of urethra.

controversial. Therapeutic options vary from immediate exploration with primary repair to placement of a suprapubic tube with delayed urethroplasty. Urethral rupture also can be treated by realigning the urethra over an indwelling urethral catheter. Primary repair or operative realignment should be reserved for urethral injuries associated with rectal laceration, a high-riding bladder, or injury to the bladder neck.

Trauma to the urethra in girls is rare because the female urethra is relatively mobile and short. Injuries may occur after surgical procedures or instrumentation. Most serious injuries involve the vesicourethral junction and result from blunt abdominal trauma in motor-vehicle accidents. The lesion generally occurs in association with pelvic fractures. The injury often extends to the vagina. Urethral injuries in the female are treated with suprapubic drainage and elective repair.

SCROTUM

Scrotal trauma may occur as a result of straddle injuries or bicycle accidents or during sporting events. The patient may present with scrotal tenderness, edema, and ecchymosis. Potential injuries include skin or dartos ecchymoses and lacerations, intrascrotal hematomas, testicular hematomas, testicular dislocation, and testicular rupture. In addition, torsion of a testicle may occur after trauma.

When inspection of the scrotum and its contents is obscured by local swelling and pain, ultrasonography is helpful to define the extent of the injury. An intratesticular hematoma may show as an echogenic or hypoechoic testicular mass. A hematocele produces a complex extratesticular fluid collection. Sonographic findings of rupture include the presence of hematocele, mixed parenchymal echogenicity, intraparenchymal hemorrhage, and disruption of the tunica albuginea or parenchyma. If the ultrasound examination is inconclusive, radionuclide scanning may provide additional information. Both ultrasonography and nuclear scintigraphy help in the diagnosis of testicular torsion (see Chapter 107).

Patients without evidence of injury to the testes who sustain intrascrotal hematomas, skin ecchymosis, or skin and dartos injury must be managed conservatively. Treatment consists of ice packs and scrotal support. Minor testicular injuries such as contusions or hematomas also can be treated conservatively. Large testicular hematomas may require surgical management. Delay in surgery may lead to ischemic necrosis, secondary infections, and disruption of testicular function.

Testicular dislocation occurs as a result of an upward blow to the scrotum. In most cases, the dislocated testis lies under the abdominal wall. Associated injuries, such as pelvic fracture, are common. Operative repair is required if closed reduction fails.

Testicular rupture with tear of the tunica albuginea and extravasation of testicular contents into the scrotal sac requires surgical exploration and repair. Testicular salvage is more likely when exploration is performed within 24 hours of the injury. Other injuries that require surgical management include tense hematoceles and torsion after trauma.

Superficial lacerations of the scrotum can be repaired using absorbable sutures. Local infiltration with lidocaine with epinephrine provides adequate anesthesia.

PENIS

The most common cause of penile trauma in infants is iatrogenic, especially at the time of circumcision. Complications include transection of the glans, urethrocutaneous fistula, deskinning of the penile shaft, and coagulation necrosis of the entire penis from electrocautery. These injuries usually require extensive surgical repair.

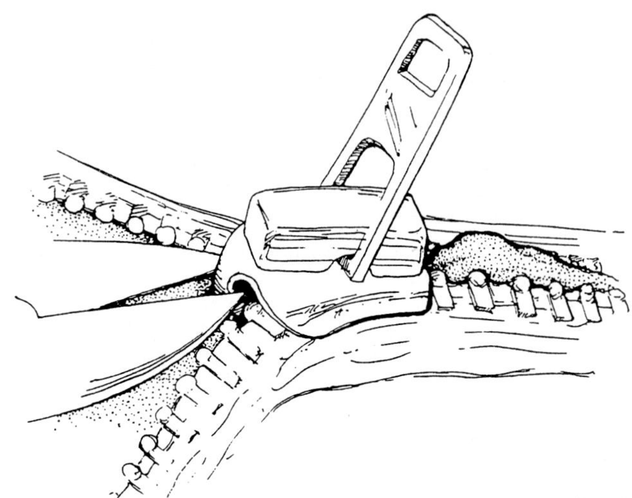

Figure 96.3. Penile zipper injury. A wire cutter may be used to cut the median bar of the zipper, releasing the two sides of the zipper and freeing the penis.

Blunt penile trauma from toilet seats falling on the glans or distal shaft has been described in toddlers. Significant injury to the corporal bodies or the urethra is rare, and patients can be managed expectantly with warm soaks. Although the child does not commonly experience urinary retention, he may be more comfortable voiding in a tub of warm water.

Tourniquet injuries can result from bands, rings, or human hair. In the infant, strangulation with a fine hair may be difficult to recognize because of local edema. The initial diagnosis may be balanitis or paraphimosis. Local or general anesthesia may be required to expose and remove the hair. Complications include urethrocutaneous fistula or loss of the penis.

Zipper entrapment of the penis or foreskin can be managed in the emergency department by cutting the median bar of the zipper with wire cutters and disassembling the zipper mechanism (Fig. 96.3). Conscious sedation may facilitate the procedure. Edema can be treated subsequently with warm soaks.

Fracture of the penis is produced by traumatic rupture of the corpus cavernosum. This injury usually occurs when the erect penis is forced against a hard surface. The patient may hear a cracking sound and develop pain, edema, and deformity of the shaft of the penis. The urethra is rarely involved. Fracture of the penis can be managed conservatively with bed rest, ice packs, and a pressure dressing. Most injuries require surgical treatment with evacuation of the penile hematoma, repair of the torn tunica albuginea, and a pressure dressing.

Superficial lacerations of the penile shaft can be repaired with absorbable sutures with the patient under local anesthesia or penile block. Lacerations extending to the corporal bodies or the urethra, as well as lacerations of the ventral surface of the penis, require urologic consultation. Diagnostic evaluation includes a retrograde urethrogram to define the extent of the injury. Injuries to the corporal bodies should be repaired primarily to prevent fibrosis and impotence. Injuries to the urethra may require urinary diversion.

PERINEUM

The mechanism most commonly associated with trauma to the female perineum is a straddle-type injury. These injuries may cause vulvar hematomas, which usually respond to treatment with ice packs and bed rest. Patients experiencing mild urinary retention may be more comfortable voiding in a tub of warm water. Massive or expanding hematomas may require evacuation.

Superficial lacerations of the perineum can be treated conservatively at home with sitz baths. Deep lacerations may extend into the rectum or urethra. Rectal penetration requires a diverting colostomy. Suprapubic cystostomy or primary repair should be performed if the urethra is disrupted.

Vaginal lacerations always must be suspected in patients with severe trauma to the external genitalia or penetration by foreign object. If a significant vaginal laceration is noted, endoscopy with sedation or general anesthesia is necessary for a full evaluation. The possibility of extension into the urethra, bladder, or rectum must be investigated. Debridement of the vaginal laceration is done, and the lacerations are repaired using fine absorbable sutures.

CHAPTER 97
Eye Trauma

Alex V. Levin, M.D.

This chapter is designed to assist the pediatric emergency physician in the diagnosis and management of basic and uncomplicated ocular injuries. It is important, however, to recognize when ophthalmology consultation is necessary. Even with the increasing number of emergency departments (EDs) that have slitlamp biomicroscopy available to the nonophthalmologist, the ophthalmologist is more expert at using the slitlamp and has experience with a wide array of diagnostic tools that allow viewing and recognition of intraocular injuries that cannot be seen with a direct ophthalmoscope.

RUPTURED GLOBE

Laceration or puncture of the cornea or sclera creates a ruptured globe. This condition can occur following trauma by projectile, sharp implement, or blunt trauma. Although severe intraocular disruption may occur, the eyeball has a remarkable ability to maintain its integrity. Immediately on laceration, the iris or choroid (which is the extension of the iris posteriorly underneath the sclera) plugs the wound. This plug may appear as a blue, brown, or black material on the surface of the sclera or at the corneal–scleral junction. The iris will come forward and plug a corneal wound. Because of this iris or choroid movement, the pupil may take on a teardrop shape, with the narrowest segment pointing toward the rupture. Hemorrhage within the anterior chamber (hyphema) often accompanies a corneal or anterior scleral laceration. With small lacerations that are plugged by iris or choroid, the eyeball does not deflate but rather takes on a remarkably normal external appearance. Subconjunctival hemorrhage for 360 degrees may obscure an underlying scleral rupture but can leave the eye fairly intact. Patients who present following trauma with this finding or with severe 360-degree conjunctival swelling without hemorrhage should be treated as if they had a ruptured globe and referred immediately to an ophthalmologist.

Management

Although the outcome in some ruptured globes, particularly small peripheral corneal lacerations, may be good, eyeball rupture is certainly an ominous sign that warrants emergent referral for ophthalmology consultation. Further ocular examination should be stopped immediately. No eyedrops should be instilled. A patch should never be used in this circumstance. A plastic shield should be placed over the eye such that the edges of the shield make contact with the bony prominences above and below the eyeball. If a commercially marketed shield is not available, the clinician should cut off the bottom of a Styrofoam or plastic cup and use it as a shield, resting it against the bony prominences.

Severe eye trauma may cause sedation or vomiting without head trauma or brain injury. If not, every attempt should be made to keep the child calm, even if sedation must be used. It must be kept in mind that crying, screaming, and Valsalva maneuvers such as vomiting can result in extrusion of intraocular contents through the rupture. Although broad-spectrum intravenous antibiotic coverage is desirable, particularly if a delay may occur before the patient sees an ophthalmologist, this treatment must be weighed against the potential aggravation of the child, which might accompany the needle puncture for catheter placement.

Even if a ruptured globe is not seen clearly on examination, any patient who has a high-risk history, severe lid swelling, and extreme resistance to examination should be given an eye shield and referred to an ophthalmologist as though a ruptured globe was confirmed.

BLOWOUT FRACTURE

Management

Some controversy exists among ophthalmologists, otorhinolaryngologists, and craniofacial surgeons regarding the urgency for radiologic evaluation and surgical intervention in the management of orbital wall fractures. About 20% of orbital fractures are associated with eyeball injury. Therefore, ophthalmology consultation for complete dilated retinal examination and slitlamp biomicroscopy is indicated in virtually every case. Axial (proptosis) or coronal displacement of the eyeball is an ominous finding because it may be a sign of orbital hemorrhage, which can cause compression of the optic nerve, requiring emergency surgical intervention.

EYELID LACERATIONS

Although eyelid lacerations are usually easy to detect, the clinician must remember that the underlying eyeball also might have been lacerated or injured. Seemingly superficial lacerations of the eyelid may be associated with penetration into the orbit or intracranial cavity, particularly when the injury was caused by a pointed implement, such as a tree branch or pencil. If possible, the eyelid should be everted to look for a conjunctival wound, indicating that the laceration is actually a complete perforation of the eyelid.

Oblique lacerations that extend into the medial canthal area (juncture of the upper and lower lids medially) may involve the

TABLE 97.1. Eyelid Lacerations

Consult ophthalmology if laceration associated with:
Full-thickness perforation of lid
Ptosis
Involvement of lid margin
Possible damage to tear drainage system
Tissue avulsion
Eyeball

proximal portion of the nasolacrimal duct. Sometimes, the lid margin puncta, which drain tears into the system, is displaced laterally as a result of the laceration. Lacerations in this area should usually be referred for ophthalmology consultation if any question persists regarding whether the tear drainage system is intact.

Lacerations of the periorbital skin and superficial eyelid skin can be managed by standard skin-closure techniques discussed elsewhere in this book. It is important, however, that sutures not grasp deep tissue within the eyelid because this could result in cicatricial eversion of the eyelid margins. Table 97.1 summarizes those findings that, when associated with eyelid lacerations, should prompt ophthalmology consultation for wound closure.

PERIORBITAL ECCHYMOSIS

Periorbital ecchymosis is usually a benign finding, although it may be associated with bony fracture or eyeball injury. Because of the loose connection of the eyelid skin and underlying tissues, dramatic ecchymosis can occur with mild blunt trauma.

Management

No treatment is routinely needed for periorbital ecchymosis. Ice packs applied to the area, with the eyelids closed, can be helpful in reducing swelling. Anticipatory guidance may be given to inform the family that the ecchymosis might persist for longer than 2 weeks. An ongoing color change from purple to green and yellow may occur as the blood is resorbed and broken down. A hyperpigmented area may be left for several weeks or months thereafter.

CORNEAL AND CONJUNCTIVAL INJURY

The conjunctiva can be abraded or lacerated, although the management of this problem is usually identical to that of corneal abrasion because the tissues heal so rapidly. Corneal or conjunctival abrasions may occur even from mild surface trauma. Self-inflicted abrasions may occur accidentally.

Corneal abrasion can be painful and may be accompanied by dramatic photophobia and resistance to opening of the eyes. Yet some children have remarkably few symptoms. They may complain of a foreign-body sensation even though no foreign body is present. A drop of topical proparacaine 0.5% or tetracaine 0.5% may have both diagnostic and temporary therapeutic usefulness. Any patient who is made more comfortable by the instillation of these drops must have an ocular surface problem (conjunctiva or cornea) as the cause of pain. The child who is crying and refusing to open the eyes may be compliant and easy to examine just a few minutes after the instillation of a topical anesthetic. Onset of action is approximately 20 seconds, and duration is approximately 20 minutes.

Topical fluorescein is used as a diagnostic agent to stain the affected area. Fluorescein is available as impregnated paper strips and as a solution combined with a topical anesthetic (Fluress, Barnes-Hind, Inc.). Considering the limited use in an ED setting, strips may be a more practical method because bacterial contamination over time may be less likely. When impregnated strips are used, they must be wet before instillation. Otherwise, the strip itself may cause a corneal abrasion, thus preventing the examiner from correctly identifying the patient's problem. Topical anesthetic or saline may be used to wet the strip. The lower eyelid should be pulled down, exposing the pink inner surface (palpebral conjunctiva) against which the strip may be placed. The solution then diffuses off the strip into the area between the lower eyelid and the eyeball (inferior fornix), where it then is displaced across the ocular surface with the next blink. The clinician must avoid placing too much fluorescein because the tear film can be so oversaturated that it may be difficult to find a small abrasion.

Fluorescein, which is orange, fluoresces yellow–green when exposed to blue light. Many modern ophthalmoscopes have a blue light. The examiner can view through the peephole of the direct ophthalmoscope, spinning the focusing dial to allow the ocular surface to be in focus with the examiner 2 to 3 inches away from the patient, inspecting the cornea and conjunctiva for an area that is stained. A Wood or Burton lamp also can be used. Some of these devices have handheld magnifying glasses attached. Although the staining may not be as dramatic, white light from a direct ophthalmoscope or penlight can be used because some blue wavelengths are incorporated in white light. Green light (red free), which is available on most direct ophthalmoscopes, may make identifying stained areas more difficult than white light.

If the staining pattern reveals one or more vertical linear abrasions, the examiner should suspect the presence of a retained foreign body under the upper lid. This foreign body may be viewed by upper lid eversion. The patient should be asked to look down repeatedly throughout this procedure. With the eye in downgaze, a cotton swab should be placed against the midbody of the upper eyelid and gently rotated downward toward the eyelashes so that the skin is rolled with the swab by friction. This procedure causes the eyelashes to turn out toward the examiner so that they may be grasped between the examiner's thumb and forefinger. It may be necessary to grab the entire lid margin in some children. If a topical anesthetic is instilled before lid eversion, this procedure is painless. After the lashes (or margin) are grabbed, they should be lifted vertically while the cotton swab is used to apply gentle downward pressure in the opposite direction. The eyelid then flips around the cotton swab. If a foreign body is identified, it can be lifted away gently by using a cotton swab or forceps. To revert the eyelid, simply have the patient look upward or massage the lid down.

Subconjunctival hemorrhage may result from blunt trauma, conjunctivitis, chemical irritation, and increased intrathoracic pressure (eg, chest trauma, suffocation). Although usually focal, the lesions may be multiple or diffuse. Hypertension, coagulopathy, or anticoagulant medications may result in subconjunctival hemorrhage out of proportion to the injury. After blunt eyeball trauma, a 360-degree subconjunctival hemorrhage may mask an underlying ruptured globe. No treatment is needed for isolated subconjunctival hemorrhages. They may take up to 2 weeks to resolve, turning yellowish in the process.

Chemical injuries of the cornea and conjunctiva also may occur. These injuries are discussed in Chapter 105.

Management

Several studies suggested that patching, especially in children with small corneal abrasions, may not accelerate healing or decrease symptoms. Although some controversy exists in this regard, many physicians prefer to apply a lubricating antibiotic ointment [eg, bacitracin, erythromycin, Polysporin (Burroughs Wellcome)] to the ocular surface, followed by a pressure patch over the closed eyelid. For patients who are in significant pain, a drop of cyclopentolate 1% can be instilled to relieve spasm of the eye's ciliary muscle. Ointments containing steroids or neomycin should not be used. If so desired, a pressure patch can be created by stacking two or three patches atop each other over the closed eyelid before applying tape. The patch should be worn overnight. For conjunctival abrasions and small corneal abrasions not involving the central cornea, the patch may be removed by the patient or parents on the following day (approximately 18–24 hours later). If the patient is asymptomatic, no follow-up is required. If pain or foreign-body sensation continues, however, the patient should be instructed to seek ophthalmologic care. A topical antibiotic ointment may be prescribed for use after patch removal two to three times daily for about 3 days. Larger corneal abrasions and those involving the visual axis should be seen the next day by an ophthalmologist.

HYPHEMA

The presence of blood between the cornea and the iris is a sign of severe ocular trauma. Although the entire anterior chamber may be filled with blood ("8-ball hyphema"), clots also may be small, requiring careful inspection for detection. Sometimes the blood is more diffuse throughout the anterior chamber or may even be microscopic, requiring slitlamp examination for detection (*microhyphema*). The size of the hyphema is directly proportional to the incidence of secondary glaucoma and is inversely proportional to visual prognosis. Patients with hyphema enter a vulnerable period 3 to 5 days after injury, when spontaneous rebleeding may occur. Patients with hemoglobinopathies are also at particular risk for ocular complications of hyphema. Therefore, all patients who are in a high-risk ethnic group should receive a screening test ("shake test") or formal hemoglobin electrophoresis at presentation unless their status is already known.

Management

All patients who have hyphema must be seen by an ophthalmologist. Although microhyphemas and perhaps some small hyphemas can be managed in select clinical situations as outpatients with careful daily follow-up, hospital admission often is recommended. The eye should be shielded, not patched, and the patient should be placed at bed rest with the head elevated 45 degrees. This position helps allow blood within the anterior chamber to settle inferiorly, thus allowing a clearance of the visual axis, improvement of vision, and a better view for the ophthalmologist looking into the eyeball. Some ophthalmologists may recommend sedation of an active or distressed child. Oral antifibrinolytics may be used to prevent spontaneous rebleeding; however, these agents should be used only under the supervision and recommendation of an ophthalmology consultant.

TRAUMATIC IRITIS

Inflammation within the anterior chamber of the eye often does not present for 24 to 72 hours after blunt trauma to the eyeball. The patient may complain of eye pain, redness, photophobia, and sometimes visual loss. The pupil on the affected side may be constricted. The ocular injection may be confined to a ring of redness surrounding the cornea (ciliary flush). Definitive recognition of traumatic iritis requires slitlamp biomicroscopy.

Management

Traumatic iritis may be an indicator that other ocular injuries have occurred. Ophthalmology consultation should be obtained in the diagnosis and management of this condition. The ophthalmologist often recommends dilating drops and topical steroids for treatment. Because of the risks associated with the use of topical steroids, they should not be prescribed except in consultation with an ophthalmologist.

TRAUMATIC VISUAL LOSS

Some techniques for the recognition of true traumatic visual loss are discussed elsewhere in this book. Occasionally, the emergency physician is faced with a child who is feigning visual loss. These situations seem to be more common after motor-vehicle accidents or other injuries in which legal action may be involved. Functional visual also can be idiopathic or associated with other overt or covert stress in the child's life. In the absence of other signs of ocular or head trauma, this diagnosis should be suspected. It then becomes necessary to "trick" the child into demonstrating that he or she actually can see. Patients who are truly acutely blind should demonstrate some degree of anxiety and a virtually incomplete inability to navigate in the new surroundings of the ED. When asked to write their names on a piece of paper, truly blind patients can do so accurately, unlike children who are functionally blind, who assume that they will be unable to write. When a mirror is held before a truly blind eye and then tilted in the vertical and horizontal planes, the eye will not follow. Any eye that truly has enough sight to recognize its own image moves involuntarily with the motion of the mirror.

Children who are feigning visual loss but not complete blindness can be more difficult to "trick." Sometimes, by placing a drop of saline or topical anesthetic in the eye while giving the child the suggestion that these "magic drops" will cause a return of vision, the child then begins to see better. The pinhole test (previously discussed) also can be used in this manner. Ophthalmology consultation is sometimes critical in discovering whether a child has truly sustained visual loss.

A rare cause of visual loss after head trauma is transient cortical visual impairment or blindness. As a result of a direct or *centre coup* occipital contusion, a child may experience acute blindness despite an otherwise normal eye examination. This centrally mediated phenomena may resolve spontaneously. Ophthalmology consultation can be useful to rule out other causes of the visual loss.

A multitude of intraocular injuries, including traumatic cataract, vitreous hemorrhage, retinal bruising (commotio retinae), retinal detachment, and optic nerve injury, can result in true visual loss or blindness. The pediatric emergency physician is the "gatekeeper" in recognizing that true intraocular injury has occurred, although in most of these circumstances, ophthalmology consultation then is required. Perhaps the best screening test for intraocular injury is the examination of the red reflex and direct ophthalmoscope.

CHAPTER 98

Otolaryngologic Trauma

Steven D. Handler, M.D., and
William P. Potsic, M.D.

The ear, nose, and throat are common sites for trauma; therefore, emergency medicine specialists must be familiar with the head and neck region because they often will be called on to evaluate this area. Although the presenting complaints may seem extremely distressing to the patient and cause considerable anxiety for the parents, the conditions prompting the visit are rarely life threatening. Many instances of trauma may be isolated to the ear, nose, or throat, but associated injuries (eg, eye, dental, central nervous system, thorax) are common and must be detected when evaluating and treating otolaryngologic trauma.

EAR

Foreign Bodies

Foreign bodies in the ear canal are common in children. Solid objects, such as stones, beads, or paper, are the most commonly encountered foreign bodies, but live insects also may also enter the ear canal. Foreign bodies should be removed as soon and as safely as possible. Most objects can be gently rolled out of the external meatus using an ear curette, or they may be grasped and removed with an otologic forceps. Round or occluding objects may be removed by irrigation of the canal with body-temperature water. [Irrigation, however, should not be performed if a tympanic membrane (TM) perforation is suspected or if a ventilating tube is in place.] The stream is directed along the side of the foreign body, forcing it to the external meatus. Before removing an insect from the ear canal, the insect should be killed by filling the ear canal with alcohol or mineral oil; the removal techniques have been described already. Objects resting against the TM are best removed by irrigation to avoid injury by manipulation.

Care must be taken to remove the foreign material without causing pain; if the removal is unsuccessful, a general anesthetic is usually necessary for removal of the object by the otolaryngologist.

Trauma

EXTERNAL EAR TRAUMA

External ear trauma is common in children because the pinna is in an exposed position on the side of the head. Reflex turning of the face to the side to avoid a blow or a fall places the ear directly in the line of injury. External blunt trauma often occurs secondary to an athletic injury, a fall, or a direct blow to the ear; the injury may result in simple ecchymosis, or it may disrupt perichondrial blood vessels with subsequent hematoma or seroma formation. These collections form a smooth bluish mass on the lateral surface of the auricle that obscures its normal contour. Hematomas and seromas must be evacuated immediately to prevent cartilage necrosis. Lacerations of the pinna should be closed using the same surgical principles applied to repairing lacerations in other end-organ areas of the body. Earrings in pierced ears may be torn from the lobule. These lacerations should be closed like all skin lacerations, reestablishing the normal anatomy.

Thermal injury of the external ear commonly occurs because the ear protrudes from the head and is exposed to burns and cold. Burns of the ear should be treated in the same manner as burns of other parts of the body (see Chapter 100). Frostbite is suspected when the ear is pale and painful on warming. The frostbitten ear should be rewarmed rapidly by applying warm, soaked cotton pledgets at 38° to 40°C (100.4°–104°F); the ear should be completely thawed and never recooled.

MIDDLE EAR TRAUMA

A slap to the side of the head (by a hand or a breaking wave) may result in perforation of the TM by sudden compression of the air in the external auditory canal, but traumatic perforation of the drum usually is caused by poking an object into the ear canal. The structures of the middle ear also may be damaged by the penetrating object. The ossicles may be fractured and a perilymph fistula may be created in the footplate of the stapes. This reaction causes immediate vertigo and a sensorineural hearing loss. The facial nerve may be injured and cause facial paralysis. Traumatic perforations of the TM must be examined carefully to be certain that the edges of the perforation do not fold into the middle ear. If they do, skin may grow into the middle ear and a cholesteatoma will develop. Clean perforations with margins that do not fold into the middle ear usually heal spontaneously in 2 to 3 weeks. The perforation should be kept clean and dry. If the ear is draining, topical otic drops (polymyxin and hydrocortisone) should be used for 10 days. Systemic antibiotics are usually unnecessary. Any perforation that does not heal within 3 weeks should be referred to an otolaryngologist for evaluation and repair.

Barotrauma to the ear may occur during an airplane trip or while scuba diving, especially if the child has an acute upper respiratory infection. A direct open communication between the middle ear and the nasopharynx normally permits prompt equalization of changes in ambient pressure. If the eustachian tube is obstructed, however, changes in ambient pressure may not be transmitted to the middle ear, and barotrauma can result. As the child descends in an airplane (or during an underwater dive), the increased ambient pressure is transmitted to the cardiovascular system and, thus, to the vessels of the mucosal lining of the middle ear. The mucosa becomes edematous and the vessels become engorged. If the eustachian tube is obstructed and has not equalized the air pressure, a large differential pressure occurs between the middle ear mucosa and its air-filled cavity. This condition results in a rupture of the blood vessels within the mucosa and bleeding into the middle ear. Serous fluid also may accumulate in the middle ear secondary to eustachian tube obstruction. Rarely, perforation of the TM occurs. These injuries usually resolve spontaneously over several weeks. Antimicrobials may be prescribed to prevent infection of the middle ear fluid or blood. Persistent symptomatic fluid may require myringotomy and ventilation tube placement. Barotrauma with acute sensorineural hearing loss or vertigo may indicate the presence of a perilymph fistula (previously described).

INNER EAR TRAUMA

Concussive injuries to the head may cause inner ear trauma by disrupting the delicate intracochlear membranes. Sensorineural hearing loss or vertigo may occur as a result of such an injury.

Occasionally, the losses from these injuries can improve spontaneously, but most are permanent. Temporal bone fractures (especially transverse) have a high incidence of cochlear disruption.

Constant exposure to loud noise or amplified sound may cause a progressive high-frequency sensorineural hearing loss. Loud blasts from explosions may cause sudden permanent sensorineural hearing loss.

Cerebrospinal Fluid Otorrhea

Cerebrospinal fluid (CSF) otorrhea can occur secondary to a temporal bone (usually longitudinal) fracture that results in a fracture through the inner ear and a ruptured TM. Manipulation or instrumentation of the external auditory canal in the presence of CSF otorrhea is discouraged because it could introduce bacteria and contribute to the development of meningitis.

FACIAL NERVE PARALYSIS

Facial nerve paralysis may occur as a result of temporal bone trauma. Transverse fractures of the temporal bone can cause disruption of the facial nerve in its intratemporal segment. Longitudinal fractures are less likely to cause facial nerve paralysis. Patients with traumatic facial nerve paralysis should be referred to the otolaryngologist for possible exploration and nerve repair.

NOSE AND PARANASAL SINUSES

Nasal Trauma

Facial trauma often occurs in children as a result of play activities, contact sports, and automobile accidents. Most of these injuries are minor.

Trauma to the nose most often causes ecchymosis and edema of the overlying skin; however, a direct blow to the nose can fracture the nasal skeleton with resultant deviation or depression of the nasal bones and septum. The deformity should be readily apparent on clinical examination, but postinjury edema may prevent its recognition for several days until the swelling has subsided (Fig. 98.1). A stepoff or bony irregularity is often detected in these patients. Radiographs of the nose are notoriously unreliable in the evaluation of nasal injuries and are not recommended in the routine management of simple nasal fractures. Epistaxis commonly accompanies nasal trauma but usually has stopped by the time the child reaches the emergency department (ED). Persistent or severe bleeding may require local pressure, topical vasoconstrictors, or nasal packing (see the section on epistaxis in Chapter 106). The presence of any associated ocular injury, such as hyphema or retinal detachment, must be detected, and ophthalmologic consultation must be obtained.

In assessing the nasal injury, the emergency physician must determine the nature and extent of trauma to the overlying skin, the nasal skeleton, and the nasal septum. A septal hematoma, if present, requires incision drainage. The amount of nasal deviation or depression should be noted. Because this condition can be masked by postinjury edema, it may be best to examine the child again in 3 to 4 days, when the swelling has subsided to allow an accurate determination of nasal deviation or depression.

If no septal hematoma or associated ocular or intracranial injuries are present, the deviated nose and septum can be reduced by the otolaryngologist when the swelling has subsided enough to permit an accurate evaluation of the nasal deformity.

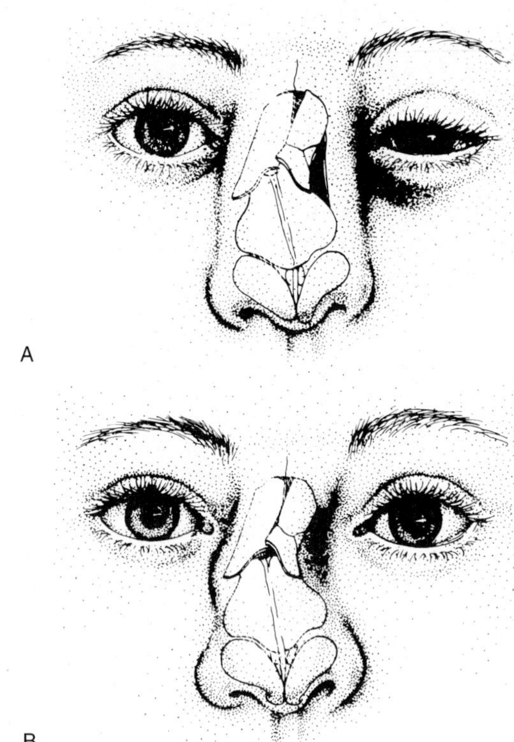

Figure 98.1. A: Postinjury edema may mask underlying nasal bone deformity. **B:** Nasal deformity manifests as edema subsides.

Septal Hematoma

The presence of a septal hematoma must be recognized as soon as possible after the injury. A septal hematoma appears as a bulging of the nasal septum into one or both sides of the nasal cavity. Accumulation of blood between the septal cartilage and its overlying mucoperichondrium deprives the cartilage of its blood supply. Otolaryngologic consultation should be obtained as quickly as possible if a septal hematoma is suspected. The hematoma is drained as soon as possible and the mucoperichondrium is packed back against the septal cartilage to restore its blood supply.

Cerebrospinal Fluid Rhinorrhea

A clear, watery rhinorrhea that occurs after nasal trauma may be CSF rhinorrhea, which would indicate a skull fracture, usually through the cribriform plate. Less commonly, the CSF originates from a temporal bone fracture and enters the nasopharynx through the eustachian tube. If the patient leans forward, allowing the nasal drainage to drip onto a piece of paper, a characteristic target pattern often appears, with a blood stain in the center of the drop and a clear halo of CSF around it. CSF is high in glucose, which can be detected with the use of a glucose oxidase test paper (used in urinalysis). Care must be taken in interpreting these tests, however, because normal nasal mucus can look like CSF, and the oxidizing substances present in nasal and lacrimal secretions may give a false-positive reaction. If CSF rhinorrhea is suspected by history or clinical examination, the child should be admitted and restricted to bed rest with his or her head elevated in an attempt to decrease the leak, and neurosurgical consultation should be obtained.

Sinus Trauma

Fractures of the paranasal sinuses may occur as isolated injuries or in association with trauma to the nose and orbital structures.

Fractures of the ethmoid sinus or anterior wall of the maxillary sinus usually occur as a result of blunt trauma to the nose or cheek, respectively. The otolaryngologist should assist the emergency physician in evaluating these injuries.

Sinus Barotrauma

A direct open communication between the paranasal sinuses and the nasal cavities normally permits prompt equalization of changes in ambient pressure. If a sinus ostia is obstructed, however, changes in ambient pressure may not be transmitted to the affected sinus cavity (most commonly the maxillary sinus, although the frontal sinus may be affected in older children and adolescents), and barotrauma can result. As the child descends in an airplane (or during an underwater dive), the increased ambient pressure is transmitted to the cardiovascular system and, thus, to the vessels of the mucosal lining of the sinus. The mucosa becomes edematous and the vessels become engorged. If the sinus is obstructed and has not equalized the air pressure, a large differential pressure occurs between the sinus mucosa and its air-filled cavity. This condition results in a rupture of the blood vessels within the mucosa and bleeding into the sinus. The child usually complains of cheek pain and may have epistaxis.

Foreign Bodies

Nasal foreign bodies are common in children. These children are usually brought to the ED with the history of putting an object into the nose, but the presence of a foreign body may often be unsuspected and may be discovered only during evaluation of a child with persistent, unilateral, foul-smelling, purulent rhinorrhea. This mode of presentation for these problems is so common that any child with a foul-smelling unilateral nasal discharge (even without a history of placing an object in the nose) should be considered to have a nasal foreign body until proven otherwise. The foreign body is usually visible on anterior rhinoscopy; however, purulent secretions may have to be suctioned from the nose before the object is seen. Radiographs are of limited value because most of the foreign bodies are radiolucent (eg, paper, cloth, sponge, food).

If the object is located in the nasal vestibule, the emergency physician may attempt to remove it. The child should be adequately restrained, and the necessary equipment, including a nasal speculum, directed light, suction, small hooks, and forceps, should be available. Otologic instruments are often useful in the removal of nasal foreign bodies. A few drops of 4% lidocaine can be placed in the nostril to provide topical anesthesia before removing the foreign body.

PHARYNX AND ESOPHAGUS

Trauma

Children may have oropharyngeal lacerations or puncture wounds when they fall with an object, such as a stick, in their mouths. If the injury is restricted to the central portion of the palate, damage to vascular or neural structures of the neck is unlikely. It is usually safe to send these children home after confirmation of absence of any retained foreign body (see the following section). Trauma to the lateral aspects of the palate or the posterior pharyngeal wall, however, may be associated with vascular injuries of the carotid artery or the jugular vein. Expanding hematoma of the neck or pharynx, continued intraoral bleeding, and diminished pulses in the neck are all signs of serious vascular injury. These children need to be admitted to the hospital and undergo an urgent angiogram and possible neck exploration. If a lateral pharyngeal or palatal puncture injury is present without signs of vascular injury, the child should be observed closely in the hospital or at home for signs of neurologic deterioration.

In treating puncture wounds of the pharynx, it is imperative to determine whether the foreign body has been recovered intact or whether a portion of the foreign body may have been left in the palatal tissues. For example, a portion of pencil lead left in the palatal tissue causes a chronic foreign-body reaction if it is not removed at the time of initial treatment and repair. Plain radiographs may not be useful in determining whether a foreign body has been left in the wound because most of the objects are radiolucent or too small to be seen. Inspecting the actual object that caused the wound to make sure that it is intact is more important. If a retained portion of the foreign body is suspected, the computed tomography scan may be required, followed by exploration of the wound, usually under general anesthesia.

CAUSTIC INJURIES

Caustic substances (lye or acid) may be ingested, causing burns anywhere from the lips to the stomach. Burns of the oral mucosa appear as patches of erythema, blebs, or ulcerated areas. Although caustic burns are usually visible in the oral cavity and pharynx, large skip areas may exist. Therefore, the absence of oral or pharyngeal burns does not rule out esophageal injury. If a history of significant caustic ingestion exists (see Chapter 78), an esophagoscopy should be performed 6 to 12 hours later to establish the presence of esophageal burns, regardless of the condition of the oral cavity and pharynx.

Caustic substances may burn the larynx when ingested and can cause rapidly progressive edema and respiratory distress. Orotracheal intubation for acute airway management should be performed in the ED if necessary. A tracheotomy should be performed as soon as possible after the intubation to minimize the possibility of laryngotracheal stenosis.

Foreign Bodies

Foreign bodies in the oral cavity and pharynx are uncommon because of the child's protective reflexes. The tongue is sensitive and can detect sharp foreign objects that then are spat out. The gag reflex often expels foreign material from the pharynx, but sharp objects, such as fish bones, pins, and pieces of plastic, may get stuck in the oral mucosa, tonsils, or pharynx. If a foreign body is visible and the patient is cooperative, the object may be removed in the ED with a clamp or forceps.

Objects of all types may lodge in the hypopharynx or esophagus. Esophageal foreign bodies generally lodge at the areas of natural narrowing of the esophagus. The most common sites are the cricopharyngeal area, thoracic inlet, arch of the aorta, and gastroesophageal junction. If the child can breathe and talk, no attempt should be made to remove the object in the ED. The safest method of removal is endoscopically by using a general anesthetic. If the child is gagging and unable to breathe, the Heimlich maneuver should be used (see Chapter 1). If this method is not effective, emergency intubation or tracheotomy may be required to bypass the obstructing object.

Lateral neck and chest radiographs reveal radiopaque hypopharyngeal and esophageal foreign bodies. Plastic and other nonradiopaque objects cause the same foreign-body sensation (something stuck in the throat) but are not visible on radiograph). Young children often have dysphagia and drooling because of painful swallowing.

If a child presents to the ED with a history of swallowing an object, such as a toy or a fish bone, and complains of a foreign-body sensation, a careful examination of the oral cavity and hypopharynx must be performed. If no foreign body is seen, plain radiographs of the neck should be obtained. Barium esophagrams are rarely helpful in pinpointing sharp foreign bodies in the esophagus but may be useful to confirm esophageal obstruction from an impacted foreign body such as a bolus of food. The ED physician can remove foreign bodies that can be seen easily in the oral cavity. Consultation with an otolaryngologist (or similarly skilled specialist) should be obtained if a foreign body is detected in the pharynx or esophagus because removal usually requires endoscopic examination under anesthesia.

If the physical examination and radiographs fail to detect a foreign body, management is determined by the child's symptoms. If the child is having significant pain, the otolaryngologist should be consulted to perform esophagoscopy in the operating room.

LARYNX AND TRACHEA

Trauma

Laryngeal trauma can occur in a variety of ways. Blunt or penetrating injuries of the larynx can result in mucosal lacerations, laryngeal hematomas, vocal cord paralysis, or fractures of the thyroid and cricoid cartilages. Proper treatment requires prompt recognition of the presence and nature of a laryngeal injury and protection of the airway. Patients with laryngeal trauma present with varying degrees of neck pain, hoarseness, hemoptysis, and airway obstruction. Physical examination of a child with blunt trauma can reveal anterior neck tenderness, crepitance, and absence of the normal prominence of the thyroid cartilage or Adam's apple. The otolaryngologist (or similarly skilled specialist) may be needed to perform an indirect examination of the larynx of the child with a suspected laryngeal injury. A direct laryngoscopy may be required when the child is in respiratory distress. The otolaryngologist should be prepared to intervene with intubation, tracheostomy, or surgical exploration of these laryngeal injuries.

Foreign Bodies

Foreign bodies may become trapped in the laryngeal inlet, causing acute upper airway obstruction. The child usually presents with severe coughing, hoarseness, and significant respiratory distress. If the child is able to phonate, air is moving through his or her larynx, indicating only partial obstruction. "Back blows" or the Heimlich maneuver should not be performed in these children because this action could cause the foreign body to lodge more firmly in the larynx and convert a partial obstruction into a complete one. The child should be taken immediately to the operating room, where the otolaryngologist (or similarly skilled specialist) can perform the direct laryngoscopy necessary to remove the foreign body. In contrast, if the child is unable to speak, the foreign body may be causing total obstruction. In this case, back blows or the Heimlich maneuver may be lifesaving. Care must be taken in performing the Heimlich maneuver in young children because of the potential hazard of liver laceration. Emergency laryngoscopy, intubation, or tracheostomy is rarely required, and only if the previously described maneuvers are unsuccessful.

Foreign bodies that pass the larynx to lodge in the trachea or proximal bronchi can present problems in diagnosis and management. A history of coughing or choking on food (eg, a peanut, raw carrot) or a toy is usually obtained. The child is often in no acute distress but may demonstrate a mild cough or wheezing or both. Inspiratory and expiratory stridor are characteristic of tracheal foreign bodies. Unilateral wheezes and decreased, or even absent, breath sounds often are seen with unilateral bronchial obstruction. Because most of the foreign bodies are radiolucent, they are not identifiable on radiographs; however, a radiographic difference in aeration of the lungs often helps detect the presence and identify the site of bronchial obstruction. Volume decrease, atelectasis, and infiltrate on the involved side may be seen on plain chest films if the bronchus is completely occluded by the foreign body. Hyperaeration (air trapping) secondary to a ball-valve effect of a foreign body partially blocking the bronchus can best be seen by comparing inspiration and expiration films. If the child will not cooperate to obtain these views, right and left lateral decubitus films often demonstrate the same phenomena. Although differentiating hyperaeration and contralateral volume loss from atelectasis and compensatory contralateral lung expansion may help to predict the location of a possible foreign body, this distinction is not as important as recognizing that any radiographic asymmetry signals a possible foreign body and requires endoscopy. A normal chest radiograph does not, however, rule out the possibility of a foreign body. If a foreign body is suspected (by history or clinical examination), the child should be admitted, and otolaryngologic consultation should be obtained to perform the endoscopy necessary for the prompt and safe removal of the object, if present.

CHAPTER 99
Dental Trauma

Linda P. Nelson, D.M.D., M.Sc.D., Howard L. Needleman, D.M.D., and Bonnie L. Padwa, D.M.D., M.D.

The care of pediatric patients with oral and maxillofacial and dental trauma should follow the basic tenets of emergency medicine. An initial general assessment includes evaluation of airway patency, breathing adequacy, and cardiovascular status [airway, breathing, and circulation (ABCs)]. Control of bleeding, assessment of the degree of shock, evaluation of neurologic status, and notation of other injuries must be done sequentially.

HISTORY

A thorough history and physical examination are paramount to any treatment considerations. Traumatic orofacial injuries can be dramatic, making a history difficult to obtain. Informants other than the patient may have to be questioned. The practitioner should always be alert to the possibility of "nonaccidental" trauma (ie, child abuse) if the history is not consistent with the observed injury. One key question is the immunization history. Many traumatic facial injuries occur with concomitant soft-tissue injuries, and the need for tetanus prophylaxis is based on the history of immunization.

PHYSICAL EXAMINATION

Extraoral Examination

The extraoral examination should start with inspection. The clinician should note the symmetry of the face in the anterior view as well as in profile. A loss of symmetry often is associated with dental infection or swelling from trauma. The child should be inspected for any nasal or orbital malalignments. The clinician should carefully note the location and nature of any swollen or depressed structures and the color and quality of the skin and should look for lacerations, hematomas, ecchymoses, foreign bodies, or ulcerations. The child should be asked to open and close his or her mouth while facing the clinician to see whether the mandible deviates during function. If the child is unable to open or close his or her mouth because of pain, the action should not be forced because it could increase the extent of injury. The clinician should inspect for lip competency (the ability of the lips to cover the teeth) because loss of competency may indicate displacement of the teeth from trauma.

Gentle digital palpation bilaterally, to feel the temporomandibular joints (TMJs), should be the next point of the examination. The clinician should feel the TMJs as the child opens and closes his or her mouth. The clinician should palpate to the orbital rim, checking to ensure that it is continuous and intact all the way to the inner canthus of the eye. The clinician then should move across the zygoma to the nose and palpate for any crepitus or mobility and move back to the preauricular region and along the posterior border of the mandible, palpating the ramus. The clinician then should move anteriorly from the angles to the symphysis, palpating for any discontinuity, mobility, swellings, or point tenderness. Finally, the clinician should palpate the major lymph nodes of the neck and note any paresthesia or hypoesthesia (numbness) of the lips, nose, and cheek, which may indicate a fracture. Figure 99.1 shows the main nerve supply to facial structures.

The clinician should listen for crepitus as the child opens and closes his or her mouth, at the same time palpating the TMJ. Crepitus may indicate TMJ pathology.

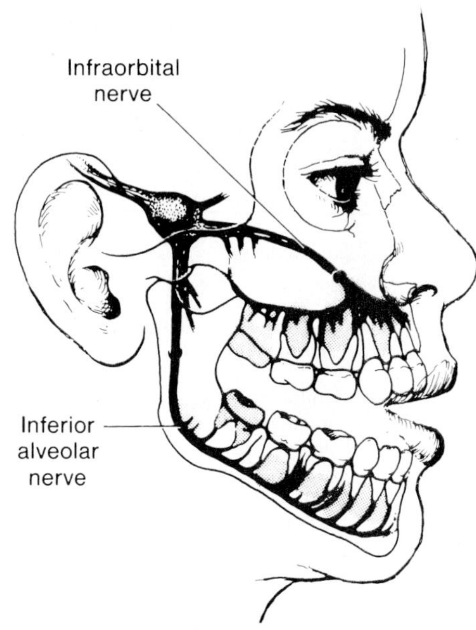

Figure 99.1. Infraorbital and inferior alveolar main nerve supplies the teeth.

Intraoral Examination

The clinician should inspect the color and quality of the lips, gingiva (gums), mucosa, floor of the mouth, tongue, and palate. The gingiva should be pink, firm, and stippled (like a grapefruit skin). The mucosa should be pink, moist, and glassy in appearance. The floor of the mouth should be flat and well vascularized. The clinician should inspect the mouth for any swellings of soft tissue that may be bluish as a result of vascularization or hematoma. Hematomas or mucosal ecchymoses in the floor of the mouth or vestibular area are highly suggestive of mandibular fractures. The clinician should note any inflamed, ulcerated, or hemorrhagic areas as well as any foreign bodies or denuded areas of bone. Traumatically displaced teeth often produce the complaint that the child's teeth do not fit together when he or she bites on the back teeth. The child should be inspected for any chipped or missing teeth. If a tooth is chipped or missing, the clinician should check for any fragments of teeth or foreign bodies in adjacent soft tissues. If the child's teeth are missing and yet no bloody socket is present, the eruption and exfoliation timetables (Table 99.1) can be helpful in determining whether the loss is normal.

Using the thumb and index finger, the clinician should palpate the alveolar ridges, evaluating for any swellings, discontinuity, or mobility of the soft tissues. This procedure should be done circumferentially in all four quadrants. The palate should be palpated for any swellings or point tenderness. The masseter muscle should be palpated with fingers placed intraorally and extraorally and rolling the muscle between the two. Using a gauze pad, the clinician should hold the tongue and lift it gently to view and examine more clearly its dorsal, ventral, and lateral surfaces. The lips should be palpated for any swellings or nodules.

Radiographs are a valuable supplement to the clinical examination; however, obtaining diagnostically perfect radiographic surveys in a child with acute orofacial or dental injuries may be difficult. Table 99.2 indicates the radiographic view that would be the preferred diagnostic aid for these injuries.

OROFACIAL AND DENTAL TRAUMA

Dental trauma occurs in a variety of forms that can be confusing to the primary care provider. The emergency physician needs to know which injuries can be managed without dental consultation, which injuries need follow-up care, and which injuries need emergency dental care.

Soft-tissue Lacerations

Management of injuries to the soft tissues of the oral cavity follows the same emergency care principles used for other soft-tissue injuries. Lip injuries swell alarmingly even after minor trauma. Lacerations of the tongue and frenum bleed profusely because of the richness of their vascularity. As with lip injuries, however, ligating specific vessels is usually unnecessary because the bleeding normally stops with direct pressure and careful suturing. Because they heal well spontaneously, frenum lacerations usually do not require suturing, especially in young children.

Suturing of the lip must be done carefully to achieve a precise approximation of the edges of the vermilion border to avoid a disfiguring scar, even with superficial lip lacerations. If necessary, the lip must be sparingly debrided and the skin closed with 5-0 or 6-0 nylon sutures. Deep lip lacerations are sutured with 4-0 chromic and then with 5-0 or 6-0 nylon for the skin and vermil-

Table 99.1A. Chronology of Eruption of the Primary and Permanent Dentition

	Maxillary	Mandible
Primary[a]	**Mean age (mo)**	**Mean age (mo)**
Central incisor	10 (8–12)	8(6–10)
Lateral incisor	11(9–13)	13(10–16)
Canine	19(16–22)	20(17–23)
First molar	16(13–19 Boys) (14–19 girls)	16(14–18)
Second molar	29(25–33)	27(23–31)
Permanent[b]	**Mean age (yr)**	**Mean age (yr)**
Central incisor	7–7.5	6–6.5
Lateral incisor	8–8.5	7.2–7.7
Canine	11–11.6	9.7–10.2
First premolar	10–10.3	10–10.7
Second premolar	10.7–11.2	10.7–11.5
First molar	6–6.3	6–6.2
Second molar	12.2–12.7	11.7–12.0
Third molar	20.5	20–20.5

[a] Mean age in month ±1 standard deviation. Reprinted from Lunt RC, Law DB. *J Am Dent Assoc* 1974;89:878, with permission.
[b] Reprinted from Baudi AR. The development and eruption of the human dentitions. In: Forrester DJ, Wagoner ML, Fleming J, eds. *Pediatric Dental Medicine.* Philadelphia: Lea & Febiger, 1981, with permission.

Table 99.1B. Sequence of Primary Tooth Exfoliation

			Mean age[a] (yr,mo)	
Rank	**Mandibular arch**	**Maxillary arch**	**Boys**	**Girls**
First	Central incisors		6.0	5.7
Second		Central incisors	6.10	6.7
Third	Lateral incisors		7.2	6.10
Fourth		Lateral incisors	7.10	7.5
Fifth	Canines		10.5	9.7
Sixth	First molars		10.8	10.2
Seventh		First molars	10.11	10.6
Eighth		Canines	11.3	10.7
Ninth	Second molars	Second molars	11.9	11.5

[a] Ages are for right side of mouth; however, exfoliation is generally bilaterally symmetric.
Reprinted from Ripa LW, Lesks GS, Sposanto AL, et al. Chronology and sequence of exfoliation of primary teeth. *J Am Dent Assoc* 1982; 105:641, with permission.

ion. If the lip laceration is through and through, debridement may be necessary. In children younger than 5 years, 4-0 chromic on the deeper mucosal aspects of the lip and 6-0 chromic on the superficial aspects are preferred. In children older than 5 years, 4-0 chromic is used on the deeper mucosal aspects of the lip and 5-0 or 6-0 nylon on the superficial edges. Most superficial tongue lacerations heal without suturing; however, deep lacerations or those that create a flap need to be sutured. When necessary, tongue lacerations usually are sutured with 4-0 chromic if superficial and 3-0 chromic in deeper wounds.

Table 99.2. Radiographic Diagnostic Aids

Radiographic view	Diagnostic aid for
Right and left lateral oblique	Fractured body and ramus of mandible
Anteroposterior view of mandible	Fracture of mandibular condyles and symphysis
Towne	Fractured condyles
Waters	Maxillary fractures
Intraoral radiographs	
Panoramic occlusal periapical/bite wing	Maxillary and mandibular fractures and related pathology; tooth fractures and pathology; alveolar fractures and pathology

Injuries to the Teeth

Traumatic dental injuries can be categorized into two groups: (1) injuries to the teeth—hard dental tissues and pulp and (2) injuries to the periodontal structures—periodontal ligaments and alveolar bones. Figure 99.2 indicates the relative positions of these structures.

Injuries to Hard Dental Tissues and Pulp

Uncomplicated tooth fractures are confined to the hard dental tissue (enamel, dentin, cementum). Clinically, there may be a jagged edge of tooth. The fracture line may appear deep, but no sign of bleeding from the central core (pulp) of the tooth is apparent. The child may complain of sensitivity, especially to cold air and fluids. Emergency treatment is aimed at protecting the pulp, even if no frank pulp exposure is noted. The dentist should be called as soon as possible to place a dressing of calcium hydroxide or glass ionomer over the exposed dentin for thermal and chemical insulation and for prevention of (pulpal) necrosis.

A complicated tooth fracture involves the pulp of the tooth. Often, bleeding is noted from the central core of the tooth. To preserve the viability of that tooth, dental pulpal treatment must be initiated immediately. Prognosis depends on the size of the exposure (<1 mm carry the best prognosis) and the time interval between the trauma and therapy (<24 hours carries the best prognosis). Thus, calling the dental consultant as soon as possible to institute pulpal therapy is important. Root fractures generally are seen after the tooth has reached full root formation, which is approximately 2 to 3 years after eruption begins (Table 99.1). These fractures usually involve maxillary anterior teeth.

In any injury resulting in fragmentation of teeth, the emergency physician should attempt to account for all the fragments. Soft-tissue lacerations, especially of the lower lip and tongue, should be evaluated clinically and, if necessary, radiographically to rule out embedded tooth fragments. Infection and poor wound healing are the sequelae of such an oversight.

Displaced Teeth

The tooth is held in the socket by slender elastic and collagen fibers collectively known as the *periodontal ligament*. These fine, slender fibers are easily injured or broken with trauma to the teeth. Clinically, the physician may note either an increase or a decrease in mobility, depending on the extent of the cortical plate fracture or displacement of the affected teeth. If asked, the child will be able to point to an injured tooth because of the tooth's heightened sensitivity. Periodontal injuries may be further subdivided into five clinical types: (1) concussion, (2) subluxation, (3) intrusion, (4) extrusion and lateral luxation, and (5) avulsion, as noted in Figure 99.3.

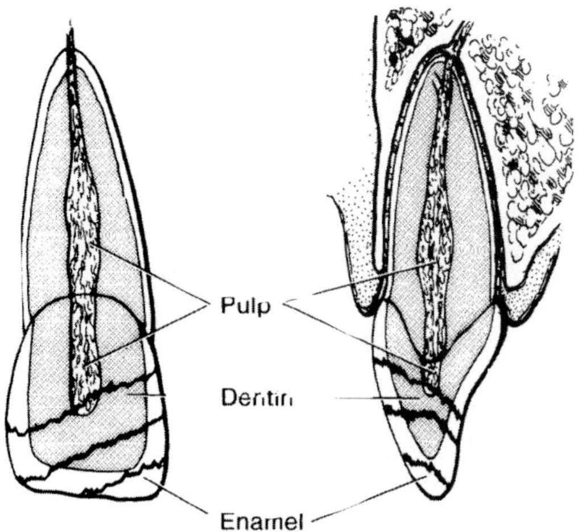

Figure 99.2. The anatomy of a tooth should be considered during a traumatic injury: enamel fracture, no emergency treatment; dentin fracture, emergency treatment as soon as convenient; and pulpal fracture, emergency treatment as soon as possible.

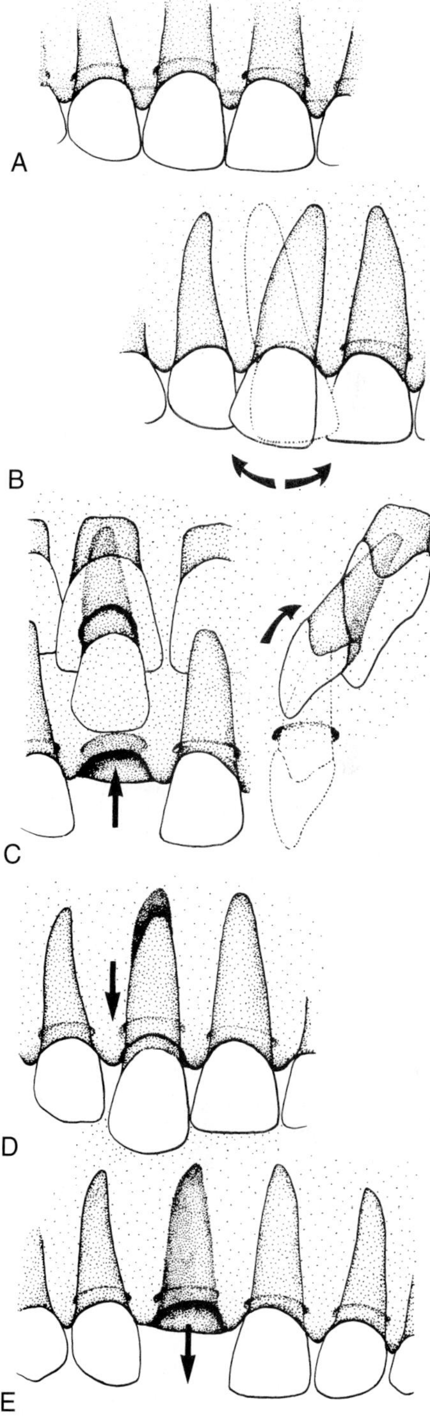

Figure 99.3. The various types of trauma to the periodontal structures. Concussion **(A):** subluxation **(B);** intrusion (if primary tooth is intruded note location of developing permanent tooth bud) **(C);** extrusion **(D);** and avulsion **(E).** Refer emergencies **B** through **E** to the dental staff as soon as possible.

Avulsion is the term used to describe a tooth that has been completely displaced from its socket. Radiographs may show the tooth to be actually intruded, ingested, or aspirated. The best prognosis exists if therapy is instituted within 30 to 60 minutes of the avulsion. The emergency physician or the parent should (as seen in Fig. 99.4) (1) find the tooth; (2) determine whether it is a primary tooth by checking the child's age and the table of tooth eruption (if it is a primary tooth, do not reimplant); (3) if it is a permanent tooth, gently rinse the tooth under running water or saline, taking care to hold the crown of the tooth and not the root (do not scrub the crown or root); (4) insert the tooth into the socket in its normal position (do not be concerned if it extrudes slightly).

A commercial product such as the 3M Save-a-Tooth Emergency Tooth Preserving System (Smart Practice, Phoenix, AZ, U.S.A.) containing Hanks is available to place the tooth in during transportation to the dental office. If none of these products is available, milk is an excellent alternative transport medium. Although saliva and saline are not ideal, they are alternative mediums that are preferred over allowing the root surface to air dry. The patient should go directly to the dentist for immobilization (splint). Dental follow-up is mandatory to prevent resorption of the root. Prophylactic pulpal therapy (endodontics) helps improve the prognosis by limiting pulpal necrosis and thus root resorption. Avulsed primary teeth are generally not reimplanted because of the close proximity of the

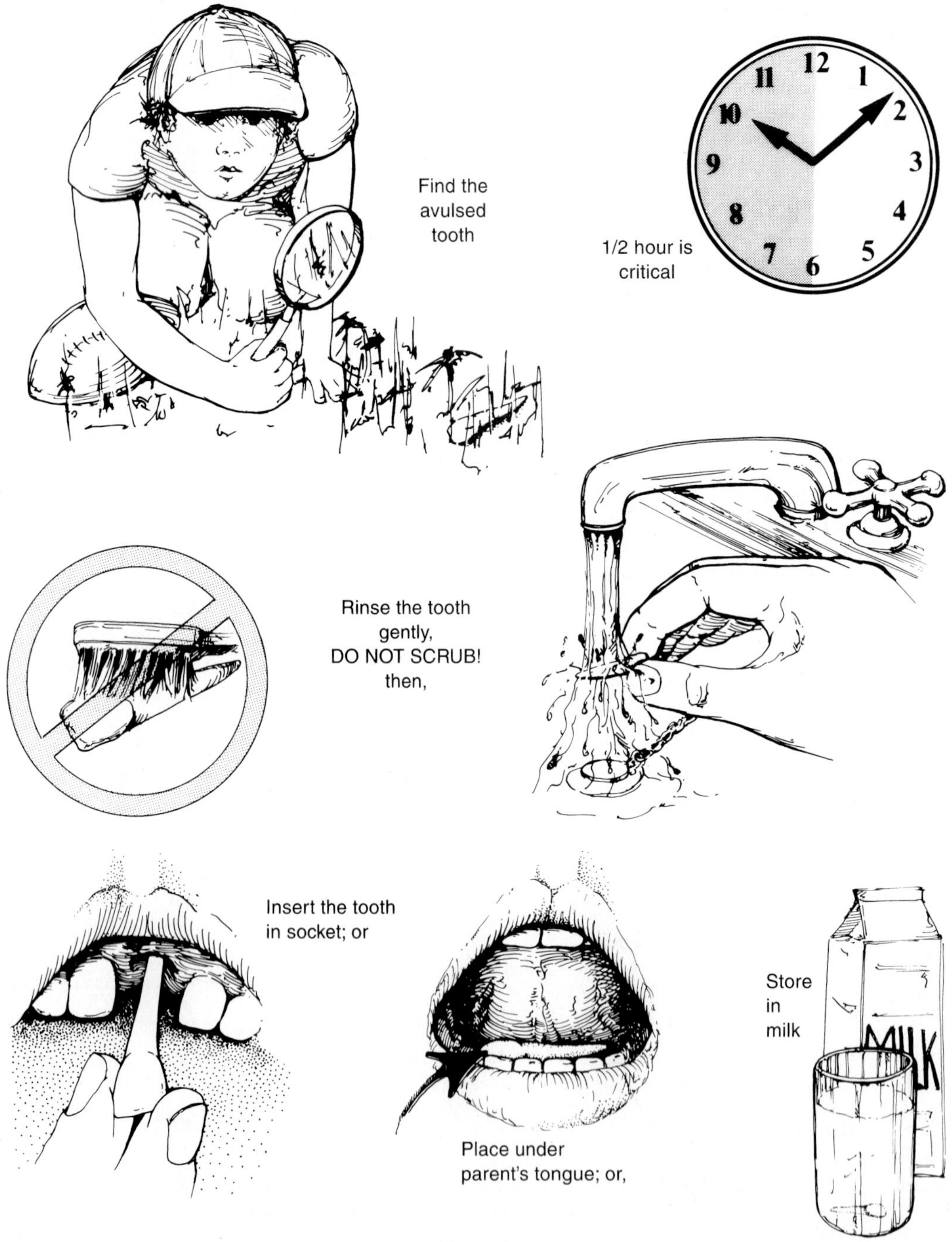
Find the avulsed tooth
1/2 hour is critical
12
1
2
3
4
5
6
7
8
9
10
11
Rinse the tooth gently, DO NOT SCRUB! then,
Insert the tooth in socket; or
Place under parent's tongue; or,
Store in milk
MILK

Figure 99.4. If a child loses or avulses a tooth. 1. Find the tooth. 2. Determine whether it is a primary or permanent tooth by checking Table 99.1. If it is a primary tooth, DO NOT REIMPLANT. 3. Gently wash but do not scrub the tooth. 4. Insert the tooth back into the socket or place in milk and take immediately to the dentist. Remember, you have only 30 minutes to preserve the vitality of the tooth.

permanent tooth and possible negative effects on development of this tooth.

Orthodontic Trauma

Orthodontic trauma often results from loose wires or ligatures that are attached to orthodontic brackets or bands. These emergencies should be seen by the dental service as soon as possible to alleviate any discomfort and soft-tissue trauma. If dental service is unavailable, the physician can bend or cut the wire away from the soft tissues with a hemostat. Softened wax can be molded over the loose wire as a temporary method or to allow the traumatized soft tissues to heal. If no discomfort is noted and no loose foreign bodies are present, the definitive treatment often can be delayed until a more convenient time.

ELECTRICAL BURNS

Electrical burns of the mouth occur when children bite on electrical cords. The saliva in the child's mouth acts as a conductor to complete the circuit. In the emergency department, the first consideration is the patient's respiratory status. Next, the patient should be assessed for the presence of shock or other injuries. Although the commissure of the mouth is most likely affected, the tongue, alveolar ridge, and floor of the mouth occasionally are involved. Most children with these injuries can be managed as outpatients. A bland, soft, cold diet is recommended initially. If refusal of food and dehydration is a problem, the child requires admission to the hospital for intravenous fluids. Meticulous oral hygiene using a toothbrush with or without toothpaste must be performed three to four times a day as well as hydrogen peroxide and water (1:1) rinses. With severe burns of the lips and mouth, severe arterial bleeding may continue 5 to 8 days after the burn occurs. The clinician should instruct the parent on the method for digitally compressing the labial artery or consider elective admission to the hospital for wound management. To prevent scarring down of the commissure, electrical burns of this area require the fabrication of an intraoral or extraoral device to separate the upper and lower segments during healing.

CHAPTER 100
Burns

Mark D. Joffe, M.D.

Modern technology has increased the exposure of children to potentially injurious thermal energy in their environment. Physicians who care for children must be prepared to treat the many different types of thermal injury. Burns and related injuries are the third leading cause of death in childhood, killing approximately 2500 children per year. Serious morbidity is three times more common than mortality, generating medical costs exceeding $1 billion per year.

A first-degree burn is characterized by redness and a mild inflammatory response confined to the epidermis, without significant edema or vesiculation. First-degree burns are not included in the calculation of burn surface area used for therapeutic decisions. These minor burns are somewhat painful, healing in 3 to 5 days without scarring (Fig. 100.1).

Most burns treated in emergency departments (EDs) are partial-thickness or second-degree burns. Superficial second-degree burns involve destruction of the epidermis and less than half of the dermis. Blistering is often present. Increased capillary permeability, resulting from direct thermal injury and local mediator release, results in edema. These injuries are usually painful because intact sensory nerve receptors are exposed. The capillary network in the superficial dermis gives these burns a pink–red color and moist appearance. Healing occurs in about 2 weeks, and scarring is usually minimal.

Deep partial-thickness burns involve the destruction of epidermis and more than 50% of the dermis. Edema can lessen the exposure of sensory nerve receptors, making some partial-thickness burns less painful and tender. Deep partial-thickness burns have a paler, drier appearance than superficial injuries. They are sometimes difficult to distinguish from areas of full-thickness injury. Thrombosed vessels often give the deep partial-thickness burn a speckled appearance. Burns evaluated immediately may appear to be partial-thickness and subsequently become full-thickness injuries, especially if secondary damage from infection, trauma, or hypoperfusion ensues. Deep partial-thickness burns can take many weeks to heal completely. Unacceptable scarring is not uncommon. Skin grafting is often necessary to optimize cosmetic results.

Full-thickness or third-degree burns involve destruction of the epidermis and all the dermis. They usually have a pale or charred color and a leathery appearance. Destruction of the cutaneous nerves in the dermis make them nontender, although surrounding areas of partial-thickness burns may cause pain. Full-thickness burns cannot reepithelialize and can heal only from the periphery. Most require skin grafting. Fourth-degree burns are those full-thickness injuries that involve underlying fascia, muscle, or bone.

MAJOR BURNS

Evaluation and Management

During the first few seconds after arrival, the physician must determine whether a burned patient requires aggressive therapy for major burns [>15% body surface area (BSA)] (Fig. 100.2). In children with severe injuries, the evaluation and initial management take place simultaneously. Smoldering clothing or other sources of continued burning must be removed. Information about the circumstances of the burn and the potential for associated injuries should be sought from prehospitalization care providers, police, or family members but should not delay the initial treatment.

Airway

There are several causes of airway obstruction in the severely burned patient. Most life-threatening burns are the result of house fires. The inhalation of hot gases can burn the upper airway, leading to progressive edema and airway obstruction. Any child with burns of the face, singed facial hairs, or hoarseness is at high risk, but airway burns can occur in the absence of these signs. Edema of the burned airway will worsen over the first 24 to 48 hours. Knowledge of the time course of airway swelling warrants intubation of the trachea for subtle signs of airway compromise that occur shortly after the injury.

Children who have jumped or fallen in house fires, have been burned in motor-vehicle accidents, or have been burned by explosions are at risk for associated cervical spine injuries. A his-

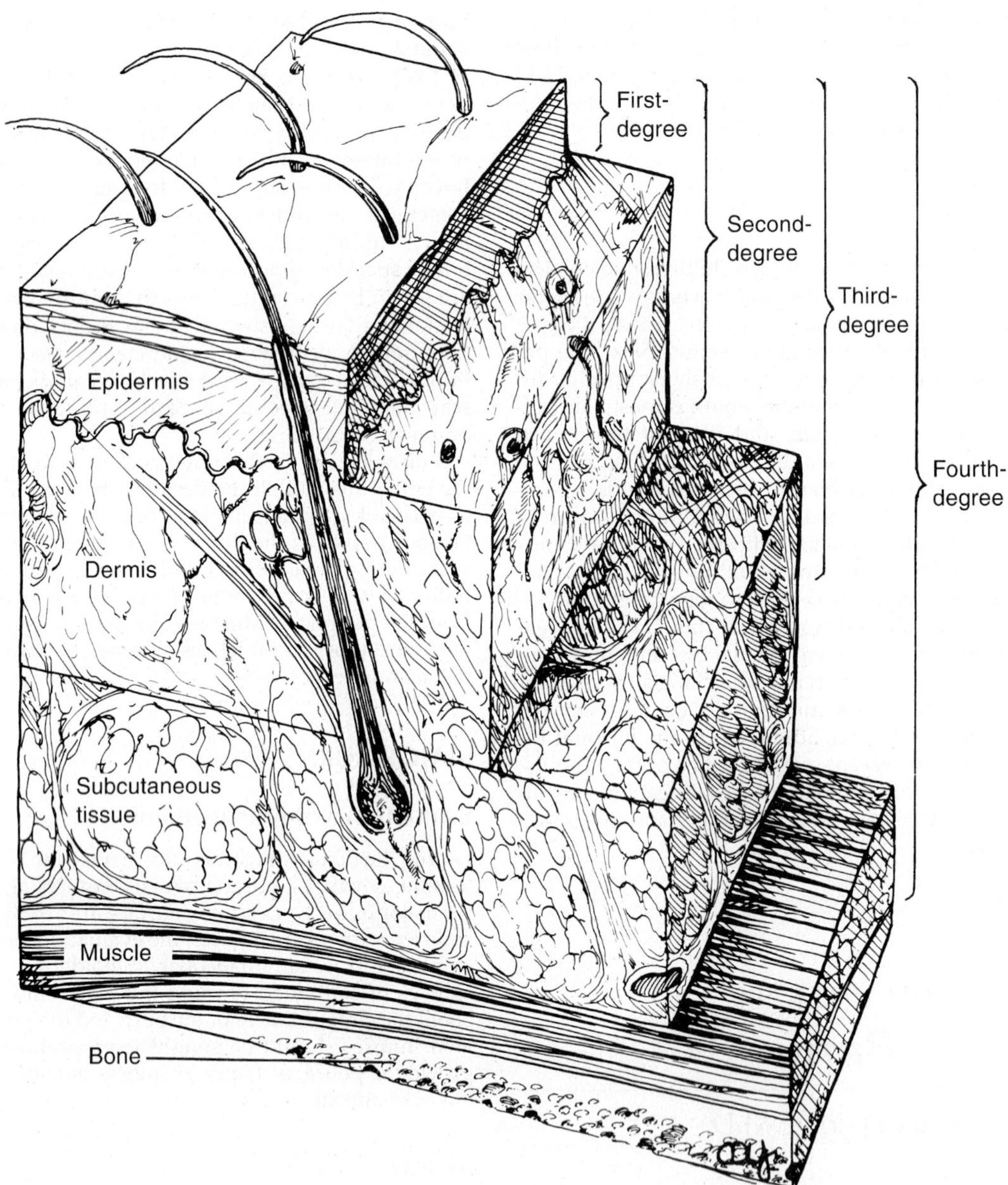

Figure 100.1. Degree of burn wound depth. First-degree burns involve only epidermis; second-degree burns extend into the dermis; third-degree burns extend into subcutaneous tissue; and fourth-degree burns extend to muscle, tendons, or bone.

tory of trauma may not be available at the time of airway management. Physicians should manage the airway with the neck in a neutral position, avoiding any flexion or extension. Radiographs can be obtained later to help to exclude cervical spine injury (see Chapter 93).

Breathing

A rapid assessment of ventilation includes respiratory effort, chest expansion, breath sounds, and color. Pulse oximetry is useful, but patients with significant levels of carboxyhemoglobin will look pink and have normal oxygen saturation as measured by a pulse oximeter. Every severely burned child should receive 100% oxygen. Arterial blood gases with cooximetry should be obtained promptly. Patients whose ventilatory status is questionable should receive careful assisted ventilation. Avoidance of high inflating pressures and application of cricoid pressure can minimize gaseous distension of the stomach and reduce the risk of regurgitation with pulmonary aspiration.

Chest radiographs may be normal initially, even if pulmonary injury has occurred. Smoke is responsible for most of the lower airway abnormalities in burned patients and management of smoke inhalation is covered in Chapter 79.

Circulation–Burn Shock

The physiology of circulatory impairment in severely burned patients is complex. Burn shock occurs in adults with burns more than 30% BSA, but it occurs in children with burns over 20% BSA. The rapid assessment of circulation includes skin color, capillary refill time, temperature of peripheral extremities, heart rate, and mental status. Blood pressure is often maintained until decompensation occurs, making it an unreliable measure of early circulatory impairment. Hypertension from increased systemic vascular resistance has been reported immediately after severe burns, particularly in pediatric patients.

Vascular access should be obtained soon after arrival of the severely burned child. Intravenous lines in the upper extremity through intact skin are preferred because they are easier to secure, but access through burned areas may be necessary.

An initial bolus of 20 mL per kilogram of Ringer lactate solution is recommended while assessment of the extent of the burns takes place. A urinary catheter should be placed and urine output monitored to assess the adequacy of fluid therapy. Major burns cause decreased splanchnic blood flow and ileus. After ensuring that the airway is protected with an endotracheal tube or an adequate gag reflex, the clinician should place a nasogastric tube. Hypothermia can occur rapidly in small children, especially in those whose skin injury impairs normal thermoregulation. Core temperature should be monitored and the child kept covered, except as necessary for examination and burn assessment. Tetanus toxoid is indicated if the child has not been immunized in the preceding 5 years; unimmunized patients require tetanus immune globulin as well.

Assessment

Major burns are three-dimensional injuries. To estimate the size of a burn, one must assess the surface area and depth of burned skin. Decisions about fluid therapy, referral, disposition, and prognosis are based on the size of the burn. After stabilization of vital functions in the primary survey, a systematic evaluation of the surface area and depth of burns follows. The "rule of nines" used to estimate burn surface area in adults cannot be applied to children with their different body proportions. Young children have relatively larger heads and smaller extremities. Areas of partial- and full-thickness injury should be recorded on an anatomic chart (Fig. 100.3) and then total percentage burn surface area computed using age-appropriate proportions. First-degree burns are not included. A child's palm (not including the fingers) is approximately 1% of BSA and can be used to estimate the extent of smaller burns (Table 100.2).

Fluid Therapy

Prompt treatment of the hypovolemia that occurs early in children with severe thermal injuries is of prime importance. The fluid status of burned children is a dynamic process that requires careful reevaluation and therapeutic adjustments. Extravasation of water and sodium through abnormally permeable capillaries continues for about 24 hours after injury. Capillary integrity then improves and intravascular volume stabilizes. Most burn centers recommend crystalloid during the first 24 hours because colloid may extravasate through the leaky capillaries and worsen interstitial edema. Once capillary integrity is restored, colloid is used for volume expansion and for preservation of serum oncotic pressure.

Several formulas for the calculation of fluid therapy exist (Table 100.1). The Parkland formula recommends 4 mL of crystalloid per kilogram of body weight per %BSA over the first 24 hours, half during the first 8 hours and half over the next 16 hours. This formula underestimates the needs of young children. Adding maintenance requirements to this volume more accurately estimates the requirements of burn victims aged younger than 5 years. The Carvajal formula uses BSA rather than weight to calculate fluid therapy and recommends 5000 mL/m^2 per %BSA, half in the first 8 hours and half over the next 16 hours, plus 2000 mL/m^2 per day as maintenance. Formulas for fluid therapy in burn patients must be used carefully in small children. The calculated volume requirements are useful to the clinician in providing an initial rate of fluid infusion. Adjustments of infusion rates are the rule, not the exception. Many pediatric burn centers prefer to follow urine output rather

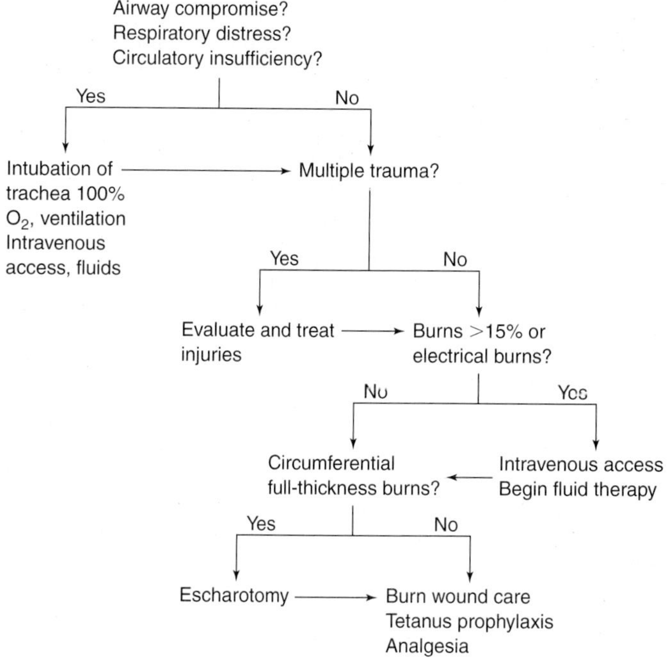

Figure 100.2. Diagnostic approach to the burn patient.

TABLE 100.1. Fluid Resuscitation Formulas

Parkland: 4 mL/kg/%BSA second- and third-degree burns, half in the first 8 h, half in the next 16 h. Add maintenance in children <5 yr old

Carvajal: 5,000 mL/m²/%BSA second- and third-degree burns, half in the first 8 h, half in the next 16 h. Add 2,000 mL/m²/d maintenance

BSA, bovine serum albumin.

than central venous pressure to assess the adequacy of fluid therapy. Children should produce at least 1 mL of urine per kilogram of body weight per hour. Oliguria, as determined by this measure, is almost always the result of inadequate fluid administration. Intrinsic renal disease sometimes is noted after electrical injuries because of myoglobinuria. Hyperglycemia may cause an osmotic diuresis and complicate care of the burned patient. Before infusions are decreased in response to excessive urine output, a measurement of blood sugar should be made.

CARE OF THE BURN WOUND

Early surgical management of some partial-thickness and most full-thickness burns with excision and grafting has been an important advance in burn treatment. In the ED, a few basic measures initiate the wound care. Burns should be covered loosely with clean sheets during the early phase of resuscitation in severe injuries. Once the cardiorespiratory status is stabilized, the wounds are uncovered and assessed for size and depth. The goals of burn wound care are to promote rapid healing and prevent infection. Cleansing with large volumes of lukewarm sterile saline reduces contamination. Loose tissue often can be wiped away with sterile gauze, simplifying and expediting burn debridement. In general, bullae should be left intact to preserve the barrier to bacterial invasion. Certain large bullae in locations that are likely to rupture may benefit from debridement.

Full-thickness burns cause a loss of skin elasticity. The burned skin cannot expand as tissue edema develops during the first 24 to 48 hours of fluid therapy. Circumferential injury can cause vascular insufficiency of the distal extremities. Assessment of blood flow with a Doppler device is useful for monitoring peripheral circulation because the usual methods of assessment, including capillary refill and temperature, may be difficult in the severely burned child. Absent flow is an indication for escharotomy. Extensive full-thickness burns of the trunk may restrict expansion of the chest and impair ventilation. Respiratory embarrassment in this setting is also an indication for escharotomy. Escharotomy involves incision through the depth of the eschar on the medial and lateral aspects of the extremities, including the hands and fingers. It is especially important to extend across the joints because at these locations the skin is tightly adherent to the underlying fascia, where vascular obstruction is likely to occur. With extensive, full-thickness thoracic burns, incision along the anterior axillary lines allows adequate chest expansion.

Pain Management

Reducing pain is an important consideration in the management of children with burns. Pain is a subjective experience that is influenced by the preceding events. Children rescued from house fires, separated from their parents, transported in ambulances, and brought to EDs are usually extremely anxious. Calm, developmentally appropriate verbal reassurance, even to preverbal children, can reduce anxiety and dramatically reduce the perception of pain (See Chapter 4).

Disposition

Guidelines for admission must be individualized when treating burned children. Hospitals, physicians, and parents have varying capabilities for managing pediatric burn patients. In general, children with burns of smaller percentages of BSA than adults require admission, especially patients younger than 2 years.

Children with partial-thickness burns greater than 10% of BSA should be admitted to a hospital. Partial-thickness injury greater than 20% of BSA warrants admission to a children's hospital or burn center. Full-thickness burns greater than 2% of BSA require inpatient treatment. Burns in certain locations are higher risk for disability or poor cosmetic outcome and should be considered for treatment in the hospital. These include greater than 1% burns of the face, perineum, hands, feet, circumferential burns, or burns overlying joints. Children with inhalation injury or associated trauma require admission with burns involving

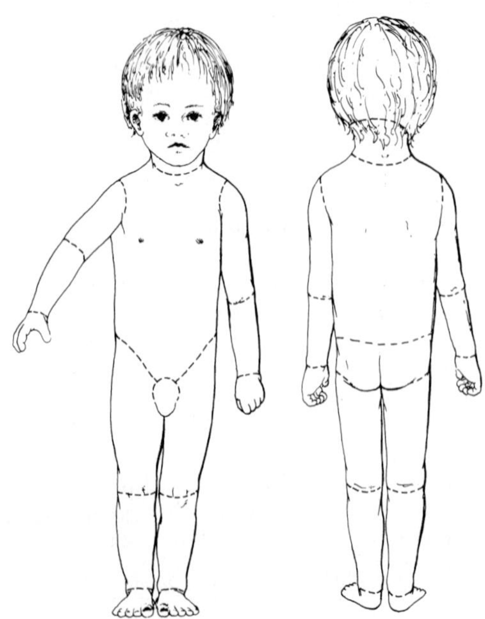

Figure 100.3. Anatomic chart for recording burn surface area.

TABLE 100.2. Estimation of Surface Area Burned Based on Age[a]

Area	Birth to 1	1–4	Age (yr) 5–9	10–14	15	Adult
Head	19	17	13	11	9	7
Neck	2	2	2	2	2	2
Ant trunk	13	13	13	13	13	13
Post trunk	13	13	13	13	13	13
R buttock	2 1/2	2 1/2	2 1/2	2 1/2	2 1/2	2 1/2
L buttock	2 1/2	2 1/2	2 1/2	2 1/2	2 1/2	2 1/2
Genitalia	1	1	1	1	1	1
R U arm	4	4	4	4	4	4
L U arm	4	4	4	4	4	4
R L arm	3	3	3	3	3	3
L L arm	3	3	3	3	3	3
R hand	2 1/2	2 1/2	2 1/2	2 1/2	2 1/2	2 1/2
L hand	2 1/2	2 1/2	2 1/2	2 1/2	2 1/2	2 1/2
R thigh	5 1/2	6 1/2	8	8 1/2	9	9 1/2
L thigh	5 1/2	6 1/2	8	8 1/2	9	9 1/2
R leg	5	5	5 1/2	6	6 1/2	7
L leg	5	5	5 1/2	6	6 1/2	7
R foot	3 1/2	3 1/2	3 1/2	3 1/2	3 1/2	3 1/2
L foot	3 1/2	3 1/2	3 1/2	3 1/2	3 1/2	3 1/2

[a] This modification by O'Neill of the Brooke Army Burn Center diagram shows the change in surface of the head from 19% in an infant to 7% in an adult. Proper use of this chart provides an accurate basis for subsequent management of the burned child.

lesser percentages of BSA. Anytime the physician suspects that the burns cannot be adequately cared for in the home, admission to the hospital is warranted.

Outpatient Management of Burns

A small minority of all burns in children will require therapy in the hospital. Once a careful assessment has led to a decision to manage a burn as an outpatient, preparations for treatment at home should begin.

A first-degree burn usually requires no therapy. Moisturizers and acetaminophen or ibuprofen can be given as needed. Partial-thickness burns are first cleansed with mild soap and water, one-quarter strength povidone–iodine solution, or saline alone. Devitalized tissue usually can be removed by wiping with gauze. Large bullae that are likely to rupture because of their location can undergo debridement. Clean partial-thickness burns of less than 2% BSA can be dressed with petrolatum gauze. Topical antibiotics are recommended for larger or more contaminated burns. Silver sulfadiazine cream (Silvadene) or bacitracin are the topical antibacterial agents of choice at most burn centers. A 2-inch layer of silver sulfadiazine is applied to the burn with a sterile tongue blade or gloved hand. Silver sulfadiazine is soothing to the burn and has few side effects. Mild bleaching of the skin may occur. Bacitracin is often chosen for burns of the face. About 5% of children are allergic to sulfa and can be treated with bacitracin or povidone–iodine ointment. Leukopenia also has been reported in patients treated with silver sulfadiazine. Mafenide acetate (Sulfamylon) is a topical antimicrobial agent that is more penetrating than silver sulfadiazine. It causes pain when applied, cannot be used in sulfa-sensitive patients, and inhibits carbonic anhydrase, which can cause a metabolic acidosis. Some experts recommend mafenide acetate for burns overlying cartilaginous structures, such as the ear and nose. Small, superficial partial-thickness burns may be treated with sterile dressings and no antibiotics.

A loose gauze dressing should be placed over the burn and secured with tape. Burns of the face can be treated with an open technique. Dressings should be changed twice each day. The parent should rinse off residual antibacterial cream with warm water and inspect the wound. Signs of infection, such as redness and tenderness around the margin of the burn, warrant immediate evaluation by a physician. A greenish material formed by serous drainage from the burn mixing with the silver sulfadiazine cream is often mistaken for purulence. If the burn is healing well, the parent should reapply the antibiotic cream and dress the wound as demonstrated by the physician or nurse in the ED. Burns should be examined by a physician every 2 or 3 days until healing is well under way. Large burns or burns of the hands, feet, perineum, or overlying joints that are managed on an outpatient basis should be referred for follow-up to a burn specialist and evaluated more frequently. Prophylactic antibiotics are not recommended.

ELECTRICAL BURNS

Burns that result when electrical current passes through the body have unique characteristics. Each year, more than 4000 ED visits are caused by electrical injuries, most in children (see Chapter 79). Electrical burns account for 3% of burn center admissions and are increasing in number. Most injuries occur in young children from contact with low-voltage (<120 V) alternating household current, often from mouthing plugs or extension cords. Severe high voltage (>500 V) injuries are seen most often in adolescent males as a consequence of risk-taking behaviors.

The initial approach to victims of electrical burns is similar to that in other severely burned children. The potential for arrhythmias requires close cardiac monitoring. Electrical burns are usually more severe than they appear. Significant deep and internal injuries may occur in patients with relatively small entrance and exit wounds. Fluid requirements are higher than predicted by formulas based on estimates of percentage of BSA because a larger portion of the injury is internal. Destruction of muscle often causes myoglobinuria. Renal failure usually can be prevented with forced diuresis and alkalinization. Electrical injury and edema within fascial compartments can cause a compartment syndrome with vascular insufficiency. Severe electrical injuries require extensive evaluation for internal injuries, which should be done at a children's hospital or regional burn center.

A common electrical injury occurs to the lips and mouth of toddlers who suck on plugs or extension cords. Deep burns at the corner of the mouth require specialized attention to prevent severe scarring and contracture. Bleeding from the labial artery 1 to 2 weeks after injury, when the eschar separates, can result in significant blood loss. In previous years, these children were hospitalized for 2 weeks, but some burn specialists now manage these children as outpatients. See also Chapter 79 for additional discussion of electrical burns, including lightning strikes.

CHEMICAL BURNS

More than 25,000 different caustic products can cause burns. Most are either acidic or alkaline. Acids cause coagulation of tissue proteins, which limit the depth of penetration. Alkali results in liquefaction and deeper injury. Caustic chemicals on the skin cause a prolonged period of burning compared with most thermal burns. Edema of the underlying tissue can make full-thickness injuries appear deceptively superficial. Treatment of caustic burns, whether acid or base, involves copious irrigation to dilute the chemical and stop the burning.

CHAPTER 101

Orthopedic Trauma

David Bachman, M.D., and
Stephen Santora, M.D.

Orthopedic trauma currently accounts for 10% to 15% of emergency department (ED) visits in urban pediatric hospitals. The number and spectrum of musculoskeletal injuries sustained by children and adolescents appear to be on the rise in recent years, in part because of the rapid growth of organized sports. As the result of a number of anatomic and physiologic differences, the array of orthopedic injuries seen in pediatrics differs greatly from that seen in adult practice. An understanding of these differences allows the emergency physician to make accurate diagnoses and to avoid complications.

FRACTURES UNIQUE TO CHILDREN

The anatomic and physiologic differences between adults and children are reflected in the number of fractures and injuries unique to the pediatric age group, including physeal fractures (Fig. 101.1), torus fractures, greenstick fractures, bowing deformities, and avulsion fractures.

FRACTURE DESCRIPTION

When obtaining an orthopedic consultation, the emergency physician must relay accurate and descriptive information to allow the orthopedist to make appropriate treatment recommendations. A clinical description should include the patient's age and sex, the mechanism of injury, the anatomic location, the status of the neurovascular structures, and the extent of associated soft-tissue injury. A careful and precise radiographic description should include the anatomic location of the fracture; the type of fracture (eg, transverse, spiral, oblique); the amount of displacement; the degree of angulation, shortening, or malrotation; the degree of comminution; and the extent of involvement of the joint and growth plate. Accurate descriptions using appropriate terminology are helpful in assisting the orthopedist in his or her recommendations (Fig. 101.2).

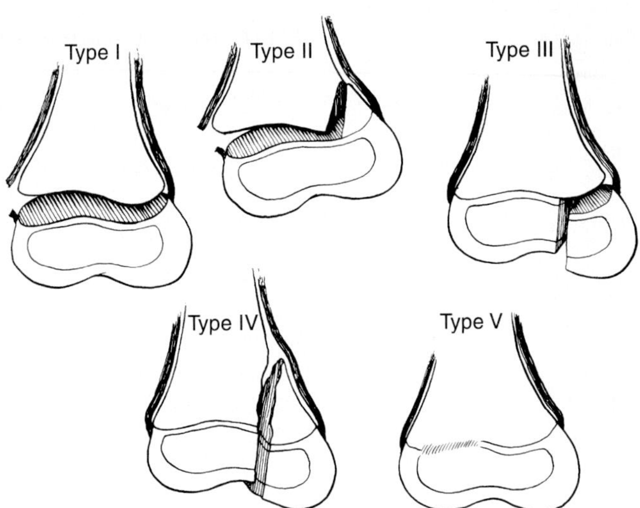

Figure 101.1. The Salter–Harris classification for physeal fractures. The prognosis for growth disturbance worsens from type I through type V.

OPEN FRACTURES

Several considerations dictate that the emergency physician approach open fractures with special concern. Such fractures generally result from high-energy accidents, namely, falls, motor-vehicle collisions, and auto–pedestrian accidents. Multiple injuries are common in such settings. The physician should not

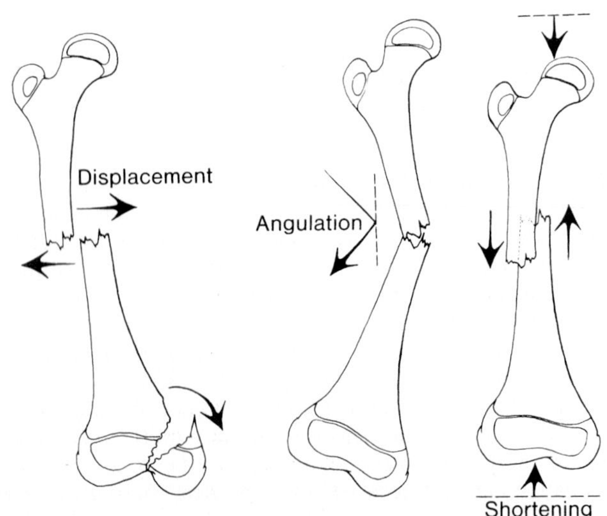

Figure 101.2. Diagrammatic representation of fracture deformities: displacement **(A)**, angulation**(B)**, overriding with shortening **(C)**.

allow an open fracture to distract from the detection and orderly management of other less apparent but potentially life-threatening injuries. A complete examination is imperative.

The incidence of complications is higher with open fractures, and a complete evaluation for neurovascular compromise and for signs of compartment syndrome should be performed. In addition, the incidence of infection is increased with open fractures. Management should include cleansing the wound, applying a sterile Betadine dressing, administering prophylactic intravenous antibiotics (eg, broad-spectrum cephalosporins), and immobilizing the fracture. Tetanus prophylaxis should be administered according to the usual guidelines. Clearly, open fractures must be regarded as true orthopedic emergencies. Surgical debridement, irrigation, and definitive care of the wound and fracture are uniformly necessary. The patient should be given nothing by mouth, and an urgent orthopedic consultation should be obtained. The laceration over a fracture should never be closed, even if the fracture is in good alignment.

COMPARTMENT SYNDROME

The compartment syndrome is a devastating fracture complication that, if left untreated, may progress to muscle necrosis and nerve palsies. It occurs when a buildup of intracompartmental pressure results in ischemia of the muscle and neurovascular tissue. The pressure initially blocks venous outflow, resulting in increased pressure in the nonelastic compartment. Eventually, the small arterioles and capillaries become occluded and irreversible muscle and nerve damage results.

The compartment syndrome can occur in the forearm, hand, thigh, leg, or foot; the most common site is the anterior compartment of the leg. The fracture need not be a severe one; indeed, the compartments are often torn with significantly displaced fractures and thus are less subject to pressure buildup. Pain, particularly pain with passive extension, is the earliest sign of the compartment syndrome. With any fracture or blunt tissue injury presenting with pain out of proportion to the injury, the compartment syndrome must be suspected. On palpation, the muscular compartment may feel hard, swollen, and tense. Other physical signs, including pulselessness, paresthesia, pallor, and paralysis, may or may not be present. Direct measurement of compartmental pressures confirms the diagnosis. When clinical and objective signs of compartment syndrome are present, a fasciotomy should be performed as soon as possible.

In the patient with multiple injuries, it is imperative to palpate every muscular compartment to rule out impending compartment syndrome. An orthopedic consultation should be obtained in every case of suspected compartment syndrome.

INJURIES OF THE UPPER EXTREMITIES

Injuries of the Shoulder Region

For purposes of this discussion, injuries of the shoulder region are grouped as follows: (1) clavicular fractures, (2) scapular fractures, and (3) shoulder dislocations.

CLAVICULAR FRACTURES

The clavicle ranks as the most commonly fractured bone in children. More than half of all clavicular fractures occur in children less than 10 years of age. In children younger than 2 years (excluding the newborn period), such fractures are uncommon and should provoke consideration of intentional trauma. For the sake of discussion, clavicular injuries can be divided into fractures of the shaft, the medial end, and the lateral end.

Fractures of the clavicular shaft result from direct trauma and from indirect forces transmitted by falls onto an outstretched hand. Most are greenstick injuries of the midshaft; the thick periosteum enveloping the clavicle prevents significant displacement or angulation. The diagnosis is usually self-evident. Typically, a child complains of shoulder pain and is cradling the arm on the injured side with the opposite one. Occasionally, the initial injury is unnoticed and comes to attention only when a lump appears as callus forms. Radiographs are confirmatory, although visualization of nondisplaced fractures may require several views. (It can be debated whether radiographs are strictly necessary when the diagnosis is self-evident on physical examination.) Despite the proximity of the brachial plexus and subclavian vessels, neurovascular injury is rare other than when a violent direct blow results in significant displacement of the fracture fragments.

Medially, strong ligaments anchor the clavicle to the sternum. Eighty percent of the growth of the clavicle occurs at the medial physis. The last epiphysis in the body to close, the medial clavicular epiphysis is rarely visible radiographically in patients younger than 18 years. Apparent dislocations of the sternoclavicular joint are invariably epiphyseal separations in children and young adults. With such fractures, either anterior or posterior displacement can occur. The direction of displacement often can be determined by direct palpation. Radiographic visualization may be difficult; special views or computed tomography (CT) scans often are required to define the degree and direction of displacement. Posterior displacement is of particular concern because compression of the mediastinal vessels and the trachea can result. If evidence of neurovascular or respiratory compromise is found, prompt orthopedic consultation and closed reduction are indicated.

Laterally, the clavicle is anchored by the coracoclavicular and acromioclavicular ligaments. Once again, fracture through the physis rather than dislocation is the rule. The usual mechanism of injury is a direct blow to the point of the shoulder. Typically, the proximal fracture fragment is displaced superiorly; the radiographic appearance suggests acromioclavicular separation. The periosteum remains whole inferiorly, however, and its ligamentous connections intact. As a result, most distal clavicular fractures heal uneventfully with no loss of joint stability.

Only rarely is orthopedic consultation or, for that matter, any follow-up necessary for a clavicular injury. Exceptions include significantly displaced midshaft fractures, for which closed reduction is occasionally desirable; posteriorly and significantly anteriorly displaced medial fractures; grossly unstable distal injuries; and all open fractures. Immobilization in a figure-of-eight dressing or a sling and swathe for 3 weeks followed by 3 weeks of restriction from sporting activities is adequate treatment for most shaft fractures. Repeat radiographs are usually unnecessary given that nonunion is extremely unusual. It is best to inform parents that a lump will appear as callus forms and may persist for as long as a year. With medial and distal fractures, a sling is recommended along with progressive motion as the pain subsides.

SCAPULAR FRACTURES

Fractures of the scapula are unusual in adolescents and rare in children. In the isolated instances in which they do occur, the usual mechanism is a severe direct blow, such as can be sustained in a fall from a height or a motor-vehicle accident. The same force that produces the scapular fracture may result in more concerning and potentially life-threatening injuries to the chest, neck, or head. Fractures of the body and neck of the scapula are usually well visualized on plain radiographs; adequate definition of glenoid injuries may require a CT scan. Although a sling and swathe are usually the only treatments necessary, orthopedic consultation is suggested given the rarity of these injuries.

SHOULDER DISLOCATIONS

Dislocations of the shoulder are unusual before physeal closure. Other than medially, the proximal humeral physis runs external to the shoulder capsule, and injuries that in an adult would cause dislocation result in fractures in children and skeletally immature adolescents. Most dislocations that do occur are anterior, as is the case with adults. Findings on physical examination include swelling and deformity with loss of the usual rounded contour of the shoulder. Palpation generally reveals displacement of the humeral head anterior to the glenoid fossa. Signs of axillary nerve injury may be present. Radiographic studies should include an axillary (Y) view in addition to the customary views of the shoulder to best define the direction of displacement. As for treatment, closed reduction of anterior dislocations can be accomplished by any of a number of techniques. Postreduction radiographs should be performed routinely in part to ensure that no fracture has occurred in conjunction with the dislocation. Given their rarity, posterior dislocations merit orthopedic consultation before reduction. The rate of chronic shoulder instability and recurrent dislocation is high; even seemingly routine anterior dislocations should be immobilized in a sling and swathe for several weeks and referred to an orthopedist for subsequent care.

Fractures of the Humerus

In this section, humeral fractures are grouped as follows: (1) proximal humeral fractures and (2) humeral shaft fractures. Supracondylar fractures are discussed under "Injuries of the Elbow."

PROXIMAL HUMERAL FRACTURES

About 80% of the growth of the humerus occurs at the proximal humeral physis. As a result, the potential for fracture healing and remodeling with fractures that involve the proximal humeral shaft and physis is remarkable. Nonunion is unheard of; malunion is rare, other than with significantly displaced or angulated injuries in older adolescents. Before adolescence, most proximal humeral fractures are metaphyseal, although Salter–Harris type I injuries are seen occasionally. With the onset of adolescence, rapid growth makes the physeal region relatively weak and thus vulnerable to injury. The incidence of proximal humeral fractures is highest in this age group; most are Salter–Harris type II injuries. Type III, IV, and V injuries are most unusual. Common mechanisms of injury include falls on an extended, adducted arm and direct blows to the shoulder.

Physical findings with proximal humeral fractures range from mild swelling to obvious deformity and shortening of the arm. Routine radiographs are generally sufficient. Care must be taken not to confuse the normal variations in the epiphyseal line with a fracture; comparison views can be useful. Conservative management is the rule. Before adolescence, as much as 50 degrees or even 70 degrees of angulation is satisfactory. In younger children, even totally displaced fractures can remodel completely. Recommendations regarding the degree of deformity acceptable in adolescents vary somewhat; 20 to 50 degrees of angulation and 50% apposition are generally tolerable. The indications for open reduction are limited. A sling and swathe for several weeks are usually the only treatments necessary. Orthopedic follow-up is recommended.

HUMERAL SHAFT FRACTURES

Fractures of the humeral shaft are much less common than those involving either the proximal or distal segments. The pattern of fracture reflects the mechanism of injury; transverse fractures result from direct blows, whereas spiral fractures are caused by indirect twisting, as with a fall. When a child younger than 3 years sustains a spiral fracture of the humerus, the strong possibility of child abuse must be considered seriously.

Many humeral fractures are obvious on physical examination, although only minimal swelling and tenderness may be present with buckle and green stick injuries. Vascular injury is relatively uncommon. On the other hand, evidence of radial nerve injury always must be sought, particularly with a fracture that involves the distal two-thirds of the humeral shaft. Physical findings suggestive of damage to the radial nerve include loss of motor strength in the extensors of the wrist and fingers and loss of sensation on the dorsum of the hand in the web space between the thumb and index finger. Of note is that, with proper fracture management, nearly all cases of radial nerve palsy resolve. As for radiographs, anteroposterior and lateral views usually suffice. A prominent vascular groove in the distal humerus is a normal finding that should not be confused with a fracture.

The thick periosteal sleeve of the humeral shaft limits fracture displacement and promotes rapid healing. A sling and swathe are all that is needed for incomplete fractures. For complete or minimally displaced fractures, application of a sugar-tong splint of the upper arm, followed by a sling to support the forearm, is recommended. Remodeling of as much as 40 degrees of angulation can be expected in younger children. Immediate orthopedic consultation is suggested for any completely displaced fracture, any fracture angulated more than 20 degrees in children and 10 degrees in adolescents, and any fracture with evidence of radial nerve injury. All humeral fractures should be referred for orthopedic follow-up within 5 days.

Injuries of the Elbow

SUPRACONDYLAR FRACTURES

Supracondylar fractures account for more than 50% of fractures of the elbow in the pediatric patients. Most of these fractures are sustained by children aged 3 to 10 years. A fall on the outstretched arm with hyperextension of the elbow is the most common mechanism. Accordingly, posterior angulation or displacement of the distal fracture fragment nearly always occurs. A direct blow to the posterior aspect of the elbow can lead to anterior angulation or displacement of the distal fragment, but such injuries are rare by comparison. With minimally displaced or nondisplaced fractures, recognition can be difficult. There may be only mild soft-tissue swelling. A suggestive history coupled with localized tenderness should prompt a radiologic examination. The radiographic findings also may be subtle. Close attention to the fat pads and the anterior humeral line, as detailed previously, facilitates diagnosis. At times, the actual fracture may be visualized only with an oblique view.

With more severe supracondylar injuries, the problem is not that of diagnosis (although a dislocated elbow may have a similar clinical presentation) but that of the recognition and prevention of complications. The complications associated with supracondylar fractures are multiple, ranging from immediate neurovascular compromise to long-term deformities and range-of-motion abnormalities. For the emergency physician, the first priorities are those of neurovascular assessment and fracture stabilization. The vascular examination should begin with palpation of the distal pulses and assessment of capillary refill. Use of a Doppler may allow detection of distal arterial flow when no pulse can be palpated. Absence of a pulse by itself is not extremely worrisome. Direct vascular injury is uncommon. In most instances, vasospasm or arterial compression has occurred instead, and arterial flow will resume with fracture reduction. On the other hand, significant muscle ischemia can be present even when pulses and capillary refill are judged to be normal. Forearm pain, pain with passive extension of the fingers, paralysis of finger extension, and paresthesias are each worrisome and should be considered evidence of an impending compartment syndrome.

Minimally displaced or nondisplaced supracondylar fractures may be immobilized in a well-padded long-arm posterior splint with the elbow at 90 degrees and the forearm in pronation or neutral rotation. Orthopedic referral for casting is suggested when the swelling subsides. Immobilization for a total of 3 weeks is adequate in most cases. All nonminimally displaced supracondylar fractures require immediate orthopedic referral.

LATERAL CONDYLAR FRACTURES

Fractures of the lateral condyle, like those of the supracondylar region, are prone to poor functional outcome if misdiagnosed or mismanaged. Unlike supracondylar fractures, lateral condyle injuries involve the articular surface; these injuries are true Salter–Harris type IV injuries. The most commonly proposed mechanism of injury is a varus stress on the elbow, as can occur with a fall on an extended and abducted arm. The lateral ligament and the common extensor tendon remain attached to the fracture fragment, which can be partially or totally avulsed from the distal humerus. Clinically, swelling, ecchymosis, and tenderness localized over the lateral aspect of the elbow should suggest a lateral condylar fracture. With severely displaced fractures, routine anteroposterior and lateral views usually provide adequate fracture definition. With less severe injuries, the fracture line and the degree of displacement may be evident only on oblique views. On occasion, stress views, an arthrogram, or CT scan may be needed to visualize adequately the extent of injury.

For minimally displaced and nondisplaced injuries, immobilization in a posterior splint with the elbow flexed to 90 degrees and the forearm in pronation (some authorities suggest supination instead) is satisfactory emergency management. Lateral condylar fractures as a group are inherently unstable and prone to displace despite immobilization; orthopedic follow-up within 3 to 4 days is essential. All fractures displaced more than 2 mm require reduction and often pinning.

MEDIAL EPICONDYLAR FRACTURES

Fractures of the medial epicondyle occur both as the result of falls directly onto the elbow and of falls onto the outstretched arm in which the elbow is subjected to a valgus stress. With the latter mechanism, the flexor muscles of the forearm avulse the medial epicondyle from the humerus. Medial epicondyle injuries are particularly common with elbow dislocations. The physical findings are those that would be expected, namely, swelling and tenderness localized to the medial aspect of the elbow. Valgus instability may be evident. Given its proximity, the ulnar nerve can sustain paresis. Oblique and comparison views may be needed on occasion. The diagnosis is particularly difficult before the onset of ossification of the medial epicondyle at 4 to 6 years of age; fortunately, it is an uncommon injury in younger children. Open reduction is almost invariably necessary for displaced fractures. Nondisplaced fractures can be placed in a posterior splint with the forearm in pronation. Orthopedic follow-up is encouraged strongly, as with most elbow injuries.

DISTAL HUMERUS PHYSEAL FRACTURES

Fractures of the entire distal humerus physis are relatively uncommon. Most such injuries take place in children younger than 2 years; nearly all the remainder of these injuries are sustained by children younger than 7 years. Recognition is both difficult and important, especially in infants, in whom this particular injury is often the result of child abuse. The proposed mechanism in abused children is forceful twisting of the arm that shears off the distal epiphysis. In children aged 5 to 7 years, a fall on an extended arm with hyperextension of the elbow usually results in a supracondylar injury but occasionally leads to a fracture of the distal humerus physis instead.

Elbow swelling without significant deformity is the usual clinical finding. When displacement is significant, the appearance may mimic that of an elbow dislocation. The latter, however, is an injury of early adolescence. Radiographic diagnosis can be difficult, particularly in infants in whom the capitellum has not yet begun to ossify. Posteromedial displacement of the ulna and radius in relation to the humerus is the most important finding. Recognition of this displacement may necessitate comparison views. Given the difficulty in recognition and the frequent need for reduction and pinning, all suspected epiphyseal separations of the distal humerus merit immediate orthopedic referral. In addition, the strong possibility of abuse needs to be considered seriously with this injury in children younger than 3 years.

OLECRANON FRACTURES

Isolated fractures of the olecranon are seen only rarely. More often than not, they occur in conjunction with another injury of the elbow, in particular a fracture or dislocation of the radial head. Various mechanisms have been described, including sudden flexion of the elbow when the triceps is strongly contracted (essentially an avulsion injury) and direct trauma. Physical findings range from swelling localized to the olecranon to a marked hemarthrosis. Elbow extension may be weak or lacking altogether. Nondisplaced fractures may be somewhat difficult to discern radiographically; fat pad abnormalities are commonplace, however, and should be viewed as presumptive evidence of a bony injury (Fig. 101.3). A nondisplaced olecranon fracture can be splinted in partial extension and referred for orthopedic follow-up. Displaced fractures often require open reduction and internal fixation. Isolated olecranon fractures almost invariably heal quickly and without significant complications.

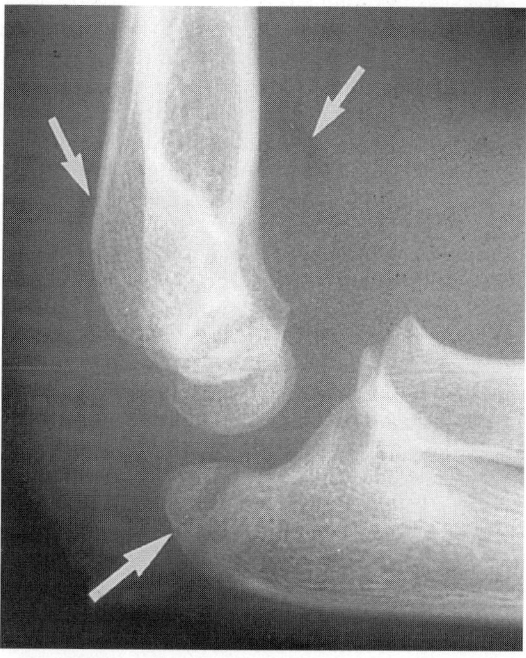

Figure 101.3. Nondisplaced fracture of the olecranon in an 8-year-old boy *(bottom arrow)*. Note the elevated fat pads *(top arrows)*.

RADIAL HEAD AND NECK FRACTURES

Falls on an outstretched, supinated arm account for most fractures of the radial head and neck. Salter–Harris types I and II and pure metaphyseal (ie, radial neck alone) injuries are the most common. Involvement of the epiphysis (ie, radial head), which is largely cartilage in childhood, is rare. The physical examination typically reveals localized swelling and ecchymosis. Tenderness overlying the proximal radius strongly suggests this diagnosis. Of note is that pain may be referred to the wrist and thus distract from the true injury. As for radiographic diagnosis, oblique and comparison views can clarify the diagnosis in uncertain cases. When the metaphysis alone is injured, a hemarthrosis may be absent and the fat pads normal. Associated fractures are common. The incidence of complications, especially loss of motion and overgrowth of the radial head, is significant. For this reason, orthopedic referral is recommended for all radial head and neck fractures. Immobilization with the elbow in 90 degrees of flexion and the forearm in neutral rotation is acceptable emergency management for minimally displaced or nondisplaced fractures. Angulation of greater than 15 degrees is an indication for immediate orthopedic consultation.

ELBOW DISLOCATIONS

The elbow is dislocated more often than any other major joint in children and adolescents. Nonetheless, it is an unusual injury. As discussed previously, the ligaments and tendons are relatively stronger than the neighboring bones (particularly the physeal plates) in children; injuries that would lead to dislocations in adults almost invariably result in fractures in the younger age group. It is not surprising, then, that dislocations of the elbow are accompanied by significant soft-tissue and bony damage. A fall on an extended or partially flexed arm with the forearm in supination is the usual mechanism of injury. Accordingly, the radius and ulna are displaced posteriorly and, in most cases, laterally. The anterior capsule is torn and the medial collateral ligament typically ruptured. Fractures of the medial epicondyle, coronoid process, olecranon, and proximal radius are the most commonly associated bony injuries.

Major neurovascular compromise often accompanies elbow dislocations. True arterial rupture is seen almost exclusively with open dislocations but has been described on occasion with closed injuries. When reduction of the dislocation fails to relieve arterial compromise, further investigation regarding the extent of vascular injury is warranted. Overall, the risk of compartment syndrome with dislocations of the elbow is such that some authors recommend hospitalization for close observation even after successful closed reduction. Nerve injury, particularly of the ulnar nerve, is even more common than vascular injury. Ulnar nerve lesions typically occur when the medial epicondyle is avulsed and then entrapped in the joint. Early recognition and appropriate treatment of such entrapment nearly always lead to complete recovery of ulnar nerve function. Median nerve entrapment is much rarer, but when it occurs, the degree of nerve damage is such that full recovery cannot be guaranteed. Moreover, recognition of median nerve injury is made difficult by the relative lack of pain and the subtlety of the initial motor and sensory deficits.

Clinical findings with dislocation of the elbow include obvious deformity and significant swelling. The forearm appears shortened. Often, the ulnar notch can be palpated posteriorly, and the humeral head can be detected as a fullness in the antecubital fossa. The importance of a thorough and well-documented neurovascular examination should be obvious from the preceding discussion. Immobilization before radiographic studies is recommended to minimize the risk of further neurovascular injury. Standard radiographic views are satisfactory. They should be inspected closely for the direction of the dislocation and for the presence of associated fractures. Although most elbow dislocations can be reduced uneventfully, the risks of entrapping a fracture fragment or a nerve in the joint space during the procedure are such that immediate orthopedic consultation is recommended. Numerous techniques for reduction have been described. Either conscious sedation or general anesthesia should be considered. If orthopedic consultation is unavailable, the child should be placed prone and the forearm allowed to hang over the side of the stretcher. The physician then should encircle the upper arm with his or her hands and use the thumbs to push the olecranon forward and downward. Whatever technique is used, hyperextension should be avoided at all times. Postreduction films are mandatory because only then will many of the associated fractures be evident. Finally, the arm should be immobilized in a posterior splint with the elbow at 90 degrees and the forearm in midpronation.

RADIAL HEAD SUBLUXATION

Of all the injuries discussed in this section, by far the most common is radial head subluxation, otherwise known as *nursemaid's elbow* or *pulled elbow*. Pathologically, radial head subluxation occurs when the annular ligament becomes partially detached from the head of the radius and slips into the radiohumeral joint, where it is entrapped. The usual mechanism is that of axial traction on an extended and pronated arm. Radial head subluxation is an injury of children a few months to 5 years of age. After 5 years of age, the strength of the annular ligament is such that the injury is uncommon.

The classic history is that of a child who cries with pain and refuses to use an arm after being pulled or lifted by that same arm. With some regularity, however, the history is one of a fall. In infants, radial head subluxation can occur when an extended arm is trapped beneath the trunk as the child is rolled over. The chief complaint is typically that the child is not using the arm; concerns about a wrist or a shoulder injury are common. Children with radial head subluxation uniformly hold the arm in pronation with the elbow slightly flexed. Much more often, the degree of distress is minimal, although supination, pronation, and elbow flexion usually elicit pain. Mild tenderness may be noted with palpation of the radial head. Significant point tenderness or swelling should suggest an alternative diagnosis (eg, a supracondylar fracture). Radiographs are not routinely recommended when the history and clinical presentation are classic.

As for treatment, various reduction techniques have been described. The most widely used is supination and flexion. If that approach proves unsuccessful, either supination or pronation with elbow extension should be attempted. When reduction succeeds, the child typically uses the arm normally within 5 to 10 minutes. The delay until normal use is longer in younger children and when there has been greater than a 4- to 6-hour period between injury and treatment. When there is no evidence of recovery, the diagnosis must be reconsidered; fractures of the elbow and clavicle in particular should be excluded because the clinical presentations can be similar. With recurrent subluxations, immobilization for a few weeks in a posterior splint with the elbow at 90 degrees and the forearm supinated is suggested. Note that even when efforts at closed reduction fail, spontaneous reduction almost invariably occurs. The need for open reduction is exceedingly rare.

Fractures of the Forearm and Wrist

FRACTURES OF THE RADIAL AND ULNAR SHAFTS

The usual mechanism of injury with forearm fractures, including those of the radial and ulnar shafts, is a fall on an outstretched hand. Direct blows account for some injuries, displaced and open shaft fractures in particular. Approximately three-quarters of all shaft fractures involve the distal third of the shaft; most of the remainder involve the midshaft. The clinical findings generally make the diagnosis self-evident. Several fracture patterns are seen; greenstick injuries are especially common.

The periosteum and remaining intact cortex limit the degree of angulation with greenstick injuries. It must be kept in mind that many greenstick fractures have a significant rotational deformity and that the degree of angulation alone should not determine the need for closed reduction. It also must be remembered that the potential for remodeling decreases with the distance from the epiphysis and with the age of the child. Less angulation is therefore accepted in midshaft fractures than in more distal injuries and in adolescents than in younger children. Although it is hard to make any absolute rules, any shaft fracture angulated more than 10 degrees merits immediate orthopedic consultation, at least by telephone. This is not to say that all such fractures will require reduction. (Another simple rule is that any forearm that looks crooked should be straightened.) Dorsal angulation is usual; immobilization with the arm in supination minimizes the tendency of the forearm muscles to cause further deformity.

Complete fractures can be particularly difficult, again because significant angulation can occur. If the ends of the bones are well opposed and angulation and rotation minimal, a well-applied sugar-tong splint is adequate initial treatment. Otherwise, immediate orthopedic referral is necessary. Closed reduction, although not always as simple as it may appear, is preferable. In children older than 10 to 12 years, adequate alignment often is obtained only with open reduction and internal fixation.

MONTEGGIA AND GALEAZZI FRACTURE DISLOCATIONS

In general, isolated fractures of the ulna do not occur. Instead, the same force that causes the ulnar fracture leads to a radial injury, in some instances a dislocation of the radial head. It is this combination of an ulnar fracture and a radial head dislocation that is known as a *Monteggia fracture*. Recognition is most important because failure to reduce the radial head dislocation results in permanent disability. Clues to the diagnosis on physical examination include elbow pain and swelling, which accompany signs of any ulnar fracture. Palpation may confirm the dislocation of the radial head, which may be displaced anteriorly, posteriorly, or laterally, depending on the mechanism of injury. A palsy of the posterior interosseous nerve, a motor branch of the radial nerve, also may be present.

If the radial head dislocation is to be recognized radiographically, the rule that a line drawn through the axis of the radius should pass through the center of the capitellum on all projections must be remembered. Once again, the need for a true lateral view that includes the elbow with all forearm studies must be emphasized. Even bowing fractures of the ulna, which may require comparison views for recognition, are associated with radial head dislocation. Any suspected Monteggia injury requires immediate orthopedic referral.

The Galeazzi fracture is a radial shaft fracture, generally at the junction of the middle and distal thirds, accompanied by disruption of the distal radioulnar joint. It is relatively rare. Physical examination reveals prominence of the distal ulna and joint instability. Radiographs are confirmatory. Once again, orthopedic consultation is necessary. The complications are few with proper management.

FRACTURES OF THE DISTAL RADIUS AND ULNA

Distal radial and ulnar fractures bear special mention, not because of any undue rate of complications, but rather because of their overall frequency. Of all the fractures that occur in childhood and adolescence, those of distal forearm are by far the most common. Except for the occasional instance of nerve entrapment at the time of reduction of a complete fracture, significant neurovascular complications are rare. Overall, the capacity for remodeling is significant. The difficulties facing the emergency physician are those of diagnosis with subtle fractures and of recognition regarding when reduction is necessary with displaced fractures.

More often than not, localized swelling and tenderness accompany distal radial fractures and can guide interpretation of the radiographic studies. Wrist pain can be the chief complaint with more proximal injuries, for example, radial head fractures. Once again, the need for studies that include the whole forearm must be reinforced. Torus fractures most often are overlooked. Often, the location of the soft-tissue swelling on the radiographs helps to highlight the position of the fracture, which may be evident on only one projection and then only as a minor irregularity in the contour of the cortex. A fracture of the ulnar styloid also should prompt a diligent search for a radial injury. Ulnar styloid fractures only rarely occur in isolation; as a rule, they are accompanied by either a torus or physeal fracture of the radius. When a torus fracture is identified, a volar splint or, if the swelling is minimal, a short arm cast for 3 to 4 weeks is recommended. Orthopedic referral is optional.

Greenstick and complete fractures are readily recognized. What must be remembered is that such fractures have a tendency to displace if not properly immobilized. The distal fragment is angulated posteriorly in most greenstick and complete fractures of the distal forearm. Angulation of greater than 10 to 15 degrees is an indication for immediate orthopedic referral. Otherwise, immobilization with orthopedic follow-up within 3 to 5 days is adequate emergency management. Although there is some disagreement, immobilization with the forearm in supination is thought to decrease the likelihood of further displacement. Accordingly, either a long arm posterior splint or a well-applied sugar-tong splint is recommended with all greenstick and complete radial and ulnar fractures. Short arm volar splints should be reserved for torus injuries.

Fractures of the Bones of the Wrist

The carpal bones are rarely fractured during childhood and adolescence. Adolescents in the later stages of skeletal maturity sustain scaphoid (navicular) fractures. Most injuries of the scaphoid in adolescence are nondisplaced fractures through the distal third of the bone. The rate of nonunion is much lower than in adults, in whom scaphoid fractures generally involve the middle third of the bone and are more often displaced. The usual mechanism is a fall on an outstretched arm with extreme hyperextension of the wrist. Physical findings that should suggest the possibility of a scaphoid fracture include snuffbox tenderness, pain with supination against resistance, and pain with longitudinal compression of the thumb. As with adults, radiographic visualization of a nondisplaced scaphoid fracture may be difficult even with special views. Should the physical signs suggest a scaphoid fracture, immobilization in a thumb spica splint or cast for 2 weeks is recommended, regardless of the radiographic findings.

METACARPAL FRACTURES

Perhaps the most commonly encountered metacarpal fracture in pediatrics is one of the distal fifth metacarpal in an adolescent who has struck someone or something with a closed fist. The equivalent of a boxer's fracture in an adult, these fractures are metaphyseal rather than physeal injuries and are typically angulated. Closed reduction is usually performed if the angulation is more than 30 to 40 degrees. Salter–Harris type I and II injuries occur on occasion, primarily in the second, third, and fourth metacarpals. Nondisplaced injuries may be immobilized in a gutter splint with the wrist neutral and the metacarpal phalangeal joints at 70 degrees and then referred. If they are not displaced or rotated, metacarpal shaft fractures can be managed similarly. Proximal metacarpal fractures of the second through fifth metacarpals are rarely displaced; recognition is more of an issue than is management; angulation is common with proximal fractures of the thumb metacarpal. When metaphyseal and Salter–Harris type II and III injuries are displaced, they require closed reduction.

PHALANGEAL FRACTURES AND DISLOCATIONS

As mentioned, distal phalanx fractures typically accompany crush injuries of the fingertip. If only the distal tuft is fractured, anatomic closure of the laceration usually results in adequate realignment of the fracture. Displaced physeal fractures merit immediate referral. Hyperflexion injuries of the distal phalanx, leading to so-called mallet-finger deformities, are also common. In the child, Salter–Harris type I or II injuries result, whereas type III injuries are the rule in adolescents. The latter group often requires open reduction and internal fixation. In either case, examination reveals an extension lag at the distal interphalangeal joint. Recognition of the tendonous disruption is important, given that proper treatment entails 6 to 8 weeks of continuous splinting in hyperextension.

Special mention should be made of the so-called gamekeeper's or skier's thumb, an avulsion of the ulnar collateral ligament of the proximal phalanx of the thumb. Localized tenderness should raise concerns about this injury and prompt an assessment of the joint for adduction stability with the metacarpal joint extended and in 30 degrees of flexion. In patients in the pediatric age range, this is a Salter–Harris type III injury. When there is evidence of only minor instability (firm endpoint, increased laxity of less than 30 degrees), thumb spica splinting for 3 to 6 weeks is generally sufficient. More severe injuries require operative intervention. Consultation is suggested when such injuries are suspected.

Despite the strength of the ligaments and tendons, hyperextension can lead to dislocations of the metacarpophalangeal and proximal interphalangeal joints in children. Dislocations of the proximal interphalangeal joints usually can be readily reduced. After a digital block, the joint should be gently hyperextended and the distal bone then pushed back into place. Both prereduction and postreduction radiographs should be scrutinized for fractures and the stability of the collateral ligaments carefully assessed. Buddy taping for 3 weeks is adequate for routine dislocation.

FRACTURES OF THE PELVIS

Avulsion Fractures

Avulsion fractures occur most commonly from sporting activities. The muscular attachments to the secondary centers of ossification (ie, the anterior superior iliac spine, the anterior inferior iliac spine, and the ischial tuberosity) can be pulled off during strong, active contractions against resistance (Fig. 101.4). Localized tenderness is usually present. The diagnosis is usually readily apparent on plain film radiographs, although on occasion bone scintigraphy may be necessary to confirm the diagnosis. Treatment is based on symptoms. Often, crutches with partial or no weight bearing for 4 to 6 weeks with slow resumption of activities are all that is required even with significantly displaced fractures. With widely separated (>2 cm) avulsion fractures of the ischial tuberosity, some researchers recommend open reduction and fixation; others continue to advocate conservative treatment.

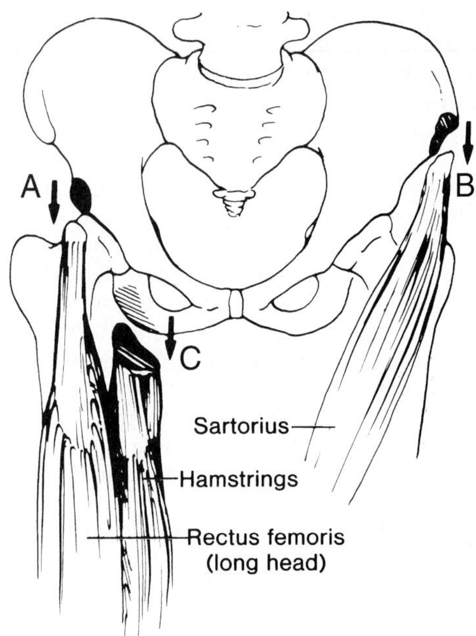

Figure 101.4. Common avulsion injuries of the pelvis: anterior inferior iliac spine **(A)**, anterior superior iliac spine **(B)**, ischial tuberosity **(C)**.

Pelvic Ring Fractures

SINGLE BREAKS IN THE PELVIC RING

Symphysis pubis diastasis, superior and inferior pubic rami fractures, and straddle fractures are classified as single breaks in the pelvic ring. These common childhood fractures often seem worse than they are. Although they are caused by high-energy accidents, they are generally stable fractures. A careful search for accompanying genitourinary and neurovascular injuries must be made. Fractures of the superior and inferior pubic rami rarely require any treatment in the child or adolescent as long as the sacroiliac joints and sacrum remain intact. One exception to this rule is a diastasis of the pubic symphysis, which often is associated with anterior disruption of the sacroiliac joint. This fracture configuration with pubic diastasis and anterior sacroiliac joint disruption is called the *open-book deformity*. If significant displacement occurs through the symphysis pubis, closed reduction with an external fixator or a pubic plate must be considered.

Double Breaks in the Pelvic Ring

Fractures of the pubic rami or symphysis pubis associated with displaced sacroiliac joint dislocations or sacral fractures are classified as *Malgaigne fractures*. The hemipelvis is unstable and displaced cephalad. This group of fractures is associated with a high incidence of complications, including genitourinary, abdominal, and vascular injuries. Life-threatening hemorrhage can occur from pelvic vein disruption. In severe cases of bleeding, emergent application of an external fixator or a pneumatic antishock garment in the ED with compression of the pelvis may slow bleeding by a tamponade effect. Angiographic embolization also should be considered in the face of persistent bleeding.

Initial treatment of the unstable pelvic fracture is bed rest. Special radiographic views consisting of an inlet and outlet view or CT scan assist the orthopedist in deciding whether to place the child or adolescent in traction or to undertake an open reduction and internal fixation of the posterior fracture–dislocation.

Acetabular Fractures

Fractures involving the acetabulum are rare in children. They often are associated with a dislocation of the hip joint. Attention should be directed toward obtaining an early congruent reduction and evaluating the stability of the hip. Acetabular fractures associated with major pelvic disruption should be treated like those involving double breaks in the pelvic ring. An orthopedic consultation should be obtained early and treatment of life-threatening complications initiated.

INJURIES OF THE LOWER EXTREMITIES

Hip Dislocation

Dislocation of the hip in children and adolescents is uncommon. It probably occurs more often than it is diagnosed, however, because of spontaneous reduction at the time of injury. A dislocation or fracture–dislocation is rather obvious if the injured limb is shortened, externally rotated, and painful. Radiographic examinations make the diagnosis. In evaluating suspected dislocations of the hips with spontaneous reduction, attention must be directed to the radiographic medial clear space of the hip. If a suspected dislocation with spontaneous reduction has occurred, the medial clear space is often wider than the normal contralateral side. The posterior labrum and capsule of the joint may be detached when a dislocation occurs. At the time of reduction (either spontaneous or after closed reduction), tissue may get trapped in the joint space, resulting in asymmetry of the joint space and an incongruent reduction. Further evaluation should consist of a CT scan or magnetic resonance imaging (MRI).

A patient presenting with a dislocated hip should undergo a closed reduction in the ED or under general anesthesia. Reduction within 6 hours of the accident is essential to decrease the incidence of osseous necrosis. The technique of closed reduction consists of hip and knee flexion to 90 degrees and axial distraction of the thigh. When closed reduction is unsuccessful or when it is suspected that tissue is trapped in the joint space, open reduction is necessary. Congruency of both hips is imperative to a good result. Complications of traumatic hip dislocation in children include osseous necrosis of the femoral head, posttraumatic arthritis, and persistent instability of the hip joint.

Proximal Femoral Physeal Fractures

Proximal femoral physeal fractures occur through the zone of provisional calcification of the proximal femoral growth plate. The degree of displacement can be mild to complete. Anatomic reduction, either by open or closed means, is essential. Unfortunately, the incidence of osseous necrosis approaches 100% in totally displaced fractures and can lead to long-term disability. In minimally displaced fractures, it may be far better to accept mild displacement than to compromise further the vascularity of the femoral head by performing a reduction.

Slipped Capital Femoral Epiphysis

Although most cases of slipped capital femoral epiphysis (SCFE) present with chronic pain, a significant percentage will present acutely. Several studies suggested that structural weakness is present in the capital femoral physis during the onset of puberty. Others identified a genetic or hormonal influence predisposing to SCFE. This malady occurs predominantly in children aged 8 to 15 years who have a male:female predominance of 2:1 to 4:1. Obese children and African Americans are particularly susceptible.

The diagnosis of SCFE should be considered in any preadolescent or adolescent complaining of hip or knee pain. The history is often one of minimal trauma, causing pain in the hip, thigh, or knee region. Vague hip or knee pain and a limp in the preceding weeks are common. The diagnosis is made by the physical and radiographic examination. Range-of-motion abnormalities of the hip, in particular, limitation of internal rotation, abduction, and flexion, are almost universal. When flexing the hip from the extended position, the examiner often notes external rotation. Range of motion in all directions may be painful.

The radiographic examination should include anteroposterior and frog-leg views of the pelvis. Changes on the anteroposterior film may be obscure. Often, the slip is seen more easily on the frog-leg view. Comparison with the normal side may assist in the diagnosis; however, 10% to 25% of slips may be bilateral.

Once a diagnosis has been made, treatment should consist of strict non–weight bearing and an urgent orthopedic consultation. Prompt pinning is required to prevent further slippage and can be performed on the night of assessment or shortly thereafter, depending on the availability of anesthesia.

Femoral Neck Fractures

Fractures of the femoral neck are relatively common. Initial treatment is traction and splinting followed by either closed or open reduction, depending on the position of the fracture. If the blood supply to the femoral head is damaged at the time of injury, osseous necrosis can occur. As would be expected, this complication is more likely with displaced than nondisplaced fractures. Overall, the incidence of osseous necrosis in this setting is 40%. Stress fractures of the femoral neck are also being reported increasingly, generally in adolescents involved in repetitive activities such as long distance running. Exercise-induced hip pain should prompt consideration of the diagnosis, which may require bone scanning or MRI study for confirmation. Early recognition is important because restriction of activity may allow healing and thus prevent progression to more complete fractures with displacement.

Intertrochanteric Fractures

Although common in adults, intertrochanteric fractures are uncommon in children and adolescents. Nondisplaced or minimally displaced fractures can be treated easily in a spica cast for 6 to 8 weeks. If significant displacement occurs, internal fixation to restore the normal anatomy may be the best approach to treatment. The incidence of complications is low in this group of patients. The rate of osseous necrosis is approximately 5%.

Fractures of the Shaft of the Femur

Femoral shaft fractures occur in all age groups, from newborns to adolescents. Each group has its specific mechanisms of injury, complications, and treatments. The following age groups are considered: (1) birth to 2 years of age, (2) 2 to 10 years of age, and (3) adolescents.

BIRTH TO 2 YEARS OF AGE

Most femoral fractures in the first 2 years of life result from either a slow twisting motion or a direct blow. A large percentage of femoral fractures in this age group result from intentional trauma. Overhead skin traction, once the cornerstone of the treatment, has fallen out of favor because of reports of neurovascular compromise and skin problems. Treatment options include immediate spica casting or a short period of Buck traction followed by spica casting. Shortening and angulation are rarely problems in this age group, although rotational deformity can occur if careful alignment is not maintained during casting.

2 TO 10 YEARS OF AGE

Femoral fractures in children aged 2 to 10 years are most often the result of high-energy motor-vehicle or vehicle–pedestrian accidents. Concomitant injuries are common. Only rarely does an isolated femur fracture cause hemodynamically significant blood loss. Neurovascular evaluation should be performed and documented at regular intervals. Initial treatment consists of traction or splinting and care of other injuries.

Distal femoral skeletal traction for several weeks followed by spica cast application has been the cornerstone of treatment in the past. Recently, early or immediate spica casting under general anesthesia has replaced traditional methods. This has reduced the hospital stay and alleviated the need for the invasive intervention of the traction pin placement. Contraindications to immediate or early spica casting are shortening greater than 2.5 cm, open fractures, and major concomitant injuries. The long-term complications of femur fractures in this age group include excessive shortening or overgrowth, malrotation, and malunions of the healing femur. It is usually desirable to leave the bone fragments overlapping by 1 cm to allow for some "overgrowth" of the healing femur. Stiffness of the knee and hip has been reported to follow prolonged spica casting treatment but is usually not a long-term complication.

ADOLESCENTS

Femur fractures in adolescents also are caused by high-energy accidents. Once again, attention to other injuries should precede treatment of the femoral fracture. Stabilization with traction splints is adequate until an orthopedic consultation can be obtained. The management of these fractures has changed over the last several years. Closed reduction and intramedullary rodding are currently recommended to improve alignment and promote an early return to activity.

Injuries of the Knee

Although relatively uncommon, fractures about the knee arguably rank as the most serious long bone injuries in children and adolescents (Fig. 101.5). The growth centers of the distal femur and proximal tibia together account for two-thirds the length of the lower extremity. Growth arrest and deformity can occur after physeal injuries about the knee; the resultant limb length discrepancies are hardly trivial problems. On the other hand, ligamentous injuries are uncommon. For purposes of discussion, pediatric knee injuries can be divided into the following groups: (1) ligamentous injuries and avulsion fractures, (2) distal femoral physeal fractures, (3) proximal tibial physeal fractures, (4) knee dislocations, and (5) patellar fractures and dislocations.

LIGAMENTOUS INJURIES AND AVULSION FRACTURES

Compared with fractures of the epiphyses and physes about the knee, ligamentous injuries are relatively uncommon before growth plate closure. Such injuries do occur, however, both in isolation and in conjunction with fractures. Most ligamentous injuries result from direct trauma to the knee, typically when a child is struck by a motor vehicle while walking or riding a bicycle. Others occur during vigorous sporting activities when the knee is subjected to significant valgus or varus stress. The medial collateral and anterior cruciate ligaments are the ones injured most often, and injury to the latter almost invariably occurs in conjunction with an avulsion of the tibial spine.

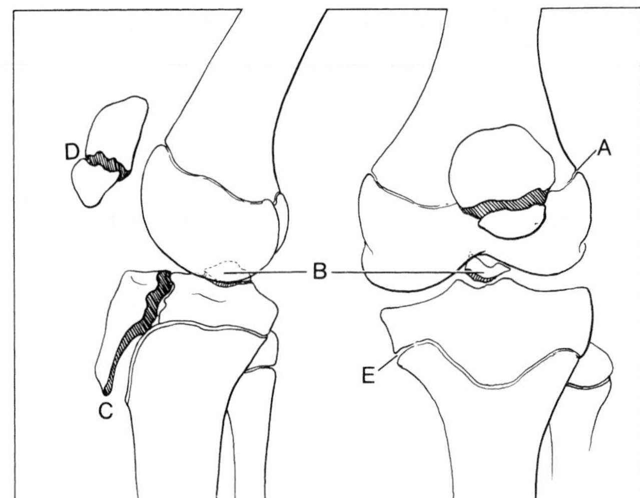

Figure 101.5. Common fractures of the knee in children: distal femoral physis **(A)**; tibial spine **(B)**; tibial tubercle **(C)**; patella **(D)**; proximal tibial physis **(E)**.

Given the propensity for knee injuries in children younger than 14 years to result in fractures rather than ligamentous injuries, radiographs should be ordered routinely for all but the most minor injuries. Stress views after adequate sedation are necessary when routine views are normal, but the history is that of a significant valgus or varus stress. Evidence of distal femoral or proximal tibial epiphyseal separation or of collateral ligament instability may thus be uncovered. Of the growth plates about the knee, the distal femoral physis is particularly vulnerable to injury. Both the medial and lateral collateral ligaments attach proximally to the distal femoral epiphysis. Their attachment to the tibia and fibula is distal to the epiphysis (Fig. 101.6). Given the relative strengths of the ligaments and the physeal plate,

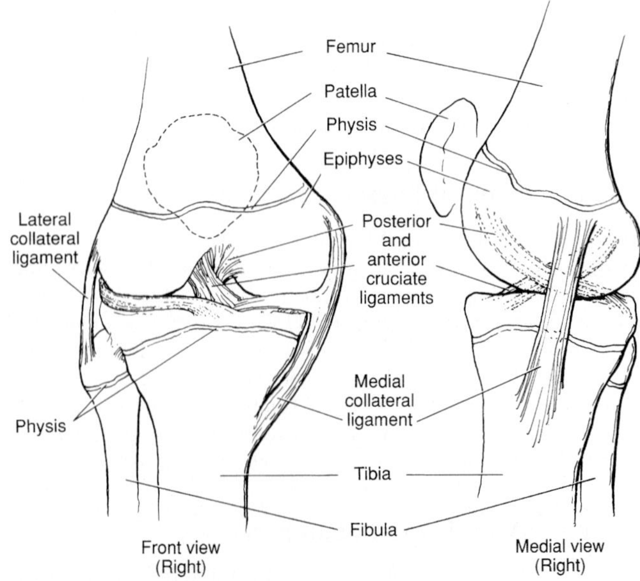

Figure 101.6. The ligaments of the knee. Proximally, both collateral ligaments attach to the epiphysis, whereas distally they attach to the tibia and fibula below the tibial epiphysis.

forceful valgus or varus stress results in distal femoral epiphysis separation rather than proximal tibial epiphysis injury or ligament rupture. Such injuries are discussed later in this chapter.

Avulsion of the tibial spine is the pediatric equivalent of an anterior cruciate ligament injury in an adult. The most commonly described mode of injury is hyperflexion of the knee during a fall from a bicycle. Significant pain and a refusal to bear weight are typical; a hemarthrosis is invariably present. Radiographic findings vary from minimal elevation of the anterior portion of the tibial spine (best seen on lateral views) to complete separation. Incomplete separations generally can be managed by closed reduction with the knee held in extension. Open repair is necessary for complete avulsions and when closed manipulation does not lead to a satisfactory reduction. Arthroscopic evaluation of all tibial spine avulsions with instability on Lachman testing (see Chapter 32) has been advocated. Such an approach allows anatomic reduction of the injury with internal fixation and is thought to lead to a better long-term outcome. Immediate management in the ED should include splinting in extension and arthrocentesis under sterile conditions when the hemarthrosis is causing severe pain.

Another uncommon but severe knee injury observed in adolescents is an avulsion fracture of the tibial tuberosity. This fracture occurs essentially exclusively in adolescents aged 12 to 17 years who are involved in vigorous sporting activities. Most such injuries occur during jumping, when the quadriceps is strongly contracted. If extension is impeded, as when a basketball player jumps to shoot but is blocked, or if the contraction of the quadriceps is particularly violent, as in high jumping, the tibial tubercle can be torn either in part or in its entirety from the proximal tibial epiphysis. The result is a Salter–Harris type III fracture. Of note is that the patient often has an antecedent history of Osgood–Schlatter disease. Once again, the severity of the injury dictates whether closed or open management is chosen.

DISTAL FEMORAL PHYSEAL FRACTURES

Historically, fractures of the distal femoral epiphysis occurred when the leg of a child was caught between the wagon and the spokes of the wheel and thus were known as *wagon-wheel injuries* during the nineteenth century. Today, they are caused by injuries during high-energy sports, motor-vehicle accidents, and falls from a great height. Overall, this injury is rare because of the undulating course of the physis and the strong perichondrial ring that surround it. Of all the fractures involving the growth plate, however, injuries of the distal femoral physis have the highest incidence of posttraumatic growth arrest.

These injuries are described according to the direction of displacement of the epiphysis and the corresponding Salter–Harris classification. Most common is medial or lateral displacement with a fracture of the adjacent metaphysis (a Salter–Harris type II injury). As already mentioned, such injuries reflect a marked valgus or varus stress. The risk of neurovascular compromise is low, but peroneal nerve damage can accompany severe medial displacement. Even with adequate reduction, the incidence of premature growth arrest is significant. Somewhat less common is an anterior displacement of the distal epiphysis caused by hyperextension. The risk of neurovascular compromise is high with this injury, which is the counterpart of a knee dislocation in an adult. Both compartment syndrome and direct compression of the neurovascular structures are well-recognized complications. Posterior displacement of the femoral epiphysis is uncommon but can occur as the result of a direct blow to the flexed knee. The preferred treatment of these injuries in the ED includes a thorough evaluation with splinting in place followed by prompt orthopedic consultation. Gentle closed reduction, often using general anesthesia, is usually successful. Postreduction remodeling cannot be assured because of the high rate of posttraumatic growth arrest associated with these injuries.

PROXIMAL TIBIAL PHYSEAL FRACTURES

Fractures of the proximal tibial physis are also rare. Hyperextension is the usual mechanism of injury. The sheer force tears the posterior periosteum and capsule of the knee, allowing a Salter–Harris fracture to occur through the growth plate. The emergency physician must recognize that the popliteal structures are tethered at this point and are therefore vulnerable to stretch or direct contusion at the time of injury. Careful sequential neurovascular examinations are mandatory. Compartment syndrome should be considered. Closed or open reduction will be necessary after stabilization. Complications after the injury include recurrent deformity, growth arrest, and limb length inequality.

KNEE DISLOCATIONS

Complete dislocation of the femorotibial joint, another hyperextension injury, is extremely uncommon in children. As a rule, hyperextension is much more likely to cause a distal femoral epiphyseal separation than is a dislocation. Given the high likelihood of neurovascular compromise or compartment syndrome in this setting, femorotibial dislocation is considered a true emergency. A reduction maneuver may be attempted in the ED with the patient under intravenous sedation. Axial traction of the tibia with slow flexion of the knee from an extended position may lead to a reduction. Following a closed reduction, an arteriogram must be obtained to rule out an intimal tear of the popliteal artery. Definitive care of the torn ligaments resulting from this injury will ultimately be necessary.

PATELLAR FRACTURES AND DISLOCATIONS

Unlike in the adult, the patella in the child is rarely fractured because of the thick covering of cartilage overlying the patella during growth and development. Fractures of the patella in adolescents are more common and present as avulsion fractures from dislocations, osteochondritis desiccans caused by overuse, symptomatic bipartite conditions, avulsion or "sleeve" fractures, and the occasional transverse displaced fracture.

Diagnosis of a patellar fracture may be difficult. A congenitally bipartite patella can be easily confused with a fracture. In this case, an accessory ossification center is located along the superior lateral margin of the patella. The margins are smooth and rounded. A comparison view of the opposite knee may assist in the diagnosis. Sleeve fractures of the patella, in particular, can easily be misdiagnosed on radiograph. The sleeve fracture occurs when the lower half of the cartilage cap is pulled free by the patellar ligament. The visible bony portion of the patella is displaced cephalad by the quadriceps mechanism. Often, a small fleck of bone is identified at the superior margin of the patellar ligament. Pain usually prevents active extension of the knee.

The preferred treatment of patellar fractures parallels that of adults. Conservative care is the cornerstone of treatment in nondisplaced fractures. Cylindrical cast treatment from 4 to 6 weeks will result in union. Fractures that are displaced more than 3 to 4 mm are best treated with open reduction and internal fixation. Complications after patellar fractures include knee stiffness, quadriceps atrophy, extensor lag, and persistent pain.

Dislocation of the patella can be classified as an acute or chronic recurrent subluxation or as a dislocation. An acute traumatic dislocation of the patella results from a force displacing the patella laterally while the foot is planted. The patella may reduce spontaneously, or it may remain dislocated. Examination of the patient reveals an acutely swollen knee with pain to palpation noted along the medial patellar retinaculum. When reduction has already occurred, displacement of the patella laterally usually elicits an apprehension sign. The patient may state that he or she feels like the knee cap is going to "pop out." When the patella remains dislocated, the diagnosis is readily apparent by clinical and radiographic examination. Reduction of a dislocated patella usually is accomplished easily with extension of the knee and a medial upward force on the lateral patella. Following reduction of an acutely dislocated patella, the physician must exclude the presence of an osteochondral fracture of the lateral femoral condyle or the medial patellar facet. Such fractures may be difficult to identify from a radiographic examination. Physical findings consistent with intraarticular loose bodies should suggest the diagnosis.

Chronic recurrent patella subluxation or dislocation is much less likely to result in osteochondral fractures. Predisposing factors include lateral femoral condyle hypoplasia, a loose medial patellar retinaculum, genu valgum, external tibial torsion, and quadriceps weakness.

The initial treatment of a dislocated patella should consist of a thorough examination, followed by closed reduction. Immobilization in an above-the-knee posterior splint or a commercially available knee immobilizer for 4 weeks is the appropriate ED management. Orthopedic referral is recommended.

Fractures of the Tibia and Fibula

Fractures of the tibia and fibula in children can be divided into the following groups: (1) proximal tibial metaphyseal fractures, (2) tibial and fibular shaft fractures, and (3) toddler's fractures. Fractures involving the distal growth plates of the tibia and fibula are discussed with ankle injuries.

PROXIMAL TIBIAL METAPHYSEAL FRACTURES

Although usually easy to manage, proximal tibial fractures can lead to two major complications, namely, compartment syndrome and progressive posttraumatic valgus deformity. As in other settings, a careful clinical evaluation followed by direct measurement of compartment pressure are the keys to the diagnosis of compartment syndrome. Progressive valgus deformity can develop after any proximal tibial injury, including greenstick and nondisplaced fractures. Deformity has been known to develop even after anatomic reduction of fracture fragments. It is speculated that stimulation of the physis from hyperemia causes asymmetric growth of the proximal tibial physis. Given the propensity for growth deformity, all fractures of the proximal tibial metaphysis should be managed by an orthopedic surgeon.

TIBIAL AND FIBULAR SHAFT FRACTURES

Fractures of the tibial and fibular shafts are the most common fractures of the lower extremity in children. The diagnosis usually is apparent by physical and radiographic examination. Most tibial and fibular fractures are stable and in acceptable alignment. Discussion with an orthopedic consultant helps to decide whether any reduction is necessary. In children, these fractures rarely persist to delayed or nonunion. Healing time is quick, averaging 6 to 8 weeks. If the neurovascular status is normal, no signs of compartment syndrome are present, and the fracture configuration is deemed acceptable, a long leg posterior splint may be applied, and orthopedic referral within the next few days arranged.

Otherwise, more immediate consultation should be sought. (Most cases of compartment syndrome result from minor closed tibial fractures; with more severe injuries, the interosseous membrane typically is torn, allowing decompression of the anterior compartment.)

The indications for open treatment of tibial and fibular shaft fractures in children include open fractures, compartment syndrome, ipsilateral femur fractures, and concomitant severe head injuries. Complications of treatment after tibial and fibular fractures include malunion, limb-length inequality, malrotation, and neurovascular deficiency.

TODDLER'S FRACTURES

Occasionally, the ED physician is asked to evaluate a young child with an acute gait disturbance, namely, a limp or a refusal to walk. The differential diagnosis is a broad one (see Chapter 36). One possibility that should always be considered is that of a toddler's fracture. Originally, the term *toddler's fracture* referred to an oblique nondisplaced fracture of the distal tibia in children 9 to 36 months of age. The term is now used more loosely.

In most cases, the history is that of a minor accident, such as a fall from a seemingly insignificant height or while walking or running. No history of injury may be recalled in some instances. The physical findings are often subtle and at best difficult to elicit unless a gentle, unhurried examination is performed while the child is calm. The degree of swelling is minimal; warmth and tenderness are more commonly detected but are not uniformly present. Gentle twisting of the lower leg will elicit pain on occasion.

Like the physical findings, the radiographic abnormalities often are subtle. The anteroposterior or lateral views may reveal a spiral or oblique fracture extending downward and medially through the distal third of the tibia. If a toddler's fracture is suspected clinically but the routine radiographic views are normal, an internal oblique projection should be ordered. Consideration also should be given to the possibility of a fracture elsewhere in the limb; fractures of the femur, the foot, and, rarely, the pelvis can also present with an acute limp. If no fracture is visualized on routine radiographs, a bone scan may be considered. Alternatively, if symptoms persist, it is certainly reasonable to repeat the plain films after 10 days, at which point subperiosteal new bone formation may be evident or enough sclerosis may have occurred at the fracture edges to render it visible. Immobilization provides symptomatic relief and promotes healing, although no treatment at all may be needed if the history suggests that the fracture occurred several weeks before actual diagnosis.

Injuries of the Ankle and Foot

ANKLE SPRAINS

Adolescents often present to the ED complaining of ankle injuries (see Chapter 30). The differential diagnosis includes ligamentous injuries; nondisplaced Salter–Harris type I fractures; osteochondral fractures of the tibia, fibula, or talus; and avulsion injuries. Once again, before growth plate fusion, physeal injuries are much more likely than ligamentous injuries. Ligamentous injuries certainly are observed in older adolescents. The most common mechanism is adduction and inversion of the foot while it is held in plantar flexion. Of the three lateral ankle ligaments, the anterior talofibular ligament is the one most commonly injured. Injury to this ligament should be suspected when palpation just anterior to the distal fibula elicits an area of maximal tenderness. Ankle sprains are graded from I to III. In grade I injuries, ligaments are stretched but not torn. Grade II injuries include partial ligament tears without loss of stability. Complete tears of the ligamentous complex with loss of stability are present in grade III injuries. Other than with minor injuries, a three-view radiographic examination should be performed. Should the stability of a ligament be in question, stress views are recommended.

Controversy exists regarding the appropriate care of ligamentous injuries. One schema is based on the severity of the ligamentous damage. Grade I mild sprains can be treated with an elastic wrap or air splint followed by ice, elevation, and compression for 72 hours. Crutches may be used until the patient is able to walk without a limp. Grade II and grade III injuries should be immobilized either in a cast or a posterior splint. (Because posterior splints break relatively easily, use of fiberglass or reinforcement with a stirrup is recommended.) Crutches are used initially. Ambulation in a cast for 3 weeks aids in initial scar formation and healing. This conservative approach with more severe sprains may help prevent recurrent ankle sprains in active athletic adolescents, as may physical therapy once the injury has healed.

DISTAL TIBIAL AND FIBULAR FRACTURES

Although any Salter–Harris type I through V fracture may occur in distal physes of the tibia and fibula, several specific injury patterns are described and discussed here. Fractures involving both the growth plate and the ankle joint often need open reduction and internal fixation to ensure adequate reduction of both the physis and the joint. Only minimal amounts of displacement can be accepted at the articular surface, or altered joint mechanics will develop with possible posttraumatic pain, stiffness, and arthritis (see also Chapter 30).

Of the fractures of the distal fibula, a Salter–Harris type I injury is the most common. Tenderness and swelling are present over the growth plate on physical examination. Often the only radiographic finding is soft-tissue swelling overlying the distal fibula. When suspicions of a Salter I injury are high, a short leg cast may be applied at the time of initial evaluation. When the diagnosis is less certain, immobilization with a repeat examination in a week to 10 days is recommended. If tenderness persists, a presumptive diagnosis of a type I fracture should be made and a walking cast applied. After 10 days, repeat radiographs may reveal periosteal changes confirming the presence of a fracture. In most cases, a total of 3 weeks of immobilization is adequate.

Although type I injuries of the tibia are uncommon, type II injuries are often observed, usually in combination with a greenstick fracture of the fibula. The mechanism of injury is plantar flexion with eversion. Closed reduction and a long leg cast application usually lead to a satisfactory recovery. Growth disturbance is unusual.

The Tillaux fracture is a Salter–Harris type III injury of the ankle joint that occurs as the medial distal tibial physis begins to close in adolescents who are nearing skeletal maturity. During external rotation of the foot, the anterior tibiofibular ligament avulses the lateral epiphysis from the medial malleolus. When displacement occurs, open reduction with internal fixation is required to ensure restoration of joint anatomy.

The triplane fracture is a complex but uncommon ankle injury that is a combination of a Salter–Harris type II fracture and a Tillaux fracture. The resultant type IV injury may appear innocuous on the anteroposterior and lateral radiographs, but the degree of growth plate damage is generally significant. Suspected triplane fractures should be evaluated by CT scan to delineate the amount of displacement at the physis and the articular surface and to determine the number of fracture fragments.

The treatment of physeal and ankle fractures depends on the type of fracture, the amount of displacement, and the patient's age. Nondisplaced fractures may be treated with a bulky posterior splint, crutches, and a referral to the orthopedist. Immediate orthopedic referral is otherwise necessary.

HINDFOOT AND MIDFOOT FRACTURES

Fractures of the foot in children are uncommon and lead to few complications. Fractures of the hindfoot, which consists of the talus and the calcaneus, are particularly uncommon. When they do occur, they are usually obvious because of swelling, pain, and occasionally deformity. "Occult" fractures of the calcaneus have been increasingly recognized in children younger than 3 years. Pain with dorsiflexion may indicate a talar neck fracture. If suspicions of a fracture are high but routine radiographs are normal, additional views or bone scintigraphy may be necessary. Because calcaneal fractures generally occur as the result of a fall from a height, associated compression fractures of the spine can occur and must be considered. Treatment of hindfoot fractures are dictated by the amount of displacement. Often, a bulky posterior splint, crutches, and no weight bearing will suffice until an orthopedic consult can be obtained. Complications include osseous necrosis of the talus and chronic pain from calcaneal fractures.

Fractures of the midfoot include the navicular; the cuboid; and the first, second, and third cuneiforms. Fractures of these bones are extremely unusual and usually form part of a more severe injury to the foot. They can be produced by blunt trauma, in which case soft-tissue damage is usually significant and a potential for neurovascular compromise results. Occasionally, an accessory ossification center on the medial side of the navicular may be confused with a fracture.

METATARSAL AND FOOT PHALANGEAL FRACTURES

Metatarsal and phalangeal fractures are common in children. The diagnosis is not difficult because pain, swelling, and occasionally a deformity accompany the fracture. Radiographic evaluations should include anteroposterior, lateral, and oblique views. The possibility of compartment syndrome must be kept in mind with crush injuries or multiple fractures in the midfoot or forefoot.

Two fractures that occur commonly at the base of the fifth metatarsal bear mentioning. The Jones fracture is a fracture at the diaphyseal–metaphyseal junction at the base of the fifth metatarsal. Although more common in adults, this type of fracture has been reported in adolescents. This fracture has a high incidence of delayed or nonunion and should be splinted and referred to an orthopedist. An avulsion fracture of the base of the fifth metatarsal at the site of attachment of the peroneus brevis is relatively common in children. This fracture occurs more proximally than the Jones fracture and has a better prognosis. The usual treatment is 3 to 6 weeks of immobilization in a weight-bearing cast. When considering the possibility of a proximal fifth metatarsal fracture, care should be taken to distinguish a fracture fragment from the accessory ossification center found in the same location.

Care of most metatarsal and phalangeal injuries is relatively straightforward. If the fracture is nondisplaced or minimally displaced with little angulation, as is the usual case, a bulky splint can be applied and crutches prescribed. Intraarticular fractures of the big toe and significantly displaced fractures of the other toes often require pinning. Buddy taping and hard-soled shoes provide adequate stabilization for most other phalangeal fractures.

CHAPTER 102

Minor Trauma—Lacerations

Steven M. Selbst, M.D., and
Magdy Attia, M.D.

Each year an estimated 12 million wounds are treated in emergency departments (EDs) in the United States. Lacerations account for 30% to 40% of all injuries for which care is sought in a pediatric ED. Broken glass, wooden furniture, asphalt or concrete, or other sharp objects cause most of these lacerations. Animal bites also account for many. More than 40% of the wounds involve a fall. Boys are the injured victims twice as often as girls. The mechanism of injury varies with the patient's age. Household items, fences, and trees most likely injure preschoolers; violent encounters injure older children.

Two-thirds of the injuries occur during warm weather months, although half of the injuries in an urban environment occur indoors. Deaths from minor lacerations are rare; however, complications occur in about 8%. Complications include infection, hypertrophic scarring or keloid formation, and poor cosmetic results.

DECISION TO CLOSE THE WOUND

Compared with adults, children are less likely to get wound infections. In children, the infection rate is about 2% for all sutured wounds. Thus, most wounds may be closed primarily, meaning the wound edges are approximated as soon after the injury as possible to speed healing and improve the cosmetic result. If primary closure is long delayed, the risk of subsequent infection increases; however, the length of time before the risk of infection becomes significant is variable. Some researchers suggest that the "golden period" for wound closure is 6 hours; however, wounds at low risk for infection (eg, a clean kitchen-knife injury) can be closed even 12 to 24 hours after the injury. In a study from a developing country where patients presented with wounds after variable delays in care, it was found that wounds of the face and scalp heal well in more than 90% of cases, regardless of the time from injury to repair.

Most wounds of the face are best closed primarily, even up to 24 hours after injury, to achieve an optimal cosmetic effect. If the wound is extensive or has a high potential for infection (eg, a dog bite on the face), thorough irrigation is essential, and in some cases, the operating room may be the best site for this. On the contrary, wounds at high risk for infection such as those in anatomic locations with poor blood supply, contaminated or crush wounds, and those involving immunocompromised hosts should be closed promptly, within 6 hours of injury. Some contaminated wounds (animal or human bites or those occurring in a barnyard) in an immunocompromised host should not be sutured, even if the patient presents immediately for care. Thus, the decision to close a wound must be individualized.

Some wounds should be allowed to heal by *secondary intention* (secondary closure), although scar formation may be more unsatisfactory. Infected wounds, ulcers, and many animal bites are best left to heal by granulation and reepithelialization. Puncture wounds to the foot, with only a small laceration and a low concern for cosmetic results, also may be left open. A small sterile wick of iodoform gauze may be placed inside the wound to keep the edges open. This gauze can be removed after 2 to 3 days, and the subsequent granulation tissue will aid healing.

If a wound is not closed initially, *delayed primary closure* (tertiary closure) should be considered after the risk of infection decreases, about 3 to 5 days later. This is recommended for selected heavily contaminated wounds and those associated with extensive damage such as high-velocity missile injuries, crush injuries, explosion injuries of the hand, and perhaps bite wounds. The wound should be cleaned and debrided and covered at the time of initial presentation and then reassessed in a few days for infection.

MANAGEMENT OF LACERATIONS

Preparing the Child and Family

It is important to reassure the child and the family that everything will be done to care for the wound appropriately and to relieve the patient's pain and anxiety. In many cases, early removal of blood and foreign material from the surface of the wound is reassuring. Also, carefully chosen words will reduce fear and pain from the procedure. The physician must honestly warn the patient of an impending painful stimulus but may leave open the possibility that it may not hurt as much as the child thinks. Appearing unhurried and confident, giving the child some control of the situation, and explaining the upcoming procedure seem to help reduce anxiety and pain. The parent(s) and child should be informed that steps will be taken to make the procedure as quick and painless as possible, such as with the use of topical anesthetics. The clinician should provide an age-appropriate empathic explanation rather than give cold, impersonal instructions about a painful procedure to reduce anxiety. Instruments that might frighten a child, such as needles and scalpels, should be prepared away from the child. The child can be allowed to listen to music or view age-appropriate, entertaining videos during the procedure to serve as a distraction (see Chapter 4).

Preparing the Wound

Appropriate use of conscious sedation and *local anesthetics* are essential for successful repair of lacerations in children (see Chapter 4).

Hair near the wound usually creates minimal difficulty during repair and generally does not need to be removed. In any case, nearby hair should not be shaved because to do so may damage hair follicles and increase infection. Instead, the hair should be clipped with scissors when necessary. Alternatively, petroleum jelly can be used to keep unwanted scalp hair away from the wound while suturing. Hair over the eyebrows should not be removed because this may lead to abnormal or slow regrowth.

It is essential to *clean the wound periphery* at the time of wound evaluation. Povidone–iodine solution (a 10% standard solution) is often used because it is a safe and effective antimicrobial with little tissue toxicity. This solution may be diluted with saline 1:10 to create a 1% solution. Use of chlorhexidine or povidone–iodine surgical scrub preparations, hydrogen peroxide, or alcohol in the wound itself is not recommended. These may be irritating to tissues, and they may increase infection by damaging white cells.

Wound irrigation is extremely important to reduce bacterial contamination and prevent subsequent infection. It is often necessary to anesthetize the wound before thoroughly cleansing. Using universal precautions, the wound should be irrigated with normal saline, about 100 to 200 mL for the average 2-cm laceration. More may be needed if the wound is unusually large or contaminated. A large syringe (20–50 mL) with a splashguard attached to the end to can be used to reduce splatter during the irrigation. With the splashguard almost touching the skin surface and the tip of the syringe about 2 cm from the wound, the clinician should apply firm pressure to the plunger. Soaking the injured body part should be avoided because this may lead to maceration of the wound and edema.

Scrubbing the wound should be reserved for particularly "dirty" wounds in which contaminants are not effectively removed with irrigation alone. It may be necessary to extract some foreign material with fine forceps if it remains adherent after copious irrigation. This will avoid tattooing of the skin and reduce the risk of infection.

In rare cases, the wound must be extended with a scalpel to allow proper exploration and cleaning. The physician should trim irregular lacerations and excise necrotic skin but should not make dramatic changes in the wound. Debridement is advantageous because it creates well-defined wound edges that can be more easily opposed. Excessive removal of tissue, however, can create a defect that is difficult to close or that may increase tension at the wound margin such that scarring is more likely. Removal of facial fat should be avoided because this may leave an unsightly depression.

Wound Closure

EQUIPMENT

Suture material must have adequate strength while producing little inflammatory reaction. Nonabsorbable sutures such as monofilament nylon (Ethilon) or polypropylene (Prolene) retain most of their tensile strength for more than 60 days and are relatively nonreactive. Thus, they are appropriate for closing the outermost layer of a laceration. With monofilament nylon, it is important to secure the knot adequately with at least four to five throws per knot. Polypropylene is useful for lacerations in the scalp or eyebrows because it is more visible and thus easier to remove. It is somewhat more difficult to control while suturing. Silk is rarely used now because of increased tissue reactions and infection.

In many cases, it is appropriate to use fine, absorbable (synthetic) sutures such as Dexon or Vicryl in deeper, subcuticular layers. These materials may elicit an inflammatory response and may extrude from the skin before they are absorbed if they are placed too close to the skin. When subcuticular sutures are used, they should be placed on the deeper surface of the dermis, and epithelial margins may be approximated with tape strips. Synthetic absorbable sutures are less reactive than chromic gut, and they retain their tensile strength for long periods, making them useful in areas with high dynamic and static tensions. Absorbable sutures are advantageous for intraoral lacerations. Some recommend using rapidly absorbable sutures (fast-absorbing gut) for skin closure of facial or scalp wounds in children because suture removal is avoided.

A 3-0 suture is recommended for tissues with strong tension, such as fascia, and 4-0 is recommended for deep tissues with light tension, such as subcutaneous tissue. Skin is best closed with 4-0 to 7-0 and oral mucosa with 3-0 to 4-0 sutures. The physician should use the finest sutures (6-0) for wounds of the face; heavier sutures for scalp, trunk, and extremities (4-0 or 5-0); and 3-0 or 4-0 for thick skin such as the sole of the foot or over large joints such as the knee.

Needles are available in a variety of forms, including cuticular, plastics, and "reverse cutting." The reverse cutting needle is used most for laceration repair. Its outer edge is sharp to allow for atraumatic passage of the needle through the relatively tough dermis and epidermal layers; this minimizes cutting of the skin where suture tension is greatest. A higher grade plastic needle (designated *P* or *PS*) should be used for repairs on the face. A small needle (such as P3) should be used for wounds that require fine cosmesis. Needles come in a variety of sizes such as 3/8 and 1/2 circle. Clinicians may develop a preference for a specific needle. In general, a 3/8 reverse cutting needle satisfies most needs.

GENERAL PRINCIPLES

Perhaps the two most important goals of suturing are to match the layers of the injured tissues and to create eversion of the wound margins so that they will flatten as the wound heals. Layers on one side of a wound should be sutured to the corresponding, matching layers on the other side. First, all layers of skin that have been injured should be identified. Then an attempt to appose each layer (muscles, fascia, subcutaneous tissue, and skin) as nearly as possible back to its original location should be made. This is achieved by carefully matching the depth of the bite taken on each side of the wound when suturing.

Proper *suture placement* should result in slight eversion of the wound so that there is not a depressed scar when remodeling takes place. Eversion may be achieved by slight thumb pressure on the wound edge as the needle is entering the opposite side. Sutures should take equal bites from both wound edges so that one margin does not overlap the opposite margin when the knot is tied. Wound-edge eversion is best achieved by taking proper bites while suturing, not by pulling the knot tightly (Fig. 102.1).

Suture placement may be deep or superficial. Deep sutures reapproximate the dermal layers of skin and do not penetrate

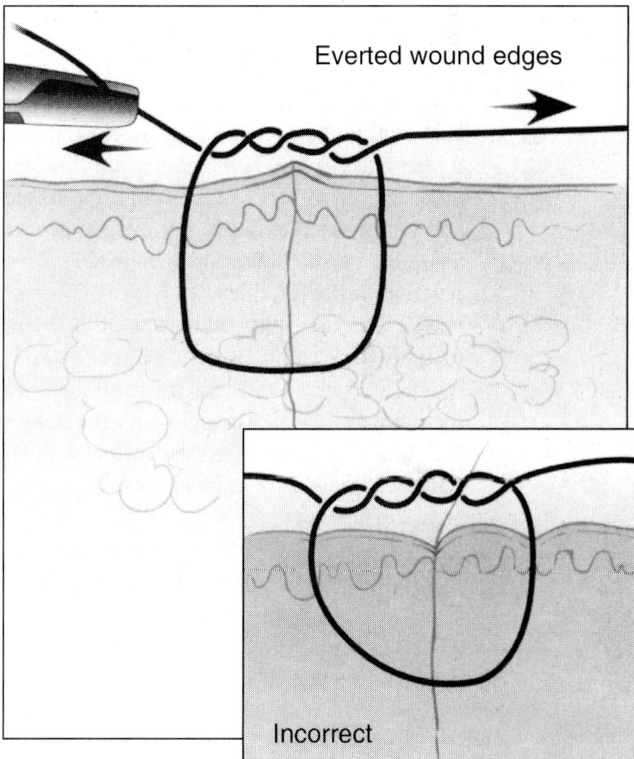

Figure 102.1. Suturing technique for wound-edge eversion.

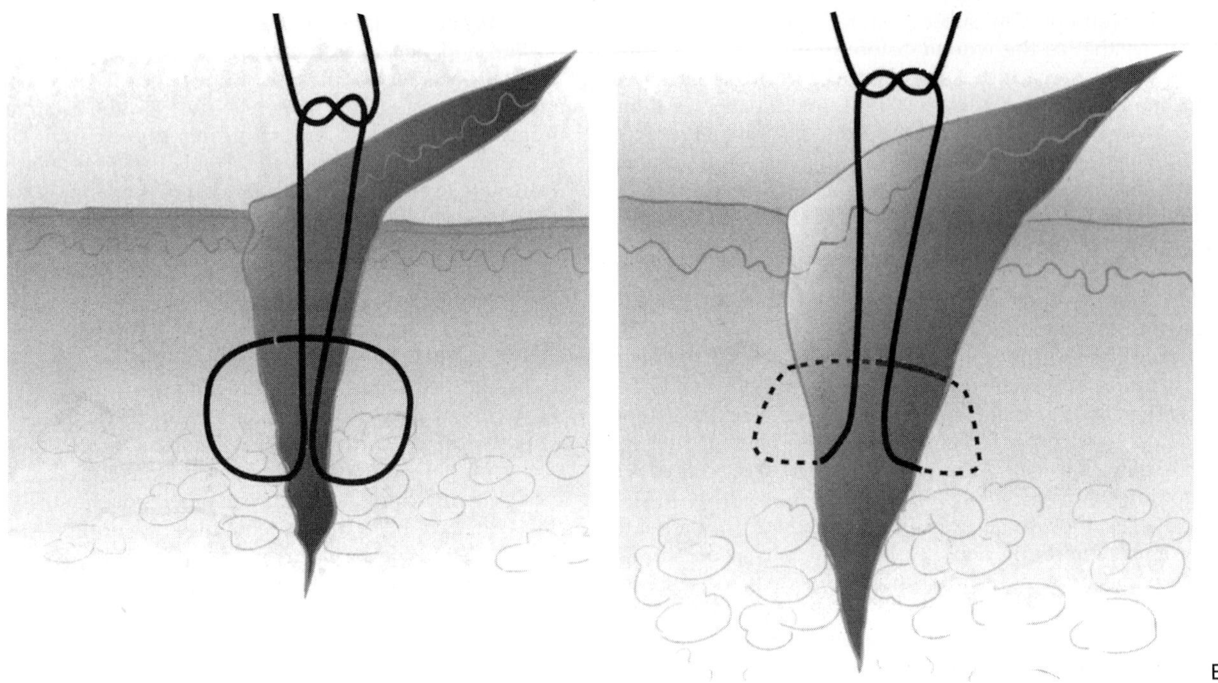

Figure 102.2. **A:** The buried subcutaneous suture. **B:** The horizontal dermal stitch.

the epidermis. They help to relieve skin tension and improve the cosmetic appearance by reducing the width of the scar. They should be avoided in wounds prone to infection because they will further increase the risk of infection. To place a deep suture, the needle is placed at the depth of the wound and removed at a more superficial level. The needle then is inserted superficially into the opposite side of the wound and exits deeply so that the knot is buried within the wound. The needle end and free end of the suture should be on the same side of the loop before the knot is tied (Fig. 102.2). The simple interrupted technique (described next) with absorbable suture material should be used.

Superficial or percutaneous sutures are passed through the dermis and epidermis and leave the knot visible at the skin surface. Skin should be closed with a minimal amount of tension. Sutures should be pulled tightly enough to approximate the wound edges, but not so tightly that they cause tissue necrosis. Sutures that seem well placed initially may begin to cut into the tissue in the next few days because of swelling and inflammation. There is no need to close the skin tightly if other layers have been well sutured. Scalp wounds are an exception. They are under considerable tension, and the knots in this location should be pulled firmly to keep the skin together. The wound will be hidden by hair, and so the skin can be pulled more tightly than elsewhere. Firm, but not strangulating, apposition of the wound will help with hemostasis as well.

To ensure proper alignment, the first suture may be placed at

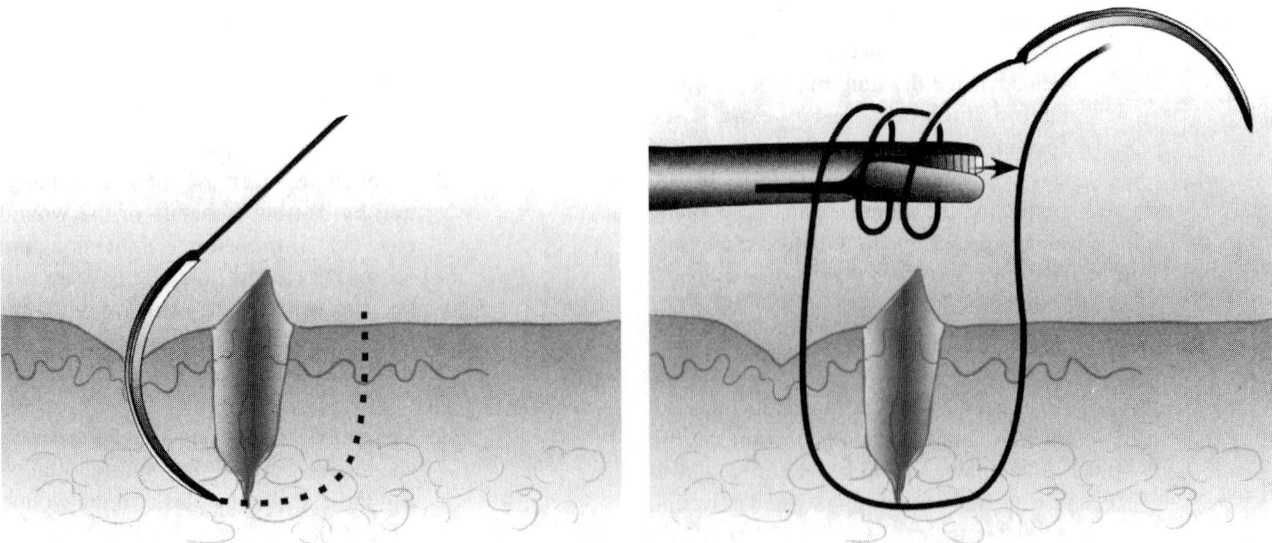

Figure 102.3. Simple interrupted skin suture secured with instrument tie.

the midpoint of the wound, with subsequent sutures then placed in a bisecting fashion lateral to the midpoint. Use of forceps to hold tissue should be encouraged because this allows the operator to pass the needle precisely through the desired points alongside the wound edge. To avoid tissue damage, the use of forceps, however, should be kept to a minimum during the repair.

SUTURE TECHNIQUE

In general, skin wounds can be repaired using interrupted suturing. To place a *simple interrupted suture,* the needle is held upside down and the wrist is pronated as the needle enters the skin at a 90-degree angle. The needle tip then will move farther away from the wound margin and penetrate deeply. Thus, more tissue is at the depth of the wound, which causes the wound to evert. Sutures should be placed about 2 mm apart and 2 mm from the wound edge on delicate areas such as the face. More sutures placed closer together decrease wound tension and leave a less noticeable scar. Larger bites should be used for body parts where cosmesis is less important.

The physician should use an instrument tie to secure the suture (Fig. 102.3). Ideally, the knots should be placed on one side of the wound. Knots placed directly over the wound increase inflammation and scar formation. On the first throw, the physician should wrap the needle holder twice to create a surgeon's knot and then wrap subsequent throws a single time. The first and second throws should be snug enough to approximate the wound edges, but not so tight that tissue is strangulated. All subsequent knots are squared to maintain the closure. Four or five throws are usually required to keep the knot from unraveling. A "loop knot" is effective in apposing the wound edge with minimal tension. This involves placing a surgeon's knot, using the instrument tie, followed by a loop. The surgeon's knot will "give" slightly if edema develops subsequently. The loop knot allows easier, painless removal of sutures because it creates a free space between the suture and the skin (Fig. 102.4).

Running or continuous sutures can be applied rapidly to close large, straight wounds or multiple wounds. With this technique, the suture is not cut and tied with each stitch. The first suture is placed at one end of the wound and a knot is tied, cutting only the end of thread not attached to the needle. The next loop is placed a few millimeters away, and continuous loops of equal bites are made to close the wound. On the final loop, the suture is not pulled through completely so that a small loop remains on the opposite side of the wound. Now the knot can be tied using the previously described loop of suture (Fig. 102.5). This type of stitch is more likely to leave suture marks if not removed in 5 days. Apposition of the edges and eversion are more difficult to achieve with this stitch, and the entire suture line can unravel if the suture breaks anywhere along the repair. This technique, however, gives the advantage of having equal tension on the wound edges.

The *vertical mattress stitch* is useful for deep wounds in which it may be difficult to tie a simple, deep, interrupted suture. It reduces tension on the wound and may close dead space within the wound. It essentially combines a deep and superficial stitch in one suture. The needle is placed deep within the wound (about 3 mm from the wound edge) and brought out to the opposite skin surface. Then it is brought across the epidermis to approximate the epidermal edges (Fig. 102.6). This stitch takes more time to accomplish and produces more cross marks, but it provides excellent wound eversion and apposition of the wound edge. A knot that is too tight will pucker the wound.

The *horizontal mattress stitch* reinforces the subcutaneous tissue and effectively relieves tension from the wound edges. It does not provide wound-edge approximation as well as the ver-

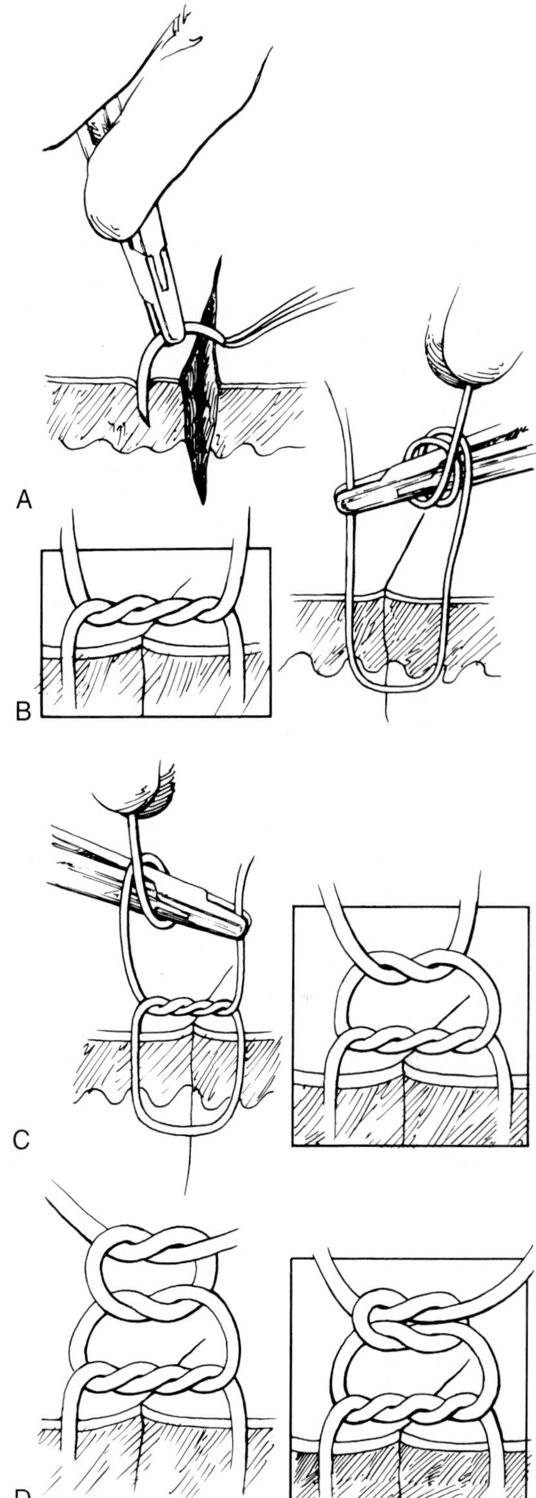

Figure 102.4. Placement of a "loop knot" in conjunction with simple sutures of the skin using an eversion technique. **A:** The needle enters the skin at a right angle in a way that allows somewhat less skin and more subcutaneous tissue to be caught in the passage of the needle. The needle should incorporate the same amount of skin and subcutaneous tissue on each side. The ideal suture material for placing a "loop knot" is 4-0 nylon. One also can use 5-0 nylon. **B:** The first knot should be a surgeon's knot drawn down gently so as barely to coapt the skin edges. **C:** The second tie should be placed so as to produce a square knot but should be drawn so as to produce an approximate 2- to 3-mm loop. **D:** The third tie should be placed so as to produce a square knot. This third tie can be secured tightly against the second tie, preserving the loop and allowing for some loosening of the surgeon's knot spontaneously as later edema develops.

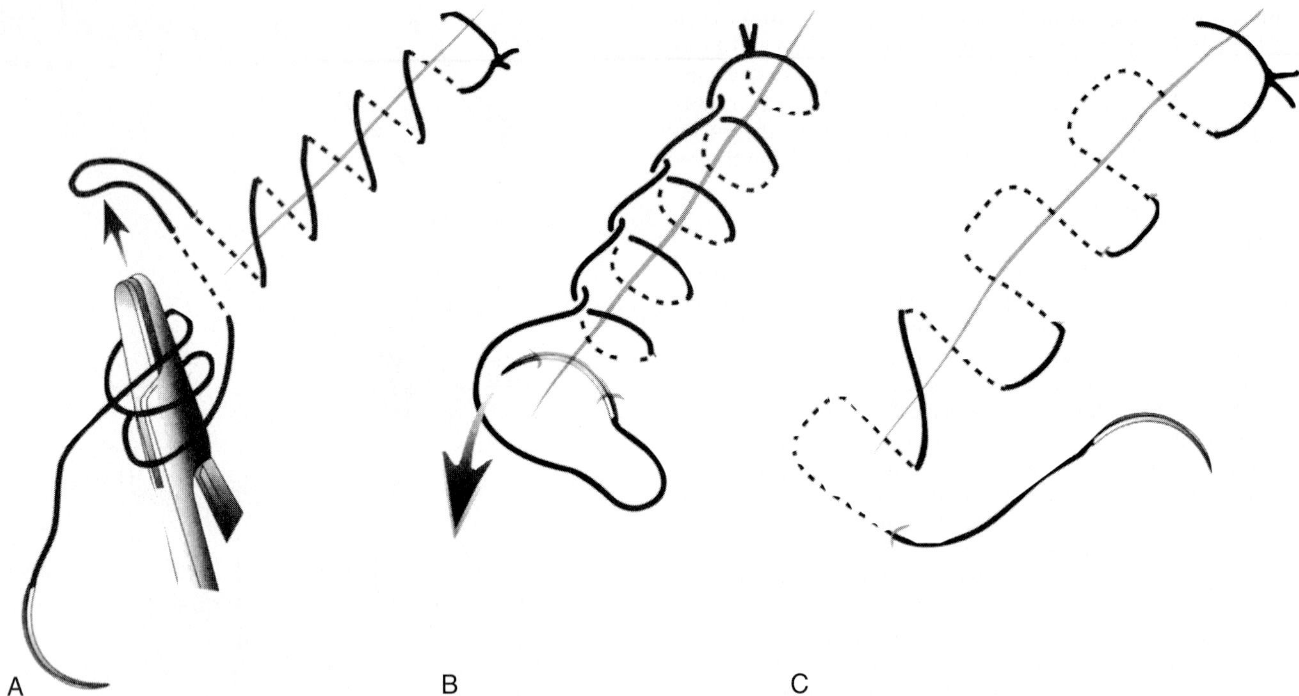

Figure 102.5. Continuous skin sutures. **A:** The simple continuous running stitch. **B:** The continuous interlocking skin stitch. **C:** The running lateral mattress stitch or continuous half-buried horizontal mattress stitch.

tical mattress stitch. The needle is passed to 1 cm away from the wound edge deeply into the wound. Then it is passed through the opposite side and reenters the wound parallel to the initial suture. To avoid "buckling" and to provide some eversion of the wound edges, the skin must be entered perpendicularly, and the wound must be entered and exited at the same depth (Fig. 102.7).

The *modified horizontal mattress stitch* (half-buried) is often used to close a flap. It is also called the *corner stitch*. It relieves intrinsic tension and vascular compromise when approximating the tip of the flap. Using 5-0 or 6-0 nylon, the physician should enter intact skin across from the apex of the flap and exit the wound just below the subcuticular plane. The needle should be brought to the tip of the flap, entering and exiting at the subcuticular plane. Then the needle is brought across the edge of the flap in the subcuticular plane and the skin is exited. A knot should be tied in the usual manner and the tip of the flap brought to the apex of the wound (Fig. 102.8).

Placing the needle in the flap edge first can also repair wounds with flaps. The edge of the flap then can be moved back and forth until proper alignment with the opposite fixed side is obtained. After the tip of the flap is sutured, the sides of the flap are brought together. For wounds with several stellate flaps, subcuticular or subcutaneous sutures should be used to hold the tips of the flap together. Then, a single suture at the tip will provide good apposition without further damaging the tip of the flap. Other interrupted sutures can be placed on the lateral margins of the wound to provide further support. If the wound has many narrow-based stellate flaps or necrotic flap tips, the wound may be better managed with excision and simpler repair (Fig. 102.9).

ALTERNATIVE WOUND-CLOSURE TECHNIQUES

Tape causes no suture marks, minimal tissue reaction, and fewer wound infections than sutures. Tape strips, cut to size, can be used to take up tension at the wound margins and can be placed between sutures. These strips are also useful as the only means to close simple lacerations that barely extend through the dermis. Multiple tangential, triangular skin flaps (eg, those created when an unrestrained passenger hits the windshield of a car) are closed well using tape strips. Likewise, old or contaminated wounds, such as dog bites on the extremities, can be loosely approximated with skin tape.

When tape is used, the wound should be cleansed as any

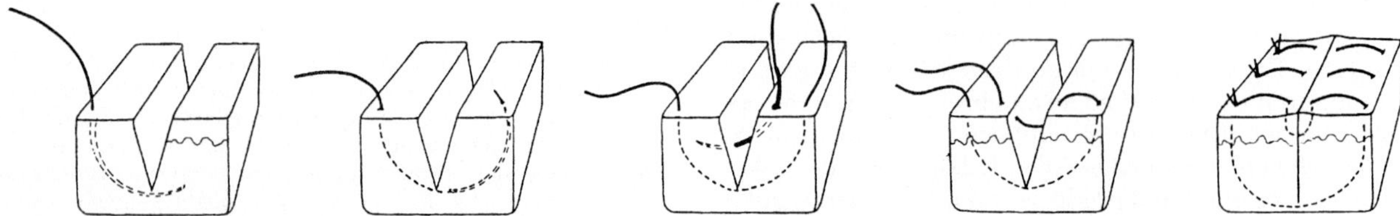

Figure 102.6. The vertical mattress suture. After initially placing a simple interrupted stitch with a somewhat larger bite, make a backhand pass across the wound, taking small, superficial bites. When the knot is tied, the edges of the laceration should evert slightly. (Reprinted from Grisham J. Wound care. In: Dieckmann RA, Fiser DH, Selbst SM, eds. *Illustrated textbook of pediatric emergency and critical care procedures*. St. Louis: Mosby, 1997:665–679, with permission.)

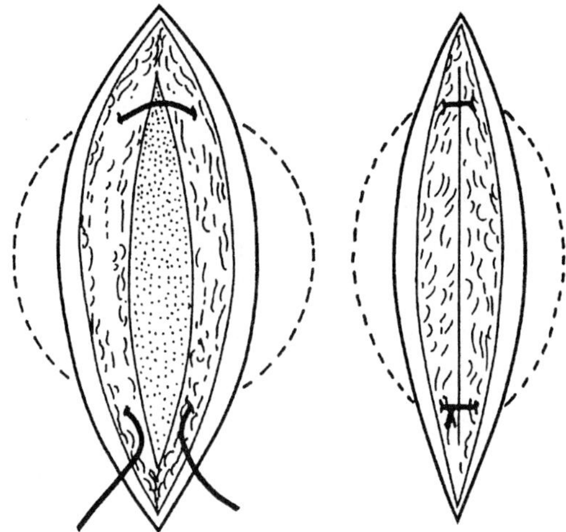

Figure 102.7. The horizontal mattress stitch is useful for closing the deep layer in shallow lacerations and in body areas with little subcutaneous tissue. Certain dyed suture materials may cause a tattooing of the skin if placed in such a shallow position. (Reprinted from Grisham J. Wound care. In: Dieckmann RA, Fiser DH, Selbst SM, eds. *Illustrated textbook of pediatric emergency and critical care procedures*. St. Louis: Mosby, 1997:665–679, with permission.)

other wound. Care must be taken to realign the dermis and epithelium properly. If the tape is pulled too tightly, the margins of the wound may overlap, causing the wound to heal with a raised ridgelike area where the overlap occurred. The tape is applied perpendicularly across the wound with some space between to allow the wound to drain. In some cases, an adhesive such as benzoin is applied to the adjacent skin (not the wound) to keep the tape strips more securely in place. Some researchers recommend leaving the taped wound uncovered because a bandage may increase moisture and cause the tape to fall off prematurely.

Staples can be applied more rapidly than sutures and have a lower rate of infection, with less of a foreign-body reaction. They are best for wounds of the scalp, trunk, and extremities when saving time is important. Therefore, they are particularly helpful when treating mass casualties. Staples are left in place for the same length of time as sutures. They are somewhat more painful to remove and should be removed with a specially designed instrument to avoid tissue damage. Staples do not allow for meticulous cosmetic repair as with sutures. Thus, they should not be used for lacerations of the face, neck, hands, or feet. They should also not be used if the patient requires magnetic resonance imaging (MRI) or computed tomography (CT).

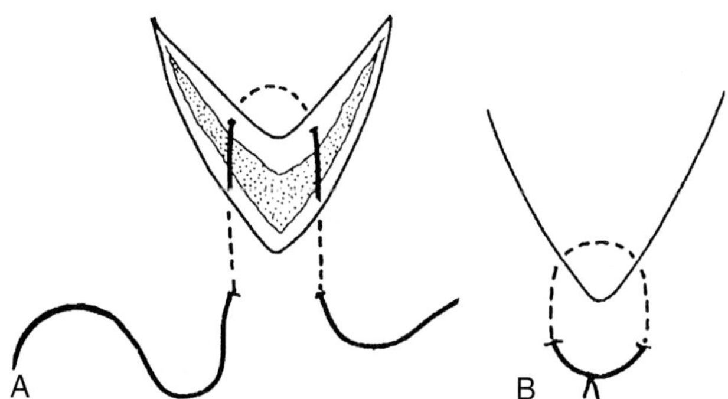

Figure 102.8. A,B: The corner stitch. Also called the *half-buried horizontal mattress stitch,* this technique allows repair of flap-type lacerations without further compromising blood flow. Additional simple interrupted sutures are placed along the sides of the flap if necessary. (Reprinted from Grisham J. Wound care. In: Dieckmann RA, Fiser DH, Selbst SM, eds. *Illustrated textbook of pediatric emergency and critical care procedures*. St. Louis: Mosby, 1997:665–679, with permission.)

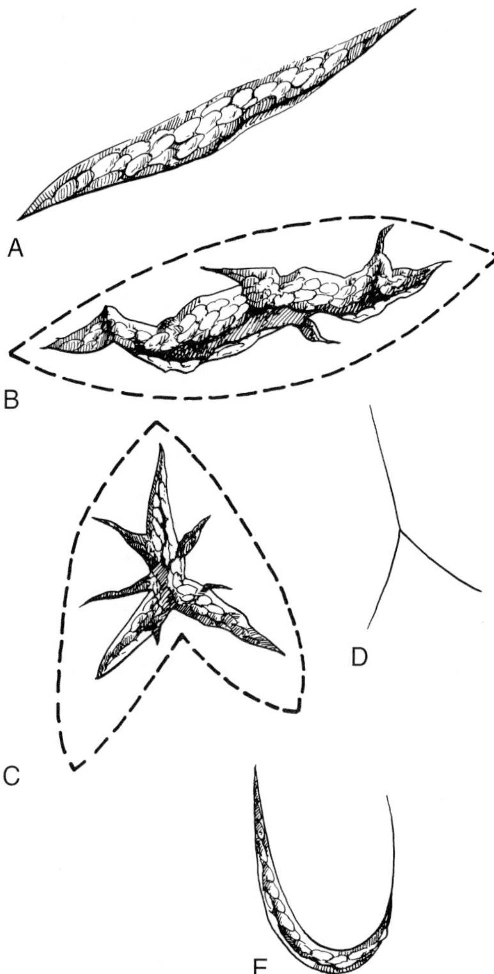

Figure 102.9. Variation in laceration injuries and suggestions for management: simple laceration **(A)**, elliptical excision of damaged wound margins **(B)**, excision and closure of stellate laceration (**C,D**), and flap-type laceration (**E**).

Tissue adhesives, or skin glues, such as cyanoacrylates (Histoacryl Blue) have been approved for use in the United States. Skin glues have been used to close wounds for many years in Europe and Canada. They allow rapid and painless closure of wounds. Anesthesia is unnecessary unless painful irrigation or exploration of the wound is anticipated. No removal is needed because the adhesives slough off after 7 to 10 days. They provide an excellent cosmetic result, comparable to sutures. One study using plastic surgeons blinded to the method of repair graded the wounds repaired with Histoacryl Blue to be cosmetically equal to sutured wounds at 2-month and 1-year follow-up visits.

Tissue adhesives act to decrease wound infections because they have antimicrobial effects against gram-positive organisms. Dehiscence rates (1–3%) are similar to those of sutured wounds. They are less expensive than sutures because little equipment is needed and personnel time is reduced. Studies have noted that patients and families of small children prefer them to sutures. Routine follow-up is not needed for uncomplicated wounds, and no long-term complications have been reported.

TABLE 102.1. Common Techniques of Wound Closure

Technique	Advantages	Disadvantages
Sutures	Greatest tensile strength Meticulous closure Low dehiscence rate	Painful Removal needed Slow application Increased tissue reaction Risk of needle stick (clinician)
Staples	Rapid application Low cost Low tissue reaction	Not for use on face (less meticulous closure)
Tissue adhesive	Rapid application Painless No removal needed Low cost No risk of needle stick (clinician)	Lower tensile strength Not for use on joints
Tape strips	Rapid application Painless Low cost Low infection risk Least tissue reaction	High risk of dehiscence Not for use in moist areas, young children

Before application of the tissue adhesive, the wound is cleaned and hemostasis achieved with dry gauze and pressure. The wound's edges are held together manually or with forceps while the tissue adhesive is applied drop-wise along the surface of the wound. The tissue adhesive should not be applied to the inside of the wound because it will act as a foreign body and inhibit healing. The wound is then held in place for about 20 to 30 additional seconds to obtain adequate bonding. One study reported that if malalignment is noted, the adhesive can be removed with forceps and reapplied without further complication. The wound is covered carefully so that bandage removal will not pull off the tissue adhesive.

Table 102.1 summarizes the advantages and disadvantages of several techniques available for wound closure.

Dressings

Dressings protect the wound from further injury and contamination. They also help to absorb secretions (not likely with small wounds) and immobilize the injured part. Some use a nonadherent sterile dressing (eg, Telfa, Xeroform) to cover the wound. This prevents the wound edges from sticking to the dressing. Then a second layer of absorbent gauze is applied, and a third layer of gauze wrap or tape is used to stabilize the other two. This protects and immobilizes the area while absorbing exudate from the wound surface.

For most simple wounds, it is adequate to cover the wound with dry sterile gauze after applying topical antibacterial ointment. Some studies indicate that topical antibiotic ointments may reduce infection and prevent scab formation by lubricating the wound edges. This allows for more rapid epithelialization of the wound.

For the face and trunk, a large bulky dressing is not practical. Thus, for small wounds in those areas, a clear plastic adhesive such as Tegaderm should be used to secure the bandage. Rolls of cotton or stretchable tube gauze can be used for larger wounds to keep the sterile dressing in place. This keeps the young child from touching the wound. Scalp wounds are usually not dressed. Patients can generally wash their hair gently after 24 hours.

For children who are active, it may be best to keep the wound covered until sutures are removed. The dressing should remain in place for 24 to 48 hours, after which epithelialization is usually sufficient to keep the wound from gross contamination. Then the bandage should be changed daily and the wound inspected. Any dressing should be changed if it becomes soiled, wet, or saturated with drainage because the wet dressing may be a source of infection.

It may be advisable to splint the wound if it overlies a joint. This is most important for active children, who are likely to resume full activity soon after the injury. Some even recommend splinting nearby joints for any large laceration of an extremity to reduce stress across the wound, even if it does not involve a joint itself. This should be done for no more than 72 hours to facilitate function. The injured extremity should be elevated to provide comfort and reduce edema.

Systemic Antibiotics

Use of prophylactic systemic antibiotics for wound management is controversial. Studies demonstrating proven benefit to use of antibiotics are lacking. They may lead to allergic reactions, growth of resistant organisms, and unnecessary expense. Thus, they are not recommended for routine use. Decontamination with proper irrigation is more efficacious than use of antibiotics to prevent wound infection. Antibiotics should be considered for heavily contaminated wounds that are at greater risk for infection. They are often used for human and cat bites (see Chapter 80), crush injuries, stellate lacerations, and very long wounds (>5 cm). Other high-risk wounds include intraoral lacerations and wounds of the hands, feet, and perineum. Similarly, open fractures, exposed joints and tendons, and any tetanus-prone wound may benefit from antibiotics. Likewise, wounds that result in exposed cartilage of the nose or ears or extensive facial wounds that may involve contamination from adjacent nasal passages are often treated with antibiotics. It may also be reasonable to use antibiotics for wounds (other than scalp lesions) when repair takes place more than 12 hours after injury. They may be justified for wounds that occurred in a contaminated environment, such as a farm or roadside. Injured immunocompromised patients may warrant antibiotics.

Usually a first-generation cephalosporin or a penicillinase-resistant penicillin is used to cover staphylococci and streptococci. Amoxicillin–clavulanic acid is recommended for wounds created by mammalian bites (see Chapter 80). Additional coverage for gram-negative organisms with an aminoglycoside may be worthwhile for heavily contaminated open fractures.

TABLE 102.2. Tetanus Prophylaxis

Prior tetanus toxoid immunization (doses)	Clean minor wound	All other wounds
Uncertain (or <3)	DTP or Td	DTP or Td and TIG or TAT
Three or more (most recent >10 yr ago)	Td	Td
Three or more (most recent within past 5 yr)	None	None
Three or more (most recent between 5 and 10 yr)	None	Td

DTP, diphtheria, tetanus, pertussis toxoid; Td, adult formulation of diphtheria, tetanus toxoid; TIG, tetanus immunoglobulin (dose: 250–500 U i.m.); TAT, tetanus antitoxin; should be used only if TIG is not available and after testing (dose: 3000–5,000 U i.m.); i.m., intramuscularly.

TETANUS

Immunization status of all injured patients should be documented in the medical record. If the wound is clean and minor and the patient has received three previous doses of tetanus toxoid, a booster of tetanus toxoid is given only if 10 or more years have passed since the last dose. If a patient has received three or more previous tetanus immunizations but the wound is not a clean, minor laceration, tetanus toxoid is indicated if the last dose was more than 5 years ago.

In many cases, the tetanus immunization record is unknown. If tetanus status is unknown and the wound is not clean or minor, tetanus toxoid and tetanus immunoglobulin (TIG) are indicated. Wounds involving massive tissue destruction and contamination also may require TIG. Patients with such wounds should be admitted to the hospital (Table 102.2).

Discharge Instructions and Suture Removal

Careful discharge instructions regarding wound care, covering the wound, when to get the wound wet, how to dry it, and so on, are extremely important. The family should be warned about signs of infection. Specifically, they should be told to return for medical care if the wound develops increasing pain, redness, edema, or wound discharge, or if the child develops a fever. Analgesics may be given for minor pain, but worsening pain should always prompt a wound check. The family should be informed that the wound was inspected for a foreign body but that there is still a possibility of a retained foreign body or an undetected injury that may require further treatment. Parents should be told that no matter how skillful the operator, every laceration leaves some scar. The appearance of the scar will change during the next several months, and the scar's appearance will not be complete for about 6 to 12 months. Patients and parents should be advised to keep the injured part elevated when possible. A sling can be provided to accomplish elevation of the upper extremities. Some recommend that healing skin not be exposed to sunlight for 6 months after injury because this could lead to permanent hyperpigmentation.

Follow-up care should be arranged for 24 to 48 hours in all but very simple wounds. The wound then can be reinspected for signs of infection, and healing can be assessed.

Wounds closed with tape strips do not require removal of the tape because these will fall off spontaneously. Skin glue also sloughs spontaneously. Nonabsorbable sutures, however, should be removed at the appropriate time, depending on the location of the injury. The importance of timely removal should be stressed to the patient and family. Sutures should be removed when fibroblastic proliferation at the wound interface is strong enough to take the place of sutures. Removing sutures too early may lead to dehiscence and widening of the scar. Sutures left in too long may create an unnecessary tissue reaction and result in visible cross-hatching ("railroad ties").

Wounds on the scalp or face are nourished by a better blood supply and generally exhibit more rapid healing. Sutures in these areas are removed more quickly than other locations to avoid unsightly tracts. When sutures are subject to considerable tension (over joints and on the hands), they should be left in longer (Table 102.3). After removal of sutures, it is often necessary to reinforce the healing wound with tape strips to prevent dehiscence.

In the first 24 to 48 hours, wound dressings should be changed only if wet or soiled. After that, bathing can be permitted as long as the wound is then patted dry and covered again. There is no proven harm to exposing the sutures to soap and water for short periods.

Table 102.4 summarizes an approach to reduce risk in managing wounds in the ED.

TABLE 102.3. Timely Suture Removal

Wound location	Time of removal (days)
Neck	3–4
Face, scalp	5
Upper extremities, trunk	7–10
Lower extremities	8–10
Joint surface	10–14

TABLE 102.4. Reducing Risk in Wound Management

1. Take thorough history.
2. Perform a careful examination.
3. Obtain a consult for complex wounds.
4. Obtain radiographs if foreign body or fracture is suspected.
5. Document carefully (inspection, irrigation, and function).
6. Communicate with parents (likely scar).
7. Arrange follow-up, recheck.

SECTION V

Surgical Emergencies

CHAPTER 103

Abdominal Emergencies

Louise Schnaufer, M.D. and
Soroosh Mahboubi, M.D.

The abdominal surgical problems most commonly found in infants and children are discussed in this chapter under the following categories: (1) diseases that produce peritoneal irritation; (2) acute intestinal obstruction; (3) chronic, partial intestinal obstruction; (4) diseases that produce rectal bleeding; (5) intraabdominal masses; (6) abdominal wall defects; and (7) foreign bodies of the gastrointestinal (GI) tract. Nonsurgical GI emergencies are covered in Chapter 82. Chapter 95 deals with major trauma to the abdominal contents. Chapter 42 reviews the diagnostic approach to the child with abdominal pain.

When the history, physical examination, and laboratory data are all available, the emergency physician must synthesize them into an overall assessment. If the physical findings are reproducible and consistent in location and character, an accurate diagnosis can often be made and appropriate treatments started. If the findings are both worrisome and equivocal, and do not fit into a comprehensive picture, the patient should be admitted for observation and reassessment. The following sections detail the cardinal symptoms and signs of the common acute surgical problems in children. Initial emergency department (ED) management is discussed, but in all cases of presumed surgical disease, the definitive treatment requires consultation with a surgeon.

DISEASES THAT PRODUCE PERITONEAL IRRITATION

The physician must perform a careful examination to elicit accurate signs of peritonitis. Tenderness is not necessarily an indication of an intraabdominal surgical problem in a child. A child with localized peritonitis may have only minimal findings, while a patient with a nonsurgical condition may have severe pain and generalized tenderness. For example, on examination, a child with severe colic caused by gastroenteritis may appear to have genuine peritoneal signs. In fact, such a child may have only exaggerated voluntary guarding of the abdominal wall, mimicking the true rigidity of peritonitis.

The well-known features of peritonitis—rigidity, spasm, involuntary guarding, and rebound—are as valid for a child as they are for an adult. In a child with abdominal pain, however, one has to be patient and gentle enough in the initial phases of the examination so that signs of peritonitis can be checked repeatedly without breaking rapport with the child. Reproducible anterior peritoneal tenderness in the same location is much more suggestive of peritonitis than deep abdominal tenderness that shifts in location with each reexamination of the child.

Acute Nonperforated Appendicitis

BACKGROUND

Acute appendicitis is one of the most common abdominal surgical conditions seen by the emergency physician or surgeon who cares for children. It occurs in all age groups and is particularly difficult to diagnose in its early states and in infants and toddlers. The emergency physician must accurately evaluate the child and promptly consult a surgeon when the diagnosis is clear or when appendicitis cannot be safely ruled out. Such consultation is especially urgent in younger children, in whom perforation can occur within 8 to 24 hours of the onset of symptoms.

CLINICAL MANIFESTATIONS

Usually the child with appendicitis complains initially of poorly defined and poorly localized midabdominal or periumbilical pain. Unfortunately, this symptom is common to many other intraabdominal, nonsurgical problems. In the young and, to a lesser extent, the older child, vomiting and a low-grade fever often occur soon thereafter. Characteristically, the pain then migrates to the right lower quadrant (Table 103.1).

Because the position of the appendix may vary in children, the localization of the pain and the tenderness on examination may also vary. An appendix that is located in the lateral gutter may produce flank pain and lateral abdominal tenderness; an inflamed appendix pointing toward the left lower quadrant may produce hypogastric tenderness. An inflamed, low-lying, pelvic appendix may not cause pain at McBurney's point but instead may cause diarrhea from direct irritation of the sigmoid colon. Often, the child with appendicitis is anorexic, suggesting the presence of nausea even if he or she is unable to verbalize this complaint. Because motion aggravates peritoneal irritation, a child with appendicitis typically prefers to lie still or, when moving, splints toward the painful area.

On examination, palpation is usually reliable in demonstrating focal peritoneal signs at the site of the inflamed appendix. If the appendix is in the pelvis or retrocecal area, however, typical anterior peritoneal signs may be absent. The physician can confirm his or her impression of point tenderness by pressing gen-

TABLE 103.1. Progression of Symptoms and Signs of Appendicitis

Nonperforated appendicitis
Poorly defined midabdominal or periumbilical pain
Low-grade fever
Anorexia
Vomiting (rare in older child)
Pain in right lower quadrant
  Localization depends on position of appendix
    Appendix in gutter → lateral abdominal tenderness
    Appendix pointing toward pelvis → tenderness near pubis may cause diarrhea
    Retrocecal appendix → tenderness elicited by deep palpation
Pain on coughing or hopping on right foot
Rectal examination: pain on palpation of right rectal wall
WBC count: 11,000–15,000/mm^3
Urinalysis: ketosis
Perforated appendix
Increasing signs of toxicity
  Rigid abdomen with extreme tenderness
  Absent bowel sounds
  Dyspnea and grunting; tachycardia
  Fever: 39°–41°C (102.2°–105.8°F)
  WBC count: >15,000/mm^3 with shift to left
  Eventual overwhelming sepsis and shock

WBC, white blood cell.

tly in each quadrant and asking the child to indicate which area is most tender. When the inflamed appendix is not close to the anterior abdominal wall, as in the case of retrocecal appendix, tenderness may be more impressive on deep palpation of the abdomen or by palpating in the flank. This impression of focal tenderness can sometimes be confirmed by shaking the child's abdomen or getting him or her to cough, which often produces a wince of pain at the involved area. Finally, a well-done rectal examination may make the difference between deciding to operate or observe the child. The examining finger should be inserted as fully as possible without touching the area of presumed tenderness. Then, when the child is relaxed and taking deep breaths, the examiner can gently stroke or indent an area high on the right rectal wall. A sudden involuntary reaction of pain confirms the presence of inflammation. In a child with a history of probable appendicitis for more than 2 or 3 days, a boggy, full mass may also be in this location, suggesting an abscess.

A complete blood count (CBC) in a child with appendicitis usually shows an elevated white blood cell (WBC) count in the range of 11000 to 15000 per mm^3 in the first 12 to 24 hours of the illness. As the appendix becomes more gangrenous, the WBC count rises further, and the differential demonstrates more and more neutrophils and an increasing number of bands. Urinalysis often shows ketosis. If the inflamed appendix lies over the ureter or adjacent to the bladder, a few WBCs may be found in the urinary sediment. The presence of numerous WBCs and bacteria on a freshly spun specimen may indicate an acute urinary tract infection. However, a child with a chronic urinary tract infection may also develop appendicitis.

If the clinical and laboratory diagnosis of acute appendicitis is convincing, no further studies are indicated.

As far as the abdominal roentgenogram is concerned, many consider it a peripheral study valid only for the demonstration of a fecalith or free air. Abdominal roentgenograms are normal in many cases of acute appendicitis. In 8% to 10% of cases, however, a calcified appendiceal fecalith can be identified on abdominal roentgenograms. Because the incidence of subsequent appendicitis with perforation is significant, it has been suggested that prophylactic appendectomy be performed on the asymptomatic child in whom a calcified fecalith is detected.

Most children with an acute nonperforated appendix show diminished air in the GI tract. This is a result of anorexia, nausea, vomiting, and diarrhea. Other roentgenographic signs of appendicitis are thickening of the cecal wall and mucosal folds with air–fluid level, indistinct psoas margins with scoliosis concave toward the right, focal obliteration of the adjacent properitoneal fat pad, or presence of air in the appendix. However, a retrocecal appendix may be filled with gas in the normal child. Ileus secondary to peritoneal irritation or an inflamed appendix crossing the terminal ileum may be seen. Rarely, a perforated appendix may produce pneumoperitoneum.

Barium enema in the diagnosis of appendicitis is no longer used because in 8% to 10% of normal children, barium does not fill the appendix. However, partial or nonfilling of the appendix with local impression on the cecum or terminal ileum, or associated with other evidence of a pelvic or right lower quadrant mass, is indicative of appendicitis. In a child with leukemia, a tender right lower quadrant mass may indicate typhlitis, an inflammatory reaction of the cecum. Differentiation of typhlitis and an appendiceal abscess in a child with leukemia, therefore, may be difficult. Today, for evaluation of uncertain appendicitis Doppler ultrasound or computed tomography (CT) is preferred.

Routine chest radiographs are not indicated unless the patient has a history of pulmonary problems, such as asthma, or unless the symptoms and signs indicate atypical right abdominal pain with splinting respirations. A chest radiograph in such a case may reveal subtle evidence of a right lower lobe pneumonia. With good hydration, these subtle findings on radiograph may develop into an early visible infiltrate in a few hours.

Unfortunately, laboratory findings do not differentiate mesenteric adenitis, which closely mimics acute appendicitis. A complete approach to the child with abdominal pain is covered in Chapter 42.

MANAGEMENT

The preoperative preparation of a patient with acute appendicitis should include blood urea nitrogen (BUN) and electrolytes if the patient has been vomiting or has had poor fluid intake for more than a few hours. If an unexpected anemia is discovered on the CBC, a cross-match should also be done. Intravenous (i.v.) fluids should be started, with emphasis on replacing the child's deficits as quickly as possible. Protracted GI losses, as with vomiting, may lead to potassium depletion. Therefore, the initial i.v. fluids should contain at least 0.5 n saline with 10 mEq of potassium chloride per 500 mL During this period, the patient and the family should be psychologically prepared for surgery.

The emergency physician must keep in mind the many variations in the way appendicitis can present. As a good rule of thumb, a patient should at least be admitted for observation if there are positive findings in two of the three classic modes of assessment: history, physical examination, or laboratory.

Perforated Appendicitis

Ideally, once the diagnosis of appendicitis is considered seriously, the patient will have surgery before the appendix has perforated. Unfortunately, some patients, particularly younger children and infants, may arrive for emergency care with an already perforated appendix because of a delay in seeking treatment or in making the diagnosis. Once the appendix has perforated, there are usually signs of generalized, rather than localized, peritonitis. In a young child, the omentum is flimsy and often incapable of walling off the inflamed appendix. As a result, perforation occurs more quickly, and secondary dissemination of the infection occurs more widely. Although the mortality from appendicitis has decreased, the incidence of perforation in children has remained the same over the last several decades.

CLINICAL MANIFESTATIONS

Within a few hours after perforation has occurred, the child begins to develop increasing signs of toxicity. First, the lower abdomen and then the entire abdomen becomes rigid with extreme tenderness. Bowel sounds are sparse to absent. In addition, there are signs of prostration such as pale color, dyspnea, grunting, significant tachycardia, and higher fever (39° to 41°C [102.2°to 105.8°F]). Rarely, the patient may develop septic shock (see Chapter 3) from the overwhelming infection caused by bowel flora.

Initially, the findings may be confused with those of pneumonia because the extreme abdominal pain may cause rapid shallow respirations and decreased air entry to the lower lung fields. There is impaired excursion of the diaphragm and respiratory failure in some cases. In infants and toddlers, the findings may also be confused with meningitis because any movement of the child (even flexion of the neck) produces pain and irritability. The high fever and other signs of prostration may be indications for a lumbar puncture. After the spinal fluid analysis is found to be normal, the suspicion of perforated appendicitis may be heightened.

The laboratory findings in the child with perforated appendicitis often suggest this diagnosis. The WBC count is significantly elevated, usually above 15000 per mm^3, with a marked shift to left; leukopenia may be seen when perforation has resulted in overwhelming sepsis and septic shock.

The radiologic evaluation of suspected perforated appendicitis should include both plain abdominal radiographs and pelvic ultrasound. The plain film of the abdomen may show free air or evidence of peritonitis. The ultrasound of the pelvis may show a complex mass with or without a calcified fecalith or free fluid within the abdominal cavity.

MANAGEMENT

Initially, the focus of therapy should be on resuscitation. There must be careful attention to airway, breathing, and circulation (see Chapter 1). The severely septic child may need positive-pressure ventilation with high concentrations of oxygen to overcome ventilatory insufficiency. Hypovolemia should be corrected with 5% dextrose in either normal saline or Ringer lactate solution. An alternative volume expander is 5% albumin solution in normal saline. An initial bolus starting at 20 mL per kg is given over 30 minutes or less until vital signs are restored and the patient produces urine. Metabolic acidosis should be treated with sodium bicarbonate, the dose being determined by the results of the serum electrolytes or, more precisely, the base deficit from an arterial blood gas.

Hypovolemia and acidosis must be treated vigorously until adequate circulation has been reestablished, as measured by the strength of the pulse, blood pressure, skin perfusion, capillary refill in the extremities, and urine output. If it is difficult to reestablish an adequate circulation, a central venous pressure catheter may be helpful in determining the amount of volume needed. Once adequate circulation has been attained, much of the acidosis may correct spontaneously as homeostatic mechanisms are restored.

Additional steps in the management include treatment of infection and further preparation of the patient for surgery. The child should receive broad-spectrum antibiotics (eg, ampicillin 200 mg per kg per day, gentamicin 6 to 7.5 mg per kg per day, and clindamycin 25 mg per kg per day) for additional anaerobic coverage. Once the emergency physician is certain that the airway can be controlled and the circulation is adequate, relief of pain can be accomplished by using narcotic agents (eg, morphine 0.1 mg per kg). The patient's fever can usually be controlled by the use of a hypothermia mattress and/or acetaminophen (10 mg per kg per dose rectally). A nasogastric tube should be placed to evacuate the contents of the stomach and to drain ongoing gastric secretions. Several units of blood or packed red cells must be prepared for the operative procedure.

Children with perforated appendicitis can deteriorate quickly. Moreover, the fever, often 40°C (104°F) or higher, may not be controlled until the intraabdominal infection is drained. Therefore, emergency resuscitation should be quickly followed by operative intervention. At surgery the appendix is removed, the area is drained, and other appropriate treatments are given. The child will recover more rapidly if this approach is taken than if prolonged medical management is instituted and surgery delayed. Rarely, the abscess may be drained with the expectation that an appendectomy will be performed later.

Meckel Diverticulitis with and without Perforation

Most patients with a Meckel diverticulum are asymptomatic or, if symptomatic, have rectal bleeding from ulceration at the junction of the ectopic gastric mucosa and the normal ileal mucosa, where the diverticulum is attached. A preoperative diagnosis of an inflamed or a perforated Meckel diverticulum is rarely made but, nevertheless, should be considered in the differential diagnosis of a perforated viscus leading to generalized peritonitis. The diagnosis is usually made in the operating room by the surgeon who finds a normal appendix, and then an exploration of the bowel finds a diseased diverticulum 20 to 25 cm of the ileocecal valve.

Primary Peritonitis

Primary peritonitis is a bacterial infection of the peritoneal cavity, usually secondary to a bloodborne or lymphborne infection. Although rare, it can occur in children with nephrosis or cirrhosis, ascites, or other etiology, and may mimic appendicitis. Primary peritonitis is usually caused by pneumococcus, group A streptococcus, or Gram-negative organisms. When peritonitis is a Gram-negative infection, the portal of entry is often the vagina. This occurs in girls from 5 to 10 years old in whom the cervix is usually open and the vaginal fluid is not yet acidic enough to retard the ascent of infection.

If the diagnosis is suspected before surgery, the patient should undergo paracentesis. The diagnosis may be confirmed by a Gram stain showing Gram-positive cocci, followed by a positive culture. It is important to remember that children with nephrosis or cirrhosis may have appendicitis unrelated to their underlying disease.

Pancreatitis

Although acute pancreatitis is common in adults, it occurs rarely in children. The most common cause is abdominal trauma. Pancreatitis produces upper abdominal or periumbilical pain, often radiating to the back. Occasionally, the presentation is that of a patient in shock. Findings that support the diagnosis include paralytic ileus, distension, and ascites. Serum or urine amylase is usually elevated. When severe, the serum calcium is also decreased. When pancreatitis occurs in a child without a history of trauma, the physician should evaluate the patient for possible congenital abnormalities of the biliary tree or pancreatic ducts, such as abnormal insertion of the main pancreatic duct or the presence of a choledochal cyst. Surgical intervention is rarely indicated in the acute phase. However, active surgical consultation from the beginning is essential, in case the patient deteriorates in spite of maximal medical therapy (see Chapter 82). Signs of deterioration or nonresponse to therapy include persistently low serum calcium, a falling hematocrit, increasing toxicity, and deterioration of the patient's coagulation profile.

ACUTE INTESTINAL OBSTRUCTION

In any child who vomits persistently, particularly if the vomitus becomes stained with bile, the diagnosis of acute intestinal obstruction must be considered. If the obstruction is high in the intestinal tract, the abdomen does not become distended; however, with lower intestinal obstruction there is generalized distension and diffuse tenderness, usually without signs of peritoneal irritation. Only if the bowel perforates or vascular insufficiency occurs will signs of peritoneal irritation be found. If complete obstruction persists, bowel habits may change, leading to complete obstipation of both flatus and stool. All patients with suspected bowel obstruction should have radiographs of the abdomen in supine, upright, and prone cross-table lateral views. In patients with acute mechanical bowel obstruction, multiple dilated loops are usually seen. Fluid levels produced by the layering of air and intestinal contents are seen in upright or lateral decubitus radiographs.

Intussusception

BACKGROUND

Intussusception occurs when one segment of bowel telescopes into a more distal segment. This is the leading cause of acute intestinal obstruction in infants and occurs most commonly between 3 and 12 months of age. The most common intussusception is ileocolic but the small bowel may intussuscept into itself. Often, it will be ileoileal at a location close to the cecum. Typically, this small bowel intussusception then prolapses through the ileocecal valve (Fig. 103.1). The intussusception continues through the colon at a variable distance, occasionally as far as the rectum, where it can be palpated on rectal examination. Colocolic intussusceptions are very rare. In infants the lead point for the intussusception may be hypertrophied Peyer patches. In children older than 2 years of age, a specific lead point, such as a polyp, a Meckel diverticulum, a duplication, or a tumor, is much more likely. A diarrheal illness, viral syndrome, or Henoch-Schönlein purpura may be a preceding illness several days to a week before the onset of abdominal pain and obstruction.

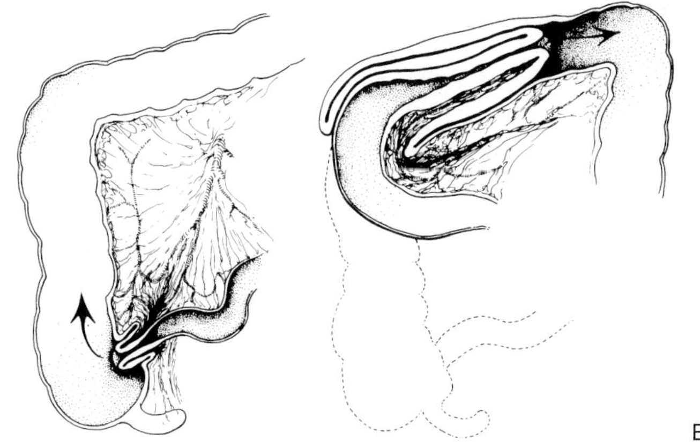

Figure 103.1. Ileocolic intussusception. **A:** Beginning of an intussusception in which terminal ileum prolapses through ileocecal valve. **B:** Ileocolic intussusceptum continuing through the colon. This can often be palpated as a mass in the right upper quadrant.

CLINICAL MANIFESTATIONS

The main manifestation of intussusception is crampy abdominal pain. This symptom may have been preceded by the symptoms and signs of a viral gastroenteritis or even an upper respiratory infection. Gradually, the child becomes more irritable and anorectic and may vomit. The pattern of pain in a child with an intussusception is often consistent and characteristic, and the diagnosis is suggested strongly if a history of episodic pain is obtained. The pain may cause the infant to cry out with intermittent spasms, but the child then appears to be perfectly comfortable or only slightly irritable between these episodes. More often, lethargy is a typical sign that occurs between the episodes of pain. The infant may become still and pale and exhibit an almost shocklike state because of the intense visceral pain. At times, patients with intussusception have been misdiagnosed as being in the postictal state.

The localized portion of the intussusception leads to either partial or complete obstruction and generalized abdominal distension. In some cases, the intussuscepted mass can be palpated as an ill-defined sausage-shaped structure if the abdomen is not too distended. This mass is most often palpable in the right upper quadrant.

As the bowel becomes more tightly intussuscepted, the mesenteric veins become compressed, while the mesenteric arterial supply remains intact. This leads to the production of the characteristic currant jelly stool, which may be passed spontaneously or found on the rectal examination. However, development of melena may occur fairly quickly, and this fact reinforces the need for a rectal examination in a child with unexplained abdominal symptoms. Once the intussusception has become tight, even the arteries are occluded by the pressure of entrapment. At this point, the bleeding lessens, but the bowel can become gangrenous and even perforate, leading to peritonitis.

MANAGEMENT

The patient should be prepared by inserting an i.v. line and a nasogastric tube. Intravenous fluids should be given to correct dehydration. Nasogastric suction minimizes the risk of vomiting and aspiration. Once blood has been sent to the laboratory for CBC, BUN, serum electrolytes, and a cross-match, the patient should be taken to the radiology department.

Plain film roentgenographic findings of intussusception are variable and depend primarily on the duration of the symptoms and the presence or absence of complications. In early cases, a normal gas pattern is seen. In the patient with symptoms longer than 6 to 12 hours, flat and upright films often show signs of intestinal obstruction, including distended bowel with air–fluid levels. Occasionally, the actual head of the intussusception can be seen on a plain film as a soft-tissue mass. If the plain film shows the presence of feces in the right colon, it is likely that the child has intussusception.

In recent years, hydrostatically controlled barium enema reduction has been a successful therapy in more than 50% of cases. Strict guidelines must be adhered to so that perforation is avoided when this method is attempted. The barium column should be no higher than 3 feet above the abdomen, and manual palpation of the abdomen during the study is contraindicated. Often an i.v. dose of morphine 0.1 mg per kg or the use of another sedative is helpful to relax the child during the study or if there is difficulty in accomplishing the reduction. The full reduction of the intussusception is confirmed only when there has been adequate reflux of barium into the ileum. Otherwise, only the ileocolic component of an ileocolic intussusception may be reduced, leaving the ileoileal intussusception unreduced. A 24-hour follow-up film should be taken to determine whether the intussusception has recurred.

Recent series have described reduction of intussusception by air insufflation rather than barium. This may be a safer method because if a perforation is present the peritoneal cavity is not contaminated with barium. Many pediatric radiology departments in the United States are now evaluating this method of air reduction.

Many youngsters with intussusception require emergency surgery, especially if the intussusception has been of long duration or the child shows evidence of gangrenous bowel, including high fever, leukocytosis, significant distension, and general toxicity. If a barium enema seems safe and appropriate, the operating room should be placed on standby and the operating team should be ready to commence immediate surgery if complications develop or if the hydrostatic reduction by barium enema is unsuccessful. Preoperative preparation and resuscitation begins in the ED and continues during the course of the barium enema. Undue delay may well result in gangrene of the entrapped bowel. The moment surgery is decided on, the patient should receive broad-spectrum i.v. antibiotics.

The recurrence rate after barium enema reduction ranges from 1% to 3%. When there is a recurrence, a second attempt at reduction may be done by barium enema. This is usually successful in most cases, but with a third episode of intussusception, an exploratory laparotomy must be done. Recurrences are more common in older children and may be caused by a lead point such as a Meckel diverticulum, an intestinal polyp, or an intraluminal tumor such as lymphoma. Therefore, it may be wise in an older child to operate with the first recurrence.

Incarcerated Inguinal Hernia

Incarcerated inguinal hernia is a common cause of intestinal obstruction in the infant and young child. Approximately 60% of incarcerated hernias occur during the first year of life. Incarceration occurs more often in girls than in boys but usually involves the ovary rather than the intestine. Often, the patient or family has no previous knowledge of the presence of a congenital hernia. Incarceration does not necessarily mean that the nonreducible portion of intestine is compromised or gangrenous. However, strangulation can occur within 24 hours of a nonreduced incarcerated hernia because of progressive edema of the bowel caused by venous and lymphatic obstruction. This obstruction then leads to occlusion of the arterial supply with resulting necrosis of the bowel and perhaps perforation.

The clinical presentation of a child with an incarcerated hernia is usually irritability, crying because of pain, vomiting, and occasionally abdominal distension. A firm, discrete mass can be palpated at the internal ring and may or may not extend into the scrotum. Occasionally, the testicle may appear dark blue because of pressure on the spermatic cord causing venous congestion, and in a prolonged incarceration, the testicle may be infarcted. Intestinal obstruction may develop quickly and an abdominal radiograph shows gas-filled loops of intestine in the scrotum.

Unless the child is extremely ill with signs of intestinal obstruction or toxic from gangrenous bowel, a manual reduction of the incarcerated hernia should be attempted. The child should be sedated with morphine 0.1 mg per kg i.v. The mother should then cuddle the baby until it relaxes and falls asleep. An older child may be placed in the Trendelenburg position to allow gravity to facilitate the reduction. Once the child is asleep, gentle manipulation of the incarcerated mass should be attempted. Mild pressure should be exerted at the internal ring with one hand, while the other attempts to squeeze gas or fluid out of the incarcerated bowel back into the abdominal cavity. If the reduction is unsuccessful, the child should be taken immediately to the operating room. After the hernia has been reduced manually, the child may be admitted for observation but not immediate repair. Rarely should a child be sent home after a manual reduction unless the parents are properly informed concerning signs of recurrence or intestinal obstruction and they are thoroughly reliable (see "Inguinal Hernias and Hydroceles" later in this chapter).

Incarcerated Umbilical Hernia

Incarceration of an umbilical hernia is rare. If present, there is a persistent and tender bulge in the umbilical hernia sac. If the incarceration is of short duration, a gentle effort might be made to reduce it manually, but it often is necessary to prepare the child for urgent surgery. At the time of surgery, the loop of incarcerated bowel should be inspected, rather than letting it drop back into the abdominal cavity, to be certain there has been no vascular impairment (see "Umbilical Hernias" p. 560).

Malrotation of the Bowel with Volvulus

BACKGROUND

Malrotation of the bowel is a congenital condition associated with abnormal fixation of the mesentery of the bowel (Fig. 103.2). Therefore, the bowel has a proclivity to volvulize and obstruct at these points of abnormal fixation. Although malrotation with volvulus usually occurs either *in utero* or during early neonatal life, malrotation can be unrecognized until childhood. This is an extraordinarily dangerous situation because a complete volvulus of the bowel for more than an hour or two can totally obstruct blood supply to the bowel, leading to complete necrosis of the involved segment. When a volvulus involves the midgut, the entire small bowel and ascending colon may be lost, making the patient dependent on i.v. hyperalimentation for survival. The only way to prevent such a catastrophe is to have a high index of suspicion for malrotation in any child with signs of obstruction and to be prepared to get a child with a presumed volvulus to the operating room immediately.

CLINICAL MANIFESTATIONS

Any child with bile-stained vomiting and abdominal pain may have malrotation with volvulus. The pain is usually constant and not crampy. Blood may appear in the stool within a few hours and suggests the development of ischemia and possible necrosis of the bowel. Clinically, malrotation can present in several different ways: first, and most dangerous, is the sudden onset of abdominal pain with bilious vomiting with no prior history of GI problems; a second is a similar abrupt onset of obstruction in a child who previously seemed to have "feeding problems" with transient episodes of bilious vomiting; third is a child with failure to thrive because of alleged intolerance of feedings. This last example may involve a child who has been fed a dozen different formulas and in whom the vomiting is chronic and generally not associated with pain.

On physical examination, there may be only mild distension of the abdomen inasmuch as the obstruction usually occurs high in the GI tract. On palpation, the physician may discern one or two prominently dilated loops of bowel. The abdomen may be diffusely tender and yet not have clear signs of peritonitis. On rectal examination, the presence of blood on the examining fin-

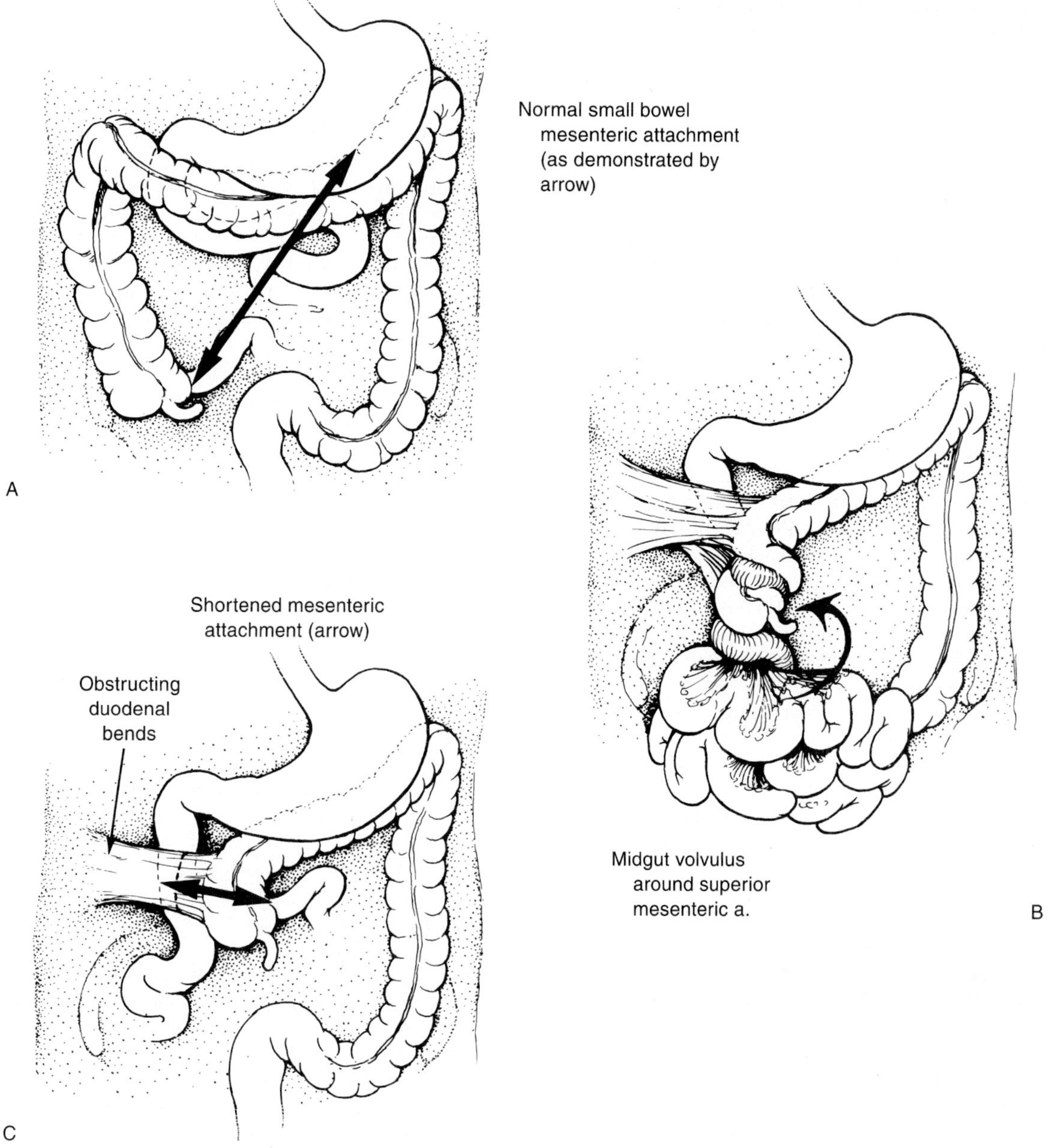

Figure 103.2. Malrotation with volvulus. **A:** Normal small bowel mesenteric attachment (as demonstrated by the *arrow*). This prevents twisting of small bowel because of the broad fixation of the mesentery. **B:** Malrotation of colon with obstructing duodenal bands. **C:** Midgut volvulus around the superior mesenteric artery caused by the narrow base of the mesentery.

ger is an alarming sign of impending ischemia and gangrene of the bowel.

MANAGEMENT

The key to management is to be suspicious of malrotation and to obtain flat and upright roentgenograms of the abdomen immediately. The presence of loops of small bowel overriding the liver shadow is suggestive of an underlying malrotation. When complete volvulus has occurred, there may be only a few dilated loops of bowel with air–fluid levels. Distal to the volvulus there may be little or no gas in the GI tract. A "double-bubble sign" is often present on an upright film because of partial obstruction of the duodenum causing distension of the stomach and first part of the duodenum.

When a child is being assessed for possible malrotation, an upper GI series is the study of choice. The ligament of Treitz is absent in the malrotation anomaly, so the C-loop of the duodenum is not present, the duodenum lies to the right of the spine, and the jejunum presents a coiled spring appearance in the right upper quadrant. The cecum is not fixed and usually assumes a position in the right upper quadrant. However, because of its mobility, the cecum on barium enema may be seen in its normal position in the right lower quadrant. Therefore, a barium enema is not the most reliable study to rule out malrotation. In the neonate, the cecum sometimes takes a high position and this could give a false impression of malrotation.

As in the case of a child with an unreduced intussusception, a child with a possible volvulus should be prepared for immediate surgery. The operating room and operating team should be on standby. Intravenous fluid and electrolyte replacement should begin immediately. A nasogastric tube should be inserted and blood cross-matched. Because this entity can present even in adulthood, every physician should understand the pathogenesis and the need for surgical therapy of malrotation. If immediate transfer to a children's hospital cannot be accomplished within an hour, a laparotomy should be performed without delay.

Pyloric Stenosis

Narrowing of the pyloric canal as a result of hypertrophy of the musculature often occurs in the first-born boy of a family. A familial incidence has been shown, particularly if the mother had hypertrophic pyloric stenosis as an infant. There is a male:female ratio of 5:1. The age of onset is usually 2 to 5 weeks. Rarely, the onset may be late in the second month of life. The cause of the muscle hypertrophy is unknown, but the symptoms, diagnosis, and therapy are well defined.

CLINICAL MANIFESTATIONS

Characteristically, the infant does well, without vomiting, for the first few weeks of life and then starts regurgitating, either at the end of feedings or a few minutes later. The infant is hungry and will eat heartily immediately after such a regurgitation. The vomiting becomes more prominent and eventually becomes more forceful; what is known as projectile vomiting. The vomitus ordinarily contains just the feeding that has been given and does not contain bile or blood. Occasionally, some mucus is in the vomitus. Infants with pyloric stenosis may also become jaundiced with the onset of the other symptoms. The hyperbilirubinemia usually improves or abates postoperatively for reasons that are unknown.

The examination of an infant is best accomplished after the infant's stomach has been emptied. With the child lying on his or her back, the examiner holds the infant's ankles and flexes the thighs at a right angle to the trunk as the mother feeds some warm sugar water with the infant's head turned to the right but not elevated. Once the infant starts to suck, the upper abdominal musculature will relax and the examiner's opposite hand can then gently palpate the upper right abdomen. Palpating under the edge of the liver in an up-and-down direction, the physician may discern a firm, fusiform, ballotable mass in the shape of an olive. If this "olive" is not felt, the stomach can be emptied with a nasogastric tube to allow easier palpation and the examination is repeated. Another diagnostic clue is the presence of prominent gastric peristaltic waves that course from left to right across the abdomen.

Serum electrolytes may be abnormal because of gastric losses. The potassium and chloride are low, and serum bicarbonate is high. This hypochloremic alkalosis may be profound with serum chlorides in the 65 to 75 mEq per L range. When dehydration becomes severe, the patient may then develop acidosis, indicating an advanced and even more dangerous metabolic imbalance (see Chapter 76).

MANAGEMENT

Infants should be hospitalized and rehydrated with appropriate fluid and electrolyte replacement. Initially, i.v. fluids should be 5% dextrose in normal saline. Potassium chloride (3 to 5 mEq per kg) should be added once urine output has been established. If hypotonic solutions are used, there is significant risk of causing hyponatremia (see Chapter 76). A volume of fluid should be used appropriate to the patient's level of dehydration.

If a pyloric "olive" or mass is palpable and clear gastric waves are visible, roentgenogram confirmation of the diagnosis is not needed. If the history of vomiting is not typical and a mass cannot be felt, real-time ultrasound is the first study to confirm the diagnosis. The real-time ultrasound scanning not only increases the accuracy of the diagnosis of pyloric stenosis but can also localize the "olive." The hypertrophic pyloric muscle is seen as a thick hypoechoic ring surrounding a central echogenic mucosal and submucosal region. The quantitative criteria for the sonographic diagnosis of hypertrophic pyloric stenosis are 1.4 cm or longer length of the pyloric canal with 0.3 cm or greater thickness of the circular muscle.

If the ultrasound study does not show a hypertrophic pylorus, an upper GI series should then be done to eliminate gastroesophageal reflux, malrotation, and antral web as diagnostic possibilities. In general, pyloric stenosis can be identified by the presence of a "string sign" in the pyloric channel, seen best on oblique projections on the upper GI series.

POSTOPERATIVE ADHESIONS

Prior abdominal surgery or peritonitis places a child at risk for intestinal obstruction from adhesions. Such obstruction can occur relatively early in the postoperative course or months or even years later. Suddenly and without warning, the child develops abdominal cramps, nausea, vomiting, and abdominal distension. Although most intestinal obstructions from adhesions do not jeopardize the vascularity of the bowel, occasionally a loop of intestine, caught under a fibrous band, can become gangrenous. Therefore, the diagnosis should be made quickly. All such patients need to be admitted to the hospital and evaluated by a surgeon who should direct the complete management.

CHRONIC PARTIAL INTESTINAL OBSTRUCTION

Any child with intermittent abdominal distension, nausea, anorexia, occasional vomiting, or chronic constipation or obstipation may have partial intestinal obstruction. A number of diagnostic considerations exist.

Chronic Constipation

Chronic constipation is probably one of the most common causes for abdominal pain, distension, and vomiting in children. The history, if available from a reliable parent, may attest to chronic constipation; however, occasionally, such a child is diagnosed only by palpating a large fecaloma through the intact abdominal wall or a hard fecal mass blocking the anal outlet on rectal examination. Such youngsters may have a history of encopresis and appear malnourished. Chapter 10 covers the diagnostic approach to the child with constipation.

These children should be disimpacted by instilling a generous amount of warm mineral oil into the rectum, followed by copious saline lavages using a large-caliber rectal tube with extra holes. Often, a gloved finger is necessary to break up a hard fecal mass and allow its evacuation.

Aganglionic Megacolon (Hirschsprung Disease)

In patients with Hirschsprung disease, the parasympathetic ganglion cells of Auerbach's plexus between the circular and longitudinal muscle layers of the colon are absent. The involved segment varies in length, from less than 1 cm to involvement of the entire colon and small bowel. The effect of this absence of ganglion cells produces spasm and abnormal motility of that segment, which results in either complete intestinal obstruction or chronic constipation.

These children have a lifelong history of constipation, so it is important to obtain an accurate account of the child's stool pattern from birth. A child with Hirschsprung disease typically has never been able to stool properly without assistance (eg, enemas, suppositories, stimulation with the finger or thermometer). Normal stooling is not possible because of the failure of the aganglionic bowel and interval anal sphincter to relax. The child usually has no history of encopresis, as one would find in chronic functional constipation. These youngsters have chronic abdominal distension and are often malnourished. Vomiting is uncommon, as are other symptoms. Complete intestinal obstruction in Hirschsprung disease is more likely to occur in early infancy and only rarely in the older age groups. Table 103.2 summarizes the pertinent diagnostic features differentiating functional constipation from Hirschsprung disease.

After flat and upright abdominal roentgenogram radiographic studies have been obtained, a properly performed barium enema with a Hirschsprung catheter is the best initial diagnostic procedure. There should be no preparation of the bowel. Ideally, the rectum should not be stimulated by enemas or digital examination for 1 to 2 days before the procedure. The key to diagnosis is seeing a "transition zone" between the contracted aganglionic bowel and the proximal dilated ganglionated bowel. Stimulation of the rectum shortly before the study may result in decompression of the proximal bowel, with loss of definition of the transition zone. When a clear-cut transition zone is seen, it is not necessary to fill the colon with barium more than 12 to 18 inches above the transition point. It is important, however, not to empty the colon of barium at the end of the study. The presence of retained barium above the transition point 24 hours later strongly suggests the diagnosis of Hirschsprung disease.

Anorectal manometry to determine the presence or absence of relaxation of the internal anal sphincter is helpful in establishing the neurogenic dysfunction of the bowel. Barium enema studies and manometry are clearly complementary in the diagnosis of Hirschsprung disease. However, rectal manometric studies are more reliable than radiologic methods for short aganglionic segments that are usually not apparent on barium enema studies. Manometric studies are not dependable in infants less than 3 weeks of age. If the barium enema and anal manometry studies indicate Hirschsprung disease, rectal biopsy is not necessary to confirm the diagnosis.

In children of all ages, an adequately performed suction mucosal biopsy of the rectum 2 cm or more above the dentate line can be reliable in diagnosing Hirschsprung disease. Because of the complicated evaluation and management of this disease, referral to a pediatric surgeon is recommended.

Duplications

Duplications occur anywhere from the mouth to the anus and produce a variety of symptoms. In the abdomen, there may be a noncommunicating cyst that gradually fills up with secretions and compresses the adjacent normal bowel, producing a palpable abdominal mass or chronic intestinal obstruction. An occasional duplication has a communication, particularly at its distal end, that produces a large mass that may be confused with the fecal mass felt with aganglionic Hirschsprung disease. Rarely, a marginal ulcer resulting from ectopic gastric mucosa may occur, and this produces painless bleeding. After appropriate radiographic diagnosis, surgery is indicated; the surgical procedures vary, depending on the locations, size, and communications of the anomaly.

Inflammatory Bowel Disease

The older child or adolescent may develop either Crohn disease or ulcerative colitis (see Chapter 82), and this must be included in the differential diagnosis of chronic intestinal obstruction. Usually, the child has a history of changing bowel habits, with mucus or blood in the stools, chronic abdominal pain, and weight loss. Chapter 82 covers inflammatory bowel disease in detail.

DISEASES THAT PRODUCE RECTAL BLEEDING

Rectal bleeding is an alarming symptom. It is important to determine the quantity of bleeding and whether the blood is on the outside of the stool or mingled with it. A "tarry" stool suggests a source of bleeding in the proximal portion of the GI tract and bright red blood a more distal origin (Fig. 103.3). Occasionally, the child will have an episode or two of blood with his bowel movements. All patients with rectal bleeding should have a rectal examination. Those with significant hemorrhage require flexible colonoscopy and a contrast enema. In some patients, no definite diagnosis may be reached despite extensive studies. In any patient with significant bleeding, however, surgical consultation is indicated. Chapters 23 and 82 further discuss the diagnosis and management of patients with GI bleeding.

Fissures

An anal fissure is probably the most common cause of bleeding, especially in infants. However, fissures may occur at any age. The child usually has a history of passing a large, hard stool with anal discomfort. Often, the child has a history of chronic constipation with progressive reluctance to pass stool because of the associated discomfort. If bleeding occurs, it usually involves streaking of bright red blood on the outside of the stool, or red blood on the toilet tissues. The diagnosis can easily be made by inspection or anoscopic examination.

TABLE 103.2. Differential Diagnosis of Functional Constipation and Hirschsprung Disease

	Functional constipation	Hirschsprung disease
Onset	>2 yrs	Birth
History	Coercive training	Enemas necessary
	Colicky abdominal pain	No abdominal pain
	Periodic volume stools	Episodes of intestinal obstruction
Encopresis	Present	Absent
Abdominal distension	Absent or minimal	Present
Rectal examination	Feces-packed rectum	Empty rectum
Barium examination	Dilated rectum	Narrow segment
Motility	Normal	Abnormal
Biopsy	Ganglion cells	No ganglion cells

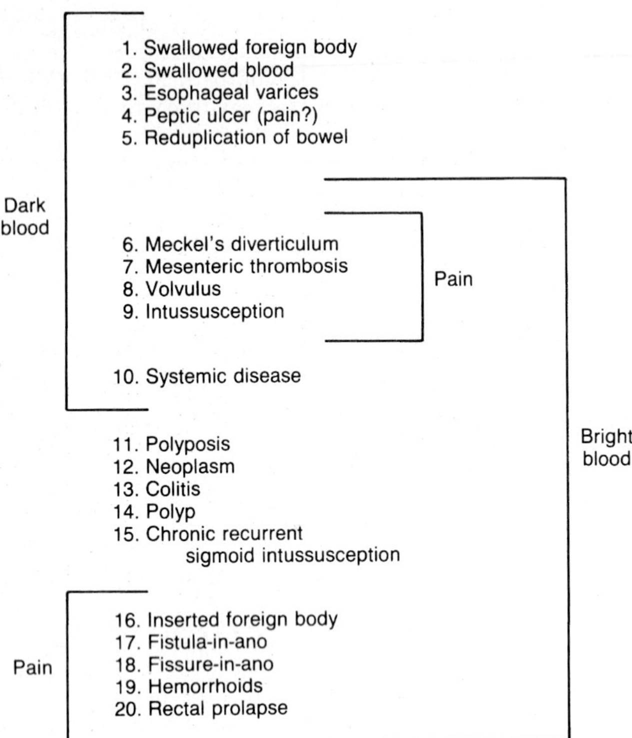

Figure 103.3. Causes of rectal bleeding in children.

Juvenile Polyps

Older infants and children can develop either single or multiple retention polyps. Usually, the polyps occur in the lower portion of the colon and can often be palpated on rectal examination. Polyps bleed, but they rarely cause massive hemorrhage. They may intermittently prolapse at the anus or on occasion come free and be passed as a fecal mass associated with bleeding. Colonic polyps may be lead points for intussusception. Usually, however, polyps are asymptomatic except for the associated bleeding. These are not premalignant lesions, and they tend to be self-limiting.

Familial Polyposis

Families with multiple adenomatous colonic polyps are rarely encountered. Bleeding is rare. More often, a colitis type of mucous discharge is present. Rectal examination and endoscopy reveal multiple "cobblestone" sessile polyps. These individuals are at risk for neoplasia because these are premalignant adenomatous polyps. The child should be referred to a pediatric surgeon and gastroenterologist for evaluation and long-term management.

Meckel Diverticulum

Two percent of the population is born with a Meckel diverticulum. This is the most common omphalomesenteric duct remnant. The diverticulum is usually located 50 to 75 cm proximal to the terminal ileum. Only 2% of persons with a Meckel diverticulum manifest any clinical problems. The most common complication of a Meckel diverticulum is a bleeding ulcer. Ectopic gastric mucosa in such patients is usually present in the diverticulum. The acid secretion produces an erosion at the junction of the normal ileal mucosa with the ectopic mucosa. Currant jelly stools are supposed to be classic for this type of bleeding, but it can be severe at times. Other modes of presentation include diverticulitis, perforation with peritonitis, or intussusception as a result of the diverticulum serving as a lead point.

Barium studies usually fail to outline a Meckel diverticulum. The imaging modality of choice for detection of ectopic gastric mucosa in a bleeding Meckel diverticulum is nuclear scintigraphy. A well-defined focal accumulation of radionuclide (99m-technetium pertechnetate) usually appears at or about the same time as activity in the stomach and gradually increases in intensity. A duplication cyst with gastric mucosa shows the same focal accumulation of radionuclide. Preoperative differentiation between two lesions as a cause of GI bleeding is not important. The accuracy of scintigraphy in detection of ectopic gastric mucosa in Meckel diverticula is approximately 95%. False-negative results may rarely occur in patients with rapidly bleeding Meckel diverticula and with those diverticula that do not contain gastric mucosa.

Henoch-Schönlein Purpura

Henoch-Schönlein purpura (see Chapter 77) is a vasculitic disorder that can produce asymptomatic rectal bleeding or abdominal pain and hematuria. Usually there is visible evidence of vasculitis on the skin surface, but a patient initially may have only abdominal pain. Occasionally, a child will develop a small bowel intussusception from a submucosal hemorrhage that is acting as a lead point. Other common manifestations are purpuric rash, fever, and joint pain (see Chapter 77).

Other Causes of Rectal Bleeding

Other causes of rectal bleeding include intestinal vascular malformations, intussusception, duplications, inflammatory bowel disease, peptic ulcer with bleeding, and portal hypertension with bleeding varices. These topics are covered elsewhere in this chapter, in Chapter 82, and in Chapter 23.

INTRAABDOMINAL MASSES

Background

Intraabdominal masses in children may be benign, but unfortunately, there are also a number of malignant ones. Abdominal masses may be silent, even after the tumor has reached a large size.

Initial evaluation in the ED may include flat and upright abdominal films. If, after such an examination, the origin of the mass is unclear or suggests a neoplasm, the patient should be admitted and a workup done without delay. Observation has no place in dealing with unexplained abdominal masses in children. The role of diagnostic imaging is to identify the precise anatomic location and extent of the pathologic process with a minimal number of procedures. It should be stressed that ultrasonography, nuclear scintigraphy, CT, and magnetic resonance imaging (MRI) have dramatically changed the traditional approach to pediatric imaging. The general location of a mass, with or without calcification, can be confirmed by plain abdominal roentgenograms. Real-time ultrasonography has become increasingly important initial imaging because it does not use radiation and yet is diagnostically accurate. Ultrasonography can differentiate a cystic flank mass that could be a hydronephrotic kidney from a solid tumor such as an adrenal neuroblastoma and thus facilitate the proper referral of the child to either a urologist or a pediatric surgeon. CT is superior to other modalities for anatomic detail and obtains an entire anatomic section of tissue, which aids in determining the precise extent of disease. CT provides anatomic and physiologic information about organs and vascular structures despite overlying gas and bones. Nuclear scintigraphy has a limited role in the evaluation of pediatric abdominal masses. Renal scintigraphy is superior to excretory urography for quantitating renal function. Angiography is indicated for an abdominal mass only if a precise knowledge of segmental vascular anatomy is required or if interventional techniques are contemplated.

Excretory urography has traditionally been the radiologic choice for abdominal masses in children. However, ultrasound and CT have forced reassessment of this classic approach. In approaching abdominal masses in infants and children, the plain film with either real-time ultrasonography and excretory urography or CT can define the origin of abdominal masses.

Sacrococcygeal Teratoma

The presacral sacrococcygeal teratoma is the most common tumor of the caudal region in children and is more common in girls than in boys (4:1). Most tumors are benign and are noted at birth. However, tumors in patients beyond neonatal age have a higher incidence of malignancy. Radiography shows a soft-tissue mass that arises from the ventral surface of the coccyx. Calcifications are present in 60% of presacral sacrococcygeal teratoma and are more common in benign tumors. Ultrasound confirms whether presacral sacrococcygeal teratomas are cystic, solid, or mixed. Tumors with more solid components are more often malignant than those with more cystic components.

Nonmalignant Intraabdominal Masses

FECALOMA

A lower abdominal mass, particularly one on the left side, is most often related to retained stool and is more often associated with chronic functional constipation than with Hirschsprung disease. If a mass is found, a careful review of the bowel habits is important. If an abdominal mass is a fecaloma, a large bolus of stool usually can be felt on rectal examination just inside the anus.

OVARIAN MASSES

Simple ovarian cysts and solid teratomas are not uncommon and may be asymptomatic even though they have reached a large size. Occasionally, the child presents with urinary complaints from the pressure on the bladder or urethra. Granulosa cell tumors of the ovary produce precocious puberty because they are hormonally active tumors. They may be malignant. The sudden onset of severe abdominal pain may indicate a torsion of an ovarian mass on a slender pedicle, with resultant infarction. Granulosa cell tumors tend to give the impression of rising up from the pelvis and on occasion lie in the midabdomen or even the upper abdomen. When they are still partially within the pelvis, they usually can be felt by rectal examination. Most ovarian masses are smooth and nontender. Radiographs may show calcification in about half of patients with teratomas. Because an occasional ovarian tumor is malignant in children, children with ovarian masses should be promptly evaluated and prepared for surgery (see Chapter 83).

OMENTAL CYSTS

Omental cysts are rare, are usually asymptomatic, and can reach gigantic size. It is often difficult to differentiate an omental cyst from ascites. There are a number of cases on record in which omental cysts have been tapped, on the assumption that they were ascitic fluid. Smaller cysts are more mobile and can be pushed freely into all quadrants of the abdomen. If a cyst volvulizes on its pedicle or has bleeding within it, it may cause abdominal pain or tenderness. Elective surgical excision is indicated.

MESENTERIC CYSTS

Mesenteric cysts can occur anywhere in the mesentery but are most common in the mesentery of the colon. They tend to be multilocular and are often discovered during a routine examination or after an episode of abdominal trauma with enlargement from bleeding. They are benign, but surgical therapy is indicated, both to confirm the diagnosis and to prevent complications. They can usually be removed with sparing of the bowel, or they can be marsupialized into the general peritoneal cavity where the fluid is absorbed.

DUPLICATIONS

GI duplications within the abdomen can occur anywhere along the greater curvature of the stomach, the lesser curvature of the duodenum, or the mesenteric side of either the small or large intestines. They can also be pararectal, rising up out of the pelvis. Duplications that produce abdominal masses are either noncommunicating, and hence gradually enlarge, or communicating in that their secretory lining has a distal communication with the true lumen of the bowel. Except for the rare occurrence of massive rectal bleeding in a child with a communicating duplication, most duplications do not present as emergencies. Instead, they present in children either as unexplained abdominal masses or with symptoms of intermittent colic, resulting from partial obstruction of the true lumen of the adjacent bowel. The exact diagnosis is often unclear until the time of laparotomy.

Malignant Intraabdominal Masses

About 50% of the solid malignant tumors seen in children occur within the abdominal cavity. They generally occur in the retroperitoneum. The most common is neuroblastoma, followed by Wilms tumor and rhabdomyosarcoma. Other unusual tumors, such as embryonal cell carcinomas (yolk sac tumor) and lymphosarcoma, also occur in young children. Chapter 89 covers oncologic emergencies. As with most malignant tumors, early diagnosis and treatment provide the best prospects for a cure. Therefore, the physician must have a high index of suspicion for malignancy in any child with a mass or unexplained GI or genitourinary symptoms.

NEUROBLASTOMA

Neuroblastoma most often occurs as a tumor in the left or right adrenal gland, but it can develop anywhere along the sympathetic chain or in the pelvis. It has even been found intrarenally. It has the ability to grow extensively, often crossing the midline of the abdomen, and enveloping key vascular and visceral structures. The best cure rates are generally in children who are less than 1 year of age at the time of diagnosis and in whom the tumor is still localized to the point of origin. In such favorable cases, the tumor can be totally excised. When widespread dissemination occurs, complete resection is unwarranted because of the risk to other vital structures.

CT is superior to ultrasonography for clearly defining morphologic details of neuroblastoma, such as calcifications, and precise extent of tumor by direct spread or lymphatic metastasis. CT with contrast enhancement demonstrates precise anatomy, as well as renal function and organ vascularity. The CT characteristics of neuroblastoma include irregular shape, irregular margins, lack of well-defined capsules, and mixed low-density center. Neuroblastoma often displaces surrounding organs and encases vessels. Prevertebral midline extension is common. There are calcifications in at least 75%. Ultrasonography has limitations in accurately determining tumor margins or local extension. Therefore, CT is the modality of choice for imaging neuroblastoma.

WILMS TUMOR

Wilms tumor is the most common intrarenal tumor seen in children. Great progress has been made in the last several decades in its management. The tumor can reach a gigantic size before its discovery. Wilms tumor should be considered in any child who has hematuria even if he or she has a history of trauma.

A solid renal mass demonstrated by ultrasound in infants and children is usually a Wilms tumor. Because of the high frequency of tumor extension into the renal veins and inferior vena cava, these vascular structures should be examined by real-time ultrasound. Venous extension is diagnosed when echogenic filling defects are identified within a renal vein, the inferior vena cava, or the right heart. Because Wilms tumors are usually large and expansive, the inferior vena cava often is extrinsically displaced by the tumor mass. CT with bolus contrast enhancement may be required for confirmation of equivocal invasion in a patient suspected of having Wilms tumor. After abdominal real-time ultrasound, excretory urography should be performed to evaluate the function of the kidneys. Angiography seldom provides additional diagnostic information. CT defines the presence of an intrarenal mass and extent of tumor, visualizes vascular structures, identifies nodal involvement, defines internal hemorrhage and necrosis, evaluates the presence or absence of liver metastases, and images the opposite kidney. Also, CT can define whether a tumor is initially nonresectable or bilateral. CT may be extremely helpful in following the response to chemotherapy. Chest CT is also performed at the initial evaluation to identify pulmonary metastases. Bone scintigraphy is helpful in diagnosing metastases. Surgical removal of Wilms tumor should not be delayed.

RHABDOMYOSARCOMA

Rhabdomyosarcoma can occur anywhere in the abdomen or pelvis where there is striated muscle. Tumors are particularly common in the pelvis, involving the prostate, uterus or vagina, and retroperitoneal structures, but they have also been found in the common bile duct and other unusual sites. These tumors can reach a large size before they become symptomatic and each must be managed individually, depending on the site of origin, extent of growth, and the degree of spread. Modern selective therapy has greatly improved the survival rate of this highly malignant tumor.

HEPATOMA

Hepatomas are fortunately rare. They are usually seen in older infants and young children. Hepatoblastoma, more common than hepatoma, is often discovered accidentally when the child is undressed for a bath. The child may feel and act well, yet the tumor is already of a formidable size when first noted. Differential diagnosis should include hemangioendothelioma, hamartoma, and renal and adrenal tumors, especially if they occur on the right side.

An important application of CT in the examination of patients with hepatomas involves a complementary role with MRI and angiography in the assessment of potential resectability.

Survival depends on both complete resection of the primary tumor before metastases have occurred and intensive prolonged chemotherapy postoperatively. As much as two-thirds of the liver may have to be removed.

ABDOMINAL WALL DEFECTS

Inguinal Hernias and Hydroceles

Indirect inguinal hernia is the most common congenital anomaly that is found in children. It is approximately 10 times more common in boys than in girls. There is a strong familial incidence.

CLINICAL MANIFESTATIONS

The child with a hernia may present in different ways. The presentation is determined by the extent of obliteration of the processus vaginalis before birth. A child may have a completely open hernia sac, which extends from the internal ring to the scrotum, or a segmental obliteration producing a sac that is narrow at its proximal end, creating a hydrocele of either the tunica vaginalis or the spermatic cord. The narrowing of the processus allows the abdominal fluid to seep into the distal portion of the sac. It then becomes entrapped and produces what is clinically recognized as a hydrocele. It is often difficult for this fluid to egress through the narrow patent processus vaginalis back into the abdominal cavity.

At the time of the embryologic closure of the processus vaginalis, many fetuses will have some fluid trapped around the testicle in the tunica vaginalis. This is called a physiologic hydrocele, which is a normal newborn finding. In such cases, the fluid gradually is absorbed in the first 12 months of life. If, however, an infant or child develops a hydrocele along the cord in the tunica vaginalis sometime after birth, it must be assumed that the processus vaginalis is still patent and in communication with the peritoneal cavity. This patent processus vaginalis represents a hernia sac. Surgical closure of the sac and drainage of the hydrocele are then indicated.

Many infants and children manifest the classic bulge in the inguinal canal that occurs during straining or crying. This is caused by a loop of intestine distending into the hernia sac. Usually, the hernia sac contents reduce into the abdominal cavity when the straining ceases. If the prolapsing loop of intestine becomes entrapped in the hernia sac, an incarceration has occurred. This is a true emergency that could eventually lead to intestinal obstruction and possibly strangulation of the bowel. Elective herniorrhaphy should be done shortly after the hernia is diagnosed.

Epiploceles (Epigastric Hernias)

If a discrete mass occurs intermittently about one-third of the distance from the umbilicus to the xiphoid, it is usually the result of a weakness of the linea alba through which properitoneal fat protrudes. This defect is called epiplocele. Such defects are fairly common in infants and usually close spontaneously. In older children, the mass may occasionally be tender. If it becomes excruciatingly tender, it is a sign that fat has become incarcerated in the hernia. Although there is no great urgency, these small midline defects should be repaired surgically when they become symptomatic.

Umbilical Hernias

Umbilical hernias are common in small infants, particularly in African-American infants. Fortunately, most of the hernias tend to close spontaneously and only rarely does incarceration occur. Umbilical hernias can be large and unsightly and families need reassurance that watchful waiting is the best course. However, if the umbilical hernia fails to close by the age of 5 to 6 years, surgical repair is indicated. Umbilical hernias may be repaired earlier if there is a large ring that shows no signs of diminishing in size over 1 to 2 years, if there is a thinning of the umbilical skin, or if an incarceration has occurred. Hernias that have a supraumbilical component tend not to close spontaneously and may be operated on at an earlier time of life.

Other Umbilical Defects

Omphalomesenteric duct remnants may persist in either of two forms. When the duct is patent from the ileum to the umbilicus, there is a release of small bowel contents via an opening in the umbilicus. A second form involves a remnant of the omphalomesenteric duct that contains a secreting mucosal patch that is attached to an opening in the center of the umbilicus. Passage of a sterile blunt probe or instillation of contrast dye under fluoroscopy via the umbilical opening will usually confirm either of these conditions. Once identified, these remnants must be excised surgically. By contrast, some infants present with umbilical granuloma in which an excessive amount of granulation tissue has built up after separation of the umbilical cord. In these patients, no opening in the granulation tissue can be seen or felt by means of a probe. These granulomas are usually best treated by application of silver nitrate to the granulation tissue (Fig. 103.4).

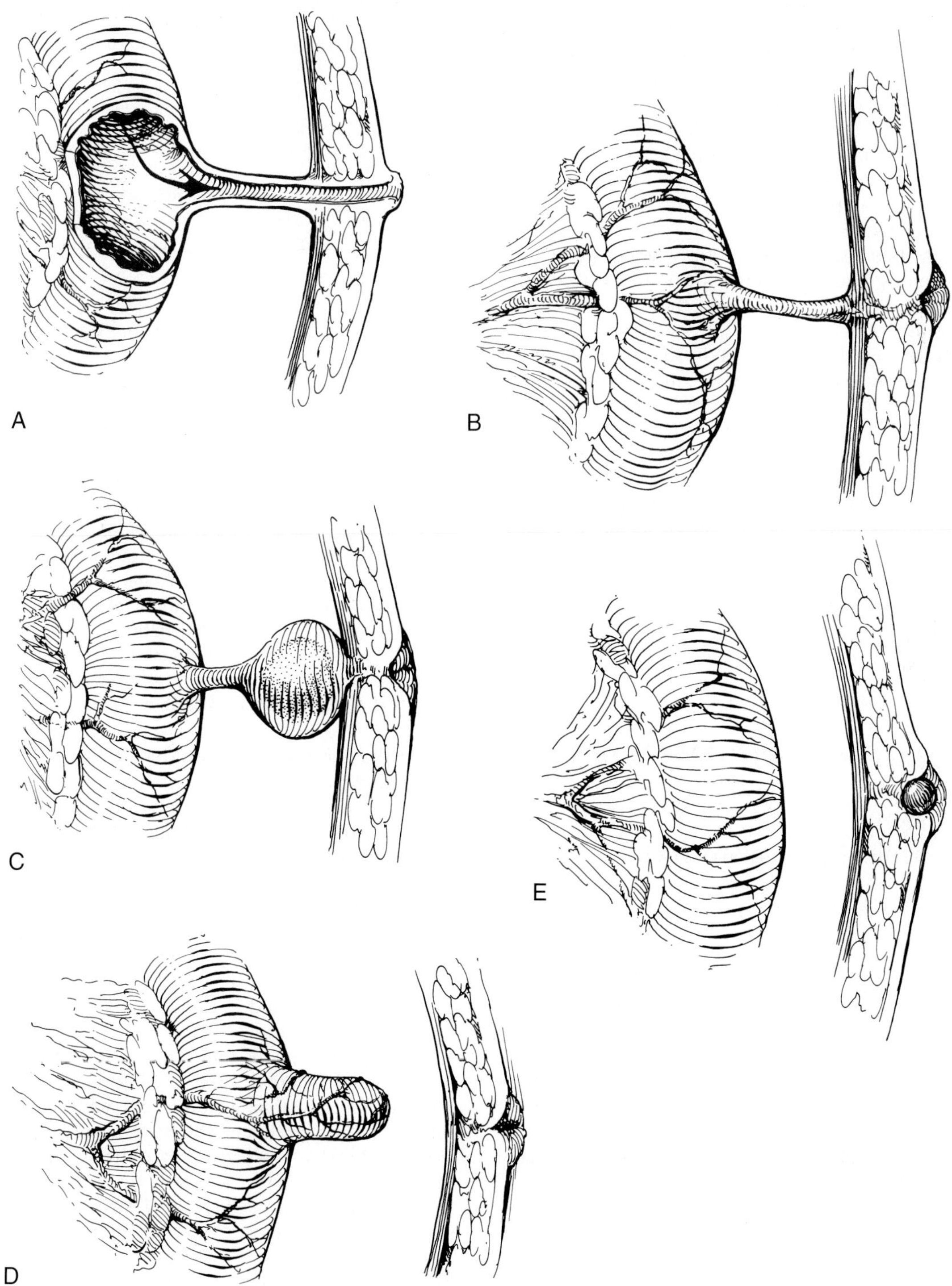

Figure 103.4. Omphalomesenteric remnants. Patent omphalomesenteric duct from terminal ileum to umbilicus **(A)**; closed omphalomesenteric duct with mucosal patch at umbilicus **(B)**; omphalomesenteric cyst below umbilicus **(C)**; Meckel diverticulum **(D)**; umbilical granuloma **(E)**.

If the urachus persists after birth, it can form a urinary fistula that drains at the umbilicus. This problem is ordinarily noted in the newborn period. Older infants or children may present with drainage at the umbilicus caused by persistence of part of the urachus even though connection with the bladder may be obliterated. These urachal remnants also require surgical excision.

FOREIGN BODIES OF THE GASTROINTESTINAL TRACT

When a child ingests a foreign body, it causes great family concern. Most swallowed foreign bodies move through the GI tract without complication. Occasionally, a foreign body lodges in the esophagus, necessitating removal. Plain film roentgenograms for suspected foreign body should focus on the suspected area initially but then expand to include the base of the skull to the anus if the object is not seen. Once an esophageal foreign body has been identified, it should be removed promptly to prevent complications such as edema, ulceration, aspiration, pneumonia, or perforation.

Foreign bodies that reach the stomach, whether pointed or sharp-edged, usually pass completely through the intestinal tract and are evacuated. Cathartics and other efforts to hurry their transit should not be used.

Occasionally, a long, thin foreign body such as a bobby pin may not be able to traverse the turn where the duodenum joins the jejunum at the ligament of Treitz. If a foreign body is trapped in this area, perforation with local or generalized peritonitis may occur. When entrapment occurs anywhere beyond the pylorus, surgical removal is indicated either to prevent or to treat local perforation. Occasionally, objects such as straight pins, toothpicks, and broom straws become entrapped in the appendix. When this occurs, the appendix should be removed.

CHAPTER 104

Thoracic Emergencies

Robert E. Kelly Jr., M.D. and
Daniel J. Isaacman, M.D.

Thoracic emergencies in children often result in life-threatening alterations in cardiorespiratory physiology. A rapid, yet organized approach to the child with a thoracic emergency may represent the difference between life and death. This chapter is aimed at guiding the emergency physician toward evaluation and stabilization of children presenting with surgical diseases involving the thorax. Congenital abnormalities usually diagnosed at birth are not included. Thoracic trauma is discussed in Chapter 94.

AIRWAY COMPROMISE

Airway compromise can occur anywhere in the respiratory tract from the nose to the alveoli. Obstructive emergencies relating to the oropharynx, larynx, and proximal trachea are discussed in Chapters 98 and 106.

TABLE 104.1. Tracheobronchial Conditions Associated with Airway Compromise

Intraluminal
Foreign bodies
Aspiration (esophageal reflux, tracheoesophageal fistula, bronchial fistula, biliary fistula, or esophageal fistula)
Mucous plugs (cystic fibrosis)
Granuloma (chronic intubation, tuberculosis)
Hemoptysis (vascular malformations, cystic fibrosis, tuberculosis, sarcoidosis, hemosiderosis, lupus)
Acute infection (tracheitis)
Mural
Tracheomalacia
Lobar emphysema
Bronchial atresia
Bronchial tumors
Extrinsic
Lymphadenopathy
Bronchogenic cyst
Cystic hygroma
Esophageal duplication
Mediastinal tumors

Compromise of the more distal tracheobronchial tree may be caused by lesions in the lumen, in the wall, or outside the wall of the bronchus. Examples of intrinsic obstruction include tumor within the bronchial lumen (eg, carcinoid tumor), foreign body, and a mucous plug. Obstruction from lesions in the wall of the bronchus include collapse from tracheomalacia and stenosis after tracheostomy. Extrinsic lesions make patients symptomatic by producing impingement on a bronchus by some adjacent structure such as a bronchogenic cyst or inflamed lymph nodes. Table 104.1 lists intraluminal, mural, and extrinsic conditions that produce airway obstruction.

CIRCULATORY IMPAIRMENT

Hemorrhage has somewhat different effects on the circulation in children than in adults. The ability of the child to support blood pressure in the face of significant blood loss has particular implications in the chest. Significant amounts of blood loss may be hidden in the large volume of the chest. It is important to recognize the early signs of shock before significant decreases in blood pressure occur, as this may represent a loss of 20% or more of the blood volume. Fortunately, nontraumatic causes of intrathoracic major blood loss are uncommon in children.

Collections of fluid in the pleural space and mediastinum, whether the result of bleeding or other causes, may produce obstruction of the venous return by *tension phenomena:* the child's mediastinum is mobile, and kinking of the great veins occurs much more easily than in adults. In a patient who requires positive-pressure ventilation, the positive inspiratory pressure inside the chest may be greater than the venous pressure returning blood to the heart.

Rarely, the heart itself can be obstructed by primary tumors such as rhabdomyosarcoma or metastatic Wilms tumor. Tamponade of the heart can be caused by pericardial effusion, hemopericardium, or, even more rarely, by pneumopericardium or pneumomediastinum. These topics are addressed in Chapter 72.

AIRWAY OBSTRUCTION

Tracheal Obstruction

Tracheal obstruction may be produced by lesions within the lumen of the trachea, in the wall of the trachea, or extrinsic to the tube. Intrinsic obstruction most commonly occurs in children because of an aspirated foreign body. Intrinsic obstruction may also occur because of a subglottic stenosis after tracheostomy. A hemangioma may also occur, but is rare. Tracheomalacia, sometimes complicating lung disease of prematurity, is characterized by a floppy trachea that collapses during expiration, when the intrathoracic trachea is compressed by the positive intrathoracic pressure. Laryngomalacia, or tracheomalacia outside the thoracic inlet, may produce obstruction during inspiration, when the negative intraluminal pressure transmitted from the chest causes the floppy wall to collapse. Tracheomalacia often occurs in infants born with tracheoesophageal fistula. Extrinsic compression may occur both from mass lesions (Table 104.1) and as a result of anomalous arteries. Bacterial tracheitis may produce sufficient inflammation that the mucosa effectively obstructs the airway.

CLINICAL FINDINGS

Tracheal compromise produces symptoms that vary from mild to severe, depending on the amount of obstruction present. When symptoms are mild, the underlying cause may not be evident. Occasional episodes of respiratory infection that are thought to result from croup or bronchitis may be the only symptom. Stridor, wheezing, or cough occur in patients with more significant obstruction, and a history of previous hospitalizations for treatment with mist tent, antibiotics, and chest percussion may be given.

Severe tracheal compromise usually is manifested by a history of stridor at rest. Progressive cyanosis and apneic episodes occur. On examination, a child with obstruction caused by extrinsic compression often has wheezing or stridor throughout the respiratory cycle. In contrast, a patient with the floppy trachea of tracheomalacia often wheezes only during expiration.

MANAGEMENT

If the patient has a life-threatening airway obstruction, he or she should receive airway management as outlined in Chapters 1 and 5. Intubation of the airway to within a short distance of the carina supports most patients with lesions extrinsic to the trachea or in the tracheal wall with a critical obstruction. Such a patient requires admission to an intensive care or other unit with ventilator capability. Lesions within the lumen will likely require endoscopic management in an operating theater.

Radiographic evaluation of the stable patient should begin with posteroanterior (PA) and lateral chest radiographs, ideally obtained at full inspiration and again at full expiration. Mass lesions will usually require computed tomography (CT) to evaluate them. Bronchoscopy is often indicated to evaluate obstructive lesions, whether in the lumen, the wall, or extrinsic to the wall of the trachea.

VASCULAR RINGS

Vascular rings are developmental anomalies of the aorta and great vessels. They may produce obstruction of the esophagus, trachea, or both. Many anatomic types of rings are produced by failure of the normal involution of the appropriate segments of the six embryologic aortic arches. The number of possible variants is at least 36; 16 or more have been seen in humans. The level of obstruction is usually at the trachea, but compression of a bronchus by the ductus arteriosus, or by a pulmonary artery sling may produce compression more distally. The reader is referred to standard texts of pediatric or thoracic surgery for further details.

Clinical Findings

Vascular rings should be suspected in infants with stridor, dysphagia, failure to thrive associated with difficult feeding, or recurrent pneumonia. The wide variety of anomalies produce varying degrees of symptoms. Esophageal obstruction produces difficulty swallowing, designated *dysphagia lusoria* by Bayford in 1794. Often, diagnosis is delayed by failure to consider these anatomic obstructions. Chest radiographs may be supplemented by a variety of diagnostic tests: angiography, echocardiography, magnetic resonance imaging (MRI), and digital subtraction angiography are needed in some combination to define the anatomy.

Management

Although a few patients with constricting anomalies improve as they grow, the usual situation is for a poor prognosis with medical therapy. Surgical treatment is usually indicated to relieve the obstruction. This is accomplished by dividing the vascular ring and preserving the blood supply to the aortic branches. This is usually accomplished by a left thoracotomy.

Bronchial Lesions

BRONCHIAL ATRESIA

Congenital bronchial atresia is a rare anomaly characterized by a bronchocele caused by a mucous-filled, blindly terminating segmental or lobar bronchus, with hyperinflation of the obstructed segment of lung. Hyperaeration is thought to result from communication via the pores of Kohn and the channels of Lambert with the normally aerated lung. First reported in 1953, a 1986 review of the literature reported a total of 86 cases.

Clinical Findings

Neonates and infants with the lesion usually are seen for respiratory distress. In older patients, a history of episodic upper respiratory infection and wheezing may be elicited. Some older patients may complain of dyspnea on exertion or unilateral chest pain. Physical findings seldom suggest the diagnosis, but often unilaterally decreased breath sounds are evident.

Management

Chest radiographs make the diagnosis most of the time. Chest CT scan is indicated to help define the anatomy. Bronchoscopy is the most efficient way to identify the atretic opening to the involved bronchus. Bronchography has been used in the past, but high-resolution CT scan can often provide the same anatomic information noninvasively.

RIGHT MIDDLE LOBE SYNDROME

The right middle lobe is anatomically predisposed to compression of its bronchus by the lymph nodes in its vicinity, which tend to encircle it. Because the right middle and lower lobes are favored sites for aspirated material, recurrent inflammation caused by pneumonia leads to adenopathy. Previously, especially in the era before antituberculous chemotherapy, this tended to result in compression of the right middle lobe bronchus alone, which produced eventual bronchiectasis. Often, right middle lobectomy was necessary. Presently, it is more common for the right middle and lower lobes to be involved together.

Clinical Presentation

Recurrent episodes of pneumonia and associated atelectasis in the right middle (and often lower) lobes occur in these patients, and are not responsive to chest percussion, postural drainage, or antibiotic treatment. The mechanical compression of the bronchus leads to a sequestered infection, which may require resection of the right middle or right middle and lower lobes. Although the need for resection is far less common than in the past, acute pneumonia in these anatomic locations should prompt a discussion of previous pneumonias and treatment. Close follow-up is indicated in such patients.

Esophagus-Related Causes of Airway Difficulties

TRACHEOESOPHAGEAL FISTULA

Tracheoesophageal fistula (TEF) occurs in children both as a congenital lesion and as an acquired problem after suppuration of mediastinal nodes. The congenital fistula is accompanied by atresia of the esophagus in more than 85% of patients. However, in about 3% of all patients with TEF, the connection between the tracheal tube and the esophagus creates the shape of the letter "H". In these patients, there is no accompanying esophageal atresia.

It is this "H-type" fistula that is most likely to be seen in the emergency department (ED). The acquired form is usually in the distal trachea or proximal bronchial tree, and is extremely uncommon.

Clinical Findings

These fistulae are notoriously difficult to diagnose. Children generally develop recurrent pulmonary infections for which no source is evident. The characteristic history of choking or gagging when swallowing that accompanies esophageal atresia with TEF may not be present.

Management

Contrast esophagram may identify the lesion. Most of these fistulae are small in diameter (much less than 1 cm), and short (also less than 1 cm), making radiographic identification difficult. Even when contrast appears in the tracheobronchial tree, it may be difficult to know whether primary aspiration of orally administered contrast is responsible. Placing a feeding tube in the esophagus and injecting contrast while pulling the tube from the lower esophagus up under fluoroscopic observation may be helpful. High-resolution CT scanning may identify the anatomy. Bronchoscopy and esophagoscopy may be both diagnostic and may aid the repair if a small catheter can be passed across the fistula to aid its identification by enabling palpation at surgery. Most such fistulae are cervical, and can be repaired without a thoracotomy.

GASTROESOPHAGEAL REFLUX

Introduction/Pathophysiology

Common causes of repetitive soilage of the tracheobronchial tree include primary aspiration of oropharyngeal secretions, often in children with impaired swallowing mechanisms, and gastroesophageal reflux (GER). GER is universal in babies, and is usually outgrown. Particularly in the neurologically impaired patient, however, GER may require medical or surgical treatment.

Clinical Presentation

GER presents with symptoms of spitting up or vomiting after eating. Aspiration may lead to presentation with recurrent pneumonia. Complications that follow prolonged GER include failure to thrive because of inadequate nutrition, esophagitis, esophageal ulceration, and esophageal stricture (Fig. 104.1). Some patients present with an acute life-threatening event (ALTE) in which laryngospasm or bronchospasm precipitated by aspiration of gastric contents produces profound hypoxia and even respiratory or cardiac arrest.

Management

Management of GER begins with establishing the diagnosis. If this is evident clinically, and the child responds to medical management, no further evaluation may be needed. Recalcitrant GER may be an indication for an upper gastrointestinal contrast study (UGI series) to establish that there is no anatomic obstruction to gastric emptying such as a duodenal web or annular pancreas. Recording the esophageal pH over a 24-hour period with a pH probe may help quantify the severity of the problem.

GER is managed by a three-tiered approach. Initially, elevating the head of the bed, thickening the feeds, and decreasing the volume of individual feeds are useful to allow gravity and mechanical effects to help. Medical management (second tier) of this problem includes efforts to decrease gastric acidity, including antacids, H_2-receptor antagonists such as ranitidine, and proton-pump inhibiting drugs. Many clinicians add prokinetic medications to improve the gastric motility such as metoclopramide. Surgical indications, the third tier, are failure of nonoperative management or occurrence of a complication that cannot be tolerated, such as esophageal stricture or repeated ALTEs without other evident cause. Presently, the favored surgical treatment in North America is fundoplication: wrapping the fundus of the stomach either partially (a Thal operation if anterior to the esophagus, or Toupet operation if posterior) or completely (the Nissen operation) around the esophagus just above the gastroesophageal junction. The procedure may be performed laparoscopically in appropriate patients.

ESOPHAGEAL WEB

Introduction/Pathophysiology/Management

Rarely, a patient presents with GER that is caused by an esophageal web (Fig. 104.2). The membranous, congenital narrowing of unclear origin is usually able to transmit liquids, and

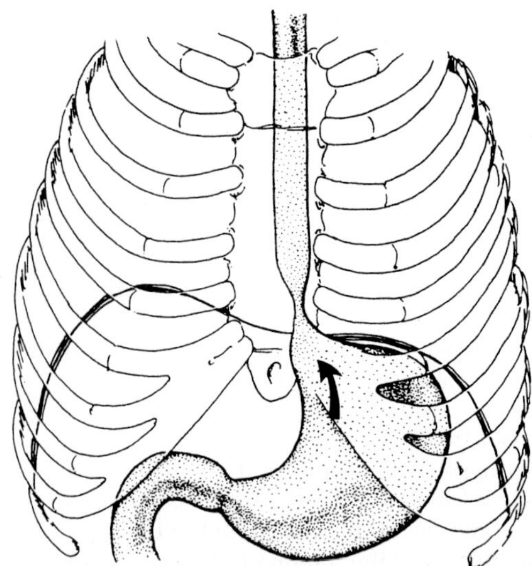

Figure 104.1. Distal esophageal stricture caused by prolonged reflux esophagitis. Note the loss of the normal angle between the esophagus and the stomach and propensity for gastric contents to reflux into the esophagus.

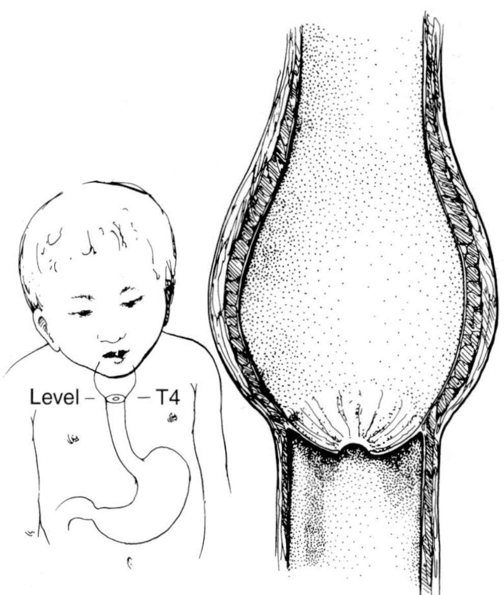

Figure 104.2. A child with chronic partial obstruction of the esophagus caused by a congenital web. Similar bulbous enlargement of the proximal esophagus can occur with any type of stricture and result in pressure on the trachea and recurrent regurgitation with aspiration.

symptoms often arise when the child begins to eat solid food. Recurrent aspiration pneumonia may also develop. An esophagram is usually diagnostic. Often, a thin membranous web may be split by a hydraulic balloon placed endoscopically across the stenosis. If this approach is unsuccessful because the lumen is too small to transmit the dilator or the tissue is unyielding, segmental esophageal resection may be necessary via thoracotomy.

CIRCULATORY IMPAIRMENT

Cardiogenic shock results from decreased cardiac preload, failure of the heart as a pump, increased afterload, or loss of heart rate. Preload may be reduced by tension pneumothorax causing kinking of the great veins bringing blood to the heart in the child's mobile mediastinum; by massive intraabdominal hemorrhage compressing the inferior vena cava; by cardiac tumor obstructing one of the atria; or by tamponade of the heart from mediastinal pressure caused by blood, pericardial fluid, or air. Hypertension resulting from coarctation of the aorta, pheochromocytoma, or other causes, may increase afterload so greatly that cardiac output is impaired. Failure of the heart as a pump occurs in viral myocarditis, or after infarction. Drug ingestions and hypoxia may slow the heart sufficiently to decrease cardiac output.

CLINICAL FINDINGS

Findings are dependent on the type of shock and the primary lesion. Whether caused by tension pneumothorax, intracardiac tumor, or tamponade, hypovolemic (or decreased preload) shock is accompanied by tachycardia. Usually blood pressure is maintained until perhaps 20% of the blood volume is lost to hemorrhage; predicting the onset of hypotension with tension pneumothorax or compressive phenomena is difficult. Characteristically, the extremities are cold and poorly perfused as peripheral vasoconstriction compensates for loss of central venous pressure. Tamponade is accompanied by muffled heart tones, often difficult to recognize in a noisy ED, especially in the setting of trauma. Distended neck veins are often present. Once tamponade has reached a critical compression pressure, it often does not respond to intravenous (i.v.) fluid. Pulsus paradoxus may not accompany acute tamponade.

Clinical findings suggestive of cardiogenic shock are discussed in Chapter 3. Septic and neurogenic shock are "warm shock" in which the extremities are well perfused because of loss of vascular tone; tachycardia commonly accompanies them. Fever in septic shock, and flaccid extremities with loss of bladder control and rectal tone in neurogenic shock may aid diagnosis.

MANAGEMENT

Intravenous support with two large-gauge peripheral catheters, electrocardiogram monitoring, pulse oximetry, and oxygen supplementation are indicated for any type of circulatory collapse. Stable patients should undergo a chest radiograph immediately. Afterward, management is directed to relieving the condition that produced shock.

If acute cardiac tamponade is suspected, emergency pericardiocentesis is indicated immediately. If the patient is not improved by pericardiocentesis, the pericardium may be filled with clotted blood that will not drain through the inserted needle. In this circumstance, pericardial drainage will require a larger opening in the pericardium. In a patient with shock and incipient cardiac arrest, a vertical subxiphoid incision should be made in the ED. After opening the linea alba, the pericardium can be opened widely enough to digitally clear hematoma from the pericardium.

PLEURAL DISEASE

The lung is covered by the densely adherent visceral pleura, which moves smoothly over the parietal pleura of the chest wall because of a thin film of pleural fluid, allowing lubricated motion of the chest during respiration, and contributing to the full expansion of the lung mechanically. When air, excess fluid, or pus comes between the two layers of the pleura, the lung tends to collapse, and consideration needs to be given to removing the interloper.

Pneumothorax

Air can collect in the pleural space acutely or chronically, statically or progressively. Because atmospheric pressure is always greater than intrapleural pressure, any mechanism that allows even momentary communication between the atmosphere outside the chest wall or the atmosphere within the tracheobronchial tree, can result in a rapid shift of air into the pleural space. Penetrating wounds of the chest are the most common cause for pneumothorax. The penetrating object (a knife, a bullet, or a doctor's needle) may cause injuries of both the parietal pleura and often the lung parenchyma. Therefore, many patients with penetrating trauma to the chest will have not only an initial pneumothorax but also an expanding pneumothorax, as more and more air leaks from the surface of the lung.

Nonpenetrating trauma to the thorax can also result in a pneumothorax. For example, a fracture of one or more ribs may result in puncture of the visceral pleura and lung, causing an escape of air from the lung into the pleural space. If the intrapleural pressure increases, air may leak out through the hole in the parietal pleura and into the chest wall tissues, resulting in subcutaneous emphysema. Another form of nonpenetrating trauma is barotrauma, which can occur in infants and children who have been ventilated with high inflating pressures via a tight-fitting endotracheal tube. A particularly hazardous form of pneumothorax occurs when severe blunt trauma to the chest results in partial or complete tear of a bronchus or the trachea.

Seemingly spontaneous episodes of pneumothorax may occur in children or adolescents. For example, a patient with one or more emphysematous blebs on the surface of the lung may develop spontaneous rupture, resulting in an acute pneumothorax often associated with nearly complete collapse of the involved lung. In patients with cystic fibrosis, spontaneous pneumothorax is the second most common pulmonary complication of this condition. Another group of children with a high incidence of spontaneous pneumothorax would be those with pulmonary metastases, for example, those with osteogenic sarcoma. Many of the metastases occur just below the pleural surface of the lung and, thus, may be the foci for the pneumothorax. Children with staphylococcal pneumonia are especially prone to develop unilateral or bilateral pneumothorax.

Two special forms of pneumothorax require emphasis because these conditions may result in the death of the patient if not recognized early and attended to rapidly. The first is a tension pneumothorax, which results not only in total collapse of the lung but also in progressive tension across the mediastinum (Fig. 104.3). The development of a progressive tension pneumothorax is a result of air accumulating in the hemithorax with each inspiration. Whether the site of entry of the air into the pleural space is through the chest wall, a torn bronchus, or an injured portion of lung, the physiologic result is a one-way valve effect, whereby air continues to accumulate in the pleural cavity with inspiration but cannot be extruded on expiration. This phenomenon continues until the intrathoracic pressure on the involved side is so high that no further air can enter the pleural space. This is often the point at which venous return from below the diaphragm is impeded and circulatory failure ensues.

The second life-threatening form of abnormal collection of air in the thorax is massive pneumomediastinum with or without an associated pneumothorax. In extreme cases, the tension produced in the mediastinum can be great enough to impair both circulation and ventilation. This phenomenon is particularly likely to occur in a patient who is receiving positive-pressure ventilation, which enhances escape of air from the bronchial tree into the mediastinum. See Chapter 94 for trauma-related causes such as rupture of a major bronchus or the trachea.

CLINICAL FINDINGS

The symptoms and signs of pneumothorax depend on the size of the pneumothorax and how rapidly it occurred. A patient with spontaneous rupture of an emphysematous bleb may complain of sudden acute pain on the involved side of the chest followed by tachypnea, pain at the tip of the ipsilateral shoulder, and a sense of shortness of breath. Such patients usually have a small to moderate pneumothorax (less than 20% of the lung volume).

In general, a patient with a pneumothorax has signs and symptoms of ventilatory impairment: dyspnea, tachypnea, pain, splinting on the involved side, agitation, increased pulse rate, diminished breath sounds, and increased resonance on the involved side, and possibly, displacement of the trachea and heart away from the involved side. See Chapter 94 for evaluation of traumatic pneumothorax.

MANAGEMENT

The essential components of management involve confirmation that a pneumothorax exists and reexpansion of the lung. If the patient's condition is not severe, an immediate upright PA and a lateral chest radiograph should be taken. These radiographs are important to determine not only the site and extent of the pneumothorax but also any complicating features such as tumor; fluid within the pleural space; or abnormalities of the lungs, diaphragm, or mediastinum.

If the child's condition is so severe that there is not time for a chest film and if a pneumothorax is suspected, immediate therapy includes (1) tamponading and obliterating any sucking or open chest wound, and (2) inserting an angiocath, percutaneous central line, or pigtail catheter into the pleural space and evacuating air. Placement of whichever tube is used is usually best done in the midaxillary line over the top of a rib about level with the nipple. Once the plastic cannula enters the pleural space, it can be advanced further inside and then attached to sterile i.v. tubing and placed to underwater seal. Alternatively, a stopcock can be attached to the same setup and an attempt made to aspirate enough air and/or fluid to improve the patient's pulmonary dynamics. In a patient with a tension pneumothorax, the insertion of the needle and catheter will immediately result in release of the tension on the mediastinum and diaphragm.

Pleural Effusion

Pleural fluid in excess amount is not a disease per se, but it indicates the presence of pulmonary or systemic illness. The classification of the fluid into *transudate,* which accumulates when the normal pressure relationships between the capillary pressure in the lung, the pleural pressure, and the lymphatic drainage pressure are disturbed, or *exudate,* an inflammatory collection, has less utility today than in previous years because of other diag-

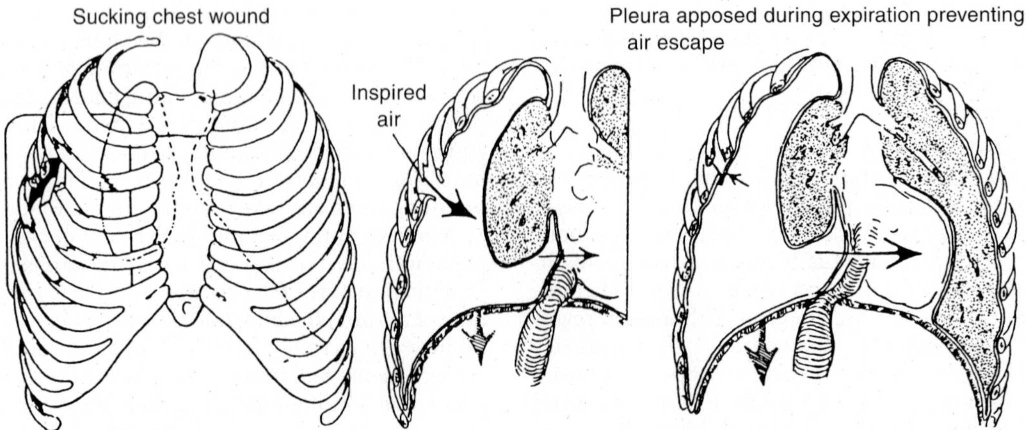

Figure 104.3. The development of a progressive tension pneumothorax as a result of air accumulating in the hemithorax with each inspiration.

nostic tools presently available. Nevertheless, an awareness that an increased pulmonary capillary pressure (as in congestive heart failure), a decreased colloid osmotic pressure (as in renal disease), increased intrapleural negative pressure (as in atelectasis), or impaired lymphatic drainage of the pleural space (eg, from surgical trauma to the thoracic duct) may result in transudative effusion is important.

CLINICAL FINDINGS

Pleuritic chest pain is a sharp, intense pain on deep inspiration that is often not present on quiet breathing. Small, sterile collections, as well as large, chronic collections, tend to be asymptomatic. Acute collections produce symptoms by compressive effects on the lung, with resultant atelectasis and right-to-left shunting, which produces oxygenation and ventilation compromise. Respiratory distress may follow, with attendant dyspnea, tachypnea, increased use of accessory muscles of respiration, and even cyanosis. Except for huge effusions, the examination, using auscultation and percussion to define the amount of fluid, is not nearly as useful as a chest radiograph.

MANAGEMENT

If the presence of a significant effusion is evident by examination and radiograph, no further radiographic studies may be needed. A CT scan, or in some institutions, an ultrasound examination of the chest helps determine whether opacity seen on a chest radiograph is parenchymal disease or pleural fluid. All patients should have a complete blood count and differential and blood culture. Analysis of the fluid itself is the most useful diagnostic test.

Aspirated fluid should be sent for cell count, differential, Gram stain, acid-fast bacillus (AFB) stain, total protein, lactate dehydrogenase (LDH), protein, specific gravity, and a complete set of cultures (aerobic, anaerobic, AFB, and fungal). The normal protein concentration is 1.5 g per dL. Classically, an exudate was said to have a total protein of more than 3.0 g per dL and a specific gravity of more than 1.016. An accuracy rate of more than 99% in classification is obtained by noting that fluid is an exudate if any one of the following criteria are present: (1) Pleural fluid protein divided by serum protein is greater than 0.5; (2) pleural fluid LDH divided by serum LDH is greater than 0.6; or pleural fluid LDH greater than two-thirds of the upper limit of normal for serum LDH. The studies ordered should clearly be tailored to the clinical setting: in patients with hemothorax with an evident cause, little is to be learned by studies of the pleural fluid. Suspected chylothorax may be identified by measurement of triglycerides and cholesterol; a fat stain such as Sudan black or oil red "O" may be performed on the fluid. Empyema can appear similar to chylothorax. Centrifuging the specimen can differentiate the two because in empyema the supernatant is clear.

Draining the pleural fluid must then be considered. Thin fluid may sometimes be managed by intermittent thoracentesis. If the underlying medical problem can be managed, the effusion may take care of itself. If not, a small-diameter tube, such as an 8-Fr pigtail percutaneous tube, may suffice. Thick fluid, such as blood, pus, and sometimes chyle, requires a large-diameter chest tube to drain it. Either tube must be attached to a pleural drainage system. When the drainage decreases significantly, to approximately 1 mL per pound of body weight per day, the drain may be removed. The drain should not be removed in the presence of an accompanying "air leak" caused by a bronchopleural connection.

Empyema

Empyema or pus within the pleural cavity is a particularly serious and, at times, life-threatening situation. The predominant organism is *Streptococcus pneumoniae* with *Staphylococcus aureus* and group A streptococcus also meriting consideration. Empyema is usually the result of septicemia or direct or lymphatic extension from an associated pulmonary infection. When empyema follows accidental trauma or surgery, other bacterial organisms may be involved.

CLINICAL FINDINGS

Empyema is most common in children 2 to 9 years of age. Presentation with a pneumonia that does not respond to antibiotic treatment for many days should lead to consideration of decubitus chest radiographs or CT scan for diagnosis. High fever is common, as are the symptoms of pneumonia: cough, pleuritic chest pain, and lassitude.

MANAGEMENT

Empyema in healthy children may respond to prolonged (3 to 4 weeks) i.v. antibiotic therapy and chest tube drainage. Recovery may be hastened to less than a week in most cases by thoracoscopic debridement of the pleural space of the infected fibrinous peel that encases the lung and prevents its full expansion in many cases. Under a general anesthetic, a fiberoptic high-resolution camera placed within the pleural space via a short (2-cm) incision between the ribs allows removal of the purulence and the fibrinous peel that often encases the lung, restricting its expansion.

Solid Pleural Lesions

Solid lesions in the pleural space occur uncommonly in children. A localized pleural-based mass should suggest neoplasm, which may be primary or metastatic. Diffuse collections usually are the sequelae of bleeding into the pleural space in the distant past or of empyema. They may encase the lung and produce restrictive lung disease.

CLINICAL PRESENTATION/MANAGEMENT

It is impossible to generalize on the mode of presentation of such rare processes. Focal lesions may be expected to be found in investigation of symptoms caused by local compression or erosion; because of the large functional pulmonary reserve of children, restrictive lung disease caused by a diffuse process is distinctly uncommon.

LUNG LESIONS

The lung is often affected in childhood illness. Asthma, pneumonia, and other conditions that do not require surgical management are addressed elsewhere in this text. Mass lesions and cystic lesions of the lung include congenital cystic adenomatoid malformation (CCAM), congenital lobar emphysema, bronchogenic cyst, congenital pulmonary arteriovenous fistula, and bronchopulmonary foregut malformations. Acquired conditions of the lung that require surgical management are distinctly uncommon because of the control of tuberculosis in North America. Bronchiectasis—the chronic dilation of the bronchi resulting from the chronic infection of the lung in cystic fibrosis, tuberculosis, or other chronic pneumonic infection—may require pulmonary resection.

Bronchogenic Cyst

Bronchogenic cysts are thought to result from aberrant budding from the primitive foregut or tracheobronchial tree. They may occur along the trachea, along the bronchi, in the lung substance, or adjacent to the esophagus.

CLINICAL PRESENTATION

Centrally located cysts may present with symptoms caused by compression of an airway. Wheezing, cough, fever, and recurrent pneumonia may result in such children. In contrast, patients with peripherally located cysts develop respiratory symptoms only 50% of the time.

MANAGEMENT

Detection of bronchogenic cysts almost always occurs radiographically. Chest radiograph often suggests the process, but CT scan is usually indicated to clarify the anatomy. Plain-film findings include a homogeneous, water-density mass without sharply defined borders. CT scanning usually shows a water-density mass as seen by Hounsfield or other density units. Cysts with turbid, mucoid fluid may appear solid on CT scan.

Treatment of bronchogenic cysts is by surgical resection. Active infection should be brought under control. Thoracoscopy may be used for some lesions, depending on the location of the mass. Asymptomatic cysts should be removed to establish the diagnosis and to prevent the complications of secondary bronchial communication, bleeding, or perforation into the pleural cavity. Carcinoma and fibrosarcomas have been reported to arise in benign-appearing bronchogenic cysts.

Congenital Cystic Disease of the Lung (Congenital Cystic Adenomatoid Malformation and Sequestration)

Grouping the several pathologic entities included in congenital cystic disease of the lung makes particular sense for the emergency physician. From a single giant unilocular cyst, to a mixed lesion composed of multiple cysts and solid tissue, or a lesion composed predominantly of solid tissue with only an occasional small cyst, these lesions are all congenital processes that present with pulmonary infection, an abnormal chest radiograph, or possibly, a mass or tension effect. Cystic adenomatoid malformations are the result of an excessive overgrowth of bronchioles and an increase in terminal respiratory structures and mucous cells lining the cyst walls. Pulmonary sequestrations arise from an accessory bronchopulmonary bud of the foregut. Histologically they are portions of pulmonary tissue; however, they are not connected with bronchi or vessels to the rest of the lung (and hence the pulmonary tissue is "sequestered"). Usually, there is a systemic rather than pulmonary blood supply. Sequestration can be intralobar (like cystic adenomatoid malformation) or extralobar.

CLINICAL FINDINGS

Recurrent respiratory infections often lead to the chest radiograph, which confirms the condition. Clinical findings may be identical to those of a lobar pneumonia. Occasionally, a lesion is discovered after failure of resolution of an empyema by chest tube placement.

MANAGEMENT

Chest radiographs in the PA, lateral, and bilateral decubitus positions should be obtained to evaluate any areas with air–fluid levels. Any pathogens identified in the sputum should be treated with appropriate antibiotics (see Chapter 74). After control of superimposed infection, the lesion should be resected to prevent recurrent infection. Attempted aspiration of the cystic lesions or placement of a chest tube is to be avoided because it may lead to spread of infection into the pleural space. When the lower lobe seems to be involved, a CT scan with i.v. contrast should be obtained to identify any possible systemic blood supply. Because the blood supply may arise from below the diaphragm, the scan should include both the chest and abdomen. Arteriography is seldom necessary with currently available imaging techniques. The CT scan will likely exclude other conditions that may be misdiagnosed, such as a diaphragmatic hernia, postpneumonic pneumatoceles, or esophageal duplication.

Congenital Lobar Emphysema

Congenital lobar emphysema, also known as infantile lobar emphysema or congenital segmental bronchomalacia, is caused by overexpansion of the air spaces of a segment or lobe of the lung. There is no significant parenchymal destruction. This entity accounts for about half of all congenital lung malformations. Bronchial obstruction caused by a variety of entities produces the condition.

CLINICAL FINDINGS

Infants with congenital lobar emphysema are often normal in appearance at birth, but develop tachypnea, cough, wheezing, dyspnea, and/or cyanosis within a few days. The onset of symptoms may be more gradual; nevertheless, 80% of patients are symptomatic by 6 months of age. The upper lobes are involved in about two-thirds of patients, and in less than 1% are the lower lobes involved. Chest radiographs show striking radiolucency in the involved lobe with mediastinal shift to the opposite side. The diaphragm is usually flattened on the affected side. It can be difficult to tell whether pulmonary markings are present at all in the involved lobe, and pneumothorax may be suspected. The compressed normal lung may be erroneously thought to be atelectatic with the emphysematous lobe compensatory.

MANAGEMENT

Treatment should be given to patients with life-threatening pulmonary insufficiency from compression of normal pulmonary tissue. If a bronchial obstruction such as a mucous plug or foreign body can be relieved, no further treatment may be necessary. Pulmonary lobectomy may be needed acutely if symptoms are progressive. The diseased lobe is evident at thoracotomy because of its overdistended state, which often pushes this part of the lung out of the chest. Lobectomy is curative if the cause of the obstruction is also relieved.

Congenital Pulmonary Arteriovenous Fistula

Congenital pulmonary arteriovenous (AV) fistula, a congenitally occurring communication between a major pulmonary artery and a vein within the lung, is usually an aneurysmal sac. Fistulae vary in size from a few millimeters to several centimeters, and can be multiple. At times, a systemic artery may also be involved. Direct right-to-left shunting leads to hypoxemia, and the size of the fistula correlates with the degree of desaturation.

CLINICAL FINDINGS

As the initial presentation of this disorder is often that of wheezing and desaturation, the child may be misdiagnosed as having asthma. Clubbing and cyanosis may suggest chronic hypoxemia. Examination of the chest may demonstrate a palpable thrill or murmurs. If there are symptoms of hemoptysis and epistaxis, one may find telangiectasias or hemangiomas of the skin and mucous membranes. Evaluation of the family may also reveal the presence of hereditary hemorrhagic telangiectasis (Rendu-Osler-Weber disease), which is present in more than half the patients with congenital pulmonary AV fistula.

MANAGEMENT

Children who are symptomatic from this condition should be evaluated by means of CT scan, contrast echocardiography, perfusion scintigraphy, and arteriograms of the pulmonary artery and aorta. Chest films may demonstrate the aneurysmal areas as rounded or lobulated discrete lesions in the parenchyma. Often, tortuous vessels trace from these rounded areas to the hilum. Resection of the fistula, often involving lobectomy, is indicated if the lesion is localized. Unfortunately, some patients have such diffuse disease that this is impossible.

MEDIASTINAL TUMORS

Mediastinal Mass

At least one-third of all mediastinal masses occur in children younger than 15 years of age. Half of these masses are symptomatic, and 50% of the symptomatic masses are malignant tumors. More than 90% of the asymptomatic masses are benign. More than 95% of biopsied mediastinal masses in children are secondary to cysts or tumors. The mediastinum is commonly divided into anterior, superior, middle, and posterior compartments (Fig. 104.4). If only the anterior and middle mediastinal compartments of children are included, between 40% and 90% of the masses are malignant or cystic in origin. Neurogenic tumors are the most common cause of mediastinal masses, with lymphomas and germ cell tumors being second and third in frequency. Infection is an uncommon cause of mediastinal node enlargement but when present, is largely caused by histoplasmosis. Thymic enlargement may mimic an anterior mediastinal mass.

CLINICAL PRESENTATION

Mediastinal masses usually present with respiratory symptoms secondary to airway obstruction or erosion. As a result, patients may present with cough, wheezing, recurrent respiratory infections, bronchitis, atelectasis, hemoptysis, chest pain, or sudden death. Dysphagia and hematemesis may occur with compression of the esophagus. Superior vena cava syndrome is a rare complication, usually in association with a rapidly growing tumor. If the recurrent laryngeal nerve is compressed as a result of the mass, hoarseness and inspiratory stridor may result. Spinal cord compression syndrome and vertebral erosion can be seen with a posterior mediastinal tumor.

MANAGEMENT

Children with tumors of the anterior or superior mediastinum should be admitted to a hospital to undergo urgent evaluation. CT scan of the chest is almost always needed to supplement plain radiographs.

When biopsy of a large mediastinal mass is necessary, the logistics of biopsy require careful, thoughtful evaluation, ideally involving the pediatrician, surgeon, and anesthesiologist. Airway compression by large mediastinal masses is often significant. If a general anesthetic is administered, the thoracic trachea may be occluded by tumor because the anesthetic eliminates the negative intrathoracic pressure caused by expansion of the chest wall. This situation can be difficult to manage; passage of a rigid bronchoscope may be necessary to stent the trachea open to allow gas exchange. Large mediastinal masses should be evaluated by CT scans to assess the likelihood of tracheal compression. MRI may be a better diagnostic tool for posterior mediastinal masses, because many of them are neurogenic in origin and extradural with extension into the spinal canal.

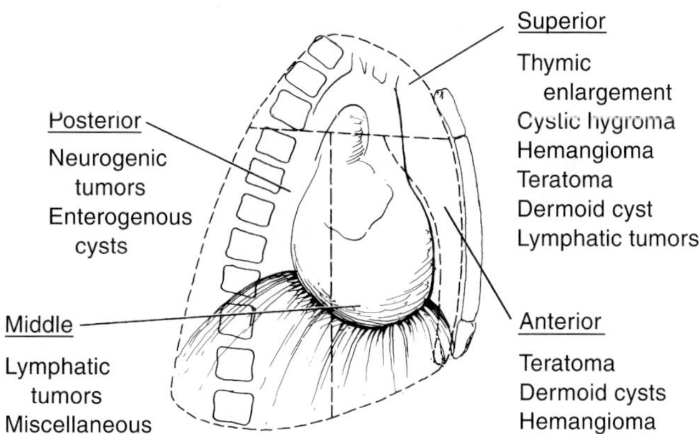

Figure 104.4. Mediastinal tumors in children. Differential diagnosis is based on anatomic location within the mediastinum.

DIAPHRAGMATIC PROBLEMS

Congenital Diaphragmatic Hernia

Congenital diaphragmatic hernia (CDH) is the presence of intestinal viscera in the chest through an opening in the diaphragm not caused by trauma. About 90% occur on the left. They occur through the foramen of Bochdalek, which is at the back of the thoracic cavity. Herniation may occur through the foramen of Morgagni, which lies just posterior to the sternum and is even more rare than the Bochdalek hernia, comprising 2% or 3% of all diaphragmatic hernias. Traumatic diaphragmatic rupture may occur through any portion of the diaphragm and may present in a delayed time frame.

PATHOPHYSIOLOGY

Most babies with congenital diaphragmatic hernia become symptomatic as newborns, when profound respiratory compromise leads to diagnosis. Until recent years, it was thought that the respiratory difficulties of babies with CDH were caused by mechanical compression of the lung by the intestinal viscera extruded through the diaphragmatic opening into the chest. It has become clear that this is not the case: pulmonary hypertension; surfactant deficiency; and a vicious cycle of hypoxia, acidosis, and intrapulmonary shunting lead to the death of about half of newborns with this diagnosis. CDH may be also identified after the neonatal period. These pathophysiologic situations are not present in older infants and children with the condition, who present with features of bowel obstruction, visceral ischemia, or pleural inflammation arising from sudden shift of abdominal viscera into the chest.

CLINICAL PRESENTATION

When CDH is found in older babies and children, identification usually is by a chest radiograph obtained for nonspecific symptoms such as fever, cough, chest or abdominal pain, or vomiting. The presence of loops of intestine on the chest radiograph may be confirmed by passing a nasogastric tube, which will often end up with its tip in the thorax. The chest radiograph may suggest pneumonia with pneumatocele formation; in fact these "pneumatoceles" may be loops of bowel. A gastrointestinal contrast study or chest and abdominal CT scan may clarify confusing findings.

Potential intestinal or visceral ischemia caused by strangulation obstruction is one of the reasons surgical repair is undertaken, and this possibility should be considered.

MANAGEMENT

Surgical repair should be undertaken soon after the diagnosis is made but may be elective in the asymptomatic patient. Because diagnosis is often made incidentally during evaluation for a condition such as pneumonia, which would increase risk of elective operation, the timing of surgery must be tailored to the individual situation.

Foramen of Morgagni Hernias

Usually asymptomatic, an opening in the diaphragm just behind the sternum allows protrusion of abdominal viscera, usually including the colon, into the pericardium (Fig. 104.5). Described by Morgagni in 1769, this defect was also noted and repaired by Larrey, Surgeon General to Napoleon, and is sometimes called Larrey's hernia. Substernal or epigastric pain and bowel obstruction resulting from the narrow neck of the sac may occur spontaneously or be precipitated by any condition that increases intraabdominal pressure.

CLINICAL FINDINGS/MANAGEMENT

A lateral chest radiograph should define the herniation as anterior, and suggest that the protrusion is not at the esophageal hiatus. A barium enema in stable patients should be considered. Surgical repair, indicated to prevent incarceration of bowel even in asymptomatic patients, may be performed through an upper abdominal incision.

Paraesophageal Hernia

Paraesophageal hernia is the protrusion of the stomach through an opening in the diaphragm that is not the diaphragmatic esophageal hiatus. It is extremely uncommon in children. When a part of the stomach migrates into the chest, it may become strangulated or kinked. Symptoms of vomiting and upper abdominal pain, tachypnea, and tachycardia may accompany the condition as the herniated stomach distends with swallowed air inside the chest.

CLINICAL FINDINGS/MANAGEMENT

Chest radiographs show an air and fluid-filled mass in the left lower chest. A nasogastric tube may not pass into the stomach

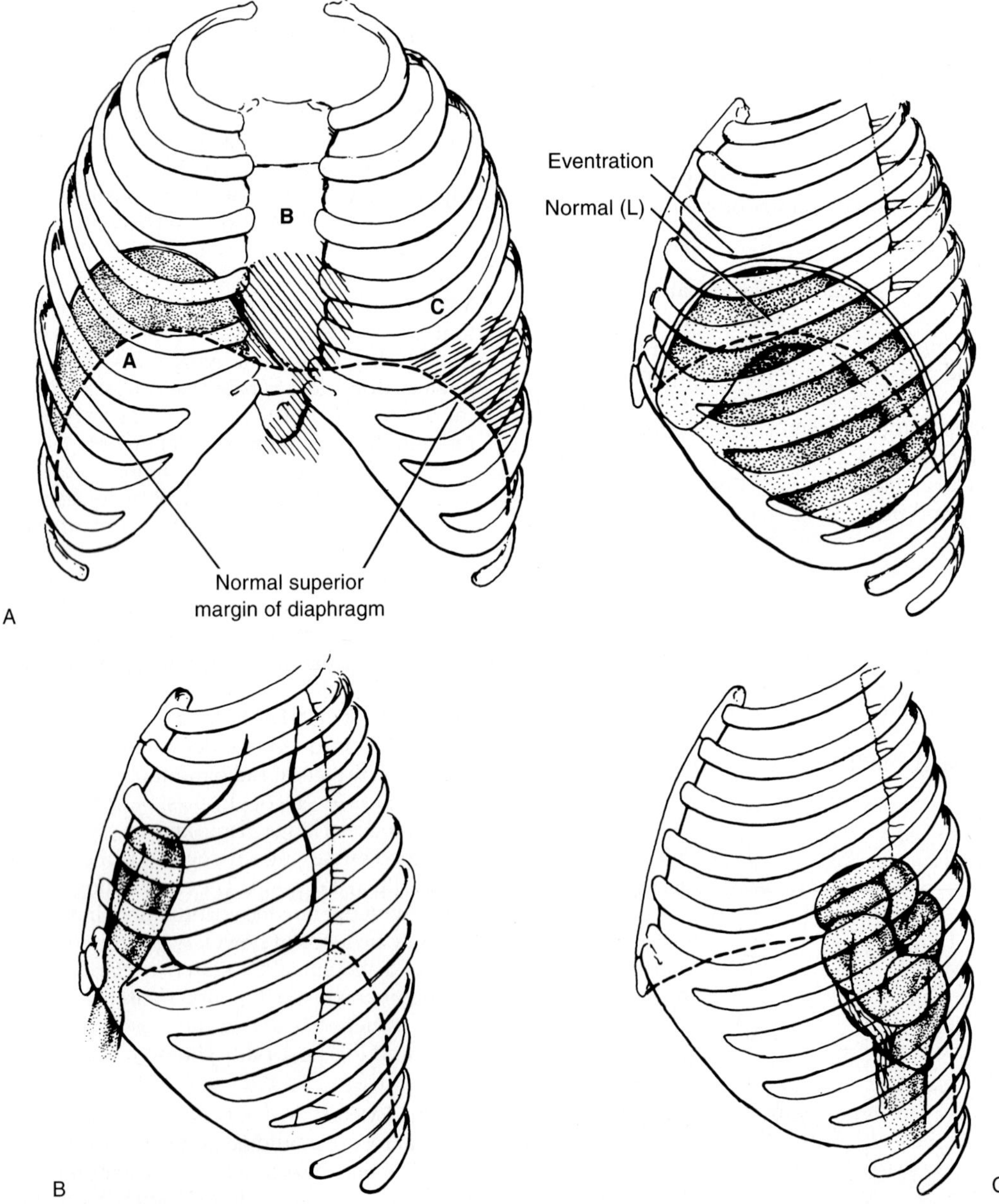

Figure 104.5. Diaphragmatic defects in infants and children. The nature of these defects are often better appreciated on a lateral view of the chest. Eventration of the diaphragm **(A)**; foramen of Morgagni hernia **(B)**; and left foramen of Bochdalek hernia **(C)**.

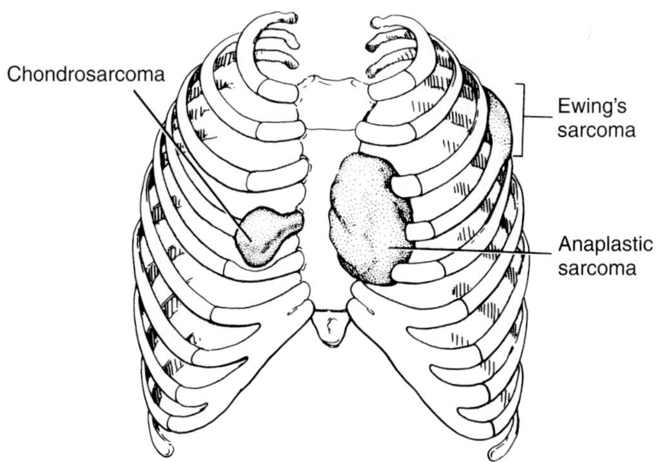

Figure 104.6. Malignant chest wall tumors in children. Most common lesions and their usual site of origin.

because of angulation of the gastroesophageal junction. Surgical consultation should be sought because immediate laparotomy is likely necessary for reduction of a potentially strangulated stomach.

CHEST WALL TUMORS

Tumors of the chest wall occurring in childhood are likely to be malignant. Tumors at this site are uncommon in adults, and rare in children. Benign tumors, arising from the ribs in many cases, include aneurysmal bone cysts, chondromas, lipoid histiocytosis, osteochondromas, and osteoid chondromas. If the clinical and radiologic picture clearly indicates a benign, self-limited process, observation may be appropriate. However, if this is unclear and there is any concern that the lesion is not benign, even a small chest mass in a child should be considered malignant. Many malignant tumors may be present at birth and have been identified early in the first year of life.

CLINICAL FINDINGS

Benign tumors of the chest wall are usually asymptomatic until trauma or fracture brings them to light. Malignancy is signaled by a rapid increase in size, pain, tenderness, or local inflammation. The site of the lesion may give a clue (Fig. 104.6). Ewing's tumor typically involves the lateral aspects of the ribs. Chondrosarcoma typically involves the costal cartilages between the sternum and the distal rib end. The sternum is a favored site for anaplastic sarcomas. These last two tumors may extend intrathoracically, as well as outside the chest cage. Chest radiographs may show pleural effusion, a mass adjacent to the pleura, or direct involvement of the lung.

MANAGEMENT

Radiographic evaluation of these areas should include a CT scan of the pertinent area, bone scans of the entire body, and a metastatic bone survey. Multiple modality, coordinated treatment is usually required involving surgery, chemotherapy, and radiotherapy. If biopsy is anticipated before definitive wide resection, the route of the biopsy should be designed to avoid compromise of the subsequent chest wall reconstruction. Preoperative chemotherapy and radiotherapy may be useful to shrink particular lesions. Resection of the tumor and even subsequent recurrences have resulted in disease-free survivals of 15 years or more.

CHAPTER 105
Ophthalmic Emergencies

Alex V. Levin, M.D.

There are a number of ocular disorders in children that may be seen by the emergency physician. Although ophthalmology consultation may be necessary in some cases, many problems can be treated by the emergency physician.

COMMON EYE EMERGENCIES

Periorbital and Orbital Cellulitis

The primary concern when making the diagnosis of periorbital cellulitis (preseptal cellulitis) is to rule out the possibility of orbital cellulitis. The cardinal signs of orbital cellulitis include decreased eye movement, proptosis, decreased vision, and papilledema. Both orbital and periorbital infection may be associated with fever, pain, swollen eyelids, and red eye. If orbital cellulitis is suspected, computed tomography (CT) scanning of the orbit is indicated. However, the diagnosis of orbital cellulitis can be made clinically if the initial CT scan taken in the first 24 to 48 hours of infection is normal and clinical signs are present. Ophthalmology consultation is indicated in all cases of suspected or proven orbital cellulitis. Surgical intervention may be required. Otorhinolaryngology consultation should also be considered when orbital cellulitis is secondary to contiguous sinus infection.

One must rule out other conditions that can simulate a periorbital cellulitis. Insect bites and allergic reactions can cause dramatic acute periorbital swelling. However, these conditions are not usually associated with fever. Often, close inspection of the skin with magnification (using the direct ophthalmoscope) can localize the site of an insect bite. Allergic swelling is often bilateral, whereas periorbital cellulitis is rarely bilateral. Underlying sinusitis can also cause periorbital swelling. Some authors have argued that CT scan evaluation of the sinuses is indicated in all cases of presumed periorbital cellulitis. Severe conjunctivitis, especially adenoviral infection and neonatal gonorrhea conjunctivitis, can also result in significant lid swelling. The presence of conjunctival discharge is helpful in making these diagnoses. Contiguous spread of conjunctival infections to the periorbital tissues can occur and one must be careful about falsely eliminating the diagnosis of periorbital infection based on the presence of conjunctivitis.

MANAGEMENT

There is some controversy about the appropriate route of antibiotic administration in periorbital cellulitis. In otherwise well children who are beyond infancy and have mild periorbital cellulitis and no systemic signs or symptoms, particularly when the cause of the cellulitis is believed to be a skin wound, intramuscular and/or oral antibiotics may be tried. The patient should be seen again (or with phone follow-up) within 24 to 48 hours, at which time improvement should be documented. If no improvement occurs, the patient should then be admitted for intravenous (i.v.) antibiotics. Periorbital cellulitis is a potentially fatal disease because complications such as meningitis may develop if inadequately treated. All cases of orbital cellulitis must be treated with i.v. antibiotics.

The choice of antibiotics should reflect the probable causative organism. Antibiotic coverage that would be used for presumed sepsis in an immunocompetent host with an unknown organism is usually appropriate. Before starting i.v. antibiotics, blood culture should be taken. Other systemic cultures (eg, cerebrospinal fluid, urine) may be indicated if signs of systemic toxicity are present. Percutaneous aspiration from the area of cellulitis is not recommended. Conjunctival cultures do not identify the causative agent of the cellulitis.

Chalazions and Styes

Chalazions (internal hordeolum) and styes (external hordeolum) represent blocked glands within the eyelids. Both may present acutely with localized lid swelling, erythema, and tenderness. Styes are associated with swelling and purulent drainage at or near the lid margin. More than one lesion may occur simultaneously and more than one lid may be involved. Acute chalazions cause swelling and redness in the body of the eyelid and may be associated with drainage on the conjunctival surface of the eyelid with or without a red eye. They may also point and drain via the skin. Chalazions may enter a chronic phase in which there is a nontender, noninflamed, mobile pea-sized nodule within the body of the eyelid. History can be helpful in establishing these diagnoses because patients often have had recurrent lesions at varying sites.

MANAGEMENT

The treatment for both chalazions and styes is essentially the same. Eyelash scrubs with baby shampoo once or twice daily are helpful in mechanically establishing drainage. Baby shampoo is applied to a washcloth and then used to scrub the base of the eyelashes. Warm compresses are also useful, but rarely tolerated well by younger children. Optimally, warm compresses should be applied four times daily for 10 to 20 minutes at each sitting. The eyelid should be closed for both lid hygiene and warm compresses. Antibiotics probably play a minimal role in the treatment of styes and chalazions. If desired, a topical antibiotic ointment (Table 105.1) can be given twice daily following eyelash scrubs.

TABLE 105.1. Pediatric Emergency Department Ophthalmic Drug Guidelines

Use	Avoid
Dilating drops	
Phenylephrine 2.5%	Scopolamine
Tropicamide 1%	Atropine
Cyclopentolate 1%	Homatropine
	Cyclopentolate 2%
Antibiotics	
Bacitracin	Neomycin
Erythromycin	Sulfacetamide
Polysporin	Aminoglycosides (except neonate)
Polytrim (trimethoprim/polymyxin B)	Quinolones
Lubricants	
Artificial tears/ointment	
Vasoconstrictors/antihistamines	
Albalon-A, Naphcon-A, Vasocon-A	
Diagnostic agents	
Topical fluorescein	
Anesthetic agents	
Proparacaine, tetracaine	Cocaine
AVOID ALL ANTIVIRALS, MIOTICS, STEROIDS,[a] and ANTIGLAUCOMA AGENTS	

[a] Including steroid-containing preparations, such as combination antibiotic–steroids.

Chemical Injury

When the child has a clear history of a noxious substance coming in contact with the ocular surface, it is important to determine whether this substance is an acid or an alkali. Alkali injuries tend to be much more severe. It is also important to determine whether particulate matter may have been deposited on the ocular surface. Smoke can also cause chemical conjunctivitis, particularly in house fires when chemicals are liberated into the air from the burning of plastics and other substances.

MANAGEMENT

Chemical injury to the eyeball is a true ocular emergency. Immediate intervention by emergency department personnel is essential to improving the patient's prognosis. Any patient with sufficient history should be immediately placed in the supine position so that ocular lavage may be started. Although a drop of topical anesthetic can make this procedure more comfortable, the physician should not wait for this to become available if it is not immediately handy. Usually, the irrigating solution itself will induce cold anesthesia. If a speculum, Desmarres retractor, or paper clip is readily available, this may be used to help obtain optimal exposure of the ocular surface. Again, the physician should not wait for these to become available. Virtually any i.v. solution can be used for ocular lavage, although normal saline solution or Ringer lactate is perhaps preferable. A standard i.v. bag and tubing set is used without a needle on the end. Rather, the solution is allowed to flow, with the system at its maximum flow rate, across the surface of the open eye from medial to lateral. If both eyes have been exposed, they should both be lavaged simultaneously with two separate setups. Lavage should be continued until the involved eye(s) has received either 2 L of fluid or until approximately 20 minutes has elapsed. Lid eversion should be performed and lavage should be continued with the lid in this position so that the conjunctiva under the upper lid may also be cleansed. Mechanical debridement should be limited to the removal of visible particles from the ocular surface.

Ophthalmology consultation is usually indicated in cases of significant chemical injury. The consultant should be notified while lavage is ongoing. In cases of minor exposure to substances that are clearly not alkaline or strongly acidic, and when the eye is not injected, an ophthalmology consultation may be deferred. However, the physician must be cautious about the absence of conjunctival injection because alkali burns can cause blanching of the conjunctiva, which is a poor prognostic sign.

Conjunctivitis

Chapter 19 provides an approach for eliminating other causes of red eyes from the differential diagnosis. Table 105.2 is designed to give some additional help in differentiating causes of conjunctivitis. The patient's age is often useful in determining a diagnosis. Neonates presenting in the first 3 days of life can have a chemical conjunctivitis caused by silver nitrate used for ocular prophylaxis perinatally. Most hospitals have now discontinued this practice and many are using erythromycin ointment. However, this is not completely effective in eliminating subsequent gonorrheal or chlamydial conjunctivitis in the neonatal period. These two forms of conjunctivitis, as well as bacterial conjunctivitis secondary to

TABLE 105.2. Differential Diagnosis of Conjunctivitis

	Bacterial	Viral (Nonherpes)	Herpetic	Chlamydial	Allergic
Discharge—purulent	+++	+/−	−	+/−	−
Discharge—clear	−	+++	+++	+/−	+++
Swollen lids	+++	+ to +++	+ to +++	+	+ to +++
Acute onset	++	++	+++	Chronic	Usually
Red eye	+++	+ to +++	Focally or diffuse ++	++	++
Cornea staining fluorescein	Nonspecific	Nonspecific	Dendrite	−	−
White cornea infiltrates	−	−	Possible	Multiple peripheral	−
Unilateral or bilateral	Uni/bi	Uni/bi	Uni	Usually bi	Usually bi
Contact history	+	+++	−	?STD	−
Preauricular node	++	+++	−	+/−	−
Other associations	Otitis media? (*H. influenzae*)	Otitis media? Malaise, fever, pharyngitis	Prior or current skin lesions Recurrent	Genital discharge	Chemosis

STD, sexually transmitted disease symptoms or contact.
Adapted from Levin AV. Ophthalmology. In: Kropt SP, ed. *The HSC handbook of pediatrics,* 9th ed. Toronto: Mosby, 1997.

enteric organisms, can be difficult to distinguish clinically. Each can present as either a mild purulent form or chronic purulent conjunctivitis. A dramatically hyperacute conjunctivitis with significant lid swelling and copious purulent ocular discharge is more characteristic of gonorrhea. In view of the risk of spontaneous corneal perforation associated with gonorrheal conjunctivitis, infants should be presumed to have this infection until proven otherwise. Immediate Gram stain should be performed looking for Gram-negative diplococci. If present, treatment for gonorrheal conjunctivitis should be started while awaiting culture results. In this age group, *Chlamydia* studies may be useful as well. Conjunctival scrapings are useful to look for inclusion bodies of chlamydial conjunctivitis. However, the sensitivity of this test depends on sampling, and the techniques may not be readily available or properly performed.

In children beyond the neonatal period, a wide range of organisms, both viral and bacterial, as well as *Chlamydia,* can cause conjunctivitis. Clinically, these entities may appear to be similar. In general, purulence is more characteristic of bacterial infections, whereas clear serous discharge is more characteristic of viral infection. Although both viral and bacterial conjunctivitis may be unilateral or bilateral, a history of multiple infected contacts argues in favor of a viral etiology. Likewise, dramatic lid swelling, associated with preauricular adenopathy; mucoid or serous discharge; and perhaps an uncomfortable, sandy, foreign body sensation that affects one eye followed closely by the other, is strongly suggestive of epidemic keratoconjunctivitis secondary to adenovirus. This fulminant viral infection is easy to recognize.

Allergic conjunctivitis is usually a hyperacute conjunctival injection associated with tearing and a blisterlike swelling of the conjunctiva (chemosis). Itching is often a prominent symptom, although this may also be a symptom of blepharitis (see Chapter 19). Conjunctival smears stained with Gram or Wright methods may reveal abundant eosinophils.

Nasolacrimal duct obstruction is often confused with conjunctivitis because discharge may be present. However, the conjunctiva is rarely inflamed, indicating the absence of true conjunctivitis.

MANAGEMENT

Until proven otherwise, and in the presence of Gram-negative diplococci, neonatal purulent conjunctivitis should be treated as gonorrheal conjunctivitis, pending the results of cultures. The patient should be admitted for i.v. antibiotic therapy with cephalosporin (ceftriaxone 25 to 50 mg per kg, maximum 125 mg, intramuscularly [i.m.] or i.v. as single dose, or cefotaxime 100 mg per kg i.m. or i.v. as single dose), particularly in areas where penicillinase-producing strains are common. Ophthalmology consultation is indicated. Saline ocular lavage on an hourly basis may be helpful in decreasing the amount of organisms having access to the cornea. Topical erythromycin ointment is helpful because it will also treat *Chlamydia.* However, topical treatment alone is insufficient for either organism. If *Chlamydia* is laboratory proven, then the child must receive a 14- to 21-day course of oral erythromycin as well. This is necessary to eradicate carriage of *Chlamydia* in the nasopharynx, which can subsequently lead to pneumonia. The mother and father should be tested.

Any of the local antibiotics suggested in Table 105.1 would be appropriate for empiric coverage in treating a presumed bacterial conjunctivitis other than gonococcal while awaiting culture results.

If the patient clearly has a viral conjunctivitis, antibiotic treatment is probably not needed. Some physicians use antibiotics to "prevent secondary infection"; however, this is not a clinically significant problem in immunocompetent children. Rather, these patients are best soothed with cool compresses and artificial tear preparations.

Allergic conjunctivitis is also helped by topical lubricants and cool compresses. The combination vasoconstrictor/antihistamine preparations listed in Table 105.1 may also be prescribed.

Any patient with a history of herpetic ocular infection and any patient who wears contact lenses and has conjunctivitis should be referred immediately for ophthalmology consultation. Herpetic corneal infection is usually painful. Patients may or may not have a history of skin lesions. Characteristic fluorescein dendritic staining patterns can be seen on the cornea or conjunctiva. However, even if there is no staining but a history of herpetic (varicella-zoster or simplex) corneal infection, urgent ophthalmology consultation is essential. However, skin lesions on the lids without any conjunctival injection does not require ophthalmology consultation.

DRUGS

Table 105.1 is designed to give emergency physicians some guidelines regarding the prescription and use of ophthalmic medications. Those drugs that should be avoided are listed because of problems with ocular toxicity, systemic toxicity, undesirable selection of resistant organisms, or the need for ophthalmology consultation and management regarding the problem that those drugs are designed to treat.

CHAPTER 106

Otolaryngologic Emergencies

William P. Potsic, M.D., and
Steven D. Handler, M.D.

The ear, nose, and throat are common sites for infection and neoplasms and may be the sources of acute pain. Therefore, emergency medicine specialists must be familiar with the head and neck region because they will be called on often to evaluate this area. Although the presenting complaints may seem extremely distressing to the patient and cause considerable anxiety for the parents, the diseases prompting the visit are rarely life threatening. This chapter includes discussion of disorders of the ear, nose, nasal sinuses, oral cavity, pharynx, esophagus, larynx, trachea, and neck.

EAR

The tympanic membrane (TM) should be evaluated for its appearance, but the examination should not stop there. Part of the middle ear contents often can be seen through a translucent ear drum (Fig. 106.1). Mobility should be assessed using the pneumatic otoscope, applying positive and negative pressure to the TM with the pneumatic otoscope fitted snugly into the ear canal. The ear pressure can be varied by squeezing a rubber bulb or blowing through tubing connected to the otoscope head.

The ear of a neonate requires special attention to perform an adequate otologic examination. The ear canal itself is narrow and collapsible. Often, the otoscopic speculum can be inserted only as positive pressure from the pneumatic bulb distends the canal ahead of the advancing speculum. The canal can be filled with vernix caseosa, which must be removed or irrigated out of the canal to permit visualization of the TM. The neonate's TM lies at a more oblique angle to the ear canal (compared with older children) and may make recognition of the TM and its landmarks more difficult.

Infections

ACUTE OTITIS MEDIA

Acute otitis media (AOM) is one of the most common head and neck infections in children and is the second most common diagnosis in the ED. It may occur as an isolated infection or as a complication of an upper respiratory infection (URI). Otitis media with effusion (OME), which is noninfected fluid in the middle ear (also called serous otitis media or secretory media), and immunodeficiency states predispose children to recurrent AOM.

The most common organisms causing acute otitis at all ages are *Streptococcus pneumoniae, Haemophilus influenzae,* and, less often, *Moraxella catarrhalis,* group A β-hemolytic streptococcus, and various upper respiratory viruses. Gram-negative organisms may occur in hospitalized patients who are younger than 8 weeks or are immunosuppressed.

Clinical Manifestations

Acute otitis media should be suspected in any child who is irritable or lethargic. The pain develops rapidly and is often severe. Spontaneous perforation of the TM with serosanguineous

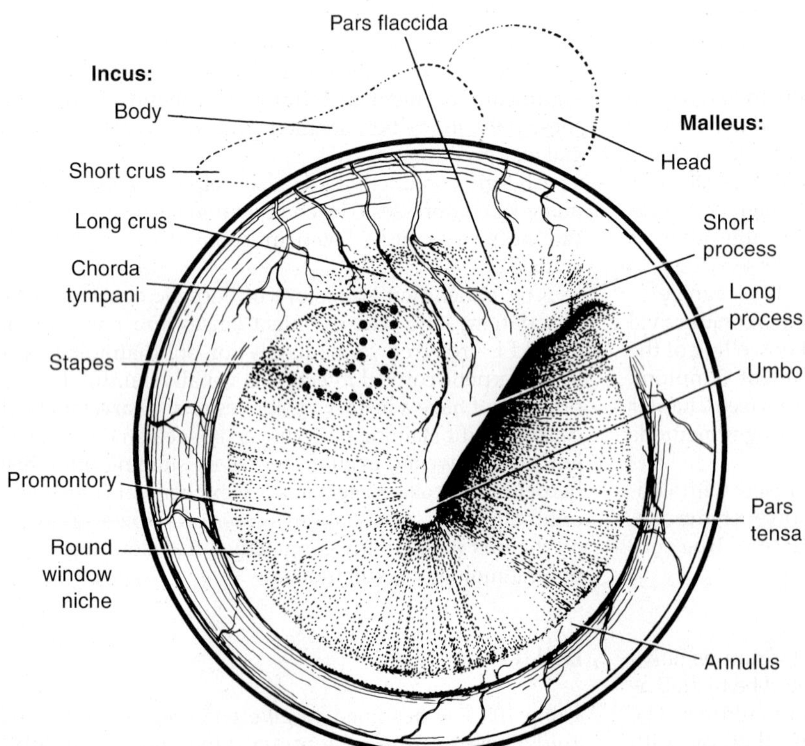

Figure 106.1. Right tympanic membrane.

drainage may occur in less than 1 hour after the onset of pain. AOM is best diagnosed by pneumatic otoscopy. The TM is hyperemic, and mobility is decreased. As the drum becomes more edematous, it bulges outward and the landmarks may become unrecognizable. Infection with *Mycoplasma pneumoniae* and other bacteria may cause blebs on the lateral surface of the drum. The vesicles of bullous myringitis are filled with clear fluid and are painful. The appearance of the TM in AOM secondary to bacterial pathogens does not differ significantly from AOM of viral etiology.

Complications

The following complications of AOM may be encountered in the ED:

1. The purulent exudate that fills the middle-ear space causes a conductive hearing loss. The congealed exudate may organize and stimulate hyalinization and calcification, leading to tympanosclerosis (white patches on the undersurface of the TM).
2. Spontaneous perforation of the TM usually produces a small hole that heals rapidly; however, large perforations may occur that do not heal even after the infection has cleared.
3. Ossicular necrosis also may occur, causing a persistent conductive hearing loss.
4. As the TM heals after a perforation, skin from the lateral surface of the TM may be trapped in the middle ear to form a cyst (cholesteatoma) that can expand and destroy the structures of the middle ear and surrounding bone.
5. Facial-nerve paralysis may occur suddenly during AOM. The nerve paralysis may be partial or complete when the child is first examined. The facial nerve usually recovers complete function if appropriate systemic (intravenous followed by oral) antibiotic therapy is administered and a wide myringotomy for drainage is carried out as soon as possible.
6. AOM can cause inflammation in the inner ear (serous labyrinthitis). This causes mild to moderate vertigo without a sensorineural hearing loss.
7. Bacterial invasion of the inner ear (suppurative labyrinthitis) causes severe vertigo and sensorineural hearing loss.
8. Pus always fills the mastoid during AOM, causing radiographic opacification, but acute suppurative mastoiditis (acute coalescent mastoid osteomyelitis) may develop, causing destruction of the mastoid air cell system. As the infection spreads to the postauricular tissues, subperiosteal collection of purulent material displaces the auricle laterally and downward from its normal position. The pus may extend through air cells to the medial portion of the temporal bone, causing sixth cranial nerve paralysis, deep retroorbital pain, and otorrhea (Gradenigo syndrome). Pus also may break through the mastoid tip and extend into the neck (Bezold abscess).
9. The most common intracranial problem associated with AOM is meningitis, which may be associated with severe sensorineural deafness and irreversible vestibular damage. Less commonly associated problems are cerebritis, epidural abscess, brain abscess, lateral sinus thrombosis, and otitic hydrocephalus. The child with overt or impending intracranial complications should be stabilized and have a computed tomographic (CT) or magnetic resonance imaging (MRI) scan.

Management

The treatment of uncomplicated AOM is oral antibiotic therapy with amoxicillin (25–80 mg per kilogram per 24 hours in three divided doses for 10 days). Systemic or local antihistamine–decongestant preparations are of no proven value. Patients with complicated AOM also should be treated with a wide inferior myringotomy for drainage, usually best performed by an otolaryngologist. Alternatively, in neonates, in immunosuppressed patients, and in patients in which antibiotic therapy is not effecting resolution of the infection, tympanocentesis may be performed for Gram stain and culture. Patients treated on an emergency basis for AOM should be referred for follow-up examination in 2 weeks after therapy is started.

EXTERNAL OTITIS

External otitis usually follows swimming and often is called *swimmer's ear*. Ear canal trauma or foreign bodies also may contribute to the development of external otitis.

Otitis externa may be localized or diffuse. Localized external otitis is the result of an abscessed hair follicle in the outer two-thirds of the ear canal. These abscesses are caused by *Staphylococcus aureus*.

Diffuse external otitis is caused by *Pseudomonas aeruginosa*, staphylococci, fungi, or a mixture of Gram-negative and Gram-positive organisms. Viral external otitis usually is caused by herpes simplex or herpes zoster.

Clinical Manifestations

External otitis usually begins with itching and fullness that progress to severe pain. The pain is worsened by chewing or by touching the ear. The external canal is red, edematous, and narrowed. The diagnosis of external otitis usually is made readily by external inspection and otoscopy. Otoscopy may be painful, and visualization of the eardrum may be impossible because of edema of the canal walls. A foul-smelling, purulent discharge is usually present. Surrounding cellulitis and regional cervical adenitis also may be present. Malignant external otitis occurs rarely in debilitated patients who have diabetes or are immunosuppressed. It may cause extensive tissue necrosis and can be rapidly fatal if not treated immediately with antibiotics and surgical debridement.

Management

If the abscess in localized external otitis is about to drain spontaneously, it should be opened where it is pointing with an 18-gauge needle, or a no. 11 scalpel blade. Drainage results in immediate relief of pain. Antibiotic therapy with an antistaphylococcal antibiotic (eg, erythromycin, dicloxacillin, or a cephalosporin) should be administered for 10 days. The treatment of diffuse external otitis is to use antibiotic eardrops containing neomycin, polymyxin, and hydrocortisone (four drops, three times daily) in the affected ear for 10 days. Before the drops are started, the pus and debris should be cleaned from the ear canal with gentle suction, a curette, or cotton-tipped applicators. If the meatus is so swollen that drops cannot enter the external canal, a wick of gauze or Merocel sponge should be advanced gently advanced into the ear canal using a forceps (Fig. 106.2) to facilitate instillation of the topical medicine. The wick should be left in place for 24 to 48 hours, by which time the canal swelling should resolve to permit entrance of the drops. Broad-spectrum systemic antibiotics should be used if cellulitis or regional cervical adenitis is present. No water should be allowed to enter the ear canal during the 10 days of therapy.

CHRONIC OTITIS MEDIA

Chronic otitis media (COM) is a persistent perforation of the tympanic membrane of more than 3 months' duration; the perforation may be acquired (from AOM or trauma) or iatrogenic (by tympanostomy tube) and may or may not be associated with active infection. When infection is present, the causative organism is usually *P. aeruginosa* or *S. aureus*, and it presents with a profuse, foul-smelling discharge. Any perforation may be asso-

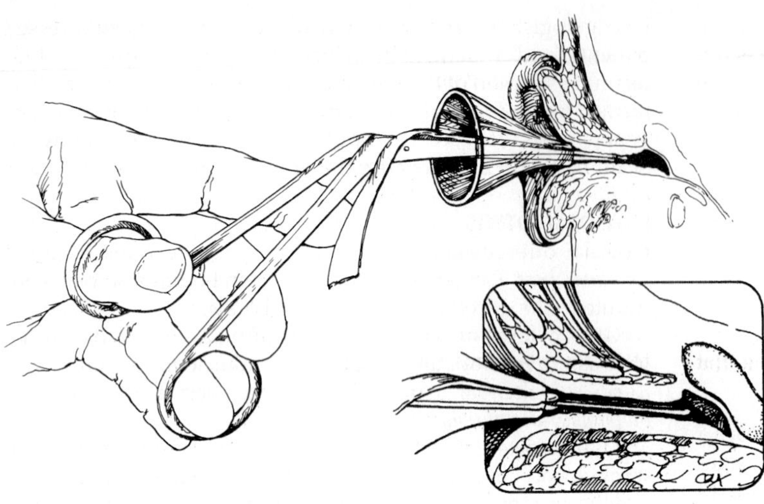

Figure 106.2. Gauze wick (1 inch) being placed in ear canal to facilitate topical treatment of otitis externa.

ciated with a cholesteatoma (white skin-lined cyst) that can destroy the structures of the ear as it expands.

Clinical Manifestations

Usually, COM is diagnosed by otoscopy. A perforation of the eardrum is readily seen and the white, pearly, flaky debris from a cholesteatoma may also be present.

Management

Dry perforations require no active treatment. When otorrhea is noted, antibiotic-containing eardrops (four or five drops, three times daily) should be placed in the ear canal. Systemic antibiotics are of limited value unless regional cellulitis or cervical adenitis is present. In those cases, an antistaphylococcal antibiotic (eg, erythromycin, dicloxacillin, or cephalosporin) should be administered for 10 days. Chronic perforation and cholesteatoma require surgical correction. All cases should be referred to an otolaryngologist for definitive management.

INFECTION OF THE PINNA

The pinna may become infected in a fashion similar to skin surfaces anywhere else on the body. Preauricular cysts and sinuses occasionally may be infected with *S. aureus* and should be treated with antistaphylococcal penicillin or cephalosporin for 10 days. If an abscess forms, it should be drained surgically. Infected preauricular sinuses or cysts require surgical excision once the acute infection has been treated.

Sudden Hearing Loss

Sudden hearing loss is not a common complaint in the emergency department (ED), but it requires prompt attention, especially if the loss is determined to be sensorineural. Sudden conductive losses almost never occur without a known antecedent event, such as head trauma, ear infection, or wax occlusion of the ear canal. History and otoscopy usually can establish the cause of the conductive hearing loss; however, the cause of sensorineural sudden hearing loss is obscure when the history is unrevealing and otoscopy is normal. Tuning fork testing helps confirm the presence of a sensorineural hearing loss.

Sudden sensorineural hearing loss that occurs after an airplane trip, scuba diving, straining, or head trauma is highly suggestive of a perilymph fistula. A perilymph fistula occurs when inner ear fluid leaks out into the middle ear through a rupture in the round window or stapes footplate (oval window). The leaking fluid causes a fluctuating sensorineural loss and vertigo. Urgent surgical exploration of the middle ear is required for repair.

Sudden sensorineural deafness may occur without a history suggestive of a fistula and without otoscopic abnormalities. This is often secondary to a viral infection of the cochlear labyrinth. Measles, mumps, and cytomegalic viral illnesses are common causes of sudden sensorineural deafness. Other viruses may injure the cochlea as well. There may be no systemic symptoms or signs of such a viral infection. These patients may have partial or complete recovery of hearing over several weeks. There is no proven effective treatment for sudden hearing loss. Aspirin has been recommended (in older children) to decrease platelet aggregation and to maintain patency of the cochlear blood vessels, and corticosteroids have been recommended by some researchers. Other treatments have been proposed (eg, cyclophosphamide, hyperbaric oxygen, inhaled CO_2), but they are of uncertain efficacy. Antivertigo medications may be prescribed for patients experiencing dizziness. All patients with a sudden sensorineural hearing loss should be referred to an otolaryngologist.

Vertigo

Sudden vertigo is a disturbing and sometimes confusing symptom. A child may be brought to the ED because the parents think he or she is having a seizure. Vertigo may follow dysfunction of any part of the vestibular system from the labyrinth to the vestibular cortex.

Vertigo may be associated with a number of conditions affecting the middle ear:

1. Serous labyrinthitis may develop in a child with OME, AOM, or COM. Pressure and infection in the middle ear may cause inner-ear inflammation and vestibular dysfunction. The conductive hearing loss and the dizziness resolve when the middle-ear pressure is normalized or the inflammation subsides.
2. Suppurative labyrinthitis may occur when bacteria invade the inner ear. Severe vertigo and a profound sensorineural hearing loss result.
3. When a cholesteatoma arises in association with COM, it may invade the bony wall of the labyrinth. Pneumatic otoscopy may produce the sensation of vertigo by transmitting the pressure directly to the inner ear.
4. A common cause of sudden vertigo is vestibular neuronitis. The origin of this entity is uncertain, and the vertigo resolves spontaneously over several weeks. There are no accompanying signs or symptoms.

5. Trauma can be associated with vertigo in several ways. Perilymph fistulae, which occur most often after barotrauma, blunt head trauma, or straining, produce vertigo that fluctuates in severity. Head trauma also may cause labyrinthine concussion or hemorrhage (hemorrhagic labyrinthitis), resulting in vertigo. Cerebral injuries involving the temporal lobe (with or without temporal bone fracture) can cause vertigo.
6. Measles and mumps may infect the inner ear and cause vertigo.
7. Meniere disease (endolymphatic hydrops) is rare in children. Its origin is unknown. The symptoms are intermittent vertigo, tinnitus, a feeling of fullness in the ear, and hearing that fluctuates.
8. Miscellaneous causes of sudden vertigo in children include benign paroxysmal vertigo of childhood and retrolabyrinthine lesions such as tumors, demyelinating diseases, and temporal lobe seizures.

Neoplasms

Neoplasms of the external ear are as varied as the tissue types of the auricle and are not difficult to diagnose because they are so visible. Neoplasms of the middle and inner ear are rare but bear mentioning because they are often missed until they are far advanced. External-canal and middle-ear tumors most often are brought to the physician's attention because of painful secondary infection that does not respond to conventional treatment of topical and systemic antibiotics. The examiner may overlook a tumor, assuming it is granulation tissue caused by an infection or related to a ventilating tube. If an ear infection does not respond to appropriate treatment or is associated with any abnormal-appearing tissue, a tumor should be suspected; otolaryngologic consultation should be made to obtain a biopsy of the abnormal tissue.

FACIAL-NERVE PARALYSIS

Facial-nerve paralysis is a frightening occurrence in children. Bell palsy (idiopathic facial paralysis) is the most common cause of facial paralysis. (See Chapter 73 for management of this presumed viral infection.) A child presenting with facial paralysis must have a careful examination to detect any other treatable cause for the nerve dysfunction. Facial paralysis secondary to AOM requires a course of systemic (24–48 hours of intravenous followed by oral) antibiotics and an urgent wide-field myringotomy for drainage. Temporal bone or facial trauma and neoplasms of the middle ear and parotid area also can present with facial-nerve paralysis. A child with a facial-nerve paralysis should be referred to an otolaryngologist for complete evaluation of the head and neck, audiogram, and radiographic imaging.

NOSE AND PARANASAL SINUSES

Infections

Infections of the nose and paranasal sinuses are most often a component of the common URI. The symptom complex of fever, nasal congestion and rhinorrhea, and headache is most often caused by a viral agent. Physical examination often reveals swollen, erythematous nasal turbinates. The rhinorrhea can be clear or white. Facial tenderness is usually absent. Viral rhinitis requires little more than supportive care with hydration, rest, and antipyretics; oral antihistamines and decongestants are thought by some to provide additional relief. Topical decongestants are to be avoided because of their tendency to cause rebound congestion as their vasoconstricting effect on the nasal mucosa wears off.

Bacterial infection of the nose and paranasal sinuses is a more serious condition and requires a careful examination and prompt treatment. Bacterial sinusitis should be suspected when the nasal discharge lasts more than 7 days and is thick yellow to yellow–green. Tenderness over the face may indicate clinical involvement of one or more of the paranasal sinuses. The diagnosis usually is confirmed radiographically. Gram stain of the material reveals many polymorphonuclear leukocytes (PMNs) and the causative organism. Because the most common organisms responsible for bacterial rhinosinusitis are *H. influenzae* and group A streptococcus, amoxicillin 25 to 50 mg per kilogram of body weight daily for 10 days is the treatment of choice.

Complications of acute sinusitis, such as orbital cellulitis, facial cellulitis or abscess, and meningitis, require admission to the hospital for appropriate intravenous antimicrobial therapy and possible operative intervention. Otolaryngologic consultation should be obtained in the evaluation of these patients with complicated acute sinusitis; surgical drainage may be needed.

Chronic Nasal Obstruction

Obstruction to the normal passage of air can occur with a variety of conditions and gives the sensation of a blocked or "stuffy" nose. Temporary partial obstruction of one nasal cavity at a time occurs normally in the nasal respiratory cycle; however, prolonged blockage is not physiologic, and the physician should search for a cause.

Although most instances of nasal obstruction cause only mild feelings of discomfort, some children present with a history of obstructive apnea (Pickwickian syndrome; see "Adenotonsillar Hypertrophy") and even cor pulmonale. A history of trauma or foreign body may lead one to the reason for the obstruction. A careful examination of the nasal cavities and pharynx is necessary to determine the cause of the obstruction. Septal deviation, nasal tumor, and turbinate hypertrophy related to allergy or infection are common causes. Adenoid hypertrophy, nasopharyngeal tumor (lymphoma, rhabdomyosarcoma), and choanal atresia (unilateral or bilateral) all can present with nasal obstruction. Flexible fiberoptic examination and radiographs (usually CT scan) of the nose and nasopharynx may be useful in the evaluation of the blocked nasal airway. If the source of the obstruction is not apparent after these maneuvers, referral should be made to an otolaryngologist to perform a complete examination of the nose and nasopharynx.

Epistaxis

Epistaxis is relatively common in children and may cause significant anxiety in both the child and the parent. Although bleeding occasionally occurs secondary to the mucosal maceration caused by URIs, nose-picking accounts for most cases of recurrent epistaxis. (A more complete discussion on the differential diagnosis is presented in Chapter 18.) The usual site of bleeding is the anterior nasal septum, Kiesselbach, or Little area (Fig. 106.3).

A complete history is an important step in the proper management of epistaxis. Site of bleeding (one or both sides of the nose), frequency, bleeding from other places, history of trauma, and family history of bleeding are important factors in this evaluation. Figure 106.4 presents an algorithm for the management of

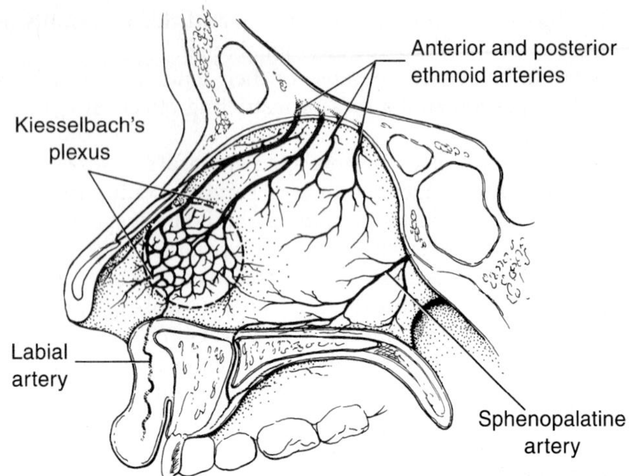

Figure 106.3. Vascular supply of nasal septum. Note confluence of vessels that forms Kiesselbach plexus.

epistaxis. A careful examination of the nose should be performed to identify the site and cause of the bleeding. Good lighting, suction, and material for cauterization and packing should be readily available. Topical vasoconstrictors such as phenylephrine (0.25%), oxymetazoline (0.05%), or epinephrine (1:1000) on a cotton pledget can be placed in the nose to shrink the nasal mucosa, allowing better visualization of the nasal cavity; vasoconstrictors may slow or even stop the bleeding. Simple pressure by squeezing the nostrils together is usually sufficient to stop most epistaxis. Occasionally, a roll of cotton placed under the upper lip will stop bleeding by compression of the labial artery. If pressure is not successful, cauterization with silver nitrate sticks or packing of the nose is performed. Absorbable packing such as oxycellulose (Surgicel) or gelatin (Gelfoam) is usually adequate for most epistaxis and has the advantage of not requiring removal.

Severe or recurrent episodes of epistaxis require the assistance of an otolaryngologist in their diagnosis and management. Epistaxis that does not stop with simple pressure or oxycellulose or gelatin packing may require a more substantial anterior nasal pack of petroleum jelly-impregnated gauze. A posterior nasal pack (using gauze or a Foley catheter) may be necessary in managing severe epistaxis that originates in the posterior nasal cavity or nasopharynx.

If the epistaxis recurs despite the above treatment, an otolaryngologist should be consulted to look for other causes for the epistaxis. Nasal septal deviation or perforation, sinusitis, tumor (nasal, nasopharyngeal or sinus), Rendu–Osler–Weber disease (hereditary hemorrhagic telangiectasia), and nasal foreign body can all present with epistaxis. Blood dyscrasias such as hemophilia, idiopathic thrombocytopenia purpura, von Willebrand disease, and those hematologic conditions associated with leukemia or the administration of chemotherapeutic agents may lead to severe epistaxis. Treatment consists of correcting the underlying hematologic problem in addition to the previously described local measures. Recurrent or severe bleeding may require more extensive cauterization or even ligation of dilated vessels on the septum.

Neoplasms

Neoplasms of the nose and sinuses are uncommon in children. They may present as mass lesions or as chronic or recurrent rhinosinusitis. When a neoplasm is suspected, the child should be referred to an otolaryngologist.

Hemangiomas are the most common benign neoplasms of the head and neck in children and often occur on the skin near or on the nose. Because hemangiomas often go through a period of rapid growth for the first 12 to 18 months of life before they begin to involute, a period of observation is recommended before corticosteroids or surgical excision is considered. Recurrent bleeding, thrombocytopenia, skin breakdown, obstruction to vision, respiratory distress, and cardiac failure are some indications for early intervention. Papillomas are viral-induced verrucous growths that are the most common neoplasms of the aerodigestive tract. When they appear in the nose, they are most often found on the nasal septum.

ORAL CAVITY, PHARYNX, AND ESOPHAGUS

Infections

STOMATITIS

The most common infectious lesion of the oral cavity is the aphthous ulcer. The ulcers are often recurrent, may appear as a single lesion or a confluence of many lesions, and can cause severe stomatitis. The exact cause of aphthous ulcerations is unknown, but it is believed to be infectious.

Herpes simplex can cause severe gingivostomatitis, whereas the pharynx is relatively spared. On the other hand, coxsackievirus infection (herpangina) causes severe ulcerative lesions of the pharynx but not the anterior mouth. These viral infections cause severe oral pain and inability to eat. They are self-limited and require only symptomatic relief (see Chapters 74 and 109).

Candida albicans oral infection (thrush) usually appears as white patches with surrounding inflammation on the oral mucosa. It often occurs in newborns, immunosuppressed patients, and patients receiving antibiotic therapy. Nystatin is an effective treatment. The dosage is 200,000 U (2 mL) four times a day for 14 days.

Acute necrotizing, ulcerative gingivitis (trench mouth) causes painful, bleeding gums. Vigorous brushing of the teeth and gums with a soft brush promotes rapid healing. Antibiotics are of limited value.

PHARYNGITIS/TONSILLITIS

Pharyngitis/tonsillitis (pharyngotonsillitis) may be caused by viral or bacterial organisms. Differentiating viral pharyngotonsillitis from an infection of bacterial origin is difficult on clinical grounds. A throat culture may be helpful in identifying an infection of bacterial origin. The degree of erythema and exudate may vary on the pharynx and tonsils. Bacterial pharyngotonsillitis is treated with a 10-day course of penicillin or amoxicillin. Patients with repeated debilitating bouts of pharyngotonsillitis that do not respond to a 6- to 8-week course of antimicrobial therapy or prophylaxis should be referred to an otolaryngologist for consideration for tonsillectomy and adenoidectomy.

Pharyngeal infections may spread to the peritonsillar area, causing cellulitis. The affected tonsil bulges forward and medially to touch the uvula. If pus localizes in the peritonsillar space, a peritonsillar abscess is formed. The peritonsillar abscess causes trismus. Suspected abscess formation requires immediate consultation with an otolaryngology specialist. Acute treatment of peritonsillar abscess requires systemic (24–48 hours of intravenous followed by oral) antibiotics and needle aspiration or incisional drainage (if possible) of the abscess. Occasionally, a "hot" or quinsy tonsillectomy may be required to treat the acute infection. Later elective tonsillectomy is indicated if there is a previous history of tonsillar or peritonsillar infections.

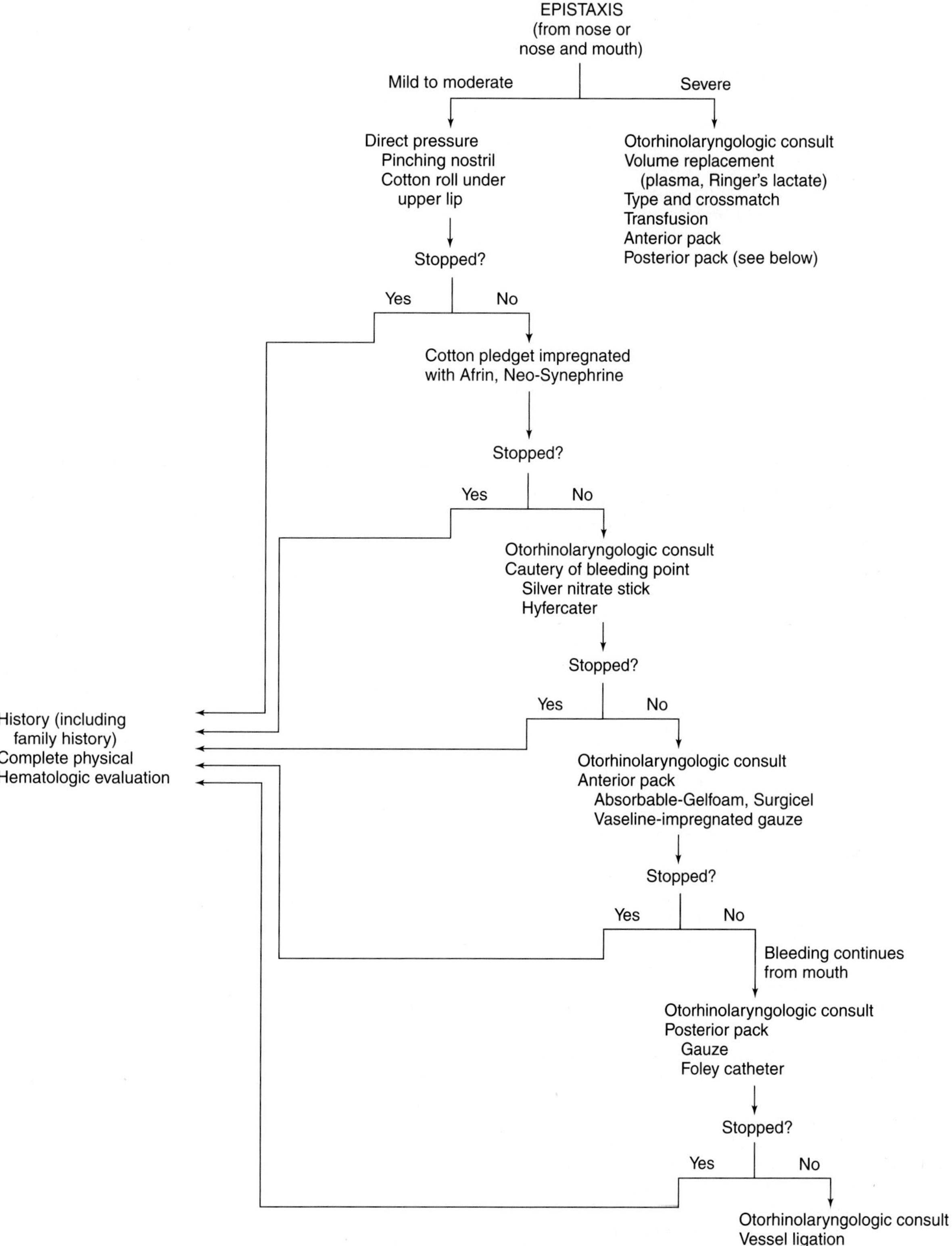

Figure 106.4. Algorithm for management of epistaxis.

RETROPHARYNGEAL AND PARAPHARYNGEAL INFECTION

Retropharyngeal and parapharyngeal lymph nodes also may be involved during pharyngitis and progress to abscess formation. Retropharyngeal abscess usually can be seen easily on the lateral neck radiograph. Peritonsillar, retropharyngeal, and parapharyngeal abscess must be treated with intravenous antibiotics and surgical drainage. (See also "Infections" under the section on "Neck and Associated Structures.")

One must always keep in mind that unusual infections like actinomycosis, mucormycosis, and syphilis may appear in the oral cavity. Actinomycosis appears with oral–cervical fistulas, and *Mucor* causes necrosis of the palate. Syphilis is visible in many ways (eg, ulceration or raised lesion) and has no one characteristic appearance.

ADENOTONSILLAR HYPERTROPHY

Lymphoid hyperplasia (enlarged tonsils and adenoids) can cause airway obstruction that can range from mild snoring to severe sleep apnea with right heart strain. Young children with obstructive sleep apnea are often in the lower 25th percentile by weight (failure to thrive). Older children with severe obstructive sleep apnea are often obese and present with daytime somnolence (Pickwickian syndrome). If right heart strain or daytime somnolence is present, a tonsillectomy and adenoidectomy may be required urgently.

Neoplasms

Benign and malignant neoplasms occur in the oral cavity, pharynx, hypopharynx, and esophagus. Benign neoplasms in the oral cavity may rise from the mucosa or underlying tissues. Minor salivary gland tumors, hemangiomas, lymphangiomas, pyogenic granulomas, and neurofibromas are found in the oral cavity, but they are rarely an emergency.

Nasopharyngeal angiofibromas occur in prepubescent males and cause nasal obstruction. They may appear in the ED with massive epistaxis. Posterior packing usually is required to control the hemorrhage that may be life threatening.

Malignant neoplasms are rare but can occur throughout the oral cavity, pharynx, and esophagus. Rhabdomyosarcoma, lymphoma, and squamous cell carcinoma (lymphoepithelioma) are the most common lesions and are rarely seen as emergencies unless there is extensive hemorrhage or a compromised airway.

Biopsy of oral, pharyngeal, and esophageal tumors is best done in the operating room where adequate exposure and control of hemorrhage is most effectively obtained.

Larynx and Trachea

INFECTIONS

Viral laryngitis is often a component of the common URI described previously in this chapter. Laryngitis manifests by a hoarse, raspy voice as a result of inflammatory edema of the vocal cords. Airway obstruction is rare in viral laryngitis. Symptomatic treatment with humidification, antipyretics, analgesics, throat gargles, and voice rest are recommended while the disease runs its natural course. When the viral infection involves the subglottic space, a more serious clinical problem appears. Laryngotracheobronchitis (croup) is a common—and potentially life-threatening—infection occurring in early childhood. The diagnosis and management of croup are discussed in other chapters of this book (see Chapters 63 and 74).

Bacterial laryngotracheobronchitis does occur, but it is not nearly as common as its viral counterpart. Children aged 3 to 6 years are more commonly affected by bacterial tracheitis compared with the infection of viral origin that usually appears in children aged less than 3 years. It may be difficult to distinguish bacterial laryngitis on clinical grounds from a similar infection of viral origin. Etiologic agents responsible for bacterial laryngitis include staphylococci and *H. influenzae.* Severe airway obstruction, a common symptom of bacterial laryngotracheobronchitis, is caused by thick, inspissated secretions that fill the trachea and are difficult for the child to clear. Treatment consists of the same measures recommended for viral laryngitis with the addition of the appropriate antimicrobial agents. The otolaryngologist usually is required to perform a direct laryngoscopy and bronchoscopy to confirm the diagnosis and to aspirate the thick secretions for therapeutic and diagnostic purposes.

Diphtheria may involve the larynx, in addition to other areas of the upper aerodigestive tract. The diagnosis is suggested by the presence of a membrane covering the pharynx and larynx that leaves a raw, bleeding surface when it is removed. The diphtheria membrane can obstruct the laryngeal airway to cause respiratory distress. Endoscopic removal of the membrane or tracheostomy may be required, in addition to antimicrobial therapy.

Bacterial infection of the supraglottic larynx can cause a symptom complex with potentially life-threatening airway obstruction. *Epiglottitis* (more appropriately called *supraglottitis*) is an infection of the supraglottic larynx that is caused most often by *H. influenzae* type b. The diagnosis and management of epiglottitis are discussed in other chapters of this book (see Chapters 63 and 74).

Neoplasms

Neoplasms of the larynx and trachea are uncommon in children. The otolaryngologist should be consulted to assist the emergency physician in the management of these patients.

The most common neoplasm of the larynx in children is the laryngeal papilloma. This is believed to be a viral-induced neoplasm that has a predilection for the upper aerodigestive tract and the larynx in particular. The disease usually is diagnosed in the child aged between 2 and 5 years and presents with persistent or worsening hoarseness and, occasionally, airway obstruction. If papillomas are suspected as the source of hoarseness in a child, the otolaryngologist should be consulted to perform the indirect or direct laryngoscopy required to confirm the diagnosis. A lateral neck radiograph may demonstrate a soft-tissue mass in the area of the larynx. The course of the disease is characterized by multiple cycles of growth and regression until a spontaneous remission occurs, usually around puberty.

Hemangiomas may occur in the larynx, primarily in the subglottic area. As with most juvenile hemangiomas, these lesions present in the second to sixth month of life and can enlarge over several months to cause significant airway obstruction. Episodes of stridor may be precipitated by a URI. Of children with subglottic hemangiomas, 50% have other cutaneous lesions. Therefore, the presence of cutaneous hemangiomas in an infant with stridor should suggest to the emergency physician the possibility of a subglottic hemangioma. If there is severe, persistent, or recurrent respiratory distress, intervention is indicated. Systemic corticosteroids, CO_2 laser or direct surgical excision, and tracheostomy are some of the modes of treatment presently being advocated.

Malignant neoplasms of the larynx are uncommon. They include rhabdomyosarcoma, chondrosarcoma, and lymphoma. These tumors are seen with varying degrees of hoarseness and respiratory obstruction.

Stridor

The differential diagnosis and emergency management of a child presenting with stridor are discussed in detail in Chapter 63.

NECK AND ASSOCIATED STRUCTURES

Infections

Cervical adenitis is the most common cause of a neck mass in a child. The lymphatic system of the neck drains the internal cavities of the head and neck (ear, nose, mouth, pharynx, sinuses, and larynx) as well as the skin and associated adnexal structures of the face and scalp. Regional cervical lymph nodes respond when there is a primary infection in any area of the head and neck. Because certain groups of nodes drain specific sites in the head and neck, the location of the swollen and infected lymph node often helps the practitioner to identify the area of the primary infection. Ear infections most often drain to the infraauricular nodes, pharyngeal infections (eg, tonsillitis) usually are seen with jugulodigastric node involvement, and posterior cervical nodes often accompany nasopharyngeal infections (eg, adenoiditis).

Cervical adenitis is uncommon secondary to a brief, uncomplicated viral URI. Tender and enlarged nodes occur more often as a result of bacterial infection of the head and neck, with the ears and throat responsible for a large portion of these. Because *Streptococcus* species are the causative agents in most bacterial infections in the head and neck, the infected lymph nodes usually contain the same organisms. Treatment with oral penicillin (or amoxicillin) usually clears the primary infection and causes regression of the enlarged lymph nodes. Culture of the nasopharynx, throat, or aspirate of the cervical node can assist the physician in the choice of antimicrobial agents.

Although most children will respond to the therapy just described, there is a small group of children whose nodes progress to suppurative cervical adenitis. Studies of children hospitalized with cervical adenitis have shown a predominance of *S. aureus* as the causative agent. This high incidence of staphylococci is probably the result of selecting patients who have not responded to oral antimicrobials effective against the more commonly occurring *Streptococcus* species. Therefore, if cervical adenitis has not responded to the primary antimicrobial treatment, agents should be added that are effective against *S. aureus* (erythromycin, dicloxacillin, clindamycin, or cephalosporins).

A child who has demonstrated rapid enlargement of cervical nodes, poor response to oral antimicrobials, cellulitis of the overlying skin, abscess formation, or signs of toxicity (high fever, malaise, dehydration) should be admitted to the hospital for treatment with intravenous fluids and antimicrobials. Surgical consultation should be obtained in the management of these complicated cases in which needle aspiration, incisional drainage, or biopsy (for possible neoplasm) may be required.

Retropharyngeal or parapharyngeal nodes are uncommonly involved with inflammatory processes that originate in the pharynx. Sore throat, dysphagia, and stiff neck are some of the symptoms that can accompany significantly enlarged pharyngeal nodes. Retropharyngeal nodes can be overlying the cervical spine during examination of the oropharynx. They also appear as widening of the retropharyngeal soft tissues on lateral neck radiographs. Parapharyngeal nodes are seldom detected clinically unless they enlarge sufficiently to deviate the tonsil and pharyngeal wall medially. Treatment of enlarged pharyngeal nodes consists of intravenous antimicrobials (usually penicillin) and observation of the child's airway. Biopsy of the mass is indicated if resolution does not occur with treatment or if a malignancy is suspected.

A collection of purulent material within the tissues of the neck, a neck abscess, requires prompt and specific treatment. The most common cause of a neck abscess is breakdown or necrosis of an infected lymph node. Purulent material may be located within a single node or may accumulate between several adjacent nodes. Once the process of cervical adenitis has progressed to the point of abscess formation, treatment involves evacuation of the infected material and the prevention of further spread of the infection. The child is hospitalized, and intravenous antimicrobials are administered that are effective against *S. aureus* (antistaphylococcal penicillin). Otolaryngologic consultation is obtained to perform a needle aspiration or incision and drainage to evacuate and culture the infected material.

Deep-neck abscesses are uncommon in children but can be extremely dangerous when they occur. Parapharyngeal abscess occurs when purulent material collects in the parapharyngeal space lateral to the pharyngeal constrictors and medial to the vascular compartment of the neck. Necrosis of parapharyngeal lymph nodes and lateral extension of a peritonsillar abscess are the two main sources of this infection. The child with a parapharyngeal abscess presents with a stiff neck, high fever, malaise, dehydration, and other signs of toxicity. The child usually has dysphagia and may not be able to swallow his or her own saliva. Physical examination reveals diffuse swelling and tenderness of one side of the neck, but fluctuance is seldom appreciated. Intraoral examination may demonstrate medial displacement of the lateral pharyngeal wall and tonsil. Lateral neck radiographs are usually not helpful in evaluating this disease process. CT or MRI scans provide the best evaluation of suspected deep-neck abscesses. If left to progress, the parapharyngeal abscess can involve the adjacent vascular structures in the neck, descend into the mediastinum, or spontaneously rupture into the pharynx, causing aspiration of purulent material.

Otolaryngologic consultation should be obtained to assist the emergency physician in the evaluation of a patient with a parapharyngeal abscess. Appropriate treatment consists of hospitalization, intravenous fluids, antimicrobials effective against *S. aureus* (antistaphylococcal penicillins, clindamycin, cephalosporins), and external drainage of the abscess.

Retropharyngeal abscess occurs as a result of the necrosis of retropharyngeal lymph nodes or secondary to perforation of the pharynx or esophagus. Purulent material collects between the retropharyngeal and prevertebral layers of the cervical fascia, also called the *danger space*. This potential space extends from the base of the skull to the mediastinum, thus allowing extensive spread of the infection. A child presents with symptoms similar to those associated with parapharyngeal abscess. Lateral neck radiographs demonstrate widening and bulging of the retropharyngeal space. Treatment consists of hospitalization, intravenous fluids, antimicrobials effective against *S. aureus*, and drainage (either intraoral or external) of the abscess.

Nontubercular mycobacterial (NTM) infection is a common cause of chronic cervical adenitis in children. Also called *atypical mycobacteria*, the ubiquitous agent is thought to gain access to the cervical lymph nodes through oral mucosal breaks (eg, teething, minor trauma). The usual presentation of NTM cervical adenitis is that of a nontender, slightly fluctuant cervical mass with overlying skin that has a characteristic violaceous hue. Chest radiographs are usually normal, and purified protein derivative (PPD) tests are most often reported as negative or intermediate in their response. NTM infections do not respond to antitubercular antibiotics. The child should be referred to an otolaryngologist to perform surgical excision that is required to cure this condition. Incision and drainage are discouraged because this will lead to a chronic draining sinus.

Salivary gland infections should be considered in the differential diagnosis of a cervical mass suspected to be infectious in origin. Both viral and bacterial agents can be responsible for the infection, with the former being more common. Mumps (endemic parotitis) is the most common salivary infection in children. Although the parotid gland is involved in more than 85% of cases, the submandibular gland also may be involved with the viral infection. The infection appears with acute painful swelling of the involved gland or glands. There is erythema around the intraoral orifice of the salivary duct, and the saliva expressed is generally clear. Treatment is supportive with clear fluids, antipyretics, and analgesics as necessary.

Bacterial infections of the salivary glands are seen with signs and symptoms similar to those associated with cervical lymphadenitis. Neonatal parotitis and, less commonly, submandibular sialadenitis usually occur in a 3- to 4-week-old child after a systemic illness has caused dehydration. The affected gland is swollen, and abscess formation may occur. Purulent material may be expressed from either the Stenson or Wharton duct by massage of the affected salivary gland. Otolaryngologic consultation should be obtained. The child is hospitalized for treatment with intravenous antimicrobials effective against *S. aureus* (antistaphylococcal penicillin) and surgical drainage of any collection of purulent material. Recurrent or chronic infections of the salivary glands usually are related to some predisposing factor such as stones, ductal stenosis, or secretory immunodeficiency. Management should include the detection and correction of these conditions.

Neoplasms

Neoplasms of the neck, both primary and metastatic, occur in children. If a cervical neoplasm is suspected, an otolaryngologist should be consulted to perform a complete examination of the head and neck, including endoscopy of the nasopharynx, larynx, and hypopharynx.

The hemangioma is the most common neoplasm of the head and neck in children. Although they are more common on the skin of the face and scalp, lesions can occur on the skin of the neck and involve deeper structures, such as the parotid gland. The diagnosis of cutaneous hemangiomas of the cervical skin is usually obvious on physical inspection; the lesions are red to reddish-purple, flat or raised, blanch with pressure, and increase in size with crying or straining. Deep-seated lesions without cutaneous manifestations may require special diagnostic aids such as CT or MRI scans and, rarely, biopsy to confirm the diagnosis.

Lymphangiomas are uncommon benign lesions of the neck. Cystic hygroma is the most common type of lymphangioma found in the neck. These lesions consist of multiple cystic spaces filled with lymph and, occasionally, blood. They appear most commonly as large lateral neck masses in neonates. The diagnosis is often obvious on physical examination of a large cystic lesion that transilluminates. The natural history of these lesions is usually one of progressive growth and enlargement. Lymphangiomas can fluctuate in size secondary to a concurrent infection of the head and neck or hemorrhage into a cyst. Small, stable, asymptomatic lesions can be managed by close observation.

Less common benign neoplasms of the neck in children include teratomas, paragangliomas (carotid body tumors, glomus tumors), neural sheath tumors (neurofibromas, neurolemmas), and thyroid and salivary gland neoplasms.

The sternocleidomastoid "tumor" of infancy is an unusual lesion that appears as a discrete mass within the substance of the sternocleidomastoid muscle in a child aged 4 to 8 weeks. The cause of this localized area of fibrosis is unknown. The lesion usually resolves with range-of-motion exercises. Surgical intervention is indicated in cases in which the fibrosis progresses to cause torticollis (see "Neck Stiffness" in Chapter 39) or if there is suspicion of a malignancy.

The most common malignant neoplasm of the neck in children is lymphoma, being almost equally divided into Hodgkin and non-Hodgkin types. The disease may be localized in the neck, or it may be a part of a more generalized disorder. Physical examination often reveals multiple firm, rubbery, unilateral, or bilateral nodes. If the diagnosis of lymphoma is suspected, otolaryngologic consultation should be obtained for a careful examination of the oral cavity, pharynx, and paranasal sinuses to look for a primary or associated lesion. This not only aids in the evaluation of the extent of the lymphoma but also may locate a site from which a biopsy can be obtained without the morbidity of a neck exploration.

Cervical lymph nodes may appear as neoplasm metastatic from a nonlymphogenous primary tumor. Thyroid carcinoma, squamous carcinoma (lymphoepithelioma) of the nasopharynx, and malignant melanoma may be seen first with enlarged cervical lymph nodes. These nodes tend to be hard and singular and may be fixed to underlying structures. Otolaryngologic consultation should be obtained for a complete examination of the head and neck to search for a primary lesion. Biopsy of the node is usually required for diagnosis.

Rhabdomyosarcoma is the most common soft-tissue sarcoma of the head and neck in children, and its frequency of occurrence in the neck is second only to that in the orbit. The child usually presents with a history of rapid enlargement of a painless neck mass. The mass itself is hard, often diffuse, and poorly mobile. Although the diagnosis of rhabdomyosarcoma may be suspected from the history and physical examination, biopsy is always required for confirmation.

Many other malignant neoplasms also can occur in the neck. These include soft-tissue sarcomas other than rhabdomyosarcoma, malignant fibrous histiocytoma, and neuroblastoma.

CHAPTER 107
Urologic Emergencies

Howard M. Snyder III, M.D.

Early in their lives, children become familiar with the act of voiding and the appearance of their genitals. Disturbances of either are a great source of concern to them and their parents. This may result in an anxious trip to the emergency department (ED), requiring the emergency physician to be familiar with the problems to be discussed in this section (see Chapter 50).

PENILE PROBLEMS

Penile Care in the Uncircumcised Male

Although the data of Wiswell and Roscelli have suggested that the presence of the foreskin may make ascending urinary infection an increased risk in newborn males, the overall low incidence of problems associated with the foreskin and the benefits from its removal lead us to continue to discourage routine circumcision. This view is common and increasing numbers of uncircumcised children are seen in EDs. Surprisingly, few physicians know how to care for uncircumcised boys. It is important to realize that, in male infants, adhesions between the glans and the foreskin are normal (Fig. 107.1). The foreskin is not normally retractable in this age group. No effort should be made to strip the foreskin back in infants because that not only produces undue pain for the child, but also may result in a raw surface, with consequent inflammation and scarring. Between ages 2 and 4, lysis of the adhesions is spontaneous in 90% of children. It is rare for the young male to have any adverse hygienic consequence

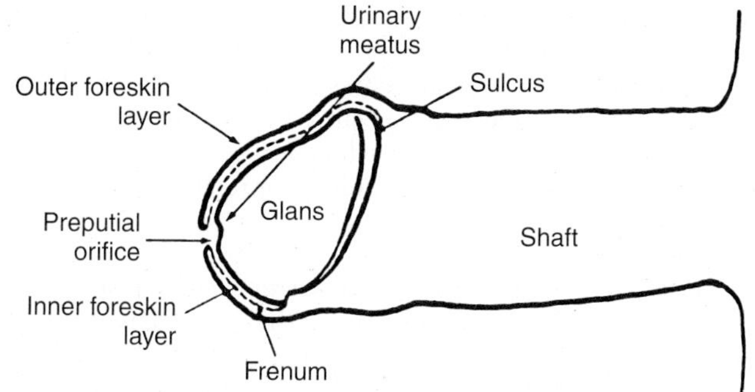

Figure 107.1. Anatomy of normal uncircumcised male. Adhesions between inner foreskin layer and glans are normal in newborns and prevent retraction of the foreskin. (Reprinted with permission from Wallerstein E. *Circumcision: an American health fallacy*. New York: Springer, 1980:201.)

from leaving the foreskin in place until spontaneous lysis of the adhesions takes place. The small, whitish lumps that may be seen and felt beneath the foreskin represent only desquamated epithelium and need not be removed. When toilet training has occurred, it is wise to teach a boy to retract the foreskin enough to expose the meatus when he voids. Not only does this facilitate better aiming, but it also avoids leaving the inner foreskin wet with urine. Ammoniacal irritation can lead to inflammatory adhesions and may create a portal of entry for a bacterial balanoposthitis. When a boy is able to retract his foreskin, usually between 4 and 6 years of age but sometimes later, he may be taught to withdraw the foreskin and carry out normal hygiene as part of bathing.

Phimosis and Paraphimosis

Phimosis exists when tightness of the distal foreskin precludes its being withdrawn to expose the glans. Although inflammation of the foreskin from severe chronic ammoniacal rash or infection may lead to scarring and a true phimosis, this is uncommon in children. More often, normal penile adhesions are confused with phimosis.

In the uncircumcised male, if the foreskin is retracted behind the glans and left in that position, venous congestion and edema of the foreskin results, making it difficult to reduce the foreskin to a normal position. This condition of a swollen, retracted foreskin is called paraphimosis. The application of ice and steady local manual compression usually reduces the edema and permits manual reduction of the paraphimosis. A local anesthetic penile block of the dorsal nerve of the penis at the base of the shaft will reduce the discomfort experienced by the child during compression of the edematous foreskin. Once a portion of the edema has been reduced, pressure on glans (like turning a sock inside out) usually permits reduction of the foreskin back to its normal position (Fig. 107.2). If manual reduction fails, a surgical division of the foreskin to permit reduction is indicated. That usually may be accomplished with sedation and local anesthetic. If surgical reduction of the foreskin is required, it should be followed a few weeks later by a circumcision. Education in the care of the uncircumcised male will reduce the incidence of this condition.

Balanoposthitis

Balanoposthitis is an infection of the foreskin that may extend onto the glans. It is a form of cellulitis and has its origin from a break in the penile skin, commonly associated with ammoniacal dermatitis. It may be the result of local trauma or may, in the older boy, be associated with poor penile hygiene. Scarring after the inflammatory reaction may lead to true phimosis. The acute infection is dealt with adequately by warm soaks and the administration of an appropriate antibiotic, usually ampicillin (50 to 100 mg per kg every 24 hours in four doses). It is unusual for a child to be unable to void as a result of this condition, although he may be more comfortable voiding while in a tub of warm water.

Penile Swelling

Although most penile swelling is painful and the result of either infection, as described previously, or trauma, to be described later, occasionally a child has isolated penile edema that is either nontender or minimally tender. This may result from an insect bite, with local edema secondary to histamine release. A history of a bite or the finding of a small punctate lesion may give the clue to diagnosis. Painless penile edema may be present with a generalized allergic reaction or as part of the manifestation of a general edematous state secondary to renal, cardiac, or hepatic problems. Here, the diagnosis is suggested by evidence of dysfunction in these organ systems on general examination. It is also important to remember that penile swelling may be caused by a strangulation injury.

Priapism

Prolonged, painful penile erection unaccompanied by sexual stimulation is called priapism. In the pediatric age group, this entity may be caused by trauma or leukemic infiltration, but it is most often seen in African-American males with sickle cell disease. A sickling crisis that involves the corporal bodies does not necessarily need to be related to symptomatic sickling elsewhere in the body. Sickling of the erythrocytes produces sludging and stasis in the erectile tissue of the corporal bodies. This stasis leads to further hypoxia, acidosis, and more sickling. The thick, dark sludge that is formed prevents detumescence of the erectile tissue and thus causes priapism. Pain results from ischemia. It is speculated that an inflammatory reaction to this material may lead to fibrosis of the erectile tissue. Impotence may result.

Although recommendations for treating priapism have ranged from ice or hot packs, estrogens, and spinal anesthesia to radiation therapy, the best treatment for priapism associated with sickle cell disease now appears to be hydration and irriga-

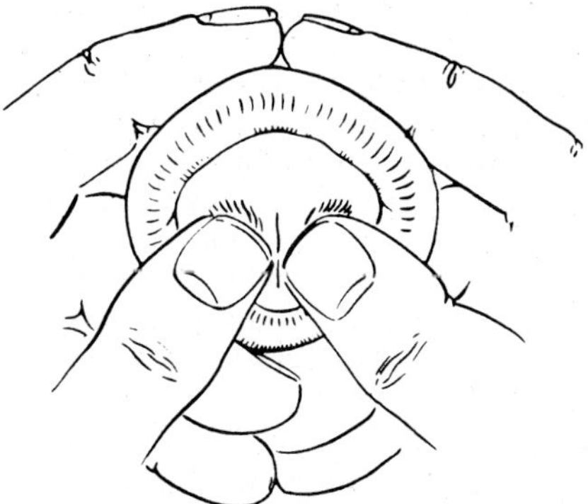

Figure 107.2. Manual reduction of paraphimosis. After a local anesthetic block of the dorsal nerve of the penis, the foreskin is manually compressed to reduce edema. The foreskin can be reduced by pressure on glans—like turning a sock inside out. (Reprinted with permission from Klauber GT, Sant GR. Disorders of the male external genitalia. In: Kelalis PP, King LR, Belman AB, eds. *Clinical pediatric urology*, 2nd ed. Philadelphia: WB Saunders, 1985:287.)

tion of the corporal bodies with saline in combination with vasoactive substances. This is best carried out with urologic consultation. Although priapism has been documented to lead to impotence in some cases, impotence is rare in priapism related to sickle cell disease, unless the patient has been subjected to a surgical procedure. It may be that the more difficult cases are the ones most likely to come to surgical treatment, and impotence thus may reflect more the basic disease, rather than the type of treatment.

Meatal Stenosis

Meatal stenosis is a problem almost exclusively of circumcised males and follows an inflammatory reaction around the meatus, usually the result of the lower edge of the meatus rubbing against a wet diaper with inflammation of the meatus resulting from mechanical and ammoniacal chemical dermatitis. Meatal stenosis is rare in the boy who has a circumcision after becoming continent. Appearances are often deceiving. The meatus may appear to be stenotic, but may be functioning adequately. Significant meatal stenosis causes spraying of the urinary stream or more commonly, dorsal deflection of the stream. Surgical treatment of the meatus is warranted only if these symptoms are present. Meatal stenosis is not a cause of frequency, enuresis, or urinary tract infection (UTI). When it is indicated, we carry out a meatotomy in our office after application of topical penile anesthesia with EMLA cream and the infiltration of a small amount of Xylocaine with epinephrine into the ventral edge of the meatus. A general anesthetic usually is neither necessary nor indicated.

Penile Trauma

DIRECT INJURY

The most common cause of direct injury to the penis comes from the toilet seat's falling on the penis of a little boy who is learning to stand at the toilet to void. Although the resulting penile edema may be notable, significant injury to the corporal bodies or urethra is rare. Although parents may be concerned that the child will be unable to void, this generally is not a problem, but the child may be more comfortable voiding in a tub of warm water. The only treatment required is warm soaks and expectant observation.

After blunt or sharp trauma, if blood is seen at the urethral meatus, urethral injury must be considered and a retrograde urethrogram carried out. Pediatric urologic consultation is appropriate, as is follow-up for possible stricture formation (see Chapter 96).

If a child is seen for a laceration of the shaft of the penis, it is important to be certain that the corporal bodies and urethra have not been injured concurrently. When a question exists, pediatric urologic consultation, retrograde urethrogram, and exploration under anesthetic may be needed. For simple lacerations of the penile skin, repair with chromic catgut suffices. It should be recalled that a child who has any form of a genital injury may be a victim of sexual abuse (see Chapter 111).

ZIPPER INJURY

Boys often seem to be in a hurry and sometimes fail to get their penis or foreskin completely back in their pants before they pull up the zipper. This results in the entrapment of penile skin or foreskin in the teeth of the zipper. The teeth may be so engaged that it is impossible to simply unzip the zipper. Often, the problem may be dealt with simply, as shown in Fig. 96.3. The median bar of the zipper may be cut with a pair of wire cutters, which will permit the two halves of the zipper to fall apart, releasing the entrapped skin. Mineral oil has also been used to allow the tissue to slide free of the metal zipper. Local infiltration of Xylocaine makes this procedure less traumatic to the child. Only rarely is a general anesthetic required. After the zipper is removed, the penis may become edematous, but generally nothing more than warm soaks is required for further treatment.

STRANGULATION

The penis may be encircled by a constricting ring formed by hair or a fiber or a thread, just as occurs with digits. Many times the cause of the problem is not immediately evident, because local edema may hide the ring of hair. The edema is produced by venous engorgement, which takes place early, after the development of this type of constriction around the penis. Once the source of the problem has been identified, therapy requires the division of the hair and the release of the constriction. This may require a general anesthetic. Pediatric urologic consultation is advisable. A urethrocutaneous fistula or even the loss of the penis has been reported, but is rare. How the hair comes to encircle the penis is generally unknown, but it should be remembered that such constriction occasionally has been reported as a form of sexual abuse.

TESTICULAR PROBLEMS

Retractile Testis

In the physical examination of the child in the ED, an empty scrotum on one or both sides is a common finding. Although the testis may be found to be truly undescended, more often it is merely a retractile testis. In a boy with a retractile testis, the active cremaster muscle attached to the small prepubertal gonad is able to draw the testis up into a position near the pubic tubercle. There is no evidence that this causes any harm to the gonad. When the testis enlarges at puberty, it will assume a scrotal position permanently because the cremaster is no longer able to draw it out of its more normal position. The diagnosis of a retractile testis is made when one is easily able to milk the testis down into a position in a dependent portion of the scrotum where the testis stays, at least briefly, after overstretch of the cremaster muscle. In an obese youngster, it may be difficult to grasp the testis to pull it down. It is worthwhile putting a youngster in a "catcher's position," in which the testis is pushed down to where it can be grasped and drawn into the scrotum. If the testis can be pulled into the scrotum but, regardless of how much the cremaster is overstretched, the testis "pops up" when released, this is a low form of a true undescended testis and not a retractile testis. This is a common diagnostic difficulty and pediatric urologic consultation should be sought if the situation is questionable.

Undescended Testis

True undescended testes are seen in 4% of newborn males. That instance decreases to 1.6% by 1 year of age, indicating that some undescended testes do descend after birth. Spontaneous descent rarely occurs after 6 months of age. Although it may be appropriate to continue for a few months to observe an infant who has an undescended testis, the child older than 6 months of age should have urologic consultation.

Testicular malignancy and infertility are increased in the male with an uncorrected undescended testis. By electron microscopy, it is possible to demonstrate degenerative changes in the undescended testis by 1 year of age. Early referral to a urologist for orchiopexy (before age 2 and preferably near age 1) appears advisable because data are now accumulating that indicate early surgery may decrease the incidence of both testicular malignancy and infertility.

Usually, an undescended testis is asymptomatic. However, in a position against the abdominal wall, it may be more subject to trauma than when freely mobile in the scrotum. The undescended testis also is malfixed and may undergo torsion more easily than a normally descended one. The boy who presents with an acutely tender groin mass with an ipsilateral empty scrotum may have a torsion of his undescended testis. The physician must consider the differential diagnosis of an incarcerated inguinal hernia or acute hydrocele of the cord. Prompt surgical treatment is required.

Varicocele

Varicoceles are abnormal dilations of the cremasteric and pampiniform venous plexuses surrounding the spermatic cord. They generally present as an asymptomatic scrotal swelling about the time of puberty and are rare in the prepubertal boy. Almost all are of congenital origin and affect the left testis. The anatomic problem is a defect in the valves of the left spermatic vein that, on the left, drains directly into the left renal vein. Why varicoceles often are not noted until a boy approaches puberty is unclear, but they are common in that age group, affecting about 15% of adolescent boys. If the varicocele does not disappear when the child lies down, it suggests a varicocele secondary to obstruction of the left renal vein, and a renal and bladder ultrasound is appropriate. Varicoceles are rarely symptomatic; a heavy or tugging sensation is occasionally reported.

Approximately 15% of these boys with a varicocele will have an adult problem with infertility, although the exact mechanism of injury to the spermatogenic elements remains to be defined.

URINARY TRACT INFECTIONS

Urinary tract infection (UTI) ranks behind upper respiratory problems as the second most common form of bacterial infection in children. Between 1% and 2% of infants and children have bacteriuria at any given time, and 5% of all girls have UTI during their school years. Most UTIs result from fecal bacteria on the perineal skin ascending the urethra. The short female urethra, with resultant ease of bacterial contamination of the bladder, accounts for the higher incidence of UTIs in girls. The uncircumcised male infant appears also to be at increased risk of ascending urinary infection because foreskin bacterial colonization may lead to increased meatal contamination.

It is now recognized that the major risk factor in the development of UTI is the physical nature of the uroepithelium lining the urethra and bladder. In some children and adults, adherence factors in the mucosa lead to recurrent episodes of symptomatic infection. In addition, some bacteria (pileated ones) have increased adherence characteristics that add to the risk of invasive infection. Because voiding dysfunction may also contribute to recurrent infection, this is another reason to consider pediatric urologic consultations, especially in the older child who persists with wetting after appropriate treatment of infection.

A UTI may be defined as the multiplication of bacteria in the urinary tract. Normally, urine from the bladder and upper urinary tract should be sterile. The concept of "significant bacteriuria" ($\geq 10^5$ organisms per milliliter of one colony type) in a cleanly voided midstream specimen is based on the statistical likelihood that this colony count is associated with the actual presence of bacteria in the bladder. A colony count of 10^5 or more organisms per milliliter of a single type suggests infected urine, with an 80% confidence level. Reliability can be increased to 95% if a second culture confirms the presence of the same bacteria type with identical antibiotic sensitivity; 10^4 to 10^5 bacteria per milliliter is an equivocal result and requires repeat culture. Less than 10^4 organisms per milliliter or the presence of several different organisms, suggests no infection or contamination of the specimen (see Chapter 74).

CLINICAL MANIFESTATIONS

Particularly in the infant, UTIs may produce nonspecific findings. The urine may be cloudy or have a foul odor. There may be a history of unexplained fevers, general irritability, or failure to thrive and gain weight normally. Gastrointestinal (GI) symptoms are common, and many times the youngster with a UTI is believed to have gastroenteritis or a food allergy. A high index of suspicion is required. If a urine culture is not obtained, the source of the child's problem will be missed.

In the older child, symptoms may point more directly at the urinary tract. Frequency, urgency, and dysuria are produced by inflammation of the bladder and urethra. A previously toilet-trained child may begin to have "accidents." Particularly in girls, hematuria may be seen. Although symptoms do not provide a completely reliable way of differentiating cystitis from pyelonephritis, the presence of systemic findings such as a high fever and malaise or abdominal/flank pain suggests renal involvement. A UTI, especially when chronic, may also have few or no symptoms. It is important to emphasize that in children, anything that irritates the urethral meatus may produce dysuria and occasionally urgency and frequency (see Chapter 46). The source of the irritation may be a tight or moist bathing suit or underwear or an ammoniacal rash. Bubble bath or other soap in contact with the urethral meatus may not only produce these symptoms, but, by producing inflammation, contributes to the ascent of bacteria up the urethra and the development of true infection.

Escherichia coli is the most commonly isolated organism responsible for UTI in children, constituting 80% to 90% of the total. This is because of the prevalence of the organism in GI tract flora, as well as its short mean-generation time, which enables it to multiply rapidly once it has entered the bladder. The other organisms commonly found can be seen in Table 107.1.

MANAGEMENT

The first step in management is to make an accurate diagnosis. The presence of pyuria does not provide an accurate criterion for the diagnosis of UTI. At least 20% of children with pyuria do not demonstrate significant bacteriuria. In any febrile illness, mobilization of the peripheral leukocyte pool may be adequate to produce the presence of white cells in the urine. Conversely, a child with bacteriuria occasionally does not demonstrate pyuria. Bacteria demonstrated by Gram stain of an unspun urine specimen are more reliably indicative of a UTI. However, it is difficult to determine whether one type of bacteria or several different contaminants are present. Thus, culture of the urine must continue to be the benchmark for the diagnosis of a UTI in children. Obtaining an adequate urine specimen for bac-

TABLE 107.1. Bacteria Commonly Causing Urinary Tract Infections

Escherichia coli	*Proteus* species
Klebsiella pneumoniae	*Pseudomonas aeruginosa*
Streptococcus faecalis (enterococcus)	*Staphylococcus epidermidis*

terial culture is the most critical step in diagnosing UTI. A cleanly voided specimen obtained as a midstream catch after washing of the periurethral area is the preferred technique in the toilet-trained child. Simple soap and water washing of the periurethral area is preferred because antimicrobial soaps or solutions may become mixed with a voided specimen and lead to a false-negative result.

In the infant, obtaining an adequate urine specimen is more difficult. Specimens collected in a plastic bag (U-bag) attached to the perineum are rapidly contaminated by perineal bacterial skin flora. If a culture from a bag is sterile, it is acceptable. However, the demonstration of bacterial growth must be confirmed by some other means before a bona fide UTI can be presumed to be present. The most reliable way to obtain a confirming specimen of urine is by suprapubic aspiration of urine from the bladder, a procedure that is not dangerous and that has a reliability approaching 100%. A specimen obtained by urethral catheterization is an acceptable alternative. If it is essential that the first specimen be the definitive one for diagnosis of UTI, as in the infant undergoing septic workup, the primary use of these techniques is justified. When symptoms strongly suggest the possibility of a UTI, beginning antibiotic therapy as soon as an adequate urine specimen for culture has been obtained is recommended. The matter of just 1 or 2 days before the institution of antibiotics may make a difference in the degree of eventual pyelonephritic scarring. If the urine culture turns out to be negative, the antibiotics may be stopped. Table 107.2 lists the most commonly used outpatient antibiotics for UTIs.

Although any of these antibiotic choices is acceptable in the initial therapy of a UTI, trimethoprim–sulfamethoxazole has become most commonly used in recent years because of its acceptance by children and high efficacy. Nitrofurantoin, although effective, can produce GI upset (lessened by taking with meals) and is less well tolerated by most children. Methenamine mandelate is not useful unless there is urinary stasis and acid urine, and accordingly has little role in most childhood UTIs. Tetracycline is not recommended for the child less than 10 years of age because of its potential for discoloration of the teeth. When the organism causing UTI is sensitive to the antibiotic selected, the urine is usually sterilized rapidly. It is advisable to repeat a culture 48 hours after starting an antibiotic. The continued presence of infection suggests inaccuracy of the sensitivity, noncompliance, or obstruction.

If a child is sufficiently toxic to warrant hospitalization, the intravenous administration of antibiotics is appropriate. The drugs of choice while cultures are pending are a cephalosporin or aminoglycoside, singly or in combination.

The duration of therapy has been a subject of recent debate. For uncomplicated cystitis, 1 to 3 days of therapy is usually adequate. For children who have not been radiographically evaluated or for any child with a congenital anomaly, a 10-day course of antibiotics continues to be recommended.

TABLE 107.2. Antibiotic Agents for Urinary Tract Infections

Drug	Oral dosage	Number of doses
Trimethoprim–sulfamethoxazole	1 mL suspension/kg/d	2
Sulfisoxazole	120 mg/kg/d	4
Nitrofurantoin	5–7 mg/kg/d	4
Amoxicillin	50–100 mg/kg/d	3
Cephalexin	50–100 mg/kg/d	4

Other factors in the treatment of UTI involve high fluid intake with regular and frequent voidings to promote bladder washout of bacteria. If the child has a history of wetting, infrequent voiding, or frequent urge episodes, the possibility of dysfunctional voiding, which can contribute to recurrent infections, should be considered and appropriate consultation obtained. Avoiding constipation helps ensure better bladder emptying. Good perineal hygiene, including wiping from front to back after a bowel movement, is important. Eliminating pinworms prevents a source of inflammation, excoriation, and secondary increase in perineal skin flora. Bubble bath, by producing inflammation at the meatus, may promote the ascent of bacteria and should be avoided. Acidification of the urine with oral Vitamin C or juices high in citric acid content may be useful to produce an acid urine in which bacteria multiply less rapidly.

UROLOGIC FOLLOW-UP AND RADIOGRAPHIC INVESTIGATION

A suppressive dose of antibiotics should be begun after the acute phase of full-dose treatment. It is customary to use one-third to one-half the dose of antibiotic used for acute treatment, usually administered in a once-a-day evening dose. Suppressive antibiotics reduce the likelihood of recurrent infection, pending urologic consultation and radiographic investigation.

The routine radiographic evaluation of a UTI is by means of a voiding cystourethrogram (VCUG), followed by an ultrasound examination of the kidneys and bladder. These studies are usually carried out about 2 to 4 weeks after the acute treatment of a UTI; however, failure of a child to respond promptly to appropriate antibiotic therapy should lead to the urgent performance of an ultrasound examination to rule out urinary obstruction. The cystogram must include a voiding phase, or significant pathology may be missed, particularly vesicoureteral reflux, which may be evident only on voiding films. In the usual child with a UTI, cystoscopy contributes little to the initial investigation; therefore, it is not recommended.

All boys should be investigated after their first UTI. In girls, Kunin's data demonstrate that after one UTI, there is an 80% likelihood of a second episode of bacteriuria and that half of these children will be asymptomatic. Thus, it appears justified to carry out radiographic studies after a first documented infection in girls as well as boys.

In approximately 50% of infants and 30% of older children, an anatomic abnormality is found in association with a UTI. The most common finding is vesicoureteral reflux. Reflux permits infected urine to ascend to the kidney, where pyelonephritic damage may occur. With linear growth of the child, many milder cases of reflux may spontaneously resolve, leaving surgical management primarily for the more severe cases. These decisions are best made in consultation with a pediatric urologist.

ACUTE URINARY RETENTION

A patient with acute urinary retention is unable to empty the bladder even though it is full. In children, as in adults, the cause may be a urethral obstruction. Congenital lesions, such as urethral valves, or acquired lesions, such as posttraumatic strictures, may lead to urinary retention. In such cases, a careful history often elicits symptoms of a weak stream or difficulty initiating the stream. Children who have any form of urethral irritation and dysuria may voluntarily retain urine. That is a different situation and needs to be separated carefully from organic obstruction causing retention. For the child with voluntary retention, gentle massage of the lower abdomen combined with a soak in a warm tub usually leads to spontaneous evacuation of the bladder. Rarely does a child's bladder become so distended, as after an outpatient surgical general anesthetic, that the child is unable to void. A simple one-time emptying of the bladder by catheterization with a feeding tube usually corrects the problem. It should be remembered that a child is able to hold urine voluntarily for longer periods than would be suspected; up to 12 hours is not unusual. Unless the child has a history suggestive of an organic obstruction or has a palpably enlarged bladder that cannot be emptied by massage and warm tub soaks, instrumenting the child's urethra should not be considered. Urologic consultation would be advisable before undertaking such maneuvers.

CHAPTER 108
Orthopedic Emergencies

Mark D. Joffe, M.D. and
John Loiselle, M.D.

OSTEOMYELITIS

Osteomyelitis is an inflammation of the bone, most commonly of infectious origin. Infection is confirmed by the presence of two of the following: pus on an aspirate of the bone, clinical findings consistent with the diagnosis, positive blood or bone aspirate cultures, and radiologic imaging. Osteomyelitis is more common in boys, and several studies have found the highest incidence among infants and preschool children. Age and underlying disorders are associated with an increased risk for contracting osteomyelitis, as well as for the particular pathogens involved.

Infection occurs by one of three routes: hematogenous, direct spread, or inoculation through a penetrating wound. Hematogenous spread is the most common route in children. A transient bacteremia is believed to be the initiating event in the infection. Bacteria enter the bone at the level of the metaphysis through the predominant vascular supply of the bone.

A less common source of osteomyelitis in children is penetration of the periosteum by local infections. Inoculation of the bone from stepping on a nail, surgical instrumentation, or intraosseous line placement, provides a third means for infection to gain entrance to the bone. With either mechanism of infection, osteomyelitis can progress to chronic osteomyelitis that may have deleterious effects on growth.

CLINICAL FINDINGS

Physical signs of osteomyelitis are age dependent. The older child is more likely to have localized infection and is more capable of expressing or identifying a site of localized point tenderness. The neonate or young infant may present with a pseudoparalysis of the affected limb. Another common, although nonspecific, finding in this age group is paradoxic irritability in which the infant exhibits pain or distress upon handling, and is more comfortable when left alone.

Fever and pain are highly sensitive findings but not universally present. Fever is described in up to 90% of children with osteomyelitis upon presentation and may be quite elevated. Pain is expressed through limp, refusal to bear weight, or a decreased range of motion when a limb is involved. Erythema and swelling are less common, but can also be observed at the site and usually suggest more advanced periosteal involvement.

DIAGNOSIS

In addition to clinical findings, the diagnosis of osteomyelitis depends on culture results. Blood cultures and bone aspirates should be obtained in suspected cases of osteomyelitis before the initiation of antibiotics. Isolation of the causative organism is important not only in diagnosis, but also in antibiotic selection and the possibility of eventual outpatient therapy. Reports of positive blood cultures range from 30% to 57%. An organism is recovered from a bone aspirate in 51% to 90% of cases. The combination identifies a pathogen in 75% to 80% of cases. Bone aspirates may remain positive for several days after antibiotic use, whereas blood cultures are often sterile within 24 hours of antibiotics.

Laboratory tests vary in sensitivity. The white blood cell (WBC) count is elevated in only one-third of the cases of osteomyelitis, whereas both the erythrocyte sedimentation rate (ESR) and C-reactive protein (CRP) are elevated in more than 90%. The latter tests are useful both in diagnosis and for monitoring the response to therapy.

The plain radiograph is the initial imaging study of choice. It is useful both in detecting early signs of osteomyelitis and excluding other diagnostic possibilities. The earliest radiograph changes suggestive of osteomyelitis include deep soft-tissue swelling with elevation of the muscle planes from the adjacent bone. These may be seen as early as 3 to 4 days after the onset of symptoms. Lytic bone changes are not detectable until 7 to 10 days. Periosteal elevation, when present, is not generally visible until 10 to 21 days after infection. A negative radiograph in the first 10 days of illness does not rule out osteomyelitis. When suspicion remains high in the setting of a negative radiograph, a bone scan should be obtained. The triple phase technetium bone scan has a reported sensitivity and specificity of more than 90%, and detects osteomyelitis within 24 to 48 hours of symptom onset. A bone aspirate preceding a bone scan will not cause a false-positive result.

Other imaging modalities, including magnetic resonance imaging (MRI), computed tomography (CT), and ultrasound, may have a limited role in certain complicated cases or to obtain further details of the infection, but they should not replace the plain film or bone scan in the acute setting.

MANAGEMENT

Initial therapy for osteomyelitis includes intravenous antibiotics. Antibiotic coverage should be based on the predominant organisms in each age group, the mechanism of infection, and Gram stain results. Suggested agents are listed in Table 108.1. Early aggressive antibiotic therapy often prevents the need for surgical intervention.

Septic Arthritis

The presence of bacterial pathogens within the articular capsule presents a true surgical emergency. Delay in the identification and treatment of an infected joint in a child can result in severe and permanent sequelae. The urgency associated with this diagnosis has given rise to the maxim, "The sun should never rise or set on an untreated septic hip."

Bacteria gain entry to the joint space through one of three means. The synovium is most commonly infected through

TABLE 108.1. Initial Antibiotic Therapy Osteomyelitis[a]

Age	Pathogens	Antibiotics
Neonate <2 mo	*Staphylococcus aureus,* group-B streptococcus, Gram-negative bacilli	Nafcillin *and* Gentamicin
<5 yr	*S. aureus,* group A streptococcus, *Streptococcus pneumoniae, Hemophilus influenzae*	Cefuroxime *or* Ampicillin/sulbactam Nafcillin *and* chloramphenicol
>5 yr	*S. aureus,* group A streptococcus, *S. pneumoniae*	Nafcillin *or* Cefazolin
Special cases		
Sickle cell disease	*S. aureus, Salmonella*	Nafcillin *and* ceftriaxone *or* Nafcillin *and* chloramphenicol
Foot puncture wound	*Pseudomonas aeruginosa, S. aureus*	*Nafcillin and* ticarcillin *or* Ticarcillin/clavulanate *or* Nafcillin *and* ceftazidime

[a] Vancomycin or clindamycin in penicillin- and cephalosporin-allergic patients.

hematogenous seeding. The role of local injury in predisposing joints to infection is unclear. Adjacent areas of infection may invade the joint, or direct inoculation can occur through penetrating injuries. Infection secondary to penetrating objects may be delayed from the actual time of injury.

Eighty to ninety percent of septic joints occur in the lower extremities. The knee and hip are most commonly afflicted. The same distribution is found in the preambulatory child. Infections involve only a single joint in more than 90% of cases. Multifocal infections are more common in neonates.

CLINICAL FINDINGS

Pain is the most common presenting complaint in the child with a septic joint. This may be expressed in many ways. The older child is better able to localize the area of discomfort. Because of the predominance of septic arthritis in the lower extremities, the younger child will often present with a limp, abnormal gait, or inability to bear weight.

Range of motion around the affected joint is dramatically reduced. Any degree of movement causes great distress and is vigorously resisted. Many orthopedic surgeons rely on this aspect of the evaluation more than any other in differentiating infection from alternative causes of joint pain.

Clinical signs are more subtle in the neonate or young infant with a septic joint. Nonspecific findings such as septic appearance, irritability, and pseudoparalysis of a limb are common presenting findings in these ages. Parents may note excessive irritability associated with diaper changes in the infant with a septic hip. The child with a septic hip will typically hold the lower extremity in abduction and external rotation in order to maximize the volume of joint space. A high degree of suspicion, close observation, and isolated manipulation of each extremity help locate the particular area of involvement.

DIAGNOSIS

The diagnosis of septic arthritis is confirmed by the presence of purulent fluid within the joint space. Arthrocentesis is a mandatory procedure in all suspected causes of septic arthritis. The level of suspicion and decision to perform this procedure is based on the degree of clinical suspicion in combination with results of laboratory tests and imaging studies. None of these in isolation are 100% sensitive in detecting or excluding septic arthritis from other conditions. A sample of synovial fluid is essential in discriminating septic arthritis from less serious inflammatory processes.

The mean WBC count is elevated in children with septic arthritis; however, more than one-half of patients will have a WBC count less than 15000 per mm^3. The ESR and CRP are more sensitive markers and are elevated in 90% to 95% of patients.

Plain radiographs may demonstrate signs of an effusion ranging from subtle blurring or displacement of fascial planes to complete dislocation of the joint. The main role of the radiograph in the evaluation is to exclude fractures or other bony abnormalities that may mimic septic arthritis. Ultrasound is increasingly used to evaluate questionable joints, especially the hip. It is much more sensitive than the radiograph in detecting a joint effusion. Some have suggested that the absence of an effusion on an ultrasound scan effectively excludes the diagnosis of septic arthritis. However, the ultrasound cannot distinguish between infected and sterile inflammatory effusions. The bone scan localizes areas of inflammation and is unaffected by prior arthrocentesis. It cannot differentiate infection from other causes of inflammation. A bone scan may be helpful in excluding osteomyelitis.

The isolation of a bacterial pathogen is important in diagnosis and in directing subsequent management. Cultures of joint fluid and blood should be performed on all patients with a possible septic joint. Cultures of the joint fluid demonstrate the highest yield, and are positive in 50% to 80% of cases. Blood cultures identify an organism in 15% to 46% of patients with septic arthritis, and are positive in many cases in which the organism is not isolated from the joint fluid.

A Gram stain should be performed on joint fluid and occasionally provides additional assistance in identifying both an infection and the infecting organism. Although elevation of the WBC count in the synovial fluid above 100000 per mm^3 is considered strong evidence of infection, the actual counts are often much lower.

MANAGEMENT

The management of septic arthritis consists of parenteral administration of antibiotics (Table 108.2), joint immobilization, and joint irrigation in selected cases. Empiric antibiotic therapy is dictated by the common organisms in the age group and results of the synovial fluid Gram stain. An antistaphylococcal agent consisting of a β-lactamase–resistant penicillin or a first-generation cephalosporin is effective in most cases. Gram-negative coverage should be added in neonates and adolescents. Until further evidence of the eradication of *Haemophilus influenzae* type b from the younger age group, appropriate coverage is recommended for children less than 5 years of age.

TABLE 108.2. Initial Antibiotic Therapy Septic Arthritis[a]

Age	Pathogens	Antibiotics
Neonate	*Staphylococcus aureus,* group B streptococcus, Gram-negative bacilli	Nafcillin *and* gentamicin or cefotaxime
≤5 yr	*S. aureus, Hemophilus influenzae,* group A streptococcus, *Streptococcus pneumoniae*	Cefuroxime *or* Ampicillin/sulbactam
>5 yr	*S. aureus,* group A streptococcus	Nafcillin
Adolescent	*S. aureus,* group A streptococcus, *Neisseria gonorrhea*	Nafcillin Ceftriaxone[b]

[a] Common pathogens and empiric antibiotic coverage by age.
[b] Empiric treatment in sexually active adolescent.

Surgical intervention for joint irrigation is generally indicated for all cases involving the hip joint, infections in which large amounts of fibrin, debris, or loculations are found within the joint space, or when the patient fails to improve after several days of intravenous antibiotic therapy. Expeditious and aggressive management limits, but does not eliminate, potential sequelae of septic arthritis.

Toxic Synovitis

Toxic or transient synovitis is a benign, self-limiting inflammatory process of the hip. It afflicts males more often than females and is the most common cause of acute hip pain in children 3 to 10 years of age. The underlying cause is unknown, although a postinfectious inflammatory response has been suggested. Its presentation can mimic that of septic arthritis of the hip, a distinction that is as crucial in management as it is difficult in diagnosis.

CLINICAL FINDINGS

The onset of symptoms is abrupt with unilateral hip pain and limp. Fever is rare, occurring in less than 10% of cases, and, when present, is usually low grade. Although patients complain of discomfort with movement of the limb, it generally remains possible to put the hip through a full range of motion. This contrasts with the septic hip in which pain and spasm are more extreme, and patients resist a full range of motion.

LABORATORY

Laboratory tests are generally useful only in attempting to distinguish toxic synovitis from more serious conditions. The WBC count and ESR are generally normal or only slightly elevated. The mean WBC count and ESR are significantly lower than in septic arthritis; however, sufficient overlap exists between values in toxic synovitis and septic arthritis such that they cannot be relied on to distinguish between them in individual patients.

Radiographs may demonstrate an effusion, but its principal role is in excluding pathologic osseous conditions. Ultrasound is more sensitive than plain films at detecting joint effusions, although accuracy declines in patients under one year of age. Reports of an effusion of the hip by ultrasound in toxic synovitis vary from 50% to 95%. Although patients often report relief of pain after aspiration, the procedure is unnecessary except to exclude the presence of a bacterial infection. When obtained, synovial fluid is sterile.

MANAGEMENT AND PROGNOSIS

Treatment occurs on an outpatient basis and emphasizes rest and analgesics. Traction is of unproven benefit and is potentially harmful. Nonsteroidal antiinflammatory medications are the first-line therapy for pain. Pain duration is typically 3 to 4 days but may last as long as 2 weeks. Exacerbations can occur if activity is resumed too early.

Radial Head Subluxation

"Nursemaid's elbow" is the most common joint injury in pediatric patients, usually occurring in children between 6 months and 5 years of age. The left elbow is more often affected because adult caretakers prefer to hold the child's left hand with their dominant right hand. Subluxation of the radial head occurs as a result of abrupt traction on a pronated hand or wrist. The annular ligament slides over the radial head and becomes interposed between the radius and capitellum. The radial head is not abnormal and the annular ligament need not tear for this injury to occur.

Subluxation of the radial head can be strongly suspected from across the room. The child holds the arm slightly flexed and against his or her body. When left alone, the child does not appear to be in significant pain. Parents may report a problem with the wrist or shoulder because, in their attempts to check these joints, inadvertent movement of the elbow causes pain. Physicians can be similarly fooled, especially when a classic history is not obtained.

The young child must be approached in a slow and nonthreatening way. Point tenderness of the clavicle, humerus, radius, and ulna can be excluded with a deliberate examination that does not move the elbow at all. True tenderness and swelling at the elbow are usually absent. When disuse of the elbow is present without pain or bony tenderness, the clinician should perform the reduction maneuver to confirm the diagnosis of radial head subluxation. Radiographs of the elbow are unnecessary unless the physician suspects another injury. Swelling and localized tenderness are usually apparent with supracondylar fractures, the next most common elbow injury in this age group.

Reduction of a subluxed radial head is one of the most gratifying procedures for physicians and parents alike. Several effective maneuvers are described. The clinician holds the elbow with his or her thumb over the radial head (Fig. 108.1). Supination of the affected arm rotates the flared aspect of the radial head, snapping the annular ligament back to its original position with a telltale click. Flexion or extension of the elbow may add to the success rate. If no click is felt, a second attempt can be made, perhaps exerting a little traction to disengage the annular ligament from between the radial head and capitellum.

Return of function after successful reduction is usually prompt, but not immediate. Toys, bottles, or interesting objects

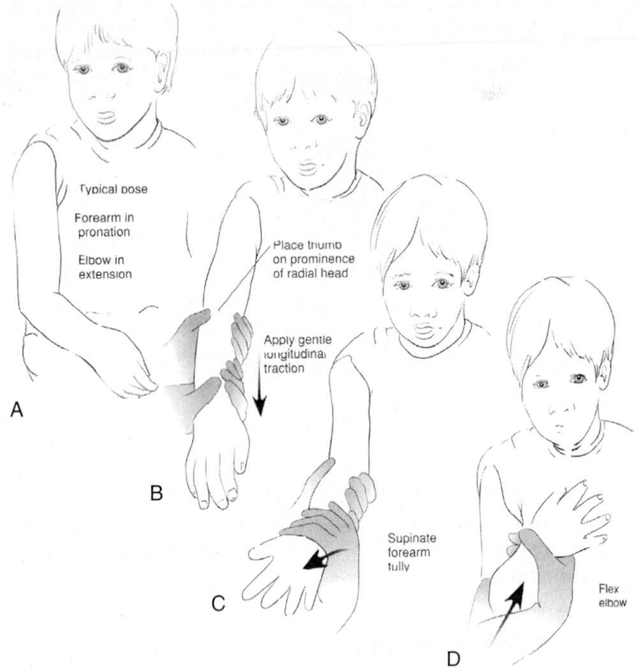

Figure 108.1. A–D: Supination–flexion maneuver for reduction of radial head subluxation (nursemaid's elbow).

can be used to encourage the child to use the affected arm. Voluntary use of the arm will return in less than 15 minutes in almost 90% of patients.

Recurrent radial head subluxations are common, occurring in about one-third of cases. Caretakers should be counseled to lift the child from the axillae, avoiding traction on the extremities.

Shoulder (Glenohumeral) Subluxation/Dislocation

Shoulder dislocation is extremely uncommon in young children. Shoulder dystocia at delivery can lead to displaced Salter I fractures. These injuries may look like dislocations because the unossified proximal humeral epiphysis remaining in the glenoid fossa is not visible radiographically. True dislocations become more common in adolescence.

Glenohumeral subluxation/dislocation may be recurrent, especially if the anterior glenoid rim is avulsed (Bankhart lesion). Patients may report that the shoulder "pops out" and reduces spontaneously. Some disturbed individuals intentionally dislocate their shoulder. Patients with recurrent shoulder dislocation need to be evaluated by an orthopedist. If a rehabilitation program is unsuccessful, a reconstructive procedure may be beneficial.

Slipped Capital Femoral Epiphysis

Slipped capital femoral epiphysis (SCFE) is the most common hip disorder in adolescent patients and should be familiar to all who care for children in this age group. It is twice as common in males as females, and more common in African-American patients. Obesity is a risk factor, although not all patients with SCFE are overweight. For unknown reasons, it is diagnosed far more often in the eastern portion of the United States, with a reported incidence of 3.41 per 100,000 in Connecticut and 0.71 per 100,000 in New Mexico. Cases are usually sporadic, but some familial tendency has been noted. Most children with SCFE are early adolescents in their growth spurt. Boys are most commonly affected between 13 and 15 years of age; girls are most commonly affected between 11 and 13 years of age because of their earlier pubertal development. SCFE onset after menarche is extremely rare.

Slippage of capital femoral epiphysis is almost always posterior and inferior relative to the proximal femoral metaphysis. Displacement anteriorly or superiorly has been reported. The epiphysis maintains a normal relationship with the acetabulum. The left hip is affected more often than the right. Radiographic evidence of bilateral SCFE is common, even though symptoms are usually unilateral. Plain radiographs document bilateral slippage in about 25% of cases; CT scans document this in approximately 50%.

Most patients with SCFE do not have identifiable endocrinologic problems. However, several hormonal abnormalities have been associated with increased risk. Elevated growth hormone and somatomedin, hypogonadism, hypothyroidism, and secondary hyperparathyroidism from renal failure (renal osteodystrophy) have been associated with SCFE. Short children receiving exogenous growth hormone therapy and tall, thin, rapidly growing children with high levels of endogenous growth hormone are both at increased risk. Children outside of the usual age range for SCFE, and those with other signs and symptoms that suggest possible endocrine abnormalities, should be referred for endocrine evaluation.

CLINICAL PRESENTATION

Pain and/or limp are the most common chief complaints in patients with SCFE. Physicians may be misled when the pain is referred to the thigh, knee, or groin. It is often dull, vague, intermittent, and chronic in nature. Many patients have had symptoms for weeks or months at the time of presentation. A history of trivial injury is sometimes obtained, perhaps causing the additional slippage that precipitates a medical evaluation. Acute onset of severe symptoms suggests acute or acute-on-chronic slippage. These patients are often unable to bear weight and may be in significant pain. Major trauma can cause SCFE, but these presentations are rare.

Examination findings in patients with SCFE include a resting position with hip flexion and some external rotation. Range of motion of the hip, especially full flexion, medial rotation, and abduction, is decreased and tender. Patients with significant displacement may have evidence of limb shortening.

DIAGNOSIS

Plain radiographs of the hip should include two views because SCFE may be missed on an anteroposterior (AP) view alone. On the AP view, widening of the physis is usually seen, even if the displacement is inapparent. The epiphysis is almost always displaced posteriorly; therefore, a frog leg or lateral view is best for documentation of the slippage. External rotation of the hip in the frog view turns the posterior aspect medially. Following the medial margin of the femur proximally reveals a step off between the metaphysis and epiphysis. New bone formation is often visible, suggesting a chronic slip. When radiographic findings are equivocal, comparison with the contralateral, asymptomatic hip should be done with caution, given the frequency of bilateral slippage with unilateral symptoms.

MANAGEMENT

Treatment of SCFE is primarily surgical. Screws are usually placed through the femoral neck into the epiphysis. Reduction of the displacement is not performed because there is some evidence that it may increase the likelihood of avascular necrosis of the femoral head and chondrolysis. Chondrolysis is the most common complication of SCFE, occurring in about 8% of patients. Pain and persistent decreased range of motion after pinning are the usual presenting symptoms.

Legg-Calvé-Perthes Disease

Legg-Calvé-Perthes disease (LCPD) is a hip disorder that generally has onset between the ages of 4 and 9 years. Males outnumber females by a ratio of 4:1. Genetic factors play a minor role. Most children with LCPD are short, with average or above-average weight. They often have delayed skeletal maturation.

LCPD begins with repeated episodes of ischemia of the femoral head, leading to infarction and necrosis. Theories about the cause of the circulatory insufficiency include increased blood viscosity and elevated intracapsular pressure caused by synovitis, but these theories remain unproven. Patients may remain asymptomatic despite varying degrees of necrosis and resorption of the femoral head. Some children recover completely without developing symptoms. Symptoms generally begin when minor trauma causes stress fracture of the subchondral bone. Rarefaction of the femoral head with subluxation and deformity may ensue. The process of reossification and remodeling takes 2 to 4 years.

The onset of symptoms in LCPD is usually insidious. Presentation as an acute emergency is rare. Mild hip pain and limp have usually been present for weeks to months before diagnosis. Pain is often referred in the distribution of the obturator nerve to the knee, anteromedial thigh, or groin. Physical findings include decreased hip abduction and medial rotation. Thigh muscle atrophy, and in advanced cases, limb shortening may also be noted.

The sequence of radiographic changes in LCPD have been described in detail. At diagnosis most patients have widening of the articular cartilage with a small, dense proximal femoral epiphysis. Subchondral fracture may be visible. Irregularity and flattening of the epiphysis develops over time. The differential diagnosis includes various bone tumors and skeletal dysplasias. As the disease progresses, anterolateral subluxation may be quantitated radiographically.

Management of LCPD requires a pediatric orthopedist who will follow and treat the child through the various stages of the disease. Prompt referral may influence long-term prognosis. Older children, obese children, girls, and those with more severe disturbance of the epiphysis on radiographs have a poorer prognosis.

Discitis

Discitis is an inflammatory condition involving the intervertebral disc space that has also been called acute osteitis of the spine, spondylitis, and spondylarthritis. The variety of diagnostic terms is an indication that the pathophysiology of this condition is poorly understood. Vertebral osteomyelitis with involvement of the disc space is a distinct diagnostic entity with different epidemiology and pathophysiology from discitis.

Discitis is a disease of childhood, with about 75% of patients being less than 10 years of age. No gender or racial predilection has been noted. The involved disc space is usually lumbar or lower thoracic. Most authorities believe discitis results from infection. A history of trauma is obtained in some patients with discitis, but whether the injury plays a role in cause or is a "red herring" is unclear. The vascular anatomy of the disc space supports the notion that organisms reach the disc space via the hematogenous route. In children, the blood supply of the disc space comes from adjacent vertebral body end plates. These vascular connections are absent in older adolescents and adults, which is consistent with the age distribution of discitis.

DIAGNOSIS

Children with discitis are a diagnostic challenge for clinicians. Symptoms are often nonspecific and vague, especially in the younger child. They have usually been present for more than 1 week at the time of diagnosis. Back pain is not always described. Limp, refusal to walk, leg pain, hip pain, and abdominal pain are common presenting complaints. Low-grade fever and irritability may be reported.

Physical findings suggesting discitis will be missed if this entity is not considered because careful examination of the spine is not performed routinely by most clinicians. Many children assume a recumbent position of comfort from which they do not want to be moved. Decreased range of motion of the spine and paravertebral muscle spasm are usually present. There is often a change in the lumbar lordosis, which may be decreased or increased. Tenderness to palpation of the disc space can usually be demonstrated. Range of motion of the hips is essentially normal, but inadvertent movement of the lumbar spine during hip examination may cause pain that is misinterpreted to suggest hip pathology. Straight leg raising may be limited by muscle spasm in the hamstrings. Neurologic assessment of the lower extremities is normal. Abnormalities in strength, sensation, and/or deep tendon reflexes suggest a spinal cord lesion, tumor, epidural abscess, or herniation of the disc (rare). Signs of discitis may vary, depending on the location of the inflamed disc. Patients with lesions of the upper spine may have meningism.

Imaging studies can be useful in the diagnosis of discitis. Plain radiographs are initially normal. Intervertebral disc space narrowing develops after 2 to 3 weeks of illness. Bone scan is the most sensitive imaging modality early in the course of this disease. Increased uptake at the level of the involved disc can confirm the diagnosis. MRI has also proven sensitive in the early phase. CT scanning can demonstrate the degree of bony erosion of the vertebral end plates and paravertebral soft-tissue involvement.

Laboratory testing plays a minor role. Elevation of the WBC count is sometimes noted at the time of diagnosis. ESRs of 40 to 60 mm per hour are usually noted in patients presenting with discitis, and decrease with resolution of the disease. Skin testing for tuberculosis, and serologic testing for brucellosis and salmonellosis are often performed. Discitis can usually be diagnosed and treated without biopsy or aspiration of the involved disc space. If the presentation is atypical, signs and symptoms severe, or response to therapy unsatisfactory, obtaining a guided needle aspiration can be helpful.

MANAGEMENT

Discitis is a self-limited disease and need not be treated aggressively. Virtually all children in reported series return to normal function in a few months. Resting the spine usually results in improved symptoms in days to weeks. Immobilization with plaster has not been shown to improve outcome over bed rest alone, but therapeutic decisions should be individualized with input from an orthopedist. Although there are no data to suggest that they speed recovery or improve outcome, antistaphylococcal antibiotics seem prudent, given the frequency of documented staphylococcal infection. When cultures demonstrate particular organisms with known antimicrobial susceptibilities, antibiotic therapy can be individualized.

SPONDYLOLYSIS AND SPONDYLOLISTHESIS

Spondylolysis and spondylolisthesis occur in 2% to 5% of children, but most are asymptomatic. In older children with low back pain, especially adolescents, it is a condition that should be considered. Spondylolysis is a defect in the pars interarticularis of the vertebral body. Spondylolisthesis is displacement of the vertebral bodies, usually involving L5 slipping anteriorly on S1. Spondylolisthesis may result from structural abnormalities of the vertebral bodies (dysplastic type) or acquired defects of the pars interarticularis (isthmic type) that allow slippage. There is a genetic predisposition to spondylolysis and spondylolisthesis. Parents of children with spondylolisthesis are found to have this condition in 28% of cases.

The cause of the defect of the pars interarticularis in spondylolysis is not fully understood. Repeated stress, such as occurs in gymnasts with frequent hyperextension of the spine, causes stress fracture. One side of the pars interarticularis fractures overtly, which adds to the stress on the contralateral side. Fracture becomes bilateral. Displacement may or may not occur. Children who play sports that stress the spine, such as gymnastics, football, rowing, diving, weight lifting, and high jumping, are at particular risk.

Patients who develop symptoms generally present during the adolescent growth spurt. Back pain worsens with activity and improves with rest, and usually has an insidious onset. Over time, there may be pain in the buttocks and posterior thighs. Symptoms radiating down the legs suggest significant nerve root irritation. Parents may describe an increase in the lumbar lordosis or a change in the child's gait.

Physical examination shows tenderness with hyperextension of the lumbar spine in the prone position, and with deep palpation. The hamstrings are usually tight, with decreased range of motion on straight leg raise and flexion of the trunk. Children seldom have motor (10%), sensory (15%), or reflex (10%) deficits in the legs.

Plain radiographs should include AP, lateral, and oblique views. The "Scotty dog" of the oblique view will have a collar on the neck if spondylolysis is present. Spondylolisthesis can be diagnosed on the lateral view, and the degree of displacement can be quantitated relative to the width of the vertebral body.

Treatment varies depending on symptoms and degree of displacement, if any. Most cases of asymptomatic spondylolysis, and spondylolisthesis with mild displacement will not progress. Children with displacement greater than 25% should avoid rough sports. Symptomatic children with displacement may benefit from immobilization. Decisions about treatment should be made in consultation with an orthopedic surgeon.

OVERUSE SYNDROMES

Overuse syndromes is a general term that encompasses a variety of injuries that result from excessive and repetitive forces on susceptible structures. Children are at unique risk for such injuries, which are particularly common in adolescent athletes. There is an increased susceptibility during the growth spurt when skeletal growth exceeds the growth of the muscle–tendon unit. This results in increased stress at the apophysis, the musculotendinous origin or insertion. In children, cartilage is interposed between tendon and bone and is most prone to injury from repetitive forces. Repetitive tensile forces at these sites result in chronic irritation and microfractures or avulsions of the apophysis. If allowed to progress, there is evidence that the repetitive microtrauma may weaken the bone and predispose to major avulsion fractures. Traction apophysitis is unique to the growing child.

General therapy for these injuries must emphasize several areas. Rest is crucial for the specific area involved until pain has completely resolved. The athlete should be actively encouraged to use alternative activities to maintain conditioning during this time. The role of inflammation in overuse injuries is controversial, but the application of ice and use of antiinflammatory agents is generally recommended. Directed stretching exercises are encouraged to reduce tension on affected areas. Biomechanics should be assessed and corrected when necessary. When returning to full activity, an appropriate training regimen should emphasize a slow gradual buildup in intensity and duration and should include explicit limitations. The sudden increase in intensity and duration of training that occurs with a change of sporting seasons is a major culprit in overuse injuries.

Little Leaguer's Elbow

Little Leaguer's elbow refers to a group of disorders resulting from repetitive valgus stress applied to the skeletally underdeveloped elbow. Its cause is a combination of excessively repetitive pitching and poor throwing biomechanics. Valgus force places tension on the medial collateral ligaments, which is translated to the medial epicondyle. A medial epicondylitis or apophysitis is the most commonly resulting lesion. An avulsion fracture of the medial epicondyle may result from an acute valgus force once the site has become weakened from repetitive microtrauma. As expected, Little Leaguer's elbow occurs most commonly in boys ages 9 to 12. Patients complain primarily of elbow pain that is exacerbated by throwing. Tenderness is localized over the medial elbow. Flexion of the wrist or finger against resistance also elicits pain. In advanced cases, extension of the elbow becomes limited.

Osgood-Schlatter Disease

Osgood-Schlatter disease is an apophysitis of the tibial tubercle. Repetitive stress imposed by the patellar tendon on its site of insertion results in a series of microavulsions of the ossification center and underlying cartilage. The condition is most common in running and jumping athletes between the ages of 11 and 15. Girls are less commonly affected than boys. Most cases are bilateral, although symptoms are commonly asymmetric.

The physical examination is notable for localized tenderness at the tibial tubercle. Any action that applies tension to the patellar tendon elicits pain. Placing the patient prone and flexing the knee so that the heel contacts the buttocks typically triggers pain at the tibial tubercle. Additional maneuvers likely to cause pain include forced extension of the knee, jumping, or squatting. In advanced cases, callus formation occurs, resulting in further prominence of the tubercle. Some experts have suggested a relationship between Osgood-Schlatter disease and acute avulsion fractures of the tibial tubercle. The diagnosis is based on the clinical features. Radiographs are not indicated in typical cases.

Management consists first and foremost of avoiding activities that place stress on the tibial tubercle. This is perhaps the most difficult instruction to enforce in young athletes. A brief period of immobilization or non–weight bearing is recommended by some as a means of ensuring compliance. Application of ice reduces pain and swelling. Nonsteroidal antiinflammatory medications are commonly recommended.

Osteochondritis Dissecans

Osteochondritis dissecans is a lesion involving separation of the osteochondral segment from underlying healthy bone. A variety of articular lesions are often lumped together under this term, including acute osteochondral fractures and epiphyseal dysplasias. This results in confounding descriptions of the natural course and outcome of the true condition. Adults are often diagnosed with osteochondritis dissecans; however, it remains primarily a condition of the adolescent age group, with the highest incidence occurring among male athletes between 12 and 16 years of age. The primary sites of osteochondritis dissecans include the medial femoral condyle in the knee, the posteromedial aspect of the talus in the ankle, and the capitellum in the elbow. It is less commonly reported in the hip, feet, and wrist. Involvement of multiple sites is rare.

CLINICAL FINDINGS

The onset of symptoms occurs over several months. Joint pain and swelling typically occur after strenuous exercise and improve over several hours with rest. When a free body is present, patients describe intermittent, abrupt locking of the joint. Locking in the knee or elbow prevents full extension of the extremity. This is in contradistinction to buckling, stiffness, or pain with extended range of motion.

The physical examination of the joint is often normal. Occasionally, a small effusion may be detectable. Lesions in the medial femoral condyle may be directly palpated and pain elicited when the knee is held in 90 degrees of flexion. The typical location of lesions in the talus are not accessible on examination. Osteochondritis dissecans in the femoral condyle may give rise to an abnormal gait with external rotation of the affected limb.

DIAGNOSIS

A plain film of the joint should be obtained, and is often diagnostic when osteochondritis dissecans is suspected. Radiographs reveal a crescentic-shaped defect within the subchondral bone. The avascular segment of subchondral bone may have increased density. A radiolucent line may demarcate the separation from the remainder of the epiphysis. A free body often includes a portion of dead subchondral bone, which appears as a radiodense object within the joint space. Standard AP and lateral views, as well as tunnel and sunrise views of the knee are recommended for lesions within the femoral condyle. Lateral, AP, and mortis views of the ankle are adequate when a lesion of the talus is suspected, and AP and lateral views of the elbow are sufficient when the capitellum is involved.

MANAGEMENT

The management of osteochondritis dissecans depends on the age and skeletal maturity of the patient, the location of the lesion, and the stage of the lesion. Conservative therapy consisting of restricted activity and relief of stress on the joint is the first-line treatment in children who have not reached skeletal maturity, and for those diagnosed at an early stage of the disease. Immobilization in a cast or non-weight bearing for lower extremity lesions is unnecessary. Patients should be followed closely by an orthopedic surgeon both for resolution of clinical symptoms and evidence of healing on serial radiographs or MRIs.

Chondromalacia Patella

Chondromalacia patella is a pathologic diagnosis referring to damage of the articular cartilage of the patella. Specific changes include softening, fissures, and erosions. Patellofemoral pain syndrome, a term often used interchangeably with chondromalacia patella, more accurately describes a constellation of symptoms, principally anterior knee pain arising from the patellofemoral joint. Whether the two conditions are actually related is the subject of debate. They share a number of symptoms and precipitating factors. Patellofemoral pain syndrome may represent the early end of the spectrum of injury, which ultimately may or may not progress to true pathologic changes within the cartilage.

Patellofemoral pain syndrome and chondromalacia patella are first seen in early adolescence. The rise in incidence tends to parallel the growth spurt. A number of underlying causes or associated factors have been identified. Malalignment of the patella and an abnormal tracking of the patella over the femoral condyles appear to be the major contributors to patellofemoral disorders.

Chondromalacia patellae and patellofemoral pain syndrome are often classified as overuse syndromes because individuals exposed to repetitive trauma are at higher risk for these disorders. Runners are particularly predisposed to develop these conditions. Poor training regimens, rapid increases in duration or intensity of training, hard or uneven running surfaces, and inadequate shoes have been blamed.

Symptoms consist mainly of anterior knee pain often described as arising from beneath or on the sides of the patella. Pain is usually of gradual onset and is exacerbated by exercise. Activities that involve loading of the knee when it is in flexion, such as climbing steps, are particularly painful.

The physical examination is notable for tenderness along the patellar margins or the posterior surface, which is accessible when the patella is manually displaced medially or laterally. Pain, and occasionally crepitus, are elicited with flexion and extension of the knee, or tightening the quadriceps while compressing the patella against the femoral condyles. Range of motion is not limited and swelling is rare. The presence of an effusion is suggestive of significant cartilaginous damage. Provocative tests that reproduce the pain include climbing steps, squatting, or knee extension against resistance.

Radiographs are generally insensitive but may show changes to the patella in advanced cases.

Treatment is conservative. More than 90% of cases of patellofemoral pain syndrome resolve after instituting a program of rest, antiinflammatory medications, and ice followed by physical therapy. Exercises that begin once the initial pain has resolved emphasize strengthening of the quadriceps muscles. Recommended exercise regimens include isometric contractions of the quadriceps with the knee in extension, straight leg raises, and knee extensions, first without and then with weights.

Sever Disease

Sever disease is a calcaneal apophysitis occurring at the insertion of the Achilles tendon at the posterior aspect of the calcaneus. It afflicts predominantly runners, jumpers, and soccer players. Sever disease is often bilateral, is more common in males, and has its peak incidence between 10 and 12 years of age.

Localized tenderness occurs at the insertion of the Achilles tendon on the calcaneus. A maneuver such as hanging the heels over the edge of a step, climbing steps, or hopping applies tension to the Achilles tendon and exacerbates the pain. Patients are often found to have a tight gastrocnemius-soleus muscle complex and limited dorsiflexion of the foot. Radiographs of the site are usually normal and are unhelpful except to exclude bony injuries such as stress fractures.

Management includes rest, ice, and antiinflammatory medications. Heel padding or lifts may be helpful in relieving tension in the area. Flexibility exercises should concentrate on both the hamstrings and the calf muscles. When therapy is initiated early in the disease, most patients are able to return to normal activity by 2 months.

Bursitis

Bursa sacs are both the shock absorbers and the ball bearings of the musculoskeletal system. They disperse forces from blows on bony prominences and reduce friction where tendons or ligaments are in frequent motion.

Trauma, either in a single blow or by repetitive forces, can inflame the bursa, which responds with increased production of synovial fluid. The bursa sac subsequently swells and a cycle of swelling, irritation, and inflammation ensues. Bursitis is most commonly an overuse syndrome seen in adolescents and adults, and is less common in young children.

Bursae are located throughout the body, but bursitis occurs only in a few. Prepatellar bursitis, commonly called "housemaid's knee" results from frequent or prolonged kneeling. Pens anserinus bursitis occurs on the lateral aspect of the knee, where the tendons of the hamstring muscles overlie the tibia. Retrocalcaneal bursitis occurs between the calcaneus and Achilles tendon and often is caused by direct pressure from ill-fitting footwear or high-heeled shoes. Olecranon bursitis most often results from a single direct blow to the elbow. Shoulder or subacromial bursitis is often associated with calcifications and produces severe pain with abduction. Other commonly affected bursae include the inferior calcaneal bursa and the trochanteric bursa.

An unusual form of bursitis is known as a popliteal or Baker cyst. This occurs in the bursa, which cushions the tendons of the gastrocnemius and semimembranous muscles from the distal femur. The presence of this condition in adults is highly suggestive of intraarticular knee damage. In children with a Baker cyst, there is often a congenitally wide opening joining the bursa sac with the knee joint itself. One-way flow of synovial fluid into the bursa produces swelling just below the popliteal fossa on the medial side. Patients with chronic inflammatory conditions of the knee, such as juvenile rheumatoid arthritis (JRA), are at increased risk of developing popliteal cysts. The swelling limits full flexion of the knee and produces the sensation of tension with extension. An arthrogram or bursagram may outline the cyst, document the articular connection, and detect ruptures of the cyst. Ultrasound is a useful noninvasive diagnostic modality. MRI is more accurate than ultrasound, but not as essential in children given the lower incidence of accompanying intraarticular injury.

Conservative therapy consisting of restricted activity, frequent application of ice, and regular use of nonsteroidal antiinflammatory medications is successful in most cases.

COMPARTMENT SYNDROMES

Compartment syndrome refers to vascular insufficiency caused by elevated tissue pressures. It usually occurs after an injury causes hemorrhage or edema within an enclosed fascial compartment. Tight circumferential bandages or casts can also limit expansion of swollen tissues and result in elevation of tissue pressures. Fluid extravasation from intravenous or intraosseous lines, especially pressure-driven extravasation, may significantly elevate compartment pressures. Direct injury to a vessel is less common as the cause of vascular insufficiency after injury. When compartment pressures approach the perfusion pressure of muscle, which is approximately 30 mm Hg, arterial inflow is reduced and veins and capillaries are collapsed. Ischemia of muscle leads to further swelling, and an ischemia–edema cycle can lead to complete cessation of tissue perfusion. Muscle necrosis is irreversible after 6 to 8 hours of tissue anoxia. Fibrosis develops and ischemic contracture results in permanent disability. The emergency physician must identify patients at risk for compartment syndromes and consult with an orthopedist, who can monitor tissue pressures and treat compartment syndromes before irreversible injuries occur.

TABLE 108.3. Compartment Syndromes

Fractures	Ischemic compartments
Supracondylar fractures of the humerus (displaced)	Deep flexor (anterior) compartment
Radius/ulna fractures (diaphyseal)	Anterior tibial and peroneal compartments
Tibia/fibula fractures (diaphyseal)	
Femur fractures	

Knowledge of the common pediatric injuries that are associated with compartment syndromes can raise the clinician's index of suspicion appropriately (Table 108.3). Displaced supracondylar fractures may lead to Volkmann contracture, which involves the distribution of the anterior interosseous artery and the flexor compartment of the forearm. Forearm fractures may also cause compartment syndromes, affecting either the flexor or extensor musculature. Fractures of the tibia and/or fibula can lead to compartment syndrome of the lower leg. Compartment syndromes may occur from crush injuries and other soft-tissue trauma that does not necessarily involve a fracture.

Compartment syndromes are diagnosed clinically by assessing the "five Ps": pain, paresthesia, pallor, paralysis, and pulselessness. All five need not be present for a compartment syndrome to exist.

Treatment of a compartment syndrome should begin when it is suspected. All circumferential bandages should be removed. If symptoms persist, orthopedic consultation should be obtained for measurement of compartment pressures. Reduction of displaced fractures can improve blood flow to affected compartments. Fasciotomy in the operating room is indicated if compartment pressures remain high.

REFLEX SYMPATHETIC DYSTROPHY

Reflex sympathetic dystrophy (RSD) is a poorly understood disorder characterized by pain, abnormal sensation, and circulatory irregularities. Over time, atrophic changes of the extremity develop. *Causalgia, algodystrophy,* and *Sudeck atrophy* are also terms that have been used for this mysterious disorder, first reported in gunshot victims during the American Civil War. The average time from onset to diagnosis of RSD in children is 1 year. Emergency physicians play an important role in the early diagnosis and treatment of RSD, which may prevent prolonged disability.

RSD is well known in adults, but children with RSD as young as 3 years have been described. The average age of children with RSD is approximately 12 years; girls outnumber boys by as much as 6:1. Most cases in children involve the lower extremity. RSD usually follows minor trauma, but some cases develop without an identified precipitant.

The pathophysiology of RSD is not understood. Early theories suggested abnormal synapses develop between sensory afferent nerves and sympathetic efferents after an injury. "Sympathetic" dystrophy may be a misnomer, however, because local epinephrine and norepinephrine levels are lower, not higher than normal, and vasodilation, not sympathetic vasoconstriction, may predominate. Theories of sympathetic receptor hypersensitivity or central, self-exciting pathways in the substantia nigra remain unproven.

Pain is usually the presenting complaint with RSD. The pain is continuous, often burning in quality, with exacerbations but no complete remissions. Abnormal sensitivity is distinctive, with severe pain provoked by normally nontender touching (allodynia). The extremity is usually swollen and cool to the touch, although warmth has also been reported. Dusky discoloration of the skin with hyperhidrosis or anhidrosis may be present. The arm or leg is not used, and atrophic muscle, skin, and bony changes develop in some patients over time. There is some evidence that demineralization of bone occurs more rapidly than would be expected from disuse alone.

Psychiatric and personality problems have been suspected in many patients with RSD, but controlled prospective studies are lacking. Factitious illness or conversion reactions may be considered, given that symptoms are out of proportion to the inciting injury.

The characteristic history and physical examination, including pain, loss of function, and evidence of autonomic dysfunction, allow for a clinical diagnosis of RSD in most cases. Thermography may document decreased temperature in the affected extremity. Treatment of RSD focuses on early mobilization of the extremity through physical therapy to avoid atrophic changes. Physiotherapy may initially exacerbate symptoms, but experienced clinicians believe it both prevents atrophy and decreases the duration of pain. The knee-jerk response to splint for comfort may be counterproductive with RSD. Referral to a pediatric pain program is advisable should symptoms persist. Intravenous regional block with guanethidine, sympathetic block, transcutaneous nerve stimulation, and, with intractable cases, sympathectomy, have all been performed, reportedly with some success.

CHAPTER 109

Dental Emergencies

Linda P. Nelson, D.M.D., M.Sc.D. and Stephen Shusterman, D.M.D.

Nontraumatic orofacial emergencies can appear suddenly and can be frightening for pediatric patients and their families. The major task in evaluating a child with a nontraumatic orofacial emergency is to identify the cause of the problem. In cases of facial swellings, the first step in treatment is determining that a tooth is the causative agent.

POSTEXTRACTION COMPLICATIONS

Hemorrhage

It is expected that any extraction site may ooze for 8 to 12 hours and perhaps longer for a permanent site. However, it is important to check the history for any prior bleeding episodes to rule out a systemic hematologic abnormality. A complete blood count and coagulation profile would be indicated.

Treatment may include:

1. Applying pressure, using folded gauze sponges that are placed over the socket with biting pressure applied for 30 minutes.
2. Physically closing the socket by suturing. Administering local anesthesia (2% Xylocaine with 1:100,000 epinephrine infiltration), the extraction site is approximated with the appropriate sutures. Alternatively, the socket may be packed with Gelfoam.
3. A possible home remedy before coming to the emergency department (ED) might include applying a tea bag to the site of the bleeding. A tea bag is dipped in hot water and allowed to cool, then placed over the socket with pressure. The tannic acid in the tea bag may accelerate or initiate coagulation.

Infection

ALVEOLAR OSTEITIS

Alveolar osteitis, or "dry socket," is a painful postoperative condition produced by a disintegration of the clot in the tooth socket. This condition usually is seen in adults and only rarely in children less than 12 years of age. It usually follows (approximately 72 hours) mandibular extractions and is painful. Emergency dental treatment is variable, but the immediate goal is relief of pain. Under local anesthesia, the socket may be debrided and then packed with 1/4-inch iodoform gauze or Bipp's paste (bismuth, iodoform, benzocaine, and petrolatum). Oral analgesic medication should be prescribed along with antibiotics.

ODONTALGIA—SIMPLE TOOTHACHE

The child with a simple toothache often complains of diffuse mouth pain and may not be able to point to a specific tooth. The emergency physician may note a grossly carious tooth or large restoration. Swelling or inflammation in the surrounding soft tissue may be present. The tooth may be sensitive to percussion and may exhibit excessive mobility. A dental consultation is necessary, especially if swelling is noted. In the case of swelling, the tooth may be opened for drainage to relieve the pressure, in a manner similar to the management of any abscess.

DENTOALVEOLAR ABSCESS

Dental abscesses are common in children because of the morphologic characteristic of the primary tooth and immature permanent tooth. In the dentoalveolar abscess, the causative factors are gross or recurrent decay, trauma, or perhaps, chronic irritation from a large restoration. Suppuration is usually confined to the bone around the tooth. If the infection is long-standing, it can perforate the thin buccal bony plate adjacent to the root of the involved tooth and spread into the subperiosteal area and then to the surrounding soft tissues. In a child, the dentoalveolar abscess usually perforates the buccal plate of bone because of the position of the tooth and the thinness of the overlying bone. If it does not drain intraorally, the infection can spread rapidly through the fascial planes of the face or neck.

The following are clinical manifestations of a dentoalveolar abscess in a child: (1) pain, (2) mobility, (3) swelling, (4) temperature elevation, (5) fistulous tracts, (6) extrusion, and (7) lymphadenopathy.

It is important that the treatment of choice for a localized dentoalveolar abscess is local in its focus (eg, drainage, moist heat). In cases of facial cellulitis with lymphadenopathy caused by acute dentoalveolar abscess, the antibiotic of choice is penicillin (or erythromycin, if there is a known allergy to penicillin). The initial dose for children who weigh more than 60 pounds (27 kg) is 1 g orally, followed by 500 mg every 6 hours until the patient can be seen by a dentist. For children who weigh less than 60 pounds (27 kg), the initial penicillin dose is 500 mg, followed by 250 mg every 6 hours.

Other factors to consider in determining the need for hospital admission include the child's ability to take fluids and the likelihood of the parent's cooperation for follow-up dental care. Obviously, if the child is toxic, a hospital admission is indicated.

As with infection elsewhere in the body, the basic surgical principles of treatment must be used: (1) establish drainage and (2) remove the cause. An abscessed primary tooth must be vigorously treated because such infections can affect the developing unerupted permanent tooth bud. A facial cellulitis can have severe systemic consequences, including cavernous sinus thrombosis, airway obstruction, brain abscess, and septicemia.

PERICORONITIS

Pericoronitis is a localized infection surrounding an erupting tooth. It is usually associated with erupting molars in the adolescent patient, although a mild form may be associated with the eruption of the first permanent molar at age 6 (Table 109.1). Symptoms usually include pain distal to the last erupted tooth in the dental arch, along with erythema and edema localized to the gingiva in the retromolar area. Lymphadenopathy, trismus, and dysphagia may accompany these symptoms. An elevated body temperature is an occasional finding.

Emergency treatment includes local curettage, oral rinses, heat, and scrupulous oral hygiene. Penicillin may be necessary (for dose, see "Dentoalveolar Abscess" earlier in the chapter) when there are systemic symptoms.

PRIMARY HERPETIC GINGIVOSTOMATITIS OR HERPES SIMPLEX VIRUS TYPE 1

Primary herpetic gingivostomatitis, or herpes simplex virus type 1 is a communicable childhood disease that is not a true dental emergency, but is a common cause of ED visits. The child is usually an infant or toddler who stops eating, drinking, or talking and is extremely irritable. The child usually has had an elevated temperature for 3 to 5 days before any clinical oral findings. A higher incidence of primary herpes has been noted after other viral illnesses. Older children may complain of headaches, malaise, nausea, regional lymphadenopathy, and/or bleeding gums. The physical examination reveals fiery red marginal gingiva with areas of spontaneous hemorrhage. Within 1 or 2 days, yellowish, fluid-filled vesicles develop on the mucosa, palate, or tongue and coalesce. The vesicles rupture spontaneously, leaving extremely painful ulcers, covered by a yellow or gray membrane and surrounded by an erythematous zone. Ulcers, especially on the lips, may become encrusted.

Viscous Xylocaine rinses and "magic mouthwash," Kaopectate and Benadryl, may be unrealistic for children in this age range. The unpleasant taste sometimes negates any benefit that the topical anesthetic gives, and makes administration difficult.

TABLE 109.1. Eruption Schedule for Specific Teeth

A. Primary teeth

	Age at eruption (mo)		Age at shedding (yr)	
	Lower	Upper	Lower	Upper
Central incisor	6	7 1/2	6	7 1/2
Lateral incisor	7	9	7	8
Cuspid	16	18	9 1/2	11 1/2
First molar	12	14	10	10 1/2
Second molar	20	24	11	10 1/2
Incisors	Range ±2 months			
Molars	Range ±4 months		Range ±6 months	

B. Permanent teeth[a]

	Age (yrs)	
	Lower	Upper
Central incisors	6–7	7–8
Lateral incisors	7–8	8–9
Cuspids	9–10	11–12
First bicuspids	10–12	10–11
Second bicuspids	11–12	10–12
First molars	6–7	6–7
Second molars	11–13	12–13
Third molars	17–21	17–21

[a] The lower teeth erupt before the corresponding upper teeth. The teeth usually erupt earlier in girls than in boys.
Modified with permission from Massler M, Schour I. *Atlas of the mouth and adjacent parts in health and disease.* The Bureau of Public Relations Council on Dental Health, American Dental Association, 1946.

ACUTE NECROTIZING ULCERATIVE GINGIVITIS, VINCENT DISEASE, TRENCH MOUTH

Acute necrotizing ulcerative gingivitis (ANUG), Vincent disease, or trench mouth is characterized by increases in the fusiform bacillus and *Borrelia vincentii,* a spirochete, which usually coexist in a symbiotic relationship with other oral flora. Adolescents complain of soreness and point-tenderness at the gingiva and often tell the physician that they feel as if they "cannot remove a piece of food that is painfully stuck between their teeth" (a wedging sensation). They may also complain of a metallic taste in their mouth and of bleeding gums. Upon examination, the breath has an obvious fetid odor. The gingivae are hyperemic and the usually triangular gingiva between the teeth is missing, or "punched out" (Fig. 109.1). Intense pain is produced with probing, and a gray, necrotic pseudomembrane may cover some areas of gingiva.

The adolescent should be advised to maintain better oral hygiene and to use frequent hydrogen peroxide mouth rinses. Diluted 1:1 with warm water, the hydrogen peroxide is vigorously swished and forced between the teeth as often as possible throughout the acute phase. Because of the rapidity of tissue destruction and sensitivity of the organisms, as well as risk of secondary infection, penicillin should be prescribed for the first week. When the acute phase is over, the patient should be sent to the dentist for a thorough debridement of the area.

ORAL AND PERIORAL PATHOLOGY PRESENTING AS DENTAL EMERGENCIES

Orofacial Neoplasms

Orofacial neoplasms in children are rare, but may be frightening to the patient and their family. Common benign and malignant neoplasms may result in emergency visits and, therefore, are included here. Identification is central to the triage process.

The oral papilloma is a benign epithelial neoplasm that is an exophytic elevation of the surface epithelium with small finger-like projections from its surface. These lesions, which rarely become malignant, constitute about 8% of all oral neoplasms in children. Slightly more than one-third of the lesions occur on the tongue and (in decreasing order of frequency) palate, buccal mucosa, gingiva, and lip. If spontaneous involution does not occur, the usual treatment is surgical removal.

The fibroma is a common smooth-surfaced lesion with a sessile base. Its consistency varies from soft to firm, and its size ranges from a few millimeters to a centimeter or more in diameter. It may become whitened secondary to the overlying hyperkeratosis caused by trauma. Fibromas occur during the first and second decades of life and are usually found on the palate, tongue, cheek, and lip. Surgical removal is sometimes indicated and recurrence is rare if the source of the irritation is removed.

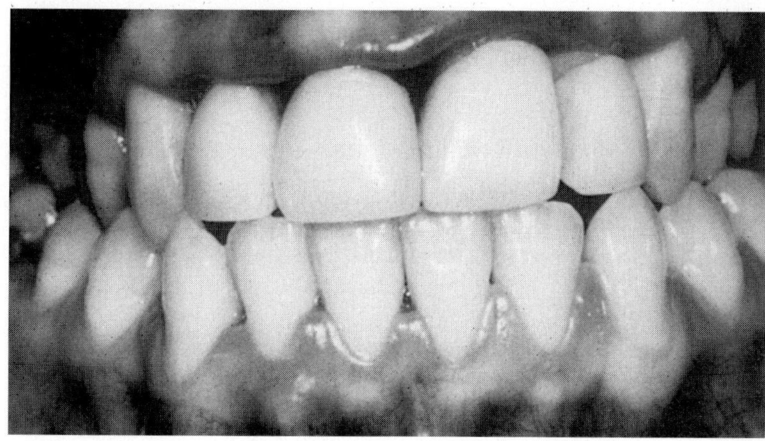

Figure 109.1. A child with typical "punched out" gingiva—pathognomonic for acute necrotizing ulcerative gingivitis. (Courtesy of Dr. Mark Snyder.)

The mucocele appears as a soft, raised, fluid-filled, and well-delineated nodule, most commonly on the lower lip. Superficial lesions appear translucent and are bluish, whereas deep-seated lesions have a normal color. A mucocele in the floor of the mouth is termed a ranula and is seen as a dome-shaped, fluid-filled lesion. Mucoceles are thought to result from severance or obstruction of a salivary gland duct, with pooling of mucin in the lamina propria. Complete excision of the mucocele or marsupialization of the ranula is indicated.

CHAPTER 110

Neurosurgical Emergencies, Nontraumatic

Dale W. Steele, M.D.

Patients with nontraumatic acute neurosurgical problems come to the emergency department (ED) with a variety of nonspecific signs and symptoms, including headache, vomiting, seizures, changes in mental status, weakness, and coma. Because headache and vomiting are common, a high index of suspicion is required.

INCREASED INTRACRANIAL PRESSURE

The functions of the buffering systems that maintain intracranial pressure (ICP) at normal levels are detailed in Chapter 92. The relatively rigid cranium contains three components: (1) brain tissue predominantly, (2) cerebrospinal fluid (CSF), and (3) blood. An abnormal increase in the volume of any of these components (by means of edema or mass lesion of the brain tissue, increased production or diminished absorption of CSF, or increased cerebral perfusion pressure related to increased blood flow) can result in elevated ICP. This closed space has limited capacity to compensate for increased volume from hydrocephalus, cerebral edema, hemorrhage, mass lesions, or pus.

A careful history must be taken with respect to the timing and severity of headaches, vomiting, changes in behavior, visual changes, and episodic decreases in level of consciousness (Table 110.1). Nighttime and morning headaches that improve on arising are always ominous suggestions of elevated ICP, as is recurrent vomiting without fever, abdominal pain, or diarrhea.

The clinical examination can help confirm the presence of intracranial hypertension, but a normal examination cannot reliably exclude it. Funduscopic examination should be performed to look for papilledema or optic atrophy. Visual fields and visual acuity should be checked. Cranial sutures may split in infants and young children with chronic elevation of ICP, resulting in a hyperresonant note when the skull is percussed, a "cracked pot" sound known as the *Macewen sign*. Cranial nerve palsy may occur, usually affecting the third and sixth nerves, resulting in dilated pupil, diplopia, and strabismus. When the fourth nerve is affected, the child may exhibit a "cock robin" head tilt. Cerebellar herniation also may cause head tilt; if herniation is bilateral, the neck may be held in an extended position.

Management

The emergency treatment of increased ICP depends on the patient's clinical state and the cause of the intracranial hypertension (Table 110.2). The first priority for all patients, however, is to follow the ABCs (airway, breathing, and circulation) of resuscitation and to prevent hypoxemia, hypercarbia, and systemic hypotension with oxygenation, ventilation, and appropriate fluid therapy. Seizures should be prevented if possible and treated aggressively when they occur because the ICP spikes during seizures aggravate intracranial hypertension. Phenytoin (15–20 mg per kilogram of body weight) and fosphenytoin are the preferred drugs.

When the clinical picture suggests intracranial hypertension, computed tomography (CT) of the head should be performed without contrast material as soon as the patient is stable. Lumbar puncture should be withheld until the scan has been read for fear of precipitating herniation. The temptation to give sedative agents to the agitated patient to accomplish head CT or to facilitate transport should be avoided. Sedative agents given without controlled ventilation may result in hypercarbia, causing an increase in cerebral blood volume and, therefore, in ICP. Sedatives also can block protective airway reflexes, increasing the risk of aspiration. Therefore, inserting an endotracheal tube before CT scan or before transport is often preferable.

Intubation should not be attempted without appropriate expertise and use of proper medications to blunt the increases in

TABLE 110.1. Signs and Symptoms of Elevated Intracranial Pressure

Symptoms	Signs
Headache	Papilledema
Nocturnal, episodic severe	Cranial nerve palsies
Vomiting	Meningismus
Stiff neck	Head tilt
Double vision	Retinal hemorrhage
Transient visual loss	Macewen's (cracked pot) signs
Gait difficulties	Decorticate/decerebrate posturing
Dulled intellect	Coma
Irritability	Progressive hemiparesis
	Bradycardia

Modified from Bruce DA. Neurosurgical emergencies. In: Fleisher GR, Ludwig S, eds. *Textbook of pediatric emergency medicine,* 3rd ed. Baltimore: Williams & Wilkins, 1993:1410, with permission.

ICP associated with the procedure. Rapid-sequence intubation (see Chapters 5 and 92) should be accomplished after preoxygenation by giving a sequence of atropine (0.02 mg per kilogram of body weight), lidocaine (1.5 mg per kilogram), and thiopental (2–5 mg per kilogram), followed by a neuromuscular blocker. Succinylcholine (1–1.5 mg per kilogram) has rapid onset and short duration, but the fasciculations related to its depolarizing effects can cause transient increases in ICP. Rocuronium (0.6–1.2 mg per kilogram) and vecuronium (0.1–0.2 mg per kilogram) are nondepolarizing blockers that provide adequate alternatives.

In the absence of signs of impending herniation, P_{CO2} should be controlled by mild hyperventilation in the range of 30 to 35 mm Hg. Prolonged excessive hyperventilation may cause cerebral ischemia. Continuous, portable capnometry may be useful as a monitor to avoid excessive hyperventilation during transport or diagnostic imaging.

Acute hyperventilation (hand ventilation) is used as an attempt to reverse the signs of acute herniation. The head of the bed should be elevated to 30 degrees, and the head should be maintained in a neutral position to promote venous drainage. Also, when the child exhibits acute herniation, drainage of CSF, either from a shunt reservoir or by a ventricular tap via an open fontanel, a split suture, or a burr hole, will allow controlled reduction of CSF volume. A ventriculostomy catheter also may be used to measure ICP directly, to direct medical therapy, and to allow drainage of CSF. Mannitol (0.25–2.0 g per kilogram) is the most useful drug to decrease acutely ICP in the deteriorating patient. Acetazolamide and furosemide have a limited role in acute management. Dexamethasone (1 mg per kilogram) is of controversial benefit, has slow onset, and appears to be most useful in treating vasogenic brain edema associated with tumors and brain abscess and nontraumatic hemorrhage. Surgical removal of collections of blood or pus may be indicated to lower ICP, as discussed later in this chapter.

TABLE 110.2. Treatment of Increased Intracranial Pressure

Prevent hypoxia and hypercarbia
Tracheal intubation/controlled ventilation
Seizure treatment and prophylaxis
Maintain adequate cerebral perfusion pressure and cerebral perfusion
Treatment of shock
Limitation of excessive hyperventilation
Decrease cerebral blood volume
Acute hyperventilation
Decrease brain tissue volume
Mannitol
Dexamethasone for vasogenic edema
Decrease cerebrospinal fluid (CSF) volume
CSF drainage
Acetazolamide
Removal of mass lesion
Surgical removal/decompression

HYDROCEPHALUS

Hydrocephalus is characterized by dilated cerebral ventricles that contain an excessive amount of CSF; this results from an imbalance between production and absorption. Production, which is accomplished in the choroid plexus, almost always remains stable and is only rarely excessive. In noncommunicating hydrocephalus, CSF in the ventricular systems is blocked from communicating with CSF in the subarachnoid spaces and basal cisterns by a congenital or acquired defect. In communicating hydrocephalus, the block in absorption is on the meningeal surfaces, outside the ventricular system. Congenital hydrocephalus may result from aqueductal stenosis or in association with Dandy–Walker or Arnold–Chiari malformations. Acquired hydrocephalus may follow bacterial meningitis. It may be secondary to tumor (particularly in the posterior fossa), or it can result from the inflammatory response to subarachnoid or intracranial hemorrhage.

Previously Undiagnosed Hydrocephalus

Children with undiagnosed hydrocephalus rarely present first to the ED, but hydrocephalus must be considered in all children with symptoms suggestive of increased ICP. A careful history should be taken of all previous illnesses and traumas. In a child with unexplained headache, chronic vomiting, and irritability, head circumference should be recorded and the fontanel, if open, evaluated. The skull should be transilluminated, and dilated scalp veins should be noted. A "cracked pot" sound may be noted on percussion if the sutures are split. The pupils and extraocular movements should be examined. Difficulty with upward gaze ("sunset" sign) may be seen. Muscular spasticity, particularly in the lower extremities, may develop as cortical motor fibers are stretched by the ventricular dilation.

MANAGEMENT

Noncontrast head CT demonstrates enlarged ventricles. The urgency with which either insertion of a ventricular shunt or ventricular drainage needs to be performed depends on the child's condition. Ventricular puncture through an open fontanel or coronal suture may be lifesaving in a child with evidence for impending cerebral herniation who is unresponsive to hyperventilation and mannitol.

Previously Shunted Hydrocephalus

Placement of CSF shunts is currently the most commonly performed neurosurgical procedure. These shunts allow diversion of CSF into another area of the body outside the brain, most commonly the peritoneal cavity, thereby relieving pressure on the brain. Unfortunately, placement of shunts is accompanied by complications, including malfunction, obstruction, infection, malposition, and migration. Children who have shunts represent a heterogeneous group with multiple causes for hydrocephalus, including congenital defects, intraventricular hemorrhage, myelodysplasia, central nervous system (CNS) infection, and brain tumor.

Shunt Malfunction

Patients with shunt malfunction commonly present with manifestations of increased ICP. Children may complain of headache (often worse in the morning), screaming episodes, lethargy, and other behavioral changes or visual symptoms. Vomiting is common. On physical examination, unilateral or bilateral cranial nerve palsies, especially a nonlocalizing sixth nerve palsy, may be present. Intermittent downward gaze (sunset sign) may be reported or observed. Swelling from CSF tracking along the shunt tract is indicative of obstruction. The fontanel may be full and tense, even when the infant is upright. Rapid enlargement in head circumference or an increase in the prominence of scalp veins may occur. Papilledema is uncommon in acute shunt malfunction. Head tilt may be seen as a result of fourth cranial nerve palsy or cerebellar tonsillar herniation.

Of particular concern are waves of severe headache with or without visual changes, loss of consciousness, decerebrate posturing, or new third nerve palsy. Although seizures are common in patients with CSF shunts, one reported series revealed that only 2.9% of ED visits for seizures in patients with shunts culminated in shunt revision. Most shunts have a pumping mechanism, but pumping the shunt correlates poorly with shunt obstruction. In one series, shunt pumping in patients with suspected shunt malfunction had a sensitivity of 18% with a positive predictive value of only 17%. The shunt should not be routinely pumped because the negative pressure generated in a small ventricle occasionally results in obstruction. If the ventricular catheter is shown on CT scan to be in the center of a dilated ventricle, however, and the shunt umbilicates on depression with slow refill, shunt obstruction is likely.

MANAGEMENT

If the history or physical examination suggests shunt malfunction, early neurosurgical consultation is strongly recommended. A plain radiographic "shunt series" should be done, consisting of anteroposterior and lateral views of the skull, neck, thorax, and abdomen. These radiographs allow the type, location, connections, and intactness of the system to be evaluated. Occasionally, split sutures on the skull film suggest increased ICP. Noncontrast head CT also should be taken and compared, if possible, with previous scans taken when the shunt was functioning. In most cases (approximately 80%), these studies identify shunt malfunction.

Shunt tap also may be useful in patients in whom the function of the shunt is questionable. This procedure should be completed under sterile conditions, and the examiner should have knowledge of the anatomy of the patient's shunt. A small but significant risk of causing a shunt infection by performing a shunt tap exists. Therefore, diagnostic shunt taps usually are performed selectively by the neurosurgical consultant.

The urgency of shunt revision depends on the patient's status. Patients with evidence of obliteration of the perimesencephalic cistern appear to be at particularly high risk for sudden deterioration. Patients with proximal obstructions may worsen quickly, and if the child suddenly deteriorates, CSF cannot be quickly withdrawn from the shunt reservoir to relieve pressure. Because fluid cannot be drawn from the shunt, the ventricle must be tapped through the fontanel, if it is open, through the sutures if they are split, or through the shunt bur hole. This latter maneuver usually damages the shunt and is therefore simply a temporizing measure to lower the ICP before operative shunt revision.

When the distal end of the shunt is blocked, the ICP can be lowered immediately by removing CSF through a shunt tap. The need for emergency shunt revision is less in this setting because the ICP can be controlled easily by tapping the shunt. Acetazolamide and dexamethasone can be used as temporizing measures if shunt revision is to be delayed but may not be effective.

In some patients, ventriculomegaly may persist despite a functioning shunt. In these patients, prior CT scans are particularly helpful. Conversely, some patients have symptoms and signs of increased ICP despite small or unchanged ventricles, which is called the "slit ventricle" syndrome. This condition may be the result of intermittent proximal obstruction, poor ventricular compliance, or overdrainage of CSF. A history of onset or worsening of symptoms with upright posture suggests overdrainage. These children require careful further evaluation, which may include ICP monitoring, to determine the functions of their symptoms.

Shunt Infection

About 70% of all shunt infections occur within 2 months of surgery. Infections are caused by low virulence organisms found in skin flora. *Staphylococcus epidermidis* accounts for approximately 75% of shunt infections, followed by gram-negative organisms and *Staphylococcus aureus*.

In the postoperative period, erythema and warmth along the course of the shunt are highly predictive of early wound infection. Later, signs of indolent infection are often variable and nonspecific. Signs of shunt malfunction occur commonly. The adage "an infected shunt is an obstructed shunt" is well remembered. Although fever raises concern for shunt infection, documented shunt infections were associated with fever in only 42% of patients in one series. Meningeal signs have been reported in only about 33% of patients. Abdominal symptoms from an associated peritonitis may predominate in cases of pseudocyst formation with distal obstruction.

MANAGEMENT

A definite diagnosis of shunt infection is made by tapping the shunt and obtaining a CSF specimen. A definite, although small, rate of infection occurs as a result of a tap, and in a patient who has the potential for bacteremia, the blood carried into the shunt reservoir on the tip of the needle may be contaminated and produce a shunt infection. Thus, shunt tap is not indicated in all children with a shunt who present with fever. Fever without localizing signs in patients in whom the current shunt was placed or revised many months to years ago and who lack signs and symptoms of shunt malfunction can be managed appropriately with close follow-up and observation without shunt tap.

STROKE

Stroke denotes a sudden onset of a persistent focal neurologic deficit, resulting from interruption of blood flow to a localized area of the brain. Pediatric stroke has a wide range of causes and risk factors distinct from those in adults, thus limiting comparison to stroke in adults.

Hemorrhagic Stroke

In children and adolescents, rupture of an arteriovenous malformation is the most common cause of spontaneous intracranial hemorrhage. (General causes of hemorrhagic stroke are listed in Table 110.3.) These lesions are within the cerebral parenchyma; therefore, when they bleed, the hematoma is intracerebral and the bleeding is arterial. Arterial intraparenchymal bleeding results in progressive surrounding edema and focal mass effect. Congenital or acquired coagulation disorders, such as severe factor VIII deficiency or severe thrombocytopenia, may result in spontaneous intracranial bleeding with minimal or no preceding head trauma.

Ruptured aneurysms are rare, accounting for only 10% of intracranial hemorrhage in children. Only rarely are congenital ruptured aneurysms seen as early as the first week of life. The bleeding occurs from an aneurysm located at branching points of the major arteries coursing through the subarachnoid space at the base of the brain. The incidence of aneurysm is increased in several inherited conditions, including autosomal-dominant polycystic kidney disease, Ehlers–Danlos type IV, neurofibromatosis type 1, and Marfan syndrome.

Other vascular abnormalities associated with intracranial bleeding include cavernous angiomas and hemangioblastoma associated with von Hippel–Lindau syndrome. Cavernous angiomas are low-flow lesions that can occur anywhere in the cerebrum, brainstem, cerebellum, or spinal cord. Because they lack large arterial feeders, onset of symptoms is usually subacute. The greatest danger is of acute hydrocephalus caused by occlusion of the fourth ventricle, resulting from posterior fossa hemorrhage or swelling.

Ischemic Stroke

Ischemic injury to the brain occurs as a result of embolism from the heart or proximal arterial circulation or from thrombosis in the arterial or sinovenous system. The most common risk factor (in about 25% of patients) is congenital heart disease.

Although it is difficult to separate risk factors from causes, several conditions have been associated with embolic or thrombotic stroke (Table 110.4). Embolic sources are primarily from the heart (dilated or abnormal chambers), from abnormal or infected heart valves, or from "paradoxical" emboli via lesions associated with right-to-left cardiac shunts. Other risk factors include congenital or acquired vascular disorders and factors that result in hypercoagulability, such as (1) oral contraceptive use; (2) anticardiolipin antibodies; and (3) deficiencies of protein S, protein C, or antithrombin III. Stroke occurs in 6% to 9% of patients with sickle cell disease (SCD). In children with SCD, most strokes are ischemic, resulting from occlusion of intracranial carotid and middle cerebral arteries.

Diagnosis of stroke syndrome in children often is delayed by the failure to consider it. Focal weakness in association with headache or after a seizure should not be dismissed as hemiplegic migraine or postictal Todd paresis. Presenting symptoms are nonspecific as to the cause, but several patterns exist. Depending on the location and nature of the intraparenchymal lesion, stroke in children may present with sudden onset of hemiplegia or hemiparesis, aphasia, and sensory symptoms. These focal signs frequently are accompanied by seizures, fever, acute change in mental status, and signs and symptoms of increased ICP. Subarachnoid hemorrhage causes sudden severe headache and meningismus caused by the breakdown of blood products in the subarachnoid space, leading to meningeal irritation. As CSF circulates, symptoms of lower back pain and radicular leg pain subsequently may predominate.

TABLE 110.3. Causes of Hemorrhagic Stroke

Secondary hemorrhage into ischemic brain
Vascular malformations
Arteriovenous malformations
Sickle cell disease
Saccular (berry) aneurysms
Hemorrhage into intracranial tumor
Coagulopathy
Hemorrhagic disease of the newborn (vitamin K deficiency)
Clotting factor deficiency (VIII, IX, XI)
Thrombocytopenia
Arterial hypertension
Renal vascular or parenchymal disease
Coarctation of the aorta
Pheochromocytoma
Illicit drugs with sympathomimetic effect
Amphetamines, cocaine

TABLE 110.4. Causes of Ischemic Stroke

Cardioembolic
Cyanotic congenital heart disease
Right-to-left shunts (e.g., patent foramen ovale)
Congenital or acquired valvular defects
Contractile dysfunction
Rhythm disturbance
Vascular disease
Sickle cell disease
Arterial dissection
Homocystinuria
Vasculitis
Moyamoya
Migraine
Thrombotic (arterial and sinovenous)
Hypercoagulable state, congenital or acquired
Hyperviscosity (polycythemia, dehydration)
Genetic/metabolic

MANAGEMENT

After initiation of supportive care to prevent secondary hypoxic ischemic injury and to ameliorate increased ICP, the next priority is to exclude an acute intraparenchymal or subarachnoid hemorrhage. Noncontrast head CT is sensitive for acute bleeding and should be obtained emergently. Noncontrast CT is a good test to exclude hemorrhagic causes of stroke, but it may be normal or near normal soon after the onset of symptoms of ischemic stroke.

If intraparenchymal hemorrhage is found, most children with bleeding from suspected rupture of an arteriovenous malformation require early angiography to localize the bleeding and the arterial feeders. Medical therapy of associated edema and increased ICP may include dexamethasone (0.5–1.0 mg per kilogram of body weight, for a maximum of 16 mg daily) and mannitol (0.25–2.0 g per kilogram). Seizures should be treated aggressively, and prophylactic administration of phenytoin (15–20 mg per kilogram) or fosphenytoin may play a role in this treatment. Coagulation defects should be corrected as appropriate (see "Coagulation Emergencies," Chapter 77).

Hemorrhagic stroke or secondary gross hemorrhage into an area of ischemic infarction may produce a rapidly expanding intracranial mass. Depending on the site of the hemorrhage, emergency surgical evacuation of the hematoma may be indicated to reverse cerebral herniation and lower ICP.

The management of ischemic stroke remains largely supportive. Acute carotid occlusion may result in significant hemispheric swelling sufficient to produce elevated ICP. Magnetic resonance imaging (MRI) permits visualization of brain infarction. Magnetic resonance angiography (MRA) yields further information about blood flow and the structure of cervical and intracranial vessels. Ultrasound can be used to evaluate the extracranial carotid circulation.

The decision to use anticoagulation must balance the likelihood of either extension of infarction or a second embolus with the risk of inducing hemorrhage. Anticoagulation is often used in children with arterial dissection, dural sinus thrombosis, or coagulation disorders; in those at high risk of embolism; or in response to progressive deterioration during the initial evaluation of a new cerebral infarction. The loading dose of heparin is 75 U per kilogram of body weight administered intravenously, followed by 20 U per kilogram per hour for children older than 1 year (or 28 U per kilogram per hour for children aged <1 year) titrated to a target activated partial thromboplastin time (aPTT) of 60 to 85 seconds. Alternately, low-molecular-weight heparin (Enoxaparin 1 mg per kilogram subcutaneously twice daily) has also been used.

Stroke in a patient with SCD is treated with simple or partial exchange transfusion to achieve a hemoglobin SS fraction of less than 30% and a hemoglobin level not greater than 10 g/dL to avoid problems of hyperviscosity.

The use of thrombolytic agents for ischemic stroke, administered intravenously, or locally utilizing angiographic catheters, is currently receiving significant attention. A single controlled trial of intravenous recombinant tissue plasminogen activator (t-PA) resulted in overall better outcomes in carefully selected adults treated within 3 hours after onset of symptoms. This therapeutic success led to the concept of stroke as a "brain attack" analogous to a heart attack. Intravenous thrombolytic therapy in children using t-PA (0.5 mg per kilogram) mostly for noncerebral thrombotic complications resulted in successful clot lysis, but at the expense of serious bleeding complications. If the diagnosis is delayed beyond 3 to 6 hours, risk of hemorrhage into ischemic infarcts clearly precludes any attempt at clot lysis. Some pediatric patients with acute ischemic stroke benefit from thrombolytic therapy when it is administered with caution, in a highly individualized manner using guidelines defined by ongoing randomized studies in adults.

SPINAL CORD COMPRESSION

Nontraumatic acute spinal cord dysfunction occurs in 4% of children undergoing treatment for cancer, usually because of spinal cord compression. Many children undergoing treatment for cancer develop back pain, which should raise concern for cord compression until proven otherwise. Spinal cord compression may be the presenting sign of neuroblastoma, lymphoma, or sarcoma. Other causes of acute spinal cord symptoms include spinal epidural and, more rarely, subdural abscess, epidural hematoma, and congenital tethered cord.

Back pain in children commonly signals an important diagnosis. A history of localized or radicular back pain or refusal to walk mandates a careful evaluation. A history of change in gait or difficulty with bowel or bladder control should be sought. Localized tenderness to palpation is commonly found, and the level of maximal spinal tenderness is usually the site of pathology. A detailed neurologic examination should be documented with attention to extremity strength, reflexes, anal tone, and evaluation of sensory level. Compression of the spinal cord above the conus may be associated with increased or absent deep tendon reflexes, an extensor Babinski reflex with symmetric (and profound) weakness, and a symmetric sensory level. Sphincter tone is spared until late, and progression is characteristically rapid. Compression of the conus medullaris results in increased knee and decreased ankle reflexes, extensor Babinski reflex with a symmetric saddle distribution of weakness, and early sphincter involvement. Compression of the cauda equina typically results in asymmetric, often mild weakness and asymmetric and radicular sensory distribution. Deep tendon reflexes are decreased with a plantar Babinski response.

Management

Evidence for progressive cord dysfunction in the presence of significant neurologic deficits mandates immediate high-dose corticosteroid therapy with methylprednisolone 30 mg per kilogram or dexamethasone 2 mg per kilogram. Plain radiographs of the spine may be helpful, but emergency MRI is necessary to view the anatomic cause and degree of spinal compression.

SECTION

VI

Psychosocial Emergencies

CHAPTER 111

Child Abuse

Stephen Ludwig, M.D.

Child abuse is the single diagnostic term used to describe a range of behaviors from somewhat harsh discipline to intentional repetitive torture. This phenomenon is complex and results from a combination of individual, familial, and societal factors. The common pathway for all these factors is parental behavior destructive to the process of normal growth, development, and well-being of the child. Abuse can be subdivided into four broad categories: (1) physical abuse, (2) sexual abuse, (3) neglect, and (4) emotional abuse. Each form of abuse has individual characteristics of family dynamics, clinical manifestations, and management.

PHYSICAL ABUSE

Background

Physical abuse is the most often reported form of child abuse. Definitions of physical abuse vary from state to state. Operationally, the definitions vary from one institution to the next, indeed from person to person. Even the definition of physical abuse is a definition in transition. Over the past century, many advances in the "rights of the children" have been made. For example, the enactment of child labor and compulsory education laws has been an important step forward. As the history of abuse is traced through the centuries, the forms and the definitions of abuse have changed. Current definitions used are likely to continue to change with time. The present widespread medical interest in abuse was stimulated by C. Henry Kempe with the introduction of the term *battered child syndrome* in 1962. As recently as 1968, the last of the 50 states enacted child abuse legislation. Many states are now using their second or third generation of child abuse laws.

There are four major types of child maltreatment: (1) physical abuse, (2) child neglect, (3) sexual abuse, and (4) emotional abuse. Physical abuse is the infliction of physical injury as a result of punching, beating, kicking, biting, burning, shaking, or otherwise harming a child. The parent or caretaker may not have intended to hurt the child, but rather the injury may have resulted from too-harsh discipline or physical punishment.

Manifestations

The manifestations of physical abuse may affect any body system. Thus, the emergency physician must be prepared to recognize a variety of signs and symptoms. Abuse also may be seen by any specialist physician. National data show neglect to be most common (Fig. 111.1).

INTEGUMENT

The skin is the most commonly injured body organ. Cutaneous injuries may be divided into nonspecific and specific traumatic lesions, burns, and hair loss. Of the nonspecific traumatic injuries, the bruise or contusion is the most commonly seen. Although bruises are also common in children who are not abused, accidental bruises usually have a different distribution and appearance. Accidental injuries occur most commonly on the extremities and forehead. As bruising moves centrally and becomes extensive, the likelihood of abuse rises. Contusions undergo recognizable stages of healing. In the first 24 hours, the size of the bruise increases slightly if careful measurements are made. The process of resolution is varied. The bruise should be dated and compared with the history provided. A prothrombin time, partial thromboplastin time, bleeding time, and platelet count should be obtained if the issue of "easy bruisability" has been offered as a possible explanation.

Other nonspecific cutaneous injuries include lacerations, punctures, and abrasions. The following criteria are important for the evaluation of any nonspecific injury: (1) the history of injury, (2) the child's age and developmental level, (3) the presence of other old or new injuries, (4) the interaction between the parents and child, and (5) the interaction between the parents and the emergency department (ED) staff.

Specific skin injuries are those that clearly reflect the method or object used to inflict the trauma. Loop-shaped marks are readily seen after a beating with an electric cord or wire. Linear

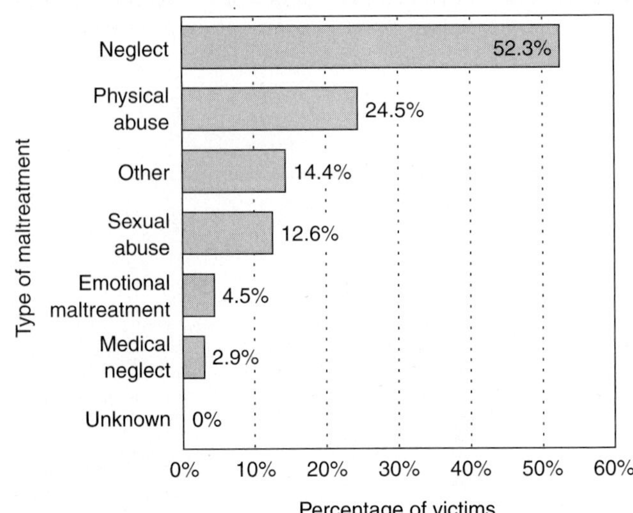

Figure 111.1. Types of maltreatment as a percentage of victims (1995) based on surveys in 49 states. $N = 1{,}000{,}502$ victims in 49 states. (*Note*: Percentages total more than 100% because some states reported more than one type of maltreatment per victim.)

marks may be seen from a belt or paddle injury. Rope burns result in circumferential marks on the wrists, ankles, or around the neck when a child has been bound. Another common specific integument lesion is a handprint on the side of the face or symmetrically on the upper arms. The lesion produced by a slap leaves ecchymotic areas in the location of the interphalangeal spaces. Human bites appear as circular lesions 1 to 2 inches in diameter. Forensic dentistry is able to match the skin lesion with the dentition of the alleged perpetrator. Some specific skin lesions are shown in Figure 111.2.

Burns of the skin can be caused by either abuse or neglect. Burns account for 5% of cases of physical abuse. In particular, tap-water scald burns that occur in an immersion pattern (Fig. 111.3A) are often the result of intentional trauma. Immersion burns are

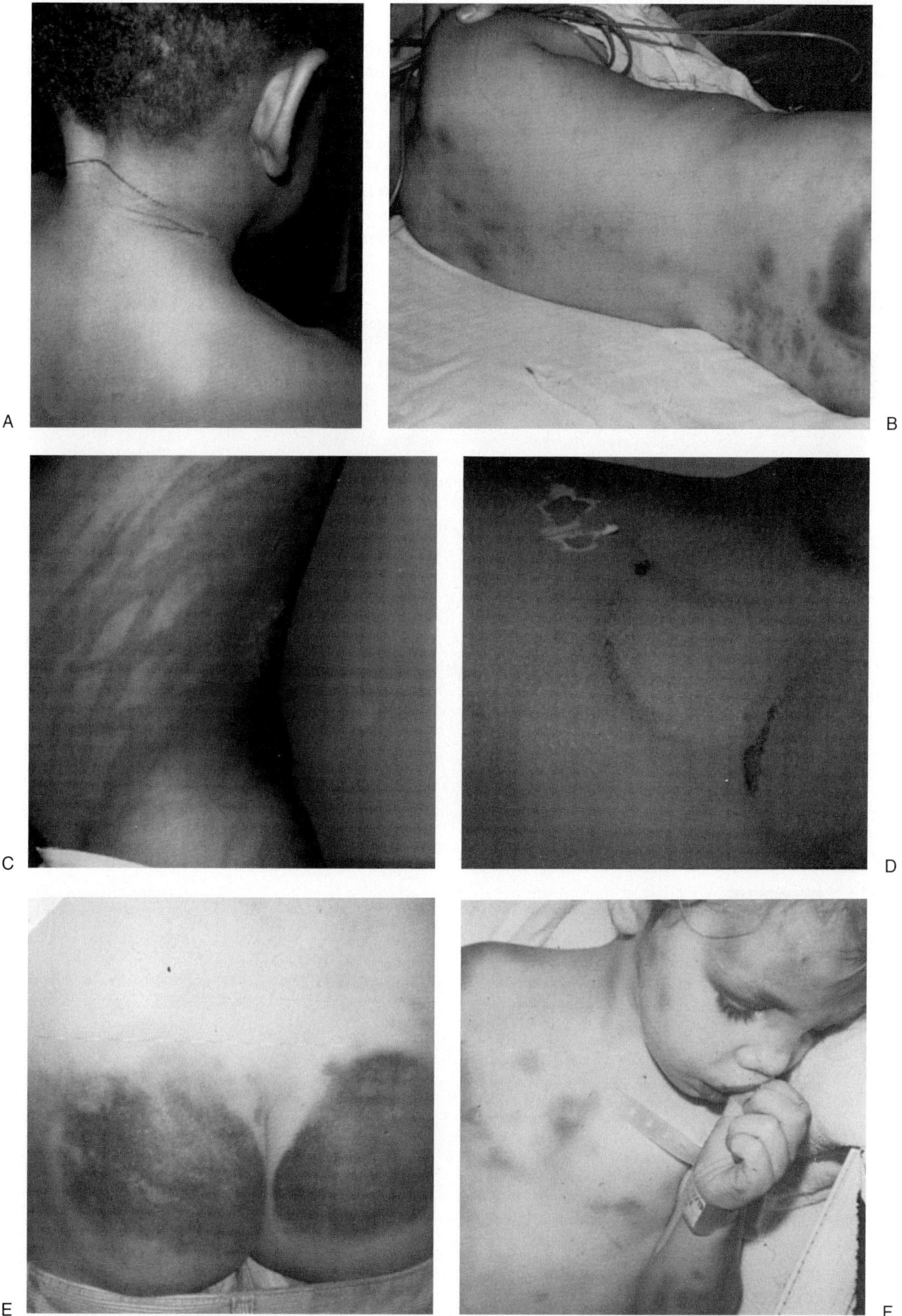

Figure 111.2. Cutaneous manifestations of child abuse. **A:** Strangulation mark. **B:** Bruises at various stages of healing. **C:** Linear loop-shaped marks. **D:** Multiple loop-shaped marks. **E:** Buttocks bruises as a cause of myoglobinuria. **F:** Multiple bruises in a central pattern.

likely to be inflicted by an abusive parent when they occur on a child who is being toilet-trained. Other indications of abuse are (1) a delay in seeking treatment, (2) a history of the child being unsupervised, and (3) the child being brought to the hospital by the parent who was not present at the time the burn occurred.

In attempting to match the physical findings of the burn with the available history, several factors must be appreciated. The extent of the burn depends on the temperature of the water, the duration of exposure, the thickness of the skin involved, and the presence or absence of clothing. Water temperature of 54°C (130°F) or higher causes a full-thickness burn with less than a 30-second exposure. Because palms and soles are thick, they are often spared. Clothing tends to keep the hot water in contact with the skin and can cause more severe burns. Burns presumably caused by falling or thrown fluids should produce a droplet or splash pattern. When the child has several small bullous lesions, the main differential diagnosis is a second-degree burn versus bullous impetigo. This differentiation is easily made by Gram stain and culture of a bulla.

Other burns occur through contact with a hot solid rather than a hot fluid. Cigarette burns are the most common of this type. If the history given is of a child brushing against a cigarette or of hot ashes falling on the child, the resulting injury should be a nonspecific first- or second-degree burn. When a cigarette is extinguished on the child's skin, the injury is a burn that is 8 to 10 mm in diameter and indurated at its margin. A healed cigarette burn is indistinguishable from any other circular skin lesion such as impetigo, abscess, or vesicles. Burns from radiators, hot plates, cigarette lighters (Fig. 111.3B), curling irons, or standard irons imprint the shape of the hot object. More recently, there have been reports of children burned by microwave ovens.

The final category of integumentary injury is injury to the hair. Traction alopecia is seen when a parent pulls the child by the hair. The scalp is usually clear, differentiating this lesion from tinea capitis, seborrhea, and scalp eczema. Alopecia areata produces a lesion in which the hair is uniformly absent. In cases of traction or traumatic alopecia, patches of broken hair remain.

A

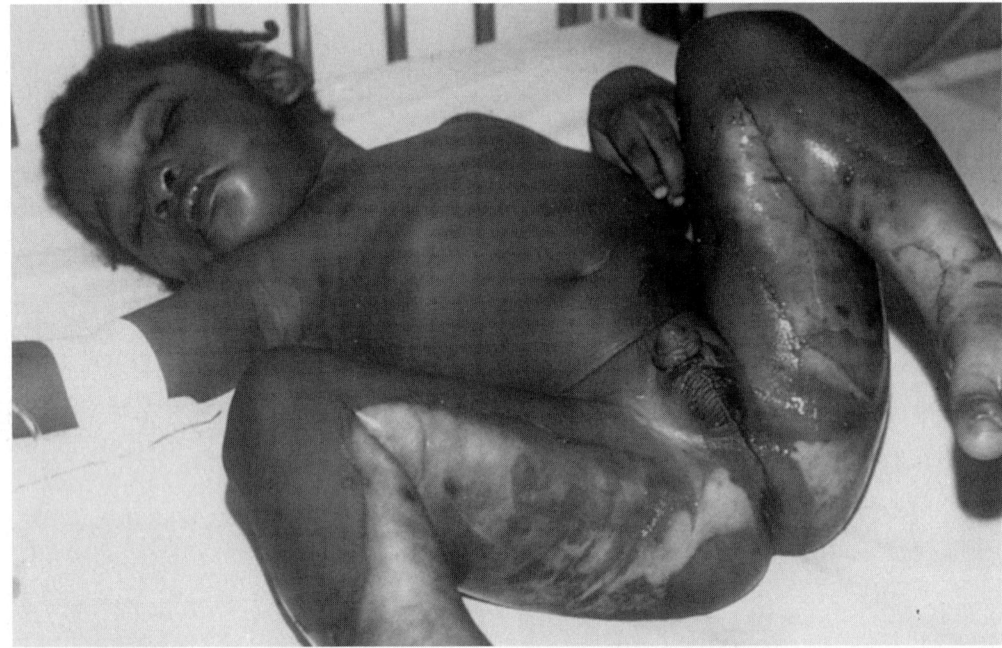

B

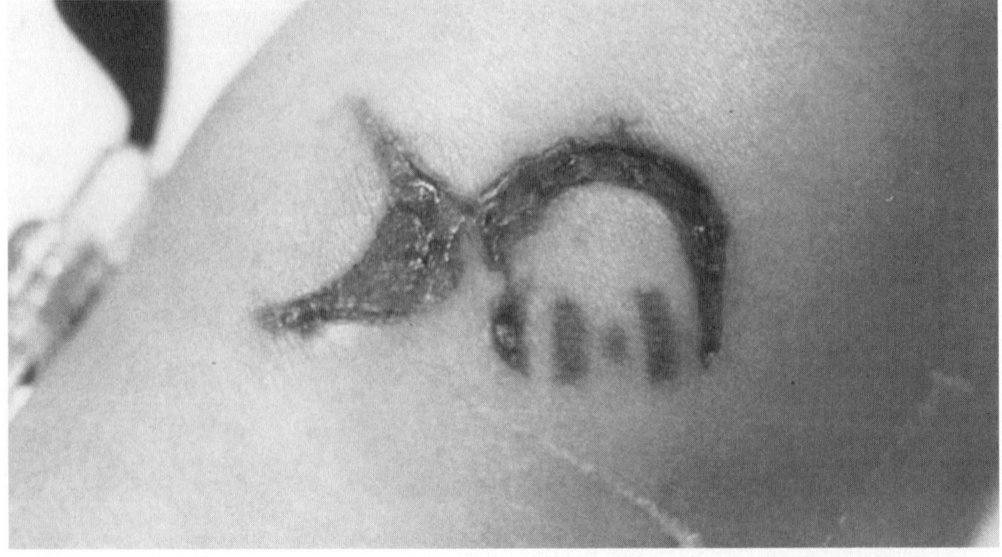

Figure 111.3. **A:** Hot-water burn in an immersion pattern. **B:** Pattern burn from cigarette lighter.

Skeletal System

The skeletal system is also commonly traumatized when children are physically abused. As previously mentioned, matching the history of injury with the physical findings is important. Considering the mobility and strength of the child is also important to identify suspicious injuries. The radiologist needs to review the patient's past radiographs to identify the child with multiple visits to the hospital for fractures. When suspicion of abuse is high, a radiographic skeletal survey should be obtained to ascertain the condition of the entire skeletal system.

Support for the use of radioisotope scans as a more sensitive and immediate way of demonstrating bone injury is increasing; however, radionuclide scans are still second-line studies. Some indications for a radiographic skeletal survey or bone scans are listed in the "Management" section of this chapter. Skeletal surveys often are performed on a young child with an obvious fracture that then reveal multiple old fractures. The skeletal survey is the preferred radiographic study because it provides information on the type, location, and age of fractures as well as presence or absence of bone diseases.

Bone injuries may be of several types, including simple transverse fractures, impacted fractures, spiral fractures, metaphyseal fractures, or subperiosteal hematomas. Radiographs of some of these injuries are shown in Figure 111.4. To explain a transverse fracture, the history should be that of direct force ap-

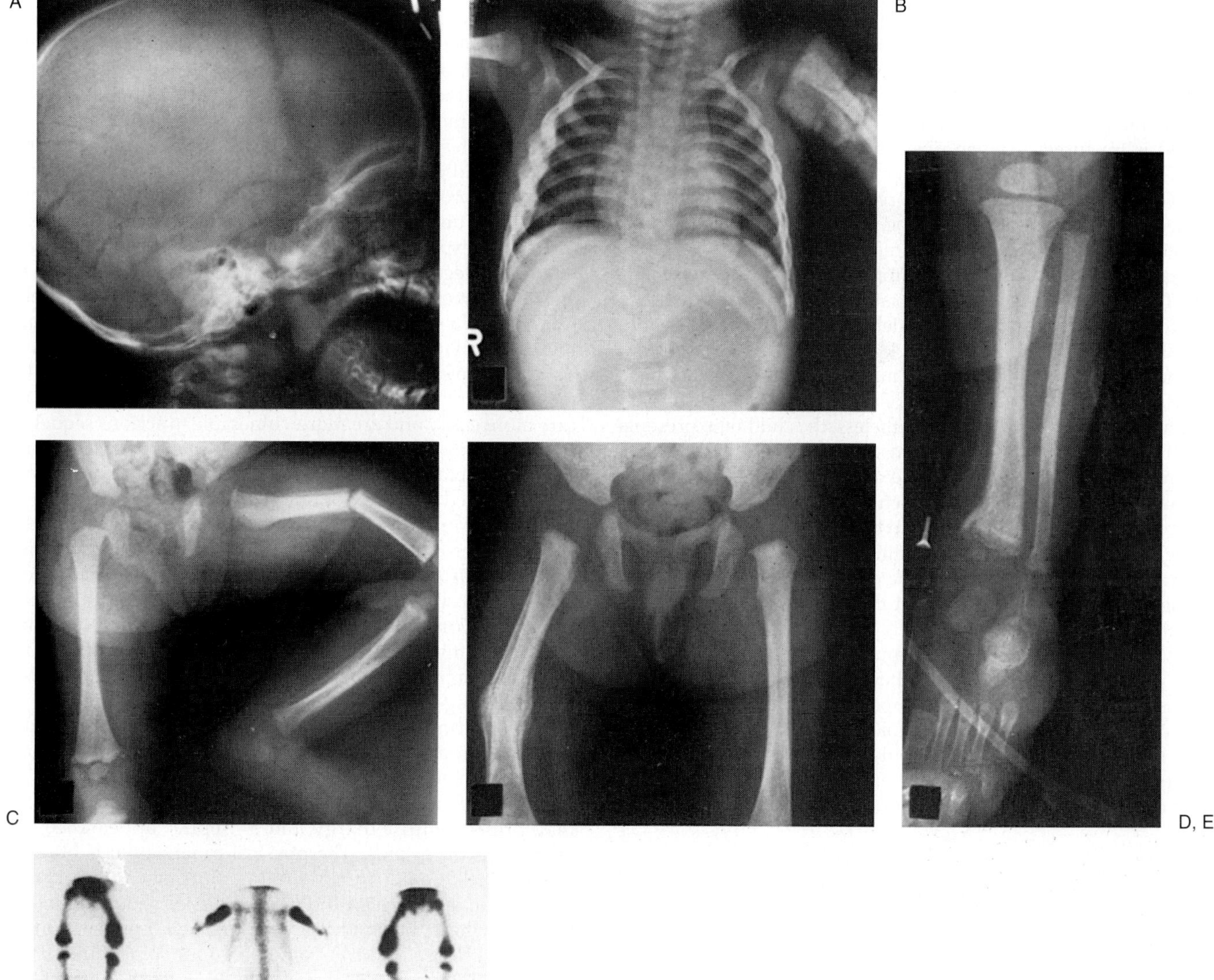

Figure 111.4. Radiographic findings of child abuse. **A:** Multiple skull fractures in an infant. **B:** Left humerus fracture and multiple old healing rib fractures. **C:** Left femur fracture and metaphyseal chip avulsion fractures of the right distal femur. **D:** Healing fracture of the right femur with callus formation and new periosteal bone formation. **E:** "Bucket-handle" deformity of healing distal tibial epiphyseal fracture. **F:** Bone scan showing multiple areas of increased uptake caused by trauma. Some of these areas appeared normal on the original radiographs.

plied to the bone. Differentiating the true cause of this type of fracture is often difficult. The impacted fracture should have an accompanying history of force along the long axis of the bone, such as the child's falling on his or her outstretched hand. In the case of a spiral fracture, a history of twisting or torque during the traumatic event should be present. Metaphyseal chip fractures occur when the extremity is pulled or yanked; the periosteum is most tightly adherent at the metaphysis, causing small bone fragments to avulse. Metaphyseal chip fractures are almost exclusively caused by abuse. Subperiosteal hematomas produce a characteristic radiograph. Elevation of the periosteum is seen as a linear opacification running parallel to the bone surface. Subperiosteal hematomas are produced by direct trauma to the bone; however, in up to 10% of small and premature infants, symmetric periosteal elevation that is not caused by abuse may occur along the tibia or humerus. The reason for this finding is unknown, but it should not be confused with abuse.

The location of the fracture is important in the identification of abuse. Fracture of a clavicle and dislocation of a radial head are common noninflicted injuries. When the femur of a young child is fractured or when ribs are fractured, the suspicion of abuse increases.

Other uncommon and therefore suspicious fractures are located in the vertebrae, sternum, pelvis, or scapulae. Uncommon fractures need to be evaluated carefully unless a clear history of significant trauma, such as an automobile injury, is reported.

The age of a fracture may be estimated from the amount of callus formation and bone remodeling seen on the radiograph. Table 111.1 lists fracture landmarks by date. Dating of fractures is not an exact science because many confounding variables, such as the child's age, location of the fracture, and nutritional status, must be considered. Nonetheless, the child who presents with an acute fracture and has a second fracture with a callus stands out as having sustained more than one episode of trauma. The usual long-bone fracture may take 8 to 10 days to form callus and several months to heal completely. In the acute stages of injury, soft-tissue swelling should be seen for 2 to 5 days. Soft-tissue swelling may be clearly seen on standard radiographs. Skull fractures or fractures of other flat bones cannot be dated in the same way.

When a young child sustains multiple fractures, the differential diagnosis must be widened beyond accidental trauma and abuse to include osteogenesis imperfecta, infantile cortical hyperostosis, scurvy, syphilis, osteoid osteoma, neoplasms, rickets, hypophosphatasia, and osteomyelitis. Table 111.2 details the distinction between child abuse and osteogenesis imperfecta. All other conditions are much more rare than abuse and can be ruled out by the appearance of the bone on the radiograph and by the levels of calcium, phosphorus, and alkaline phosphatase in the serum.

TABLE 111.1. Dating Fractures

0–10 Days
Soft-tissue edema
Joint fluid
Visible fracture fragments
Visible fracture lines
10 Days–8 wk
Periosteal new bone (layered)
Callus (first subtle and then heavy)
Bone resorption along fracture line makes fracture line more visible
Metaphyseal fragments often more visible
8 wk and over
Periosteal new bone matures, becomes thicker
Callus formation becomes more dense and smoother
Metaphyseal fragments are incorporated into metaphyseal callus and become smoother
Fracture line less visible and then invisible
Deformities and cortical bumps persist

CENTRAL NERVOUS SYSTEM

Injuries to the central nervous system (CNS) are the main cause of child abuse deaths. These injuries may be subdivided into two categories: direct trauma and shaking injuries. Direct trauma is inflicted by striking the child with an object or by dropping or throwing the child against a wall or onto the floor. The extent of the resulting trauma depends on the amount of force used, the surface contacted, and the child's age. The child may be brought to the ED with a small subgaleal hematoma or in coma. Injuries may vary from scalp contusions to intracerebral hematomas.

Often a young infant will have a history of falling off a bed or dressing table. The precise extent of injury from this type of fall is unknown, but several reports suggest that even uncomplicated skull fractures are as uncommon as 1% to 2% of cases. If the injury is more severe and the only history is of a fall from less than 8 to 10 feet, abuse should be suspected. Another scenario is that of a child who sustained trauma 1 week before the ED visit. The visit is prompted when the parent notices a soft spot on the child's cranium. This sequence may occur when the initial scalp hematoma expanded so rapidly that it had a bony consistency. Only with degradation and softening of the mass does the parent now perceive the hematoma. Although a delay in seeking treatment is a well-recognized red flag for child abuse injuries, this case provides a plausible exception. In all children younger than 1 year of age who have a history of head trauma, skull radiographs are recommended. Infants tend to sustain skull fracture more easily and are more vulnerable to serious sequelae. If a fracture does exist and abuse is suspected, a skeletal survey should be obtained. Chapter 92 describes the diagnostic methods to be used for more serious head injuries.

Shaking injuries characteristically cause serious CNS damage without evidence of external trauma. The infant's relatively large head size and weak neck muscles are predisposing factors for whiplash injury. Whether the injury is caused by shaking alone or shaking followed by an impact is controversial. In most fatal cases, minor bruising to the scalp is apparent, although such scalp injuries may not be apparent until the scalp is reflected during the autopsy.

The shearing and contusive forces that result from shaking the infant produce this type of injury. Specific lesions that occur include hematomas, subarachnoid hemorrhages, or brain contusions, particularly in the frontal and occipital lobe. The child may present with lethargy and a "septic" appearance, with seizures, or in a coma. The physical examination is otherwise unremarkable except for retinal hemorrhages (Fig. 111.5A). Occasionally, bruises on the upper arms or shoulders indicate the sites where the child has been grasped. Lumbar puncture produces grossly bloody or xanthochromic spinal fluid. If computed axial tomography is available, it shows the characteristic findings of occipital contusion and intrahemispheric blood (Fig. 111.5B). This form of abusive behavior by the parent usually is triggered by the infant's persistent crying. Occasionally, excessively rough forms of play or misguided resuscitative efforts may result in shaking injuries.

GASTROINTESTINAL SYSTEM

Gastrointestinal (GI) injuries are relatively uncommon abuse manifestations but, similar to CNS injuries, account for a significant percentage of fatal injuries. Of all GI injuries, mouth trauma is perhaps the most common. Small infants may sustain a tear of the frenulum resulting from "bottle jamming." In the older child, dental trauma may be a sign of abuse.

TABLE 111.2. Osteogenesis Imperfecta Versus Child Abuse

Finding	Osteogenesis imperfecta	Child abuse
Incidence	Rare	Common
Positive family history	Common	Common
Blue sclerae	Common	Rare
Abnormal teeth	Common	Rare
Hearing impairment	Common	Uncommon
Osteoporosis	Common	Rare
Abnormal fracture healing	Common	Rare
Wormian bones	Common	Rare
Joint laxity	Common	Rare
Short stature	Common	Occasional
Fracture recurrence in protected environment	Common	Rare
In utero fracture	Occasional	Rare
Biochemical studies	Abnormal	Normal

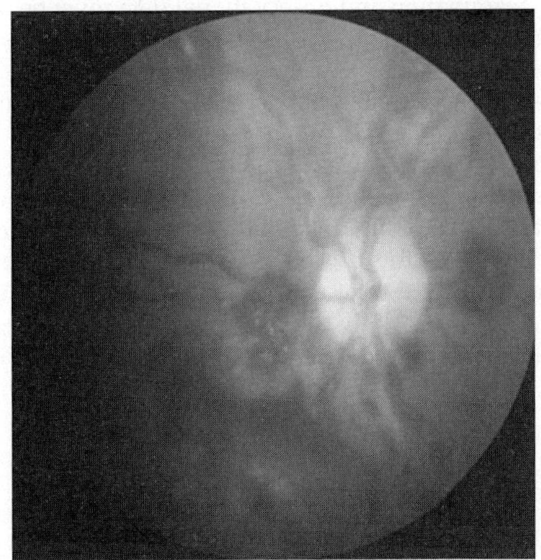

A

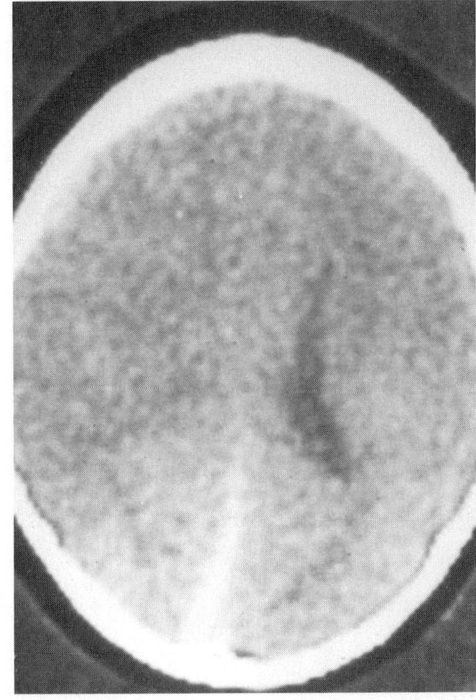

B

Figure 111.5. Manifestations of the whiplash shaking injury. **A:** Retinal hemorrhages as seen on fundoscopic examination. **B:** Computed tomogram showing intrahemispheric subdural bleeding and right cortical brain swelling.

Other GI system manifestations are more medically serious and generally result from blunt trauma to the abdominal contents. Rupture of the spleen or laceration of the liver causes the child to present with elevated liver enzymes, with an acute abdomen, or in shock, with no external source of bleeding and with absent or only minor bruising of the abdominal wall. The identification and management of these emergencies are covered in Section IV. A less acute presentation is the afebrile child with persistent bilious vomiting from a duodenal hematoma with small-bowel obstruction. Documenting an elevated serum amylase or lipase or increased liver enzymes is important in providing tangible evidence of abdominal trauma in cases that lack any radiographic finding or abdominal wall bruising. Elevation of the serum amylase may also identify those cases that should be followed for possible development of a pancreatic pseudocyst.

CARDIOPULMONARY SYSTEM

Abuse may be manifested in cardiac or pulmonary trauma with no injuries that are characteristically induced by abuse. Pulmonary contusion, pneumothorax, hemothorax, cardiac tamponade, and myocardial contusion all may occur occasionally. Specifics of identification and management of these problems are covered in Chapter 94.

GENITOURINARY SYSTEMS

Common genitourinary complaints, such as hematuria, dysuria, urgency, frequency, and enuresis, may be the initial sign of abuse. These problems may result from direct trauma, sexually transmitted infections, or emotional abuse. Some aspects of genitourinary manifestation are covered subsequently under the "Sexual Abuse" section. As for direct trauma, any part of the genitourinary system may be involved, from the renal parenchyma to the urethral meatus. Penile trauma that does not have an adequate explanation may be an alerting sign of abuse. Traumatic hematuria is managed as described in Chapter 96.

A life-threatening renal manifestation may be the occurrence of rhabdomyolysis and myoglobinuria. With extensive deep soft-tissue and muscle trauma, myoglobin may be liberated in quantities sufficient to cause acute renal failure. Such children have dark or tea-colored urine that tests positive for blood with urine dipstick but has no visible red blood cells on microscopic examination. Serum myoglobin levels confirm the diagnosis, and the serum creatine phosphokinase reaches extremely high values. Before using hypertonic intravenous contrast materials in the child with heme-positive urine, myoglobinuria should be considered and ruled out. The patient with possible myoglobinuria and acute renal failure must not be given potassium-containing intravenous solutions.

SENSORY

All the sensory organs are vulnerable to physical abuse, including ocular, nasal, and otic injuries. The eye may sustain several different forms of injury, including periorbital ecchymosis, corneal abrasion, subconjunctival hemorrhage, hyphema, dislocated lens, retinal hemorrhages, or detached retina. Each of these lesions is discussed in Chapters 97 through 99. A careful history of injury is important when treating any of these conditions. Injury to the nose may result in simple hemorrhage or fracture and disfigurement of the nasal structures. The external ear may show evidence of contusion. In particular, ecchymosis on the internal surface of the pinna may result from "boxing" the ear and crushing it against the skull.

A direct blow to the ear also can cause hemotympanum and perforation of the tympanic membrane. In such cases, hemotympanum on the basis of basilar skull fracture should also be considered. The presence of discoloration behind the ear (Battle sign) may be a further indication of a basilar skull fracture. Chapter 92 deals specifically with these aspects of emergency care.

UNUSUAL MANIFESTATIONS

Rarely, the emergency physician is confronted by one of the unusual abuse manifestations. Cases of toxic and nontoxic ingestions, electrolyte disorders such as hyponatremia and hypernatremia, foreign bodies, bathtub drowning, and multiple serious infections may be the result of abuse. In all these situations, the parent actively abuses the child by feeding, instilling, or injecting harmful substances or objects into the child's body. Some children with a toxic ingestion reveal that their parents forced them to ingest the substance. The most common toxic ingestants of this type are alcoholic beverages that are given to or forced on the child to either quiet the child or to demonstrate "manly" qualities. Other drugs may be used to poison the child. Most recent reports are of cocaine ingestions.

Several cases of parents who have placed their children on high-salt, water-only, or pepper diets as a form of punishment have been reported. Such children may present with signs of hypernatremia or hyponatremia, possibly with seizures. Foreign bodies have been found in every orifice as well as under the skin and in fingernail beds. Several cases of Munchausen syndrome by proxy have occurred in which a parent has inflicted illness on the child rather than feigning or inducing illness (Table 111.3). Cases of fictitious fever, hematuria, and even sepsis have resulted from this form of abuse. Although rare, the unusual manifestations of abuse should be considered when more common causes of these problems cannot be identified.

Management

The management of a child abuse case is difficult unless the emergency physician has a previously prepared, well-structured protocol. If reports of abuse are not a daily occurrence, an institutional policy serves as an important guide to the mechanics of management. Consultants from different disciplines, such as nursing and social work, provide invaluable assistance. A multidisciplinary approach simplifies the initial decision making and subsequent case management. The steps in the protocol are shown in Figure 111.6.

TABLE 111.3. Characteristics of Munchausen Syndrome by Proxy

Difficult to understand medical situation with recurrent episodes
Failure of other centers to arrive at diagnosis; doctor shopping
Unsupportive or "absent" marital relationship
Compliant, cooperative, overinvolved mother
Medical knowledge in parent's background
Findings abort with surveillance of child
Findings correlate to presence of parent
Extensive medical care in parent's background

SUSPECTED ABUSE

The first step is to decide whether a reasonable likelihood of abuse exists. Many shades of suspicion make the term *abuse* imprecise. Although every traumatic injury should be suspected as abuse, the physician has the onerous task of deciding how much suspicion is necessary to take some action (ie, report). To establish the level of suspicion, data are gathered by obtaining a complete history, performing a thorough physical examination, comparing the history and physical examination, observing interactions, and obtaining laboratory studies and radiographs. Then the physician can formulate a differential diagnosis and assign a rank to abuse. Indications of abuse in the history and physical examination and observational data must be used like building blocks that are added until they achieve a certain threshold of suspicion. As demonstrated in Figure 111.7, when the threshold is reached, a report of suspected abuse must follow. In the example of case 1, all the building blocks must be used to build a level of suspicion; in case 2, the physical injury is sufficient to make the diagnosis.

A detailed history is always important. As in many other medical situations, this process is initiated by asking some general open-ended questions about "what happened?" If the child has sufficient verbal skills, the first questions are directed at him or her. General inquiries then must be followed with specific re-

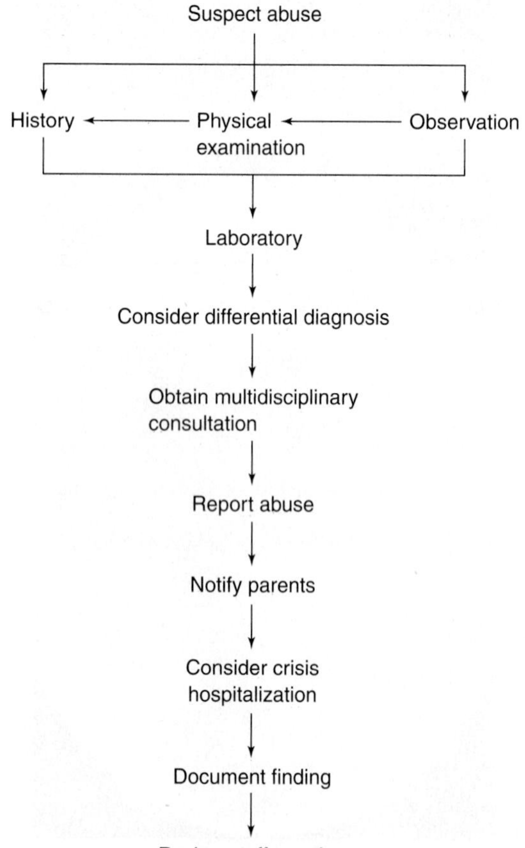

Figure 111.6. Procedure for emergency department management of suspected physical abuse.

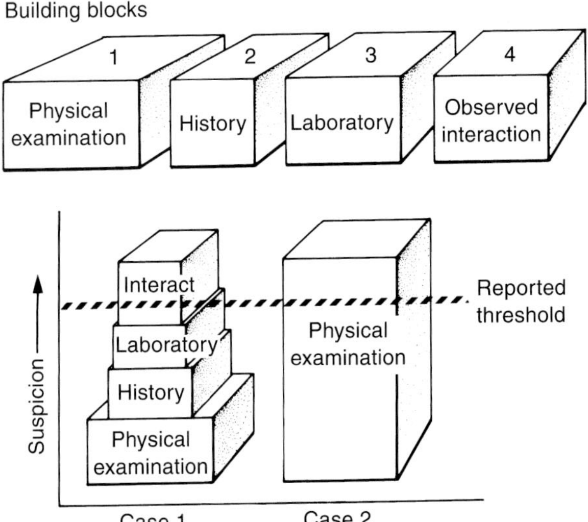

Figure 111.7. Building a level of suspicion.

quests for information; however, a harsh interrogation only alienates the family. Some specific historical indications are listed in Table 111.4.

After completion of the history and physical examination, the next step is to compare them. Does the stated history match the physical findings? Does the history make sense? Does the history correlate with the developmental level of the child? Answers to these important questions may add further elements of suspicion.

This step of comparing history and physical examination is completed subconsciously by most practitioners. Physicians often attempt to match the patient's degree of symptoms with the presence or absence of physical findings, particularly in patients with psychosomatic complaints. In child abuse cases, this step should be a conscious and well-defined step because it is vital to establishing suspicion. In some cases, a lack of consistency is obvious, such as a parent's claim that burns on the child's buttocks occurred when the child inserted his or her finger into an electric socket. Other situations may be less clear, such as the injury being attributed to hot plastic seat covers on an automobile. Although the latter explanation has in fact been reported as a case of accidental injury, it rarely explains burns on the buttocks.

Laboratory data and radiographs are other sources of indicators of abuse. The laboratory studies used are few and, for the most part, document the obvious or rule out other disease states. Biochemical, hematologic, and urinary studies that are used appear in Table 111.5 along with their indications. Radiographs document a specific bony or soft-tissue injury. They may provide a comprehensive and longitudinal record of osseous injury at any site in the skeletal system. Although no precise indications for ordering a skeletal survey exist, some relative indications are (1) any child younger than 1 year presenting with a fracture, (2) any child with severe or extensive fractures, (3) any child who has a history of more than one fracture, and (4) a history in the child or the family of "soft" or easily broken bones.

During the time occupied by the history, physical examination, and performance of laboratory studies, the physician should be cognizant of the interactions among family members and between the parents, the child, and the ED staff. Such awareness often uncovers subtle indicators of abuse. The observation of parents arguing vehemently on the way to the radiology department may be a clue. The parent who appears to be distant from both the child and the physician is also suspect. Although the parent who is intoxicated or incoherent never fails to gain staff attention, such persons are in the minority of abusive parents. Observation of the child is important as well. All abused children are not withdrawn, passive, and depressed. On the contrary, some are competent, outgoing, or "pseudomature."

The final step in establishing a threshold level of suspicion is to review the differential diagnosis. At this point in the management scheme, the physician must add up the indicators and arrive at a judgment. If the process does not lead to a clear determination, most state laws imply that reporting suspected abuse is more prudent than not reporting at all. Physicians are asked to report suspected, not proven, abuse. The major differentiation is between accidental and nonaccidental trauma. The other elements of the differential diagnosis are all uncommon diseases, including (1) bone diseases such as osteogenesis imperfecta, osteoid osteoma, hypophosphatasia; (2) hematologic disorders such as idiopathic thrombocytopenic purpura and hemophilia; (3) neoplasms; (4) metabolic disorders such as rickets or scurvy; (5) infections such as syphilis or osteomyelitis; and (6) syndromes in which pain sensation is absent, such as spina bifida or congenital indifference to pain. All these diseases occur with much less frequency than abuse but deserve consideration; simple laboratory and radiographic studies confirm or deny these diagnoses.

TABLE 111.4. Historical Indicators of Abuse

Is the history one of inflicted injury?
Is there an absence of history, a "magical" injury?
Could the injury have been avoided by better care and supervision?
Are there inconsistencies or changes in the history?
Is there a history of repeated injury or hospitalization?
Was there a delay in seeking medical care?
Does the history overestimate or underestimate the injury?
Is there a medical history of prematurity, failure to thrive, failure to receive adequate medical care such as immunization?

MULTIDISCIPLINARY CONSULTATION

If consultation with a nurse, social worker, or physician with more extensive experience in the management of child abuse is available, it should be obtained. The advantages of consultations are many. They allow for (1) information sharing, (2) joint decision making, (3) planning, and (4) mutual support. Planning an approach to the family and subsequent case management is useful. This brief consultation enables the physician to be more secure in making decisions about matters that are generally unfamiliar and often value-laden. Joint interviewing is not only time efficient, but it gives the family a uniform approach from the professional staff.

REPORTING

Once the suspicion of abuse has been established and consultations obtained, the next step is reporting. Although laws vary from state to state, most have common elements. The emergency physician should become familiar with his or her current state law. The definition of abuse is central to each of the reporting laws. A stated age defines a child. The laws also specify who must report (*mandated reporters*) and who may report (*nonmandated reporters*). For most mandated reports, the law requires a specific penalty (as well as malpractice liability) for failure to report and provides protection from liability if the report of suspected abuse is shown to be unfounded once investigated. Finally, the law dictates to whom and how the report should be made. Generally, reports are made to child protective services (CPS) agencies, to police departments, or to some combination of law enforcement and social work personnel. Many states now have statewide central registries for receiving reports.

TABLE 111.5. Laboratory/Diagnostic Evaluation of the Physically Abused Child

Radiographic skeletal survey
- Method of choice for screening abused children for bony injury
- For all children <2 yr old with suspected physical abuse
- Of limited use in children >5 yr
- For children 2–5 yr old, use clinical findings

Radionuclide bone scan
- Adjunct to skeletal survey
- Most useful if there is high suspicion of bony injury and skeletal survey is negative

Computed tomography (CT) scan
- Provides sliced views through internal organs, such as brain and abdominal organs
- Essential part of the evaluation of seriously injured children
- Initial test used for children with suspected shaking impact syndrome
- Abdominal trauma

Magnetic resonance imaging (MRI)
- More sensitive than CT for many injuries
- Can provide images in multiple planes
- Generally used as an adjunct to CT in the acute-care setting

Blood tests for easy bruising/bleeding
- Complete blood count
- Prothrombin time
- Partial thromboplastin time
- ± Bleeding time

Screening tests for evidence of abdominal trauma
- Liver
  - Alanine aminotransferase (ALT, SGPT)
  - Aspartate aminotransferase (AST, SGOT)
- Pancreas
  - Amylase
  - Lipase
- Kidney
  - Urinalysis

Toxicology screens
- For children with unexplained neurologic symptoms or symptoms compatible with ingestion
- Variance among laboratories in drugs tested in "tox screen"
- Screening of urine *and* blood and/or gastric contents
- Consideration of blood alcohol levels for children with altered mental status

From the US Advisory Board on Child Abuse and Neglect, US Department of Health and Human Services.

NOTIFYING THE PARENTS

An important, but often avoided, step in case management is notification of the parents. This step is often forgotten because it is a difficult interpersonal task; nonetheless, it must be done. Nothing makes parents more resistant to change than completing a "routine" ED visit, only to later receive notification that the physician has filed a suspected child abuse report. Some specific guidelines are helpful in avoiding this breech of trust. The overall approach to the parents must be based on concern for the child. Concern for the child, not accusation, should be stressed. The physician should not confront the parents or attempt to seek an admission of guilt. Many times, the parent in the ED may not be the abusive parent and may know as little about the episode as the hospital staff. The physician should explain the requirement for a mandated reporter to report all suspected cases; however, stating the requirement should not be used as an excuse. The desire to report also should be stated.

In many states, the reporter is required to report all injuries that are not fully explained. This requirement also may be stated to the parent. Using the words *child abuse report* is important. This situation is not a time to "soft pedal"; however, child abuse does represent a range of behaviors, from the parent who too vigorously disciplines to the parent who sadistically tortures. Parents often have not seen themselves as abusers, and an explanation of the range of abuse is helpful in demonstrating how a child abuse report applies to them. Parents are fearful of what a child abuse report means and of what will happen. Therefore, the consequences of the report should be explained (eg, "a social worker will call and come visit you in 1 or 2 days"). The physician's natural fear is that the parent will have a dramatic and hostile reaction.

CRISIS HOSPITALIZATION

In some cases of abuse, the family crisis is at such an acute level that hospitalization is necessary. The physician must ask, "Is the home safe?" If the child's environment poses a potential danger, the child should be admitted, no matter what the extent of injury. Some state laws include protective custody sections that allow physicians virtual police powers in detaining a child for protection. In other states, the physician may need to obtain parental consent for admission.

This task is also difficult. As with reporting, the approach to the parents must be honest but not accusatory. The reasons for admission are to observe the child and allow time to evaluate the possibility of such an injury happening again. The focus must be the physician's concern for the child's health. In hospitalizing the child, the physician also makes a statement about the seriousness of the situation and the depth of his or her concern. Most hospitals do not have the resources to hospitalize every abused child, nor is it necessary or advisable to do so in every case. Factors that favor sending the child home are (1) a concerned relative or neighbor who is available to support the family, (2) a solution to the inciting crisis, (3) parental acceptance of responsibility, (4) prompt (<24 hours) CPS or police response, (5) a first episode or minor degree of abuse, and (6) an alternative environment (eg, grandmother's house). If the physician is unable to hospitalize the child and has lingering doubts, a specific agreed-on return appointment for the next day may be a solution. If the family is unable to keep the appointment, there should be grave concern, and emergency CPS or police involvement should be requested.

DOCUMENTATION

Throughout each step of case management, documentation is important. The record of this visit is both a medical and a legal document. A precise description of the injuries enhances the document's value, and small sketches are also helpful. Photographs are invaluable in documenting extensive injuries. Some states require parental permission for photographs, whereas other jurisdictions allow photographs to be taken without parental consent. Photographs may be used in court to illustrate, for a judge or jury, injuries that would be difficult for most witnesses to describe. Even if the photographs are not admissible in court, they refresh the memory of the physician for testimony. Often, court proceedings may not take place for several months after the ED visit. If photographs are taken, their quality must be good. Poor-quality photographs can damage a case by failing to show all of the pertinent findings.

SEXUAL ABUSE

The sexually abused child is another difficult psychosocial emergency for the emergency physician. The state-of-the-art method in identifying and managing cases of sexual abuse has developed rapidly in the last decade. Most child abuse centers are reporting dramatically increasing numbers of sexually abused children. The Children's Hospital of Philadelphia currently sees more than ten times the number of sexually abused children than were reported 10 years ago. The number of sexual abuse cases reported now equals the number of physical abuse cases. Of all societal taboos, those that prohibit incest are the strongest. This belief leads to denial and makes even basic recognition of the problem more difficult.

As with the physically abused, the sexually abused child engenders a great deal of emotion from the health care professionals in the ED. Treatment issues for both the child and the abuser are more complex. Working in a multidisciplinary fashion with nursing and social work staff is important. The effects of this form of abuse may clearly be profound but may not be expressed as symptoms for many years. Prompt diagnosis, humane emergency management, and referral to long-term treatment resources are the goals of the emergency physician. Many centers have adopted strategies to use the ED for recognition and screening of acute (<72 hours) episodes of sexual abuse as well as developing programs for comprehensive evaluation outside the ED.

Background

CAPTA defines sexual abuse as (1) employment, use, persuasion, inducement, enticement, or coercion of any child to engage in, or assist any other person to engage in, any sexually explicit conduct or any simulation of such conduct for the purpose of producing any visual depiction or such conduct; or (2) rape, and in cases of caretaker or interfamilial relationships, statutory rape, molestation, prostitution, or other form of sexual exploitation of children, or incest with children.

Sexual abuse includes fondling a child's genitals, intercourse, incest, rape, sodomy, exhibitionism, and commercial exploitation through prostitution or the production of pornographic materials. Many experts believe that sexual abuse is the most underreported form of child maltreatment because of the secrecy or "conspiracy of silence" that so often characterizes these cases. Traditionally, sexual abuse has been more the domain of police and other law enforcement personnel.

The true incidence of sexual abuse is unknown. There is a recent documented upward trend in number of reports. The National Center on Child Abuse/Neglect estimates that the current annual incidence of sexual abuse is between 75,000 and 250,000 cases per year. Most estimates do not include children who are victims of pornographic exploitation and child prostitution.

Clinical Manifestations

The manifestations of sexual abuse may occur at a time shortly after the abuse has occurred or at a time more distant from the event. The manifestations may be influenced by a single episode or by a pattern of repeated encounters. Finally, the manifestations may depend on the child's age and maturity. The manifestations may be divided into four categories, as shown in Table 111.6. These categories are specific physical findings, specific behavioral manifestations, nonspecific physical complaints, and nonspecific behavioral complaints.

SPECIFIC PHYSICAL COMPLAINTS

Bruising on the upper thigh, lower abdomen, or genitalia is a rare finding in childhood sexual abuse. The child is not usually

TABLE 111.6. Identification of Sexual Abuse

Physical complaints	Behavioral complaints
Specific	Specific
Genital injury	Explicit descriptions of sexual contact
Bruises	Inappropriate knowledge of adult sexual behavior
Lacerations	Compulsive masturbation
Rectal laceration, fissures	Excessive sexual curiosity, sexual acting out
Sexually transmitted disease	Nonspecific
Pregnancy	Excessive fears, phobias
Nonspecific	Refusal to sleep alone, nightmares
Anorexia	Runaways
Abdominal pain	Aggressive behavior
Enuresis	Attempted suicide
Dysuria	Any abrupt change in behavior
Encopresis	
Evidence of physical abuse in genital area	
Vaginal discharge	
Urethral discharge	
Rectal pain	

injured because he or she is often used for stimulation, masturbation, or genital contact that involves no force. Nonetheless, a physical injury to the genitalia should elicit a suspicion of sexual abuse. For children with even small vaginal lacerations, a detailed history of injury should be obtained. Straddle injuries do produce genital trauma and are the most common form of accidental genital injury to young girls. In boys, accidental penile trauma may occur from zipper accidents or from a toilet seat that falls. Beyond these common accidental situations, the emergency physician should scrutinize the history given. The premenstrual child who presents with vaginal hemorrhage may be bleeding from a vaginal laceration that is not visible on external examination. Accidental injuries such as straddle injuries can be seen. Prompt surgical or gynecologic consultation should be obtained to identify and repair unseen sites of trauma.

The presence of sexually transmitted disease in a prepubertal child is a specific finding of sexual abuse until proven otherwise. Studies by Branch and Paxton and others have shown that when instances of prepubertal gonorrhea were carefully investigated for cause, the source of the infection was through sexual contact, most often in the child's home or in a relative's home. Gonorrhea may occur in the genitourinary tract, rectum, or oropharynx. When gonorrhea is culture proven, it should be pursued as sexual abuse, according to the Centers for Disease Control and Prevention. The American Academy of Pediatrics has issued guidelines for the diagnosis of gonorrhea. Parents may bring their child to the ED for the complaint of vaginal discharge. Gonorrhea also may appear in cases of less well-defined symptoms, such as vaginal pain, itching, urinary frequency, or enuresis. Recent studies indicate that only children with vaginal discharge need to be cultured.

The Centers for Disease Control and Prevention indicate in their treatment guidelines that "Any sexually transmitted infection in a child should be considered as evidence of sexual abuse until proven otherwise." At present, knowledge about sexually transmitted diseases is limited. Any sexually transmitted disease in a prepubertal child is suspicious of abuse; however, basic understanding about disease transmission places these infections in three categories (Table 111.7). In the first category are infections that virtually always are transmitted through sexual contact, for example, syphilis and gonococcal infections. In the second category are infections that to the best of clinical knowledge are usually transmitted sexually. It must be noted, however, that exact scientific information is not present. For example, Kaplan reported six cases of genital herpes simplex, but in only four cases could sexual abuse be documented. Category three includes diseases that are suspicious of abuse but that may be transmitted by nonsexual contact. The pregnant adolescent may be a victim of incest. The physician should try to obtain a specific history of conception. Often, the focus of case management centers on how the adolescent plans to notify her parents or whether she considers abortion or adoption as options. If the issue of paternity is not pursued, instances of sexual abuse escape detection.

SPECIFIC BEHAVIORAL COMPLAINTS

The most common clinical manifestation of sexual abuse is a positive history. The child who gives a clear detailed story of sexual encounter with an adult has a specific behavioral manifestation. Reports of suspected sexual abuse can be based on history alone because children do not fabricate such allegations. Most children who are not abused are not knowledgeable in the details of sexual encounters. Thus, when a child offers the specifics of an encounter, he or she must be believed. The detail of the history varies with the child's age and language development, but even children aged 3 or 4 years are able to make simple yet credible statements about someone touching their genitals.

Some children manifest behaviors in their play or in their conversation that indicate that they have been exposed to sexual experiences, perhaps abused. These signs are less specific than a clearly stated history but are significant enough to require further explanation. For example, the young child who discusses urogenital contact may be demonstrating a specific behavioral manifestation. Children who wish to fondle their parents' genitals as an expression of affection are cause for concern. These behaviors are usually learned. All children manifest sexual curiosity and may engage in some form of masturbation, but when either of these behaviors appears in excess, it deserves investigation. Sexual abuse may be the cause.

Recently, several films, videotapes, books, and school programs were developed as prevention tools in sexual abuse situations. These instructional materials are also helpful in opening discussions between parents and children and thereby promote disclosure of past events experienced by the child.

NONSPECIFIC PHYSICAL COMPLAINTS

The physician should keep sexual abuse in the differential diagnosis for many complaints. Sexual abuse may be related to cases that present with pain in the abdomen, thighs, or genitals; dysuria; pain on defecation; hematuria; or hematochezia. Abuse may manifest as a change in habits, such as urinary frequency, enuresis, constipation, or encopresis; other complaints may be vaginal discharge or chronic sore throat. The cause of each of these complaints may be any number of things. For example, in studying a group of children with enuresis, sexual abuse is an uncommon cause of the complaint. Nonetheless, sexually abused children are regularly brought to the ED with nonspecific complaints. If sexual abuse is not considered, it goes unnoticed.

NONSPECIFIC BEHAVIORAL COMPLAINTS

The final group of clinical manifestations includes unexplained changes in the child's behavior. In this group are relatively minor behavioral changes, such as the recent acquisition of nightmares or phobias, or major changes, such as school truancy and adolescent runaways. Children who bear no physical evidence of their abuse and in whom no physical symptoms develop may express themselves behaviorally. Many children demonstrate change in one or more of the important spheres of their life: at

TABLE 111.7. Sexually Transmitted Diseases and Their Probability of Being Caused by Child Sexual Abuse

Always	Usually	Possibly
Neisseria gonorrhoeae	Herpes simplex	Condylomata
Syphilis	*Chlamydia trachomatis*	Scabies
	Trichomoniasis	Pediculosis
		Gardnerella vaginalis

home, in school, or with peers. This situation is exemplified by a 5-year-old girl who begins avoiding contact with her father and other male relatives after an abusive episode with a male friend of the family. A sudden change in school performance unexplained by the teacher, social withdrawal, and isolation are also nonspecific behavioral manifestations. Similar to the nonspecific physical complaints, these behavioral complaints may be caused by several other things as well. Sexual abuse is likely to produce a behavioral change in children old enough to comprehend the wrongness and shamefulness of the situation.

Management

The primary goals in case management of the sexually abused child are to identify and report the abuse and to avoid the secondary abuse phenomenon. *Secondary abuse phenomenon* refers to the physical examination that is so overzealous that it assumes a rape-like quality in the mind of the child. Also to be avoided are parental or staff reactions that make the child feel responsible or blamed for the abuse. Many centers have moved to performing a screening function. If the child has been abused in the past 72 hours or more and no acute symptoms (eg, bleeding, signs of sexually transmitted disease) are present, the child is referred to a sexual assault center, provided such a community service exists. In places where no center is functioning, the entire evaluation must be done in the ED. The following sections offer techniques in management to identify suspected sexual abuse and to gather enough documentation for legal purposes in a manner that is humane for the child and supportive for the family.

INTERVIEWING THE PARENT

Parents may present the problem of sexual abuse either directly or indirectly. For the parent who is direct (ie, "my child's been abused"), it is important to provide a controlled, quiet environment because he or she will be upset and angry. It may be necessary to limit what is said in front of the child. With such parents, the interviewer's tasks are calming, limiting, and clarifying. In an example of the indirect presentation, the parent brings the child for complaints such as those detailed in the sections on nonspecific physical or behavioral manifestations. With this parent, the task of the interviewer is to bring the possibility of sexual abuse into the open. Once the topic is nominally broached, it becomes apparent that the parent has often already given it consideration. With both types of parents, exploring both their concerns and their information in detail is important.

INTERVIEWING THE CHILD

Beyond standard history taking from the parents, the emergency physician must always obtain a history from the child. This task is difficult for several reasons: (1) the child's level of language development, (2) the child's level of psychosexual development, (3) the desire not to contaminate what may be important evidence, (4) the apprehension of the child and the parent, and (5) the awkwardness and apprehension felt by the interviewer in discussing sexual matters with a child. The first steps are for the physician to obtain a quiet, private place and to decide whether he or she wishes the parent or parents to be present. If possible, the physician may wish to defer the comprehensive examination to a more appropriate time and place. Based on previous history taking from the parents, the physician can gauge the parents' level of emotional composure. This criterion is useful to decide whether parents should be present. If the parents are excluded, another third party (eg, a nurse or social worker) should be present. An initial discussion of topics, other than the alleged abuse, comforts the child and encourages him or her to talk to the interviewer. Information about school, peers, and family adjustment is important in looking for nonspecific behavioral manifestations, and this preliminary conversation also helps in evaluating the child's developmental level.

In focusing the conversation on the abuse, one technique may be to ask the child why his or her parents brought him or her to the hospital. Another approach that is more appropriate for younger children is to establish common vocabulary by asking the child the term used for his or her genitalia. Children offer a rich variety of terms and may have no understanding of the words *vagina* and *penis.* One 4-year-old girl stated, "He tried to put his pencil in my pocketbook." In eliciting and using common language, the physician gets to the point of the interview more easily.

If the parental history and surrounding circumstances are credible, inquiries should be phrased to obtain the details of the abuse rather than to ask the child to make the initial allegation. For example, the physician may want to directly ask, "How did Uncle Tommy touch your pee pee (vagina)?" rather than "Did Uncle Tommy touch you?" If questions are phrased in a yes-or-no format, a one-word response will be given. Obtaining detail is important to add credibility to the history. The history is also important in guiding the physician to significant aspects of physical examination, evidence collection, and treatment.

EMOTIONAL SUPPORT

Throughout the interview and in all contacts with the child, the rightness of his or her decision to discuss the abuse should be stressed. A child experiences conflict about revealing a secret, especially a long-standing secret. The patient may also feel conflict in sensing that his or her actions may be provoking a great deal of emotional turmoil. Often, the child has a relationship with the perpetrator and realizes that this admission may alter or end the relationship. At times, the child is aware or is made aware of getting the perpetrator "in trouble." It is important to reaffirm the importance of what the child has revealed and focus the wrongdoing on the perpetrator. The child may have been threatened not to tell. Thus, bringing the nature of the threats into the open and offering protection to the child are important concerns. Finally, many children have fears about the abuse. The physician may anticipate and address these fears based on the child's development.

PHYSICAL EXAMINATION

The physical examination may be a point of significant trauma for the child. The examination should be conducted in a standard fashion with all parts of the body examined. The position of the child depends on age and comfort. Many young children want to be examined while sitting in their parent's lap. In examining the genitalia of young girls, two positions are recommended. One is a frog-leg posture while sitting on an adult lap. Alternatively, the child can lie prone with knees tucked under the thorax (ie, the knee–chest position).

In the prepubertal girl, only the external genitalia need be examined. If even minimal vaginal bleeding appears to be coming from a more internal source, exploration and possible surgical repair are best done with the child under general anesthesia in the operating room. Examination in the ED should be deferred. In the pubertal child, a full genital examination should be performed. This examination may be modified if it is a girl's first speculum examination and it proves too difficult. Chapter 83 details physical examination techniques.

Examination of the rectum and oropharynx needs to be performed carefully, particularly if the history suggests that these were sites of sexual contact. Other physical findings to note carefully are any contusions, abrasions, or lacerations in nongenital areas. Common sites for these signs of trauma are the upper thighs, buttocks, and upper arms. Figure 111.8 shows some of the visible findings of child sexual abuse.

If the physical examination proves too traumatic for the child, the physician is faced with a significant dilemma. The choices are to traumatize the child further or to perform an incomplete examination and collect inadequate evidence. As with all dilemmas, the best choice is not obvious. Physically or psychologically traumatizing the child should be avoided. Often, no physical evidence is present, and the history, if detailed enough, may be sufficient. The guiding principle should be primum *non nocere* ("first do no harm").

TABLE 111.8. Evidence for Child Sexual Abuse

Child's history in detail
History of observers
Documentation of general physical examination; note signs of force (e.g., bruises)
Documentation of genital injury (colposcopy)
Documentation of sexual contact
Presence of sperm or semen (e.g., on patient's clothing, linens)
Sexually transmitted disease
Pregnancy
Foreign material
Documentation of perpetrator
Sperm: motile/nonmotile
Seminal fluid
Genetic marker (blood group antigens)
Acid phosphatases
P30 glycoprotein
Blood
Hair analysis
DNA matching

Adapted from De Jong (personal communication).

EVIDENCE COLLECTION

The type of evidence to be collected, the collection methods used, and the procedures for processing the results vary by locale. The specimen-collecting procedures at the Children's Hospital of Philadelphia have been reviewed by the Philadelphia Police Department and District Attorney. The protocol is listed in Table 111.8. Whatever the specifics of a particular jurisdiction, some general principles should be followed. Establishing a standard protocol is important so that each new case does not force the emergency physician to reformulate the entire process. The ED should have on hand either standard "rape kits" or some modification thereof. The kits should contain all the necessary tubes, slides, swabs, and supplies. Evidence collection should be performed with another health care professional present, either a nurse or a social worker. A standard for marking the specimens should be established, including the patient's name and medical record number. Finally, the protocol should include a procedure for a specified person to take the specimens to the laboratory and to have them received officially or logged in by the laboratory. This detail becomes important in the court proceedings against the perpetra-

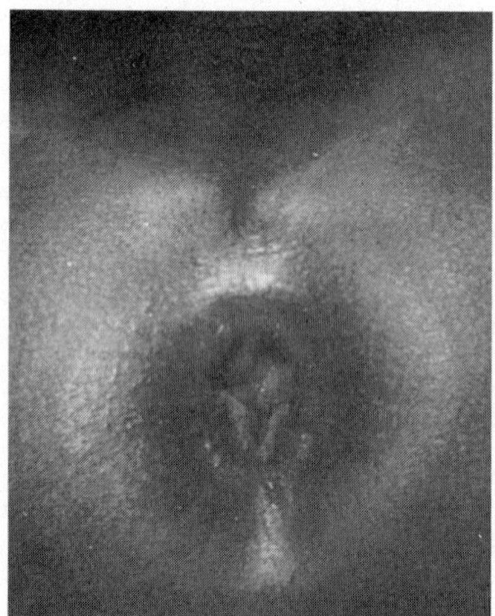
A

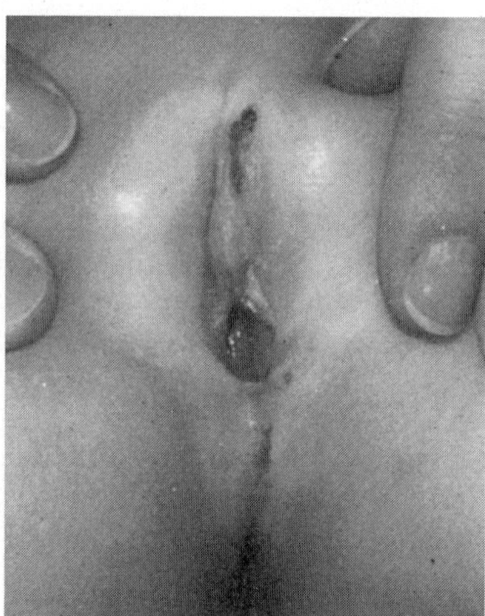

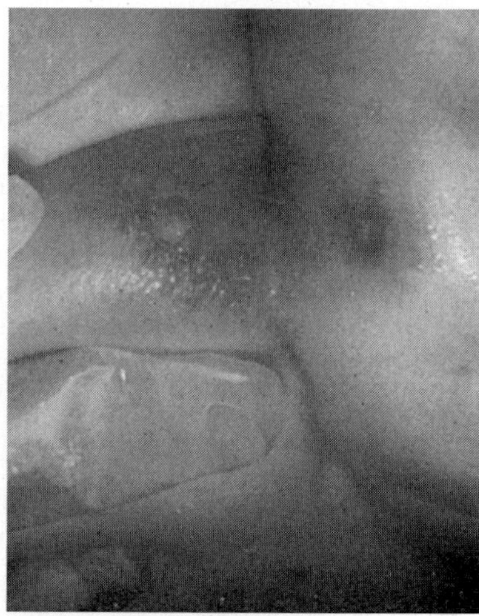
B, C

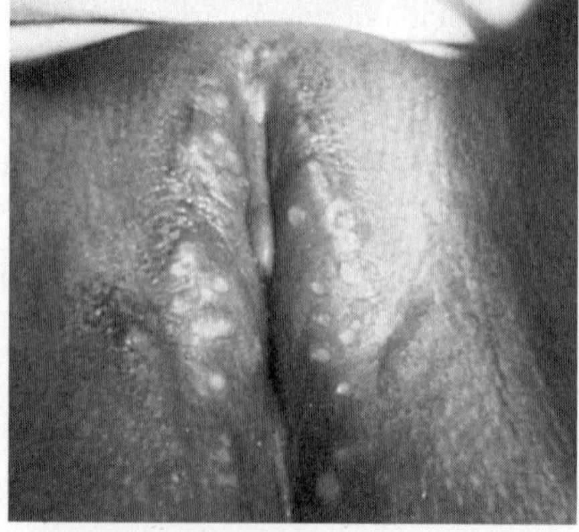
D

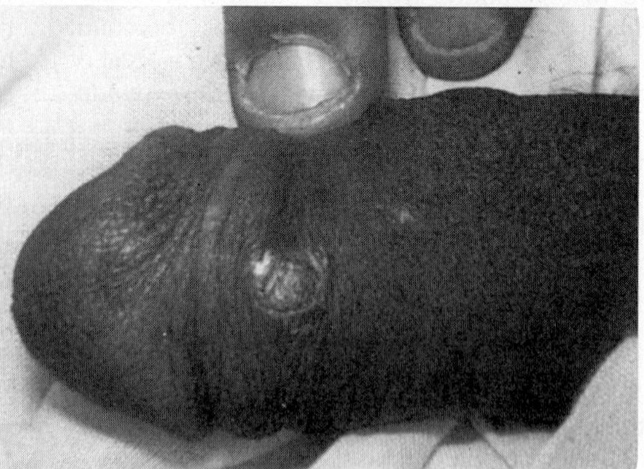
E

Figure 111.8. Physical signs of child sexual abuse. **A:** Rectal dilation and multiple lacerations after sodomy. **B:** Multiple vaginal and paraclitoral lacerations. **C:** Herpes virus infection in perirectal area. **D:** Herpes virus vaginitis. **E:** Syphilis in a sexually abused adolescent.

tor. For example, nothing is less satisfying than seeing an alleged perpetrator go unconvicted because the hospital cannot be legally sure that a positive gonorrheal culture belongs to the victim in question.

CONSIDER A DIFFERENTIAL DIAGNOSIS

In any consideration of abuse, the physician must always consider the question, "What else could it be?" There may be plausible explanations, such as accidental injuries to the genitals as in straddle injuries. Other important alternatives to consider are (1) infections such as streptococcal, *Haemophilus influenzae* and monilial; (2) congenital anomalies such as hydrometrocolpos, hemangioma, and perineural clefts and pits; (3) foreign bodies of the rectum and vagina; and (4) dermatologic conditions such as lichen sclerosus et atrophicus, diaper dermatitis, contact dermatitis, Ehlers–Danlos syndrome, and phytodermatitis. Perhaps the most common mistaken perineal finding is prolapsed urethra, which appears as a hemorrhagic mass covering the upper vaginal area.

DOCUMENTATION

Careful record keeping cannot be stressed too strongly. As with the collection and processing of evidence, ED records can make or break a case. All aspects of record keeping mentioned in the section on physical abuse apply. In particular, what the child said in his or her own words should be recorded carefully. Such questions may be the mainstay of any legal actions to be taken. Good records not only help the police and lawyers involved but also help the physician review the case before a hearing that may not take place for 6 months. In some jurisdictions, legal provisions allow videotaping patient interviews. This tool is particularly helpful to the victim in that he or she may not have to repeat the history so many times. It may also be helpful to the physician by serving as another form of documentation. When such tapes are shown during court proceedings, they are most helpful.

Diagnosis

The diagnosis of sexual abuse should be based on a composite of the history, physical examination, and laboratory findings. Many centers have begun to use a four-category classification of assessment developed by Adams and Harper (Table 111.9) using a classification of physician findings noted in Table 111.10.

REPORTING

In most jurisdictions, sexual abuse is a criminal offense. Thus, all cases are reported to the police department. In some jurisdictions, when the abuse has occurred in the home or during a time when parental supervision was lax, a civil report to the CPS agency may also be required. This detail needs to be specified according to local guidelines and included in an ED procedure. In the event of a criminal (police) report, a civil (child abuse) report, or both, the parent needs to be informed that such reports are being made. The physician or social worker must spell out the practical consequences of the reports for the parent.

PREPARING THE PARENT

Beyond notifying the parent about reporting the sexual abuse, additional preparation must be given. Many workers believe that, for the young child, the parental reaction to sexual abuse may have as important a role as the abuse itself in producing subsequent manifestations. Long-term follow-up studies of sexually abused children performed using a case–control methodology show that the sexually abused child is at long-term risk for a variety of psychological and behavioral consequences. Parents need to be aware of this correlation. All parents will be upset. All parents will be angry. Some parents may express disbelief or the feeling that "this could not be happening to me." Parental reactions vary, depending on whether the abuse is intrafamilial or extrafamilial. Social worker consultation and collaboration for this aspect of case management are essential.

TABLE 111.9. Overall Assessment of the Likelihood of Sexual Abuse

Class 1: No evidence of abuse
Normal examination, no history, no behavioral changes, no witnessed abuse
Nonspecific findings with another known cause, and no history or behavioral changes
Child considered at risk for sexual abuse but gives no history and has nonspecific behavior changes
Class 2: Possible abuse
Class 1, 2, or 3 findings in combination with significant behavioral changes, especially sexualized behaviors, but child unable to give history of abuse
Presence of condyloma or herpes 1 (genital) in the absence of a history of abuse, and with otherwise normal examination
Child has made a statement, but not detailed or consistent
Class 3 findings with no disclosure of abuse
Class 3: Probable abuse
Child gives a clear, consistent, detailed description of molestation, with or without other findings present
Class 4 or 5 findings in a child, with or without a history of abuse, in the absence of any convincing history of accidental penetrating injury
Culture-proven infection with *Chlamydia trachomatis* (child >2 years of age) in a prepubertal child. Also culture proven herpes type 2 infection in a child, or documented *Trichomonas* infection
Class 4: Definite evidence of abuse or sexual contact
Finding of sperm or seminal fluid in or on a child's body
Witnessed episode of sexual molestation (This also applies to cases in which pornographic photographs or videotapes are acquired as evidence.)
Intentional, blunt penetrating injury to the vaginal or anal orifice
Positive, confirmed cultures for *Neisseria gonorrhoeae* in a prepubertal child or serologic confirmation of acquired syphilis

Reprinted from *Adolesc Pediatr Gynecol* 1992;5:73–75, with permission of Springer-Verlag.

TABLE 111.10. Proposed Classification of Anogenital Findings in Children

Normal (class 1)
- Periurethral bands
- Intravaginal ridges or columns
- Increased erythema in the sulcus
- Hymenal tags, mounds, or bumps
- Elongated hymenal orifice in an obese child
- Ample posterior hymenal rim (1–2 mm wide)
- Estrogen changes (thickened, redundant hymen)
- Diastasis ani/smooth area at 6 or 12 o'clock in perianal area
- Anal tag/thickened fold in midline

Nonspecific findings (class 2)[a]
- Erythema of vestibule or perianal tissues
- Increased vascularity of vestibule or hymen
- Labial adhesions
- Rolled hymenal edges in the knee–chest position
- Narrow hymenal rim, but at least 1 mm wide
- Vaginal discharge
- Anal fissures
- Flattened anal folds
- Thickened anal folds
- Anal gaping with stool present
- Venous congestion of perianal tissues, delayed in examination
- Fecal soiling

Suspicious for abuse (class 3)[b]
- *Enlarged hymenal opening—greater than 2 standard deviations from non-abused study*
- Immediate anal dilation of ≥15 mm with stool not visible or palpable in rectal vault
- Immediate, extensive venous congestion of perianal tissues
- Distorted, irregular anal folds
- Posterior hymenal rim <1 mm in all views
- Condyloma acuminata in a child
- Acute abrasions or lacerations in the vestibule or on the labia (not involving the hymen) or perianal lacerations

Suggestive of abuse/penetration (class 4)
- Combination of two or more suspicious anal findings or two or more suspicious findings
- Scar or fresh laceration of the posterior fourchette with sparing of the hymen
- Scar in perianal area (must take history into consideration)

Clear evidence of penetrating injury (class 5)
- Areas with an absence of hymenal tissue (below the 3 to 9 o'clock line with patient supine), which is confirmed in the knee-chest position
- Hymenal transections or lacerations
- Hymenal laceration extending beyond (deep to) the external anal sphincter
- Laceration of posterior fourchette, extending to involve hymen
- Scar of posterior fourchette associated with a loss of hymenal tissue between 5 and 7 o'clock

[a] Findings that may be caused by sexual abuse but may also be caused by other medical conditions. History is vital in determining significance.
[b] Findings that should prompt the examiner to question the child carefully about possible abuse. May or may not require a report to protective services in the absence of a history.
Modified from Adams JA, Harper K, et al. Examination findings in legally confirmed child sexual abuse: it's normal to be normal. *Pediatrics* 1994;94:310–317, with permission.

Hospitalization

Two indications for hospitalizing the sexually abused child are (1) severe injury requiring treatment and (2) an unsafe home. Outpatient management of sexual abuse victims is always preferable. The rationale is to avoid victimizing the child twice. If an adult man has been the intrafamilial perpetrator, he should be removed from the home so that the child may return. Children who are hospitalized because the home is unsafe believe that they are being sent away for their wrongdoing. Another message hospitalization may transmit is that the parent is incapable of providing protection. Both messages are harmful to the child's psychological adjustment.

Treatment

Whether the child is hospitalized or discharged from the ED, three additional issues should be considered: (1) gonococcal prophylaxis, (2) human immunodeficiency virus (HIV) testing, and (3) pregnancy prevention. If the abuse has occurred less than 48 hours before the hospital visit, gonococcal prophylaxis is recommended. Within this period, cultures for *Neisseria gonorrhoeae* may prove negative, even if a true infection is incubating. In abuse that has occurred more than 48 hours before the visit, the choices are either to treat all children prophylactically or to culture the genitalia, anus, and throat and await culture results. This choice depends in part on the reliability of the microbiology laboratory in recovering *N. gonorrhoeae* (which is a fastidious organism) and the ability to provide follow-up treatment for positive cultures. Recommended treatment regimens are shown in Table 111.11 (see also Chapter 83).

Testing for HIV is already an issue on the minds of most parents of sexual abuse victims. Transmission of HIV during child sexual abuse contacts has been reported. Routine testing for HIV may depend on the nature and extent of sexual contact, regional rates of HIV infection, ability to test the alleged perpetrator, and

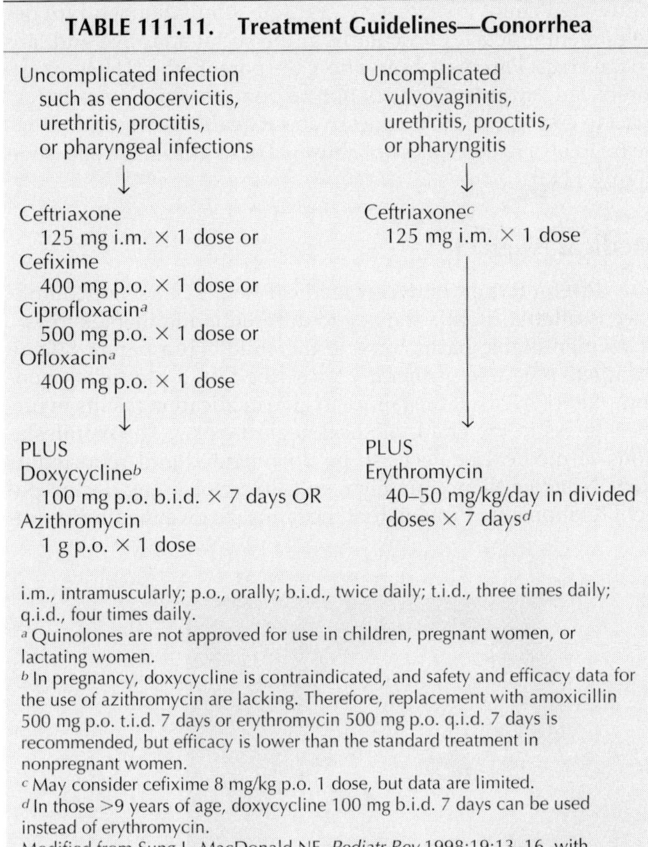

TABLE 111.11. Treatment Guidelines—Gonorrhea

Uncomplicated infection such as endocervicitis, urethritis, proctitis, or pharyngeal infections	Uncomplicated vulvovaginitis, urethritis, proctitis, or pharyngitis
↓	↓
Ceftriaxone 125 mg i.m. × 1 dose or Cefixime 400 mg p.o. × 1 dose or Ciprofloxacin[a] 500 mg p.o. × 1 dose or Ofloxacin[a] 400 mg p.o. × 1 dose	Ceftriaxone[c] 125 mg i.m. × 1 dose
↓	↓
PLUS Doxycycline[b] 100 mg p.o. b.i.d. × 7 days OR Azithromycin 1 g p.o. × 1 dose	PLUS Erythromycin 40–50 mg/kg/day in divided doses × 7 days[d]

i.m., intramuscularly; p.o., orally; b.i.d., twice daily; t.i.d., three times daily; q.i.d., four times daily.
[a] Quinolones are not approved for use in children, pregnant women, or lactating women.
[b] In pregnancy, doxycycline is contraindicated, and safety and efficacy data for the use of azithromycin are lacking. Therefore, replacement with amoxicillin 500 mg p.o. t.i.d. 7 days or erythromycin 500 mg p.o. q.i.d. 7 days is recommended, but efficacy is lower than the standard treatment in nonpregnant women.
[c] May consider cefixime 8 mg/kg p.o. 1 dose, but data are limited.
[d] In those >9 years of age, doxycycline 100 mg b.i.d. 7 days can be used instead of erythromycin.
Modified from Sung L, MacDonald NE. *Pediatr Rev* 1998;19:13–16, with permission.

parental desires for testing. All HIV testing should be preceded by written consent and should be done in a manner that results in proper notification, counseling, and follow-up. See Chapter 75 for more on HIV infections.

Most children can be eliminated from consideration for pregnancy prophylaxis if they have not yet reached menarche. Another group may be eliminated based on the nature of the abuse. If the abuse took the form of fondling, and no ejaculate was produced by the perpetrator, prophylaxis does not need to be used. In the pubertal child not using contraception, in whom active penetration occurred at a midmenstrual cycle time, pregnancy prophylaxis should be offered. Documenting that the patient does not have an existing pregnancy is always important. The Children's Hospital of Philadelphia's current therapy is a single-day treatment with oral contraceptive pills.

Referral and Follow-up

All sexually abused children need some form of referral and careful follow-up care. Initially, referral may be to the hospital social worker for monitoring of the child's symptoms and the family's ability to cope with this stress. In some locales, volunteer self-help groups organized for women who have been raped may provide support to the child victim and parent. Referral for more in-depth mental health counseling depends on the (1) symptoms manifested by the child, (2) the state of the family organization, (3) the length of time the abuse has occurred, and (4) the child's age. In general, the older the child and the longer the abuse has occurred, the more likely he or she may have or may develop a serious mental health problem. All children should be referred to mental health services. Follow-up health care visits should be arranged with an informed and sympathetic practitioner who can continue the humane and supportive care initiated in the ED.

False Allegation and Unfounded Reports

At times, the emergency physician is called on to establish the diagnosis of sexual abuse without adequate data. Two situations may be at play: a false allegation or an unfounded report. False allegations refer to situations in which a complaint of child sexual abuse is being used by one adult against an estranged wife or husband. These situations are extremely difficult to manage from the ED. Beyond taking a detailed history and performing a physical examination to rule out acute injury, these cases are best referred to a child abuse center. False allegations often are identified by weekend presentation, lack of both history from the child and physician findings, upcoming custody hearing, and bitter divorce situation. Unfounded reports often occur because of undue parental concern stimulated by a media presentation or public discussion of sexual abuse or an unwarranted fear stemming from a parent's own childhood sexual abuse experience. Historical indications by the child or physical findings may be absent. Unfounded reports also should be referred to the local child sexual abuse center for further evaluation if parental concerns cannot be satisfied.

NEGLECT

Child neglect is by far the most prevalent form of child abuse. When neglect is blatant, it is easily recognized and reported. More often, neglect is not obvious and goes undetected for long periods. Although the manifestations of neglect are less dramatic than those of physical abuse, the long-term effects may be more destructive to the child. The indolent nature of child neglect makes it a serious public health problem. For the ED staff, neglect cases are difficult because they require that certain value judgments be made. The balance between supporting the independent rights of the child and maintaining the privacy and sanctity of family rights is delicate. With neglected children, the questions are (1) how much the family should be doing, (2) how much they are capable of doing, (3) how much support from the community or society they require, and (4) how much support or help are they willing to accept on behalf of their child. As with the other forms of child abuse, the management of child neglect cases is made easier by working with a multidisciplinary team. In the ED, the team would generally consist of the physician, nurse, and social worker. Particularly in situations in which the line between adequate child care and neglect needs to be drawn, the diversity of personal and professional opinions adds credibility to decision making and lessens the burden on the single practitioner.

Failure to Thrive

The term *failure to thrive* has been used as a diagnostic term to group several diseases and disorders that result in growth failure. Growth failure is generally measured in weight, length, and head circumference compared with standard growth curves for these parameters. *Growth failure* may be defined as measurements that fall below two standard deviations for age or patterns that cross percentile lines (ie, move two standard deviations) and do not follow the normal lines of growth. Patients diagnosed as having failure to thrive may be subcategorized into three groups: (1) organic, (2) nonorganic, and (3) mixed group. *Organic* refers to children whose failure to thrive is based on a physical cause such as congenital heart disease, renal disease, or a genetic abnormality. *Nonorganic* refers to the group whose growth failure is environmentally related. When these children are hospitalized and fed standard diets, they grow rapidly and thrive. The group of patients with nonorganic failure to thrive includes a substantial number of neglected children who may be brought to the ED for care. The mixed group refers to patients who have a combination of physical and environmental factors. An example might be a physical condition that so overstresses a family that the family members cannot function and thus neglect the child in some aspect of the feeding process.

In recognizing patients with nonorganic failure to thrive, the following factors are suggestive. History: (1) an idealized feeding history; (2) a chief complaint and history that do not identify the child's growth pattern as a problem; (3) no description of losses, such as vomiting or diarrhea; and (4) failure to give a history of a schedule or scheduled pattern of feeding (eg, the infant eats about every 4 hours). Physical examination: (1) measurements in which weight is more depressed than length, which is more depressed than head circumference; (2) other signs of neglect such as poor hygiene, diaper rash, and flat and balding occiput; (3) dull, apathetic facies; (4) body posture of an understimulated child; (5) excessive oral self-stimulation; and (6) developmental delay, particularly in the social adaptive and language areas. Parental observation: the parent who (1) has an uninterested attitude; (2) does not respond to child's needs (eg, react to crying); (3) lacks concern about health issues; and (4) appears to be a drug or alcohol abuser. These factors are shown in Figure 111.9.

Medical Neglect

The differentiation between medical neglect and noncompliance is often difficult. The key to differentiating them is to ask, "Has identifiable harm come to the child?" If a parent fails to complete a course of therapy prescribed by a physician, noncompliance exists. If the failure to give medication results in further illness in the child, medical neglect exists. The manifestations of medical neglect can be documented and reported as such. Noncompliance merely results in a worsening doctor–patient relationship. Proving that the failure to give medication, at-

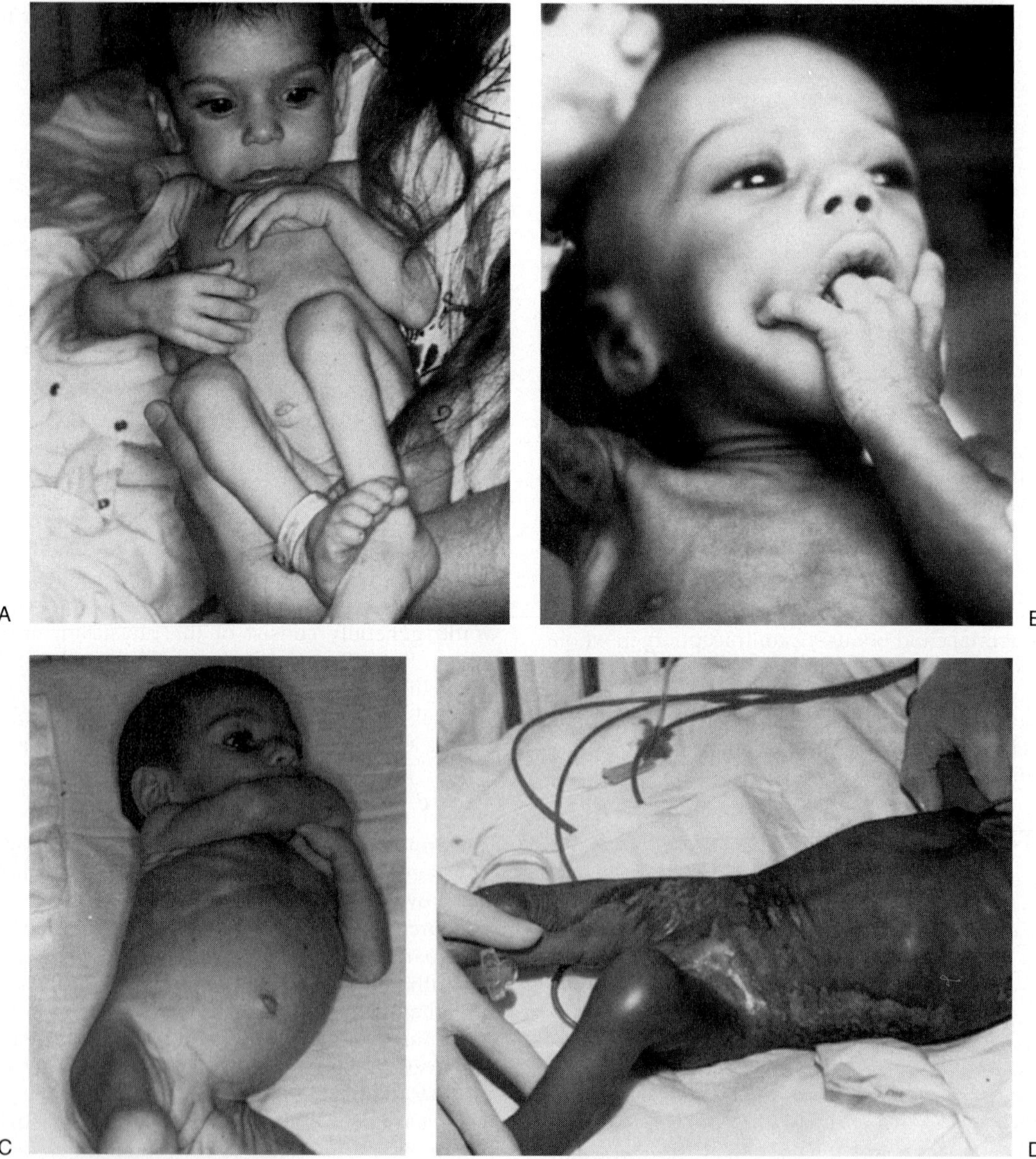

Figure 111.9. Physical signs of failure to thrive. **A:** Dull, apathetic eyes that avoid eye contact. **B:** Oral self-stimulatory behavior. **C:** Wasted extremities and protuberant abdomen. **D:** Severe diaper rash as a sign of overall neglect.

tend follow-up appointments, or obtain a procedure directly resulted in damage to the child's health may be difficult. Intervening variables, such as the complexity of the disease (eg, the exacerbations of an asthma attack) or the proven efficacy of the treatment often exist. The ED is often the central place for identifying the manifestations of medical neglect. Good documentation of prescribed treatments and good communication with the source of the child's ongoing health care are important.

Abandonment

Local jurisdictions may dictate the length of time a child must be without supervision before he or she is declared legally abandoned. These cases often come to the ED as the result of a neighbor's call or the initiative of a relative who is aware of the neglect. At times, the situation becomes apparent as the ED attempts to obtain permission to treat a child and has difficulty locating a parent or responsible adult. Manifestations of abandonment include (1) physical findings such as excessively dirty diapers, poor hygiene, or hoarse cry; (2) excessive hunger documented by unusual intake; and (3) dehydration as documented by urine specific gravity or blood urea nitrogen. Other manifestations may relate to lack of supervision and protection and may include burns, ingestions, or repeated accidents. Children with all these manifestations may be brought to the ED for treatment. Good case management results in their identification.

Truancy

Truancy as a manifestation of neglect may be less commonly recognized in the ED. The section on school avoidance (see Chapter 112) details many of the aspects of this complex psychosocial emergency. The emergency physician may recognize truancy as a neglect problem when the truant child presents with multiple somatic complaints. As the complaints are explored and no organic basis is found, the parent may be instructed to return the child to school. A failure to comply with this aspect of treatment constitutes medical neglect. For the child who makes frequent visits to the ED, neglect needs to be considered.

Management

The management of cases of child neglect follows the principles detailed in the "Physical Abuse" section. The steps are to (1) suspect and recognize neglect manifestations, (2) obtain multidisciplinary consultation, (3) report the neglect, (4) inform the parents, (5) determine the need for hospitalization, and (6) arrange follow-up. These steps are reviewed in the following sections to underscore those aspects unique to neglect.

EMOTIONAL ABUSE

Emotional abuse is the form of child abuse that most seriously and most often affects children. With every episode of physical or sexual abuse, a negative psychological message is being inflicted. The child is told, "You are bad!" and often comes to believe this statement. When the bruises, burns, and broken bones are healed, psychological injury may remain untreated. The neglected child also feels devalued and unloved. Emotional abuse always accompanies other forms of abuse and at times is inflicted independently.

Yet this form of abuse is the least well understood. Furthermore, a report of suspected abuse is rarely based solely on emotional abuse. Gathering enough objective data to prove that emotional abuse has occurred is difficult. Courts and legal authorities remain unconvinced that a given parental behavior or set of behaviors can be shown to be responsible for effects in the child. Emotional abuse rarely results in a psychosocial emergency. More often, similar to neglect, it is a chronic impediment to normal growth and development.

Manifestations

Emotional abuse manifests in many forms, including children who are excessively withdrawn and passive and those who are aggressive and act out. The manifestations are so varied that it is difficult to identify any constant characteristics of the emotionally abused child. To identify emotional abuse, the physician must witness family interactions on repeated occasions; however, the emergency physician does not often have the opportunity for such comprehensive evaluation.

Rarely, more direct presentations of emotional abuse may be seen in the ED. Some children may seek hospital asylum because of excessive fear of their parents. Adolescent "runaways" may include a subset of children who are emotionally abused (see Chapter 112). Developmental delay may be recognized in the ED, but the cause of the delay can rarely be identified. Finally, children with drug or alcohol abuse may be in a high-risk group for prior emotional abuse. The effects of emotional abuse closely parallel the findings in children with substance abuse (eg, poor self-image, difficulty in establishing relationships).

Another group of emotionally abused children frequently seen in the ED is youngsters caught in the conflict between estranged parents. These victims have been called "yo-yo" children because they are pulled between arguing parents. Sometimes one parent will virtually kidnap a child. These presentations to the ED are based on one parent's attempt to document the poor parenting or neglect of the other. The misuse of the child as a pawn in the marital dispute constitutes emotional abuse. Despite the credibility and motivation of the parent in the ED, emotional abuse should be reported to remove the child from the middle.

Management

The management principles for emotional abuse are the same as those for other forms of abuse. To substantiate emotional abuse, documentation of behavior must be precise. The physician, nurse, and social worker must record observed interactions in behavioral terms using a minimum of subjective assessments and personal conclusions. Recording significant statements from the parents and child is good documentation. Citing a pattern of abuse or repeated episodes of abuse may be necessary to strengthen a report.

It is often difficult and painful for parents to see themselves as emotionally abusive. Thus, informing the parent in a constructive and sensitive way is also difficult. The informant must keep the discussion focused on the child and must not be accusatory. Child welfare agencies and the family court system also have difficulty in identifying and treating emotional abuse. As the rights of children become more well established and standards for child care more widely accepted, management of cases of emotional abuse will become less difficult.

CHAPTER 112
Psychiatric Emergencies

Gordon R. Hodas, M.D., and
John Sargent, M.D.

In contemporary American society, the emergency department (ED) of the hospital has become a major community resource. It is open 24 hours each day, professionally staffed, and used by the community for assistance in dealing with many physical, social, and emotional problems. The ED is the setting for the initial evaluation of a variety of difficulties of children and their families, including acute and chronic illnesses with their emotional sequelae, psychophysiologic conditions, family crises, and the entire spectrum of emotional and behavioral disorders.

Table 112.1 lists the major categories of the mental status examination. These categories are described as they apply to emergency psychiatric assessment.

MENTAL STATUS EVALUATION CATEGORIES

Orientation

The level of consciousness and orientation of the child are the first areas of assessment. The child not under the influence of drugs or with severe organic illness should be oriented in all spheres: person, place, time, and situation.

Appearance

The physical appearance of the child reveals important information about both the way the child feels about and cares for himself or herself and the supervising care by the family. The examiner should carefully observe factors such as physical size, personal hygiene, choice of clothes, neatness, grooming, posture, and gait.

Memory

The child's memory can be evaluated while the examiner is listening to the history and through direct questioning. Impairment of memory in a child is a strong indication that his or her emotional and behavioral disturbance may have an organic cause.

Cognition

Intelligence, fund of knowledge, and the ability to think and reason are evaluated while talking with the child. Intelligence and fund of knowledge need be categorized only as adequate or inadequate for the child's age.

TABLE 112.1. Childhood and Adolescent Psychiatric Emergencies: Child Mental Status Examination

Orientation	Speech
Appearance	Affect
Memory	Thought content and process
Cognition	Insight and judgment
Behavior	Strengths
Relating ability	Synthesis of evaluation

Behavior

The child's behavior can be observed throughout the visit. Activity level may be at the appropriate age level and goal-directed, it may be too rapid and random (*hyperactive*), or too slow and diffuse (*psychomotor retarded*). The child may appear well focused or may be distractible. Behavioral tendencies are revealed in the child's talking with the examiner and in interactions with various family members. Psychotic youngsters may respond to people as objects and use objects in nondirected, bizarre ways. Nonpsychotic children may behave in angry, aggressive ways that usually can be distinguished from the behavior of psychotic children by its negative or resistant nature. The child's ability to control his or her behavior in response to the examiner's or the family's request should be carefully noted.

Relating Ability

The child's capacity to relate to the examiner is a key element in the mental status evaluation. In a sense, the examiner is a window to the outside world, and the degree to which a positive relationship can develop during the assessment suggests the child's current capacity for forming relationships in general. The examiner should be concerned with what occurs at any moment during the evaluation and, even more important, how the interaction evolves during the course of the visit.

Speech

Speech includes elements such as spontaneity, coherence, articulation, and vocabulary. As such, the category of speech overlaps with the capacity to relate, the quality of thought processes, and the level of intelligence. Poor vocabulary and articulation may suggest mental retardation, psychosocial deprivation, specific language disabilities, or combinations of these.

Affect

The child's affect, as the external manifestation of predominant feeling states, is assessed informally during the course of the interview. Fluctuations of affect according to changes in content and interactions should be observed carefully observed, with more serious concern raised by children whose affect does not change as different subjects are discussed. Depressed children may show both sad and angry affect, which suggests the way in which the child sees both self and the external world. Some angry children express their anger directly, even in the form of rage. Other children become so well defended that their affect appears flat and constricted.

Thoughts

Thoughts include both thought processes and thought content. Evaluation of the preceding categories necessarily yields much information on thinking. Thought process involves the coherence and goal directedness of verbal communication. Evasiveness and guardedness must be distinguished from the looseness of associations of the psychotic child or adolescent. Loose associations have no logical coherence or connection with previous statements. Flight of ideas, as found in bipolar disorder, involves rapid shifting from one topic to another, often triggered by the patient's ongoing monologue. Thought content involves the major themes that emerge as the child talks spontaneously and responsively to the examiner. Thorough screening also involves determining the possible presence of psychotic phenomena (hallucinations, delusions, grandiosity, and ideas of reference) and present or past tendencies toward suicide or homicide.

Insight and Judgment

Insight involves the degree of recognition and acknowledgment of current problems by the child. A child with a high degree of insight also can identify possible precipitating factors. Judgment involves the child's ability to think before acting. Over the course of the interview in the ED, the examiner can assess these elements informally.

Strengths

The purpose of any child's mental status examination is not only to screen for possible deficits but also to search for strengths and areas of competence in the child. Thus, the examiner must determine areas of interest, competence, and motivation of the child. These strengths may go undiscovered unless specifically looked for. Thus, the role of the evaluation extends beyond assessment; it also involves, through the identification of strengths, the beginnings of positive interventions.

Synthesis

After the component parts of the mental status examination have been determined, the physician should integrate them into a comprehensive picture of the child. For example, a 14-year-old boy presents to the ED fully alert and oriented but disheveled and malnourished. His cognitive abilities appear to be intact, but his actions are slow and labored. The child's thinking shows no evidence of incoherence, but themes of disappointment emerge from the conversation. The boy relates to the physician in a withdrawn manner and appears to be preoccupied. The data from this mental status examination suggest that the adolescent described is depressed. This impression should then be integrated with historical, medical, and family information as the examiner plans appropriate treatment.

FAMILY EVALUATION

Physicians, while performing emergency assessments, explaining results of evaluations, and developing treatment plans, typically deal with both the ill child and his or her family. Recommendations depend in part on the physician's impression of the family and of how effectively the family will carry out the required treatment. To assess families, the physician needs to have an organized framework to guide the evaluation process (Table 112.2). The goal of a family evaluation for childhood psychiatric emergencies is to determine the methods that the family uses to help its members when distressed, the adequacy of these efforts, and the possibilities for new alternatives that will help the family cope successfully with the current crisis. Just as it is important to know the child's mental status, the emergency physician also must determine the mental status of the rest of the family. This task can be accomplished as the physician observes the family members and listens to their presentation of the history.

Hierarchy and Leadership in the Family

The family is a social system that requires acknowledged leadership that is consistent and whose direction is followed. In many families, grandparents live nearby and help with the children, but they are expected to defer to the parents' plans and approaches. In other families, however, especially single-parent families, a grandparent may function as caretaker while the parent is away at work and the parenting responsibility is shared. For effective collaboration to occur, the specific roles for each caretaker must be explicit and agreed on.

TABLE 112.2. Child Adolescent Psychiatric Emergencies: Family Assessment

Signs of competence and strength	Danger signs with parents/caretakers
Level of concern	Psychosis
Verbal communication	Intoxication/drug abuse
Problem-solving ability	Depression
Relationships	Violence
Parents and child	History of abuse (physical, emotional, sexual) or neglect
Parents or caretakers	
Parents and physician	

The emergency physician should be concerned when either excessive closeness or excessive distance characterizes the relationship between parent and child. An overly close relationship between parent and child may interfere with the parent's ability to establish and enforce rules. The parent may hold back either because he or she is unable to become angry with the child or because he or she fears upsetting the child by taking a firm stand.

The emergency physician can assess an overly close parent–child relationship in several ways. He or she can suggest that child and parent not sit so close to each other or can have the child switch seats with another family member. The physician can ask parental permission to speak with the child in the presence of the family, with only the child speaking for himself or herself. The physician can point out the nature of the overly close relationship to the other parent and ask whether this situation is of concern to the less involved parent. When these interventions fail, psychiatric consultation is in order.

Excessively distant relationships exist in some disorganized families when parents are so involved with their own problems that the needs of the child are overlooked. In such families, the child is given more autonomy or responsibility than is appropriate for his or her age, and rules are either nonexistent or enforced inconsistently. Such families may be unable to focus on the child's problem.

In responding to an underinvolved family, the emergency physician should create an intensely serious mood and emphasize the gravity and danger of the situation. The physician can appeal to positive parental instincts, conveying a belief that the parents want to do what is best for their child. In some cases, this approach creates a tone that enables family members to respond actively to the child's distress. In other situations, however, the caretakers remain unresponsive. When this happens, psychiatric consultation is required, and hospitalization may be necessary.

Protectiveness Versus Autonomy

All relationships can be placed on a continuum of involvement, with intimacy at one pole and disengagement at the other. Effective parenting requires avoidance of the extremes and the capacity to shift from one position to another at different times and in different situations. As previously described, some families have an overly close relationship between the child and one parent.

Underinvolved families, on the other hand, provide insufficient protection and support for the child. The child learns not to expect parental support and may present as undersocialized, with a conduct disorder or as depressed and possibly suicidal. The may may also present as an overwhelmed "little adult."

With overprotective families, the emergency physician can assess the family's flexibility by suggesting that the child speak for himself or herself and that the parents increase their expectations. When the overprotectiveness is rigid and severe, the physician may request psychiatric consultation as a way of initiating ongoing therapy for the family.

Conflict Resolution Versus Conflict Avoidance

All families have disagreements among their members. In some families, disagreements are acknowledged and confronted directly, whereas in others potential conflict is consistently avoided. Other families disagree openly but are unable to reach a constructive resolution. The capacity of the family for conflict resolution is an important area for the emergency physician to assess because unresolved disagreements typically lead to chronic hostility, undermining of relationships, and ineffective parenting.

The emergency physician should request psychiatric consultation when inability to resolve conflict has seriously impaired the functioning of the family and the child. Psychiatric involvement should also be sought when patterns of conflict avoidance occur in conjunction with other aspects of family adaptational problems described in this section.

Capacity for Problem Solving

Families in crisis usually try to solve their problems by attempting the same solutions over and over again. They perceive other remedies as currently inaccessible or impossible. As a result, the family's repertoire of behaviors becomes extremely limited and responses to problems become stereotyped and rigid. As the physician pursues historical information and observes the family, he or she looks for signs of flexibility and strength.

Relating to the Physician

The emergency physician should rely substantially on his or her overall impression of the family and how members relate to him or her. Do family members maintain eye contact with the physician, or do they avoid looking at her or him and display guardedness or a sense of hostility? Families who accept the physician's expression of interest and concern are more likely to benefit from the ED visit. Families that are suspicious of the physician's motives and unresponsive to his or her input probably gain less from emergency interventions. Emergency physicians need to recognize that those families that antagonize them the most may also be the families most in need of the physician's (and the psychiatrist's) interventions.

Using Social Support

Some families come to the ED feeling isolated, overwhelmed, and exhausted. Often, such families have not used all of the family and community resources available to them. Effective crisis intervention for psychiatric emergencies involves not only emergency treatment but also effective disposition planning for the family. The ED staff should determine what community resources are available, or potentially available, to the family. The parents should be asked about relatives or neighbors who might be able to help them. Families who have previously mobilized community supports should be commended by the emergency physician for their competence and resourcefulness. This support by the physician often stimulates the family to recognize its capacity to address the crisis.

Integration

In following the aforementioned guidelines for family evaluation, the emergency physician obtains the necessary data for understanding the family in crisis. By integrating the history, the physical examination, the child's mental status, and the family assessment, the emergency physician is better able to understand the nature of the current crisis and the appropriate responses. However, effective intervention involves more than understanding. The emergency physician needs to offer information and recommendations in a respectful manner that conveys his or her recognition of the family's competence and its desire to help the child.

DEPRESSION

The appreciation of depression in children and adolescents as a highly significant problem has increased greatly in recent years. *Depression* can refer to the symptom of feeling sad but most appropriately describes a symptom complex or syndrome that includes cognitive and physiologic components in addition to affective ones. Depression implies more than momentary sadness and involves a pervasive inflexibility of sad mood, accompanied frequently by self-deprecation and suicidal ideation. Depression also implies a change in functioning from an earlier state of relatively good adjustment, rather than a temperamental or personality type.

Considerable evidence suggests that a genetic predisposition exists for depression, particularly severe depression. Depressive episodes may be triggered by environmental events of significance to the child.

The depressed child typically experiences a profound sense of helplessness, feeling unable to improve an unsatisfactory situation. The child may be experiencing frustration and failure at home, at school, and with peers. Negative outcomes reinforce the child's negative self-image, which contributes in circular fashion to more negative outcomes.

Clinical Manifestations

Depression appears differently at different stages of development. In infancy, depression is usually the result of the loss of the mother or a lack of nurturance, and it is seen as a global interference of normal growth and physiologic functioning. Thus, some of the manifestations of depression in infancy include apathy and listlessness, staring, hypoactivity, poor feeding and weight loss, and increased susceptibility to infection.

During latency, depression can appear as part of a syndrome, or it may be masked by other symptoms. Petti described the two key features in childhood depression as dysphoric mood and self-deprecatory ideation. *Dysphoric mood* is manifested by looking or feeling sad and forlorn, being moody and irritable, and crying easily. *Self-deprecatory* thoughts are reflected by low self-esteem, feelings of worthlessness, and suicidal ideation. Depression in this age also can appear as other common symptoms, including multiple somatic complaints, school avoidance or underachievement (including learning-disabled children or children with attention deficit disorder), angry outbursts, runaway behavior, phobias, and fire-setting.

Depression during adolescence is more similar to adult-onset depression. The major symptom is a sad, unhappy mood or a pervasive loss of interest and pleasure. Other symptoms may include a change in appetite, a change in a sleep behavior, and psychomotor retardation or agitation. Also present in many depressed teenagers are loss of energy, feelings of worthlessness or excessive guilt, decreased ability to concentrate, indecisiveness, and recurrent thoughts of death or suicide. Depressed teenagers also may present with somatic complaints, academic problems, promiscuity, drug or alcohol use, aggressive behavior, and stealing. Many teenagers with behaviors such as these are unaware of their depression because it is not on the surface.

Others simply deny the painful depressive affect. In talking with these patients about their lives at home, at school, and with peers, the underlying depression usually becomes apparent.

Management

Once any initial medical concerns have been dealt with, the three major goals in the management of depression involve (1) determining suicidal potential, (2) uncovering acute precipitants, and (3) making an appropriate disposition.

The emergency treatment of depression can usefully be thought of as the prevention of suicide attempts. The task of the physician is to determine carefully whether any suicide attempts have been made and whether suicidal ideation is present. The physician should not be hesitant about asking the child about suicidal deeds, thoughts, or wishes. Such questions represent a positive confrontation of the problem of depression and are unlikely to catalyze a subsequent suicide attempt. In fact, questions about suicide actually may provide a sense of relief for the depressed child.

The physician should attempt to determine possible acute precipitants of the current depression to guide subsequent recommendations. The duration of the depression should be determined as well as the family response. Assessing overall adjustment at home, in school, and with peers is important, as is looking for the strengths of child and family for use in the treatment plan.

When suicidal ideation is present, the emergency physician should request psychiatric consultation. A decision then can be made jointly regarding outpatient or inpatient treatment. Whether or not suicide is an imminent danger, the task of the physician is to create a sense of hope that things will improve. To achieve this goal, the physician must form a solid doctor–patient relationship with child and family. Outpatient management can be used when adequate social support is present.

Psychotropic medication, although not approved by the Federal Drug Administration (FDA) for use in children and adolescents, has been increasingly used in the treatment of childhood and adolescent depression. As an acute intervention, however, the emergency physician should not prescribe antidepressant medication because its desired mood-elevating effects generally require up to 1 month to take effect, and the act of prescribing medication in the ED may decrease the likelihood of successful referral for follow-up mental health treatment.

The emergency physician should be familiar with commonly used antidepressants, which are sometimes used adjunctively in the treatment of depression. In recent years, use of the selective serotonin reuptake inhibitors (SSRIs) has displaced the tricyclic antidepressants as first-line medications. SSRIs include Prozac (fluoxetine), Paxil (paroxetine), Zoloft (sertraline), and Luvox (fluvoxamine). Advantages of these agents over tricyclic antidepressants include a decreased likelihood of cardiotoxicity, the absence of anticholinergic side effects, and the relative safety of these medications when used in overdose. These medications all require approximately 1 month to take effect. Another commonly prescribed antidepressant is Wellbutrin (bupropion), which is chemically distinct from other agents. A side effect of potential concern with Wellbutrin involves seizures.

Because the older tricyclic antidepressants are still prescribed at times for children and adolescents, and may more commonly be prescribed to a parent by a family physician, emergency physicians should be familiar with these medications, which include Tofranil (imipramine), Elavil (amitriptyline), Pamelor (nortriptyline), Norpramin (desipramine), and Anafranil (clomipramine). If the emergency physician learns that any of these medications have been used in overdose, especially in doses exceeding 10 mg per kilogram of body weight of the child, the possibility of cardiac arrhythmias should be considered. Other common side effects of tricyclic antidepressants are drowsiness and those resulting from the anticholinergic effects of these drugs, which include dry mouth, constipation, and blurred vision. Cardiac arrhythmias are reportedly less common with Sinequan (doxepin), Ascending (amoxapine), and Ludiomil (maprotiline), none of which are tricyclic compounds. Drowsiness and variable amounts of anticholinergic effects may occur (see Chapter 78).

Suicide Attempts

Suicidal behavior involves thoughts or actions that may lead to self-inflicted death or serious injury. A distinction is made between suicidal ideation and suicidal attempts in which a deliberate attempt to take one's own life has occurred.

The increasing trend toward suicidal behavior by children and adolescents is alarming. Table 112.3 provides information on the nature and scope of this problem.

A factor that complicates the discussion of suicide in children is their differing conceptions of death at various ages. Up to age 5, death is seen as a reversible process in which the activities of life still occur. From 5 to 9 years, the irreversibility of death is beginning to be understood but death is personified rather than seen as an independent event. It is not until about age 9 that death is seen as irreversible in the adult sense of being both final

TABLE 112.3. Childhood and Adolescent Suicide: Nature of the Problem

Adolescent suicide is now epidemic
44% rise in suicide rate, adolescents aged 15–19, since 1970
6,000 completed adolescent suicides, 1984
Estimated 400,000 adolescent attempts, 1983 (1:50–1:100 attempts succeed)
Suicide is the third leading cause of death, aged 15–24 yr (after accidents, homicides)
Childhood suicide is also a serious problem
Younger children attempt suicide as a result of depression ???and/or poor judgment
Increase in attempted and completed suicides, children aged 6 yr and older
Suicide attempts via ingestions (children aged 5–14 yr) 5 times more common than all forms of meningitis
12% of all pediatric emergency department visits result from childhood and adolescent suicide attempts
Additional data
Girls *attempt* at least 3 times more often than boys
Boys *succeed* at least 2 times more often than girls
80% of attempts are pill ingestions
More lethal means—gun, knife, jumping, running into car—more common with boys
Many car "accidents" are not accidents

TABLE 112.4. Characteristics Associated with Childhood and Adolescent Suicide Attempts

Positive family history	Active wish to die
Hopelessness	Depression
Low self-esteem	Anger/wish for revenge

TABLE 112.5. Childhood and Adolescent Suicide: High-Risk Situations for Suicide Attempts

Suicide attempt just made	Aggressive violent behavior
Suicidal threat made	Psychotic child
"Accidental" ingestion	Significant withdrawal by child
Child complains of depression	
Medical concerns, but child appears depressed	

TABLE 112.6. Assessing Childhood/Adolescent Suicide Attempts: Four Major Dimensions

Medical lethality	Impulsivity
Suicidal intent	Strengths/supports

TABLE 112.7. Childhood and Adolescent Suicide: Assessing Medical Lethality

Vital signs
Level of consciousness
Evidence of drug/alcohol intoxication (e.g., pupils, smell on breath)
Need for emesis, lavage, or catharsis
Acute medical complications (cardiac, respiratory, renal, neurologic)
Indications for medical hospitalization, including intensive care
Residual abnormalities

TABLE 112.8. Childhood and Adolescent Suicide: Assessing Suicide Intent

- Circumstances of suicide attempt
  - Nature of suicide attempt (pills versus violent means)
  - Use of multiple methods
  - Method used to extreme (all versus some pills ingested)
  - Suicide note written
  - Secrecy of attempt (attempt concealed versus revealed)
  - Premeditation (long-planned versus impulsive attempt)
  - History of prior attempts
- Child self-report
  - Premeditation of attempt
  - Anticipation of death
  - Desire for death
  - Attempt to conceal attempt
  - Nature of precipitating stresses
- Child's mental status
  - Orientation/cognitive intactness
  - Presence/absence of psychosis
  - Manner of relating to physician
  - Current suicidality
    - Response to being saved/being unsuccessful in attempt
    - Active plan for another attempt
    - Readiness to discuss stresses
    - Readiness to accept external and family support
- Nature of orientation toward future

and inevitable. Even then, however, the child may imagine his or her own death as being reversible. Under such circumstances, a suicide attempt may have a different meaning from that for an adult, for whom suicide corresponds to a definite end of one's life.

CLINICAL MANIFESTATIONS

In latency-aged children, certain risk factors have been identified that distinguish children with suicidal behavior from other children with emotional problems (Table 112.4). Teicher has offered a longitudinal perspective of adolescent suicide attempts, which are usually not simply impulsive acts. Before the suicide attempt, problems have been present in the family for at least 5 years. These problems include a parent or close relative attempting suicide, many residential and environmental changes, and unexpected separations from meaningful relationships (divorce, separation, or death). With the onset of adolescence, an escalation phase occurs in which frustration results from the teenager's desire for autonomy and the belief that his or her parents do not understand. The teenager withdraws or rebels, becoming alienated from his or her parents at a time when they are really still needed. The scene is then set for the final stage, in which some precipitating event leads to the suicide attempt. The precipitating event may be a peer rejection, the breakup of a romance, an unwanted pregnancy, or problems in school. (It was found that 36% of children attempting suicide were not enrolled in school at the time of the suicide attempt.)

Table 112.5 indicates the high-risk situations for suicidal behavior in which direct questioning about suicide should occur.

The dichotomy sometimes drawn between suicide "attempts" and suicide "gestures" is ill conceived. All suicidal behavior should be regarded as suicide attempts, which are best evaluated by appreciating the medical lethality of the act, the suicidal intent of the child, the impulsivity of the act, and the strengths and supports within the family (Table 112.6). The lethality of a suicide attempt by itself may be misleading because suicidal children may miscalculate, causing at times greater harm than was intended and at other times less harm than was intended (Table 112.7). The physician cannot conclude, however, that attempts with low lethality are not serious attempts until he or she has specifically asked about and assessed the child's suicidal intent, that is, just how seriously the child wanted to end his or her life (Table 112.8).

In addition to asking directly about suicidal intent ("When you took those pills, what were you hoping would happen?"), the physician should gather as much information as possible about the attempt itself to help infer the degree of suicidal intent on the part of the child. Did the child take all of the pills that were available? Did he or she expect to wake up? Did he or she tell anyone after taking the pills? Did he or she leave a suicide note? Now that he or she is awake, is the child pleased or displeased to be alive? Does he or she intend to try again?

Children who threaten suicide without making an actual attempt should also be questioned carefully about suicidal in-

TABLE 112.9. Childhood and Adolescent Suicide: Assessing Impulsivity

Evidence of impulsive suicide attempt	Evidence of impulsivity during interview
History of prior impulsive behaviors	

TABLE 112.10. Childhood and Adolescent Suicide: Assessing Strengths and Supports

Strengths and assets of child	Nature of external supports
Ability to relate to physician	Outpatient psychiatrist/family physician
Ability to rely on parents in crisis	Extended family
Ability to acknowledge problem	Neighbors/other significant adults
Positive orientation toward future	Religious community
Strengths and assets of family	Self-help groups
Commitment to child	
Ability to unite during crisis	
Problem-solving abilities	
Capacity to supervise child (support *and* limits)	
Ability to use external supports	

tent. How long has the child considered suicide? What methods are planned? When will this take place? Has the child ever made previous attempts? How about other family members? Psychotic and depressed children, especially when the parents appear unable to supervise the child, should elicit particular concern.

Assessment of the child's level of impulsivity is also important (Table 112.9). Does the attempt appear to have been impulsive rather than planned? Is there a history of prior impulsive behaviors? Is there evidence of impulsivity during the ED interview?

The physician should ask the child and family about possible precipitating events to determine what changes in the environment may be needed. The strengths of the family should be assessed to determine whether sufficient social support exists to allow for outpatient management (Table 112.10).

EVALUATION FOR HOSPITALIZATION

No universally agreed-on criteria have been established for when to hospitalize a child with suicidal behavior and when to manage him or her on an outpatient basis. Garfinkel and Golombek identified seven areas to assess to determine whether hospitalization is indicated (Table 112.11).

In general, any suicide attempt deserves a thorough assessment by the emergency physician and a complete psychiatric consultation. Hospitalization should be used in the circumstances listed in Table 112.12): (1) when the physician has had difficulty in gaining the cooperation of the child and the family, (2) the child has made a serious suicide attempt, (3) the child is continuing to be actively suicidal, (4) the child is unwilling or unable to provide a no-suicide commitment to the parents, (5) the child is psychotic, (6) the family appears unable to provide necessary supervision and support to the child, and (7) the child and family rapidly deny the significance of a serious suicide attempt.

INITIATING TREATMENT

The critical goal in dealing with suicidal behavior in a child is to create a context for living, an immediate response to the crisis that increases the likelihood that the child remains alive. The emergency physician creates a context for living through his or her thorough assessment of child and family, the eventual disposition, and the encouragement of family and child to increase communication and develop alternative solutions to problems that have arisen.

Although a no-suicide commitment is not always sufficient to avoid psychiatric hospitalization, sending any child home when an earnest no-suicide commitment has not been given and accepted is potentially hazardous.

If inpatient treatment is required, the child and family should be informed about how the hospital operates and what to expect. The goals of the hospitalization should be discussed and the active role of the family in the treatment emphasized. In many states, voluntary consent forms need to be signed. In instances in which the child or parents do not agree to hospitalization, involuntary commitment may need to be used, although every effort should be made to enlist the concurrence of the parents first. When possible, the child and family should be accompanied to the psychiatric hospital by the consultant psychiatrist or an involved social worker so that the transition to the psychiatric facility is made smoother.

Outpatient psychotherapy can begin immediately with emergencies that occur during the workday. When outpatient treatment cannot begin until the next day, the physician should give the family a therapist's name or the name of the "intake person" at the mental health agency. This information personalizes the agency and increases the chances that the family will follow through. The family should be instructed to use the physician's name as the source of referral and should be reassured that the physician will contact the agency before the family's call. At least one parent and the child, if an adolescent, should be asked to sign a release of confidentiality to authorize communication between the physician and the mental health agency. This release also enables the agency or the psychiatrist to contact the family if the family fails to follow through in making an appointment to be seen. Any discussion of suicide must contain careful consideration of prevention (Table 112.13 & Table 112.14).

TABLE 112.11. Areas to Assess Following a Suicide Attempt

Social set	Stress
Intent	Mental status
Method	Support
History	

TABLE 112.12. Indications for Psychiatric Hospitalization Following Childhood/Adolescent Suicide Attempt

- Failure of rapport among physician, child, and family
- Serious suicide attempt (lethality and intent)
- Continuing active suicidality
- Inability to provide no suicide commitment to parents
- Psychosis of child
- Divisive/disturbed family, incapable of support and supervision
- Rapid denial of significance of suicide attempt

TABLE 112.13. Prevention of Childhood and Adolescent Suicide: Guidelines for Parents

Understand nature of parent–child dilemma during adolescence
Maintain physical contact—be around, combat tendency toward isolation
Maintain emotional contact—stay involved, show positive regard
Listen to child before responding—promote safety in talking
Respond to child, once child has finished—take child seriously, do not dismiss or attack
Encourage choices by adolescent
Acknowledge child and provide respect

TABLE 112.14. Prevention of Childhood and Adolescent Suicide: Warning Signs for Parents

Withdrawal (peers, parents, siblings)
Somatic complaints
Irritability
Crying
Diminished school performance
Sad or anxious appearance
Significant loss (rejection by peer group, break-up of romance, poor grades, failure to achieve important goal)
Major event or change within family
Casual mention of suicide or being "better off dead"
Explicit suicide threat
Minor, seemingly unimportant suicide "gestures"
Apparent "accidents"
Other unusual behavior pattern—housebound behavior, breaking curfew, running away, drug or alcohol abuse, bizarre or antisocial actions

PSYCHOSIS

Psychosis is the term used to describe severe disturbances in a patient's mental functioning. It is manifested by significant aberrations in cognition, perception, mood, impulses, and reality testing. Thoughts and feelings are not well integrated and acted on, perceptions may become distorted so that the world is seen as threatening, and mood may become ecstatic or despondent. Behavior also may become extremely agitated and potentially violent or excessively withdrawn to the point where the patient does not recognize and attend to his or her physical needs.

Psychosis in children and adolescents can be divided into two groups based on cause: organic psychosis and psychiatrically based psychosis. Psychiatrically based psychosis in children and adolescents has four major causes: (1) autism with onset before 30 months of age, (2) other pervasive developmental disorders with onset between 30 months and 12 years of age, (3) adult-type schizophrenia with onset in adolescence, (4) acute reactive psychosis, and (5) bipolar or manic–depressive illness with onset in late childhood or adolescence. Emergency management of organic psychosis and the four major types of psychiatrically based psychosis is described in the following sections.

Organic Psychosis

Differentiation of organic psychosis as a separate class does not imply that other (psychiatrically based) psychosis is completely independent of brain processes. On the contrary, all psychosis is assumed to be associated with aberrant brain function. The term *organic psychosis* merely implies that the cause of the aberrations in mental functioning is known and resolution of the psychosis depends on improvement in the underlying organic problems. Psychiatrically based psychoses, on the other hand, are those in which specific organic causes have not yet been determined (Table 112.15). The causes of organic psychoses can be acute or chronic illnesses, trauma, or intoxications with an exogenous substance (Tables 112.16 through 112.18).

TABLE 112.15. Organic versus Psychiatrically Based Psychosis: Major Differentiating Features

Assessment feature	Organic psychosis	Psychiatrically based psychosis
History		
Nature of onset	Acute	Insidious
Preillness history	Prior illness/drug use	Prior psychiatric history (self or family)
Medical evaluation		
Vital signs	May be impaired	Usually normal
Level of consciousness	May be impaired	Normal
Pathologic autonomic signs	May be present	Normal
Laboratory studies	May be abnormal	Normal
Mental status evaluation		
Orientation	May be impaired	Intact
Recent memory	May be impaired	Intact
Cognitive/intellectual functioning	May be impaired	Intact
Nature of hallucinations	Usually not auditory (e.g., visual, tactile)	Auditory
Response to support and medication	Often dramatic	Often limited

TABLE 112.16. Causes of Organic Psychosis

Medical conditions (acute and chronic)
Trauma (acute and chronic)
Prescribed medications (toxicity/side effects/withdrawal)
Drug intoxications
  Accidental, including misuse of proprietary medication
  Drug abuse/experimentation
  Alcohol abuse (alone or with drugs)
  Deliberate suicide attempt

TABLE 112.18. Exogenous Substances That Cause Psychosis Following Ingestion of Significant Quantity

Alcohol	Quaalude
Barbiturates	Anticholinergic compounds
Antipsychotics (e.g., phenothiazines)	Heavy metals
Amphetamines	Cocaine and crack
Hallucinogens—LSD, peyote, mescaline	Corticosteroids
Marijuana	Reserpine
Phencyclidine (PCP)	Opiates (e.g., heroin, methadone)

CLINICAL MANIFESTATIONS

The child or adolescent with an organic psychosis presents to the ED in an agitated and confused state. The child's orientation to time and place is often disturbed, and he or she may be highly distractible, with significant disturbance of recent memory. Evidence of bizarre and distorted thoughts is apparent, and disconnected ideas may be juxtaposed. The child also may have significant difficulty controlling behavior and may persist in activities without regard for personal safety.

The child with an organic psychosis may experience visual hallucinations, which may be frightening in nature. Tactile hallucinations may be present. Auditory hallucinations, more common in schizophrenia and manic–depressive illness, are rare in organic psychoses but may occur. As a result of impaired reality testing, organically psychotic children and adolescents are often extremely difficult to control and may strike out at family or staff when attempts are made to control their behavior.

A complete medical history helps determine whether the organic psychosis is a concomitant feature of an already existing chronic illness (eg, lupus cerebritis), a result of medication prescribed to treat an ongoing disease (eg, steroids for lupus erythematosus), or a result of a drug ingestion (eg, amphetamine psychosis). Typically, an acute intoxication or drug ingestion causes the acute onset of psychosis and represents an abrupt change from the child's previous psychological functioning. The possibility of alcohol use must also be considered in the cause of organic psychosis, and the history should explore the possibility of trauma.

The physical examination is often extremely helpful in both differentiating organic from psychiatrically based psychosis and in determining the underlying cause of an acute organic psychosis. Fever is likely to be present in infections, and tachycardia often is associated with chronic illness or intoxication. The general physical examination gives indications of pulmonary, cardiac, liver, or autoimmune disease, and the neurologic examination assists in the diagnosis of central nervous system (CNS) disease. Abnormalities of reflexes or of motor, sensory, or coordination systems always require complete neurologic evaluation. Signs of increased intracranial pressure may be indicative of a cerebral vascular accident, CNS tumor, or cerebral edema. Signs of autonomic dysfunction, such as pupillary abnormalities, are often indicative of acute intoxication.

In instances of suspected organic psychosis, laboratory evaluation should include a complete blood count, urinalysis, serum electrolytes, calcium, blood urea nitrogen, blood glucose, and complete drug and alcohol screens. Serum, urine, and gastric aspirate should be obtained for toxicology screening. Other laboratory and radiologic studies depend on abnormalities noted in the history and physical examination. If CNS disease is suspected, skull radiographs, computed tomography, and a lumbar puncture may be necessary. Liver function studies, thyroid studies, and other specialized and specific laboratory tests may be obtained as required.

MANAGEMENT

Management of the child or adolescent with organic psychosis involves several steps (Table 112.19). First and foremost is diagnosing the underlying cause. Medical treatment then is pursued as indicated for the specific organic condition. Any child with a suspected organic psychosis should be admitted to a medical inpatient unit for diagnostic evaluation and treatment. This treatment is especially important because organic psychosis may be a transitory condition in a child or adolescent whose illness or intoxication is progressive and life threatening.

TABLE 112.17. Medical Conditions That May Lead to Psychosis

Central nervous system lesions
  Tumors
  Brain abscess
  Cerebral hemorrhage
  Meningitis or encephalitis
  Temporal lobe epilepsy
Cerebral hypoxia
  Pulmonary insufficiency
  Severe anemia
  Cardiac failure
  Carbon monoxide poisoning
Metabolic and endocrine disorders
  Electrolyte imbalance
  Hypoglycemia
  Hypocalcemia
  Thyroid disease (hyperthyroidism and hypothyroidism)
  Adrenal disease (hyperadrenalism and hypoadrenalism)
  Uremia
  Hepatic failure
  Diabetes mellitus
  Porphyria
Rheumatic diseases
  Systemic lupus erythematosus
  Polyarteritis nodosa
Infections
  Malaria
  Typhoid fever
  Subacute bacterial endocarditis
Miscellaneous conditions
  Wilson disease
  Reye syndrome

TABLE 112.19. Guidelines for Management of Acute Adolescent Psychosis

Diagnose underlying cause.
Request *immediate psychiatric consultation,* with all psychiatrically based psychosis.
Use *medical hospitalization,* if clinically indicated, with organic psychosis.
Request *psychiatric consultation* with psychotic drug intoxications, either immediately or when mental status stabilizes.
Use *quiet room, family* and *friends,* and *constant medical supervision.*
Avoid administration of antipsychotic medication for psychiatrically based psychosis, in emergency department, when possible.
Use *restraints* if necessary.
Recognize clinical variations of *extrapyramidal reactions* to antipsychotic medications

Other important components of the management of a psychotic child involve controlling the child's behavior, preventing injury to himself or herself or others, and alleviating the child's fear and anxiety. Antipsychotic and sedative medications affect the child's neurologic status and therefore should be used only when the medical diagnosis is known with certainty and when it is clear that the medication will not worsen the underlying disease process or potentiate the intoxication. (Specific medications and dosages for psychosis are discussed under "Management"; see Table 112.20.) In most instances, when direct behavior control is essential, the child should be placed in arm and leg restraints. While in restraints, the patient should be attended by staff or family members and provided with frequent orienting statements and explanations of the need for restraint.

AUTISM AND OTHER PERVASIVE DEVELOPMENTAL DISORDERS OF CHILDHOOD

Autism

According to the current psychiatric diagnostic nomenclature (*the Diagnostic and Statistical Manual, or DSM* IV), autism is one specific type of pervasive developmental disorder (PDD) of childhood. The major differentiating feature between autism and other forms of PDD is the age of onset. Autism always has an onset before 30 months of age. Children with autism have a generalized lack of responsiveness to other people and a failure to develop normal attachment behavior. They do not develop relationships and instead play alone, often showing stereotyped behavior and using objects in bizarre, inappropriate ways. The autistic child becomes extremely upset if objects in his or her environment are disturbed or changed. Language development is impaired or absent. Only 30% of autistic children have an IQ (intelligence quotient) greater than 70. Some autistic children have underlying illnesses, such as maternal rubella syndrome or previous encephalitis or meningitis, but in many cases the cause is unknown. Many autistic children have coexisting seizure disorders. The course of infantile autism is generally chronic, with two-thirds of all autistic children remaining severely handicapped throughout life.

In general, acute psychiatric hospitalization is rarely necessary with autism. In instances of extremely disturbing behavior or acute agitation, sedation with either diphenhydramine (1 mg per kilogram of body weight) or chloral hydrate (30 mg per kilogram) may be helpful. If the parents are distressed by their child's immediate behavior and the child is receiving psychiatric treatment, phone contact with the psychiatrist may be helpful to both the emergency physician and the family. In the absence of ongoing care, a psychiatric consultation should be requested.

Other Pervasive Developmental Disorders

Pervasive developmental disorder of childhood is a generic term that includes other developmental impairments in which an incapacity to form reciprocal relationships with others results in severe, sustained impairment of attachment and social relationships. Other features may include extreme anxiety and severe emotional reactions to minor difficulties, with inappropriate affect and extreme mood lability. Abnormalities of speech, hypersensitivity to sensory stimuli, peculiar posturing, and self-mutilation also may occur. PDD other than autism has onset after 30 months and before 12 years of age.

The term *PDD* incompletely incorporates entities such as childhood schizophrenia, symbiotic psychosis, and atypical psychosis, as well as other recently added conditions. One type of PDD with which the emergency physician should be familiar is Asperger disorder. Children with this disorder typically have normal or above average intelligence and a well-developed capacity for speech and language. The impairment is in the capacity to form reciprocal relationships, and emotional rigidity, idiosyncratic thinking, and intense pursuit of a narrow range of interests may be present.

When necessary, the same acute pharmacologic approaches for children with autism are also relevant for other PDDs. Low-

TABLE 112.20. Antipsychotic Medications

Generic name	Brand name	Estimated equivalent dosage (mg)	Total daily dosage
Phenothiazines			
Chlorpromazine	Thorazine	100	50–1,000
Thioridazine	Mellaril	100	50–800
Trifluoperazine	Stelazine	5	5–30
Fluphenazine	Prolixin	2	1–20
Butyrophenone			
Haloperidol	Haldol	2	2–40
New atypical neuroleptics			
Clozapine	Clozaril	75	300–450
Risperidone	Risperdal		1–6
Olanzapine	Zyprexa		2.5–17.5
Quetiapine	Seroquel		150–300

dose thioridazine, a sedating neuroleptic, also may be used. With the acute exacerbation of a child with PDD, psychiatric hospitalization may be necessary, both to provide assistance to the parents and to develop or modify a comprehensive treatment program.

SCHIZOPHRENIA

Symptoms of schizophrenia involve impairment of basic psychological processes, including perception, thinking, affect, capacity to relate, and behavior (Table 112.21). Impaired thought content includes delusions (strongly held beliefs involving the self with no basis in reality), such as delusions of persecution and external control. For example, an adolescent with schizophrenia may think others can read and insert thoughts into his or her mind. Significantly illogical thinking occurs. Speech often is characterized by loose associations, in which ideas shift from one subject to another entirely unrelated subject without the speaker recognizing that the topics are not connected. Auditory hallucinations are common and may include direct commands for suicide or for violence to others. Affect may be blunted and flat or inappropriate and bizarre. Sudden and unpredictable changes in mood may occur. These teenagers may appear extremely agitated or may be withdrawn, speaking only in monosyllables and describing only concrete objects. Schizophrenic patients typically have significant distortions of their identity and their abilities and demonstrate behavior that is not goal directed.

The history often reveals a prodromal phase that includes social withdrawal, peculiar behavior, failure to look after one's appearance, and significant reduction in performance in school or work. This phase is followed by an acute phase in which the previously described symptoms develop, sometimes as a result of an acutely stressful event. The overall course of schizophrenia is often chronic and associated with remissions and exacerbations. Exacerbations often occur when treatment, including medication, is suspended. Other persons, however, experience a schizophrenic-like acute psychosis and recover completely with appropriate treatment, experiencing no further deterioration.

Management

The management of an acute schizophrenic episode always should take place in collaboration with psychiatric consultation. Patients with suicidal or homicidal ideation should receive psychiatric hospitalization. Psychotic patients from disorganized home environments also should be hospitalized for initial treatment. In general, the approach to the psychotic patient in the ED depends on the condition of the patient and the anticipated site of the ongoing treatment. For agitation and dangerousness, approaches include reassurance and a quiet setting, psychotropic medication, and physical restraint. Medication involves a choice between a calming, sedating medication such as diphenhydramine or use of an antipsychotic medication. If the child requires an additional psychiatric assessment at a site different than the ED, such as at a designated psychiatric emergency facility as a precondition for psychiatric hospitalization, antipsychotic medication should be used sparingly, if at all, at the pediatric ED.

A conservative approach involves a single dose of 5 to 10 mg of haloperidol orally or intramuscularly for adult-sized adolescents (approximately 70 kg) or 2 to 5 mg of haloperidol (orally or intramuscularly) for smaller children. A more aggressive approach involves the use of these same doses, administered every 3 to 60 minutes up to a maximum dose of 40 mg, until the patient's state of agitation lessens or until he or she becomes sedated. The patient's vital signs, general condition, and possible side effects should be monitored frequently. If the patient does not respond to this latter medication regimen, inpatient psychiatric hospitalization is necessary. If significant improvement occurs, suicidal and homicidal tendencies are absent, and side effects do not occur, the patient can be considered for discharge to outpatient psychiatric treatment with careful follow-up. This is possible as long as the parents or caretakers are well organized, appreciate the child's condition, and feel capable of managing the child at home.

Commonly used antipsychotic medications, their trade names, relative potency, and usual dosage ranges are listed in Table 112.20.

TABLE 112.21. Acute Schizophrenia in Adolescence: Most Common Features

Flat affect (Patient uninvolved and without emotion)
Auditory hallucinations
(Physician: "Have you been hearing voices even when no one is there?")
Thoughts spoken aloud
(Physician: "Can other people read your mind? Can you read their minds?")
Delusions of external control
(Physician: "Is anyone trying to kill you? ... trying to control your mind or your body?")

ACUTE REACTIVE PSYCHOSIS

Acute reactive psychosis, a relatively uncommon psychiatrically based psychosis, involves a time-limited loss of reality caused by the accumulated effects of externally imposed traumatic events. Although vulnerability may vary from child to child, children and teenagers can develop acute psychotic symptoms in response to trauma. The diagnosis of reactive psychosis can be made partly by history, but only after a complete medical and psychiatric evaluation has eliminated organic and other psychiatrically based psychoses. The acuteness of the clinical presentation and its precipitating events differentiates acute reactive psychosis from posttraumatic stress disorder.

The clinical picture of acute reactive psychosis varies, in some instances resembling schizophrenia and in others a less defined disorganized state characterized by loss of contact with reality, panic, and specific hallucinations (usually auditory or visual).

Different traumatic experiences, including physical or sexual abuse, rape, homelessness, and running away, may elicit a reactive psychosis. All such situations impose stress on the child and also can disrupt usual patterns of living. Confronted with a new environment and a new reality, the child's familiar cues are absent and confusion or frank psychosis may occur.

MANIC–DEPRESSIVE OR BIPOLAR DISORDER

Manic–depressive or bipolar disorder occurs in approximately 0.5% of the population. Onset is usually before 30 years of age and occurs during late childhood and adolescence. Because depression is discussed in detail elsewhere in this chapter, this section deals only with manic psychosis, most commonly observed in adolescence, and with the childhood form of bipolar disorder.

Clinical Manifestations

The patient with mania has a distinct period of predominantly elevated, expansive, and irritable mood (Table 112.22). The child has a significant decrease in need for sleep, high distractibility, hyperactivity and pressured speech, and emotional lability. These patients also exhibit what is called *flight of ideas*—a nearly continuous flow of accelerated speech with abrupt changes from topic to topic, usually based on understandable associations, distractions, or plays on words. Unlike the loose associations of the schizophrenic, the flight of ideas of a manic patient retains logical connection from one idea to the next but moves quickly from one topic to another. The manic patient may at times have a remarkably inflated self-esteem, with uncritical self-confidence and significant grandiosity. This grandiosity also may include delusional ideas. The individual may be aggressive and combative. He or she may go on buying sprees or pursue other reckless behaviors. Sleep patterns may be significantly impaired, with the individual reporting limited or no need to sleep.

Bipolar disorder that occurs in childhood and early adolescence usually looks different from the later adolescent and adult form just described. The child typically presents in the beginning with depression rather than mania and with remarkable shifts in mood, involving sudden changes from depressed to irritable or happy and then back to irritable or depressed. These changes can be disorienting to parents, who cannot understand why the child changes so much and so dramatically, possibly even several times the same day. The sudden shifts in mood and functioning are the reason that childhood bipolar disorder is often referred to as "rapid cycling."

Management

When an adolescent is suspected of having manic–depressive illness or an acute manic episode, psychiatric consultation should be obtained and psychiatric hospitalization initiated. Involuntary commitment may be necessary. Because the treatment of mania often includes the long-term use of lithium carbonate, which takes time to take effect and requires careful blood monitoring to assure therapeutic levels, psychiatric hospitalization is necessary. Initial emergency treatment of the agitated manic patient may require the use of restraints and the acute administration of antipsychotic agents, such as haloperidol, in doses equivalent to those used for schizophrenic adolescents. The physician should be aware that some patients receiving lithium may present with signs of lithium overdose, including nausea, vomiting, muscle weakness, ataxia, tremor, slurred speech, blurred vision, and confusion or somnolence.

POSTTRAUMATIC STRESS DISORDERS

In part to acknowledge the accumulated effect of stress on individuals and also to avoid more invasive diagnoses, psychiatry has invoked the concept of posttraumatic stress disorder (PTSD) with increasing frequency in recent years. Used in the 1970s and 1980s to explain some of the maladjustments of some Vietnam War veterans, PTSD can also occur in childhood and adolescence, typically based on the experience of severe trauma during earlier years. Either the reemergence of the old trauma (or the emergence of a new similar one) or the recollection of the original trauma can activate a PTSD.

A summary of the official description of PTSD in the psychiatric nomenclature (*DSM*-IV) is helpful in understanding this concept:

The person has been exposed to a traumatic event in which the person experienced, witnessed, or was confronted with an event that involved actual or threatened death or serious injury or a threat to the physical integrity of self or others. The person's response involved intense fear, helplessness, or horror, or, in children, disorganized or agitated behavior. In addition, the traumatic event is persistently reexperienced in one or more ways, there is persistent avoidance of stimuli associated with the trauma and numbing of general responsiveness, and there are persistent symptoms of increased arousal.

TABLE 112.22. Acute Mania in Adolescence: Most Common Features

Pressured speech	Euphoria
Grandiosity	Anxiety/irritability
Apparent	Combativeness/panic
Rapid shifts of emotion	

DISSOCIATIVE DISORDERS

Some children develop a dissociative disorder in response to extreme trauma. In a dissociative disorder, the child separates the usually integrated functions of identity, memory, and consciousness. As a result, the child's affect appears split off from the rest of the person. Specific symptoms vary, but in most cases, the child appears distant, even weird, but is not psychotic. Dissociative disorders occur most commonly in females, with sexual abuse a common original trauma.

The function of dissociative reactions is believed to decrease the child's awareness of emotional pain caused by the trauma. The process of splitting off the affect from the body may help a severely traumatized child deal with and survive the assault. This response probably begins at the time of the trauma, especially if it occurs repeatedly and then is continued afterward as a form of coping; however, a consequence is that the child may continue to split off full emotional responsiveness to daily experiences, creating a profound isolation. This process may continue into adulthood.

The emergency physician may encounter a child with depersonalization, a feeling of detachment from one's self or a feeling of being an automaton or in a dream. Another dissociative response is *psychogenic amnesia*, the sudden inability to recall important personal information (or even know one's own identity). Some runaway adolescents may present with a *psychogenic fugue*, another dissociative disorder. In a fugue state, the individual leaves home unexpectedly with no apparent justification and may at times assume a partial or complete new identity.

The most extreme—and increasingly common—form of dissociative disorder is multiple personality disorder (MPD). In this condition, the child has two or more personalities and appears puzzling to parents, teachers, and physicians. At least two of these personalities recurrently take full control of the child's behavior, with the child unaware of the process. Children with MPD are aptly described as erratic, inconsistent, even mercurial. The emergency physician should consider the possibility of MPD or other dissociative disorders in all children and adolescents who present in a confused and confusing way.

CONDUCT DISORDERS

A child with a disorder of conduct engages in repetitive, socially unacceptable behavior, without evidence of medical or other psychiatric disorder. The diagnosis of conduct disorder implies a continuing pattern of disruptive or deviant behavior rather than isolated antisocial acts. The behavior may involve violence and aggression (eg, vandalism, mugging, assault, and rape), or it may involve behavior that is socially unacceptable but nonaggressive (eg, truancy, running away, lying, stealing, substance abuse). Therefore, a disorder of conduct involves more serious behavior than ordinary mischief and pranks of children and adolescents. Because violent and other unacceptable behaviors may be performed by children with medical illnesses and intoxications, these causes must be ruled out before the diagnosis of conduct disorder can be made.

Society disagrees about whether to regard children and adolescents with conduct disorders as psychiatrically impaired and needing treatment or as delinquent and needing detention or incarceration. Probably only a small percentage of violent and aggressive children are brought to the ED for psychiatric evaluation. Many are taken by police to detention centers and others engage in their unacceptable behavior without receiving legal or medical attention.

Clinical Manifestations

Children with conduct disorders typically have poor adjustment at home and in the community. Peer relationships are superficial, based more on what the child can get from the other person than on a sense of empathy. The child thinks primarily about himself or herself, trying to manipulate situations to personal advantage without significant concern for the feelings and needs of others. The child with a conduct disorder is unlikely to extend himself or herself for others when no immediate advantage can be gained. When the child is apprehended, little sense of remorse or guilt is exhibited, but rather the child exhibits a sense of anger at being detected and detained. Such children rarely accept responsibility for their own actions and instead tend to blame others for their mistakes.

The child or adolescent with a conduct disorder shows low frustration tolerance, irritability, and temper outbursts. He or she may be reckless in behavior and project an image of "toughness." Smoking, drinking, drug use, and precocious sexual activity all may occur. In addition to possible legal difficulties, the child may have other problems, including school suspensions, drug dependence, sexually transmitted disease, pregnancy, and physical injury from accidents and fights.

In addition to inconsistent limit setting, families of children with conduct disorders tend to be poorly organized, with the roles and expectations of various family members often unclear. Parental separations and divorce, mental illness, and alcohol or drug abuse also may be factors. Parental criminality and incarceration occur in some families. Families with aggressive and impulsive children often do not know how to effectively use social service resources and may consider themselves helpless in controlling their child and in dealing with the world at large.

Management

The goals for managing aggressive and disruptive children in the ED are (1) to ensure the safety of the child, family, and staff; (2) to rule out possible medical conditions and severe psychiatric disorders before making the diagnosis of conduct disorder; and (3) to gather sufficient information to make an appropriate disposition.

The safety of the child and staff and control of the child's unacceptable behavior must be achieved in the ED. In many instances, the disruptive behavior occurred and ended before the child's coming to the ED and gaining the child's cooperation is not a problem. In other instances, however, the child may remain combative and aggressive in the ED. Dealing with such a problem requires the presence of adequate security staff and a quiet space where attempts to control the patient do not disrupt the remainder of the ED.

Involuntary hospitalization may be necessary when the child's condition continues to pose a threat to himself or herself or others or when overt homicidal or suicidal ideation is present. When the child is not suicidal or homicidal and refuses to make a commitment to work in psychotherapy, and when the family does not support the proposed psychiatric hospitalization, problematic behaviors are more likely to continue and the child may eventually enter the juvenile justice system.

ATTENTION DEFICIT HYPERACTIVITY DISORDER

Attention deficit hyperactivity disorder (ADHD) refers to a syndrome found in school-aged children, characterized by a pervasive difficulty in maintaining attention and goal-directed behavior. The condition, previously called *hyperkinetic syndrome* and *minimal brain dysfunction*, has been relabeled as ADHD because the primary source of difficulty is believed to be inattention. ADHD has an incidence between 5% and 10% of school-aged children, occurring ten times more often in boys than girls. It is presumed to have an underlying neurologic cause. Some cases of ADHD may be inherited, whereas others may be a consequence of prenatal or perinatal difficulties or of unknown cause. ADHD occurs in up to 50% of latency-aged children receiving psychiatric treatment, making it the most common cause of chronic behavioral problems for this age group. The peak age range for referral of ADHD children is between the ages of 8 and 10 years.

Clinical Manifestations

Although some children with attentional problems present without hyperactivity, most children have hyperactivity in association with inattention and impulsivity and therefore fit within the full ADHD umbrella. Wender described the various possible components of the ADHD picture. Attentional difficulties occur both at home and in school and are often more severe in school. The child has difficulty fixating attention. This problem manifests itself as an inability to persist for long periods in any activity and, in extreme form, may involve a frenetic movement from activity to activity. Rather than persisting in schoolwork and other tasks, the child often appears not to be listening to the teacher, and discipline may be a problem.

Impulsivity is another essential characteristic of ADHD. The child has difficulty with self-control, exhibiting behaviors that get him or her in trouble with parents, siblings, teachers, and peers. At home, the child typically has outbursts and temper tantrums, and enforcement of discipline may be difficult. Lack of self-control may also manifest through stealing, lying, playing with matches, and other forms of acting out.

Hyperactivity is usually part of the clinical picture, although some children with a subtype of attentional problems are inattentive but not hyperactive or impulsive.

The child with ADHD may be labile, with fluctuations in mood and a tendency toward overreaction and temper tantrums, but such responses are not always extreme. Appreciating the low self-esteem and possible depression that may be present in these children, as a result of academic failure, conflicts at home, and peer and sibling rejection, is important. In acute situations, the depression may find expression as suicide attempts or violent behavior.

Management

The principal responsibility of the emergency physician is to recognize the possibility of ADHD in children who present with other problems—including depression, mood instability, and conduct disorder—and to consider the diagnosis. The physician is then in a position to clarify the meaning of this disorder with the family and to restore hope for the child's improved behavior and adaptation by making a psychiatric referral when indicated. The history is the most reliable diagnostic indicator. Once a presumptive diagnosis is made, appropriate referral and treatment can follow.

The treatment approach to ADHD should be comprehensive and multimodal and is best managed by a child psychiatrist who has a long-term relationship with the child and family.

Index

Note: Page numbers followed by f indicate figures; page numbers followed by t indicate tables.